WALLACH'S
Interpretation *of*
Diagnostic Tests

Pathways to Arriving at
a Clinical Diagnosis

TENTH EDITION

Edited by

Mary A. Williamson, MT (ASCP), PhD
Vice President, Scientific Affairs & Laboratory Operations
ACM Medical Laboratory
Rochester, New York
Former Assistant Professor
Department of Pathology
University of Massachusetts Medical School
Worcester, Massachusetts

L. Michael Snyder, MD
Professor
Department of Medicine and Pathology
University of Massachusetts Medical School
UMass Memorial Medical Center
Worcester, Massachusetts
Chief Medical Officer
Quest Diagnostics MA, LLC
Marlborough, Massachusetts

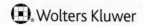
. Wolters Kluwer

Philadelphia • Baltimore • New York • London
Buenos Aires • Hong Kong • Sydney • Tokyo

Executive Editor: Rebecca Gaertner
Senior Product Development Editor: Kristina Oberle
Production Project Manager: Alicia Jackson
Design Coordinator: Joan Wendt
Senior Manufacturing Coordinator: Beth Welsh
Marketing Manager: Stephanie Manzo
Prepress Vendor: SPi Global

Printed in China

Library of Congress Cataloging-in-Publication Data
Wallach's interpretation of diagnostic tests. — Tenth edition / edited by Mary A. Williamson,
L. Michael Snyder.
     p. ; cm.
  Includes bibliographical references and index.
  ISBN 978-1-4511-9176-9 (paperback : alk. paper)
  I. Williamson, Mary A., editor. II. Snyder, L. Michael, editor.
  [DNLM: 1. Clinical Laboratory Techniques. 2. Diagnostic Techniques and Procedures.
QY 25]
  RB38.2
  616.07'56—dc23
                                                                        2014012353

Care has been taken to confirm the accuracy of the information presented and to describe
generally accepted practices. However, the authors, editors, and publisher are not responsible
for errors or omissions or for any consequences from application of the information in this
book and make no warranty, expressed or implied, with respect to the currency, completeness,
or accuracy of the contents of the publication. Application of this information in a particular
situation remains the professional responsibility of the practitioner; the clinical treatments
described and recommended may not be considered absolute and universal recommendations.

The authors, editors, and publisher have exerted every effort to ensure that drug selection
and dosage set forth in this text are in accordance with the current recommendations and
practice at the time of publication. However, in view of ongoing research, changes in govern-
ment regulations, and the constant flow of information relating to drug therapy and drug
reactions, the reader is urged to check the package insert for each drug for any change in
indications and dosage and for added warnings and precautions. This is particularly important when the recommended agent is a new or infrequently employed drug.

Some drugs and medical devices presented in this publication have Food and Drug
Administration (FDA) clearance for limited use in restricted research settings. It is the
responsibility of the health care provider to ascertain the FDA status of each drug or device
planned for use in his or her clinical practice.

RRS1405

I am deeply grateful to my parents Priscilla and
Thomas Williamson for their unconditional love. Sincere thanks
to Joanne Saksa for her gracious hospitality and warmest gratitude to
Brenda DeMay, for her unconditional love and continually
encouraging me to challenge myself.

I am most indebted to Dr. L. Michael Snyder, a true mentor
throughout the years who has taught me that anything is possible—
even the Boston Red Sox can win the World Series! Special thanks
to all of the authors for their hard work and commitment,
especially Liberto Pechet, a true gentleman.
Mary A. Williamson, MT(ASCP), PhD

To my wife Barbara, and children Cathe, Lizzy,
and John for their tireless understanding and
support throughout the years.

To my assistant Suzanne O'Brien for her dedication
and help with the textbook.

I would also like to acknowledge Dr. Mary Williamson, for
without her commitment, dedication and hard work,
we would not have met the target date for completion of
the tenth edition.
L. Michael Snyder, MD

Contributors

M. Rabie Al-Turkmani, BPharm, PhD
Assistant Professor
Department of Pathology
University of Massachusetts Medical School
Associate Director, Immunology,
    Immunoassay & Hematology
    Laboratories
UMass Memorial Medical Center
Worcester, Massachusetts
Scientific Director,
Quest Diagnostics MA, LLC
Marlborough, Massachusetts

Vishesh Chhibber
Medical Director, Transfusion Medicine
North Shore University Hospital
Hofstra North Shore-LIJ School of Medicine
    North Shore-LIJ Health System
Manhasset, New York

**Marzena M. Galdzicka, PhD,
MP(ASCP)^CM, DABCC**
Clinical Assistant Professor
Department of Pathology
University of Massachusetts Medical School
Shrewsbury, Massachusetts
Scientific Director,
Quest Diagnostics MA, LLC
Marlborough, Massachusetts

Edward I. Ginns, MD, PhD, DABCC
Professor of Neurology, Pathology, Pediatrics
    and Psychiatry
Director, Lysosomal Disorders Treatment and
    Research Program
University of Massachusetts Medical School
Shrewsbury, Massachusetts
Scientific Director,
Quest Diagnostics MA, LLC
Marlborough, Massachusetts

Amanda J. Jenkins, PhD
Associate Professor
Department of Pathology
University of Massachusetts Medical School
Director, Toxicology
UMass Memorial Medical Center
Worcester, Massachusetts
Scientific Director,
Quest Diagnostics MA, LLC
Marlborough, Massachusetts

Charles R. Kiefer, PhD
Associate Professor
Department of Pathology
University of Massachusetts Medical School
Director, Andrology Laboratory
Director, Clinical Assay Research
UMass Memorial Medical Center
Worcester, Massachusetts

Patricia Minehart Miron, PhD
Clinical Associate Professor of Pathology and
    Pediatrics
University of Massachusetts Medical School
Director, Cytogenetics
UMass Memorial Medical Center
Worcester, Massachusetts
Scientific Director,
Quest Diagnostics MA, LLC
Marlborough, Massachusetts

Michael J. Mitchell, MD
Clinical Associate Professor
Department of Pathology
University of Massachusetts Medical School
Director, Microbiology
UMass Memorial Medical Center
Worcester, Massachusetts
Scientific Director,
Quest Diagnostics MA, LLC
Marlborough, Massachusetts

Liberto Pechet, MD
Professor Emeritus
Departments of Pathology and Medicine
University of Massachusetts Medical School
Worcester, Massachusetts

Lokinendi V. Rao, PhD
Clinical Associate Professor
Department of Pathology
University of Massachusetts Medical School
Laboratory Director, UMass Memorial
   Clinical Laboratories
UMass Memorial Medical Center
Worcester, Massachusetts
Scientific Director,
Quest Diagnostics MA, LLC
Marlborough, Massachusetts

Craig S. Smith, MD
Assistant Professor
Department of Medicine
University of Massachusetts Medical School
Director, Cardiac Intensive Care
Division of Cardiology
UMass Memorial Medical Center
Worcester, Massachusetts

L. Michael Snyder, MD
Professor
Department of Medicine and Pathology
University of Massachusetts Medical School
UMass Memorial Medical Center
Worcester, Massachusetts
Chief Medical Officer,
Quest Diagnostics MA, LLC
Marlborough, Massachusetts

Juliana G. Szakacs, MD, MSW
Director of Pathology and Laboratory
   Medicine
Harvard Vanguard Medical Associates
Boston, Massachusetts

Mary A. Williamson, MT (ASCP), PhD
Vice President, Scientific Affairs &
   Laboratory Operations
ACM Medical Laboratory
Rochester, New York
Former Assistant Professor
Department of Pathology
University of Massachusetts Medical School
Worcester, Massachusetts

Hongbo Yu, MD, PhD
Associate Professor
Department of Pathology
University of Massachusetts Medical School
Director, Hematopathology and
   Hematopathology Fellowship Program
Director, Flow Cytometry Laboratory
UMass Memorial Medical Center
Worcester, Massachusetts

Tribute to Jacques Wallach

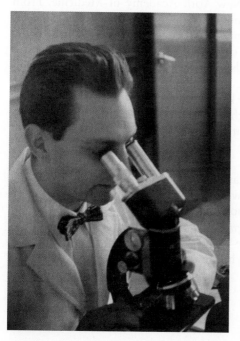

Jacques Wallach, pathologist, educator, and author of this book left us on August 10, 2010. He was 84. Forty years before that, he wrote the first edition, widely recognized as a necessary resource for both busy house staff and seasoned clinicians alike. It was the product of his vast experience as a clinical pathologist, his unquenchable thirst for medical knowledge, and his passion for teaching. He devoted tireless hours of research toward updating this book seven times since then. Several hundreds of thousands of copies have been distributed in numerous translations throughout the world.

As a resident in Internal Medicine in the mid-1980s, my first encounter with this book came in the early hours before our daily morning report, as my fellow house officers scurried to review the overnight admissions prior to presenting these cases to the Department Chief. The ensuing hour was usually punctuated by moments when one or more of us incurred the Chief's wrath for failure to accurately appreciate the patient's disorder or appropriately intervene. In an effort to avoid a similar fate, each of us would keep a copy of the book in an overfilled pocket of our lab coat to review quickly prior to this daily inquisition. Years later, I witnessed many students and house officers under my supervision do same, often secretly racing each other to the passage contained therein that would earn them the sought after recognition of their peers.

In the years that followed, I saw the third edition of the book become the fourth, fifth, and so on, never really appreciating the work that Jacques put into each update. Like many of us, however, I did appreciate the place that each update had among my collection of those clinical books, which were always kept within easy reach and never seemed to collect any dust in my personal medical library.

When I first met Jacques, I was impressed by his dedication and commitment to medical education. He taught pathology at Albert Einstein, Rutgers, and SUNY Downstate and consulted for Children's Specialized Hospital in Mountainside, South Amboy Memorial Hospital, Kings County Hospital in Brooklyn, and for the Bronx Zoo. He also wrote *Rheumatic Heart Disease* (1962) and *Interpretation of Pediatric Tests* (1983) as well as over 40 articles for peer review medical journals. He was a Fellow of the American College of Physicians, the American Society of Clinical Pathologists, the College of American Pathologists, and the New York Academy of Medicine. From 1975 to 1985, he donated his time and expertise in pathology to laboratories around the world. His office was crammed with countless notes he made while researching, scrolled on small pieces of paper, and filed between the pages of dozens of medical books and journals, waiting their turn to adorn the pages of his next book. It was like he realized that clinicians and patients around the world depended on him to unlock the keys to their own medical mysteries, and he did not take that responsibility lightly. More recently, Jacques asked me to join his small list of distinguished contributors and lend some assistance in my own area of expertise. To contribute in some small way to his labor of love was truly an honor.

As the devoted teacher, nothing was more rewarding to Jacques than being able to impart the wisdom he had worked hard to accumulate to the pupil looking for guidance. This ninth edition and all subsequent editions, now entitled *Wallach's Interpretation of Diagnostic Tests*, represent his legacy and his ongoing gift to physicians around the world who continue to use his guidance everyday to care for their patients. I have no doubt that nothing would have made him happier.

ANTHONY G. AUTERI, MD

Preface

In the 10th edition of Wallach's, the authors continue to modify the content and organization based on feedback from readers as well as attempting to keep pace with a rapidly changing health care environment. Since the main focus of the textbook is to stress the most efficient use of clinical lab testing, we have changed the format so that the first section will now be devoted to disease states. Moreover, we have extended the presentation of the patient's chief complaints and physical findings format to additional chapters such as pulmonary, cardiac, and neurologic disease states. We have added chapters on HLA, Transfusion Medicine, and OBGYN and updated the chapters on Molecular Diagnostics and Cardiology.

The second section will now list the individual lab tests in alphabetical order stressing the integration of the clinical laboratory results in the clinical decision-making process. When appropriate, tests will include the sensitivity, specificity, and positive and negative probability. Infectious disease assays as before are listed separately.

We have enhanced the index to make it easier for the reader to locate the subjects of interest. In addition, we have created a robust electronic version, which will include "hypertexting" of tests mentioned in the disease section referring back to the individual test section. This textbook does not include references to pathophysiology or therapy. However, common pitfalls and limitations of testing as well as identifying appropriate tests for specific clinical presentations are addressed.

As in previous editions, this textbook is geared to the primary care physician, subspecialists, physician's assistant, nurse practitioner, as well as medical and nursing students. The 10th edition is not an exhaustive catalogue of disease states but a practical guide. We would appreciate continued feedback about changes we have instituted and further comments.

L. MICHAEL SNYDER, MD

GARY LAPIDAS

MARY A. WILLIAMSON, MT (ASCP), PHD

Preface to the First Edition

Results of laboratory tests may aid in
  Discovering occult disease
  Preventing irreparable damage (e.g., phenylketonuria)
  Early diagnosis after onset of signs or symptoms
  Differential diagnosis of various possible diseases
  Determining the stage of the disease
  Estimating the activity of the disease
  Detecting the recurrence of disease
  Monitoring the effect of therapy
  Genetic counseling in familial conditions
  Medicolegal problems, such as paternity suits

This book is written to help the physician achieve these purposes the least amount of
  Duplication of texts
  Waste of patient's money
  Overtaxing of laboratory facilities and personnel
  Loss of physician's time
  Confusion caused by the increasing number, variety, and complexity of tests
    currently available. Some of these tests may be unrequested but performed
    as part of routine surveys or hospital admission multitest screening.

In order to provide quick reference and maximum availability and usefulness,
    this handy-sized book features
  Tabular and graphic style of concise presentation
  Emphasis on serial time changes in laboratory findings in various stages of
    disease
  Omission of rarely performed, irrelevant, esoteric, and outmoded labora-
    tory tests
  Exclusion of discussion of physiologic mechanisms, metabolic pathways,
    clinical features, and nonlaboratory aspects of disease
  Discussion of only the more important diseases that the physician encoun-
    ters and should be able to diagnose

This book is not
  An encyclopedic compendium of clinical pathology
  A technical manual
  A substitute for good clinical judgment and basic knowledge of medicine

Deliberately omitted are

Technical procedures and directions

Photographs and illustrations of anatomic changes (e.g., blood cells, karyo-types, isotope scans)

Discussions of quality control

Selection of a referral laboratory

Performance of laboratory tests in the clinician's own office

Bibliographic references, except for the most general reference texts in medicine, hematology, and clinical pathology and for some recent references to specific conditions

The usefulness and need for a book of this style, organization, and contents have been increased by such current trends as

The frequent lack of personal assistance, advice, and consultation in large commercial laboratories and hospital departments of clinical pathology, which are often specialized and fragmented as well as impersonal

Greater demand for the physician's time

The development of many new tests

Faculty and administrators still assume that this essential area of medicine can be learned "intuitively" as it was 20 years ago and that it therefore requires little formal training. This attitude ignores changes in the number and variety of tests now available as well as their increased sophistication and basic value in establishing a diagnosis.

The contents of this book are organized to answer the questions most often posed by physicians when they require assistance from the pathologist. There is no other single adequate source of information presented in this fashion. It appears from numerous comments I have received that this book has succeeded in meeting the needs not only of practicing physicians and medical students but also of pathologists, technologists, and other medical personnel. It has been adopted by many schools of nursing and of medical technology, physician's assistant training programs, and medical schools. Such widespread acceptance confirms my original premise in writing this book and is most gratifying.

A perusal of the table of contents and index will quickly show the general organization of the material by type of laboratory test or organ system or certain other categories. In order to maintain a concise format, separate chapters have not been organized for such categories as newborn, pediatric, and geriatric periods or for primary psychiatric or dermatologic diseases. A complete index provides maximum access to this information.

Obviously, these data are not original but have been adapted from many sources over the years. Only the selection, organization, manner of presentation, and emphasis are original. I have formulated this point of view during 40 years as a clinician and pathologist, viewing with pride the important and growing role of the laboratory but deeply regretting its inappropriate utilization.

This book was written to improve laboratory utilization by making it simpler for the physician to select and interpret the most useful laboratory tests for his clinical problems.

J.W.

Contents

CHAPTER 1

FALTs: Factors Affecting Laboratory Tests

Lokinendi V. Rao

Laboratory testing is an integral part of modern medical practice. Although clinical laboratory testing accounts for only 2.3% of annual health care costs in the United States, it plays a major role in the clinical decisions made by physicians, nurses, and other health care providers for the overall management of disease. More than 4,000 laboratory tests are available for clinical use, and about 500 of them are performed regularly. The number of Clinical Laboratory Improvement Amendments (CLIA)-certified laboratories has grown to exceed more than 200,000. The laboratory medicine workforce comprises pathologists, doctoral-level laboratory scientists, technologists, and technicians, who play a vital role in the health care system.

The health care system is increasingly dependent on reliable clinical laboratory services; however, as part of the overall health care system, these laboratory evaluations are prone to errors. Laboratory medicine comprises more than just the use of chemicals and reagents for the measurement of various analytes for clinical diagnosis purposes. Interference by both endogenous and exogenous substances is a common problem for the test analysis. These substances play a significant role in the proper interpretation of results, and such interference is adverse to patient care and adds to the cost of health care. It would be an oversimplification to conclude that each variable will always produce a specific effect; it depends on the person, the duration of exposure to that variable, and the time between initial stress, the sample collection, and the degree of exposure. Awareness that many factors occurring outside the laboratory in and around the patient may affect the test result before the sample reaches the laboratory or even before the sample is collected is very important. These factors can be minimized when the clinician takes a good history and when there is a good communication of such information between the laboratory and the physician.

 # WHAT CAUSES ABNORMAL TEST RESULTS (BESIDES DISEASE)?

The total testing process defines the preanalytic, analytic, and postanalytic phases of laboratory testing and serves as the basis for designing and implementing interventions, restrictions, or limits that can reduce or remove the likelihood of errors. Over the last several years, there has been a remarkable decrease in error rates, especially analytic errors. Evidence from recent studies demonstrates that a large percentage of laboratory errors occur in preanalytic and postanalytic steps. Errors in the preanalytic (61.9%) and postanalytic (23.1%) processes occurred much more frequently than occurrences of analytic errors (15%). About one fourth of these can have consequences to the patient either in delay of the test result or life threatening.

PREANALYTIC ERRORS

Preanalytic factors act on both the patient and the specimen before analyses. These factors may be divided further into those acting in vivo (biologic or physiologic) and those acting in vitro (specimen handling and interference factors).

PHYSIOLOGIC FACTORS

Some physiologic factors are beyond our control. They include age, sex, and race, and so on, and can be managed by placing appropriate reference limits. Others factors such as diet, starvation, exercise, posture, diurnal and seasonal variations, menstrual cycle, and pregnancy must be considered in the interpretation of the test results. Age has noticeable effect on some test results and the need for establishing appropriate reference intervals. In newborns, the composition of blood is affected by the maturity of the infant at birth. At birth, RBC and hemoglobin values are higher than adults due to low levels of oxygen in the uterus. They continue to decrease and level out to adult values about the age of 15. Adult values are usually taken as the reference for comparison with those of the young and the elderly. The concentration of most test constituents remains constant between puberty and menopause in women and between puberty and middle age in men. The plasma concentrations of many constituents increase in women after menopause. Hormone levels are affected by aging. However, changes in concentrations are much less pronounced than an endocrine organ's response to stimuli. Until puberty, there are few differences in laboratory data between boys and girls. After puberty, the characteristic changes in the levels of sex hormones become apparent.

In addition to the commonly known hormonal changes during the menstrual cycle, there is a preovulatory increase in the concentrations of aldosterone and renin. Coincident with the ovulation, serum cholesterol levels are lower than at any other phase of the menstrual cycle. In pregnancy, a dilutional effect is observed due to the increase in mean plasma volume, which in turn causes hemo-dilution. Normal pregnancy is characterized by major physiologic adaptations that alter maternal blood chemistry and hematology laboratory values. In addition, there are time-related fluctuations in the levels of certain analytes. Many analytes—such as cortisol, thyrotropin (TSH), growth hormone, potassium, glucose, iron, and proinflammatory cytokines—exhibit diurnal variation. Hormones such as luteinizing hormone (LH), follicle-stimulating hormone (FSH), and testosterone released in short bursts lasting barely 2 minutes make accurate measurements problematic. Seasonal changes also affect certain analytes like vitamin D (higher during summer), cholesterol, and thyroid hormones (higher during winter). Changes in the levels of some of the constituents in blood occur when measured at sea level as opposed to measurement at a higher altitude. Hematocrit, hemoglobin, and C-reactive protein (CRP) can be higher at high altitude. Levels of plasma renin, transferrin, urinary creatinine, creatinine clearance, and estriol decrease with increasing altitude.

The dietary effect of laboratory test results is complex and simply cannot be separated into the categories of "fasting" and "nonfasting" status of the patient. A significant variation in some routine tests after a regular meal showing that fasting time needs to be carefully considered when performing tests to prevent spurious results. Clinically significant differences are observed within 1–4 hours for triglycerides, albumin, ALT, calcium, iron, LDH, phosphorus, magnesium, lymphocytes, RBC, hemoglobin, hematocrit, etc. The type of diet (high fat, low fat, vegetarian, malnutrition), length of time since last meal, and test-specific dietary concerns can affect some tests. Consumption of caffeine, bran, serotonin (consumption of fruits and vegetables such as bananas, avocados, and onions), herbal preparations (e.g., aloe vera, Chinese rhubarb, senna, quinine, and quinidine), recreational drug use, ethanol, and smoking can induce both short- and long-term effects that alter the results of several analytes. Differentiations of the effects of race from those of socioeconomic conditions are difficult. Carbohydrate and lipid metabolism differ in blacks and whites. Glucose tolerance is less in blacks, Polynesians, and Native Americans in comparison to whites.

Physical stress and mental stress influence the concentrations of many plasma constituents, including cortisol, aldosterone, prolactin, TSH, aldosterone, cholesterol, glucose, insulin, and lactate. With blindness, the normal stimulation of the hypothalamic–pituitary axis is reduced. Consequently, certain features of hypopituitarism and hypoadrenalism may be observed. In some blind individuals, the normal diurnal variations of cortisol may persist; in others, it does not. Fever provokes many hormonal responses as does shock and trauma. The stress of surgery has been shown to reduce the serum triiodothyronine (T_3) levels by 50% in patients without thyroid disease.

Transfusions and infusions can also significantly affect the concentration of certain laboratory values. For persons receiving an infusion, blood should not be obtained proximal to the infusion site. Blood should be obtained from the opposite arm. A minimum of 8 hours must elapse before blood is obtained from a subject who has received fat emulsion. For patients receiving blood transfusions, the extent of hemolysis and with it increased levels of potassium, lactate dehydrogenase (LDH), and free hemoglobin are released progressively to the age of the transfused blood.

Exercise such as running up and down several flights of stairs or strenuous activity such as working out in a gymnasium or marathon running the night before the specimen collection can affect the results obtained for several analytes. To minimize preanalytic variables introduced by exercise, subjects should be instructed to refrain from strenuous activity on the night before testing and not to exert themselves by walking a long distance, running, or climbing stairs before blood specimen collection. In addition, the muscle damage associated with trauma of surgery will increase the serum activity of enzymes originating in skeletal muscles, and this activity may persist for several days.

The plasma and extracellular volumes decrease within a few days of the start of bed rest. With prolonged bed rest, fluid retention occurs and plasma protein and albumin levels may be decreased by an average of 0.5 and 0.3 g/dL, respectively. As a result, concentrations of bound protein are also reduced. Changes in posture during blood sampling can affect the concentrations of several analytes measured in serum or plasma. Change in posture from a supine to an erect or sitting position can result in a shift in body water from intravascular to interstitial compartments. As a result, the concentrations of larger molecules that are not filterable are increased. These effects are accentuated in patients with a tendency for edema, such as in cardiovascular insufficiency and cirrhosis of the liver.

SPECIMEN HANDLING FACTORS

Among controllable preanalytic variables, specimen collection is most critical. Unacceptable specimen collection due to misidentification, insufficient volume to perform test, incorrect whole blood-to-anticoagulant ratio, and specimen quality (hemolysis, clots, contaminated, collected in wrong container) accounts for the majority of preanalytic errors. Hemolysis, lipemia, and icteric samples have variable effects on assays and depend upon testing method and analyte. The time and temperature for storage of the specimen and the processing steps in the preparation of serum or plasma or cell separation can introduce preanalytic variables.

Pneumatic tube systems of various lengths are routinely used in many hospitals to transport blood collection tubes to the testing laboratory. Significant differences between plasma but not serum levels of LDH are observed when blood collection tubes are transported through pneumatic tube systems. The application of a tourniquet, by reducing the pressure below the systolic pressure, maintains the effective filtration pressure within the capillaries. As a result, small molecules and fluid are transferred from the intravasal space to the interstitium. Application of tourniquet for longer than 1 minute can result in hemoconcentration of large molecules that are unable to penetrate the capillary wall. To minimize the preanalytic effects of tourniquet application time, the tourniquet should be released as soon as the needle enters the vein. Avoidance of excessive fist clenching during phlebotomy and maintaining tourniquet application time to no more than 1 minute can minimize preanalytic errors.

Various salts of heparin, ethylenediaminetetraacetic acid (EDTA), and sodium citrate are used widely in the clinical laboratory. Heparin is the preferred anticoagulant for blood specimens for electrolyte levels and other routine chemistry tests. Obvious differences in the results of certain analytes between serum and heparinized plasma are related to the consumption of fibrinogen and the lysis of cellular elements during the process of clotting. EDTA is the commonly used anticoagulant for routine hematologic determinations. It functions as anticoagulant by chelating calcium ions, which are required for the clotting process. Citrate has been used as an anticoagulant for collection of blood specimens intended for global coagulation tests such as prothrombin time (PT) and partial thromboplastin time (PTT). A laboratory that has been using one of the concentrations (3.2% or 3.8%) to perform PT determination for patients receiving oral anticoagulant therapy should not interchange the formulations. Doing so will affect the international normalized ratios (INRs) that are used to report the results of PT. Sodium fluoride and lithium iodoacetate have been used alone or in combination with anticoagulants such as potassium oxalate, EDTA, citrate, or lithium heparin for blood collection. In the absence of glycolytic inhibitors, a decrease in the glucose level of as much as 24% can occur in 1 hour after blood collection in neonates, in contrast to a 5% decrease in healthy individuals when specimen is stored at room temperature. The anticoagulant-to-blood ratio is critical for some laboratory tests. In general, collecting of blood specimens to less than nominal volume increases the effective molarity of the anticoagulant and induces osmotic changes affecting cell morphologic features. Furthermore, the binding of analytes such as ionic calcium or magnesium to heparin can be enhanced when the effective concentration of unfractionated heparin increased beyond the normal 14.3 U/mL of blood. In addition, stability of various analytes are significantly reduced in plasma (Lithium Heparin) compared to serum tubes when plasma is stored, but not separated from the gel after centrifugation.

Virtually, all drugs may affect the results of clinical laboratory tests that includes both in vivo (pharmacologic) and in vitro (interferences and methodologic) effects. The problem of drug interference is complex, and physicians are generally aware of main therapeutic effects of drug, but many secondary effects are ignored. Some of the examples are increase in liver enzymes with Dilantin and barbiturates, increase in fibrinogen, transferrin, amylase, etc. following oral contraceptives and contrast agents (gadolinium) decreasing total calcium levels.

In coagulation, testing knowledge or access to the patient history may be necessary, as many medications such as anticoagulant therapies (warfarin, heparin, and direct thrombin inhibitors), blood product, and component transfusion and coagulation factor replacement therapies all impact coagulation test results. Over-the-counter drugs (aspirin) have prolonged effect on platelet function studies. In addition, the patient's physiologic state plays a role.

The quality of the specimens submitted to the microbiology laboratory is critical for optimal specimen evaluation. The general techniques of specimen collection and handling that have been established both to maximize the yield of organisms and isolate relevant pathogens from specimens obtained from different body sites should be reviewed with clinical laboratory prior to obtaining the specimen. In addition, valid interpretation of the results of culture can be achieved only if the specimen obtained is appropriate for processing. As a result, care must be taken to collect only those specimens that may yield pathogens, rather than colonizing flora or contaminants. Specific rules for the collection of material vary, depending on the source of the specimen, but several general principles apply. Prompt transport of specimens to the microbiology laboratory is essential to optimize the yield of cultures and the interpretation of results. Delays in processing may result in the overgrowth of some microorganisms or the death of more fastidious ones. Samples for bacterial culture should ideally arrive in the microbiology laboratory within 1 to 2 hours of collection. If a delay is unavoidable, most specimens (with the exception of blood, cerebrospinal fluid, joint fluid, and cultures for *Neisseria gonorrhoeae*) should be refrigerated until transported.

ANALYTIC ERRORS

Clinical laboratories have long focused their attention on quality control methods and quality assessment programs dealing with analytic aspects of testing. Total analytic error (or measurement error) refers to assay errors from all sources arising from the data collection experiment. Some error is expected, because not all components of measuring are the same. There are four major types of experimental error: random (not predictable), systematic (one direction), total (random and systematic), and idiosyncratic (nonmethodologic).

Errors due to analytic problems have been significantly reduced over time, but there is evidence that, particularly for immunoassays, interference may have a serious impact on patients. Paraproteins can interfere in chemical measurements when they form precipitates during the testing procedure. Heterophilic antibodies are human antibodies that can bind animal antibodies. They can cause problems in immunoassays, particularly immunometric assays, where they can form a bridge between the capture and detection antibodies, leading to false-positive results in the absence of analyte or if analyte is also present, a false increase in measured concentrations. Very rarely, heterophilic antibodies can also lead to false-negative or falsely low results.

Very high hormone levels can interfere with immunoassay systems, resulting in falsely low analyte determinations. This is attributable to the "hook effect," which describes the inhibition of immune complex formation by excess antigen concentration. There are proteins that are well known to form aggregates with immunoglobulins or high molecular weight proteins. Clinically relevant proteins that can have "macro" forms—including amylase, creatinine kinase, LDH, and prolactin—can elevate the results when using certain laboratory tests, yet the patient lacks clinical disease related to elevated analyte concentration.

Immunoassay interference is *not* analyte specific and is variable with respect to time. In some patients, this interference can lost for a long time and in some for only a short time. This interference affects lots of assays but not all of them. In addition, a different manufacturer's test kits have different cross-reactions with interference compounds, and the test results vary from lab to lab.

Incorrect results can also occur as a result of a large number of biologically common phenomena causing analytic variation. These include cold agglutinins, rouleaux, osmotic matrix effects, platelet agglutination, giant platelets, unlysed erythrocytes, nucleated erythrocytes, megakaryocytes, red cell inclusions, cryoproteins, circulating mucin, leukocytosis, in vitro hemolysis, extreme microcytosis, bilirubinemia, lipemia, and so on.

DIAGNOSTIC TEST VALUES

Before a method is used routinely, method evaluation protocols must ensure that the measurement procedure meets defined criteria, for example, the accuracy, precision, and stability required in meeting the laboratory's patient population needs.

Four indicators are most commonly used to determine the reliability of a clinical laboratory test. Two of these, accuracy and precision, reflect how well the test method performs day to day in a laboratory. The other two, sensitivity and specificity, deal with how well the test is able to distinguish disease from the absence of disease.

The accuracy and precision of each test method are established and are frequently monitored by the clinical laboratory. Sensitivity and specificity data are determined by research studies and clinical trials. Although each test has its own performance measures and appropriate uses, laboratory tests are designed to be as precise, accurate, specific, and sensitive as possible.

ACCURACY AND PRECISION

"Accuracy" (*trueness*) refers to the ability of the test to actually measure what it claims to measure and is defined as the proportion of all test results (both positive and negative) that are correct. *Precision* (*repeatability*) refers to the ability of the test to reproduce the same result when repeated on the same patient or sample. The two concepts are related, but different. For example, a test could be precise but not accurate if on three occasions it produced roughly the same result but that result differed greatly from the actual value determined by a reference standard.

Sensitivity is defined as the ability of the test to identify correctly those who have the disease. It is the number of subjects with a positive test who have the disease divided by all subjects who have the disease. A test with high sensitivity has few false-negative results. *Specificity* is defined as the ability of the test to identify correctly those who do not have the disease. It is the number of subjects who have a negative test and do not have the disease divided by all subjects who do not have the disease. A test with high specificity has few false-positive results. Sensitivity and specificity are most useful when assessing a test used to screen a free-living population. These test characteristics are also interdependent (Figure 1-1): an increase in sensitivity is accompanied by a decrease in specificity and vice versa.

Predictive values are important for assessing how useful a test will be in the clinical setting at the individual patient level. The *positive predictive value* (PPV) is the probability of disease in a patient with a positive test. Conversely, the *negative predictive value* (NPV) is the probability that the patient does not have disease if he has a negative test result.

PPV and sensitivity of tests are complementary in their examination of true positives. Given that the test is positive, PPV is the probability that the disease is present, in contrast to sensitivity, which is given that the disease is present, the probability that test is positive. Likewise, NPV and specificity are complementary in their examination of true negatives. Given that the test is negative, NPV is the probability that the disease is absent. This is in contrast to specificity, which is given that the disease is absent, the probability that test is negative (see Figure 1-1 for more information). Predictive values depend on the prevalence of a disease in a population. A test with a given sensitivity and specificity can have different predictive values in different patient populations. If the test is used in a population with high disease prevalence, it will have a high PPV; the same test will have a low PPV when used in a population with low disease prevalence.

Is disease actually present?

		Yes	No
		True Positive	**False Positive**
	Yes	A	B
Does my test indicate		**False Negative**	**True Negative**
that disease is present?	No	C	D

Sensitivity = A/(A+C)
Specificity = D/(B+D)
PPV   = A/(A+B)
NPV   = D/(C+D)

Figure 1–1   *Sensitivity, specificity, and predictive values in laboratory testing. NPV, negative predictive value; PPV, positive predictive value.*

Likelihood ratios (LRs) are another way of assessing the accuracy of a test in the clinical setting. They are also independent of disease prevalence. LR indicates how much a given diagnostic test result will raise or lower the odds of having a disease relative to the probability of the disease. Each test is characterized by two LRs: positive LR (PLR) and negative LR (NLR). PLR tells us the odds of the disease if the test result is positive, and NLR tells the odds of disease if the test result is negative.

$$PLR = Sensitivity / (1 - Specificity)$$
$$NLR = (1 - Sensitivity) / Specificity.$$

An LR >1 increases the odds that the person has the target disease, and the higher the LR, the greater this increase in odds. Conversely, an LR ratio <1 diminishes the odds that the patient has the target disease.

RECEIVER OPERATING CHARACTERISTIC (ROC) CURVES

ROC curves allow one to identify the cutoff value that minimizes both false positives and false negatives. An ROC curve plots sensitivity on the y axis and 1 – specificity on the x axis. Applying a variety of cutoff values to the same reference population allows one to generate the curve. The perfect test would have a cutoff value that allowed an exact split of diseased and nondiseased populations (i.e., a cutoff that gave both 100% sensitivity and 100% specificity). It would plot as a right angle with the fulcrum in the far upper left corner (x = 0, y = 1). This case, however, is very rare. For most cases, as one moves from the left to right on the ROC curve, the sensitivity increases and the specificity decreases.

Calculation of the area under the ROC curve allows comparison of different tests. A perfect test has an area under the curve (AUC) equal to 1. Therefore, the closer the AUC is to 1, the better the test. Similarly, if one wants to know the cutoff value for a test that minimizes both false positives and false negatives (and hence maximizes both sensitivity and specificity), one would select the point on the ROC curve closest to the far upper left corner (x = 0, y = 1).

However, finding the right balance between optimal sensitivity and specificity may not involve simultaneously minimizing false positives and false negatives in all situations. For example, when screening for a deadly disease that is curable, it may be desirable to accept more false positives (lower specificity) in return for fewer false negatives (higher sensitivity). ROC curves allow a more thorough evaluation of a test and potential cutoff values but are not the ultimate arbiters of how to set sensitivity and specificity.

POSTANALYTIC ERRORS

Approximately 70–80% of the patient chart or medical record is composed of laboratory test results. Postanalytic errors are dependent on the design and development of those processes and procedures that will ensure correct and timely notification of these test results to the patient's medical record with right reference range and appropriate interpretation of the test result. Manual and telephone reporting should be discouraged as this reporting is subject to transcription errors at the receiver end. The introduction of a hospitalized computer order entry system has eliminated some errors, but it has not eliminated the risk of mismatching the patients.

 ## REFERENCE INTERVALS

The term "reference values" has essentially replaced the obsolete term "normal values." Laboratory tests are commonly compared to a reference interval before health care providers make physiologic assessments, medical diagnosis, or management decisions. These comparisons may be cross-sectional or longitudinal. A cross-sectional comparison is comparison of an analyte result for a single patient with the interval of results for that analyte obtained from a group of apparently healthy individuals. This is referred to as the "population-based" reference interval. Another example of a cross-sectional comparison is when a single patient result is compared with a fixed value or cutoff value. There are two types of population-based reference intervals. The most common type is derived from a reference sample of persons who are in good health (health associated). The other type of reference interval has been termed "decision based" and defines specific medical decision limits that clinicians use to diagnose or manage patients. Longitudinal comparisons are when a patient's most recent value is compared with previous values for the same analyte. This may help detect a change in health status.

Comparison of patient results with a population-based reference interval or with the cutoff values is used for diagnostic or screening purposes. The reference value change over a period of time is used for monitoring patients. Both healthy reference limits and disease-associated reference limits are important for the clinical interpretation of the laboratory test results and vary from laboratory to laboratory. These variations may be caused by preanalytic processing procedures, populations of healthy individuals, inherent random biologic variations, analytic platforms, or analytic imprecision that was present when reference intervals were determined.

Decision limits for optimally classifying patients into "disease" versus "healthy" categories are difficult to define. Most diseases are not homogenous distributions but represent a continuum of mild and severe forms. Various statistical tools and models have been developed to formalize the medical decision process, but most of the models do not include the methodologic differences in laboratory test values. The major utility of healthy reference intervals for clinicians is to provide a rough assessment of the possibility that a test value on a specific patient is difficult for the values normally found in similar healthy subjects. The guidelines for medical decision making use a standard 95% reference interval. By defining the healthy reference interval to include central 95% of matched healthy subjects, there is less than a 1 in 20 chance for a value outside the reference interval to be found in a matched healthy subject. Conventionally, a common limit of acceptability is based on the mean of population data ±2 standard deviation (SD), because this encompassed roughly 95% of the observations expected to be "normal." With this convention, it must be remembered that 5% (usually 2.5% on the low side and 2.5% on the high side) of results can be expected to fall outside the ±2 SD limit, even in a "normal" healthy population. This is best illustrated in the use of multitest chemistry profiles for screening of persons known to be free of disease. The probability of any given test being abnormal is about 2–5%, and the probability of disease if a screening test is abnormal is generally low (0–15%). The frequency of abnormal single tests is 1.5% (albumin) to 5.9% (glucose) and up to 16.6% for sodium. Based on statistical expectations, when a panel of eight tests is performed in a multiphasic health program, 25% of the patients have one or more abnormal results; when the panel includes 20 tests, 55% have one or more test abnormalities.

In terms of qualitative test reports (e.g., positive, negative), optimal decision limits (cutoff) can be determined with ROC curve analyses. If false-positive labeling leads to a more harmful outcome, the decision limits should be moved away from the ROC optimum in a direction to minimize false-positive diagnoses. Likewise, if false-negative labeling is more dangerous, the decision limits should be moved to minimize the false-negative diagnoses. Although decision limits are better tools than reference values for deriving diagnostic value from laboratory tests, they have some drawbacks. First, decision limits will not address the degree of deviation of a test result above or below the decision limit. A test result slightly above the limit will be regarded as positive the same as a result far above the decision limit, and a test result slightly below the cutoff limit will be reported as negative.

PERFORMING THE RIGHT TEST AT THE RIGHT TIME FOR THE RIGHT REASON

As with the absolute value of a result, a test result or change in sequential results must be interpreted in the context of the clinical situation, recent changes in patient management, and historical results. Excessive repetition of tests is wasteful, and the excess burden increases the possibility of laboratory errors. Appropriate intervals between tests should be dictated by the patient's clinical condition. Negative laboratory values (or any other type of tests) do not necessarily rule out a clinical diagnosis. Tests should be performed only if they will alter the patient's diagnosis, prognosis, treatment, or management. Incorrect test values or isolated individual variation in results may cause Ulysses syndrome and result in loss of time, money, and peace of mind.

SECTION 1

DISEASE STATES

SECTION 1

DISEASE STATES

CHAPTER 2

Autoimmune Diseases

M. Rabie Al-Turkmani

This chapter provides the latest information on the diagnosis of systemic autoimmune diseases. Each entry is organized with a brief definition of the disease, information regarding clinical presentation, and laboratory findings. The chapter also provides a list of common organ-specific autoimmune diseases, with an indication to where these diseases are discussed elsewhere in this book.

Autoimmune disease is the pathologic result of autoimmunity, whereby the immune system attacks the person's healthy body tissues. Autoimmunity is caused by the inappropriate activation of T cells or B cells, or both, in the absence of a definite cause. B lymphocytes can produce autoantibodies, which may interfere with a cellular function (e.g., Graves disease, myasthenia gravis) or cause tissue damage, either directly or by forming immune complexes that are deposited in tissues or blood vessels. T lymphocytes may aggregate in tissues (or a tissue) with resultant destruction.

There are more than 80 different autoimmune disorders, and more than one autoimmune disorder can be manifested by one patient. These disorders can be classified as systemic, affecting multiple organs or tissues (e.g., connective tissue autoimmune diseases such as systemic lupus erythematosus, Sjögren syndrome, or scleroderma), or organ specific, targeting one particular organ.

Multiple factors contribute to the development of autoimmune diseases:

- Genetic susceptibility, mostly due to linkage to particular HLA molecules
- Environmental triggers (e.g., drugs, chemicals)

- Infectious agents (e.g., *Mycoplasma pneumoniae*, HIV)
- Loss of regulatory T cells
- Defects in cytokine production

 ORGAN-SPECIFIC AUTOIMMUNE DISEASES

Organ-specific autoimmune diseases involve a particular organ or tissue of the body in which the target autoantigen is found. Examples of these autoimmune diseases and their target organs:

- Adrenal glands (e.g., autoimmune adrenal insufficiency). See Chapter 6, Endocrine Diseases
- Bile ducts (e.g., primary biliary cirrhosis). See Chapter 5, Digestive Diseases
- Blood cells: RBC (e.g., autoimmune hemolytic anemia), WBC (e.g., autoimmune neutropenia), platelets (e.g., immune thrombocytopenic purpura). See Chapter 9, Hematologic Disorders
- Blood vessels (e.g., autoimmune vasculitis). Discussed in this chapter and in Chapter 3, Cardiovascular Disorders
- Gastrointestinal tract (e.g., celiac disease, Crohn disease, ulcerative colitis). See Chapter 5, Digestive Diseases
- Kidney (e.g., anti–glomerular basement membrane antibody disease). See Chapter 12, Renal Disorders
- Liver (e.g., autoimmune hepatitis). See Chapter 5, Digestive Diseases
- Nervous system (e.g., myasthenia gravis [a disorder of the neuromuscular junction], multiple sclerosis, Guillain-Barré Syndrome, autoimmune autonomic failure). See Chapter 4, Central Nervous System Disorders
- Pancreas: type 1 diabetes mellitus (see Chapter 6, Endocrine Diseases), autoimmune pancreatitis (see Chapter 5, Digestive Diseases)
- Thyroid gland (e.g., Hashimoto thyroiditis, Graves disease). See Chapter 6, Endocrine Diseases

 SYSTEMIC AUTOIMMUNE DISEASES

FELTY SYNDROME

❏ **Definition**
- Felty syndrome is characterized by the triad of long-standing, aggressive rheumatoid arthritis (RA), neutropenia, and splenomegaly.
- It develops in a minority of patients with RA (<1%).

❏ **Who Should Be Suspected?**
- Patients typically present with general malaise, fatigue, loss of appetite, and unintentional weight loss. Some patients have recurrent infections, such as respiratory or skin infections, attributed to the neutropenia.
- The syndrome is more common in women >30 years of age and in patients with a family history of RA.

❏ **Laboratory Findings**
- Neutropenia (<2,000 granulocytes/μL) is required for diagnosis. WBC count is usually <2,500/μL.

- Elevated levels of rheumatoid factor (RF) and anti–cyclic citrullinated peptide (anti-CCP) antibodies (high titers).
- Antinuclear antibodies (ANAs), antihistone antibodies, and antineutrophil cytoplasmic antibodies (ANCAs) are found in more than two thirds of patients.
- Anti-glucose-6-phosphate isomerase antibody titer is elevated in the majority of patients.
- Anemia and thrombocytopenia may develop or be aggravated by splenomegaly (hypersplenism).
- Erythrocyte sedimentation rate (ESR) and C-reactive protein (CRP) are very elevated.
- Circulating immune complexes and immunoglobulin levels are higher than those found in RA.
- Peripheral blood smear review and bone marrow aspirate or biopsy may be indicated to exclude other causes of neutropenia.

MIXED CONNECTIVE TISSUE DISEASE

❑ **Definition**

- Mixed connective tissue disease (MCTD) represents an overlap syndrome with features of systemic lupus erythematosus (SLE), systemic sclerosis, and polymyositis.
- The disease can be serious with development of kidney, cardiovascular, gastrointestinal, and central nervous system manifestations. Pulmonary disease is associated with the highest mortality.

❑ **Who Should Be Suspected?**

- Presenting symptoms are often nonspecific, such as fatigue, myalgia, arthralgia, and low-grade fever. In the early stages of disease, 90% of MCTD patients have Raynaud phenomenon, arthralgia, swollen hands, fingers with "sausage-like" appearance, and muscle weakness. Other common symptoms that may develop gradually include swollen joints, esophageal dysfunction, sclerodactyly, and calcinosis.
- MCTD usually develops in the second or third decade of life, and is more common in women than men.

❑ **Laboratory Findings**

- Positive ANA, with a high-titer speckled pattern (>1:1,000 and often >1:10,000) using the indirect fluorescent antibody test (IFA).
- Presence of high titers of anti-U1 ribonucleoprotein (anti-RNP) antibodies, especially antibodies to the 68 kDa protein, is highly suggestive of an MCTD diagnosis and separates it as an independent disease.
- Anti-SSA/Ro, anti-single-stranded DNA (ssDNA), anti-Smith (Sm), and anti-double-stranded DNA (dsDNA) antibodies have also been detected, but they are not specific for MCTD.
- Antiphospholipid antibodies have been reported in patients with MCTD, with a lower frequency than that found in SLE. Anticardiolipin antibodies (ACAs) are present in approximately 15% of MCTD patients.
- Elevated ESR and CRP.

- Positive RF and anti-CCP antibodies in approximately 50% of the patients.
- Anemia, leukopenia, and hypergammaglobulinemia may present.

Suggested Reading

Ortega-Hernandez OD, Shoenfeld Y. Mixed connective tissue disease: an overview of clinical manifestations, diagnosis and treatment. *Best Pract Res Clin Rheumatol.* 2012;26(1):61–72.

POLYMYALGIA RHEUMATICA

❏ Definition

- Polymyalgia rheumatica (PMR) is an inflammatory rheumatic disorder characterized by morning stiffness and pain in the muscles of the shoulders, neck, back, hip, and thighs.
- The 2012 European League Against Rheumatism (EULAR)/American College of Rheumatology (ACR) classification criteria for PMR use a scoring algorithm that applies to patients >50 years of age, presenting with new bilateral shoulder pain (not better explained by an alternative diagnosis) and elevated CRP/ESR. The elements of this algorithm include the following:
  - ▼ Morning stiffness for more than 45 minutes (2 points)
  - ▼ Hip pain/ limited range of motion (1 point)
  - ▼ Absence of rheumatoid factor and/or anti–citrullinated protein antibody (2 points)
  - ▼ Absence of peripheral joint pain (1 point)
- A score of 4 or more has 68% sensitivity and 78% specificity for distinguishing PMR patients. Ultrasound findings of bilateral shoulder abnormalities or abnormalities in one shoulder and hip were found to significantly improve both sensitivity and specificity of the clinical criteria.

❏ Who Should Be Suspected?

- The disease is almost exclusively found in individuals >50 years of age. Patients typically present with general malaise, fatigue, as well as aches and morning stiffness in the shoulder, hip girdles, neck, lower back, and knees. Loss of appetite, unintentional weight loss, and depression are also common findings.
- PMR develops in nearly 50% of patients with giant cell arteritis (GCA), and 15–30% of patients with PMR eventually develop GCA.

❏ Laboratory Findings

Laboratory finding are nonspecific.

- ESR is markedly elevated (>40 mm/hour, but values >100 may be seen). However, some patients with mild disease may have only slight elevations of ESR.
- CRP is elevated and considered a more sensitive marker than ESR.
- Serologic tests such as RF, ANA, and anti-CCP antibodies are typically negative.

Suggested Reading

Dasgupta B, Cimmino MA, et al. 2012 provisional classification criteria for polymyalgia rheumatica: a European League Against Rheumatism/American College of Rheumatology collaborative initiative. *Ann Rheum Dis.* 2012;71(4):484–492.

POLYMYOSITIS, DERMATOMYOSITIS, AND INCLUSION BODY MYOSITIS

❑ Definition

- Polymyositis (PM), dermatomyositis (DM), and inclusion body myositis (IBM) are related inflammatory myopathies that share common features, including muscle weakness and inflammatory infiltrates on a muscle biopsy.
- PM and DM are characterized by a subacute onset of symmetric proximal muscle weakness, common involvement of other organ systems such as lung and skin, a strong association with autoantibodies, and responsiveness to immunosuppression. Both are widely accepted as having an autoimmune basis. Cutaneous involvement is the primary clinical feature distinguishing patients with DM from those with PM.
- In contrast to PM and DM, patients with IBM typically have slowly progressive weakness in both proximal and distal muscles, rarely have other extramuscular involvement or autoantibodies, and most often do not respond to immunosuppressive therapies. A muscle biopsy showing the presence of typical inclusion bodies is diagnostic for IBM.

❑ Who Should Be Suspected?

- Patients with PM and DM typically present with progressive proximal muscle weakness and evidence of muscle inflammation. They may also have constitutional symptoms and evidence of involvement of other organs (e.g., interstitial pulmonary disease, polyarthritis). DM patients can be differentiated by having specific cutaneous signs such as Gottron papules or heliotrope eruption.
- Patients with IBM generally have a more insidious onset compared to PM and DM, and more prominent distal muscle weakness.
- PM and DM can occur at any age, with peak incidence between the ages of 40 and 50, whereas IBM mainly affects individuals >50 years of age.

❑ Laboratory Findings

Diagnosis of the three conditions is based on clinical manifestations, serum muscle enzymes, autoantibodies, EMG findings, and muscle biopsy. The latter is the definitive test for establishing the diagnosis of IBM, and in PM or DM patients presenting with atypical clinical or laboratory findings.

- Muscle enzymes:
  - ▼ Levels of the muscle enzyme creatine kinase (CK) are greatly elevated in PM and DM patients (typically >10 folds the upper limit of normal but may be >50 folds), and to a lesser extent in patients with IBM.
  - ▼ Other muscle enzymes including lactate dehydrogenase (LDH), aldolase, aspartate aminotransferase (AST) and alanine aminotransferase (ALT) are also elevated. Similar to CK, elevations are less profound in IBM than in PM or DM.
- ANA test is positive in up to 80% of patients with DM or PM.
- Myositis-specific antibodies are positive in 30% of patients with PM or DM. The most common antibodies are those against histidyl-tRNA synthetase

(anti-Jo-1), and titers of these antibodies have been found to correlate with disease activity. Other myositis-specific antibodies include anti-Mi-2 and anti–signal recognition particle (anti-SRP) antibodies. Presence of other connective disease conditions associated with myositis is suggested when another type of autoantibodies is positive (e.g., anti-SSA/Ro, anti-SSB/La, anti-Sm, or anti-RNP).

- ESR is normal or mildly increased.
- Myoglobin is elevated in the serum and urine.

Suggested Reading

Mammen AL. Dermatomyositis and polymyositis: clinical presentation, autoantibodies, and pathogenesis. *Ann N Y Acad Sci.* 2010;1184:134–153.

PSORIATIC ARTHRITIS

❏ Definition

- Psoriatic arthritis (PsA) is a type of arthritic inflammation that occurs in approximately 15% of patients with psoriasis. It can affect any joint in the body causing pain, swelling, and stiffness. CD8+ T cells and T-cell-derived cytokines play a central role in the pathogenesis of PsA.
- The Classification Criteria for Psoriatic Arthritis (CASPAR) require the presence of joint, spine, or entheseal inflammatory disease plus a minimum score of 3 points from the following five categories (98.7% specificity and 91.4% sensitivity):
  - ▼ Current psoriasis (2 points); personal or family history of psoriasis (1 point)
  - ▼ Typical psoriatic nail dystrophy (1 point)
  - ▼ Negative rheumatoid factor (1 point)
  - ▼ Current dactylitis or history of dactylitis (1 point)
  - ▼ Hand or foot plain radiography demonstrating juxta-articular new bone formation (1 point)

❏ Who Should Be Suspected?

- Most patients who develop PsA have skin symptoms of psoriasis first (erythematous papule and plaques with a silver scale), followed later by arthritis symptoms characterized by pain, tenderness, and stiffness in the joints and back.
- Several HLA types have been identified to be associated with PsA, suggesting a genetic predisposition. This is also indicated by the presence of a family history of psoriasis and psoriatic arthritis in up to 40% of patients.

❏ Laboratory Findings

Laboratory finding are not specific.

- ESR and CRP are elevated in approximately 50% of cases; levels correlate with the number of involved joints.
- RF is negative.
- Anemia of inflammation, hypergammaglobulinemia with increased IgA levels, and hypoalbuminemia have been reported in some cases.

- Hyperuricemia, related to either increased skin cell turnover or metabolic defect, is found in nearly 20% of patients.
- HLA testing can be helpful: HLA Cw6 is the most important allele for susceptibility to early-onset psoriasis; HLA-B17 may be associated with a more severe phenotype.

Suggested Reading

Cantini F, Niccoli L, Nannini C, et al. Psoriatic arthritis: a systematic review. *Int J Rheum Dis.* 2010;13(4):300–317.

REACTIVE ARTHRITIS

❑ Definition

- Reactive arthritis, formerly known as Reiter syndrome, is an autoimmune spondylarthritis that develops 1–4 weeks after an infection with a pathogen elsewhere in the body. Most often, causing pathogens are urogenital (e.g., *Chlamydia*) or enteric (e.g., *Campylobacter, Salmonella, Shigella,* or *Yersinia*).

❑ Who Should Be Suspected?

- A likely patient is a young adult (20– 40 years of age) who develops postinfectious asymmetric oligoarthritis (affecting most often the knees, ankles, and heels), enthesitis, dactylitis, and lower back pain. In addition, patients may have extra-articular signs including urinary (urethritis, balanitis, dysuria, prostatitis in men, cervicitis, salpingitis or vulvovaginitis in women), ocular (conjunctivitis or anterior uveitis), and/or constitutional (malaise, fever, weight loss) symptoms.

❑ Laboratory Findings

Diagnosis is primarily clinical.

- Culture and serology tests are helpful in identifying the infectious etiology of the disease in only a fraction of cases since pathogens may no longer be retrievable by the time arthritis develops. Nevertheless, a trial to identify the following pathogens by stool or urine cultures, or in some cases by serology, should be attempted:
  - ▼ *Chlamydia,* especially *Chlamydia trachomatis* and *Chlamydia pneumoniae*. PCR for urinary *Chlamydia* DNA has high sensitivity.
  - ▼ *Yersinia enterocolitica* and *Yersinia pseudotuberculosis*.
  - ▼ *Salmonella* of various serovars.
  - ▼ *Shigella,* especially *Shigella flexneri* and *Shigella dysenteriae*.
  - ▼ *Campylobacter,* especially *Campylobacter jejuni*.
  - ▼ *Clostridium difficile*.
  - ▼ Possibly other organisms (e.g., HIV, *Escherichia coli, Mycoplasma genitalium*).
- HLA-B27 is positive in approximately half of the patients and seems to be associated with a more sudden and severe onset of symptoms as well as increased likelihood to have chronic (long-lasting) disease.
- Elevated ESR and CRP during the acute phase of disease.

- RF is negative.
- Synovial fluid analysis shows elevated WBC count, predominantly neutrophils, and may help distinguish reactive arthritis from other forms of arthritis.

RETROPERITONEAL FIBROSIS

❑ Definition

- A rare disease characterized by the presence of fibrosclerotic tissue in the retroperitoneum, often leading to encasement of the ureters and, less frequently, blood and lymphatic vessels.
- About two thirds of the cases are idiopathic, while the remaining cases are secondary to a variety of causes, including drugs (e.g., beta-blockers, methyldopa, hydralazine, analgesics), tumors (e.g., Hodgkin disease and non-Hodgkin lymphoma, sarcomas, carcinomas), infections (e.g., TB, histoplasmosis, actinomycosis), radiation, or surgery.
- Idiopathic retroperitoneal fibrosis is part of the disease spectrum of chronic periaortitis, which is characterized by inflammation and fibrosis surrounding the aorta and iliac arteries. It has also been suggested that idiopathic retroperitoneal fibrosis is a manifestation of either a systemic autoimmune disorder or IgG4-related disease.

❑ Who Should Be Suspected?

- Most patients present with abdominal, lower back, or flank pain. In addition, up to one half of patients complain of constitutional manifestations such as fever, weight loss, fatigue, and night sweats. Renal failure due to obstruction of the ureters develops in more than 40% of patients, and new-onset hypertension has been reported in approximately one third of patients.
- The idiopathic disease most commonly occurs in individuals 40–60 years of age. Men are affected two to three times more than women.

❑ Laboratory Findings
Diagnosis is established by imaging studies.

- ESR and CRP are elevated in approximately one half to two thirds of patients.
- Anemia of chronic inflammation (normochromic, normocytic) is a frequent finding and can also be related to renal dysfunction.
- Leukocytosis, eosinophilia, hyperferritinemia, or hypergammaglobulinemia may be present in some patients.
- ANA test is positive in up to 60% of cases.
- Serum IgG4 levels are frequently elevated in patients with IgG4-related disease.
- Blood urea nitrogen (BUN) and creatinine can be elevated; levels are variable depending on the presence and size of urinary obstruction. Urine sediment is often normal.

Suggested Reading
Pipitone N, Vaglio A, Salvarani C. Retroperitoneal fibrosis. *Best Pract Res Clin Rheumatol.* 2012;26(4):439–448.

RHEUMATOID ARTHRITIS

2

❑ Definition

- Rheumatoid arthritis (RA) is a chronic inflammatory arthritis characterized by progressive, symmetric joint swelling, tenderness, and destruction, leading in some cases to severe disability and premature mortality. The potential of synovitis to cause cartilage damage and bone erosion is characteristic for the disease. In addition to joints, RA may affect many other tissues and organs (e.g., lungs, pleura, pericardium, sclera), but the joints are usually most severely affected.

- Given the presence of autoantibodies, RA is considered an autoimmune disease, and it is the most common type of autoimmune arthritis. Autoimmunity and the overall systemic and articular inflammatory load drive the destructive progression of the disease.

- According to the 2010 ACR/EULAR criteria, classification of RA is based on the confirmed presence of synovitis in at least one joint, absence of an alternative diagnosis that better explains the synovitis, and achievement of a total score of 6 or greater (of a possible 10) from the individual scores in four domains:

  ▼ Number and site/size of involved joints (score range 0–5)

  ▼ Serologic abnormality, based on serum levels of RF and anti–citrullinated protein antibody (score range 0–3)

  ▼ Elevated acute-phase response, based on CRP and ESR (score range 0–1)

  ▼ Symptom duration (< or ≥6 weeks; range 0–1)

❑ Who Should Be Suspected?

- Candidates are individuals presenting with fatigue, weakness, anorexia, and slowly progressive pain and swelling of the joints. Involvement of the small joints of the hands or feet should raise suspicion of RA. Early symptoms may also include fatigue, muscle pain, low-grade fever, weight loss, and numbness and tingling of the hands.

- Onset of RA most often occurs between the fourth and sixth decades of life but can also be seen in the pediatric population (juvenile rheumatoid arthritis) as well as the elderly. Women are three times more likely to develop RA than are men.

- Sixty to seventy percent of RA patients of European ancestry carry the *HLA-DR4* gene compared to 30% in the general population, indicating a genetic predisposition.

❑ Laboratory Findings

There is no pathognomonic test for RA. Tests for diseases that can mimic RA (hemochromatosis, SLE, systemic sclerosis, sarcoidosis) may be indicated.

- RF is positive in approximately 80% of patients within one year of presentation, but in only 30% at the onset of arthritis. In the absence of RF (15–20% of cases), the disease is called seronegative RA.

- Anti–citrullinated protein antibody, tested as anti-CCP or anti–mutated citrullinated vimentin, is more specific for RA than RF. Anti-CCP antibodies are found in 60–70% of RA cases and have approximately 95% specificity.

- ANA test is positive in 25–50% of patients.

- Synovial fluid analysis reveals an inflammatory pattern with increased WBC counts (2,000–50,000/µL in affected joints), with a predominance of neutrophils. Total hemolytic complement, C3, and C4 are markedly reduced.
- ESR and CRP are elevated.

Suggested Reading

Aletaha D, Neogi T, Silman AJ, et al. 2010 rheumatoid arthritis classification criteria: an American College of Rheumatology/European League Against Rheumatism collaborative initiative. *Arthritis Rheum.* 2010;62(9):2569–2581.

SJÖGREN SYNDROME

❏ Definition

- Sjögren syndrome (SjS) is an inflammatory, autoimmune disease in which the exocrine glands, mainly the salivary and lacrimal glands, are attacked and destroyed by the immune cells.
- The syndrome is divided into primary SjS (not associated with other diseases), or secondary SjS, which is associated with other autoimmune rheumatic conditions, principally rheumatoid arthritis (most common) or SLE. In both primary and secondary SjS, decreased exocrine gland function leads to the "sicca complex," characterized by dry mouth (xerostomia) and dry eyes (keratoconjunctivitis sicca).
- The American-European Consensus Group criteria for classification of SjS were developed in 2002. In 2012, new criteria were proposed by the American College of Rheumatology and the Sjögren's International Collaborative Clinical Alliance. Using the later criteria, classification of SjS, which applies to individuals with signs/symptoms that may be suggestive of SjS, will be met in the presence of at least two of the following three objective features:
  - ▼ Positive serum anti-SSA/Ro and/or anti-SSB/La *or* positive rheumatoid factor and ANA titer ≥1:320
  - ▼ Labial salivary gland biopsy exhibiting focal lymphocytic sialadenitis with a focus score ≥1 focus/4 mm²
  - ▼ Keratoconjunctivitis sicca with ocular staining score ≥3 (assuming that the individual is not currently using daily eye drops for glaucoma and has not had corneal surgery or cosmetic eyelid surgery in the last 5 years)

❏ Who Should Be Suspected?

- SjS patients typically present with complaints of ocular symptoms, such as persistent dry eyes for more than 3 months and oral symptoms of dryness (e.g., the need to drink water to be able to swallow food). This may be associated with vague symptoms such as fatigue and myalgia.
- SjS can affect people of any age, but symptoms usually appear between the ages of 45 and 55. It affects 10 times as many women as men, and about half of SjS patients also have rheumatoid arthritis or other connective tissue diseases, such as lupus.
- Occasionally, other tissues or organs may be involved. As a result, extraglandular manifestations develop, and they may include pain and stiffness in

the joints, even in the absence of rheumatoid arthritis or lupus, rashes on the arms and legs related to vasculitis, or inflammation in the lungs, liver, and kidneys.

❏ Laboratory Findings

- Positive ANA test, with high titers and a fine speckled staining pattern by IFA, is found in two thirds of patients.
- Anti-SSA/Ro and Anti-SSB/La antibodies are frequently detected in the serum of patients with SjS, and their presence supports the diagnosis. These antibodies are also detected in patients with SLE.
- RF is frequently positive because of the association of SjS with rheumatoid arthritis.
- CRP and ESR are typically elevated.
- Other laboratory tests are indicated to evaluate systemic and extraglandular involvement, and they include serum electrolytes, anticardiolipin antibodies, lupus anticoagulant, cryoglobulins, liver function tests, and urinalysis.
- Imaging studies and specific diagnostic tests of the glands can help with the diagnosis. Tests commonly used include Schirmer test to measure tear production, rose bengal test to assess the damage to epithelial cells in the cornea and conjunctivae, and tear breakup time test to measure overall lacrimal function.

Suggested Reading

Shiboski SC, Shiboski CH, Criswell L, et al. American College of Rheumatology classification criteria for Sjögren's syndrome: a data-driven, expert consensus approach in the Sjögren's International Collaborative Clinical Alliance cohort. *Arthritis Care Res.* 2012;64(4):475–487.

SYSTEMIC LUPUS ERYTHEMATOSUS

❏ Definition

- SLE is a chronic autoimmune disease characterized by multisystem involvement and a variable clinical course. A prominent feature of SLE is the production of a number of antinuclear antibodies. The autoantibodies and immune complexes bind to various tissues, with resulting damage.
- According to the ACR classification criteria for SLE, a person is said to have SLE if any four or more of the following 11 criteria are present, serially or simultaneously, during any interval of observation:
  - ▼ Malar rash
  - ▼ Discoid rash
  - ▼ Photosensitivity
  - ▼ Oral ulcers
  - ▼ Nonerosive arthritis, involving two or more peripheral joints
  - ▼ Pleuritis or pericarditis
  - ▼ Renal disorder, manifested by persistent proteinuria or cellular casts
  - ▼ Neurologic disorder: seizures or psychosis
  - ▼ Hematologic disorder: hemolytic anemia, leukopenia, lymphopenia, or thrombocytopenia

▼ Immunologic disorder: anti-dsDNA antibody, anti-Sm antibody, or positive finding of antiphospholipid antibodies

▼ Positive antinuclear antibody at any point in time and in the absence of drugs

❏ Who Should Be Suspected?

- Likely patients are individuals presenting with constitutional symptoms (fatigue, fever, weight loss) associated with features of multisystem or, in some cases, a single organ involvement. These features may include rash, photosensitivity, arthralgia or arthritis, anemia, serositis, nephritis, mild peripheral edema, or neurologic symptoms such as seizures, psychosis, or peripheral nephropathy.

- SLE affects 10 times as many women as men. Disease onset commonly occurs between 20 and 40 years of age.

- A variant of lupus, called drug-induced lupus erythematosus, may be the result of treatment with procainamide, hydralazine, chlorpromazine, quinidine, or, more recently, anti-TNF alpha. Patients typically present with skin and joint manifestations but rarely have renal or neurologic features. It is a self-limited condition in most cases, and symptoms usually recede after discontinuing the drug.

❏ Laboratory Findings

Supportive laboratory studies are mandatory for the diagnosis.

- ANA test is positive with high titers (1:160 or higher) in >98% of SLE patients during the course of disease. ANA staining pattern can be homogenous (common), rim (specific), speckled, or nucleolar. Rheumatoid diseases other than SLE may also be associated with a positive ANA, but usually in lower titers (e.g., Sjögren syndrome, scleroderma, rheumatoid arthritis). If ANA is repeatedly negative, SLE can be excluded in the vast majority of suspected patients.

  ▼ Anti-double-stranded DNA (anti-dsDNA) antibodies are highly specific for SLE. They are present in 70% of SLE patients but in less than 0.5% of healthy population or patients with other autoimmune diseases. These antibodies have been found to be associated with renal involvement (lupus nephritis), and their titers fluctuate with the activity of SLE, allowing for following the course of disease.

  ▼ Anti-Smith (anti-Sm) antibodies are very specific (96%) but lack sensitivity (25%). They are associated with renal disease and occur more frequently in African American and Asian patients than in Caucasians with SLE.

  ▼ Antibodies to U1 ribonucleoprotein (anti-RNP) coexist with anti-Sm antibodies in patients with SLE, but they are less specific. These antibodies are associated with myositis, Raynaud phenomenon, and less severe lupus. They are also present in mixed connective tissue disease and systemic sclerosis.

  ▼ Anti-SSA/Ro and, less frequently, anti-SSB/La antibodies are detected in some SLE patients. These antibodies are frequently detected in patients with Sjögren syndrome. Presence of anti-SSA/Ro antibodies in patients with SLE is associated with lymphopenia, photosensitivity, neonatal lupus, complement deficiency, and subacute cutaneous lupus. In addition, their presence with anti-SSB/La antibodies during pregnancy confers a 1–2% risk of congenital heart block in the offspring.

▼ Anti–ribosomal P protein (anti-Ribo-P) antibodies have been reported in SLE patients with neuropsychiatric manifestations.

▼ Antihistone antibodies are present in >95% of patients with drug-induced lupus, especially with the disease associated with procainamide, hydralazine, chlorpromazine, and quinidine, whereas other autoantibodies are uncommon. Antihistone antibodies are also present in up to 80% of patients with idiopathic SLE.

▼ See Figure 2-1.

- Antibodies associated with the antiphospholipid syndrome (anticardiolipin antibodies, anti-β2 glycoprotein 1 antibodies) and lupus anticoagulant are frequently positive in SLE patients and associated with venous or arterial thrombosis. Approximately one third of patients with antiphospholipid syndrome have SLE.

- Although RF is not specific for SLE, its presence correlates with active inflammatory arthritis.

- Anemia may be that of chronic inflammation or autoimmune hemolytic.

- Thrombocytopenia, neutropenia, or lymphopenia are usually immune in origin.

- Serum complement C3 and C4 levels are decreased in parallel with disease activity.

- ESR and CRP are often elevated in active disease.

- Renal function studies are indicated to assess renal involvement.

- Presence of cryoglobulins may correlate with disease activity.

Suggested Reading

Rahman A, Isenberg DA. Systemic lupus erythematosus. *N Engl J Med.* 2008;358:929–939.

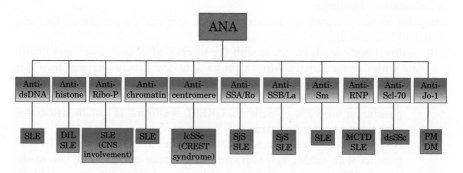

Figure 2–1 *Role of antinuclear antibodies in the diagnosis of connective tissue diseases. ANA, antinuclear antibodies; CNS, central nervous system; DIL, drug-induced lupus erythematosus; DM, dermatomyositis; dsDNA, double-stranded DNA; dsSSc, diffuse cutaneous scleroderma; lcSSc, limited cutaneous scleroderma; MCTD, mixed connective tissue disease; PM, Polymyositis; Ribo-P: ribosomal P protein; RNP, U1 ribonucleoprotein; SjS, Sjögren syndrome; SLE, systemic lupus erythematosus; Sm, Smith.*

SYSTEMIC SCLEROSIS (SCLERODERMA)

❑ **Definition**

- Systemic sclerosis (SSc) is a complex, progressive disease characterized by extensive fibrosis, vascular alterations, and multiple system involvement.
- SSc is subcategorized into two distinct subtypes, depending on the extent of skin involvement:
  - ▼ Limited cutaneous scleroderma (lcSSc): fibrosis is mainly restricted to the hands, arms, and face. Patients typically display features of the CREST syndrome (calcinosis, Raynaud phenomenon, esophageal motility dysfunction, sclerodactyly, and telangiectasia).
  - ▼ Diffuse cutaneous scleroderma (dsSSc): rapidly progressive and affects large areas of the skin and one or more internal organs. Sclerosis skin is found on the chest, abdomen, or upper arms or shoulders.
- Patients with scleroderma plus evidence of SLE, rheumatoid arthritis, polymyositis, or Sjögren syndrome are considered to have overlap syndrome.

❑ **Who Should Be Suspected?**

- SSc patients typically present with fatigue, weakness, arthralgias, and thickening and tightness of the skin, either restricted or diffuse. They can also have Raynaud phenomena and signs of multiple internal organ involvement.
- Extracutaneous organ involvement can lead to dysfunction or failure of almost any internal organ including the musculoskeletal system (e.g., arthralgia, myalgia), lungs (e.g., pulmonary fibrosis, interstitial lung disease), kidneys (e.g., proteinuria, decreased GFR, scleroderma renal crisis, hypertension), heart (e.g., ventricular dysfunction), gastrointestinal tract (e.g., dysphagia, heartburn), and the nervous system (e.g., headache, seizures). Lung involvement is the leading cause of death in SSc patients.
- Women are at much higher risk for scleroderma than are men, with a ratio of ≥3:1.

❑ **Laboratory Findings**

Diagnosis of SSc is based on clinical findings, and can be confirmed (but not excluded) by serology.

- Autoantibody levels correlate with the severity of disease, and titers fluctuate with disease activity. More than 95% of SSc patients have at least one autoantibody.
  - ▼ ANA test, with low titers and a nucleolar or speckled pattern by IFA, is positive in 60–90% of patients. CREST syndrome is usually associated with the centromere pattern.
  - ▼ Anti–topoisomerase I (anti-Scl-70) antibodies are present in 30–70% of patients with dcSSc, and they are highly specific, but occur late in the disease. When positive, they suggest higher risk of severe interstitial lung disease, cardiac, or renal involvement.
  - ▼ Anticentromere antibodies in moderate titers are highly specific but have only moderate sensitivity. They are typically associated with lcSSc and found in the majority of patients with CREST syndrome.

▼ Anti-RNA polymerase III antibodies are specific for SSc and have moderate sensitivity. They are associated with extensive skin involvement and scleroderma renal crisis.

▼ Anti-β2-glycoprotein 1 and anticardiolipin antibodies may be positive. Anti-β2-glycoprotein 1 antibodies have been found to be independently associated with macrovascular disease and mortality in SSc patients.

▼ Antibodies to U3-RNP (antifibrillarin) are detected in dcSSc patients and associated with increased risk of pulmonary hypertension, scleroderma renal disease, and skeletal muscle involvement.

▼ Anti-PM/Scl autoantibodies indicate associated myositis.

▼ Antibodies to RNA polymerase II may be found in SSc and SLE patients.

▼ RF is positive in 30% of patients. When present in high titer, it suggests overlap disease.

■ Serum and urine protein electrophoresis may be indicated to exclude monoclonal gammopathies in patients with symmetrical skin induration but no Raynaud phenomenon.

■ Eosinophilia is common.

■ ESR may be normal, mildly increased, or greatly increased.

■ Skin biopsy is rarely necessary.

Suggested Reading

Gabrielli A, Avvedimento EV, Krieg T. Scleroderma. *N Engl J Med.* 2009;360(19):1989–2003.

 AUTOIMMUNE VASCULITIS

See Vasculitis (Chapter 3, Cardiovascular Disorders).

EOSINOPHILIC GRANULOMATOSIS WITH POLYANGIITIS (CHURG-STRAUSS SYNDROME)

❏ **Definition**

■ Eosinophilic granulomatosis with polyangiitis (EGPA), also referred to as Churg-Strauss syndrome (CSS) or allergic granulomatosis and angiitis, is a multisystem vasculitis affecting small and medium-sized blood vessels and characterized by asthma, allergic rhinitis and sinusitis, eosinophil-rich inflammation, and peripheral blood eosinophilia.

■ EGPA has three phases:

▼ Prodromal (allergic) phase: characterized by airway inflammation (asthma and allergic rhinitis).

▼ Eosinophilic phase: peripheral eosinophilia and eosinophilic infiltration of multiple organs, especially the lungs and gastrointestinal tract.

▼ Vasculitic phase: systemic vasculitis that can be life threatening and is often associated with vascular and extravascular granulomatosis.

■ See Table 2-1.

TABLE 2–1. The American College of Rheumatology 1990 Criteria for the Classification of Vasculitis

Eosinophilic Granulomatosis with Polyangiitis (Churg-Strauss Syndrome)	Giant Cell (Temporal) Arteritis	Granulomatosis with Polyangiitis (Wegener Granulomatosis)	Henoch-Schönlein Purpura	Hypersensitivity Vasculitis	Polyarteritis Nodosa	Takayasu Arteritis
Presence of at least 4 of 6 criteria (sensitivity of 85%; specificity of 99.7%)	Presence of at least 3 of 5 criteria (sensitivity of 94%; specificity of 91%)	Presence of at least 2 of 4 criteria (sensitivity of 88%; specificity of 92%)	Presence of at least 2 of 4 criteria (sensitivity of 87%; specificity of 88%)	Presence of at least 3 of 5 criteria (sensitivity of 71%; specificity of 84%)	Presence of at least 3 of 10 criteria (sensitivity of 82%; specificity of 87%)	Presence of at least 3 of 6 criteria (sensitivity of 91%; specificity = 98%)
1) Asthma	1) Age at disease onset ≥50 years	1) Nasal or oral inflammation (e.g., oral ulcers or purulent or bloody nasal discharge)	1) Palpable purpura (not related to thrombocytopenia)	1) Age at disease onset >16 years	1) Weight loss ≥4 kg	1) Age at disease onset <40 years
2) Eosinophilia >10%	2) New headache	2) Abnormal chest radiograph showing the presence of nodules, fixed infiltrates, or cavities	2) Age ≤20 at disease onset	2) Medication was taken at the onset of symptoms that may have been a precipitating factor	2) Livedo reticularis	2) Claudication of the extremities (especially the upper extremities)
3) Neuropathy, mono or poly	3) Temporal artery tenderness to palpation or decreased pulsation	3) Urinary sediment showing microhematuria (>5 red blood cells per high-power field) or red cell casts	3) Diffuse abdominal pain, worse after meals, or the diagnosis of bowel ischemia, usually including bloody diarrhea	3) Palpable purpura (does not blanch with pressure and is not related to thrombocytopenia)	3) Testicular pain or tenderness	3) Decreased brachial artery pulse
4) Pulmonary infiltrates, nonfixed	4) Elevated erythrocyte sedimentation rate ≥50 mm/h by the Westergren method	4) Histologic changes showing granulomatous inflammation within the wall of an artery or in the perivascular or extravascular area (artery or arteriole)	4) Histologic changes showing granulocytes in the walls of arterioles or venules	4) Maculopapular rash	4) Myalgias, weakness or leg tenderness	4) Blood pressure difference between arms >10 mm Hg
5) Paranasal sinus abnormality	5) Abnormal artery biopsy, showing vasculitis characterized by a predominance of mononuclear cell infiltration or granulomatous inflammation, usually with multinucleated giant cells			5) Biopsy demonstrating granulocytes around an arteriole or venule	5) Mononeuropathy or polyneuropathy	5) Bruit over subclavian arteries or aorta
6) Extravascular eosinophils					6) Development of hypertension with diastolic blood pressure >90 mm Hg	6) Arteriographic narrowing or occlusion of the entire aorta, its primary branches, or large arteries in the proximal upper or lower extremities, (changes usually focal or segmental)
					7) Elevated blood urea nitrogen (>40 mg/dL) or creatinine (>1.5 mg/dL)	
					8) Evidence of infection with hepatitis B virus	
					9) Characteristic arteriographic abnormalities	
					10) Biopsy of a small- or medium-sized artery containing polymorphonuclear neutrophils	

Adapted from the website of the American College of Rheumatology (www.rheumatology.org).

2

❑ Who Should Be Suspected?

- Candidates are patients with asthma that is poorly controlled and a necrotizing eosinophilic vasculitis. In addition to pulmonary and sinus involvement, organs commonly affected by EGPA include the skin, kidneys, peripheral nervous system, gastrointestinal tract, and cardiovascular system. Cardiac involvement accounts for approximately one half of deaths attributable to EGPA.
- EGPA frequently occurs in patients between 40 and 60 years of age.

❑ Laboratory Findings

Diagnosis relies on a combination of tissue biopsy (eosinophilic infiltrates, necrosis, and eosinophilic giant cell vasculitis) and laboratory testing.

- Leukocytosis with peripheral blood eosinophilia (>1,500 cells/µL; usually in the 5,000–9,000 range) is found in approximately 90% of patients. Eosinophilia may be missed in some cases due to spontaneous fluctuations or corticosteroid therapy preceding the diagnosis.
- Circulating ANCAs are present in 40–60% of EGPA cases. The majority of ANCA-positive patients have antibodies against myeloperoxidase (MPO), with a perinuclear staining pattern (p-ANCA).
- Elevated serum IgE during the vasculitic phase.
- Hypergammaglobulinemia and markedly elevated ESR and CRP.
- Complement components (C3, C4, CH50) may be normal or elevated.
- Normochromic, normocytic anemia.
- Proteinuria and microscopic hematuria can be present.

GIANT CELL ARTERITIS

❑ Definition

- Giant cell (temporal) arteritis is a chronic systemic vasculitis of the large- and medium-sized vessels, involving especially the cranial branches of the arteries that originate from the aortic arch.
- Visual impairment is a major complication of the disease, and failure to make the diagnosis may lead to irreversible visual loss.
- See Table 2-1.

❑ Who Should Be Suspected?

- Candidates are patients with severe bitemporal headache, visual disturbances (primarily partial, transient monocular visual loss), jaw claudication, and symptoms of polymyalgia rheumatica (30–50% of cases). Other frequent manifestations of systemic inflammation can be present and they include fatigue, general malaise, fever, anorexia, weight loss, and night sweats.
- This disorder mainly affects individuals >50 years or age and is extremely rare in younger people. The incidence rises markedly with increasing age, peaking in the eighth decade of life.

❑ Laboratory Findings

Diagnosis is mainly clinical. Laboratory studies are pertinent, but not specific.

- Increased ESR (≥50 mm/h, mean 88 mm/h).
- Thrombocytosis with platelet counts >400,000/µL and CRP levels >2.45 mg/dL have been found to be to the strongest laboratory predictors of a positive temporal artery biopsy.
- Increased levels of IgG and complement.
- Mild to moderate normocytic, normochromic anemia in approximately 50% of patients.
- Mildly abnormal liver function tests, particularly increased aspartate aminotransferase (AST) and alkaline phosphatase (ALP) levels in nearly one third of patients.
- Increased interleukin-6 (IL-6); levels are related to disease activity.
- Biopsy of the involved arterial segment (commonly the temporal artery) and imaging studies can support the diagnosis.

Suggested Reading

Borchers AT, Gershwin ME. Giant cell arteritis: a review of classification, pathophysiology, geoepidemiology and treatment. *Autoimmun Rev.* 2012;11(6–7):A544–A554.

GRANULOMATOSIS WITH POLYANGIITIS (WEGENER GRANULOMATOSIS)

❑ **Definition**

- Granulomatosis with polyangiitis (GPA), also referred to as Wegener granulomatosis (WG), is a multisystem autoimmune disease characterized by granulomatous inflammation and vasculitis of small and medium-sized vessels. The disease is often associated with the presence of ANCAs and most commonly affects the upper and lower respiratory tracts and kidneys.
- Microscopic polyangiitis is another ANCA-associated vasculitis that is similar to GPA and can be distinguished by the absence of granuloma formation.
- See Table 2-1.

❑ **Who Should Be Suspected?**

- Likely candidates are patients presenting with constitutional symptoms (e.g., fever, malaise, arthralgia, weight loss) and severe upper respiratory findings including sinusitis, persistent rhinorrhea, purulent or bloody nasal discharge, nasal ulcers, cough, dyspnea, and hemoptysis. Renal disease is also common in GPA patients and characterized by asymptomatic hematuria. Other involved organs include the skin (50% of patients), eyes (e.g., conjunctivitis, corneal ulceration, retinal vasculitis), nervous system, or other internal organs. There is a high incidence of deep venous thrombosis in GPA patients.
- Both genders are equally affected, and the disease is far more common in white individuals.

❑ **Laboratory Findings**

- Approximately 90% of patients with active disease have ANCAs, with mostly a cytoplasmic staining pattern (c-ANCA). In most cases, antibodies associated with this pattern are directed against proteinase-3 (PR3) located in the azurophilic granules of neutrophils. Few GPA patients may have anti-MPO

2

antibodies, which are typically associated with a perinuclear staining pattern (p-ANCA). This MPO-ANCA pattern is primarily associated with microscopic polyangiitis and eosinophilic granulomatosis with polyangiitis (Churg-Strauss syndrome).

- Positive RF (low titers), negative ANA, and mild hypergammaglobulinemia, especially of the IgA class, are frequently found in GPA.
- Urinalysis and serum creatinine measurements reflect the degree of renal involvement. Microscopic hematuria and proteinuria are common.
- Elevated CRP and ESR.
- Mild normochromic, normocytic anemia is present in nearly half of the patients.
- Diagnosis must be confirmed by biopsy of the pulmonary (highest yield), upper airway, or renal tissue.

HENOCH-SCHÖNLEIN PURPURA

- See Chapter 3, Cardiovascular Disorders; see also Henoch-Schönlein Purpura Nephritis in Chapter 12, Renal Disorders.
- See Table 2-1.

HYPERSENSITIVITY VASCULITIS

❑ Definition
- Hypersensitivity vasculitis (HS) is a vasculitis of small vessels of the skin, which can be idiopathic or secondary to drug treatment or infections.
- See Table 2-1.

❑ Who Should Be Suspected?
- HS patients present with skin lesions, palpable purpura, and/or petechiae that might follow the initiation of drug therapy or infection (e.g., hepatitis C infection with cryoglobulinemia). Other findings include fever, urticaria, and arthralgia.
- Visceral organ involvement is uncommon.

❑ Laboratory Findings
Diagnosis is based on clinical findings and the history of offending drug treatment or infection. Skin biopsy typically shows leukocytoclastic vasculitis.
- Decreased complement levels and increased ESR are present.
- Presence of mixed cryoglobulinemia in the serum can be found in patients chronically infected with hepatitis C virus.

POLYARTERITIS NODOSA

❑ Definition
- This systemic necrotizing arteritis affects medium-sized muscular arteries, with occasional involvement of small muscular arteries.
- See Table 2-1.

❏ **Who Should Be Suspected?**

- Candidates are middle-aged or elderly individuals presenting with nonspecific symptoms of fatigue, arthralgias, weakness, or fever. These symptoms can be associated with signs of multisystem involvement such as hypertension, renal insufficiency, neurologic dysfunction, skin lesions, muscle involvement, or abdominal pain.
- The condition is more common in men than women and may be preceded by hepatitis B or C infection.

❏ **Laboratory Findings**

Diagnosis is based on clinical manifestations and confirmed by biopsy of involved organs. Laboratory studies are not diagnostic.

- Elevated ESR and CRP.
- Serologic tests are useful to rule out other autoimmune disorders and narrow down the differential diagnosis. ANCA test is usually negative in polyarteritis nodosa patients.

TAKAYASU ARTERITIS

- See Chapter 3, Cardiovascular Disorders.
- See Table 2-1.

CHAPTER 3

Cardiovascular Disorders

Craig S. Smith

This chapter focuses on the common presenting symptoms and conditions of cardiovascular disorders and the differential diagnoses to be considered in the evaluation of the patient. Chest pain, dyspnea, syncope/sudden cardiac death, hypertension, and dyslipidemia are discussed and further subdivided by clinical presentation and diagnostic approach.

CHEST PAIN

CHEST PAIN: ACUTE CORONARY SYNDROMES

❑ **Definition**

- Chest pain accounts for over 6 million annual emergency department visits and 3 million hospital admissions in the United States. The differential diagnosis for chest pain is broad and ranges from benign musculoskeletal conditions to life-threatening emergencies.
- The prevalence of chest pain etiology varies greatly by location of the patient interaction. Acute coronary syndromes account for <2% of outpatient chest pain visits as opposed to 15% of emergency room visits. Of central importance in the evaluation of the patient with chest pain is a thorough history and physical supported by ancillary testing to determine if emergent treatment is required.
- Initial clinical assessment is focused on immediate threats to life: acute coronary syndrome, aortic dissection, pulmonary embolism, tension pneumothorax, pericardial tamponade, and mediastinitis (esophageal rupture).
- Evaluation of the patient with chest pain should differentiate non-cardiac from cardiac etiologies. Acute coronary syndrome (ACS) is a unifying term representing the potentially life-threatening syndrome of myocardial ischemia that results from a disparity between coronary blood flow and myocardial oxygen demand most often due to atherosclerosis, vasoconstriction, or thrombus with superimposed myonecrosis. ACS syndromes present as unstable angina (UA), or myocardial infarction either with ST-segment elevation on ECG (STEMI) or without (NSTEMI).
- NSTEMI and unstable angina comprise two thirds of ACS.
- Immediate recognition of ACS in patients presenting with chest pain is important as the diagnosis triggers both triage and treatment decisions.
- It is prudent to have a low threshold for the diagnosis of ACS, which is made from the clinical characteristics of the presenting symptoms, ECG findings and the presence of myonecrosis as reflected by an elevation of cardiac biomarkers. These diagnostic tools also provide risk assessment, which may dictate therapy, management strategy and placement.
- NSTEMI patients have an intermediate risk of acute complications when compared to unstable angina (lower) and STEMI patients (higher), approaching a 5% 30-day mortality rate.

❑ **Etiology**

- Cardiac sources of chest pain:
  1. *Ischemic/coronary heart disease*—acute coronary syndromes (STEMI, NSTEMI, UA), stable angina pectoris
  2. Ischemic/nonatherosclerotic—aortic stenosis, hypertrophic cardiomyopathy, severe systemic hypertension, right ventricular hypertension, aortic regurgitation, severe anemia, coronary vasospasm, anatomical abnormalities
  3. *Inflammatory*—pericarditis, infectious and autoimmune vasculitis
  4. *Hyperadrenergic states*—stress CM, severe hypertension, pheochromocytoma
  5. *Chest pain syndromes*—mitral valve prolapse, psychosomatic

- Noncardiac sources: GI (GERD, esophageal rupture, esophagitis, esophageal motility/achalasia, referred pain—biliary colic, appendicitis), pulmonary (pneumonia, pulmonary embolism, pulmonary hypertension, sarcoidosis, effusion, pneumothorax, pleuritis, serositis), aortic syndromes, musculoskeletal, psychosomatic

❑ **Who Should Be Suspected of ACS?**

- Consideration of the pretest probability of coexisting coronary artery disease should influence the diagnosis of ACS.
- ACS should be considered a working diagnosis subject to reevaluation.
- Unstable angina (UA) and NSTEMI are closely related clinical conditions with similar pathophysiology but differing severity. NSTEMI is usually characterized by ischemic chest discomfort at rest, absence of ST-segment elevation on a 12-lead ECG, and positive necrosis biomarkers.
- As an elevation of cardiac biomarkers may not be detectable for 12 hours, UA and NSTEMI may be initially indistinguishable. However, the distinction is important to make for early acute management. Increasing evidence supports early aggressive anticoagulation and mechanical revascularization as superior to conservative medical therapy for NSTEMI patients.
- Unstable angina presents as three scenarios: ischemic discomfort at rest (approximately 20 minutes' duration), new-onset discomfort at mild exercise threshold in the last 6 weeks, or progression of previously stable angina to easily evoked with ordinary physical activity or increased in severity (Canadian Cardiovascular Society Class III).
- UA should be differentiated from *stable angina pectoris*. While similar in character, stable angina pectoris represents short-lived chest discomfort elicited from states of higher cardiac demand that is relieved with rest and is without a crescendo pattern as described above.
- Because of a lack of objective data for diagnosis, unstable angina is the most subjective of the ACS diagnoses. Nevertheless, history/exam, ECG, and cardiac biomarkers on presentation can be utilized to formulate a likelihood of an ACS diagnosis.
- Elderly, diabetic, and female patients are more likely to present with ACS symptoms that do not include chest pain. Rather, symptoms may include dyspnea, diaphoresis, emesis, or hypotension.
- While ACS syndromes are mediated through platelet activation, at present, use of platelet aggregation assays (P2Y12, etc.) and measurement of immature platelet forms are not recommended for the diagnosis of ACS.
- The inflammatory markers/mediators of CRP, serum amyloid A, and IL-6 have been shown to risk stratify UA and NSTEMI patients but cannot be recommended for routine use in clinical diagnosis or guiding therapy for ACS patients at this point in time.

❑ **Who Should Be Suspected of an MI?**

- A diagnosis of NSTEMI implies ischemia severe enough to cause myocardial damage as evidenced by a release of cardiac biomarkers of necrosis. While the presence of objective markers of injury makes a diagnosis of MI less prone to error than UA, abnormal values must be interpreted in a clinical context to avoid false-positive interpretation.

▪ Due to the increasing sensitivity of newer-generation biomarkers of myonecrosis, a universal definition of *myocardial infarction* was adopted in 2007 and specifies that one of the following criteria be met in a clinical setting consistent with myocardial ischemia:
1. Detection of *rise and/or fall* of cardiac biomarkers (preferably troponin) with at least one value above the 99th percentile of the upper reference limit (URL), together with evidence of myocardial ischemia with at least one of the following:
   ● Symptoms of ischemia
   ● ECG changes indicative of new ischemia (new ST-T changes or left bundle branch block, LBBB)
   ● Development of pathologic Q waves on ECG
   ● Imaging evidence of new loss of viable myocardium or new regional wall motion abnormality
2. Sudden or unexpected cardiac death, often with symptoms suggestive of myocardial ischemia, and accompanied by presumably new ST elevation, or new LBBB, and/or evidence of fresh thrombus by coronary angiography and/or at autopsy, but death occurring before blood samples could be obtained or at a time before the appearance of cardiac biomarkers in the blood.
3. For percutaneous coronary intervention (PCI), patients with normal baseline troponin, an elevation >3× 99th percentile URL is defined as a PCI-related MI. It is important to note the threshold for characterizing NSTEMI post-PCI is higher than in spontaneously presenting NSTEMI (3× 99th percentile). This is due to the fact the 99th percentile is reached in up to 50% of PCI patients but does not carry the same prognosis as chest pain patients. In fact, only 5–8× 99th percentile elevations of CK-MB carry negative long-term prognosis.
4. For coronary bypass patients with normal troponin, an increase of biomarkers >5× 99th percentile URL with pathologic Q waves, new LBBB, or angiographically documented new graft or native coronary artery occlusion or loss of a viable myocardium by imaging has been designated bypass-related MI.
5. Pathologic findings of acute myocardial infarction.
▪ Once the criteria for MI are met, a clinical classification of MI has been established to recognize different etiologies of myocardial necrosis. Each etiology differs in both short- and long-term mortality rates. The classifications are
1. Type 1 MI: spontaneous MI related to ischemia from a primary coronary event such as atherosclerotic plaque erosion, rupture fissure, or dissection with accompanying thrombus
2. Type 2 MI: ischemia/necrosis related to increased oxygen demand or decreased supply such as in coronary spasm, embolism, anemia, arrhythmia, hypertension, and hypotension
3. Type 3 MI: sudden cardiac death meeting criterion as listed above
4. Type 4 MI: PCI-related MI with further classification as type 4a or type 4b
   ● Type 4a MI: MI directly related to procedure
   ● Type 4b MI: MI due stent thrombosis as documented by angiography or autopsy
5. Type 5 MI: coronary bypass related

- Type 1, 3, and 4b MIs have the highest short- and long-term mortalities and must be triaged and treated aggressively upon presentation. Prognosis for type 2, 4a, and 5 MIs is generally more favorable.
- MI classification is almost always based entirely on clinical context with supporting imaging/autopsy findings if needed. A notable exception may be the use of point of care platelet assays (see Chapter 16: Platelet Function Assay). *High on-treatment platelet reactivity* in a recently stented patient may suggest suboptimal antiplatelet therapy or genetically determined resistance to treatment, greatly increasing the risk of stent thrombosis (type 4b MI).
- Any type of MI classification can present as either STEMI or NSTEMI depending upon the severity of ischemic insult.

❑ Diagnosis

The diagnosis of ACS depends on the likelihood of coronary atherosclerosis, characteristics of the chest pain, abnormalities on ECG, and levels of serum markers of cardiac injury. A rapid assessment of chest pain patients (Figure 3-1) is required to initiate appropriate and potentially lifesaving treatment and may need to be revisited until a final diagnosis is confirmed.

- The *physical examination* of patients with uncomplicated ACS is usually normal but has the goal of evaluating for precipitating factors (uncontrolled hypertension, anemia, thyrotoxicosis, sepsis), assessing hemodynamic consequences of ACS (CHF, third heart sound, new mitral regurgitant murmur, shock), revealing comorbid conditions that impact treatment decisions (malignancy), and ruling out other chest pain etiologies. A targeted initial exam should evaluate for unequal extremity pulses and aortic regurgitation (aortic dissection), a pericardial rub (pericarditis), pulsus paradoxus (tamponade), or reproducible chest pain with palpation (musculoskeletal).
- The *ECG* should be performed first and within 10 minutes of first medical contact and reviewed for ischemic findings as ECG changes have both diagnostic and prognostic implications.
  - ▼ ST-segment deviation (depression or elevation) is the most specific sign of ischemia.
  - ▼ T-wave changes are the most sensitive.
- ST-segment elevation of >1 mm in two contiguous precordial or two adjacent limb leads that is persistent and accompanied by symptoms consistent with ACS (>30 minutes) should be considered for immediate mechanical or pharmacologic reperfusion due to the poor short-term prognosis of STEMI. This category also includes ECG changes of hyperacute T waves, new LBBB, or posterior MI (may require posterior leads for diagnosis).
- If STEMI (or equivalent) is excluded, the presence of ST-segment depressions and T-wave abnormalities should be assessed.
  - ▼ Horizontal or downsloping depressions of ≥0.05 mV are important indicators of ongoing ischemia.
  - ▼ T-wave inversions or "pseudonormalizations" may aid diagnosis, particularly with symptoms, but are less sensitive for ischemia.
- As ACS is highly dynamic, serial ECGs (every 20–30 minutes) and clinical reassessment should be performed if the initial ECG is nondiagnostic and the patient remains symptomatic.

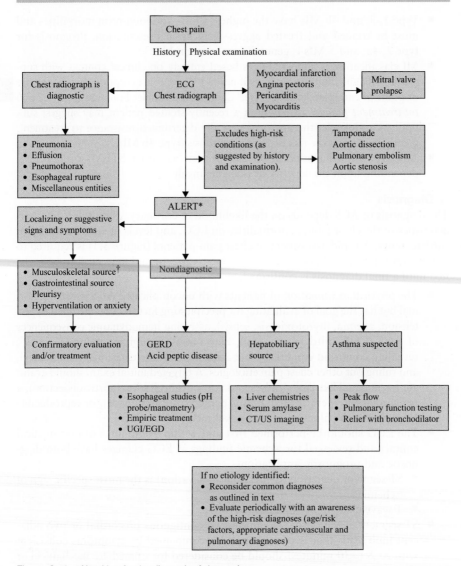

Figure 3–1 *Algorithm for the diagnosis of chest pain.*
*This algorithm is intended to direct the workup in patients with chest pain of unclear etiology.
†Many of these patients will be discovered to have musculoskeletal syndromes that are diagnosed through a detailed history and physical examination. Musculoskeletal diagnoses to specifically consider include overuse syndromes, costochondritis, pectoral girdle syndrome, and xiphodynia. CT, computed tomography; ECG, electrocardiogram; EGD, esophagogastroduodenoscopy; GERD, gastroesophageal reflux disease; UGI, upper gastrointestinal series; US, ultrasound.

- Continuous ECG monitoring should be performed in all UA/NSTEMI patients admitted to the hospital for surveillance of arrhythmias and ongoing ischemia.
- *Cardiac biomarkers*, along with the ECG, remain a cornerstone for the diagnosis of MI. Cardiac troponin T and I are preferred markers given the

myocardial specificity. CK-MB is the next favored biomarker and is released more rapidly with ischemia than troponin, although it lacks the former's absolute tissue specificity (see Chapter 16, Troponin limitations).

- Most NSTEMI patients have troponin elevation within 4–6 hours after symptom onset. Initially negative biomarkers should be remeasured within 8–12 hours after symptom onset.
- New "high-sensitivity" troponin assays increase sensitivity with an associated loss of specificity, particularly in low-risk patients and must be interpreted in the clinical context.
- Even without ACS as an etiology, however, an elevation in troponin >99th percentile portends a worse prognosis when compared to patients without elevation.
- *Cardiac imaging* is emphasized in the definition of acute MI and can aid in clinically indeterminate cases. Because of its widespread availability and mobility, echocardiography is often used to differentiate myocardial ischemia from nonischemic etiologies of chest pain. Regional wall motion abnormalities can help distinguish ischemia from perimyocarditis, valvular heart disease, cardiomyopathy, pulmonary embolism, or ascending aortic dissection. Wall thickness (or lack thereof) may aid in determining if MI is acute or subacute/old. While MRI is validated for these purposes as well, its availability, cost, and time make it less efficient for acute chest pain evaluation.

❑ Laboratory and Additional Testing

While the diagnosis of MI is in part dependent upon laboratory testing, cardiac biomarkers and supplemental imaging may also be utilized for risk stratification and delivery of cost-effective care based on patient risk.

- The diagnosis of STEMI is made by clinical history, ECG findings, and, if needed, cardiac imaging. It should not be dependent upon the results of cardiac biomarker assays given the time-dependent nature of reperfusion therapy efficacy in this high-risk population. Stat renal function and CBC to assess for anemia and baseline platelet levels are recommended in patients presenting with STEMI. Cocaine history/tox screen should be considered.

Up to 25% of hospital admissions are due to symptoms consistent with ACS, yet up to 85% of these patients do not have ACS as a final diagnosis. Serial biomarkers with stress testing may help identify low- and intermediate-risk patients who may be safely *discharged home* to continue a cardiovascular evaluation as an outpatient. Based on history, exam, ECG, and laboratory testing, risk assessment may be performed. The presence of ischemic symptoms, hypotension, dynamic ECG changes, heart failure, or advanced age indicates high-risk ACS, and these patients admitted as either NSTEMI (positive biomarkers) or high-risk UA (negative markers).

- The distinction between NSTEMI and UA is determined by the presence or absence of detectable biomarkers of necrosis. Troponin is widely accepted as the "gold standard" for cardiac myonecrosis and appears in serum 4 hours after onset of ischemia and peaks in 8–12 hours. Patients with negative biomarkers within 6 hours of chest symptoms should have a second set obtained 8–12 hours after symptom onset.

- At conclusion of two biomarker evaluations (observed for 8–24 hours post-symptoms), the decision for admission (positive biomarkers) or noninvasive provocative testing (normal biomarkers without high-risk clinical features) may be made (Figure 3-2).
- There are a number of *abbreviated biomarker strategies* (<6 hours) to potentially discharge low-risk patients home earlier than current practice. Due to superior release kinetics, initially CK-MB was used for these protocols. CK-MB has fallen out of favor due to superior troponin sensitivity for MI. Troponin-based protocols incorporate assays performed 2 hours apart combined with either risk model assessment (TIMI score) or potentially imaging modalities (CT). While these strategies show promise, due to the use of point-of-care testing, they require institution-specific customization of cutoff thresholds of troponin as point-of-care testing has lower sensitivity than central laboratory troponin assays (which result more slowly).
- The role of very high-sensitivity troponin for rapid assessment (not approved yet in United States) shows promise due to superior sensitivity and earlier detection (hs-TnT 100% sensitivity for MI within 4–6 hours after symptoms or 0–2 hours after ED presentation).

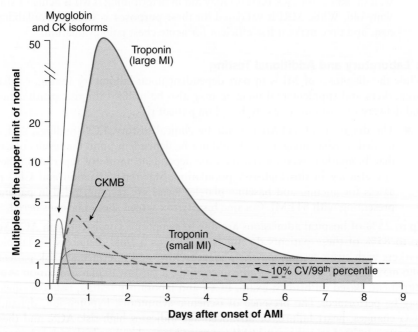

Figure 3–2 *Graph of temporal expression of cardiac biomarkers. Anderson JL, Adams CD, Antman EM, et al. ACC/AHA 2007 guidelines for the management of patients with unstable angina/non–ST elevation myocardial infarction: a report of the American College of Cardiology/American Heart Association Task Force on Practice Guidelines (Writing Committee to Revise the 2002 Guidelines for the Management of Patients With Unstable Angina/Non–ST Elevation Myocardial Infarction) developed in collaboration with the American College of Emergency Physicians, the Society for Cardiovascular Angiography and Interventions, and the Society of Thoracic Surgeons endorsed by the American Association of Cardiovascular and Pulmonary Rehabilitation and the Society for Academic Emergency Medicine. J Am Coll Cardiol. 2007;50(7):e1–e157.*

■ Assessment of platelet reactivity at this point in time cannot be recommended for the diagnosis of ACS.

Without positive biomarkers, low-risk patients (age < 70, no rest pain, pain <2 weeks without prolonged episodes, normal ECG, no prior CAD or diabetes mellitus) may be discharged home and additional evaluation performed as an out-patient. Appointment should be made within 72 hours for evaluation. Intermediate-risk patients without high-risk features require in-hospital triage with provocative noninvasive imaging. The sensitivity and specificity of stress testing can be combined with pretest risk to give a prognosis of coronary heart disease.

■ *Exercise treadmill testing* should be considered first, particularly in low-risk groups; low sensitivity, predictive value, and inability to identify and quantify ischemic areas when compared with imaging modalities; cannot interpret ECG if LBBB, ventricular paced rhythm, LVH hypertrophy, and conduction abnormalities. Duke prognostic treadmill score establishes the risk of death from CAD; combined with imaging (SPECT, MRI, or echo) to improve sensitivity and specificity in women and those with confounding baseline ECGs.

■ The advantage of echocardiography over SPECT (single-photon emission computed tomography) is lack of radiation exposure but carries higher false-negative results at submaximal heart rates. SPECT has higher positive-negative predictive values over treadmill testing alone.

■ *Cardiac MRI* has excellent spatial resolution without radiation; similar to SPECT, may assess myocardial viability (unlike SPECT can differentiate peri-carditis). Stress MRI can be performed with dobutamine or adenosine; difficulty imaging irregular heart rhythms and patients with metal implants. No large comparative studies published yet.

■ *Cardiac CT* (64 slice) has excellent negative predictive value (>90%), slightly diminished positive predictive value (80%). Rapid acquisition but requires lower heart rates for image analysis with a tendency to overestimate disease severity; provides only anatomic, not functional information (i.e., culprit lesion). At present, no consensus for use of CT as a "triple rule out"—CAD, aortic dissection, PE in the rapid assessment of chest pain.

Suggested Readings

Anderson JL, Adams CD, Antman EM, et al. ACC/AHA 2007 guidelines for the management of patients with unstable angina/non–ST elevation myocardial infarction: a report of the American College of Cardiology Foundation/American Heart Association Task Force on Practice Guidelines. *J Am Coll Cardiol.* 2007;50:e1–e157.

Body R, Carley S, McDowell G, et al. Rapid exclusion of acute myocardial in patients with unde-tectable troponin using a high-sensitivity assay. *J Am Coll Cardiol.* 2011;58:1332–1339.

McCaig L, Burt C. National Hospital Ambulatory Medical Care Survey: 2003 Emergency Department Summary. In: *Advance Data from Vital and Health Statistics.* Atlanta, GA: Centers for Disease Control and Prevention, 2005.

Than M, Cullen L, Aldous S, et al. 2-Hour accelerated diagnostic protocol to assess patients with chest pain syndromes using contemporary troponins as the only biomarker: the ADAPT trial. *J Am Coll Cardiol.* 2012;59:2091–2098.

Thygesen K, Alpert JS, White HD; on behalf of the Joint ESCIACCFI AHA/WHF Task Force for the Redefinition of Myocardial Infarction. Universal definition of myocardial infarction. *J Am Cardiol.* 2007;50:2173–2195.

CHEST PAIN: NONATHEROSCLEROTIC ISCHEMIA

❏ **Definition**

- Approximately 5% of patients with acute myocardial infarction do not have atherosclerotic coronary disease, increasing to 20% in patients under the age of 35. Necropsy studies in these individuals often demonstrate luminal narrowing, leading to ischemia via several mechanisms: internal narrowing by obstructions or encroachment by adjacent structures.
- Ischemia may also result from dynamic changes in an otherwise normal arterial wall (spasm and anomalous arteries) or an imbalance in oxygen supply and demand (type 2 MI).
- Over 50% of fatal MIs without coronary disease likely represent coronary vasospasm.

❏ **Who Should Be Suspected?**

- Diagnosis is often made by exclusion via cardiac imaging due to overlap of symptom presentation with ACS.
- Young age (<35 years) and lack of coronary risk factors raise the suspicion of congenital coronary anomalies or congenital coronary aneurysm. A careful history to exclude cocaine use (supported by tox screen if needed) is mandatory in STEMI patients without significant atherosclerotic risk factors, as is rheumatic history.
- Coronary spasm has also been described with patients receiving chemotherapeutic drugs such as 5-fluorouracil, and those talking herbal medicines. A careful medical reconciliation should be performed on all chest pain patients and review of "vasospastic potential" performed, and this includes use of estrogen replacement therapy (coronary dissection).
- Hypercoagulable/malignancy history should be reviewed, and subtherapeutic INR for patients on Coumadin should be assessed for the possibility of coronary embolism.

❏ **Presentation/Findings**
Congenital Coronary Anomalies

- Present in 1–2% of the general population but 4% of autopsies for MI. When coronary arteries arise from the contralateral sinus of Valsalva, the anomalous artery may course between the great vessels. States of increased cardiac output may cause either compression or torsion of the proximal coronary artery resulting in ischemia, infarct, or sudden cardiac death.
- Diagnosis is made by imaging based on ACS risk profile of presentation. Cardiac catheterization (high-risk patients) demonstrates interarterial course of anomalous vessel. Direct visualization with cardiac CT or MRI is an advantage when considering these modalities for stress testing in younger populations but must be balanced by cost consideration. Surgical bypass for high-risk anatomy is the preferred treatment.

Myocardial Bridges ("Tunneled" Epicardial Arteries)

- Congenital in origin: The course of the epicardial coronary artery dives below the myocardium and is compressed in systole. As the majority of coronary blood flow occurs in diastole, tachycardia with resulting shortened diastolic filling period is often required to produce ischemia. Length of the tunneled arterial segment may not play a significant role in risk.

- Diagnosis made by direct visualization by angiography or CT/MRI. The presence of a myocardial bridge does not necessarily imply ischemia is present.

Coronary Aneurysm

- Congenital (more common in right coronary artery) or acquired (infection/inflammation): Turbulent flow in the aneurysm may predispose to thrombus formation and ACS. Acquired aneurysm may be the result of atherosclerosis (50%) or syphilis, mycotic emboli, Kawasaki disease, or lupus. Appropriate serologies should be sent when aneurysm is identified by imaging (see Chapter 2, Autoimmune Diseases and Chapter 11, Infectious Diseases).

Embolism

- Coronary artery emboli should be considered in any patient presenting with ACS (usually STEMI) in the setting of atrial fibrillation, active infective endocarditis, prosthetic heart valve, known LV thrombus, or left-sided cardiac tumor (right-sided tumors require a right-to-left shunt to be present). Initial triage is performed as dictated by ACS algorithm, and diagnosis often made angiographically. Coronary embolism most often involves the LAD and may resolve spontaneously with anticoagulation.
- Embolism or spasm should be considered for angiographically normal arteries in the setting of MI.

Spontaneous Coronary Artery Dissection

- Occurs from vessel wall hematoma between media and adventitia in the absence of trauma or iatrogenic causes. Most diagnosed with autopsy and occur in LAD or left main artery.
- Described in young women with risk factors among whom 25–30% are pregnant or in the postpartum period. Likely etiologies include hormonal impairment of collagen synthesis. Oral contraceptive use also associated with dissection. Thrombolytic therapy should not be given in postpartum patients with STEMI due to increased chance of propagation of hematoma.
- Men are more likely to be older and have right coronary involvement with coronary risk factors. Systemic hypertension is not a risk factor for dissection.
- Other associated conditions include cocaine or cyclosporine use, hypertrophic cardiomyopathy, Marfan or Ehlers-Danlos syndrome, and immune-mediated diseases such as rheumatic arteritis, autoimmune thyroiditis, hepatitis C infection, sarcoidosis, systemic lupus erythematosus, Kawasaki arteritis, and eosinophilic coronary arteritis.
- A careful family history of connective tissue disease, lab assessment for eosinophilia, ESR, ANA, and thyroid evaluation should be performed if coronary dissection is suspected.

Coronary Artery Spam

- Spasm that occurs within epicardial coronary arteries usually occurs at sites with non–flow-limiting luminal narrowing by atherosclerotic plaque.

An abundance of smooth muscle cells is usually present in necropsy studies at the known sites of spasm.

■ Hyperadrenergic conditions associated with spasm include pheochromocytoma, cocaine, amphetamine, and ecstasy use. This includes dobutamine infusion for stress testing. Epicardial spasm can be seen in inflammatory conditions of thyrotoxicosis, allergic angina, as well as administration of fluorouracil, capecitabine, sumatriptan, and bromocriptine.

■ Diagnosis of spasm is usually made with angiography. Provocative challenge during catheterization with ergotamine is no longer performed due to risk of MI/death from refractory spasm. Potential offending medications or behaviors should be stopped immediately.

■ Epicardial spasm should be differentiated from *Syndrome X*, or microvascular spasm. This syndrome carries a benign prognosis but presents with angina-like pain. Stress testing often reveals signs of ischemia with normal epicardial arteries on invasive testing (coronary flow reserve—which can be assessed invasively is often abnormal). Pain is likely due to either microvascular spasm or abnormal pain perception (sympathetic predominance).

Hypertrophic Obstructive Cardiomyopathy
■ See Dyspnea/CHF section.

Suggested Readings

Angelini P, Trivellato M, Doris J, et al. Myocardial bridges: a review. *Prog Cardiovasc Dis.* 1983;26:75–88.

Chetlin MD, Virami R. Myocardial infarction in the absence of coronary atherosclerotic disease. In: Virmani R, Forman MB (eds). *Nonatherosclerotic ischemic heart disease.* New York, NY: Raven Press; 1989:1–30.

CHEST PAIN: INFLAMMATORY

Chest pain may occur due to an inflammatory response to immune-mediated or infectious triggers without necessarily predisposing to ischemic insult. Pericardium, myocardium, or direct coronary artery involvement may occur. Ischemia may occur when coronary arteries are involved as a direct result of the inflammatory process (necrosis and aneurysm formation) or via wall thickening and luminal narrowing, rupture of the vessel wall, or from thrombosis due to hypercoagulable state or accelerated atherosclerosis.

VASCULITIS

❑ **Definition**
■ Vasculitis describes a heterogeneous group of disorders that are characterized by leukocyte migration in the vessel wall resulting in damage of blood vessels, which leads to tissue ischemia and necrosis.
■ Epicardial coronary vasculitis is relatively rare but can be life threatening. Coronary arteries are involved through either direct extension or hematogenous spread.

- Cardiac manifestations are rarely predominant in vasculitis and are just as likely to occur as a result of other organ involvement or treatment side effects of this systemic process.
- Heart failure due to direct myocardial involvement, ischemic cardiomyopathy, or valvular involvement in vasculitis is more common than ACS-like presentation.
- Size and shape of both arteries and veins are affected due to a primary process or secondary to an underlying pathology.

□ **Classification By**
Etiology
- Primary: polyarteritis nodosa, Wegener granulomatosis, giant cell arteritis, hypersensitivity vasculitis (see Chapter 2, Autoimmune Diseases)
- Secondary
  - ▼ Infections: bacteria (e.g., septicemia caused by gonococcal organisms or *Staphylococcus*), mycobacteria, viruses (e.g., CMV, hepatitis B), *Rickettsia* (e.g., Rocky Mountain spotted fever), spirochetes (e.g., syphilis, Lyme disease)
  - ▼ Associated with malignancy (e.g., multiple myeloma, lymphomas)
  - ▼ Connective tissue diseases (e.g., RA, SLE, Sjögren syndrome)
  - ▼ Diseases that may simulate vasculitis (e.g., ergotamine toxicity, cholesterol embolization, atrial myxoma)

Size of Involved Vessel (Noninfectious Vasculitis)
- Large vessel: dissection of aorta (dissecting aneurysm), Takayasu arteritis, giant cell (temporal) arteritis
- Medium-sized vessel: polyarteritis nodosa (or small), Kawasaki disease, primary granulomatous CNS vasculitis
- Small vessel: ANCA-associated vasculitis (Wegener granulomatosis, Churg-Strauss syndrome, drug-induced, microscopic polyangiitis), immune complex–type vasculitis (Henoch-Schönlein purpura, cryoglobulinemia, rheumatoid vasculitis [or medium], SLE, Sjögren syndrome, Goodpasture syndrome, Behçet syndrome, drug-induced serum sickness), paraneoplastic vasculitis (lymphoproliferative, myeloproliferative, carcinoma), inflammatory bowel disease
- Any size vessel (pseudovasculitis): antiphospholipid syndrome, emboli (e.g., myxomas, cholesterol emboli, bacterial or nonbacterial endocarditis), drugs (e.g., amphetamines)

□ **Who Should Be Suspected?**

- Patients may present with fatigue, weakness, fever, myalgias, arthralgia, headache, abdominal pain, hypertension, nosebleeds, palpable purpura, and/or mononeuritis.
- Coronary artery imaging (angiography, MRI, CT) that reveals a "string-of-pearls" sign sequential proximal coronary aneurysms that is suggestive of a primary or secondary vasculitic process. A focused rheumatic history should be performed in all patients with this angiographic finding.

❏ **Laboratory Findings**

The gold standard in the diagnosis of most vasculitides is based on pathologic findings in a biopsy of the involved tissue.

- Hematology: ESR is increased in 90% of cases, often to very high levels; CRP correlates with disease activity even better than ESR. Normochromic anemia of chronic disease, thrombocytosis, and mild leukocytosis occur in 30–40% of patients; eosinophilia may occur but is not a feature. Leukopenia or thrombocytopenia occurs only during cytotoxic therapy.
- Urinalysis: hematuria, proteinuria, and azotemia.
- Core laboratory: serum globulins (IgG and IgA) are increased in ≤50% of cases. Serum C3 and C4 complement levels may be increased. RF may be present in low titer. ANA positive in vasculitis secondary to connective tissue disorders. ANCA determination provides valuable information and is highly specific for the diagnosis of small-vessel vasculitides, particularly Wegener granulomatosis.
- Imaging studies: arteriogram, MRI, and ultrasound.
- Considerations.
- c-ANCA (anti-proteinase 3; coarse diffuse cytoplasmic pattern) is highly specific (>90%) for active Wegener granulomatosis. Sensitivity is >90% in systemic vasculitic phase, approximately 65% in predominantly granulomatous disease of respiratory tract, and approximately 30% during complete remission.
- ELISA titer does not correlate with disease activity; a high titer may persist during remission for years. c-ANCA is also occasionally found in other vasculitides (polyarteritis nodosa, microscopic polyangiitis [e.g., lung, idiopathic crescentic and pauci-immune GN], Churg-Strauss vasculitis).
- p-ANCA (against various proteins [e.g., myeloperoxidase, elastase, lysozyme; perinuclear pattern]) occurs only with fixation in alcohol, not formalin. A positive result should be confirmed by ELISA. The test has poor specificity and 20–60% sensitivity in a variety of autoimmune diseases (microscopic polyangiitis, Churg-Strauss vasculitis, SLE, inflammatory bowel disease, Goodpasture syndrome, Sjögren syndrome, idiopathic GN, chronic infection). However, pulmonary small vessel vasculitis is strongly linked to myeloperoxidase antibodies.
- Both p-ANCA and c-ANCA may be found in non–immune-mediated polyarteritis and other vasculitides.
- Atypical pattern (neither c-ANCA nor p-ANCA; unknown target antigens) has poor specificity and unknown sensitivity in various conditions (e.g., HIV infection, endocarditis, CF, Felty syndrome, Kawasaki disease, ulcerative colitis, Crohn disease).

ANTIPHOSPHOLIPID ANTIBODY SYNDROME

See Chapter 9, Hematologic Disorders.

HENOCH-SCHÖNLEIN PURPURA

❏ **Definition**

- Henoch-Schönlein purpura is a self-limited hypersensitivity systemic vasculitis of the small vessels. It involves the skin and to variable degrees joints, kidneys, and GI tract. The small vessel and renal involvement is caused by IgA deposition.

❑ Who Should Be Suspected?

- This condition is seen more commonly in children (90% of cases), but it may affect adults as well.
- In adults, renal disease is common. The renal picture may vary, with minimal urinary abnormalities occurring for years. Patients may present with palpable purpura without thrombocytopenia or a coagulopathy and acute abdominal pain, or with purpura and joint symptoms.

❑ Laboratory Findings

Diagnosis is made clinically; there are no pathognomonic laboratory findings.

- Histology: renal or skin biopsy supports the diagnosis; it shows focal segmental necrotizing GN that becomes more diffuse and crescentic with IgA and C3 deposition.
- Urinalysis: RBCs, casts, and slight protein in 25–50% of patients. The renal picture varies from minimal urinary abnormalities for years to end-stage renal disease within months. Gross hematuria and proteinuria are uncommon.
- Hematology: coagulation tests are normal.
- Core laboratory: BUN and creatinine may be increased.

Suggested Reading

Trapani S, Micheli A, Grisolla F, et al. Henoch Schönlein Purpura in childhood: epidemiological and clinical analysis of 150 cases over a 5-year period and review of the literature. *Semin Arthritis Rheum.* 2005;35:143–153.

KAWASAKI SYNDROME (MUCOCUTANEOUS LYMPH NODE SYNDROME)

❑ Definition

- Kawasaki syndrome is a variant of childhood polyarteritis of unknown etiology, with a high incidence of coronary artery complications.

❑ Laboratory Findings

- Histology: diagnosis is confirmed by histologic examination of the coronary artery (same as for polyarteritis nodosa).
- Hematology: anemia (approximately 50% of patients). Leukocytosis (20,000–30,000/μL) with shift to left occurs during 1st week; lymphocytosis appears thereafter, peaking at the end of the 2nd week, and is a hallmark of this illness. Increased ESR.
- CSF findings: increased mononuclear cells with normal protein and sugar.
- Urinalysis: increased mononuclear cells; dipstick negative.
- Joint fluid findings: increased white blood cell (WBC) count (predominantly PMNs) in patients with arthritis.
- Core laboratory: laboratory changes due to AMI. Acute-phase reactants are increased (e.g., CRP, α-1-antitrypsin); these usually return to normal after 6–8 weeks.

TAKAYASU SYNDROME (ARTERITIS)

❑ **Definition**

- Takayasu syndrome is the term for granulomatous arteritis of the aorta. Temporal arteritis and rheumatic disease may also be associated with aortitis.
- Greater incidence in young to middle-aged Asian females. Coronary involvement occurs in 15–25% of cases. Involvement is usually in segments and rarely diffuse.
- Average age of onset is 24 years, and the diagnosis should be considered in individuals of <40 years with acute myocardial infarction.
- Diagnosis is established by characteristic arteriographic narrowing or occlusion or histologic examination. Laboratory tests are not useful for diagnosis or to guide management.

❑ **Laboratory Findings**

Findings are due to involvement of coronary or renal vessels.

- Hematology: increased ESR is found in approximately 75% of cases during active disease but is normal in only 50% of cases during remission. WBC count is usually normal.
- Core laboratory: serum proteins are abnormal, with increased γ globulins (mostly composed of IgM). Female patients have a continuous high level of urinary total estrogens (rather than the usual rise during the luteal phase after a low excretion during the follicular phase).

THROMBOANGIITIS OBLITERANS (BUERGER DISEASE)

- Thromboangiitis obliterans is very rare and is the vascular inflammation and occlusion of medium and small arteries and veins of limbs; it is related to smoking and occurs mostly in males. Histology shows characteristic inflammatory and proliferative lesions. Coronary involvement is uncommon. Laboratory tests are usually normal.

INFECTIOUS (SECONDARY) VASCULITIS

❑ **Definition**

- Various microorganisms may cause vasculitis of any size vessel by either hematogenous spread or direct extension of cardiac structures involved (pericardium, valves).
- Most important infections of the coronary arteries are syphilis, tuberculosis, and syphilitic arteritis.

❑ **Who Should Be Suspected?**

- Tuberculosis coronary arteritis occurs mainly in patients with preexisting pericardial or myocardial tuberculosis.
- Syphilitic arteritis can involve the first 3–4 mm of the left and right coronary arteries with an obliterative arteritis.

- When a nonviral infectious angiitis occurs, it is almost always accompanied by myocarditis with abscesses and pericarditis.

❑ **Laboratory Findings**

- Core lab blood work, cultures, and PCR analysis should be dictated by systemic clues to the underlying infectious process.

THROMBOPHLEBITIS, SEPTIC

❑ **Definition**

- Thrombophlebitis is vascular inflammation due to a blood clot.

❑ **Laboratory Findings**

Findings are due to associated septicemia, complications (e.g., septic pulmonary infarction), and underlying disease.

- Hematology: increased WBC count (often >20,000/µL), with marked shift to left and toxic changes in neutrophils. DIC may be present.
- Core laboratory: azotemia.
- Culture: positive blood culture (*Staphylococcus aureus* is the most frequent organism; others are *Klebsiella, Pseudomonas aeruginosa*, enterococci, *Candida*).

PERICARDITIS (ACUTE) AND PERICARDIAL EFFUSION

❑ **Definition**

- The pericardium is a double-walled sac that surrounds the heart. The inner visceral pericardium is normally separated from the outer, fibrous parietal pericardium by a small volume (15–50 mL) of fluid, a plasma ultrafiltrate. Inflammation of the pericardium results in pericarditis, with or without an associated pericardial effusion.
- Common causes of pericardial inflammation include infection, uremia, trauma, malignancy, hypersensitivity, and autoimmune diseases. Viral infections (coxsackie- and echovirus) are by far the most common and are usually self-limited.
- Cardiac tamponade is more likely to present as dyspnea in its mild form with additional precordial discomfort and hypotension/shock more likely with severe tamponade.
- When presenting as chest pain, myocarditis is often due to concomitant pericarditis. Myocardial involvement alone more often presents as dyspnea and dilated cardiomyopathy (see Dyspnea section), although younger patients are more likely to present.

❑ **Who Should Be Suspected?**

- Any recent trauma victim in shock, post-MI patients, patients with comorbid conditions predisposed to effusion (neoplasm, chronic inflammatory disease), patients with chest pain after a viral prodrome.

- Typical signs and symptoms of acute pericarditis include chest pain (often pleuritic and worse with inspiration and supine position), pericardial friction rub (pathognomonic), ECG changes (e.g., ST elevation, PR depression), and pericardial effusion.
- Not all patients will manifest all of these features; the presence or absence of an effusion does not exclude the diagnosis.

❑ **Diagnostic and Laboratory Findings**

- *Echocardiography*: Most useful imaging technique for the evaluation of acute pericarditis and is critical for patients if tamponade is suspected. Small pericardial effusions, undetectable by routine examinations, may be detected, providing support for the diagnosis of pericardial disease. Typically >1 cm of effusion is required for safe performance of pericardiocentesis. Doppler-derived flow-velocity measures of mitral and tricuspid flow may assist in diagnosing tamponade, but it is ultimately a clinical diagnosis based on inspiratory decline in systolic arterial pressure exceeding 10 mm Hg (pulsus paradoxus), which can be also seen in COPD and pulmonary embolism. The absence of any chamber collapse on echocardiography has a high negative predictive value for tamponade (92%), although the positive predictive value is low (58%). Abnormalities of right heart venous return (expiratory diastolic reversal) are more predictive but cannot be obtained in one third of patients.
- *Electrocardiography*: ECG abnormalities may support a diagnosis or suggest alternative diagnoses, such as myocardial infarction or early repolarization abnormalities. There are several important distinguishing characters of pericarditis ECGs from that of STEMI patients. There is upward concavity of ST elevations (compared with downward for ischemic) that rarely exceeds 5 mm with PR-segment depression (not in aVR) that is not present with repolarization abnormalities. T-wave inversions may persist with tuberculuous, uremic, or neoplastic pericarditis. Electrical alternans suggests large effusion.
- *Chest x-ray*: Generally normal but may detect specific abnormalities, like increased cardiac silhouette with effusions (water-bottle heart), pleural effusion, or evidence of underlying etiology (TB, fungal disease, pneumonia, neoplasm).
- *Chest CT and MRI* detect effusions with high sensitivity and specificity and may provide useful information pertinent to performing pericardiocentesis (hematocrit of effusion, loculations, pericardial thickening). Often, concern of tamponade makes echocardiography the imaging modality of choice for clinically tenuous patients due to its mobility.
- *Tuberculin skin test or interferon-gamma release assay*: Evaluation to rule out TB is recommended for all patients. Additional diagnostic testing for TB, like AFB cultures, should be performed on patients at increased risk on the basis of epidemiologic and clinical factors.
- *Cultures*: Cultures of blood and other potentially infected specimens should be submitted for patients with significant fever, signs of sepsis, or systemic or local infection.
- *Histology*: Pericardiocentesis (and occasionally pericardial biopsy) should be performed for patients with clinically significant tamponade or persistent effusions. Pericardiocentesis is recommended for patients in whom pyogenic,

tuberculous, or malignant pericardial disease is suspected. As most forms of pericarditis are viral in etiology, the diagnostic yield of routine pericardiocentesis has a low diagnostic yield (7%).

- Recommended tests for pericardial fluid include
  - ▼ Histopathologic and cytologic examination of tissue and fluid.
  - ▼ Bacterial and mycobacterial stains and culture.
  - ▼ Triglyceride concentration for chylous fluid.
  - ▼ Adenosine deaminase and *M. tuberculosis* PCR, if tuberculous pericarditis is suspected.
  - ▼ Other specific diagnostic tests, like fungal cultures or PCR, are performed based on clinical suspicion.
  - ▼ Core laboratory: CBC, electrolytes, tests of renal function and thyroid function, and plasma troponin concentration. ANA titers, anti-dsDNA, and serum complement are recommended for patients when an autoimmune cause is suspected. Note: protein, glucose, LDH, RBC count, and WBC count cannot distinguish exudative from transudative effusions and are usually noncontributory in establishing a diagnosis.
  - ▼ Serology: HIV should be considered. Pericardial disease is relatively common in HIV-infected patients. Furthermore, HIV infection predisposes patients to mycobacterial infections. Viral diagnostic testing, including serology, has low diagnostic yield and is not routinely recommended.

Suggested Readings

Ben-Horin S, Bank I, Shinfeld A, et al. Diagnostic value of the biochemical composition of pericardial effusions in patients undergoing pericardiocentesis. *Am J Cardiol.* 2007;99:1294–1297.

Hidron A, Vogenthaler N, Santos-Preciado JI, et al. Cardiac involvement with parasitic infections. *Clin Microbiol Rev.* 2010;23:324–349.

Lange RA, Hillis D. Acute pericarditis. *N Engl J Med.* 2004;351:2195–2202.

Levy PY, Cory R, Berger P, et al. Etiologic diagnosis of 204 pericardial effusions. *Medicine (Baltimore).* 2003;82:385–391.

CHEST PAIN: HYPERADRENERGIC STATES

- Syndromes of catecholamine excess may cause chest pain from increased heart rate and peripheral vasoconstriction, resulting in a mismatch of oxygen supply and demand. Severe presentations may result in type 2 MI.
- Autoregulation of tissue blood flow and cardiac output are able to adapt to a wide range of perturbations in hear rate and blood pressure, particularly those that are chronic in nature. Symptoms are more likely to occur during periods of acute changes induced by either exogenous administration of catecholamines (cocaine, methamphetamines) or intrinsic paroxysmal episodes (stress cardiomyopathy, pheochromocytoma).

❏ Definition

- *Cocaine intoxication*: Chest pain is the most common reason for cocaine users to seek medical attention with 64,000 ED visits per year in the United States (50% admitted). Six percent of chest pain episodes are MI. Aortic dissection is a rare consequence of cocaine use. Cocaine is both sympathomimetic and thrombogenic and accelerates atherosclerotic deposition—as a result, ischemic damage can manifest as either type I MI (ruptured plaque) or type 2 MI (either severe epicardial spasm or increased oxygen demand).

- *Methamphetamine intoxication*: Biologic effects are similar to cocaine but with less vasoconstriction; more likely to produce tachyarrhythmias rather than chest pain.
- *Pheochromocytoma*: A rare form of secondary hypertension in 0.05% of hypertensive patients. It should be considered in patients with chest pain who lack coronary risk factors and who have characteristic symptoms or who worsen after beta-blocker administration (must rule out cocaine ingestion) (see Chapter 6, Endocrine Diseases).
- *Stress-induced (takostubo) cardiomyopathy*: Transient dysfunction of the LV apex and/or mid-ventricle that mimics acute MI but is without obstructive coronary disease or clear epicardial (LAD) spasm. Pathogenesis is uncertain but likely is catecholamine mediated as it is often triggered by acute medical illness or emotional stress, occurs in the context of significantly elevated plasma catecholamines and mimics LV dysfunction seen in other hyperadrenergic states such as pheochromocytoma, neurologic injury, and exogenous administration of supraphysiologic doses of catecholamines (iatrogenic or intentional). Potentially mediated through direct toxic effect causing myocyte stunning or microvascular spasm. In several large registries, stress-induced cardiomyopathy accounts for 1–2% of all ACS inpatient admissions.

❏ Who Should Be Suspected?

- Often indistinguishable from symptoms of ACS, a hyperadrenergic etiology of chest pain should be a diagnosis of exclusion. In young individuals without coronary risk factors, cocaine exposure should be assessed immediately (beta-blockade therapy contraindicated).
- Stress-induced cardiomyopathy has a predilection for postmenopausal women for unclear reasons, although men are affected at a much lower rate. Early genetic studies have not yielded any polymorphism associated with the disease. Prevalence is 1–2% of hospital admissions for ACS. It should be suspected in postmenopausal women with ACS after a physical or emotional stressor with clinical presentation or ECG findings out of proportion to cardiac biomarker elevation.

❏ Diagnosis

- Exogenous catecholamine diagnosis is made via history or toxicology screening.
- Pheochromocytoma.
- Stress-induced cardiomyopathy: Four necessary criteria are required for diagnosis by the Mayo Clinic criteria—(1) transient hypokinesis, akinesis, or dyskinesis of the left ventricular midsegment with or without apical involvement most often in the setting of a stressor (physical or emotional). Wall motion abnormalities usually extend beyond the distribution of a single coronary artery; (2) absence of obstructive coronary disease or plaque rupture; (3) new ECG changes (ST-elevation or T-wave inversion) or modest troponin elevation; (4) absence of pheochromocytoma or myocarditis.

- If ST-segment elevations are present or the clinical presentation is consistent with high-risk ACS, confirmation of a diagnosis should not delay decision to proceed to mechanical revascularization. A lack of angiographic findings of a "culprit" stenosis will suggest the diagnosis along with wall motion abnormalities seen by ventricular imaging.

❑ Laboratory Findings

- Positive tox screen for intoxication syndromes (see pheochromocytoma).
- Serial cardiac troponins may help differentiate between ACS.
- At present, stress-induced cardiomyopathy is a diagnosis of exclusion from overlapping clinical syndromes.

Suggested Readings

Simpson RW, Edwards WD. Pathogenesis of cocaine-induced ischemic heart disease. *Arch Pathol Lab Med.* 1986;110:479–484.

Wittstein I, Thiemann D, et al. Neurohumoral features of myocardial stunning due to sudden emotional stress. *N Engl J Med.* 2005;325:539–548.

CHEST PAIN: NONCARDIAC ETIOLOGY

ACUTE AORTIC SYNDROMES

❑ Definition

- Acute aortic syndromes encompass the related entities of aortic dissection, intramural aortic hematoma, and penetrating aortic ulcer. As these conditions may be imminently life threatening, a high clinical suspicion must be present to ensure prompt diagnosis and treatment.
- The Stanford model of classification is the most widely used and is based on anatomical location. Type A is involvement of the ascending aorta, and type B is a dissection not involving the ascending aorta.
- Intramural hematoma accounts for 13% of acute aortic syndromes.
- Aortic rupture is rare outside of trauma but may be seen more commonly in type A dissections.

❑ Who Should Be Suspected?

- Aortic dissection occurs in the general population of 16.3 and 9.1 per 100,000 in men and women, respectively, with a mean age of 63.
- A classic presentation of "aortic chest pain" is cataclysmic in onset of described as sharp or tearing and may radiate to the chest, jaw, back, or abdomen depending on aortic area involved. Clinical signs of poor prognosis include syncope (cerebral malperfusion), cardiac effusion and tamponade, abdominal pain, and paraplegia (compromised spinal cord perfusion).
- Most common in men older than 60 with hypertension, smoking, and atherosclerosis as risk factors.
- Other acquired risk factors are pregnancy, cocaine/amphetamine use, and inflammatory arthritis (Takayasu, giant cell arteritis, Behchet's, relapsing polychondritis, SLE, *not* syphilis-induced aortitis).
- Younger populations with aortic syndromes should be suspected of genetic contributions that weaken the medial layer of the aortic ("cystic medial

degeneration" or loss of elastin fibers). These include bicuspid aortic valve (most common genetic defect), Marfan syndrome (1:5,000 general population), Ehlers-Danlos syndrome type IV (autosomal dominant, but one half of cases are not inherited), aberrant right subclavian artery, aortic coarctation, Noonan syndrome, and Turner syndrome.

❑ **Diagnosis**

- Physical examination: Patients often present acutely ill and accompanied by hypertension. Aortic dissection typically associated with physical signs of murmur of aortic regurgitation (short duration and low pitch), loss of a peripheral pulse (usually femoral), or difference in upper extremity blood pressures. Signs of cardiac tamponade (pulsus paradoxus and elevated jugular venous pressure) should also be assessed.
- Imaging studies:
  - ECG: often abnormal, but nondiagnostic. Presence of Q waves or ST elevations (<4%) suggests type A dissection involving the coronary artery ostium (more likely RCA). Avoid thrombolytics.
  - Chest x ray: abnormal in most cases (>85%) with widened mediastinum and angulation of aortic border.
  - Transesophageal echocardiography: Sensitivity and specificity of 99% and 88%. Doppler may be used to discriminate true from false lumen. Cannot distinguish full arch or abdominal aorta but provides detailed information of aortic valve and pericardial involvement.
  - CT: 64 slice CTA near 100% accuracy. Rapid acquisition and ED availability make CTA the first imaging choice for suspected aortic syndromes. Requires echo for detailed cardiac information.
  - MRI: Superior spatial resolution improves accuracy for intramural hematomas and aortic ulcers. Provides cardiac information as well (10% of hematomas will progress to dissection, ulcer depth of >1 cm and >2 cm diameter portend worse prognosis. Small ulcers may be managed conservatively with serial imaging).

❑ **Laboratory Findings**

- D-dimer (by-product of fibrin degradation) is 99% sensitive for detection of dissection, but nonspecific. Elevation occurs only after dissection; hence, it is not useful as a predictor.
- Aneurysm-related mRNA signature tests show promise for detection and monitoring purposes but are not yet available for clinical use.
- It is recommended that a STAT 64 slice CT with D-dimer is obtained in any patient with suspected aortic dissection.
- If aortitis is noted on imaging studies, serologic evaluation for giant cell arteritis, HLA-B27, syphilis, and tuberculosis (infectious aortitis) should be performed.

Suggested Readings

Baverman AC. Acute aortic dissection: clinician update. *Circulation.* 2010;122:184–188.

Hiratzka LF, Bakris GL, Beckman JA, et al. 2010 ACCF/AHA/AATS/ACR/ASA/SCA/SCAI/SIR/STS/SVM Guidelines for the diagnosis and management of patients with thoracic aortic disease. *J Am Coll Cardiol.* 2010;55:e27–e129.

Wang YY, Barbacioru CC, Shiffman D, et al. Gene expression signature in peripheral blood detects thoracic aortic aneurysm. *PLoS One.* 2007;2:e1050.

CHEST PAIN: MUSCULOSKELETAL

Potential life-threatening cardiovascular and pulmonary conditions are considered first in the evaluation of any patient with chest pain; however, there are a number of isolated chest wall syndromes and systemic conditions that may manifest as chest pain.

3

❏ Who Should Be Suspected?

- Patients whose chest pain is persistent, lasting hours to days, and is sharp and localized
- Pain that is exacerbated with movement
- Individuals with no clear cardiovascular or pulmonary etiology of symptoms
- Isolated chest wall syndromes: Costochondritis (no swelling, point tenderness), Tietze syndrome (young adults with swelling at second or third rib), sternalis (palpation causes bilateral radiation of pain), xiphoidalgia, sternoclavicular subluxation (usually dominant side, often in middle-aged women), fractures, and chest wall syndrome due to herniated disc
- Systemic chest pain syndromes: fibromyalgia, rheumatoid arthritis, ankylosing spondylitis, psoriatic arthritis, and sickle cell disease/crisis

❏ Laboratory and Imaging

- Diagnostic approach should first exclude cardiac, pulmonary, and abdominal etiologies either by exam or by focused testing. Older patients should receive ECG, CBC, urinalysis, and chest radiograph given the higher likelihood of atypical presentation of ACS and infectious processes.
- Exclusion of a systemic rheumatic process should be performed. ESR is a nonspecific test for inflammatory conditions. The presence of back stiffness should be evaluated with lower-back radiographs and HLA-B27 antigen to assess for spondyloarthropathies.

❏ Psychogenic/Psychosomatic

Several large registries have identified up to one third of patients presenting to emergency departments with chest pain have a psychiatric disorder. Panic disorder is a particularly common diagnosis, although appropriate clinical and laboratory evaluation for organic disease must be performed before symptoms are attributed to psychiatric disorders. Hyperventilation may cause ST and T-wave changes on ECG and result in nonanginal chest pain. Furthermore, elevations of heart rate and blood pressure may precipitate true ischemia in individuals with preexisting coronary atherosclerosis.

Suggested Readings

Evans DW, Lum LC. Hyperventilation: an important cause of pseudoangina. *Lancet.* 1977;1:155.
Wuslin LR, Yingling K. Psychiatric aspects of chest pain in the emergency department. *Med Clin North Am.* 1991;75:1175.

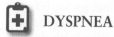 DYSPNEA

As dyspnea is a nonspecific presenting symptom for a number of clinical syndromes, the selective use of diagnostic testing and laboratory assessment can aid in the differentiation of cardiac from noncardiac etiologies. Most common cardiac etiologies include CAD, congestive heart failure (CHF), valvular disease, and arrhythmia. Individuals with a moderate coronary risk profile who report exertional symptoms should undergo appropriate risk stratification (see stress testing above). Over the past several decades, the prevalence and incidence of congestive heart failure have increased dramatically with CHF now accounting for the largest cost of Medicare. Diagnostic testing is an important adjunct to the clinical diagnosis of CHF to help identify reversible etiologies or precipitants, monitor treatment response, aid in prognosis, and screen for potential heritable conditions.

CONGESTIVE HEART FAILURE

❑ Definition

- Heart failure (HF) is the inability of the cardiac output to meet the metabolic demands of the body due to an impaired ability of the ventricle to fill or eject blood. It is a clinical syndrome that occurs at the end stage of a number of structural or functional cardiac disorders.
- The nonspecific symptoms of HF are due to either excess fluid accumulation (dyspnea, orthopnea, ascites, edema) or poor cardiac output (fatigue, weakness) either with exertion, or, when severe, at rest.
- It is important to recognize that HF includes symptoms not only from systolic dysfunction but from HF with preserved ejection fraction (HFpEF), which is predominant in the elderly.
- At 40 years of age, the lifetime risk of CHF in both men and women is 1 in 5 (without MI, it is 1 in 9 for men and 1 in 6 for women).
- In developed countries, CAD accounts for 60–75% of symptomatic cases of HF and has surpassed hypertension as an etiologic factor in HF (although hypertension continues to have a higher attributable risk in the general population due to its prevalence).
- Both the prevalence and incidence of CHF increase with age, roughly doubling with each decade of life to >50% in individuals over 70 years of age. Women are more likely than men to have CHF with preserved systolic function.

❑ Who Should Be Suspected?

- History alone is insufficient to make a diagnosis of HF given the nonspecific presenting symptoms. Chronic HF is more likely to present with anorexia and fatigue with decreased prevalence of rales on exam (sensitivity of 15%) due to increases in pulmonary vascular resistance and capacitance.
- However, history (particularly functional limitation) is essential for assessing HF severity, which is critical for prognosis, staging, and appropriateness of advanced treatment options.
- Dyspnea has high sensitivity for HF (87%) but low specificity (51%). Signs of right-sided congestion are the most sensitive exam findings for HF with JVP of >12 mm Hg and hepatojugular reflux at 65% and 85%, respectively. A finding of a displaced apical impulse on exam in patients with dyspnea has the best combination of sensitivity, specificity, and predictive value for systolic HF.

- Large registries have identified the following risk factors as having the largest population attributable risk for heart failure: CAD, cigarette smoking, hypertension, obesity, diabetes, and valvular heart disease.
- Special consideration should be given to individuals with a familial history of cardiomyopathy. A detailed history dating back three generations should be obtained to determine age of onset, inheritance pattern, and lethality along with possible nongenetic risk factors. As upward of 30 cardiomyopathy genes have been identified, current guidelines recommend referral to genetic counseling whenever appropriate. Testing (and screening frequency) of the proband and family members will be determined by the type of cardiomyopathy. Mode of inheritance is usually dominant with antibodies present in 30% of patients and first-degree relatives. Common screening measures of relatives include echocardiography, treadmill testing, Holter monitor (hypertrophic), and/or cardiac MRI in addition to disease-specific genetic testing.

❑ Diagnostic and Laboratory Findings

- *Electrocardiogram*: A normal ECG has a 98% negative predictive value for systolic dysfunction. Dilated cardiomyopathy (DCM) often presents with conduction abnormality (first-degree AV block, LBBB, fascicular block, or nonspecific QRS widening). Low limb lead voltage with loss of precordial R waves suggests infiltrative cardiomyopathies (amyloidosis) and with LVH suggests idiopathic dilated cardiomyopathy.
- ECG with tachyarrhythmia such as atrial fibrillation/AVNRT may suggest tachycardia-induced cardiomyopathy (typically requires 120–200 bpm for prolonged periods). Heart block, often complete, is seen with cardiac sarcoid or Lyme carditis.
- *Chest radiography*: Useful to differentiate CHF from pulmonary disorders. Cardiomegaly, cephalization of pulmonary vessels, Kerley B lines, effusions, and valvular calcification are associated with CHF. Diagnostic sensitivity of x-ray findings is high (83%), with lower specificity (68%).
- *Coronary angiography/stress imaging*: Coronary angiography is a Class I ACC/AHA recommendation for patients presenting with HF and angina-like symptoms unless the patient is not a candidate for revascularization. It is also recommend in young patients with systolic HF to exclude congenital coronary anomalies. Noninvasive stress imaging to detect ischemia or myocardial viability is reasonable (Class IIa) in HF patients with established CAD.
- *Viability testing* (PET with FDG, MRI, SPECT, Dobutamine stress echocardiogram): Over 80% of ischemic HF demonstrates viability, but only modest benefit seen with revascularization in the only randomized trial to date.
- *Right heart (pulmonary artery) catheterization*: Not recommended (Class III) to be performed routinely in HF patients due to lack of evidence in guiding medical therapy. Class I (recommended) to guide therapy when intracardiac filling pressures cannot be established by clinical measures or for worsening renal function. Also recommended for the consideration of advanced treatment options (Class II a).
- Initial *laboratory evaluation* for patients with HF include a complete blood count to assess for anemia or infection that may mimic, or worsen, HF-associated dyspnea. Blood urea nitrogen and creatinine may help

differentiate states of volume overload due to renal disease, or if HF is confirmed, demonstrate cardiorenal syndrome as a consequence of low-output HF. Urinalysis in CHF is notable for mild albuminuria (<1 g/day) with isolated RBCs and WBCs, hyaline, and granular casts (less common). Specific gravity is high (>1.020) as opposed to primary renal disease. Hyponatremia generally indicates HF, although may be reflective of excessive diuresis (along with potassium depletion). Lowered serum sodium is a powerful predictor of HF mortality.

- Liver function tests may be altered due to hepatic congestion and is often accompanied by elevated INR with signs of right heart failure. Primary liver dysfunction is also associated with a dilated cardiomyopathy. Serum albumin and total protein are decreased in HF. The presence of elevated total protein may indicate HF due to infiltrative disease (amyloid, sarcoid).
- ESR may be decreased due to decreased serum fibrinogen.
- *BNP or NT-proBNP* is suggested in evaluation of all patients in whom CHF is suspected when the diagnosis is uncertain and is a class I indication to support the diagnosis of decompensated HF in hospitalized patients. Both have similar concentrations in normals but are significantly elevated in HF (NT-proBNP are fourfold higher). Natriuretic peptides are elevated in both systolic and diastolic heart failure and aid in the diagnosis with similar accuracy for both conditions.
  - ▼ A number of factors affect natriuretic peptide levels including age, renal function, nutritional state, and gender. Natriuretic peptides are also known to be elevated in sepsis, atrial fibrillation, pulmonary hypertension, valvular heart disease, coronary artery disease, and other conditions that may present with dyspnea. Elevated levels alone should not be used as the sole determinant for the presence of CHF nor exclude the presence of other diseases.
- There are little data directly comparing BNP to NT-proBNP, but both have been show to aid in diagnosis and prognosis of HF, as well as assessing efficacy of HF therapy and predicting readmission rates. An NT-proBNP level of >900 pg/mL has equivalent accuracy of a BNP >100 pg/mL for diagnosis (predictive accuracy of 83%). Values below this have a very high negative predictive value for HF as a cause of dyspnea.
- Natriuretic peptides may be utilized for both diagnostic and prognostic value. Independent of other clinical factors, BNP quartiles are predictive of in-hospital mortality with risk varying more than three- to fourfold on the basis of the patient's initial BNP. Values >840 pg/mL conferred a twofold increase in hospital mortality in one large registry.
- Biomarkers of myocardial necrosis are also found in HF patients (in some studies 30%), often without overt ischemia or CAD. Given the close association of CAD and HF, markers of cardiac injury should be assessed in all patients with acute dyspnea and may be deployed in a multimarker strategy for risk stratification (class I recommendation). Elevated concentrations of cardiac troponin (0.5 µg/L) have been shown to be predictive of morbidity and mortality in HF patients at every level of admission BNP. With the use of a BNP >840 pg/mL threshold, the presence of positive troponin I >0.5 µg/L identifies patients at highest risk for in-hospital mortality (up to fivefold risk).

- *Echocardiography*: Remains the gold standard cardiac imaging in HF and should be performed in all patients with new onset heart failure. Diagnosis for systolic dysfunction approaches a specificity of 100% (sensitivity 80%). Echocardiography meets professional society appropriateness criteria when performed for patients with dyspnea due to suspected cardiac etiology or when chest x-ray or serum BNP are concerning for cardiac disease. The diagnosis of CHF can be aided by assessment of ventricular size and function (right- and left-sided systole and diastole). Clues to the etiology of HF such as CAD (focal wall motion abnormalities—nonspecific), valvular disease, pericardial findings (constriction, effusion with tamponade), intracardiac shunts, amyloid, as well as duration of HF (atrial size) may be gleaned from initial images. Furthermore, cardiac output, pulmonary pressures, and hemodynamic status may be derived from tissue Doppler to aid treatment decisions and predictor prognosis.
- *Cardiac magnetic resonance (CMR)*: Expense and lack of portability limit use, but with use of gadolinium can differentiate viability/perfusion, fibrosis, and inflammation. CMR can identify hypertrophic cardiomyopathy (HCM), arrhythmogenic right ventricular cardiomyopathy (ARVC), and cardiac amyloid and may obviate the need for endomyocardial biopsy in some cases of myocarditis.
- *Cardiac CT*: Can establish the likelihood of coronary disease contribution to heart failure either by direct imaging of coronary arteries or through calcium scores via EBCT.

Given the similar clinical presentation of heart failure with preserved or reduced left ventricular ejection fraction, additional testing and differential diagnosis is often driven by echocardiographic (or other imaging modality) findings.

SYSTOLIC DYSFUNCTION/DILATED CARDIOMYOPATHY (DCM)

- In developed countries, systolic dysfunction *with* heart failure is most likely due to coronary disease, hypertension, or valvular disease. These common etiologies are often apparent upon initial history and diagnostic evaluation. Idiopathic cardiomyopathy accounts for approximately 30% of cases of symptomatic cases.
- Patients with DCM by echocardiography *without* signs of heart failure have significantly different distribution of etiologies. Coronary disease and hypertension account for only 10–15% of cases with 50% deemed idiopathic. Myocarditis, infiltrative disease, peripartum cardiomyopathy, HIV infection, Chagas disease, connective tissue disease, substance abuse, doxorubicin exposure, and nutritional abnormalities must be considered.
- If the cause of dilated cardiomyopathy is not apparent after initial evaluation, additional laboratory testing is warranted. These include thyroid function tests (especially elderly with atrial fibrillation), Ferritin and TIBC (hemochromatosis), pheochromocytoma evaluation (see Chapter 7, Genitourinary System Disorders), thiamine, carnitine and selenium (nutritional deficiency), evaluation for Chagas disease, Lyme disease, HIV serologies, and evaluation for myocarditis or inherited diseases predisposing to DCM.

MYOCARDITIS

- Myocarditis is an inflammatory disease of heart muscle due to infectious and noninfectious etiologies with potential long-term sequela of DCM. Most common etiology in developed countries is viral infection (Coxsackie, echovirus, adenovirus, HIV, CMV, parvovirus B19), with rheumatic carditis, *Trypanosoma Cruzi* (more likely to present as chronic cardiomyopathy), and bacterial infections still contributing substantially to cases in the developing world.

☐ Who Should Be Suspected?

- Clinical presentation of myocarditis is highly variable with most cases likely asymptomatic. Chest pain most commonly is pleuritic in nature due to concomitant pericarditis, although may mimic chest pain of acute coronary syndromes. Sinus arrhythmias predominate over AV block or ventricular tachycardia.
- Chest symptoms are often preceded by a viral prodrome with tachycardia out of proportion to fever.
- Myocarditis should be suspected when unexplained LV dysfunction or arrhythmias are present, particularly in the young. CAD, valvular disease, congenital abnormalities must be excluded with a careful history of toxin and autoimmune disease taken. Myocarditis associated with autoimmune disease (giant cell myocarditis), unlike most other etiologies, is a rapidly progressive disease that is often fatal. Ventricular arrhythmias are more common with this variant of myocarditis.
- Recent vaccination should raise the possibility of a hypersensitivity myocarditis.

☐ Laboratory and Other Findings

- ECG: neither sensitive nor specific for diagnosis. Most commonly will reflect changes with pericarditis (see Pericarditis above) but may mimic ST elevation MI. Widened QRS and Q waves carry a poor prognosis, with diffuse low voltage seen with myocardial edema particularly ominous.
- Viral serology should not be used for diagnosis with positive and negative predictive values of 25% and 49%, respectively.
- Core laboratory: Elevation of cardiac biomarkers occurs in less than half of all acute cases but does predict mortality in patients hospitalized with fulminant myocarditis (CK-MB >29 ng/mL sensitivity of 83%). Acute-phase reactants are elevated (ESR, CRP, mild leukocytosis). If clinically appropriate, serology for toxoplasmosis, Chagas disease, trichinellosis, and Lyme carditis may be sent in addition to those for autoimmune disease, fat aspirates for amyloidosis, and ferritin (hemochromatosis).
- *Endomyocardial biopsy* with histopathologic confirmation remains the gold standard for diagnosis but is little used given the mild course of most viral myocarditis. In practice, it is used to differentiate giant cell, lymphocytic, and hypersensitivity myocarditis in fulminant heart failure. A diagnosis of GCM is critical as it can be ameliorated with immunosuppressive therapy and/or transplantation. Biopsy sensitivity for GCM is approximately 85%.
- *Cardiac MRI* is increasingly utilized for diagnosis with sensitivity of 88% and even higher when combined with biopsy. It should be performed only

if the CMR result will change management (minority of cases). Proposed diagnostic criteria for myocarditis are based on pattern and distribution of gadolinium enhancement.

- *Stress-induced (Takotsubo) cardiomyopathy*: Acute but rapidly reversible LV dysfunction in the absence of flow-limiting coronary disease. The ventricular pattern of wall motion abnormality in this form of stunning involves distal portion of the LV (apical ballooning) with basal hypercontractility. Typically effects older women and is precipitated by intense psychological stress. ECG may mimic ST elevation MI with low-level troponin positivity. While hemodynamic perturbations and shock may be present, almost all patients recover completely in 1–4 weeks.

- *Inherited syndromes*: DCM can be associated with various inherited neuromuscular diseases in addition to genetically determined HF as noted above. These include hereditary hemochromatosis, sideroblastic anemia, myotonic dystrophy, and muscular dystrophies.

- *Left ventricular noncompaction*: A congenital cardiomyopathy (0.05%) where the apical portion of the ventricle with deep intratrabecular recesses that occur in embryogenesis. Presentation usually includes DCM with heart failure, but thromboemboli, arrhythmias, and sudden cardiac death may occur. Diagnosis is made with echo, with genetic testing available for some recognized etiologies (X-linked).

- *Toxins/medications*: Exposure to alcohol (80 g/day in men and 40 g/day in women over a number of years), cocaine, cobalt, and arsenic and deficiencies of selenium and thiamine may cause DCM. Common medications include antiretrovirals, chloroquine, and anthracyclines. A cumulative dose >450 mg/m^2 of anthracycline greatly increases the chance of cardiotoxicity. While diagnosis is definitely made with biopsy, often history alone is sufficient for diagnosis.

- *Valvular*: Diagnosed by exam and echocardiography. Due to valvular abnormalities, systolic dysfunction occurs out of proportion to increases in wall stress. Most commonly seen in left-sided regurgitant lesions (mitral regurgitation, aortic regurgitation >aortic stenosis).

- *Autoimmune*: Autoimmunity likely plays a role in myocarditis but can also result in a DCM from cardiac antigens of troponin, myosin (α,β chains), and beta-1 adrenoreceptor. Presence of antiheart antibodies is increased in families with DCM, but at present, no recommendations exist for routine screening. Systemic lupus erythematosus commonly involves the heart, but with varied clinical presentation ranging from coronary disease/vasculitis to cardiomyopathy. Involvement is almost uniformly secondary. Celiac disease, however, may not present with classic GI symptoms, but rather iron deficiency with DCM only. Endomysial antibody screening is reasonable in such patients.

HEART FAILURE WITH PRESERVED EJECTION FRACTION (HF$_p$EF)

❏ **Definition**

- Clinical history, presentation, and physical findings are essentially indistinguishable from HF with reduced ejection fraction.

- As many as half of all patients presenting with HF will have normal/near normal ejection fraction.
- Diastolic HF is the predominant etiology of HFpEF, which also encompasses a mixed group of clinical syndromes that includes cardiac infiltrative disease, valvular heart disease, right ventricular cardiomyopathy, and hypertrophic cardiomyopathy.

❏ **Who Should Be Suspected?**

- Risk factors for HFpEF due to diastolic dysfunction include older age (>50% of HF patients over 70 years), female (2:1), hypertension, and diabetes mellitus.
- HF presentation in a younger patient with preserved EF suggests etiology other than diastolic HF.
- If clinical signs of severe venous congestion are present (ascites, hepatomegaly) out of proportion to left-sided symptoms, infiltrative CM, pulmonary hypertension, or constrictive pericarditis should be considered.
- Early systolic flow murmurs and bounding pulses suggest high output failure and a venous hum or thrill an AV fistula or malformation as etiology of HF.
- Amyloid should be considered with low ECG voltage and LV hypertrophy on echocardiogram.
- Dynamic outflow tract murmur along with ECG hypertrophy without history of hypertension accompanies both aortic stenosis and hypertrophic cardiomyopathy. Echocardiography will aid in the differentiation of both conditions.

❏ **Diagnostic and Laboratory Findings**

- Core laboratory: similar to HF with reduced EF. CBC, renal function, liver, and thyroid serologies to rule out confounding clinical syndromes.
- *BNP and NT-proBNP*: Should be measured early if the diagnosis of HF is uncertain. Both are elevated in diastolic HF. There is no threshold to differentiate systolic from diastolic HF, but BNP and NT-proBNP tend to be higher in HF with LV dysfunction. Acute HF diagnostic thresholds are BNP >100 pg/mL and NT-proBNP >300 pg/mL and are independent predictors of adverse events.
- If troponin is >99th percentile upon presentation, etiologies of coronary disease, infiltrative cardiomyopathy (amyloid), and myocarditis should be considered.
- *Echocardiography*: HFpEF is defined as EF ≥ 50%. Patients with mildly reduced EF (40–49%) should be evaluated and treated as HF with reduced EF (see Congestive Heart Failure above). Differential diagnosis of HFpEF can be performed with echocardiography, differentiating between CAD (regional wall motion abnormalities), amyloid/infiltrative disease, hypertrophic CM, constrictive pericarditis, and mitral/aortic regurgitation. Doppler criteria including mitral inflow, pulmonary venous velocity, and mitral annular motion by tissue Doppler can effectively diagnose presence of abnormal diastolic function.
- *Hypertrophic cardiomyopathy (HCM)*: Diagnosed by unexplained increase in LV wall thickness (13–60 mm) with a nondilated LV chamber. Obstruction of the LV outflow track or systolic anterior motion of the mitral valve with

concomitant mitral regurgitation may or may not be present. HCM is the most common genetic cardiomyopathy (1:500) with diverse clinical presentation and course. Echocardiography or CMR may be used for diagnosis. LV wall thickness may be noncontiguous. Commercially available genetic testing may be performed to confirm diagnosis (not prognostic) but should be performed in at-risk relatives to help define screening frequency (echo) and participation in competitive sports (ACC/ESC recommended). Extreme LV hypertrophy on imaging (≥30 mm), nonsustained ventricular tachycardia on ECG, and failure to augment blood pressure with exercise increase the risk of sudden cardiac death and warrant consideration of ICD.

■ *Amyloid cardiomyopathy*: Typically presents as right-sided failure with frank pulmonary edema rare. Anginal may occur from small vessel involvement. Cardiac involvement varies with type of amyloidosis, with 50% in AL (primary) amyloidosis and 5% in secondary (AA) amyloidosis. HF with heavy proteinuria, periorbital purpura, and significant hepatomegaly should raise suspicion. TTR mutation (autosomal dominant) amyloid is present in patients of African descent (3.5%) and presents as late-onset heart failure. LV wall thickening is usually out of proportion to degree of hypertension (>15 mm) and should not be attributed to hypertensive heart disease. Syncope is common, particularly exertional, but high-grade AV block is unusual in AL amyloid (common in TTR). Echo findings of increased wall thickness and reduced ECG voltage are unique to amyloidosis and carry a 72% and 91% sensitivity/specificity. CMR has similar excellent diagnostic yield. BNP may be significantly elevated prior to the onset of heart failure due to amyloid infiltration. Definitive diagnosis requires tissue biopsy—may be from endomyocardial biopsy or fat pad aspirate in other cardiac diagnostic criteria are present.

■ *Right ventricular dysfunction*: Most common etiologies of preserved left ventricular function with isolated RV dysfunction include RV myocardial infarction, tricuspid regurgitation, and pulmonary disorders (embolus, pulmonary hypertension—see Chapter 13, Respiratory Disease). *Arrhythmogenic right ventricular cardiomyopathy* (ARVC) is a rare (1:5,000) autosomal dominant disorder with incomplete penetrance characterized by electrical instability and heightened risk of sudden cardiac death. There is no definitive diagnostic test, but rather, diagnosis requires an integrated assessment of electrical, functional, and anatomic abnormalities. Most commonly, monomorphic VT with a LBBB pattern is seen with focal wall motion abnormalities of the right ventricle in the absence of coronary artery disease. Differential diagnoses may include Brugada syndrome, and endomyocardial biopsy may be required to differentiate between focal infiltrative disorders such as sarcoid and amyloid.

Suggested Readings

Bonow RO, Maurer G, et al. Myocardial viability and survival in ischemic left ventricular dysfunction. *N Engl J Med*. 2001;364:1617–1625.

Fonarow GC, Peacock W, et al. Admission B-type natriuretic peptide levels and in-hospital mortality in acute decompensated heart failure. *JACC*. 2007;49:1943–1950.

Fonarow GC, Peacock W, et al. Usefulness of B-type natriuretic peptide and cardiac troponin levels to predict in-hospital mortality from ADHERE. *Am J Cardiol*. 2008;101:231–237.

Friedrich MG, Sechtem U, et al. Cardiovascular magnetic resonance in myocarditis: a JACC white paper. *JACC.* 2009;53:1475–1487.

He J, Ogden LG, et al. Risk factors for congestive heart failure in US men and women: NHANES 1 epidemiologic follow-up study. *Arch Intern Med.* 2001;161:996.

Hershberger RE, Lindenfeld J, et al. Genetic evaluation of cardiomyopathy—a Heart Failure Society of America practice guideline. *J Card Fail.* 2009;15:83–97.

Loyd-Jones DM, et al. Lifetime risk for developing congestive heart failure: the Framingham Heart Study. *Circulation.* 2002;106:3068–3072.

Maisel AS, McCord J, et al. Bedside B-type natriuretic peptide in the emergency diagnosis of heart failure with reduced or preserved ejection fraction. Results from the Breathing Not Properly Multinational Study. *JACC.* 2003;41:2010.

Park JP, Song J-M, et al. In-hospital prognostic factors in patients with acute myocarditis. *JACC.* 2009;53:A144–A197. (Abstract 1042–1178).

Roger Vl, et al.; on behalf of the American Heart Association Statistics Committee and Stroke Statistics Subcommittee. Heart disease and stroke statistics 2011 update: a report from the American Heart Association. *Circulation.* 2011;123:e18–e209.

Yancy C, Jessup M, et al. 2013 ACCF/AHA guideline for the management of heart failure: a report of the American College of Cardiology Foundation/American Heart Association task force on practice guidelines. *Circulation.* 2013;128:e240–e327.

PERICARDIAL CONSTRICTION

❏ Definition

- Effusion and tamponade (see above) remain the most common cause of dyspnea due to pericardial disease; however, constriction of the pericardial space due to fibrosis of the inelastic pericardium is an important contribution to dyspnea as surgical pericardiectomy is potentially curative.
- Pericardial constriction is typically chronic but may present acutely.
- Effusive–constrictive pericarditis is a variant that presents often as tamponade but exhibits hemodynamic constriction after pericardiocentesis (ventricular interdependence).

❏ Who Should Be Suspected?

- Patients with fatigue and dyspnea in the context of clinical evidence of right-sided failure and congestion. Anorexia and abdominal distention are frequent. It is not uncommon for patients to have undergone hepatobiliary evaluation prior to diagnosis.
- Exam may be notable for a pericardial knock (diastole) and prominent X and Y descent of the jugular venous pulsation especially during inspiration (Kussmaul sign).
- May be confused with restrictive/infiltrative CM or HF. Presence of pericardial thickening and calcification on imaging make the diagnosis more likely, but 18% of patients have normal findings.
- May occur after any pericardial inflammatory process, but rare after pericarditis. Post–cardiac surgery or radiation therapy (Hodgkin lymphoma or breast cancer) accounts for a large percentage of patients (up to 30%). Direct pericardial infections (tuberculous or purulent pericarditis), connective tissue disease, and pericardial involvement of neoplasms are far more likely to cause constriction than pericarditis from viral etiologies.

- In cases where cirrhosis is initially suspected, but no etiology is found via serologic testing. JVP is rarely elevated in cirrhotic patients, and if present, will not persist after pericardiocentesis as it will in constrictive pericarditis.

❏ Diagnostic and Laboratory Findings

- BNP/NT-proBNP are less elevated than with HF or restrictive cardiomyopathy.
- Echocardiography may establish the diagnosis with respiratory variation in mitral inflow and hepatic vein reversal and pericardial thickening. Biatrial enlargement is more common in myocardial disease than in constriction.
- While often not required for diagnosis, catheterization remains the gold standard of diagnosis demonstrating ventricular interdependence with respiratory maneuvers, which is >90% sensitive and specific for constriction.

 ## SYNCOPE AND SUDDEN CARDIAC ARREST

SYNCOPE

Syncope is a common chief complaint, accounting for up to 6% of all hospital admissions from the emergency department, with one third of people experiencing syncope at some point during their lifetime. While most often self-limited and not associated with poor prognosis, the cardiovascular assessment of patients with syncope must distinguish potentially life-threatening etiologies from benign causes that require no further evaluation or treatment.

❏ Definition

- Syncope is the paroxysmal and transient loss of consciousness associated with an absence of postural tone with rapid and complete recovery.
- Causes of syncope can be divided into several categories that include arrhythmias, cardiovascular structural abnormalities, orthostatic and neurally mediated responses, cerebrovascular events, and metabolic derangements.
- Syncope must be distinguished from cardiac arrest requiring cardiopulmonary resuscitation and/or cardioversion. The latter warrants extensive evaluation for coronary artery disease, structural heart disease, and possible arrhythmogenic triggers. The two entities are not unrelated, however, with up to one quarter of patients with cardiac syncope with high-risk features having subsequent cardiac arrest at 1 year.

❏ Who Should Be Suspected?

- A transient, complete loss of consciousness and postural tone with spontaneous complete recovery without sequelae is likely to be syncope as opposed to a nonsyncopal event with apparent loss of consciousness. Differential of the latter includes seizure, hemorrhage, pulmonary embolism, subarachnoid hemorrhage, and metabolic (hypoglycemia/hypoxia) (Figure 3-3).
- Unlikely seizure disorders, patients rarely experience prolonged disorientation or confusion after syncope.
- Syncope occurring with exercise or chest pain should be aggressively evaluated for life-threatening causes such as aortic stenosis, hypertrophic cardiomyopathy, coronary artery disease, and dysrhythmias.

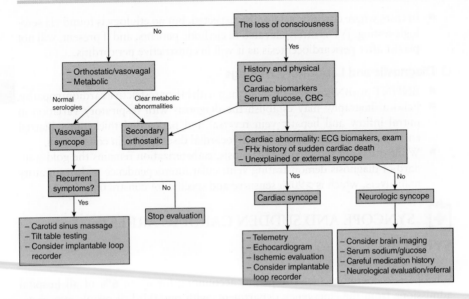

Figure 3–3 *Evaluation of syncope.*

- In both young and elderly patients, orthostatic and neutrally mediated syncope is the most frequent etiology (50–60%) as compared to arrhythmia or structural cardiac disease (20–25%). However, young patients should be screened for family history of sudden cardiac death and the ECG scrutinized for high-risk features (see Diagnostic Testing below). Elderly patients are at a greater risk of adverse outcomes after a syncopal episode, but mortality risk appears to be driven more from the presence of underlying heart disease than age-related risk alone.
- A complete list of all medications (prescription and nonprescription) should be obtained in all patients.

❑ **Laboratory and Other Diagnostic Testing**

- A comprehensive medical history, characterization of the syncopal event with associated triggers, is essential and may yield a diagnosis in up to half of all cases without testing.
- Extensive routine laboratory screening is not supported by evidence and rarely yields an etiology. Serum glucose should be assessed, particularly in patients with altered mental status. Electrolyte and renal function should be screened to assess for abnormalities that might cause or aggravate arrhythmias. Complete blood count to assess for anemia is reasonable.
- *Plasma BNP* may aid in distinguishing cardiac from noncardiac syncope but is not yet endorsed by professional society guidelines. A large prospective study (released after most current guidelines) utilizing a risk-stratification admission algorithm if any of the following were present: BNP ≥300 pg/mL, bradycardia ≤50 bpm, fecal occult blood, anemia with ≤9 g/dL, chest pain, Q waves on ECG, or oxygenation saturation ≤94% had a sensitivity of 87% and specificity of 66% with negative predictive value of 98.5%.

3

- An *electrocardiogram* should be performed in all patients with syncope and is central to risk stratification of patients with syncope. The presence of high-risk features should dictate hospital admission and further evaluation, not the diagnosis of syncope. ECG high-risk features include bifascicular block, QRS ≥ 0.12 seconds, Mobitz I second-degree AV block, sinus bradycardia (≤ 50 bpm), or sinus pause ≥ 3 seconds without chronotropic medications, evidence of preexcitation (Wolf-Parkinson-White syndrome), long or short QT intervals, Brugada syndrome (RBBB with ST elevation V1–V3), and Q waves. Clinical high-risk features that require hospitalization are the presence of cardiac structural disease, family history of sudden cardiac death, severe anemia, palpitations at the time of syncope, exertional syncope, electrolyte disturbances, and severe comorbidities.
- ECG is diagnostic for arrhythmia-related syncope if the following are present: sinus bradycardia ≤ 40 bpm or persistent sinus pauses ≥ 3 seconds, alternating left and right bundle branch blocks, pacemaker/ICD malfunction with pauses, Mobitz II or third-degree AV block, ventricular tachycardia.
- Low-risk patients should not undergo further evaluation unless episodes are recurrent.
- *Echocardiography* is recommended when underlying structural heart disease (i.e., hypertrophic cardiomyopathy, aortic stenosis, dilated cardiomyopathy) is known or is suspected by exam or secondary findings and will help in risk stratification. Only the presence of severe aortic stenosis, obstructive tumor (atrial myxoma), aortic dissection, and cardiac tamponade are considered diagnostic echocardiographic findings for syncope.
- Exercise testing is appropriate with exertional syncope and may reveal arrhythmogenic etiologies. Coronary ischemia rarely presents as syncope, but stress testing is recommended in patients with prior coronary artery disease presenting with syncope.
- Twenty-four– to forty-eight– hour Holter monitors are not recommended for outpatients, as the sensitivity is low (1–3%). Patients with symptoms on a frequency of ≤ 4 weeks can be considered for external event recorders or implantable loop recorders.
- Invasive electrophysiological study (EPS) is expensive and of very low diagnostic yield (3%) in syncope without structural heart disease. In patients with structural heart disease, EPS is positive in 50% and should be performed in individuals with known coronary disease and high-risk ECG features.
- For orthostatic or neutrally mediate syncope, tilt table testing may be performed. This should be done in patients with only intermediate suspicion as the sensitivity is variable (25–75%) but specificity is high 90%, with negative tilt table testing having excellent reproducibility (>90%).

Suggested Readings

Kapoor WN. Evaluation and outcome of patients with syncope. *Medicine (Baltimore)*. 1990;69:160.

Reed MJ, Newby DE, Coull AJ, et al. The ROSE (risk stratification of syncope in the emergency department) study. *J Am Coll Cardiol*. 2010;55:713.

Strickberger SA, Benson DW, Biaggioni I, et al. AHA/ACC Scientific Statement on the evaluation of syncope: from the American Heart Association Councils on Clinical Cardiology, Cardiovascular Nursing, Cardiovascular Disease in the Young, and Stroke, and the Quality of Care and Outcomes Research Interdisciplinary Working Group; and the American College of Cardiology Foundation: in collaboration with the Heart Rhythm Society: endorsed by the American Autonomic Society. *Circulation.* 2006;113:316.

Task Force for the Diagnosis and Management of Syncope, European Society of Cardiology (ESC), European Heart Rhythm Association (EHRA), et al. Guidelines for the diagnosis and management of syncope (version 2009). *Eur Heart J.* 2009;30:2631.

SUDDEN CARDIAC ARREST

❑ Definition

- The sudden cessation of cardiac activity and hemodynamic collapse due to sustained ventricular arrhythmia.
- Formal definition has been difficult to define due to the fact up to one third of cases not witnessed. Absence of noncardiac pathology and presumed sudden loss of pulse are the most agreed upon criteria.
- Up to 15% of overall mortality in industrialized countries, with ≥300,000 cases/year.

❑ Who Should Be Suspected?

- Risk factors for sudden cardiac arrest (SCA) are driven largely by risk factors for coronary artery disease and structural heart disease, the most frequent cause of SCA in patients over 35 years of age (80%). The presence of known cardiac structural disease raises the risk of SCA six- to eightfold and is the index presentation of coronary disease in 15% of patients. Valvular disease and hypertrophic cardiomyopathy each account for 5% of cases in adults.
- In contrast, hypertrophic cardiomyopathy accounts for 48% of SCA in patients ≤35 years.
- In structurally normal hearts (5–10% of all SCA), the most common inherited arrhythmogenic diseases contributing to SCA include long- and short-QT syndromes, Brugada syndrome, Wolf-Parkinson-White syndrome, ARVC (see above), and catecholaminergic polymorphic VT. These conditions may account for 10–12% of SCA in young patients, and 5% in adult populations.

❑ Laboratory and Diagnostic Testing

- Potentially reversible causes of SCA should be immediately assessed in survivors and include assessment of electrolytes (particularly hypokalemia and hypomagnesemia, hypocalcemia), ischemia (ECG and troponins), arterial blood gas, recreational drugs, and medication lists scrutinized for proarrythmogenic effects (reference www.qtdrugs.org).
- Electrolyte abnormalities may be the result of hemodynamic derangement and resuscitative efforts. Attribution of primary etiology of SCA to electrolyte disturbance is appropriate only if other etiologies are excluded.
- It is essential that survivors of SCA undergo a full evaluation of structural heart disease including, but not limited to, ECG, cardiac catheterization and echocardiography.
- Cardiac MRI is indicated if a structural abnormality is uncertain after initial assessment and is particularly useful for the diagnosis of myocarditis, cardiac

infiltrative disease (amyloid and sarcoid) and arrhythmogenic right ventricular cardiomyopathy.

- Electrophysiology testing is not routinely performed in survivors of SCA, but may be useful in patients whose evaluation reveals no clear etiology of SCA. Inducible arrhythmias are a nonspecific finding and lack of inducible rhythm does not confer low risk for recurrence.
- First- and second-degree relatives of SCA patients should be screened for cardiovascular disease and considered for genetic testing. Risk of SCA increases 1.57-fold in family members, and up to 9.4-fold if maternal and paternal history of SCA is present.
- OTC ≥ 440 ms in males and ≥460 ms in females should be screened for inherited long QT syndrome by family history and potentially genetic testing. Given the number of genes identified in long QT syndromes and uncertainly over the functional significance of some reported variants, referral to an experienced testing center is recommended. Genetic testing in long QT syndrome has a yield of 40% positive genotype at a cost of $13,000 per diagnosis (in contrast, EP study >$50,000).
- Genetic evaluation for suspected cases of Brugada syndrome (SCN5A mutations) and catecholaminergic polymorphic ventricular tachycardia (RyR2 gene) has high yield and may impact clinical treatment and recommendations to patients and family members.

Suggested Readings

Bai R, Napolitano C, Bloise R, et al. Yield of genetic screening in inherited cardiac channelopathies: how to prioritize access to genetic testing. *Circ Arrhythm Electrophysiol.* 2009;2:6–15.

Priori SG, Blomstrom-Lundqvist C, et al. Update of the guidelines on sudden cardiac death of the European Society of Cardiology. *Eur Heart J.* 2003;24:13–15.

 HYPERTENSION

❑ Definition

- The NHANES national survey from 2005 to 2008 estimates that 30% of adults in the United States have hypertension, and most (>90%) have essential or primary hypertension.
- An individual is considered to have hypertension based on the average of two or more blood pressure readings following an initial assessment (Table 3-1).
- Using ambulatory blood pressure monitoring, a patient is hypertensive if average BP for 24 hours is above 135/85 mm Hg, daytime is >140/90 mm Hg, or nighttime is >125/75 mm Hg.
- *Secondary hypertension* is high BP caused by an identifiable and potentially curable disorder.
- *Hypertensive crisis* encompasses hypertensive urgency and emergency. Hypertensive urgency is DBP > 120 mm Hg with end-organ damage. Hypertensive emergency is acute or worsening end-organ damage associated with elevated BP, regardless of level. The term *malignant hypertension* is reserved for hypertensive emergency with papilledema or retinal hemorrhage.
- A 20 mm Hg increment of SBP or 10 mm Hg of diastolic BP in middle-aged and elderly persons is associated with a twofold increase in mortality from

TABLE 3–1 Blood Pressure Classification Suggested by the Joint National Committee

Classification	Systolic Pressure (mm Hg)		Diastolic Pressure (mm Hg)
Normal	<120	And	<80
Prehypertension	120–139	Or	80–89
Stage 1 hypertension	140–159	Or	90–99
Stage 2 hypertension	≥160	Or	≥100

The Seventh Report of the Joint National Committee on Prevention, Detection, Evaluation, and Treatment of High Blood Pressure. *Hypertension*. 2003;42:1206.

CVD throughout the BP range. This relationship is strongly correlated and continuous.

❑ Who Should Be Suspected?

▪ Mild to moderate essential hypertension is usually asymptomatic. The physical exam and history should focus on the need for a secondary hypertension work up (including the degree of difficulty achieving acceptable BP control) and the presence and severity of end-organ damage.

▪ Common essential hypertension risk factors are family history (2× risk), African descent, obesity, excessive alcohol or salt intake, physical inactivity, dyslipidemia, and personality traits of depression, time urgency/impatience.

▪ Secondary hypertension should be considered for severe or resistant hypertension (high BP despite treatment from three medications in different classes including diuretic), an acute rise in previously stable BP, <30 years old non-black patients with no family history, malignant hypertension, or findings from screening data.

▪ If secondary hypertension is suggested, a number of conditions need to be considered including primary renal disease, renovascular disease, sleep apnea, coarctation of the aorta (young children), pheochromocytoma, primary aldosteronism, oral contraceptive use, and thyroid and parathyroid disease.

▪ Malignant hypertension is associated with neurologic symptoms due to intracerebral or subarachnoid bleeding (headache, nausea, vomiting, somnolence, confusion, seizures, coma) and/or visual disturbance (retinal hemorrhages and exudates or papilledema).

❑ Laboratory Findings

▪ Most patients with presumed primary (essential) hypertension should undergo a limited evaluation due to poor diagnostic yield and high likelihood of false positive results.

▪ *Core laboratory:* hematocrit, urinalysis, routine blood chemistries, GFR, lipid profile and ECG (assess for LVH). Urine microalbumin or echocardiography could be considered.

▪ Considerations:
  ▼ When hypertension is associated with decreased serum potassium, rule out antihypertensive medication, Cushing syndrome, primary aldosteronism

(also with slight hypernatremia), and diuretic administration. Consider plasma aldosterone to renin ratio (also elevated in obesity).

▼ Increased calcium is seen with hyperparathyroidism. Vascular reactivity and day–night blood pressure regulation play a role in hypertensive response.

- Laboratory findings due to administration of some antihypertensive drugs, such as

  ▼ Oral diuretics (e.g., benzothiadiazines): hyperuricemia, hypokalemia, or hyperglycemia or aggravation of preexisting DM; less commonly, bone marrow depression, aggravation of renal or hepatic insufficiency, cholestatic hepatitis, or toxic pancreatitis.

  ▼ Hydralazine: syndrome may not be distinguishable from SLE. ANA may be found in ≤50% of asymptomatic patients.

  ▼ Methyldopa: ≤20% of patients may have positive direct Coombs test, but relatively few have hemolytic anemia. When the drug is discontinued, Coombs test may remain positive for months, but anemia usually reverses promptly. Abnormal liver function tests indicate hepatocellular damage without jaundice. Rheumatoid factor (RF) and SLE tests may occasionally be positive.

  ▼ Monoamine oxidase inhibitors (e.g., pargyline hydrochloride): wide range of toxic reactions, most serious of which are blood dyscrasias and hepatocellular necrosis.

- Renovascular hypertension is the most common correctable cause of secondary hypertension. Less than 1% of patients with mild hypertension, between 10% and 45% with malignant hypertension. Correlates with peripheral arterial disease.

- 2005 ACC/AHA guidelines propose diagnostic testing if

  ▼ Laboratory testing clues are present for secondary hypertension.

  ▼ Severe hypertension after 55 years of age (>180 mm Hg SBP, >120 mm Hg DBP).

  ▼ Unexplained kidney deterioration with antihypertensive therapy.

  ▼ Severe hypertension with diffuse atherosclerosis, unexplained atrophic kidney, or recurrent flash pulmonary edema.

  ▼ Abdominal bruit that lateralizes to a side (sensitivity of 40%, specificity up to 99%).

- Renovascular imaging studies: angiography, magnetic resonance angiography, CT angiography, and Doppler ultrasound (least invasive imaging test for renal artery stenosis).

Suggested Readings

Aram VC, Bakris GL, Black HR, et al.; the National High Blood Pressure Education Program Coordinating Committee. The Seventh Report of the Joint National Committee on Prevention, Detection, Evaluation, and Treatment of High Blood Pressure. *JAMA*. 2003;289:2073–2082.

Egan BM, Zhao Y, Axon RN. US trends in prevalence, awareness, treatment, and control of hypertension, 1988–2008. *JAMA*. 2010;303:2043.

Hirsch AT, Haskal ZJ, Hertzer NR, et al. ACC/AHA 2005 Practice Guidelines. *Circulation*. 2006;113:e463.

Papadakis MA, McPhee SJ. *Current Medical Diagnosis and Treatment 2009*. New York: McGraw-Hill Professional, 2008.

HYPERLIPIDEMIA

❑ Definition

- Hyperlipidemia is an elevation of lipids (cholesterol, cholesterol esters, phospholipids, and triglycerides) in the bloodstream; is a risk factor for coronary heart disease (CHD); and promotes atherosclerosis. Lipids are transported as lipoproteins in the body; there are five major types: chylomicrons, VLDLs, intermediate-density lipoproteins (IDLs), LDLs, and HDLs. The protein portions of the lipoprotein are referred as apolipoprotein, of which there are six major classes (A, B, C, D, E, and H) and numerous subclasses (AI, AII, AIV, AV, B48, B200, CI, CII, CIII, and CIV).

- The diagnosis of primary hyperlipidemia is made after the secondary causes are evaluated and ruled out or attempt is made to treat or eliminate the underlying cause. Secondary causes of dyslipidemia and associated lipid changes include some underlying disease, organ failure, or some drugs. It is not uncommon to have some overlap, with dyslipidemia being attributed to both primary and secondary causes (Table 3-2).

- Historically, primary dyslipidemias, such as the familial dyslipidemias, have been grouped according to the electrophoretic activity. The primary dyslipidemias are associated with overproduction and/or impaired removal of lipoproteins. A potentially more useful presentation of primary lipidemias is to classify them according to the principal lipid abnormality (Table 3-3).

TABLE 3–2 Diseases That May Cause Dyslipidemia and Associated Lipid Changes

Cause	Changes
Diabetes mellitus	TG↑, HDL-C↓
Hypothyroidism	LDL-C↑
Acromegaly	TG↑
Anorexia nervosa	LDL-C↑
Lipodystrophy	TG↑, HDL-C↓
Glycogen storage disorders	TG↑
Nephrotic syndrome	Mixed hyperlipidemia (LDL-C↑ predominates)
Chronic renal failure	TG↑
Obstructive liver disease	LDL-C↑, lipoprotein X↑
Alcohol	TG↑
Immunoglobulin excess: paraproteinemia	Mixed hyperlipidemia
Medications	
β-Adrenoceptor antagonists (selective)	HDL-C↓, TG↑
Thiazide diuretics	LDL-C↑, TG↑ or no change
Glucocorticoids	LDL-C↑ or no change, TG↑ or no change, HDL-C↑
Cyclosporine	LDL-C↑, TG↑
Interferons	TG↑
Antiviral medications (HIV protease inhibitors)	TG↑, LDL-C↑, HDL-C↓
Exogenous estrogens	TG↑, HDL-C↑, LDL-C↓
Retinoic acid derivatives	LDL-C↑, TG↑, HDL-C↓

HDL-C, high-density lipoprotein–cholesterol; LDL-C, low-density lipoprotein–cholesterol; TG, triglyceride; ↑, increased levels; ↓, decreased levels.

TABLE 3–3 Classification of Familial Dyslipidemias According to Predominant Lipid Abnormality and Etiology

Increased Cholesterol	Increased Triglyceride	Increased Cholesterol and Triglyceride	Decreased HDL	Increased HDL
Familial hypercholesterolemia	Familial hypertriglyceridemia	Familial combined hyperlipidemia	Familial hypoalphalipoproteinemia of unknown genetic defect	Familial hyperalphalipoproteinemia of unknown etiology
Polygenic hypercholesterolemia	Deficiency of lipoprotein lipase	Familial dysbetalipoproteinemia	Apoprotein A1 deficiency	CETP deficiency
Familial defective apoprotein B100	Deficiency of apoprotein CII		LCAT deficiency	Apoprotein A1 overexpression
Familial combined hyperlipidemia			Fish-eye disease	
			Tangier disease	

CETP, cholesteryl ester transport protein; HDL, high-density lipoprotein; LCAT, lecithin–cholesterol acyltransferase; TG, triglyceride.

❏ Who Should Be Suspected?

- There are typically no symptoms associated with hyperlipidemia, and it tends to be discovered during routine examination or evaluation for atherosclerotic cardiovascular disease. Detection of cholesterol disorders and other CHD risk factors occurs primarily through clinical case findings. On occasion, symptoms can include xanthomas around the eyes, Achilles tendons, and the extensor tendons of the hands, particularly with familial forms of the disorder.
- Individuals with higher lipid levels may develop lipemia retinalis (white appearance of the retina), arcus senilis (white discoloration of the peripheral cornea), or pancreatitis.

❏ Laboratory Findings

- Core laboratory: Standard lipid profile—total cholesterol (TC), LDL cholesterol, HDL cholesterol, and triglycerides (TGs)—should be obtained at least once every 5 years in adults age 20 and older.
  - ▼ Low-risk persons: Further testing is not required if the HDL-cholesterol level is ≥40 mg/dL and TC is <200 mg/dL.
  - ▼ High-risk persons: Lipoprotein measurement is recommended as a guide to clinical management. More frequent measurements are required for persons with multiple risk factors or, in those with 0–1 risk factors, if the LDL level is only slightly below the goal level.
- Apolipoprotein (LpA): Elevated in the presence of concomitant hypercholesterolemia or hypoalphalipoproteinemia—may aid in risk assessment for CHD.
- Lipoprotein electrophoresis: Shows a specific abnormal pattern in <2% of Americans; may be indicated if serum TG >300 mg/dL; fasting serum is lipemic; or if significant hyperglycemia, impaired glucose tolerance, or glycosuria is present. There is increased serum uric acid >8.5 mg/dL and/or strong family history of premature CHD.
- Molecular tests: Pharmacogenomic studies have shown a genetic predisposition for individuals to develop heart disease.
- Considerations:
  - ▼ If lipid screen is normal, further testing should be performed with consideration paid to the measurement of Lp(a) and apolipoproteins B and A-I. A standard serum lipid profile consists of total cholesterol, TG, and HDL-cholesterol.
  - ▼ Measure serum TC, HDL cholesterol, and TG after a 12- to 13-hour fast to minimize the influence of postprandial hyperlipidemia (total and HDL cholesterol can be measured in fasting or nonfasting individuals because the difference is clinically insignificant). Average results of two or three tests; if a difference of ≥30 mg/dL appears, repeat tests 1–8 weeks apart and average the results of three tests.
- Use TC for initial case finding and classification and monitoring of diet therapy. Do not use age- or sex-specific cholesterol values as decision levels.
- Consider values in association with clinical risk factors (e.g., age, gender, obesity, smoking, hypertension, and family history).

DISORDERS OF LIPID METABOLISM

ACID LIPASE DEFICIENCIES

❏ **Definition**
- Acid lipase deficiencies are characterized by the inability to hydrolyze lysosomal TG and cholesteryl esters.

❏ **Laboratory Findings**
- Decreased acid lipase in lymphocytes or fibroblasts
- Increased serum TG, LDL-C, and cholesterol esters

METABOLIC SYNDROME

- Metabolic syndrome is a condition of interrelated risk factors of metabolic origin, chief of which is insulin resistance, dyslipidemia, and hypertension that confer elevated cardiovascular risk.
  - The most common definition of metabolic syndrome requires abdominal obesity (waist circumference >88 cm in women and >102 cm in men), elevated blood pressure (SBP >130 mm Hg, DBP >85 mm Hg or antihypertensive medication), Low HDL-C (<40 mg/dL men, <50 mg/dL women), elevated fasting triglycerides of >150 mg/dL or nonfasting >400 mg/dL and impaired fasting glucose of 100 mg/dL or greater.
  - Prevalence is 33.7% in men and 35.4% in women from data from 1999 to 2002.
  - Metabolic syndrome may contribute up to 12–17% of all cardiovascular disease.
  - Direct measurement of LDL-C is recommended for the diagnosis of metabolic syndrome.
  - At present, CRP is not part of the definition of metabolic syndrome but does appear to add predictive risk of coronary events and may impact treatment decisions. Increased levels of fibrinogen, plasminogen activator inhibitor-1 and other coagulant factors are seen in patients with metabolic syndrome, but are not required for diagnosis.

ATHEROGENIC DYSLIPIDEMIA

- TG >150 mg/dL, HDL-C <40 mg/dL in men and <50 mg/dL in women, with small dense LDL particles.
- Abnormalities in fibrinolysis and coagulation.
- Exclusion of other causes of dyslipidemia (e.g., cholestasis, hypothyroidism, chronic renal failure, nephrotic syndrome).

HYPERALPHALIPOPROTEINEMIA (HDL-C EXCESS)

- This condition is inherited as a simple autosomal dominant trait in families with longevity, or it may be caused by alcoholism, extensive exposure to chlorinated hydrocarbon pesticides, or exogenous estrogen supplementation.

- It occurs in 1 in 20 adults with mildly increased TC levels (240–300 mg/dL) secondary to increased HDL-C (>70 mg/dL). LDL-C is not increased, and TG is normal.

SEVERE HYPERTRIGLYCERIDEMIA (TYPE I) (FAMILIAL HYPERCHYLOMICRONEMIA SYNDROME)

❑ Definition
- Hypertriglyceridemia is a rare autosomal recessive trait due to deficiency of lipoprotein lipase (LPL) or apo C-II or circulating inhibitor of LPL.
- There is marked heterogeneity in causative molecular defects.

❑ Laboratory Findings
- Core laboratory: changes due to fatty liver (increased serum transaminase)
- Persistent very high TG (>1,000 mg/dL) with marked increase in VLDL and chylomicrons.
- Deficiency of apo C-II is shown by isoelectric focusing or two-dimensional gel electrophoresis of plasma.

FAMILIAL HYPERCHOLESTEROLEMIA (TYPE II)

❑ Definition
- Familial hypercholesterolemia is inherited as an autosomal dominant disorder. Homozygous patients are very rare (1 per million).
- Clinical manifestations include increased TC (xanthomata, corneal arcus, CAD that causes death usually before age 30 years). Heterozygous patients present with premature CAD; tendinous xanthomas and corneal arcus are often present.

❑ Laboratory Findings
- Homozygous
- TC is very high (600–1,000 mg/dL) with corresponding increase in LDL.
- Neonatal diagnosis requires finding increased LDL-C in cord blood; serum TC is unreliable. Because of marked variation in serum TC levels during the 1st year of life, diagnosis should be deferred until 1 year of age. Prenatal diagnosis of homozygous fetus can be made by estimation of binding sites on fibroblasts cultured from amniotic fluids; useful when both parents are heterozygous.
- Heterozygous
- Increased serum TC (300–500 mg/dL) and LDL (two to three times normal) with similar change in a parent or first-degree relative; serum TG and VLDL are normal in 90% and slightly increased in 10% of these cases.
- Gene frequency occurs in 1 in 500 in the general population, but 5% in survivors of acute myocardial infarction (AMI) <60 years old. Plasma TG is normal in type II-A but increased in type II-B. This is not the most common cause of phenotype II-A.
- LDL receptors in fibroblasts or mononuclear blood cells are <25% in homozygous and 50% of normal levels.

POLYGENIC HYPERCHOLESTEROLEMIA (TYPE IIA)

❑ **Definition**

- Polygenic hypercholesterolemia can be diagnosed only after secondary causes of hypercholesterolemia and autosomal dominant traits have been excluded.
- Premature CAD occurs later in life than with familial combined hyperlipidemia. Xanthomas are rare.

❑ **Laboratory Findings**

- Persistent TC elevation (>240 mg/dL) and increased LDL without familial hypercholesterolemia or familial combined hypercholesterolemia.
- In type IIB disease, both LDL and VLDL are increased.

FAMILIAL COMBINED HYPERLIPIDEMIA (TYPES IB, IV, V)

❑ **Definition**

- Familial combined hyperlipidemia occurs in 0.5% of general population and 15% of survivors of AMI <60 years old. Premature CAD occurs later in life (after age 30 years) than with familial hypercholesterolemia.
- Xanthomas are rare. Patients are often overweight.

❑ **Laboratory Findings**

- There may be any combination of increased LDL-C and VLDL and chylomicrons; HDL-C is often low.
- Different family members may have increased serum TC or TG or both.

FAMILIAL DYSBETALIPOPROTEINEMIA (TYPE III)

❑ **Definition**

- Familial dysbetalipoproteinemia occurs in 1 per 5,000–10,000 persons.
- Atherosclerosis is more common in peripheral than coronary arteries. Tuberous and tendinous xanthomas and palmar and plantar xanthomatous streaks are present.

❑ **Laboratory Findings**

- Diagnosis by combination of ultracentrifugation and isoelectric focusing that shows abnormal apoprotein E pattern.
- Abnormality of apoprotein E with excess of abnormal lipoprotein (beta mobility—VLDL); TC > 300 mg/dL plus TG > 400 mg/dL should suggest this diagnosis.
- VLDL cholesterol-to-TG ratio = 0.3 (normal ratio = 0.2).

❑ **Familial Hypertriglyceridemia (Type IV)**

- Familial hypertriglyceridemia is an autosomal dominant condition present in 1% of general population and 5% of survivors of AMI < 60 years of age. The distinction from familial combined hyperlipidemia is made only by extensive family screening.
- There is elevated TG (usually 200–500 mg/dL) and VLDL with normal LDL-C and decreased HDL-C.

ABETALIPOPROTEINEMIA (BASSEN-KORNZWEIG SYNDROME)

❑ **Definition**

- Abetalipoproteinemia is a rare autosomal recessive disorder in which the liver and intestine cannot secrete apo B.
- It should be ruled out in children with fat malabsorption, steatorrhea, failure to thrive, neurologic symptoms, pigmented retinopathy, and/or acanthocytosis.

❑ **Laboratory Findings**

- Hematology
  - ▼ Abnormal RBCs (acanthocytes) are present in the PBS; may be 50–90% of RBCs and are characteristic. Decreased RBC life span may vary from severe hemolytic anemia to mild compensated anemia. Abnormal pattern of RBC phospholipids.
  - ▼ ESR is markedly decreased (e.g., 1 mm/hour).
- Core laboratory
  - ▼ Marked decrease in serum TG (<30 mg/dL) with little increase after ingestion of fat, and in TC (20–50 mg/dL). Chylomicrons, LDL-C, VLDL, apo B-48, and apo B-100 are absent; HDL-C may be lower than in normal persons.
  - ▼ Low serum carotene levels.
  - ▼ A variant is normotriglyceridemic abetalipoproteinemia in which patient can secrete apo B-48 but not apo B-100, resulting in normal postprandial TG values but marked hypocholesterolemia; associated with mental retardation and vitamin E deficiency.
  - ▼ There may be decrease of serum β-lipoprotein and cholesterol. Plasma lipids are normal in heterozygotes.
  - ▼ Low serum fat-soluble vitamin (A, K, and E) levels.
- Histology: Biopsy of small intestine shows characteristic lipid vacuolization, but this is not pathognomonic (occasionally seen in celiac disease, tropical sprue, juvenile nutritional and megaloblastic anemia).

HYPOBETALIPOPROTEINEMIA

❑ **Definition**

- Hypobetalipoproteinemia is an autosomal dominant disorder with increased longevity and lower incidence of atherosclerosis.
- At least one parent will show decreased β-lipoprotein.

❑ **Laboratory Findings**

- There is a marked decrease in LDL-C and LDL-C-to-HDL-C ratio.
- Homozygous patients have decreased serum TC (<50 mg/dL) and TG and undetectable or trace amounts of chylomicrons, VLDL, and LDL.
- Heterozygotes are asymptomatic and have serum TC, LDL-C, and apo B values that are 50% of normal (consistent with codominant disorder); may also be caused by malabsorption of fats, infection, anemia, hepatic necrosis, hyperthyroidism, AMI, acute trauma.

TANGIER DISEASE

❑ **Definition**

- Tangier disease is a rare autosomal recessive disorder caused by mutations at chromosome 9q31 causing a defect in the metabolism of apo A, in which there is a marked decrease (heterozygous) or absence (homozygous) of HDL.
- Deposits of cholesterol esters in reticuloendothelial cells cause enlarged liver, spleen, and lymph nodes; enlarged orange tonsils; and small orange-brown spots in rectal mucosa. Patients may have premature CAD, mild corneal opacification, and neuropathy in homozygous type.

❑ **Laboratory Findings**

- Plasma levels of apo A-I and apo A-II are extremely low.
- In homozygotes, HDL-C is usually <10 mg/dL and apo A-I is usually <5 mg/dL.
- In heterozygotes, HDL-C and apo A-I are approximately 50% of normal. Serum TC (<100 mg/dL), LDL-C, and phospholipids are decreased; TG = 100–250 mg/dL. Pre-β-lipoprotein is absent.

LECITHIN–CHOLESTEROL ACYLTRANSFERASE DEFICIENCY (FAMILIAL)

❑ **Definition**

- Lecithin–cholesterol acyltransferase deficiency is a very rare autosomal recessive disorder of adults.
- It is associated with premature CAD, corneal opacities, and glomerulosclerosis.

❑ **Laboratory Findings**

- Serum TC is normal but cholesterol esters are virtually absent. Plasma free cholesterol is extremely increased. HDL-C is low.
- Normochromic anemia with large RBCs that are frequently target cells.
- Proteinuria

❑ **High HDL-C Lipidemia**

- High HDL-C is a rare autosomal recessive disorder causing cholesteryl ester transfer protein gene defects.
- It may be due to active lifestyle, drugs (e.g., estrogens, alcohol, phenytoin, phenobarbital, rifampicin, griseofulvin).

❑ **Low HDL-C Lipidemia**

- Familial hypoalphalipoproteinemia (autosomal dominant disorder with HDL-C).
- It may be due to deficiency of apo A-I and apo C-III, abetalipoproteinemia, hypobetalipoproteinemia (<30 mg/dL in women and <40 mg/dL in men), or drugs (isotretinoin, anabolic steroids).

Suggested Reading

Hachem S, Mooradian A. Familial dyslipidaemias: an overview of genetics, pathophysiology and management. *Drugs.* 2006;66(15):1949–1969.

ATHEROSCLEROSIS

❑ Definition

- Atherosclerosis is the condition in which the atheroma (plaque) is the characteristic lesion found in the intima of medium-sized and large arteries as an inflammatory response to injury. The plaques contain lipids, smooth muscle cells, connective tissue, inflammatory cell, and other extracellular constituents.
- Atherosclerosis is responsible for almost all cases of coronary heart disease.
- Plaque stability is variable and can rupture, triggering in situ thrombosis or embolization, leading to potential acute ischemic events.

❑ Who Should Be Suspected?

- Atherogenesis occurs over years and is initially asymptomatic until ischemia is clinically manifested. Clinical manifestation is dependent on the particular circulatory bed affected. Manifestations include myocardial infarction and angina, intermittent claudication and gangrene, stroke, mesenteric ischemia or renal artery stenosis, aneurysms, and arterial dissection.
- Risk factors for atherosclerosis include age, gender, cigarette smoking, DM, endothelial dysfunction, dyslipidemia, hypertension, and family history.
- Risk assessment models and guidelines derived from these risk factors allow for the matching of intensity of management to the degree of cardiovascular risk. This is critical given the prevalence of established risk factor in the general population and the substantial cost associated with escalating medical therapy. The most well established risk model continues to be the Framingham Risk Score, which serves as the foundation for prevention treatment guidelines (see http://framinghamheartstudy.org/risk/hrdcoronary.html)
- Adjunctive risk assessment tools such as C-reactive protein, other circulating inflammatory biomarkers, and subclinical atherosclerosis imaging (CT, carotid intimal thickness or CIMT) have emerged within the past decade and have been cautiously included in recommendations for risk assessment in asymptomatic adults (level of evidence B: no randomized trials based on management).
- CRP (along with CT scanning and CIMT) is currently recommended (Class IIa) for asymptomatic moderate-risk individuals in whom lipid lowering therapy is considered based on atherosclerotic risk alone (i.e., LDL-C < 130 mg/dL not on medication).
- Individuals with evidence of peripheral arterial disease, symptomatic carotid disease, asymptomatic carotid disease >50%, diabetes mellitus, and/or abdominal aortic aneurysm are considered to have a coronary heart disease risk equivalent and warrant aggressive preventive therapy akin to established coronary atherosclerosis. In these patients, subsequent lipid assessment is required for titration of therapy. Adjunctive testing for the diagnosis of coronary atherosclerosis (CRP/imaging) is not justified.

❑ Laboratory Findings

- Core laboratory: Lp(a) and homocysteine are increased.
- Elevated CRP (if first result is >3.0 mg/L, repeating the test at least 2 weeks later when patient is in metabolically stable state free of infection or acute illness is recommended). Persistent values >3.0 mg/L define a high-risk category. The Reynolds Risk Score incorporates CRP into initial risk assessment (http://www.reynoldsriskscore.org). Overall the modest strength of CRP inclusion into risk assessment points argues against a causative role in atherosclerosis.
- Coronary artery calcium scores exceeding 100 AU (Agatston units) or 75th percentile are considered high risk for coronary events, as are any carotid plaque or IMT exceeding 75th percentile.

Suggested Readings

Faxon DP, Fuster V, Libby P, et al. Atherosclerotic vascular disease conference: writing group III: pathophysiology. *Circulation*. 2004;109:2617–2625.

Greenland P, Alpert JS, Beller GA, et al. 2010 ACCF/AHA guidelines for assessment of cardiovascular risk in asymptomatic adults: a report of the American College of Cardiology Foundation/American Heart Association Task Force on Practice Guidelines. *J Am Coll Cardiol*. 2010;56:e50–e103.

Lloyd-Jones DM. Cardiovascular risk prediction: basic concepts, current status, and future directions. *Circulation*. 2010;121:1768–1777.

CHAPTER 4

Central Nervous System Disorders

Juliana G. Szakacs

4

In the 10th edition, this chapter has been updated to present the laboratory workup of neurologic diseases by primary presenting symptomatology and expanded to provide a thorough differential diagnosis. Please remember that many disorders overlap in their presenting signs, and these will be cross-referenced when possible. Evaluation of the nervous system requires a multidisciplinary approach to the patient and, where appropriate, pertinent clinical findings, radiologic procedures, and laboratory tests have been included to aid in the diagnosis. Please see the e-book version for the figures referenced in this chapter.

 # DISORDERS OF COGNITION AND DEMENTIA

INTELLECTUAL DISABILITY

❑ Definition

Intellectual disability (ID) is defined by the DSM-IV[1] as significant subaverage intellectual function, significant limitations in adaptive functioning, and onset before 18 years. It is an unchanging encephalopathy that may be due to a number of disorders that affect brain development and function.

❑ Clinical Presentation

Developmental screening with standard screening tools should be performed at every well-child visit. A comprehensive history and physical should include measurements of height, weight, and head circumference, including growth velocity, dysmorphic features, neurologic and sensory development, and a detailed observation of behavior.

❑ Causes

Prenatal

Genetic causes are the most common forms of ID in the prenatal group. Current testing for fetal trisomies and a number of other known genetic disorders is routinely carried out as part of the prenatal screen. Amniotic fluid or chorionic villi sampling may be used for microarray or chromosomal analyses, and maternal blood may now be tested by cell-free DNA methods. Chromosomal disorders resulting in ID include Down syndrome; trisomy 18; fragile X; autosomal recessive genes PRSS12, CRBN, CC2D1A, TUSC3, GRIK2, and SYNGAP1; autosomal dominant genes STXBP1, SYBGAP1, and SCN2A; cri-du-chat syndrome; and Klinefelter syndrome[2-4] (See Chapter 10 Hereditary and Genetic Diseases).

Nongenetic prenatal causes include the following:

- CNS malformations
- Congenital infections (e.g., syphilis, rubella, toxoplasmosis, CMV) resulting in hydrocephalus (see eBook Figure 4-1)

- Metabolic abnormalities (e.g., DM, eclampsia, placental dysfunction)
- Environmental toxins or teratogens (alcohol, lead, mercury, hydantoin, and valproate) and radiation exposure
- Metabolic abnormalities (congenital hypothyroidism)
  - ▼ Amino acid metabolism (e.g., phenylketonuria, maple syrup urine disease, homocystinuria, cystathioninuria, hyperglycemia, argininosuccinicaciduria, citrullinemia, histidinemia, hyperprolinemia, oasthouse urine disease, Hartnup disease, Joseph syndrome, familial iminoglycinuria)
  - ▼ Lipid metabolism (e.g., Batten disease, Tay-Sachs disease, Niemann-Pick disease, abetalipoproteinemia, Refsum disease, metachromatic leukodystrophy) resulting in abnormal storage disorders (see eBook Figure 4-2)
  - ▼ Carbohydrate metabolism (e.g., galactosemia, mucopolysaccharidoses)
  - ▼ Purine metabolism (e.g., Lesch-Nyhan syndrome, hereditary orotic aciduria)
  - ▼ Mineral metabolism (e.g., idiopathic hypercalcemia, pseudopseudohypoparathyroidism, and pseudohypoparathyroidism)
- Other syndromes (e.g., tuberous sclerosis, Louis-Bar syndrome)

Perinatal

- Infections (e.g., syphilis, rubella, toxoplasmosis, CMV, HIV, HSV)
- Kernicterus
- Prematurity (see eBook Figure 4-3)
- Anoxia, hypoxia
- Trauma (CNS hemorrhage) (see eBook Figure 4-4)

Postnatal

- Poisoning (e.g., lead, arsenic, carbon monoxide)
- Infections (e.g., meningitis, encephalitis)
- Metabolic abnormalities (e.g., hypoglycemia, malnutrition)
- Postvaccinal encephalitis
- CVA
- Trauma (CNS hemorrhage)
- Hypoxia
- Psychosocial deprivation

❏ Laboratory Findings

Genetic Studies

Children with global developmental delay have a 4% incidence of abnormal cytogenetic studies. A karyotype should be routinely performed on all affected patients even if dysmorphic features are not present. Additional factors that should prompt genetic testing include family history of multiple miscarriages, unexplained infant death, parental consanguinity, or developmental regression or loss of milestones.[5-7]

Chromosomal microarray analysis identifies subtelomeric chromosomal rearrangements, which may be seen in an additional 5% of children with ID. FISH may be used if microarray diagnosis is not available or if a specific telomeric disorder such as cri-du-chat syndrome is suspected.[2]

Down syndrome (trisomy 21) is the most common form of inherited ID followed by fragile X syndrome, caused by an abnormal expansion mutation of a CGG triplet repeat in the fragile X mental retardation 1 (FRM1) gene. Testing for fragile X mutations should be considered in male and female patients, especially in those with a family history of ID.[8] Because Down syndrome often presents with nonspecific global developmental delay in young children, there should be a low threshold for this investigation.[5]

Metabolic studies: ID is a clinical feature of some inborn errors of metabolism; these may be identified by newborn screening.

Thyroid screening: Congenital hypothyroidism may result in ID; thyroid testing is not indicated unless clinical features suggest dysfunction.

Lead screening: Lead is the most common environmental neurotoxin. At concentrations >10 µg/dL (0.48 µmol/L), it has been associated with cognitive deficits. Children should be screened at 1–2 years of age. Risk factors for increased levels of lead include living in a community where >12% of children have blood lead levels of >10 µg/dL and living in a house built before 1950.[9]

References

1. American Psychiatric Association. *Diagnostic and Statistical Manual*, 4th ed. Washington, DC: APA Press; 1994.
2. Kaufman L, Ayub M, Vincent JB. The genetic basis of non-syndromic intellectual disability: a review. *J Neurodev Disord*. 2010;2:182.
3. Miller DT, Adam MP, Aradhya S, et al. Consensus statement: chromosomal microarray is a first-tier clinical diagnostic test for individuals with developments disabilities or congenital anomalies. *Am J Hum Genet*. 2010;86:749.
4. de Ligt J, Willemsen MH, van Bon BW, et al. Diagnostic exome sequencing in persons with severe intellectual disability. *N Engl J Med*. 2012;367:1921.
5. Moeschler JB, Shevell M. Clinical genetic evaluation of the child with mental retardation or developmental delays. *Pediatrics*. 2006;117:2304.
6. Ropers HH. Genetics of intellectual disability. *Curr Opin Genet Dev*. 2008;18:241–250.
7. Shevell M, Ashwal S, Donley D, et al. Practice parameter: evaluation of the child with global developmental delay: report of the Quality Standards Subcommittee of the American Academy of Neurology and The Practice Committee of the Child Neurology Society. *Neurology*. 2003;60:367.
8. Hagerman PJ. The fragile X prevalence paradox. *J Med Genet*. 2008;45:498.
9. American Academy of Pediatrics Committee on Environmental Health. Screening for elevated blood lead levels. *Pediatrics*. 1998;101:1072.

DEMENTIA

❑ Definition

According to the DSM-IV,[1] dementia is defined by impairment of memory and at least one other cognitive domain such as aphasia, agnosia, apraxia, or executive function. It must also represent a decline in the patient's prior ability and interfere with daily life.

❑ Clinical Presentation

The most common form of dementia is Alzheimer disease followed by vascular dementia, frontotemporal dementia, Lewy body disease, Parkinson disease, and progressive supranuclear palsy. These must be differentiated from depression, delirium, and drug or alcohol effects. Disorders that present with no other neurologic symptoms include Alzheimer disease, depression, delirium, and drug effect. Disorders that present with other neurologic symptoms in addition to dementia include neurosyphilis, Huntington disease, hepatic encephalopathy, Creutzfeldt-Jakob disease, Parkinson disease, progressive supranuclear palsy, toxic and alcoholic disorders, endocrine abnormalities, and malignancies.

Reference

1. American Psychiatric Association. *Diagnostic and Statistical Manual*, 4th ed. Washington, DC: APA Press; 1994.

ALZHEIMER DISEASE

❑ Definition

Alzheimer disease (AD) is the insidious onset of dementia due to cortical atrophy with accumulation of plaques containing abnormal proteins and fibrillary tangles in the neurons. The dominant abnormal protein is Aβ peptide, a form of amyloid.

❑ Clinical Presentation

AD is the most common cause of dementia in the elderly. It begins insidiously and progresses over 5–10 years to severe cortical dysfunction. The incidence of AD doubles every 5 years, starting at 1% in the 60- to 64-year-old age group and rising as high as 40% in the 85- to 89-year-old age group. In patients older than 60 with dementia, the usual causes are AD 60–80%, vascular dementia 10–20%, dementia with Lewy Bodies 10%, frontotemporal dementia 10%, and Parkinson disease with dementia 5%.[1] Recent studies now suggest that patients with some types of cancer may have a decreased risk of AD.[2] Laboratory testing should be performed to rule out treatable causes of dementia; definitive diagnosis of AD is not currently possible, although newer biomarkers are becoming more useful in suggesting the diagnosis.

❑ Laboratory Findings

Initial screening for patients with dementia should include B_{12} and thyroid studies to rule out deficiencies. Routine screening labs such as CBC, electrolytes, glucose, renal, and liver functions have not been shown to be helpful in the general population. Screening for neurosyphilis should be undertaken if there is increased suspicion, and testing for RBC folate in alcoholics may be of help in the differentiation of these disorders. In patients with multiple myeloma or breast or prostate cancer, ionized calcium may also be helpful. In patients with rapidly progressing disease or who are under the age of 60, the American Academy of Neurology recommends the following tests: serology, CSF, and EEG.[3] The gold standard for the diagnosis of AD is the histologic finding of plaques and fibrillary tangles in the brain on biopsy or at autopsy (see eBook Figure 4-5).

Genetic Testing

Early-onset (<60 years) AD has been associated with three genes seen in approximately 60% of these cases and is transmitted as an autosomal dominant. APP (amyloid precursor protein) on chromosome 1q (also seen in Down syndrome) and PSEN1 (presenilin 1) on chromosome 14q are the more common genes affected, and PSEN2 (presenilin 2) on chromosome 1q is rare. Commercial testing for these genes is not available, and in order to fully rule out abnormalities, full gene sequencing would be needed as numerous mutations have been found. APP mutations increase the production of amyloidogenic Aβ or alter the ratio of Aβ42 to Aβ40. PSEN1 mutations in AD most likely are involved in the γ-secretase cleavage of APP. PSEN2 is similar to PSEN1, affecting cleavage of APP, and also enhances apoptotic activity, leading to neurodegeneration.[4]

The APOE ε4 gene allele has been associated with both late-onset AD and vascular dementia. The APOE lipoprotein is involved in cholesterol homeostasis and neuronal protection in the brain. It may also participate in Aβ deposition. APOE ε4 may be measured in the serum, and increased levels have been associated with late-onset AD and atherosclerotic vascular disease.[5] Genetic testing for late-onset AD is controversial due to the significant number of both false positives and false negatives; in addition, APOE ε4 is a susceptibility gene, and 40% of patients with AD do not carry the APOE ε4 gene.[6] Testing for the APOE ε4 allele is available through commercial laboratories. An increased number of APOE ε4 alleles is associated with a greater risk of disease; risk is also dependent on age, gender, and race.

4

Blood and CSF Testing
Biomarkers including increased levels of tau protein and decreased levels of Aβ40 and 42 in the CSF and plasma may either predict development of or suggest a diagnosis of AD.[7–9]

References

1. Hebert LE, Scherr PA, Bienas JL, et al. Alzheimer disease in the US population: prevalence estimates using the 2000 census. *Arch Neurol.* 2003;60:1119.
2. Musicco M, Adorni F, DiSanto S, et al. Inverse occurrence of cancer and Alzheimer disease: a population-based incidence study. *Neurology.* 2013;81(4):322–328.
3. Knopman Ds, DeKosky ST, Cummings JL, et al. Practice parameter: diagnosis of dementia (an evidence based review). Report of the Quality Standards Subcommittee of the American Academy of Neurology. *Neurology.* 2001;56:1143.
4. Campion D, Dumanchin C, Hannequin D, et al. Early-onset autosomal dominant Alzheimer disease: prevalence, genetic heterogeneity, and mutation spectrum. *Am J Hum Genet.* 1999;65:664.
5. Kivipelto M, Helkala EL, Laakso MP, et al. Apolipoprotein E epsilon 4 allele, elevated midlife total cholesterol level, and high midlife systolic blood pressure are independent risk factors for late-life Alzheimer disease. *Ann Intern Med.* 2002;137:149.
6. Myers RH, Schaefer EJ, Wilson PW, et al. APOE ε4 association with dementia in a population-based study: the Framingham study. *Neurology.* 1996;46:763.
7. Galasko D, Clark C, Chang L, et al. Assessment of CSF levels of tau protein in mildly demented patients with Alzheimer's disease. *Neurology.* 1997;48:632.
8. Kahle PJ, Jakowec M, Teipel SJ, et al. Combined assessment of tau and neuronal thread protein in Alzheimer's disease CSF. *Neurology.* 2000;54:1498.
9. Sunderland T, Linker G, Mirza N, et al. Decreased beta-amyloid1-42 and increased tau levels in cerebrospinal fluid of patients with Alzheimer disease. *JAMA.* 2003;289:2094.

VASCULAR DEMENTIA

❑ Definition
First described by Binswanger and Alzheimer, vascular dementia or vascular cognitive impairment is a heterogeneous group of cerebrovascular disorders resulting in dementia. Three pathologic entities contribute to this disorder: cortical infarcts, lacunar infarct, and chronic subcortical ischemia.[1] Vascular dementia is the second most common form of dementia in the United States and Europe.

❑ Clinical Presentation
The clinical presentation varies depending on the location of the underlying lesion. Patterns of dementia may be divided into cortical or subcortical ischemic injury with the most severe being those in which there is damage to the region of the thalamus.[2]

Conditions related to vascular dementia include cerebral amyloid angiopathy, which is caused by the deposition of amyloid in the cerebral vessels resulting in hemorrhage or infarct; cerebral autosomal dominant arteriopathy with subcortical infarcts and leukoencephalopathy (CADASIL), which is caused by a mutation in the NOTCH3 gene resulting in leukoencephalopathy, subcortical infarcts, migraines, and psychiatric symptoms; and mixed dementia of cerebrovascular disease and AD, which is seen in 35–50% of patients with AD.[1]

❏ Laboratory Findings

Diagnosis is made by neuroimaging (MRI is significantly more sensitive than CT). When evidence of CNS infarction is found, additional testing to determine the stroke subtype or etiology should be undertaken, including carotid artery Doppler, echocardiogram, and Holter monitor. Patients should be screened for hypertension, diabetes, and hyperlipidemia. If a patient has a history suggestive of CADASIL, genetic testing for the NOTCH3 gene is commercially available (see eBook Figure 4-6).

References

1. Kalaria RN. Cerebrovascular disease and mechanisms of cognitive impairment: evidence from clinicopathological studies in humans. *Stroke.* 2012;43:2526.
2. Benitsy S, Gouw AA, Porcher R, et al. Location of lacunar infarcts correlates with cognition in a sample of non-disabled subjects with age-related white-matter changes: the LADIS study. *J Neurol Neurosurg Psychiatry.* 2009;80:478.

FRONTOTEMPORAL DEMENTIA

❏ Definition

Frontotemporal dementia (FTD) results from degeneration of the frontal or temporal lobes resulting in personality, language, and behavior abnormalities. It is a group of disorders with onset in the 45–65 age range that may progress to global dementia. This entity was once called Pick disease, but this diagnosis is now reserved for a subset of patients who exhibit Pick bodies (abnormal protein deposition within cells) on autopsy or biopsy.

❏ Clinical Presentation

FTD appears to be associated with genetic abnormalities more frequently than AD, the symptoms progress more rapidly, and FTD patients are less likely to demonstrate memory loss on initial examination.[1,2] Three variants of FTD are based on the functional aspects of the frontal lobe. These include a behavioral variant, several progressive aphasia variants, and semantic dementia. A smaller group of patients will also have motor impairment.

Recent genetic abnormalities have been identified that are associated with FTD. These include mutations in the MAPT gene on chromosome 17 that encodes the tau protein (tau protein repeats are found in the deposition of Pick bodies) and an abnormal form of TARDBP called pathologic TDP43, which is the major disease protein in ubiquitin-positive, tau-, and alpha-synuclein–negative frontotemporal dementia.[3]

❏ Laboratory Findings

The diagnosis is primarily made by clinical assessment, neuropsychologic testing, and neuroimaging with MRI. Laboratory tests to rule out treatable forms of dementia (B_{12}, thyroid, syphilis, electrolytes) should be considered. There is no definitive test for diagnosis of FTD, but genetic testing for some known mutations is now available. Caution should be taken in interpretation of negative tests since not all mutations underlying FTD have been identified.[4]

References

1. Snowden JS, Neary D, Mann DM. Frontotemporal dementia. *Br J Psychiatry.* 2002;180: 140–143.
2. Rosen HJ, Hartikainen KM, Jagust W, et al. Utility of clinical criteria in differentiating fronto-temporal lobar degeneration from Alzheimer disease. *Neurology.* 2002;58:1608.
3. Hardy J, Parastoo M, Bryan JT. Frontal temporal dementia: dissecting the aetiology and patho-genesis. *Brain.* 2006;26(4):830–831.
4. Goldman JS, Rademakers R, Huey ED, et al. An algorithm for genetic testing of frontotemporal lobar degeneration. *Neurology.* 2011;76:475.

DEMENTIA WITH LEWY BODIES

❏ Definition
Dementia with Lewy bodies (DLB) is a degenerative dementia that also presents with at least two of the following three clinical features: cognitive fluctuations, visual hallucinations, or parkinsonism.[1]

❏ Clinical Presentation
In contrast to AD, DLB presents early on with alterations in attention, visual, and executive functions and only later with memory deficits. It is characterized by cortical atrophy with less hippocampal atrophy than that seen in AD and by the presence of Lewy bodies, clumps of alpha-synuclein, and ubiquitin protein in neurons of the cortex, on autopsy (see eBook Figure 4-7). DLB is not thought to be a familial disorder; however, recent association with the PARK11 gene has been described.[2]

❏ Laboratory Findings
Diagnosis of DLB is made by clinical assessment, neuropsychologic testing, neuroimaging (MRI), and screening laboratory studies to rule out treatable forms of dementia (B_{12}, thyroid, syphilis, electrolytes). No specific test for definitive diagnosis of DLB is available. EEG may be helpful to rule out seizure or Creutzfeldt-Jakob disease. Genetic testing is not currently recommended.

References

1. McKeith IG, Dickson DW, Lowe J, et al. Diagnosis and management of dementia with Lewy bodies: third report of the DLB Consortium. *Neurology.* 2005;65:1863.
2. Bogaerts V, Engelborghs S, Kumar-Singh S, et al. A novel locus for dementia with Lewy bodies: a clinically and genetically heterogeneous disorder. *Brain.* 2007;130(9):2277.

PARKINSON DISEASE DEMENTIA

❏ Definition
Parkinson disease (PD) when severe may present with dementia as a symptom surpassing the functional effects of the motor features (see also Disorders of Movement) and is then classified as Parkinson disease dementia.

❏ Clinical Presentation

The differential diagnosis from Alzheimer disease and other degenerative dementias is made by a history of motor dysfunction predating the dementia in PD. Dementia in PD may be as high as 41%, and therefore, differentiation from other dementias should be undertaken for proper treatment.[1] In addition, Parkinson disease may coexist with Alzheimer disease or vascular dementia as all three are fairly common. Research continues to determine if Parkinson disease dementia and dementia with Lewy bodies may represent different presentations of the same disease.[2]

The risks for dementia in PD include an older age of onset, longer duration, and severity of parkinsonism. Genetic risk factors have been described; these include mutations on chromosome 1P in the ATPase gene, which is associated with juvenile parkinsonism with dementia[3]; multiplication-type mutations of the alpha-synuclein gene; APOE ε4 and APOE ε2[4]; and the microtubule-associated protein tau (MAPT) H1/H1 gene, which has been implicated in more rapid onset of dementia.[5]

❏ Laboratory Findings

The diagnosis of PD dementia is primarily made by clinical assessment and history. Dementia usually occurs in the setting of well-established parkinsonism, while in DLB, dementia may occur at the same time as the development of motor signs, and in AD, motor symptoms only develop very late in the course of disease[6]. Neuropsychiatric testing may assist in the diagnosis, but no published clinical criteria for PD dementia exist. Neuroimaging with MRI may reveal more atrophy with dementia than in PD without dementia but is not diagnostic[7]. Lab tests should be performed to exclude other treatable causes of dementia (CBC, electrolytes, glucose, thyroid studies, and renal and liver functions). The diagnosis of PD dementia is suggested when dementia occurs at least 1 year after the development of established parkinsonism.

References

1. Mayeux R, Denaro J, Hemenegildo N, et al. A population-based investigation of Parkinson's disease with and without dementia: relationship to age and gender. *Arch Neurol.* 1992;49:492.
2. Lippa CF, Duda JE, Grossman M, et al. DLB and PDD boundary issues: diagnosis, treatment, molecular pathology, and biomarkers. *Neurology.* 2007;68:812.
3. de Lau LM, Schipper CM, Hofman A, et al. Prognosis of Parkinson disease: risk of dementia and mortality: the Rotterdam Study. *Arch Neurol.* 2005;62:1265.
4. Huang X, Chen P, Kaufer DI, et al. Apolipoprotein E and dementia in Parkinson disease: a meta-analysis. *Arch Neurol.* 2006;63:189.
5. Burton EJ, McKeith IG, Burn DJ, et al. Brain atrophy rates in Parkinson's disease with and without dementia using serial magnetic resonance imaging. *Mov Disord.* 2005;20:1571.
6. Portet F, Scarmeas N, Cosentino S, et al. Extrapyramidal signs before and after diagnosis of incident Alzheimer disease in a prospective population study. *Arch Neurol.* 2009;66:1120.
7. Melzer TR, Watts R, MacAskill MR, et al. Grey matter atrophy in cognitively impaired Parkinson's disease. *J Neurol Neurosurg Psychiatry.* 2012;83:188.

HUNTINGTON DISEASE

Huntington disease (HD) is a neurodegenerative disease presenting with choreiform movements, psychiatric disorder, and dementia (see HD in the section on Disorders of Movement).

DISORDERS OF ALTERED MENTAL STATE

COMA AND STUPOR

❑ Definition
Coma is defined as unconsciousness lasting for more than 6 hours. There is no response to external stimuli, including pain and no voluntary movements. Stupor is defined as a decreased level of consciousness in which there is only response to pain.

4

❑ Clinical Presentation
Patients with coma or stupor are poorly or nonresponsive to external stimuli. The causes are many and can be divided into several etiologic categories (see "Causes" below). The goal of diagnostic testing is to identify treatable conditions including infection, metabolic abnormalities, seizures, intoxications/overdose, and surgical lesions as rapidly as possible. Diagnosis is made on physical and neurologic examination, history, neuroimaging, and laboratory testing.[1,2]

❑ Causes
Poisons, Drugs, or Toxins
- Sedatives (especially alcohol, barbiturates)
- Enzyme inhibitors (especially salicylates, heavy metals, organic phosphates, cyanide)
- Other (e.g., paraldehyde, methyl alcohol, ethylene glycol)

Cerebral Disorders
- Brain contusion, hemorrhage, infarction, seizure, or aneurysm
- Brain mass (e.g., tumor, hematoma, abscess, parasites)
- Subdural or epidural hematoma
- Venous sinus occlusion
- Hydrocephalus
- Hypoxia
- Decreased blood O_2 content and tension (e.g., lung disease, high altitude) (see eBook Figure 4-8)
- Decreased blood O_2 content with normal tension (e.g., anemia, carbon monoxide poisoning, methemoglobinemia)
- Infection (e.g., meningitis, encephalitis)
- Postictal state
  - ▼ Vascular abnormalities (e.g., subarachnoid hemorrhage, hypertensive encephalopathy [see eBook Figure 4-9], shock, acute myocardial infarction, aortic stenosis, Adams-Stokes disease, tachycardias)
- Metabolic abnormalities, such as hyponatremia with central pontine myelinolysis (see eBook Figure 4-10)
- Acid–base imbalance (acidosis, alkalosis)
- Electrolyte imbalance (increased or decreased sodium, potassium, calcium, magnesium)
- Porphyrias
- Aminoacidurias

- Uremia
- Hepatic encephalopathy
- Other disorders (e.g., leukodystrophies, lipid storage diseases, Bassen-Kornzweig syndrome)
- Nutritional deficiencies (e.g., vitamin B_{12}, thiamine, niacin, pyridoxine)

Endocrine Disorders
- Pancreas (diabetic coma, hypoglycemia)
- Thyroid (myxedema, thyrotoxicosis)
- Adrenal (Addison disease, Cushing syndrome, pheochromocytoma)
- Panhypopituitarism
- Parathyroid (hypofunction or hyperfunction)

Psychogenic Conditions That May Mimic Coma
- Depression, catatonia
- Malingering
- Hysteria, conversion disorder

Initial workup must be based on the clinical presentation. Rapid evaluation of treatable lesions, especially surgical, may improve survival. Conditions that may be mistaken for coma or stupor include the locked-in syndrome, akinetic mutism, and psychogenic unresponsiveness. In children, also consider complete paralysis with lesions of the brain stem, botulism, and Guillain-Barré syndrome.

❑ Laboratory Findings
Diagnosis is made on clinical examination, history, and urgent CT scan to rule out possible structural abnormalities such as papilledema, focal neurologic changes, acute stroke, expanding mass lesion, or herniation syndrome.

In patients with fever, a lumbar puncture should be performed to rule out bacterial meningitis or viral encephalitis. Neuroimaging prior to lumbar puncture in a comatose patient is recommended to avoid precipitating transtentorial herniation.[3] CSF may exclude subarachnoid hemorrhage (absence of xanthochromia) when CT is normal and may help in the diagnosis of demyelinating, inflammatory, and neoplastic disease with evaluation of glucose, cytology, and OCB.

Blood tests to exclude treatable causes of coma and stupor include the following:

- CBC
- Serum electrolytes, calcium, magnesium, phosphate, glucose, BUN, and creatinine
- Liver and renal function tests
- Ketones, lactose, and osmolarity to rule out diabetic coma
- ABG
- PT and PTT
- Drug screen to include ethanol, acetaminophen, salicylates, opiates, benzodiazepines, barbiturates, cocaine, amphetamines, ethylene glycol, and methanol

If the initial screening is unrevealing, additional testing should include the following:

- Blood cultures
- Thyroid and adrenal function tests

- Blood smear: to screen for thrombotic thrombocytopenic purpura and hemolysis
- LDH, D-dimer, and fibrinogen to rule out DIC
- Antiphospholipids if a coagulation problem is suspected
- Carboxyhemoglobin if carbon monoxide poisoning is suggested

References

1. Goldman L, et al. *Cecil Medicine. Coma and Other Disorders of Consciousness*, 24th ed. Philadelphia, PA: Saunders Elsevier; 2012.
2. Plum F, Posner JB. *The Diagnosis of Stupor and Coma*, 4th ed. Philadelphia, PA: FA Davis; 1995.
3. Hasbun R, Abrahams J, Jekel J, et al. Computed tomography of the head before lumbar puncture in adults with suspected meningitis. *N Engl J Med.* 2001;345:1727.

4

REYE SYNDROME (ACUTE TOXIC–METABOLIC ENCEPHALOPATHY)

❏ Definition
Reye syndrome is an acute toxic noninflammatory encephalopathy with fatty changes of the liver and kidney. Rarely, fatty changes are also seen in the heart and pancreas.

❏ Clinical Presentation
The syndrome occurs typically in children recovering from influenza, varicella, or nonspecific viral illness and is associated with the use of aspirin. Reye syndrome presents with nausea, vomiting, headache, and delirium with frequent progression to coma. Since aspirin was identified as a major precipitating factor for the development of Reye syndrome, this complication has virtually disappeared.[1] The differential diagnosis includes sepsis, meningitis, brain tumor, and intracranial hemorrhage and in small children shaken baby syndrome. Imaging studies should be undertaken to rule out intracranial hemorrhage or mass and sinus thrombosis.

❏ Laboratory Findings
- The diagnostic criteria for Reye syndrome include a markedly increased CSF pressure with no other abnormalities.
- Screening tests to eliminate other etiologies include CBC, glucose, electrolytes, BUN, creatinine, calcium, magnesium, and phosphate.
- Serum AST, ALT, or ammonia may be three times greater than the upper limit of normal.
- On biopsy of the liver, noninflammatory, panlobular fatty changes are seen.

Reference
1. Belay ED, Bresee JS, Holman RC, et al. Reye's syndrome in the United States from 1981 through 1997. *N Engl J Med.* 1999;340:1377.

SEIZURES

❏ Definition
Seizures represent a sudden change in behavior as a result of brain dysfunction.

❑ Clinical Presentation

Patients present in one of three major groups: *epileptic* (resulting from electrical hypersynchronization of neuronal networks in the cerebral cortex), *provoked* (resulting from metabolic abnormality, drug or alcohol withdrawal, and acute illness or neurologic disorders such as stroke), and *nonepileptic* events (imitators of epilepsy such as syncope, psychological disorders, migraine, and transient ischemic attack).

Conditions associated with seizure activity include the following:

- Brain tumors, abscess, and space-occupying lesions
- Circulatory disorders such as thrombosis, hemorrhage, embolism, hypertensive encephalopathy, vascular malformations, and angiitis
- Hematologic disorders such as sickle cell anemia, leukemia, and TTP
- Metabolic abnormalities such as DM, hyperthyroidism
- Porphyria, eclampsia, and renal failure
- Drugs that may induce seizures such as crack cocaine, amphetamines, ephedrine, and other sympathomimetics
- Allergic disorders including drug reactions and postvaccinal reactions
- Disorders in amino acid metabolism such as phenylketonuria and maple syrup urine disease
- Disorders in lipid metabolism such as the leukodystrophies and lipidoses
- Glycogen storage diseases
- Infections, meningitis, encephalitis, and postinfectious encephalitis (measles, mumps)
- In the fetus–maternal infection with rubella, measles, and mumps
- Degenerative brain diseases

The diagnosis of seizure requires an excellent history and evaluation of the events leading up to the seizure and the behavior during the seizure and after the seizure. The primary goal is to determine whether the event was a seizure and if so whether it was epileptic or due to a treatable or preventable cause. Electroencephalography (EEG) may be diagnostic in epileptic seizures. It may also determine whether a patient has generalized or partial seizures. Neuroimaging (MRI) should be performed to rule out structural abnormalities in the brain.[1]

❑ Laboratory Findings

Laboratory diagnosis is directed at determining an underlying cause of a provoked or nonepileptic seizure. Most important are blood tests for electrolytes, glucose, calcium, magnesium, hematology studies, renal function tests, liver function tests, and toxicology screens. Testing for underlying conditions should be performed as indicated by the history and physical examination. A lumbar puncture is helpful if there is an acute infectious process involving the CNS or the patient has a history of cancer. In other circumstances, the test may be misleading, since a prolonged seizure can cause CSF pleocytosis.[2]

Carbohydrate metabolism abnormalities may result in seizures with hypoglycemia (glucose <40 mg/dL) or hyperglycemia (glucose >400 mg/dL). Electrolyte imbalance results in neurologic change when sodium is <120 or >145 mEq/L, calcium is <7 mg/dL, or magnesium is low. Hyperosmolality (serum osmolality >300 mOsm/L) may also result in seizure activity.

Laboratory tests that may help to differentiate between seizures and syncope or psychogenic abnormalities include creatinine phosphokinase (CPK), cortisol, white blood cell count, LDH, CO_2, and ammonia. CPK may be elevated following generalized seizures but not usually after a partial seizure.[2]

References

1. Krumholz A, Wiebe S, Gronseth, G, et al. Practice Parameter: evaluating an apparent unprovoked first seizure in adults (an evidence-based review): report of the Quality Standards Subcommittee of the American Academy of Neurology and the American Epilepsy Society. *Neurology.* 2007; 69:1996.
2. Petramfar P, Yaghoobi E, Nemati R, et al. Serum creatine phosphokinase is helpful in distinguishing generalized tonic-clonic seizures from psychogenic nonepileptic seizures and vasovagal syncope. *Epilepsy Behav.* 2009;15:330.

4

DELIRIUM

❏ Definition

According to the DSM-IV, delirium is defined as having four key features: disturbance of consciousness, change in cognition, development over a short period of time, and an etiology due to medical illness, substance abuse, or intoxication or medication effect. Additional features that may accompany delirium include psychomotor disturbances and emotional disturbances.[1]

❏ Clinical Presentation

In elderly patients and in patients with medical illness, delirium and confusional states are not uncommon. The diagnosis of delirium requires that the practitioner recognize that delirium is present, a thorough history and physical examination, neurologic examination, and testing to determine the underlying etiology. The differential diagnosis includes sun downing, nonconvulsive status epilepticus, dementia, primary psychiatric illness, and focal syndromes such as Wernicke aphasia, Anton syndrome, and brain tumor particularly in the frontal lobe.

❏ Laboratory Findings

Targeted testing is recommended based on the history and physical. General screening tests should include electrolytes, creatinine, glucose, calcium, CBC, and urinalysis. Appropriate drug levels should be ordered. Delirium may occur even with therapeutic drug levels of digoxin, lithium, or quinidine. Blood and urine toxicology screens should be considered. Blood gas analysis to rule out hypoxia, respiratory alkalosis (which may be seen in sepsis, hepatic failure, or cardiopulmonary disease), and metabolic acidosis is helpful. Liver function tests may be contributory in patients with a history of alcoholism or liver disease. Thyroid function and vitamin B_{12} may be helpful in patients with a history of cognitive decline over several months.[2]

Suggested Readings

1. American Psychiatric Association. *Diagnostic and Statistical Manual,* 4th ed. Washington, DC: APA Press; 1994.
2. Plaschke K, von Haken R, Scholz M, et al. Comparison of the confusion assessment method for the intensive care unit (CAM-ICU) with the Intensive Care Delirium Screening Checklist (ICDSC) for delirium in critical care patients gives high agreement rate(s). *Intensive Care Med.* 2008;34:431.

DISORDERS WITH FOCAL NEUROLOGIC DEFICITS (NEUROPATHIES)

Disorders of the peripheral nerve system include polyneuropathies, mononeuropathies, and mononeuropathy multiplex (multiple mononeuropathies). The etiology of each of these is varied and includes systemic illnesses, toxins, or genetic abnormalities. The distinction between central nervous system disorders and peripheral nerve or muscle diseases can be made on clinical assessment with help from various diagnostic modalities including EEG, EMG, blood tests, genetic testing, and muscle or nerve biopsy. The involvement of a single limb, especially if with pain, suggests a peripheral neuropathy. This section reviews the major categories and several of the more common individual disorders.

POLYNEUROPATHY (NEURITIS/NEUROPATHY, MULTIPLE)

❏ Definition
Polyneuropathy is a generalized, homogeneous process affecting multiple peripheral nerves. Polyneuropathy must be distinguished from mononeuropathy, mononeuropathy multiplex (multifocal neuropathy), and disorders of the CNS.

❏ Clinical Presentation
Patients may present with symmetric distal sensory loss, burning, or weakness. Etiologies vary and include medication side effects or manifestations of systemic disease (DM, alcoholism, and HIV). The rate of progression of the polyneuropathy and type (axonal or demyelinating) can help identify its etiology. Polyneuropathy may also be difficult to distinguish from central nervous system disorders such as brain tumor, stroke, or spinal cord lesion.

The etiology of polyneuropathy varies and includes infections, metabolic and immune disorders, neoplasms, postvaccinal effect, and rare genetic disorders such as Charcot-Marie-Tooth.

❏ Laboratory Findings
Initial diagnosis includes obtaining a history of the disease and its progression, physical examination with neurologic testing, and electromyography and nerve conduction studies. Based on EMG studies, a decision can be made as to whether the disorder is axonal or demyelinating. Laboratory tests are recommended by the American Academy of Neurology for each of these categories.[1]

Screening for predominantly axonal disorders:

- Serum glucose
- Serum protein electrophoresis and immunofixation
- B_{12} level
- ANA
- ESR
- RPR
- Glycohemoglobin
- Urine/blood for heavy metals
- Urine/blood for porphyrins
- RF

- Sjögren syndrome testing (anti-Ro, anti-La antibodies)
- Lyme testing
- HIV
- Methylmalonic acid and homocysteine levels (in patients with borderline low serum B_{12} levels)
- Hepatitis screen (for types B and C)

Screening for predominantly demyelinating disorders:

- Serum protein electrophoresis and IEP
- Urine protein electrophoresis
- Hepatitis screen (for types B and C)
- Anti–myelin-associated glycoprotein (MAG) testing (in patients with predominantly sensory symptoms)
- Anti-GM1 test (in patients with predominantly motor symptoms)
- HIV
- Genetic testing for Charcot-Marie-Tooth disease
- Lumbar puncture

Findings of the CSF:

- The CSF is usually normal; however, in approximately 70% of patients with diabetic neuropathy, the CSF protein is increased to >200 mg/dL.
- In inflammatory demyelinating polyneuropathies, increase in CSF protein with minimal elevation in CSF white cells (albuminocytologic dissociation).
- In some cases of chronic uremia, the CSF protein is 50–200 mg/dL.
- In collagen vascular disease (polyarteritis nodosa has nerve involvement in 10% of patients), the CSF is usually normal.
- In neoplasms (leukemia, multiple myeloma, carcinoma), the CSF protein is often increased and may be associated with an occult primary neoplastic lesion outside the CNS.
- In alcoholism, the CSF is usually normal.

Additional laboratory tests to rule out infectious disorders:

- Leprosy
- Diphtheria: CSF protein is 50–200 mg/dL
- EBV (mononucleosis associated: CSF shows increased protein and up to several hundred mononuclear cells)
- Lyme disease

Additional laboratory information that may be contributive:

- Serum and urine for toxicity to drugs and chemicals (lead, arsenic, etc.)
- Blood tests for vitamin deficiencies, pregnancy, and porphyria

Biopsy:

Nerve biopsy may be useful in diagnosing the underlying cause of the neuropathy especially in cases that are difficult to differentiate between axonal and demyelinating etiologies. Nerve biopsy may also help to diagnose amyloidosis, leprosy, vasculitis, and sarcoidosis.[2] Skin biopsy may be helpful in disorders that affect small unmyelinated nerve fibers, such as in pain, numbness, and paresthesias.[3]

References

1. England JD, Gronseth GS, Franklin G, et al. Practice Parameter: evaluation of distal symmetric polyneuropathy: role of laboratory and genetic testing (an evidence-based review).

Report of the American Academy of Neurology, American Association of Neuromuscular and Electrodiagnostic Medicine, and American Academy of Physical Medicine and Rehabilitation. *Neurology.* 2009;72:185.
2. England JD, Asbury AK. Peripheral neuropathy. *Lancet.* 2004;363:2151.
3. McCarthy BG, Hsieh ST, Stocks A, et al. Cutaneous innervation in sensory neuropathies: evaluation by skin biopsy. *Neurology.* 1995;45:1848.

DIABETIC POLYNEUROPATHY

❏ Definition
Diabetic polyneuropathy is primarily a symmetrical neuropathy affecting the distal lower extremities. There is loss of vibratory sensation and impairment of pain, light touch, and temperature sensation.[1]

❏ Clinical Presentation
Patients with diabetes may present with a number of different neuropathies including symmetric polyneuropathy, autonomic neuropathy, radiculopathies, mononeuropathies, and mononeuropathy multiplex.

❏ Laboratory Findings
The differential diagnosis includes metabolic disorders such as uremia, folic acid deficiency, hypothyroidism, and acute intermittent porphyria. Other entities in the differential should include alcohol, heavy metal toxicity, and exposure to hydrocarbons. Collagen vascular diseases such as periarteritis nodosa and lupus may also cause symmetric polyneuropathy. Also in the differential is infection with leprosy or inflammatory disorders such as sarcoidosis. Rare disorders including paraneoplastic syndromes, hematologic malignancy, amyloidosis, and hereditary neuropathies may also be considered.

In a patient with known diabetes, the diagnosis is based on clinical findings and physical examination using one of a number of testing tools.[2,3] When the presentation is atypical electrodiagnostic, testing may be helpful. Laboratory testing should include screening to rule out vitamin B_{12} deficiency, hypothyroidism, and uremia.

References
1. Partanen J, Niskanen L, Lehtinen J, et al. Natural history of peripheral neuropathy in patients with non-insulin-dependent diabetes mellitus. *N Engl J Med.* 1995;333:89.
2. Dyck PJ, Kratz KM, Lehman KA, et al. The Rochester Diabetic Neuropathy Study: design, criteria for types of neuropathy, selection bias, and reproducibility of neuropathic tests. *Neurology.* 1991;41:799.
3. Dyck PJ, Albers JW, Andersen H, et al. Diabetic polyneuropathies: update on research definition, diagnostic criteria and estimation of severity. *Diabetes Metab Res Rev.* 2011, Jun 21. doi: 10.1002/dmrr.1226. [Epub ahead of print]

CRANIAL NERVE NEUROPATHY, MULTIPLE

❏ Definition
Neuropathies of the cranial nerves are most commonly due to local compression of the nerve by trauma, infection, or tumor; vascular and collagen vascular disorders; and some metabolic diseases.

❏ Laboratory Findings

Laboratory findings may be helpful to determine the underlying etiology:

- Peripheral blood for glucose, HgbA1c, BUN, creatinine, AST, and ALT may reveal a metabolic disorder (DM, renal failure, chronic liver disease, myxedema, and porphyria).
- Serology and/or culture may be helpful in identification of infection (herpes zoster, benign polyneuritis associated with cervical lymph node TB, or Lyme disease).
- Tissue biopsy of the nerve or adjacent soft tissues may diagnose sarcoidosis and tumors (meningioma, neurofibroma, carcinoma, cholesteatoma, chordoma).
- Imaging studies are most useful for the detection of trauma and aneurysms.

4

MONONEUROPATHY

❏ Definition

Mononeuropathy is defined as the focal dysfunction of a single nerve and may be due to trauma or compression such as carpal tunnel syndrome. Mononeuropathy multiplex is the involvement of several noncontiguous nerves.

❏ Clinical Presentation

Patients present with various symptoms such as pain, paresthesias, or weakness relating to the nerve that is involved. Mononeuropathy may be due to a systemic vasculitic process that affects the vasa vasorum resulting in multiple infarcts. Other causes of mononeuropathy include

- DM
- Infections (e.g., HIV, diphtheria, herpes zoster, leprosy)
- Sarcoidosis
- Polyarteritis nodosa
- Tumor (leukemia, lymphoma, carcinomas)
- Trauma
- Serum sickness
- Bell palsy
- Idiopathic
- Drugs, toxic substances
- Chronic renal failure
- Thyroid disorders

The diagnosis of a mononeuropathy is based on history, neurologic examinations over time evaluation of progression, electrodiagnostic studies, somatosensory potentials, and neuroimaging (MRI).

❏ Laboratory Findings

Blood tests:

- Fasting glucose and glycohemoglobin in patients with possible diabetic amyotrophy, idiopathic radiculopathy, or polyneuropathy
- Lyme titers in patients with polyradiculopathy, especially in endemic areas
- Genetic tests for hereditary neuropathy with predisposition to pressure palsy for patients with multiple mononeuropathies (usually affecting at least two to three extremities) and Chédiak-Higashi syndrome

Lumbar puncture: Evaluation of CSF is warranted in patients with unusual presentations. CSF should be examined for evidence of inflammation, elevated CSF protein, and serologic testing for Lyme disease, syphilis, and CMV. Cytologic evaluation for tumor cells may be warranted.

FACIAL PALSY (BELL PALSY)

❑ Definition
Bell palsy is the loss of function of cranial nerve VII resulting in facial paralysis.

❑ Clinical Presentation
Patients with Bell palsy typically present with the sudden onset (usually over hours) of unilateral facial paralysis and comprise approximately 50% of patients with facial nerve palsy.[1] Current research suggests that herpes simplex virus is the etiologic agent causing neural inflammation, demyelination, and palsy.[2] Other infectious agents associated with facial palsy include herpes zoster, CMV, Epstein-Barr virus, adenovirus, rubella virus, mumps, influenza B, HIV, and coxsackie virus.[3]

Lyme disease may produce bilateral palsy. Early negative blood serology does not exclude the diagnosis. A lymphocyte pleocytosis in the CSF is suggestive, and the finding of specific oligoclonal IgG in the CSF is a sensitive indicator.[4] Rickettsial and Ehrlichia infection have also been found in patients with facial palsy.[5,6]

Bacterial infections such syphilis, leprosy, diphtheria, catscratch disease, *M. pneumoniae,* and nonspecific local inflammation including otitis media have also been known to cause facial palsy as have some parasitic infections such as malaria. Granulomatous disease such as sarcoidosis should be considered, especially in patients with bilateral facial palsy.

Trauma, tumor (acoustic neuromas [see eBook Figure 4-11], tumors invading the temporal bone), cholesteatoma, and Paget disease of bone should be suspected if the onset of facial palsy is gradual. These can be diagnosed on imaging.

Drug reaction, particularly to dental injections, may cause local facial neuropathy, diagnosed on history. Postvaccinal effect and Guillain-Barré syndrome may cause bilateral facial palsy.

Melkersson-Rosenthal syndrome, a granulomatous disorder of unknown etiology, may display recurrent facial palsy.[7]

❑ Laboratory Findings
Testing should be designed to rule out causes of underlying diseases, serology for herpes simplex, HIV, and other viruses; Borrelia; Ehrlichia; and other agents as appropriate by history. If collagen vascular disease is suspected, an ANA test may be of help. Bell palsy may occasionally present with a slight increase in cells in the CSF.

References
1. Peitersen E. The natural history of Bell's palsy. *Am J Otol.* 1982;4:107.
2. Peitersen E. Bell's palsy: the spontaneous course of 2,500 peripheral facial nerve palsies of different etiologies. *Acta Otolaryngol Suppl.* 2002;(549):4–30.
3. Morgan M, Nathwani D. Facial palsy and infection: the unfolding story. *Clin Infect Dis.* 1992;14:263.
4. Markby DP. Lyme disease facial palsy: differentiation from Bell's palsy. *BMJ.* 1989;299:605.

5. Bitsori M, Galanakis E, Papadakis CE, et al. Facial nerve palsy associated with Rickettsia conorii infection. *Arch Dis Child*. 2001;85:54.
6. Lee FS, Chu FK, Tackley M, et al. Human granulocytic ehrlichiosis presenting as facial diplegia in a 42-year-old woman. *Clin Infect Dis*. 2000;31:1288.
7. Levenson MJ, Ingerman M, Grimes C, et al. Melkersson-Rosenthal syndrome. *Arch Otolaryngol*. 1984;110:540.

HEMIANOPSIA, BITEMPORAL

4

❑ Definition
Bitemporal hemianopsia is the loss of vision in the temporal fields due to a mass lesion causing compression of the optic chiasm.

❑ Clinical Presentation
Patients present with decreased vision in the temporal fields. The most common cause is pituitary adenoma (see eBook Figure 4-12), but any mass lesion may be causative, including metastatic tumor, sarcoidosis, Hand-Schüller-Christian disease, meningioma of sella (see eBook Figure 4-13), craniopharyngioma (see eBook Figure 4-14), and aneurysm of the circle of Willis.

Diagnosis is predominantly made by neuroimaging. Biopsy may help identify tumor type.

OPHTHALMOPLEGIA

❑ Definition
Internuclear ophthalmoplegia is an impairment of horizontal eye movement. There is weak adduction of the affected eye and abduction nystagmus of the contralateral eye. It is the result of a lesion in the medial longitudinal fasciculus.

❑ Clinical Presentation
Patients may present with a number of causative disorders including MS (approximately 30% of cases and most common in younger patients, also tends to be bilateral),[1,2] cerebrovascular disorders (infarction is most common in older patients), infection, trauma, and tumor.

Diagnosis is based on physical findings and neuroimaging with MRI and specialized neural ophthalmologic techniques such as oculographic recording.[2] The differential diagnosis includes oculomotor nerve palsy.

❑ Laboratory Findings
Testing is directed at identifying the causative disease. Tests to rule out DM, vasculopathies, multiple sclerosis, myasthenia gravis, hyperthyroidism, infection, and drug toxicities will be of help.[3]

References
1. Frohman EM, Zhang H, Kramer PD, et al. MRI characteristics of the MLF in MS patients with chronic internuclear ophthalmoparesis. *Neurology*. 2001;57:762.
2. Frohman EM, Frohman TC, O'Suilleabhain P, et al. Quantitative oculographic characterisation of internuclear ophthalmoparesis in multiple sclerosis: the versional dysconjugacy index Z score. *J Neurol Neurosurg Psychiatry*. 2002;73:51.
3. Keane JR. Internuclear ophthalmoplegia: unusual causes in 114 of 410 patients. *Arch Neurol*. 2005;62:714.

OCULOMOTOR NERVE PALSY

❑ **Definition**

Oculomotor nerve palsy may result from lesions of the third cranial nerve (oculomotor nerve) anywhere along its path.

❑ **Clinical Presentation**

The diagnosis varies by patient age, type of diplopia, and lid involvement. The most common causes include intracranial aneurysm, ischemia, trauma, and migraine. Ischemic diabetic third nerve palsies are the most common etiology in adults. Traumatic third nerve palsy arises only from severe blows to the head. Ophthalmoplegic "migraine" has been reclassified as a cranial neuralgia by the International Headache Society in 2004.[1]

The differential diagnosis includes MS (may mimic pupil-sparing ophthalmoplegia) and orbital inflammation or fracture. The diagnosis rests on complete history, and neurologic exam and neuroimaging with MRI, MRA, or CTA to rule out aneurysm.[2]

❑ **Laboratory Findings**

Laboratory testing can help in the diagnosis of diabetes and vasculopathies (glucose, hemoglobin A1c, sedimentation rate). Testing to exclude myasthenia gravis should be performed in younger patients.

References

1. Headache Classification Committee of the International Headache Society. The International Classification of Headache Disorders. *Cephalalgia*. 2004;24:1.
2. Jacobson DM, Trobe JD. The emerging role of magnetic resonance angiography in the management of patients with third cranial nerve palsy. *Am J Ophthalmol*. 1999;128:94.

TRIGEMINAL NEURALGIA (TIC DOULOUREUX)

❑ **Definition**

Trigeminal neuralgia is a sudden, usually unilateral, severe, brief, stabbing, recurrent pain in the distribution of one or more branches of the fifth cranial (trigeminal) nerve.

❑ **Clinical Presentation**

Eighty to ninety percent of cases are caused by compression of the trigeminal nerve root, by an artery or vein, leading to demyelination.[1] Compression may also be caused by vestibular schwannoma (acoustic neuroma), meningioma, epidermoid, or other cyst. Saccular aneurysm or arteriovenous malformations are rare causes of compression. MS may cause demyelination of one or more of the trigeminal nerve nuclei resulting in pain.

❑ **Laboratory Findings**

Diagnosis is performed predominantly by neuroimaging (CT or MRI) and electrophysiologic testing. Laboratory findings may assist in identifying MS or herpes zoster. Tissue biopsy may be needed in the diagnosis of schwannoma (see eBook Figure 4-11), meningioma (see eBook Figures 4-13 and 4-15), and cysts.

Reference

1. Love S, Coakham HB. Trigeminal neuralgia: pathology and pathogenesis. *Brain*. 2001;124:2347.

RETROBULBAR NEUROPATHY (OPTIC NEURITIS)

❑ Definition
Retrobulbar neuropathy is a disorder of the optic nerve resulting in pain behind the affected eye, impaired vision, and rarely blindness.

❑ Clinical Presentation
Patients with retrobulbar neuropathy may present with a number of causative disorders including MS (demyelinating optic neuritis), ischemia (arteritic or nonarteritic ischemic optic neuropathy), infectious (West Nile virus, catscratch disease, toxoplasma, *Tuberculosis*, and *Cryptococcus*), tumors, and medications (chloramphenicol, ethambutol, isoniazid, penicillamine, phenothiazines, phenylbutazone, quinine, and streptomycin).[1,2] Postviral infectious optic neuritis may also occur. Less common causes include sarcoidosis and autoimmune diseases such as lupus, Sjögren syndrome, and Wegener granulomatosis.[3] Retrobulbar neuropathy is associated with MS, which ultimately develops in 30–50% of patients with optic neuritis. Ischemic optic neuropathy is the most common etiology in older patients.[4] There are two hereditary forms of optic neuropathy: Leber hereditary optic neuropathy and Kjer disease.[5,6]

The diagnosis is based on the elimination of underlying disorders by history and examination including funduscopic evaluation. Neuroimaging (MRI) may help confirm the presence of acute demyelinating disease and MS. Visual-evoked responses may be helpful in determining demyelination.

❑ Laboratory Findings
Laboratory testing including sedimentation rate, ANA, angiotensin-converting enzyme levels, and serologic test for Lyme disease should be obtained. Lumbar puncture is helpful to rule out multiple sclerosis. CSF may be normal or reveal increased protein and $\leq 200/\mu L$ lymphocytes. Oligoclonal bands may be present. Other testing should be performed to rule out possible infectious agents, toxins, and genetic disorders based on the history of the individual patient.

References
1. Balcer LJ. Clinical practice. Optic neuritis. *N Engl J Med.* 2006;354:1273.
2. Lee AG, Brazis PW. Systemic infections of neuro-ophthalmic significance. *Ophthalmol Clin North Am.* 2004;17:397.
3. Rabadi MH, Kundi S, Brett D, et al. Neurological pictures. Primary Sjögren syndrome presenting as neuromyelitis optica. *J Neurol Neurosurg Psychiatry.* 2010;81:213.
4. Hayreh SS. Posterior ischaemic optic neuropathy: clinical features, pathogenesis, and management. *Eye (Lond).* 2004;18:1188.
5. Lamirel C, Cassereau J, Cochereau I, et al. Papilloedema and MRI enhancement of the prechiasmal optic nerve at the acute stage of Leber hereditary optic neuropathy. *J Neurol Neurosurg Psychiatry.* 2010;81:578.
6. Alexander C, Votruba M, Pesch UE, et al. OPA1, encoding a dynamin-related GTPase, is mutated in autosomal dominant optic atrophy linked to chromosome 3q28. *Nat Genet.* 2000;26:211.

AUTONOMIC NEUROPATHY

❑ Definition
Autonomic neuropathy is a group of diseases or syndromes affecting the parasympathetic and/or the sympathetic nerves. It can be hereditary or acquired.

❏ Clinical Presentation

A wide range of symptoms affecting many different organ systems can occur, including the cardiovascular, GI, GU, pulmonary, and neuroendocrine systems. The most common cause of autonomic neuropathy is DM[1] (see also Polyneuropathy and the section on Autoimmune Disorders of the CNS).

Disorders that may cause autonomic dysfunction include amyloidosis, Guillain-Barré syndrome, hereditary neuropathies, infections (e.g., Chagas disease, HIV, botulism, diphtheria, and leprosy), toxicities including drugs (vincristine, cis-platinum, Taxol, thallium, and heavy metals), collagen vascular disease (e.g., Sjögren disease, systemic lupus, RA), porphyria, uremia, alcoholic neuropathy, hepatic disease, paraneoplastic syndromes, Lambert-Eaton syndrome, and medications (antihypertensives, tricyclics, MAO inhibitors, and dopamine agonists).[2]

❏ Laboratory Findings

Laboratory testing to determine the causative disease or toxin should be based on the presenting symptoms and history of the patient to rule out the preceding disorders. All patients with diabetes should be screened for autonomic neuropathy with a complete history and physical examination, including evaluation of heart rate, respiratory rate, response to the Valsalva maneuver, and evaluation for orthostatic hypertension.

References

1. Boulton AJ, Vinik AI, Arezzo JC, et al. Diabetic neuropathies: a statement by the American Diabetes Association. *Diabetes Care*. 2005;28:956.
2. Freeman R. Autonomic dysfunction. In: Samuels M, Fesky S, eds. *The Office Practice of Neurology*, 2nd ed. Philadelphia, PA: Churchill Livingstone; 2003;14:141–145.

PSEUDOTUMOR CEREBRI

❏ Definition

Pseudotumor cerebri is idiopathic intracranial hypertension.

❏ Clinical Presentation

Patients present with headache and papilledema. The CSF is normal except for increased opening pressure. The primary means of diagnosis is one of exclusion and consists of neuroimaging to rule out a mass lesion or ventricular obstruction, funduscopic exam to rule out papilledema, and visual field testing to determine the severity of optic nerve involvement.[1]

❏ Laboratory Findings

Laboratory findings may help in the diagnosis of "secondary pseudotumor cerebri," which is due to an underlying condition. Lumbar puncture should be performed only after neuroimaging to measure the opening pressure and to evaluate for cell count, differential, and glucose and protein levels. Culture and cytology may be indicated based on the clinical situation. Obesity has been associated with increased CSF opening pressures.[2]

Testing may be helpful to rule out Addison disease, infection, and metabolic disorders including acute hypocalcemia and other electrolyte disturbances, empty sella syndrome, and pregnancy. Testing for drugs that may be implicated in secondary pseudotumor cerebri includes psychotherapeutic drugs, sex hormones and oral contraceptives, and a reduction in dosage of corticosteroids. Immune diseases may be implicated, including SLE, polyarteritis nodosa, and serum sickness. Other conditions that may be tested for as the symptoms warrant include sarcoidosis, Guillain-Barré syndrome, head trauma, various anemias, and chronic renal failure.

References

1. Friedman DI, Jacobson DM. Diagnostic criteria for idiopathic intracranial hypertension. *Neurology.* 2002;59:1492.
2. Corbett JJ, Mehta MP. Cerebrospinal fluid pressure in normal obese subjects and patients with pseudotumor cerebri. *Neurology.* 1983;33:1386.

DISORDERS OF MOVEMENT

PARKINSON DISEASE

❑ Definition

Parkinson disease (PD) is a progressive neurodegenerative disorder resulting from the loss of dopaminergic cells in the substantia nigra.

❑ Clinical Presentation

Patients present with rest tremor, rigidity, bradykinesia, and gait disturbance. In the late stages, PD may result in dementia (see Dementia). The differential diagnosis includes essential tremor, dementia with Lewy bodies, cortical basal degeneration, progressive supranuclear palsy, and multiple system atrophy. It must also be distinguished from secondary parkinsonism due to drugs, toxins, head trauma, infections, cerebrovascular disease, and metabolic disorders.[1]

The diagnosis is based on clinical evaluation, there are no specific physiologic or blood tests to confirm the diagnosis. Neuroimaging is usually not helpful in distinguishing PD from other syndromes with motor disorders. MRI may be performed to exclude structural abnormalities of the brain. Olfactory dysfunction is seen early in PD, and testing may help to establish the diagnosis.[2] At autopsy, gross sectioning of the brain stem through the substantia nigra reveals the loss of pigmentation. Microscopy demonstrates loss of neurons and Lewy Bodies (see eBook Figures 4-7 and 4-16).

References

1. Tolosa E, Wenning G, Poewe W. The diagnosis of Parkinson's disease. *Lancet Neurol.* 2006;5:75.
2. Katzenschlager R, Zijlmans J, Evans A, et al. Olfactory function distinguishes vascular parkinsonism from Parkinson's disease. *J Neurol Neurosurg Psychiatry.* 2004;75:1749.

PROGRESSIVE SUPRANUCLEAR PALSY

❑ Definition

Progressive supranuclear palsy (PSP) is a neurodegenerative disorder resulting in the loss of neurons and glia in the basal ganglia, brain stem, cerebral cortex, dentate nucleus, and upper spinal cord.

❑ Clinical Presentation

Patients present with symptoms similar to Parkinson disease. Symptoms more specific to PSP include vertical supranuclear gaze palsy and unexplained falls due to postural instability. A genetic susceptibility has been suggested, but no genetic abnormality has been found to be causative. The diagnosis of PSP is made on clinical examination.

❏ Laboratory Findings

As in PD, laboratory and imaging studies are not definitive and should be performed to rule out treatable forms of disease (encephalitis, dopaminergic drug use, tumors, and Whipple disease). Blood, urine, and CSF are normal in PSP. Recent studies suggest that there may be biomarkers for PSP including a low homovanillic acid level in the CSF and decreased levels of tau protein.[1,2] Pathologic evaluation of the brain at autopsy will identify globose neurofibrillary tangles within neurons and glia predominantly in the basal ganglia typical for PSP[3] and midbrain and cerebral cortical atrophy with hypopigmentation of the substantia nigra and locus ceruleus.[4] The abnormal filaments are composed of 4R tau.[5,6]

References

1. Mendell JR, Engel WK, Chase TN. Modification by L-dopa of a case of progressive supra-nuclear palsy. With evidence of defective cerebral dopamine metabolism. *Lancet.* 1970;1:593.
2. Urakami K, Wada K, Arai H, et al. Diagnostic significance of tau protein in cerebrospinal fluid from patients with corticobasal degeneration or progressive supranuclear palsy. *J Neurol Sci.* 2001;183:95.
3. Williams DR, Lees AJ. Progressive supranuclear palsy: clinicopathological concepts and diagnostic challenges. *Lancet Neurol.* 2009;8:270.
4. Hauw JJ, Daniel SE, Dickson D, et al. Preliminary NINDS neuropathologic criteria for Steele-Richardson-Olszewski syndrome (progressive supranuclear palsy). *Neurology.* 1994;44:2015.
5. Kumar V, Abbas AK, Fausto N, et al. *Robbins and Code Trend Pathologic Basis of Disease*, 8th ed. Philadelphia, PA: Saunders Elsevier; 2004:1318.
6. Takahashi M, Weidenheim KM, Dickson DW, et al. Morphological and biochemical correlations of abnormal tau filaments in progressive supranuclear palsy. *J Neuropathol Exp Neurol.* 2002;61:33.

HUNTINGTON DISEASE

❏ Definition

Huntington disease (HD) is a neurodegenerative disease inherited as autosomal dominant and is caused by a repeat expansion in the huntingtin gene on chromosome 4p. The disease exhibits variable penetration rates in affected families but is fully penetrant when the repeat size is >38.[1]

❏ Clinical Presentation

Patients present with choreiform movements, psychiatric disorder, and dementia. The differentiation from other neurodegenerative dementias is made based on the preexistence of choreiform movements and/or psychiatric illness and from other movement disorders by the manner of abnormal movements.

❏ Laboratory Findings

The diagnosis of HD is based on a familial history, clinical assessment, and genetic testing. Genetic screening is also available for family members who wish to know their risk of disease. Testing for the CAG repeat length is now commercially available with good sensitivity and 100% specificity based on a cutoff of >38 repeats for HD.[2] Neuroimaging is no longer recommended.

References

1. Richards RI. Dynamic mutations: a decade of unstable expanded repeats in human genetic disease. *Hum Mol Genet.* 2001;10:2187.
2. Kremer B, Goldberg P, Andrew SE, et al. A worldwide study of the Huntington's disease mutation. The sensitivity and specificity of measuring CAG repeats. *N Engl J Med.* 1994; 330:1401.

DYSTONIA

4

❑ Definition

Dystonia is a movement disorder with sustained muscle contractions. It may be hereditary or acquired.

❑ Clinical Presentation

Patients present with twisting repetitive movements and abnormal posture. Classification is by age of onset, anatomic distribution, and etiology. In primary dystonia, there are no neurologic symptoms in addition to the dystonic findings while in secondary dystonia, additional findings such as spasticity, ataxia, muscle weakness, ocular or cognitive impairment, or seizures may be present.[1,2]

A genetic etiology has been determined for dystonia with the two most common mutations the TOR1A gene in DYT1 dystonia and the THAP1 gene in DYT6 dystonia representing early-onset and late-onset dystonia, respectively.[3,4] Dopa-responsive dystonia presents in early childhood with focal dystonia and is frequently due to an autosomal dominant DYT5 dystonia caused by mutation in the GTP cyclohydrolase-1 gene.[5] Segawa syndrome, an autosomal recessive form, is due to a mutation in the tyrosine hydroxylase gene.[6]

The diagnosis of dystonia is predominantly made on clinical examination with special attention to evaluation of the movement disorders.

❑ Laboratory Findings

Genetic testing for the DYT1 dystonia gene is available for early-onset dystonia, and in some areas, DYT5 dystonia genetic testing may be obtained. Other tests may help to exclude secondary dystonia these include neuroimaging with MRI or CT to evaluate the basal ganglia, CBC, electrolytes, renal and liver function tests, ANA, ceruloplasmin, serum copper and 24-hour urinary copper to rule out Wilson disease, and sedimentation rate.

References

1. Geyer HL, Bressman SB. The diagnosis of dystonia. *Lancet Neurol.* 2006;5:780.
2. Phukan J, Albanese A, Gasser T, et al. Primary dystonia and dystonia-plus syndromes: clinical characteristics, diagnosis, and pathogenesis. *Lancet Neurol.* 2011;10:1074.
3. Bressman SB, Sabatti C, Raymond D, et al. The DYT1 phenotype and guidelines for diagnostic testing. *Neurology.* 2000;54:1746.
4. Fuchs T, Gavarini S, Saunders-Pullman R, et al. Mutations in the THAP1 gene are responsible for DYT6 primary torsion dystonia. *Nat Genet.* 2009;41:286.
5. Trender-Gerhard I, Sweeney MG, Schwingenschuh P, et al. Autosomal-dominant GTPCH1-deficient DRD: clinical characteristics and long-term outcome of 34 patients. *J Neurol Neurosurg Psychiatry.* 2009;80:839.
6. Segawa M, Nomura Y, Nishiyama N. Autosomal dominant guanosine triphosphate cyclohydrolase I deficiency (Segawa disease). *Ann Neurol.* 2003;54 (Suppl 6):S32.

TOURETTE SYNDROME

❏ **Definition**
Tourette syndrome (TS) is an inherited neuropsychiatric disorder of unknown etiology resulting in motor and phonic tics with an onset in childhood.

❏ **Clinical Presentation**
Patients present with sudden, repetitive movements and sounds. The disorder may be chronic or transient. It has a genetic component that is complex and has been associated with a mutation in the gene SLITRK1 on chromosome 13.[1] This gene appears to be involved in dendritic growth. Patients with TS also frequently have comorbid conditions including attention deficit disorder, obsessive–compulsive disorder, obsessive–compulsive behavior, learning disorders, and oppositional defiant disorder.[2]

❏ **Laboratory Findings**
The diagnosis of TS is predominantly made on the clinical examination and history. Neuroimaging is not helpful. No laboratory tests are available for the positive diagnosis of TS; however, drug testing to rule out secondary tics should be performed especially for cocaine and dopamine receptor blocking agents. Review of a blood smear may rule out neuroacanthocytosis, which has been associated with tics.

References
1. Abelson JF, Kwan KY, O'Roak BJ, et al. Sequence variants in SLITRK1 are associated with Tourette's syndrome. *Science.* 2005;310:317.
2. Freeman RD, Fast DK, Burd L, et al. An international perspective on Tourette syndrome: selected findings from 3,500 individuals in 22 countries. *Dev Med Child Neurol.* 2000;42:436.

CEREBRAL PALSY

❏ **Definition**
Cerebral palsy is a nonprogressive dysfunction of the cerebral motor regions resulting from perinatal jaundice or asphyxia.[1]

❏ **Clinical Presentation**
Patients present in childhood with chorea and muscle tone abnormalities, abnormal reflexes, and coordination. The diagnosis is made primarily based on history and physical findings.

❏ **Laboratory Findings**
Testing that may help to rule out alternative causes such as abnormal development of the brain and infarcts includes MRI, cranial ultrasound, and CT scan. EEG may also be used to rule out seizure. Laboratory testing with PT, PTT, Protein C and S, and antithrombin may rule out coagulopathy as a basis for stroke that may mimic cerebral palsy.

Reference
1. Kuban KC, Leviton A. Cerebral palsy. *N Engl J Med.* 1994;330:188.

SYDENHAM CHOREA

❑ Definition
Sydenham chorea is a sequela of acute rheumatic fever.

❑ Clinical Presentation
Sydenham chorea is the most common acquired form of chorea in childhood. The onset is usually 1–8 months following the infection and may be insidious or abrupt.[1] The diagnosis is made by clinical evaluation. No specific laboratory testing currently exists although initial testing for streptococcal infection and ASO titers may be helpful.

Reference
1. Eshel G, Lahat E, Azizi E, et al. Chorea as a manifestation of rheumatic fever—a 30-year survey (1960–1990). *Eur J Pediatr.* 1993;152:645.

LESCH-NYHAN SYNDROME

❑ Definition
Lesch-Nyhan syndrome is an inherited X-linked recessive trait resulting in hyperuricemia.

❑ Clinical Presentation
Patients present early on with mental retardation, delayed development, extrapyramidal motor symptoms, and self-mutilating behavior and also severe gout and renal disorders. A genetic mutation is found in the hypoxanthine–guanine phosphoribosyltransferase enzyme gene and results in deficient enzymatic activity. A large number of mutations of this gene have been reported.[1]

❑ Laboratory Findings
Molecular genetic testing with sequence analysis of the entire coding region is available for Lesch-Nyhan syndrome as both a carrier test and prenatal test.

Reference
1. Mak BS, Chi CS, Tsai CR, et al. New mutations of the HPRT gene in Lesch-Nyhan syndrome. *Pediatr Neurol.* 2000;23:332.

ESSENTIAL TREMOR

❑ Definition
Essential tremor (ET) is defined as an isolated tremor with no other physiologic or psychological symptoms. It is common and may be seen in up to 5% of the population.[1]

❑ Clinical Presentation
Patients present with a tremor on exertion of the affected muscle group. Mental or physical stress may worsen the symptoms. Most common are tremors of the hands or arms, but the head, neck, jaw, and other body parts may be affected. There is a complex genetic inheritance of ET with a dominant form revealing linkage to genetic loci on chromosomes 2P, 3q13, and 6p23.[2] In one study, neuropathologic changes noted in the brains of patients with ET at autopsy have revealed brain

stem Lewy bodies and degenerative changes in the cerebellum.[3] A separate study revealed loss of pigmented neurons in the locus ceruleus.[4]

❑ Laboratory Findings

Commercial genetic testing is not currently available for ET although this is a common form of motor disorder that should be distinguished from other progressive and treatable disorders such as Parkinson disease and metabolic disorders. Screening laboratory tests for thyroid disease (TSH and free T4), diabetes, and drug levels (sympathomimetic drugs and stimulants), caffeine, and alcohol may rule out causes for nonessential tremor.

References

1. Louis ED, Ottman R, Hauser WA. How common is the most common adult movement disorder? Estimates of the prevalence of essential tremor throughout the world. *Mov Disord.* 1998;13:5.
2. Shatunov A, Sambuughin N, Jankovic J, et al. Genomewide scans in North American families reveal genetic linkage of essential tremor to a region on chromosome 6p23. *Brain.* 2006;129:2318.
3. Louis ED, Faust PL, Vonsattel JP, et al. Neuropathological changes in essential tremor: 33 cases compared with 21 controls. *Brain.* 2007;130:3297.
4. Shill HA, Adler CH, Sabbagh MN, et al. Pathologic findings in prospectively ascertained essential tremor subjects. *Neurology.* 2008;70:1452.

RESTLESS LEG SYNDROME

❑ Definition

Restless leg syndrome (RLS) is a motor disorder in which patients feel the need to move their legs to alleviate discomfort. It may be primary or secondary. The primary, idiopathic form of this disorder is associated with a familial component in patients with onset before age 40. RLS has been shown to be associated with genetic variants of BTBD9 and MEIS1, both of which influence expression of the disorder and are involved in iron homeostasis.[1,2] RLS may also be associated with a number of medical disorders including iron deficiency, renal disease, diabetes, multiple sclerosis, Parkinson disease, pregnancy, rheumatic disease, and venous insufficiency.

❑ Clinical Presentation

Patients present with an irresistible urge to move, most commonly when at rest or trying to sleep, because of unpleasant sensations in the legs of other body parts. The diagnosis of RLS is primarily made on clinical evaluation and history. Genetic testing is currently not commercially available. Underlying medical disorders that may be causative should be ruled out with appropriate testing.

References

1. Winkelmann J, Schormair B, Lichtner P, et al. Genome-wide association study of restless legs syndrome identifies common variants in three genomic regions. *Nat Genet.* 2007;39:1000.
2. O'Keeffe ST, Gavin K, Lavan JN. Iron status and restless legs syndrome in the elderly. *Age Ageing.* 1994;23:200.

AMYOTROPHIC LATERAL SCLEROSIS (ALS)

❑ Definition

Amyotrophic lateral sclerosis (ALS) is a progressive neurodegenerative disorder that may be familial resulting in muscle weakness and death.

❑ Clinical Presentation

Patients with ALS present with upper and lower motor neuron dysfunction beginning in the cranial/bulbar, cervical, thoracic, or lumbosacral regions. There is steady progression of the disease over years, spreading to the other regions, resulting in weight loss and muscle wasting. Familial ALS accounts for 5–10% of all ALS cases (see eBook Figure 4-17).

Diagnosis is made on clinical history and examination. Sensory and motor nerve conduction studies and electromyography may help support the diagnosis when features of acute and chronic denervation and reinnervation are present. Neuroimaging may exclude other possible diagnoses.

❑ Laboratory Findings

Creatine kinase may be elevated up to 1,000 U/L due to denervation.

Evaluation of the CSF may rule out Lyme disease, HIV infection, chronic inflammatory demyelinating polyneuropathy, malignancy, and paraneoplastic syndromes secondary to lymphoma or breast cancer.

Familial ALS genetic testing is commercially available. Mutations occur in the SOD1, TARDBP, FUS, FIG4, ANG, Alsin (ALS2), VAPB, OPTN, and SETX genes (see Chapter 10 Hereditary and Genetic Diseases).

Muscle biopsy may rule out myopathy. In ALS, there is chronic denervation and reinnervation.

AUTOIMMUNE DISORDERS OF THE CNS

PRIMARY AUTOIMMUNE AUTONOMIC FAILURE

❑ Definition

Primary autoimmune autonomic failure (also known as autoimmune autonomic ganglionopathy, acute panautonomic neuropathy, or acute pandysautonomia) is an autoimmune disorder possibly due to anti-ganglionic acetylcholine receptor antibodies (AChRs) causing dysfunction of efferent sympathetic and parasympathetic pathways.

❑ Clinical Presentation

Patients present with orthostatic hypotension, anhidrosis, decreased production of saliva and tears, erectile dysfunction, and impaired bladder emptying. This disorder is responsive to plasma exchange. Antibodies to ganglionic AChR are present in about two thirds of all subacute cases and in one third of chronic cases.[1–3]

The differential diagnosis should include secondary causes of autoimmune autonomic failure. These are DM, amyloidosis, paraneoplastic syndromes, Lambert-Eaton syndrome, botulism, syphilis, HIV infection, collagen vascular disease, and porphyria.[4]

❑ Laboratory Findings

Testing varies according to the presentation and history of autonomic symptoms. Testing should be directed to differentiate between acute inflammatory demyelinating polyneuropathies (Parkinson disease, drug or toxin exposure, and hereditary etiologies) from primary autoimmune autonomic failure. Detection of antibodies binding to ganglionic nicotinic AChRs is performed by radioimmunoprecipitation and is diagnostic.[1] There may also be decreased plasma norepinephrine levels.

Tests that rule out disorders that may cause autonomic symptoms include

- Glycosylated hemoglobin to test for diabetes
- Anti-Hu antibody titers, which may be used to test for paraneoplastic syndromes
- Anti-calcium channel antibody titers for Lambert-Eaton myasthenic syndrome
- Stool for botulinum by culture and detection of toxin for botulism
  - ▼ Serum and urine protein electrophoresis to evaluate myeloma due to amyloidosis, or genetic testing to evaluate for familial amyloidosis
- Rapid plasma reagin (RPR) or syphilis antibody screen
- HIV serology
  - ▼ ANA levels, ESR, and other autoimmune tests (e.g., rheumatoid factor [RF] and Sjögren syndrome, SS-A and SS-B antibodies) to evaluate for collagen vascular disease
- Urinary porphyrins and erythrocyte porphobilinogen deaminase levels for porphyria

References

1. Klein CM, Vernino S, Lennon VA, et al. The spectrum of autoimmune autonomic neuropathies. *Ann Neurol.* 2003;53:752.
2. Sandroni P, Vernino S, Klein CM, et al. Idiopathic autonomic neuropathy: comparison of cases seropositive and seronegative for ganglionic acetylcholine receptor antibody. *Arch Neurol.* 2004;61(1):44–48.
3. Schroeder C, Vernio S, Birkenfeld AL, et al. Plasma exchange for primary autoimmune autonomic failure. *N Engl J Med.* 2005;353:1585.
4. Vernino S, Freeman R. Peripheral autonomic neuropathies. *Continuum Lifelong Learning Neurol.* 2007;13(6):89–110.

GUILLAIN-BARRÉ SYNDROME

❑ Definition
Guillain-Barré syndrome (GBS) is the name given to a group of heterogeneous disorders comprising the acute immune-mediated polyneuropathies. There are several variant forms including the acute inflammatory demyelinating polyradiculoneuropathy (AIDP), seen in the United States and Europe, and the acute motor axonal neuropathy (AMAN) and acute sensory motor axonal neuropathy (AMSAN), which are usually seen in China, Japan, and Mexico[1]

❑ Clinical Presentation
The usual presentation is that of an acute monophasic paralyzing illness following an infection.[2] In 70% of cases, it is reversible, but 10% of patients die and 20% have residual defects. Dysautonomia occurs in 70% of patients, and severe autonomic dysfunction is occasionally associated with sudden death.[3,4]

A number of glycolipid antibodies have been found to be the underlying cause of GBS. These include antibodies against GQ1b, which is a ganglioside component of nerve seen in the Miller-Fisher variant, and antibodies to GM1, GD1a, GalNac-GD1a, and GD1b, which are associated with axonal variants.[5] Electromyography and nerve conduction studies may be helpful in diagnosing GBS by revealing the predominantly demyelinating polyneuropathy of AIDP or the axonal neuropathy of AMAN or AMSAN.

❑ Laboratory Findings

The CSF shows albumin–cytologic dissociation with normal cell count and increased protein (average 50–100 mg/dL). The protein increase parallels increasing clinical severity, and the increase may be prolonged. The CSF may be normal at first.

Commercial testing for antibody to GQ1b is now available and may be useful in the diagnosis.[6] A biopsy of the nerve will show evidence of demyelination and remyelination.

Laboratory findings due to associated disease may be present (e.g., evidence of recent infection with *Campylobacter jejuni* in 15–40% of cases and CMV in 5–20% of cases; EBV and *Mycoplasma pneumoniae* in <2% of cases in developed countries, other viral and rickettsial infections, immune disorders, DM, exposure to toxins [e.g., lead, alcohol], neoplasms). No agent was identified in ≤70% of cases.[7]

References

1. McKhann GM, Cornblath DR, Griffin JW, et al. Acute motor axonal neuropathy: a frequent cause of acute flaccid paralysis in China. *Ann Neurol.* 1993;33:333.
2. Ropper AH. The Guillain-Barré syndrome. *N Engl J Med.* 1992;326:1130–1136.
3. Zochodne DW. Autonomic involvement in Guillain-Barré syndrome: a review. *Muscle Nerve.* 1994;17:1145–1155.
4. Köller H, Kieseier BC, Jander S, et al. Chronic inflammatory demyelinating polyneuropathy. *N Engl J Med.* 2005;352:1343–1356. Review.
5. Nagashima T, Koga M, Odaka M, et al. Clinical correlates of serum anti-GT1a IgG antibodies. *J Neurol Sci.* 2004;219:139.
6. Chiba A, Kusunoki S, Obata H, et al. Serum anti-GQ1b IgG antibody is associated with ophthalmoplegia in Miller Fisher syndrome and Guillain-Barré syndrome: clinical and immunohistochemical studies. *Neurology.* 1993;43:1911.
7. Sivadon-Tardy V, Orlikowski D, Rozenberg F, et al. Guillain-Barré syndrome, greater Paris area. *Emerg Infect Dis.* 2006;12:990.

MULTIPLE SCLEROSIS

❑ Definition

Multiple sclerosis (MS) is an inflammatory disorder of the brain and spinal cord resulting in the loss of myelin, which insulates the neurons. It is the most common autoimmune demyelinating disease of the CNS.

❑ Clinical Presentation

Patients present with distinct episodes of neurologic deficits separated in time. It is caused by an inflammatory demyelination of distinct foci of white matter that are separated in space. Women are twice as likely to be affected as men, and the disease is rare in children or in patients >50 years of age. At autopsy, histology of the brain reveals multifocal areas of demyelination with loss of oligodendrocytes and astroglial scarring (see eBook Figure 4-18). Diagnosis should not be made by CSF evaluation alone unless there are *multiple clinical lesions in time* (by clinical history) and *anatomic location* (by MRI, evoked potentials, or physical examination). The diagnosis of MS is most commonly made using the McDonald criteria, which have undergone recent revision and require both MRI and CSF findings for definitive diagnosis.[1,2]

❏ Laboratory Findings

CSF changes are found in >90% of patients with MS.[3] The opening pressure, glucose, and albumin levels are normal, and leukocyte count is normal in two thirds of patients. Less than 5% of patients have a white blood cell (WBC) count >50 cells/μL. Cells are predominantly T lymphocytes. There are two significant CSF tests that are positive in MS: oligoclonal bands (OCBs) and the IgG index.[1]

❏ Oligoclonal IgG Bands

The qualitative test of IgG on unconcentrated CSF is the single most informative test. It has a greater sensitivity and specificity than the quantitative IgG test. A diagnosis of MS can be made when oligoclonal bands are found in the CSF, which are not seen in the serum, consistent with intrathecal synthesis. The test is best performed using isoelectric focusing (IEF) with immunodetection by blotting or fixation run with a simultaneous serum sample on an adjacent track with positive and negative controls. A diagnostic study will show one of five recognized staining patterns of oligoclonal banding[4,5]:

- Type 1: No OCBs in CSF and serum samples
- Type 2: OCBs in CSF but not serum, indicating intrathecal IgG synthesis
- Type 3: OCBs in CSF with additional identical OCBs in CSF and serum but still indicating intrathecal IgG synthesis
- Type 4: Identical OCBs in CSF and serum, indicating a systemic immune reaction with a normal or abnormal blood–CSF barrier and passive transfer of OCBs to the CSF
- Type 5: Monoclonal bands in CSF and serum, indicating the presence of a monoclonal gammopathy

If results are equivocal, negative, or show only a single band on IEF and the clinical suspicion for MS is high, the lumbar puncture and CSF analysis should be repeated. Ninety percent of patients with MS have OCBs in their CSF, at least two of which are *not* present in simultaneously examined serum. Rarely, patients with MS may have normal CSF immunoglobulins and lack OCBs. Positive results also occur in ≤10% of patients with noninflammatory neurologic disease (e.g., meningeal carcinomatosis, cerebral infarction) and ≤40% of patients with inflammatory CNS disorders (e.g., neurosyphilis, viral encephalitis, progressive rubella encephalitis, subacute sclerosing panencephalitis, bacterial meningitis, toxoplasmosis, cryptococcal meningitis, inflammatory neuropathies, and trypanosomiasis).

OCBs are not known to correlate with severity, duration, or course of MS, and they persist during remission. With steroid treatment, the prevalence of OCBs may be reduced by 30–50%. The evaluation of light chains may help in cases of equivocal oligoclonal IgG patterns.[4,5]

IgG Index

The immunoglobulin level, predominantly IgG, is elevated in the CSF relative to other proteins in MS. This finding is expressed as the IgG index (the normal value is less <0.66). It is an indication of IgG synthesis in the CNS. An increase in *production* of IgG is expressed as the ratio of CSF to serum albumin to rule out increased IgG due to disruption of the blood–brain barrier. Ninety percent of MS patients have an index of >0.7. CSF IgM and IgA may also be increased but are not useful for diagnosis.[1,3]

The CSF IgG does not correlate with duration, activity, or course of MS. It may also be increased in other inflammatory demyelinating diseases (e.g., neurosyphilis, acute GBS), 5–15% of patients with miscellaneous neurologic diseases, and a few normal persons. Recent myelography is said to invalidate the test. The CSF IgG synthesis rate (3.3 mg/day) is increased in 90% of MS patients and 4% of non-MS patients.[3] PCR demonstrates an expansion of B-cell clones.

Other Useful Tests

The presence of *myelin basic protein* indicates recent myelin destruction. It is increased in 70–90% of patients with MS during an acute exacerbation and usually returns to normal within 2 weeks. A weakly reactive result (4–8 ng/mL) indicates an active lesion >1 week old. Normal is <1 ng/mL. Myelin basic protein is useful for following the course of MS but not for screening; it may be helpful very early in the course of MS before OCBs have appeared or in approximately 10% of patients who do not develop these bands. It does not predict progression.[1] It is frequently increased in other causes of demyelination and tissue destruction (e.g., meningoencephalitis, leukodystrophies, metabolic encephalopathy, SLE of the CNS, brain tumor, head trauma, amyotrophic lateral sclerosis, cranial irradiation and intrathecal chemotherapy, and 45% of patients with recent stroke) and other disorders (e.g., diabetes mellitus, chronic renal failure, vasculitis, carcinoma of vasculitis, immune complex diseases, and pancreas). It is falsely increased by CSF contamination with blood. It is associated with certain histocompatibility antigens (e.g., Caucasian patients with B7 and Dw2 antigen).[2]

The *albumin index* (ratio of albumin serum to CSF) is a measure of integrity of the blood-to-CSF barrier. Use of this index can prevent false misinterpretation of increased CSF IgG concentrations. An increase indicates CSF contaminated with blood (e.g., traumatic tap) or increased permeability of the blood–brain barrier (e.g., aged persons, obstruction of CSF circulation, diabetes mellitus, SLE of CNS, GBS, polyneuropathy, cervical spondylosis).[1]

CSF total protein is usually normal or may be mildly increased in approximately 25% of patients and is not a very useful test by itself. Decreased values or values >100 mg/dL should cast doubt on the diagnosis of MS.

CSF gamma globulin is increased in 60–75% of patients regardless of whether the total CSF protein is increased. Gamma globulin ≥12% of CSF total protein is abnormal if there is not a corresponding increase in serum gamma globulin but may also be increased in other CNS disorders (e.g., syphilis, subacute panencephalitis, meningeal carcinomatosis) and may also be increased when serum electrophoresis is abnormal due to non-CNS diseases (e.g., RA, sarcoidosis, cirrhosis, myxedema, multiple myeloma).

Peripheral blood studies and routine CSF tests yield no changes of diagnostic value. Antimyelin antibodies initially were thought to be a marker of MS and progression of disease. However, subsequent evidence suggests that these antibodies are not associated with an increased risk of progression or with MS disease activity.[6,7]

Natalizumab (Tysabri) a recombinant humanized IgG4kappa monoclonal antibody that is used in the treatment of recurring MS and Crohn disease. Tysabri antibodies that block the efficacy of the drug may develop. Testing for Tysabri antibodies is commercially available.

References

1. McDonald WI, Compston A, Edan G, et al. Recommended diagnostic criteria for multiple sclerosis: guidelines from the International Panel on the diagnosis of multiple sclerosis. *Ann Neurol.* 2001;50:121–127.
2. Polman CH, Reingold SC, Banwell B, et al. Diagnostic criteria for multiple sclerosis: 2010 Revisions to the McDonald criteria. *Ann Neurol.* 2011;69(2):292–302.
3. McLean BN, Luxton RW, Thompson EJ. A study of immunoglobulin G in the cerebrospinal fluid of 1007 patients with suspected neurological disease using isoelectric focusing and the Log IgG-Index. A comparison and diagnostic applications. *Brain.* 1990;113(Pt 5):1269.
4. Barclay L. New guidelines for standards for CSF analysis in MS. *Arch Neurol.* 2005;62: 865–870.
5. Freedman MS, Thompson EJ, Deisenhammer F, et al. Recommended standard of cerebrospinal fluid analysis in the diagnosis of multiple sclerosis: a consensus statement. *Arch Neurol.* 2005;62:865.
6. Lampasona V, Franciotta D, Furlan R, et al. Similar low frequency of anti-MOG IgG and IgM in MS patients and healthy subjects. *Neurology.* 2004;62:2092.
7. Kuhle J, Pohl C, Mehling M, et al. Lack of association between antimyelin antibodies and progression to multiple sclerosis. *N Engl J Med.* 2007;356:371.

 NEOPLASTIC DISORDERS OF THE CNS

BRAIN TUMOR

❏ Definition
Brain tumors are a diverse group of neoplasms, both malignant and benign, with varying growth rates and symptoms. A large number of mass lesions within the intracranial vault are metastatic, arising from malignancies in other organs, or hematologic (leukemia or lymphoma).

❏ Clinical Presentation
Patients may present with headache, seizure, nausea and vomiting, syncope, cognitive dysfunction, weakness, loss of sensation, and aphasia. Suspicion for intracranial neoplasm should be followed by neurologic testing and neuroimaging including CT, MRI, PET, and single-photon emission computed tomography (SPECT) scanning.[1] Definitive diagnosis of an intracranial mass lesion is made on biopsy. Frozen-section or smear evaluation of tumoral tissue can be made in the operating room, which will allow the neurosurgeon to proceed with definitive resection if possible (see eBook Figure 4-19).

❏ Laboratory Findings
Evaluation of the CSF may help in the diagnosis. The CSF is usually clear, but it may occasionally reveal xanthochromia or be frankly bloody if there is hemorrhage into the tumor. The WBC count may be increased ≤150 cells/µL in up to 75% of patients and normal in others. Protein is usually increased. Protein is particularly increased with meningioma of the olfactory groove and with acoustic neuroma.

Tumor cells may be demonstrable in up to 40% of patients with all types of solid tumors, but failure to find malignant cells does not exclude neoplasm.[2]

Atypical WBCs may be seen in leukemia or lymphoma. Tumor antigens/markers may indicate the source of some metastatic tumors. Glucose may be decreased if cells are present. Oligoclonal bands may be present in patients with tumor and are nonspecific.

Brain stem gliomas, which are characteristically found in childhood, are usually associated with normal CSF. The CSF is usually normal in "diencephalic syndrome" of infants due to glioma of the hypothalamus.

References

1. Sun D, Liu Q, Liu W, et al. Clinical application of 201Tl SPECT imaging of brain tumors. *J Nucl Med.* 2000;41:5.
2. Marton KI, Gean AD. The spinal tap: a new look at an old test. *Ann Intern Med.* 1986; 104:840.

GLOMUS JUGULARE TUMOR (JUGULOTYMPANIC PARAGANGLIOMA)

❑ Definition

This tumor arises from the jugular and tympanic paraganglia within the ear and is the most common tumor of the middle ear.[1] It is a slow-growing, vascular tumor, with blood supply from the external and/or internal carotid artery.

❑ Clinical Presentation

It is most common in women and may result in hearing loss with pulsing/ringing in the ear, dizziness, and ear pain.

❑ Laboratory Findings

The diagnosis is made by neurophysiologic testing and CT or MRI. Blood and urine tests for endocrine workup (urinary and/or plasma fractionated metanephrines and catechol amines) should be performed. Evaluation of the CSF may reveal an increase in protein.

Reference

1. Michaels L, Soucek S, Beale T, et al. Jugulotympanic paraganglioma. In: Barnes L, Eveson JW, Reichart P, Sidransky D, eds. *World Health Organization Classification of Tumours. Pathology and Genetics Head and Neck Tumours.* Lyon, France: IARC Press; 2005:362–366.

LEUKEMIC INVOLVEMENT OF THE CENTRAL NERVOUS SYSTEM

See Chapter 9, Hematologic Disorders.

❑ Laboratory Findings

Intracranial hemorrhage is the principal cause of death in leukemia (may be intracerebral, subarachnoid, or subdural). It is more frequent when the WBC count is >100,000/μL and with rapid increases in the WBC count, especially in blast crises. The platelet count is frequently decreased. Often there is evidence of bleeding elsewhere. At autopsy, the tumor may be identified in the arachnoid, meninges, and perivascular regions (see eBook Figure 4-20).

Evaluation of the CSF may be diagnostic. There may be intracranial hemorrhage and infiltration of leukemic cells into the meninges and fluid. The CNS is involved in 5% of patients with ALL at diagnosis and is the major site of relapse.

PCR is used to detect minimal residual cells that are not recognized morphologically. Involvement of the CSF by AML is less common than ALL and CLL, and plasmacytoid leukemias are very rare.[1]

The CSF may show an increased opening pressure and protein level. The glucose may be decreased to <50% of the blood level. Abnormal cells may be identified by cytochemical, immunohistochemical, immunofluorescent, or flow cytometric techniques to help diagnose leukemia. Malignant cells are found in 60–80% of patients with meningeal involvement.[2]

Evaluation of the CSF may also help in identifying complicating meningeal infection (e.g., various bacteria, opportunistic fungi).

References

1. Peterson BA, Brunning RD, Bloomfield CD, et al. Central nervous system involvement in acute nonlymphocytic leukemia. A prospective study of adults in remission. *Am J Med.* 1987;83:464.
2. Shihadeh F, Reed V, Faderl S, et al. Cytogenetic profile of patients with acute myeloid leukemia and central nervous system disease. *Cancer.* 2012;118:112.

LYMPHOMATOUS INVOLVEMENT OF THE CENTRAL NERVOUS SYSTEM

See Chapter 9, Hematologic Diseases.

❑ Laboratory Findings

Cytologic evaluation of the CSF may provide sufficient diagnostic material to avoid brain biopsy in some patients. The meninges are involved in <30% of patients with malignant lymphoma. Involvement is most prevalent in diffuse large cell ("histiocytic"), lymphoblastic, and immunoblastic lymphoma and occurs in 30–50% of patients with Burkitt lymphoma and 15–20% of patients with non-Hodgkin lymphoma.[1] Hodgkin disease seldom involves the CNS.

Evaluation of the CSF often reveals an elevated protein and a lymphocyte-predominant pleocytosis. The glucose level is usually normal but may be decreased if there is leptomeningeal disease. Abnormal cells found in the CSF may be differentiated by immunohistochemistry, immunofluorescence, or flow cytometry. PCR may also be used for identification of clonality. The demonstration of neoplastic lymphocytes in the CSF on cytologic evaluation or flow cytometry is sufficient for the diagnosis of CNS lymphoma.[2]

References

1. Fischer L, Martus P, Weller M, et al. Meningeal dissemination in primary CNS lymphoma: prospective evaluation of 282 patients. *Neurology.* 2008;71:1102.
2. Abrey LE, Batchelor TT, Ferreri AJ, et al. Report of an international workshop to standardize baseline evaluation and response criteria for primary CNS lymphoma. *J Clin Oncol.* 2005;23:5034.

SPINAL CORD TUMOR

❑ Definition

Spinal cord tumors occur within the cord parenchyma or membranes adjacent to the cord. They may be primary or metastatic. Primary spinal cord tumors account for 2–4% of all primary CNS tumors. Extradural tumors are usually metastatic and can cause spinal cord compression.[1] Tumors arising within the dura, outside of the spinal cord, are termed intradural–extramedullary and comprise the nerve sheath tumors and meningiomas. Tumors arising within the spinal cord itself are called intramedullary tumors, predominantly gliomas (astrocytomas or ependymomas).[2,3]

❑ Clinical Presentation

Patients present with progressive symptoms that vary based on the location of the compression of the cord and spinal nerve roots. Symptoms range from pain to loss of sensation or motor function and decreased sensitivity to heat or cold and bowel or ladder dysfunction.

❑ Laboratory Findings

Evaluation of the CSF reveals increased protein. The level may be very high and is associated with xanthochromia when there is a block of the subarachnoid space. The protein concentration is higher with complete block in cord tumors located at lower levels. Tumor cells may be demonstrable. Definitive diagnosis is made on tissue evaluation at biopsy (see eBook Figure 4-21).

References

1. Duong LM, McCarthy BJ, McLendon RE, et al. Descriptive epidemiology of malignant and nonmalignant primary spinal cord, spinal meninges, and cauda equina tumors, United States, 2004–2007. *Cancer.* 2012;118(17):4220–4227.
2. Kim MS, Chung CK, Choe G, et al. Intramedullary spinal cord astrocytoma in adults: postoperative outcome. *J Neurooncol.* 2001;52:85.
3. Reimer R, Onofrio BM. Astrocytomas of the spinal cord in children and adolescents. *J Neurosurg.* 1985;63:669.

CONGENITAL DISORDERS OF THE CNS

NEURAL TUBE DEFECTS

❑ Definition

Neural tube defects (NTD) are due to a failure of the closure of the embryonic neural tube. They are second only to cardiac malformations as the cause of congenital anomalies. The supplementation of folic acid for all pregnant women has decreased the incidence of NTD markedly in the United States. Neural tube defects range from the most severe (anencephaly) to mild spinal defects (spina bifida) (see eBook Figure 4-22).

❑ Clinical Presentation

The risk factors for NTD include folic acid deficiency, certain drugs (valproic acid, carbamazepine, and methotrexate), diabetes, obesity, and hyperthermia. Genetic factors may be associated with NTD, and fetuses with NTD have a high rate of karyotypic abnormalities. Trisomy 18 is the most common chromosomal abnormality found in NTD.[1]

❑ Laboratory Findings

Screening for NTD in all pregnant women should include alpha-fetoprotein(AFP) in the maternal serum. Screening should occur between 15 and 20 weeks, and results are expressed as multiples of the median (MoM) for each gestational week. Values >2.0–2.5 MoM are abnormal. AFP is more reliable for open neural tube defects, and the detection rate for anencephaly has been reported as high as 95%.[2] Care should be taken in the interpretation of this test as it is affected by gestational age, maternal weight, maternal diabetes, multiple gestation, and race. In addition to laboratory testing, ultrasound is an excellent means for the identification of NTD.

References

1. Kennedy D, Chitayat D, Winsor EJ, et al. Prenatally diagnosed neural tube defects: ultrasound, chromosome, and autopsy or postnatal findings in 212 cases. *Am J Med Genet.* 1998;77:317.
2. Wang ZP, Li H, Hao LZ, et al. The effectiveness of prenatal serum biomarker screening for neural tube defects in second trimester pregnant women: a meta-analysis. *Prenat Diagn.* 2009;29:960.

 # TRAUMA AND VASCULAR DISORDERS OF THE CNS

CENTRAL NERVOUS SYSTEM TRAUMA

Laboratory findings vary depending on the type of brain injury (e.g., contusion, laceration, subdural hemorrhage, extradural hemorrhage, subarachnoid hemorrhage). There may also be laboratory findings due to complications of the brain injury (e.g., pneumonia, meningitis).

Basilar skull fracture results in the disruption of the barriers between the sinonasal cavity and the anterior and middle cranial fossae and subsequent leak of CSF into the nasal cavity or ear (see eBook Figure 4-23). This communication with the CNS can lead to infectious complications, resulting in morbidity and mortality.[1]

❏ Laboratory Evaluation for CSF Rhinorrhea

Beta-2-transferrin is produced by neuraminidase activity within the CNS; it is found in the CSF, perilymph, and aqueous humor. Immunofixation electrophoresis with anti-transferrin-precipitating antibody is performed to differentiate CSF desialated transferrin from nasal secretions. The assay has a high sensitivity and specificity. This is currently the recommended laboratory test for identifying the presence of CSF in sinonasal fluid.[2,3]

Testing for the glucose content in rhinorrhea with the use of glucose oxidase paper is not recommended for the following reasons: reducing substances in lacrimal gland secretions and nasal mucus may cause false-positive results and meningitis may lower the glucose level in the CSF leading to a false-negative result. The test is not specific for the side or site of leak.

Beta-trace protein, also known as prostaglandin D synthase, has been used to diagnose CSF rhinorrhea in multiple studies, with a sensitivity of 92% and specificity of 100%. It is synthesized primarily in arachnoid cells, oligodendrocytes, and the choroid plexus, but it is also present in the testes, heart, and serum, and it is nonspecific for CSF. Prostaglandin D synthase may also be altered in renal failure, MS, cerebral infarction, and certain CNS tumors. This test is not specific for the side or site of leak and can be difficult to collect if the leak is intermittent.[4]

References

1. Lindstrom DR, Toohill RJ, Loehrl TA, et al. Management of cerebrospinal fluid rhinorrhea: the Medical College of Wisconsin experience. *Laryngoscope.* 2004;114(6):969–974.
2. Porter MJ, Brookes GB, Zeman AZ, et al. Use of protein electrophoresis in the diagnosis of cerebrospinal fluid rhinorrhoea. *J Laryngol Otol.* 1992;106(6):504–506.
3. Ryall RG, Peacock MK, Simpson DA. Usefulness of beta 2-transferrin assay in the detection of cerebrospinal fluid leaks following head injury. *J Neurosurg.* 1992;77(5):737–739.
4. Pretto Flores L, De Almeida CS, Casulari LA. Positive predictive values of selected clinical signs associated with skull base fractures. *J Neurosurg Sci.* 2000;44:77.

ACUTE EPIDURAL HEMORRHAGE

❑ Definition

Epidural hemorrhage (bleeding between the dura and skull) is a rare but serious complication of head injury. It is most commonly due to an injury of the arteries predominantly the middle meningeal artery. It is found in up to 4% of patients surviving injury and up to 15% of autopsy series (see eBook Figure 4-24).[1,2]

❑ Clinical Presentation

Patients usually present with a lucid interval following the head injury. Expansion of the hematoma eventually causes pressure on the brain with shift of the tissues. Symptoms include abnormalities of cranial nerve III function or weakness of the extremities on the contralateral side. Severe bleeds may progress to transtentorial or uncal herniation and death.

Epidural hemorrhage may also be due to nontraumatic etiologies including: infection, coagulopathy, vascular and congenital malformations, and tumors. Rarely, it may occur during hemodialysis, pregnancy, and cardiac surgery.[3,4] It may also occur in the epidural space of the spinal cord following spinal procedures.[5]

Lumbar puncture is contraindicated in cases where epidural hemorrhage is suspected, due to the risk of herniation. Diagnosis is primarily based on neuroimaging with unenhanced CT. Differentiation of epidural versus subdural hematoma can be made on imaging as epidural hematoma will not cross suture lines and has a lens-shaped appearance.

❑ Laboratory Evaluation

CSF is usually under increased pressure; it is colorless unless there is associated cerebral contusion, laceration, or subarachnoid hemorrhage in which case it will be xanthochromic or bloody.

References

1. Bullock MR, Chesnut R, Ghajar J, et al. Surgical management of acute epidural hematomas. *Neurosurgery.* 2006;58:S7.
2. Mayer S, Rowland L. Head injury. In: Rowland L, ed. *Merritt's neurology.* Philadelphia, PA: Lippincott Williams & Wilkins; 2000:401.
3. Szkup P, Stoneham G. Case report: spontaneous spinal epidural haematoma during pregnancy: case report and review of the literature. *Br J Radiol.* 2004;77:881.
4. Takahashi K, Koiwa F, Tayama H, et al. A case of acute spontaneous epidural haematoma in a chronic renal failure patient undergoing haemodialysis: successful outcome with surgical management. *Nephrol Dial Transplant.* 1999;14:2499.
5. Sokolowski MJ, Garvey TA, Perl J II, et al. Prospective study of postoperative lumbar epidural hematoma: incidence and risk factors. *Spine.* 2008;33:108.

SUBDURAL HEMATOMA

ACUTE

❑ Definition

Acute subdural hematoma is most commonly due to the shearing effect on the bridging veins between the brain and the dural sinus during trauma. Occasionally, it may also be due to arterial injury or low CSF pressure. It is a complicating factor in up to 20% of severe traumatic brain injuries (see eBook Figure 4-25).[1]

❏ Clinical Presentation

Most patients develop coma following injury, but some have a transient "lucid interval" after the acute injury, followed by a progressive neurologic decline to coma.[2] Lumbar puncture is contraindicated due to the risk of herniation. The diagnosis is readily made on CT of the brain with subdural hematomas appearing as crescent-shaped lesions as opposed to the lens-shaped lesion of the epidural hematoma.

❏ Laboratory Findings

CSF findings are variable: clear, bloody, or xanthochromic, depending on recent or old associated injuries (e.g., contusion, laceration).

CHRONIC

❏ Definition

Chronic subdural hematoma develops over days or weeks following minor injury that may not have been recognized by the patient. The bleed is slow and may be recurrent.

❏ Clinical Presentation

Chronic subdural hematoma is more commonly seen in the elderly and may present with the insidious onset of cognitive impairment, headaches, light-headedness, apathy, somnolence, or seizures. Symptoms may only appear weeks after the initial injury and may be transient or fluctuating.[3] Diagnosis is based on CT imaging with membranous encapsulation visualized surrounding the hematoma. Lumbar puncture is contraindicated due to the risk of herniation.

❏ Laboratory Findings

CSF is usually xanthochromic, and the CSF protein content is 300–2,000 mg/dL. Anemia is often present in infants.

References

1. Bullock MR, Chesnut R, Ghajar J, et al. Surgical management of acute subdural hematomas. *Neurosurgery.* 2006;58:S16.
2. Victor M, Ropper A. Craniocerebral trauma. In: Victor M, Ropper A, eds. *Adams and Victor's Principles of Neurology,* 7th ed. New York: McGraw-Hill; 2001:925.
3. Kaminski HJ, Hlavin ML, Likavec MJ, et al. Transient neurologic deficit caused by chronic subdural hematoma. *Am J Med.* 1992;92:698.

STROKE

❏ Definition

Stroke or cerebrovascular accident is the loss of function of an area of the brain due to vascular compromise. Stroke or ischemia of the brain may be transient or permanent. The causes include intracerebral (see eBook Figure 4-26) or subarachnoid hemorrhage (see eBook Figure 4-27) and thrombotic or embolic ischemia (see eBook Figure 4-28). The American Heart Association data review of strokes finds that the majority of strokes are due to ischemia (87%), followed by intracerebral hemorrhage (10%) and subarachnoid hemorrhage (3%).[1]

❏ Clinical Presentation

The presenting signs depend on the size and location of the infarct. Risk factors include hypertension, trauma, drugs, smoking alcoholism, atherosclerosis, and vascular malformations.

The diagnosis of stroke is made on history, physical examination, and neurologic imaging (CT or MRI) to identify hemorrhagic versus thrombotic (or embolic) stroke and rule out mass lesion. If the blood pressure is normal, berry aneurysm, hemorrhage into tumor, angioma, or coagulopathy should be considered. Rapid diagnosis is important for the treatment of the patient as thrombolysis must be initiated within the first 4.5 hours after the initial event.[2]

In hemorrhagic stroke, the most common causes include ruptured berry aneurysm (45% of patients), hypertension (15% of patients), angiomatous malformations (8% of patients), and less commonly brain tumor and blood dyscrasia. Ischemic causes of stroke include thrombosis or embolism in 80% of patients.[3,4]

A genetic basis for increased risk of stroke probably exists, but a definite gene has not yet been identified, nor is genetic testing commercially available. Risk is increased in patients with a family history of stroke, and following a stroke in one twin, a monozygotic second twin has a higher risk of stroke than a fraternal twin. Studies in Iceland have found three loci revealing significant association with ischemic stroke (PITX2, ZFHX3, and HDAC9).[5] In patients with sickle cell anemia, studies have shown an increased risk for stroke is associated with SNPs in the ANXA2, TGFBR3, and TEK genes.[6] A number of biochemical markers in both blood and CSF have been studied with the hope of providing prognostic or predictive value in stroke patients. A meta-analysis of all reported biochemical tests in blood and CSF concluded that the combined results were not sufficiently predictive for clinical use.[7,8]

❏ Laboratory Findings

Blood testing at the time of suspected stroke should include CBC, PT and PTT, thrombin time or ecarin clotting time (for patients taking a thrombin or factor Xa inhibitor), and lipid panel. A hypercoagulable panel including lupus anticoagulant (LA), anticardiolipin antibodies (ACAs), protein C, protein S, and factor V Leiden should also be obtained. Testing to rule out SLE may be indicated. Additional tests may include a fibrinogen level, ESR, serology for Lyme disease, and HIV, and toxicology to rule out cocaine and other drugs.

References

1. Go AS, Mozaffarian D, Roger VL, et al. Heart disease and stroke statistics—2013 update: a report from the American Heart Association. *Circulation.* 2013;127:e6.
2. Arnold M, Nedeltchev K, Brekenfeld C, et al. Outcome of acute stroke patients without visible occlusion on early arteriography. *Stroke.* 2004;35:1135.
3. MacMahon S, Peto R, Cutler J, et al. Blood pressure, stroke, and coronary heart disease. Part 1, Prolonged differences in blood pressure: prospective observational studies corrected for the regression dilution bias. *Lancet.* 1990;335:765.
4. Kawachi I, Colditz GA, Stampfer MJ, et al. Smoking cessation and decreased risk of stroke in women. *JAMA.* 1993;269:232.
5. Traylor M, Farrall M, Holliday EG, et al. Genetic risk factors for ischaemic stroke and its subtypes (the METASTROKE collaboration): a meta-analysis of genome-wide association studies. *Lancet Neurol.* 2012;11:951.
6. Flanagan JM, Frohlich DM, Howard TA, et al. Genetic predictors for stroke in children with sickle cell anemia. *Blood.* 2011;117:6681.
7. Zandbergen EG, de Haan RJ, Stoutenbeek CP, et al. Systematic review of early prediction of poor outcome in anoxic-ischaemic coma. *Lancet.* 1998;352:1808.
8. Zandbergen EG, de Haan RJ, Hijdra A. Systematic review of prediction of poor outcome in anoxic-ischaemic coma with biochemical markers of brain damage. *Intensive Care Med.* 2001;27:1661.

CEREBRAL EMBOLISM

❑ Definition
Embolism is caused by particles of debris or tissue that originate distally (from vessel walls, the heart, or tumors) and travel through the circulation resulting in the blockage of arterial blood flow to the brain. Unlike thrombosis, which involves the local vessel, local therapy in embolic stroke is only temporizing. The source of the embolic fragment must be identified and treated, or additional events may occur. There are four categories of embolic stroke: those with known cardiac source, those with a possible cardiac or aortic source, those with an arterial source, and those with an unknown source (see eBook Figure 4-29). Cerebral embolism is the most common cause of stroke in the elderly.

❑ Clinical Presentation
Embolic stroke should be suspected if the change is sudden with maximal deficit at the onset, if the infarct is large, if there is a known cardiac or large arterial lesion, if the infarct is or becomes hemorrhagic on CT, if there are multiple lesions, and if clinical findings improve quickly. It is more common in patients with strokes of the posterior circulation. Atrial fibrillation, cardiac murmurs, and enlargement are risk factors for embolus of cardiac origin. A possible cardiac source should always be considered even in young patients. If the patient is febrile, septic emboli and endocarditis should be suspected. Small vessel (lacunar) stroke is most commonly seen in patients with hypertension, DM, or polycythemia. Patent foramen ovale is also a risk factor for venous to arterial embolism.

The diagnosis of embolic stroke is primarily made on clinical examination and neuroimaging (MRI and CT scan). Cardiac evaluation with EKG and echocardiography is also helpful. Doppler studies of the large vessels of the neck and aorta may show lesions in these regions. Additional imaging studies to rule out myxoma of the left atrium, fat embolism in fracture of long bones, and air embolism in the neck, chest, or cardiac surgery may be indicated.[1]

❑ Laboratory Findings
Laboratory tests should be performed to try to determine any underlying disorder and should include blood cultures to rule out bacterial endocarditis, hypercoagulable panel to rule out nonbacterial thrombotic vegetations on heart valves (lupus anticoagulant, anticardiolipin, prothrombin mutation, factor V Leiden mutation), and cardiac enzymes to rule out underlying myocardial infarction with mural thrombus.[2,3]

Lumbar puncture with evaluation of the CSF reveals findings similar to cerebral thrombosis. Hemorrhagic infarction develops in one third of patients, usually producing slight xanthochromia. Some patients may have grossly bloody CSF (10,000 RBCs/μL). Septic embolism (e.g., bacterial endocarditis) may cause increased WBC (CSF WBC count ≤200/μL with variable lymphocytes and PMNs), increased RBC (CSF RBC count ≤1,000/μL), slight xanthochromia, increased protein, normal glucose, and negative culture.

References
1. DeRook FA, Comess KA, Albers GW, Popp, RL. Transesophageal echocardiography in the evaluation of stroke. *Ann Intern Med.* 1992;117:922.

2. Jauch EC, Saver JL, Adams HP Jr, et al. Guidelines for the early management of patients with acute ischemic stroke: a guideline for healthcare professionals from the American Heart Association/American Stroke Association. *Stroke.* 2013;44:870.
3. Markus HS, Hambley H. Neurology and the blood: haematological abnormalities in ischaemic stroke. *J Neurol Neurosurg Psychiatry.* 1998;64:150.

INTRACEREBRAL HEMORRHAGE

4

❏ Definition
Intracerebral hemorrhage (ICH) is defined as bleeding into the brain parenchyma and has many etiologies (see eBook Figure 4-30).

❏ Clinical Presentation
ICH is the second most common cause of stroke following ischemic stroke. It is the cause of up to 15% of all first time strokes, with a higher incidence in Asians, Hispanics, and African Americans.[1] The risk for ICH is increased in patients with hypertension, amyloidosis, vascular malformations, and berry aneurysm. Risk also increases with age, alcohol intake, and African American ethnicity. Etiologies of ICH include hypertensive vasculopathy, septic emboli, brain tumor, infection, vasculitis, bleeding disorders (including anticoagulants), and drugs such as cocaine and amphetamines.[2]

The diagnosis of intracranial hemorrhage is made by neurologic imaging (CT or MRI).

❏ Laboratory Findings
Lumbar puncture reveals an increased CSF WBC count (15,000–20,000/µL), higher than in cerebral infarct (e.g., embolism, thrombosis). All patients should have a platelet count, PT, and PTT to establish bleeding potential. Tests that may be helpful include an elevated ESR in vasculitis and urinalysis, which may reveal transient glycosuria or concomitant renal disease. Additional tests may be obtained to rule out causes of intracerebral hemorrhage such as leukemia, aplastic anemia, polyarteritis nodosa, SLE, and other coagulopathies.

References
1. Flaherty ML, Woo D, Haverbusch M, et al. Racial variations in location and risk of intracerebral hemorrhage. *Stroke.* 2005;36:934.
2. Gebel JM, Broderick JP. Intracerebral hemorrhage. *Neurol Clin.* 2000;18:419.

BERRY ANEURYSM (SACCULAR ANEURYSM)

❏ Definition
A berry or saccular aneurysm is a rounded dilation of an artery in the brain. The wall of the aneurysm is weaker than the normal vessel and therefore at risk for rupture with increased pressure (see eBook Figure 4-31).

❏ Clinical Presentation
Most subarachnoid hemorrhages are due to ruptured saccular aneurysms. The incidence of saccular aneurysms is approximately 5% among the general population.[1] The risk of rupture varies with aneurysm size, and most subarachnoid hemorrhages due to aneurysm rupture occur in the 40- to 60-year-old age group,

with a slight increase in women over men. African Americans have a higher incidence than Caucasians.[2,3] Patients with subarachnoid hemorrhage due to aneurysm rupture present with severe headache, nausea, vomiting, vision loss, or loss of consciousness.

Risk factors for saccular aneurysm include smoking, hypertension, genetic diseases (adult dominant polycystic kidney disease, aldosteronism, Ehlers-Danlos syndrome), family history, and sympathomimetic drugs such as phenylpropanolamine and cocaine, and decreased estrogen as is seen in postmenopausal women. A number of studies have looked at the evidence for a candidate gene associated with aneurysmal subarachnoid hemorrhage including the elastin gene on chromosome 7q.[4]

The diagnosis of saccular aneurysm rupture is made by identification of symptomatology and laboratory tests. The most common presenting symptom is sudden severe headache. CT scan will identify subarachnoid clot.

❏ **Laboratory Findings**

Lumbar puncture reveals increased opening pressure and elevated RBC count that does not decrease between tubes 1 and 4. In early subarachnoid hemorrhage (<8 hours after onset of symptoms), the test for occult blood may be positive before xanthochromia develops. Xanthochromia is an indicator that blood has been in the CSF for at least 2 hours.[5] Bloody CSF clears by the 10th day in 40% of patients and is persistently abnormal after 21 days in 15% of patients, and approximately 5% of cerebrovascular episodes due to hemorrhage are wholly within the parenchyma, resulting in normal CSF findings.[6]

References

1. Broderick JP, Brott T, Tomsick T, et al. The risk of subarachnoid and intracerebral hemorrhages in blacks as compared with whites. *N Engl J Med.* 1992;326:733.
2. Rinkel GJ, Djibuti M, Algra A, et al. Prevalence and risk of rupture of intracranial aneurysms: a systematic review. *Stroke.* 1998;29:251.
3. de Rooij, NK, Linn, FH, van der Plas JA, et al. Incidence of subarachnoid haemorrhage: a systematic review with emphasis on region, age, gender, and time trends. *J Neurol Neurosurg Psychiatry.* 2007;78:1365.
4. Farnham JM, Camp NJ, Neuhausen SL, et al. Confirmation of chromosome 7q11 locus for predisposition to intracranial aneurysm. *Hum Genet.* 2004;114:250.
5. UK National External Quality Assessment Scheme for Immunochemistry Working Group. National guidelines for analysis of cerebrospinal fluid for bilirubin in suspected subarachnoid haemorrhage. *Ann Clin Biochem.* 2003;40:481.
6. Beetham R, UK NEQAS for Immunochemistry Working group. Recommendations for CSF analysis in subarachnoid haemorrhage. *J Neurol Neurosurg Psychiatry.* 2004;75:528.

CEREBRAL VEIN OR SINUS THROMBOSIS

❏ **Definition**

Cerebral venous sinus thrombosis is the presence of clot within the sinus.

❏ **Clinical Presentation**

Cerebral vein and dural sinus thromboses are an uncommon cause of stroke. They are more likely to occur in neonates and children than adults and more likely in women than in men.[1,2] The causes of thrombosis include prothrombotic conditions in 85% of cases (oral contraception, pregnancy, malignancy), infection (e.g., otitis, mastoiditis, sinusitis, meningitis), and head injury. Genetic disorders may also be implicated, including antithrombin III deficiency, protein C and protein S deficiency, factor V Leiden mutation, and prothrombin gene mutation.[3] Collagen vascular and inflammatory diseases (e.g., SLE, sarcoidosis, and Wegener granulomatosis) may also be causative.

Venous thrombosis results in elevated venous pressure followed by leakage into the surrounding parenchyma and resultant impairment of CSF reabsorption leading to increased intracranial pressure. Patients may present with headache that increases over several days, motor weakness, paresis, or seizures. Thromboses of the cerebral veins and sinuses may produce focal hemorrhagic infarcts, which can be seen on neuroimaging (see eBook Figure 4-32).

The diagnosis of cerebral vein thrombosis is made predominantly by neurologic imaging (CT or MRI).

❏ **Laboratory Findings**

Laboratory tests are nonspecific but may give clues to the etiology. Routine hematology, coagulation (PT, PTT), and chemistry tests are recommended and give an idea of underlying cause. Evaluation of an underlying hypercoagulable state with antithrombin, Protein C and S, factor V Leiden, prothrombin mutation, lupus anticoagulant, anticardiolipin, and anti-beta2 glycoproteins may be helpful. An elevated D-dimer may support the diagnosis but will not exclude it if negative.[4]

Lumbar puncture for evaluation of CSF to rule out infection is required. Up to 50% of patients may have CSF findings. The CSF may reveal normal or mildly increased protein to ≤100 mg/dL. The CSF cell count may be normal or ≥10 WBC/µL during the first 48 hours and rarely ≥2,000 WBC/µL transiently on the 3rd day. Red cells may be increased.

Additional blood tests may be informative. An increased CRP and ESR are risk factors for development of stroke, and an increased CRP is associated with a poorer short-term prognosis. Hematologic disorders (e.g., polycythemia, sickle cell disease, thrombotic thrombocytopenia, and macroglobulinemia) may be identified (see Chapter 9, Hematology).

Vasculitis (e.g., polyarteritis nodosa, Takayasu syndrome, dissecting aneurysm of aorta, syphilis, meningitis; see Chapter 3, Cardiovascular Disorders) and hypotension (e.g., myocardial infarction, shock) are other potential causes of cerebral vein thrombosis.

References

1. de Veber G, Andrew M, Adams C, et al. Cerebral sinovenous thrombosis in children. *N Engl J Med*. 2001;345:417.
2. Stam J. Thrombosis of the cerebral veins and sinuses. *N Engl J Med*. 2005;352:1791.
3. Marjot T, Yadav S, Hasan N, et al. Genes associated with adult cerebral venous thrombosis. *Stroke*. 2011;42:913.
4. Crassard I, Soria C, Tzourio C, et al. A negative D-dimer assay does not rule out cerebral venous thrombosis: a series of seventy-three patients. *Stroke*. 2005;36:1716.

HYPERTENSIVE ENCEPHALOPATHY

❏ **Definition**

Hypertensive encephalopathy is usually associated with a blood pressure of ≥180/120 mm Hg and is an acute, life-threatening disorder presenting with signs of cerebral edema (see eBook Figure 4-33).

❑ Clinical Presentation

Clinical symptoms are characterized by the insidious onset of headache, nausea, and vomiting. If not treated, patients progress to mental confusion, seizures, and coma. Although these symptoms differ from the abrupt onset of stroke, an MRI scan should be obtained, which may reveal edema in the parieto-occipital regions (reversible posterior leukoencephalopathy) or in the pontine region (hypertensive brain stem encephalopathy).[1,2]

❑ Laboratory Findings

Findings on laboratory tests are due to changes in other organ systems and to underlying conditions such as cardiac, renal, and endocrine disorders and toxemia of pregnancy. Testing may also reveal changes that may occur due to progressive disorders following hypertensive encephalopathy such as focal intracerebral hemorrhage. The CSF frequently shows increased pressure and protein ≤100 mg/dL.

References

1. Kitaguchi H, Tomimoto H, Miki Y, et al. A brain stem variant of reversible posterior leukoencephalopathy syndrome. *Neuroradiology.* 2005;47:652.
2. Hinchey J, Chaves C, Appignani B, et al. A reversible posterior leukoencephalopathy syndrome. *N Engl J Med.* 1996;334:494.

THROMBOPHLEBITIS OF CAVERNOUS SINUS

❑ Definition

Thrombophlebitis or inflammation of the vein results from infected or septic thrombosis of the venous sinus

❑ Clinical Presentation

Septic dural sinus thrombosis has become a rare disease since the advent of antibiotics. Patients present with headache, occasionally eye swelling or diplopia, and alterations in mental status. The diagnosis is primarily made by imaging studies; however, lumbar puncture can be supportive, differentiating periorbital cellulitis from septic cavernous sinus thrombosis.

❑ Laboratory Findings

Laboratory findings that may be helpful include the CBC where an elevated peripheral WBC count may suggest an acute bacterial infection or other causes of venous thromboses such as sickle cell disease, polycythemia, or dehydration. The CSF reveals inflammatory cells in 75% of cases with increased neutrophils or mononuclear cells, elevated protein, normal glucose, and a negative culture. Thirty percent of patients have a CSF finding consistent with bacterial meningitis with a positive culture.[1]

Culture of the CSF may reveal organisms associated with septic cavernous sinus thrombosis. *Staphylococcus aureus* is seen in 70% of all infections and is associated with facial infection or sphenoid sinusitis, and MRSA is becoming more frequent.[2] Streptococci (including *Streptococcus pneumoniae, Streptococcus milleri,* and viridans group streptococci) are less commonly found. Anaerobes are most often found with accompanying sinus, dental, or tonsillar infections.[3,4] Fungal pathogens have been less commonly reported and include *Mucor, Rhizopus,* and *Aspergillus.*[5,6]

References

1. Southwick FS, Richardson EP Jr, Swartz MN. Septic thrombosis of the dural venous sinuses. *Medicine (Baltimore)*. 1986;65:82.
2. Naesens R, Ronsyn M, Druwé P, et al. Central nervous system invasion by community-acquired methicillin-resistant *Staphylococcus aureus*. *J Med Microbiol*. 2009;58:1247.
3. Cannon ML, Antonio BL, McCloskey JJ, et al. Cavernous sinus thrombosis complicating sinusitis. *Pediatr Crit Care Med*. 2004;5:86.
4. Watkins LM, Pasternack MS, Banks M, et al. Bilateral cavernous sinus thromboses and intraorbital abscesses secondary to *Streptococcus milleri*. *Ophthalmology*. 2003;110:569.
5. Chitsaz S, Bagheri J, Mandegar MH, et al. Extensive sino-orbital zygomycosis after heart transplantation: a case report. *Transplant Proc*. 2009;41:2927.
6. Devèze A, Facon F, Latil G, et al. Cavernous sinus thrombosis secondary to non-invasive sphenoid aspergillosis. *Rhinology*. 2005;43:152.

4

SPINAL CORD INFARCTION

❏ Definition
Spinal cord infarction may result from occlusion of the anterior spinal artery, the posterior spinal artery, or the Brown-Séquard syndrome in which no defined vascular pattern can be determined.

❏ Clinical Presentation
Symptoms of paresis either unilateral or bilateral occur with infarction of the anterior spinal artery and loss of touch, proprioception, and vibratory sense with infarction of the posterior spinal artery. Venous infarction may also occur and is usually associated with vascular malformations.[1] The differential diagnosis includes transverse myelitis, compression, and acute polyneuropathy. Diagnosis is made primarily by neuroimaging (MRI) and vascular imaging (CTA or MRA).

❏ Laboratory Evaluation
A lumbar puncture should be performed in younger patients to rule out infectious or inflammatory etiologies. In spinal infarct, the CSF may be normal or may show mild pleocytosis with WBC <100 and elevation in protein (<119 mg/dL).[2,3] CSF testing should include cell count, glucose, protein, gram stain, and culture. Infectious agents such as Lyme, herpes, varicella, coxsackie, EBV, and CMV should be ruled out with serology. In addition, OCB should be performed on CSF and serum to rule out MS. Blood and urine toxicology should be performed to rule out cocaine. Additional blood tests to rule out hypercoagulable state and collagen vascular disease may be of benefit.

References

1. Mohr JP, Benavente O, Barnett HJ. Spinal cord ischemia. In: Barnett HJ, Mohr JP, Stein BM, et al., eds. *Stroke Pathophysiology, Diagnosis, and Management*. Philadelphia, PA: Churchill Livingstone; 1998:423.
2. Cheshire WP, Santos CC, Massey EW, et al. Spinal cord infarction: etiology and outcome. *Neurology*. 1996;47:321.
3. Sandson TA, Friedman JH. Spinal cord infarction. Report of 8 cases and review of the literature. *Medicine (Baltimore)*. 1989;68:282.

CNS VASCULITIS

❏ Definition
Vasculitis is an inflammation of the vessels that may occur within the central nervous system, and most commonly it is due to collagen vascular disease but may also be due to infection, atherosclerosis, embolic disease, malignancy, and drugs.[1] Primary angiitis of the central nervous system is a rare disorder of unknown etiology presenting predominantly in men and may occur at any age (see eBook Figure 4-34).[2] Giant cell arteritis is one of the more common forms of vasculitis.

❏ Clinical Presentation
Patients may present with various neurologic symptoms depending on the area of the brain affected and the severity of the disease. In giant cell arteritis, patients present with neurologic symptoms of headache and visual disturbances. Amyloid angiopathy (see Vascular Dementia) may also occur in the central nervous system.[3] The differential diagnosis of vasculitis is broad, and diagnostic testing includes clinical examination and history, neuroimaging such as MRA or CTA, and evaluation of the blood and CSF.

❏ Laboratory Evaluation
Blood work should include a sedimentation rate and C-reactive protein, which may be elevated in collagen vascular diseases, infection, and temporal arteritis. These are normal in primary angiitis. Serologic evaluation should be carried out to rule out syphilis, Lyme disease, catscratch disease, tuberculosis, herpes virus, hepatitis B and C virus, HIV, and cysticercosis. Rheumatologic studies should be performed to rule out collagen vascular disease (ANA, rheumatoid factor, antineutrophilic cytoplasmic antibody).

A lumbar puncture with analysis of the CSF should be performed to rule out infection (cell count and culture), malignancy (cytology), or hemorrhage with evidence of xanthochromia.

If the diagnosis cannot be made with less invasive means, a biopsy should be performed. Biopsy will help in the diagnosis of giant cell arteritis. Vascular changes include loss of the internal elastic lamina and inflammatory infiltrates of the vascular wall by histiocytes, giant cells, and lymphocytes.

References
1. Calabrese LH, Duna GF, Lie JT. Vasculitis in the central nervous system. *Arthritis Rheum.* 1997;40:1189.
2. Calabrese LH, Mallek JA. Primary angiitis of the central nervous system. Report of 8 new cases, review of the literature, and proposal for diagnostic criteria. *Medicine (Baltimore).* 1988;67:20.
3. Fountain NB, Eberhard DA. Primary angiitis of the central nervous system associated with cerebral amyloid angiopathy: report of two cases and review of the literature. *Neurology.* 1996;46:190.

 PARANEOPLASTIC SYNDROMES AFFECTING THE CNS

❏ Definition
A group of disorders resulting from an immunologic response to a shared antigen between a tumor and antigens normally expressed by the nervous system are classified as paraneoplastic neurologic syndromes.

❏ Clinical Presentation

Patients present with muscle weakness and autonomic dysfunction. Both humoral and cell-mediated immune response is believed to be involved in these disorders. Antibodies can be detected in both the serum and CSF of patients with these disorders. A group of antibodies have been identified associated with small cell lung carcinoma (SLCL), and additional antibodies have been associated with other tumors including thymoma, breast and GYN carcinomas, Hodgkin lymphoma, teratoma, melanoma, and other lung cancers. In addition, several antibodies may occur either with or without an associated carcinoma; these include the Lambert-Eaton myasthenic syndrome (LEMS) and myasthenia gravis (see Sections on LEM and Myasthenia gravis below).

❏ Laboratory Evaluation

Screening for patients suspected of having a paraneoplastic neurologic syndrome requires evaluation of both serum and CSF for antibodies.[1] Patients with small cell lung carcinoma may have multiple antibodies with or without symptoms. Some patients without an underlying carcinoma may also have antibodies causing neurologic disease. Paraneoplastic symptoms and antibodies may be present years before a malignancy is diagnosed. The identification of antibodies in a patient does not necessarily predict symptomatology.

The well-characterized paraneoplastic antibodies that most often are found in the symptomatic patients include anti-Hu, anti-Yo, anti-Ri, anti-Tr, anti-CV2/CRMP5, anti-Ma 1 and 2, anti-amphiphysin, and anti-recoverin.[2]

Small cell lung carcinoma is the tumor most commonly associated with paraneoplastic neurologic syndromes and include LEMS and autonomic neuropathy (anti-VGCC antibody), cerebellar ataxia and encephalomyelitis (associated with several antibodies), sensory neuropathy (anti-Hu antibody), retinopathy, and opsomyoclonus.[3]

In addition to evaluation of antibodies in the CSF, spinal fluid should be evaluated for malignant cells by cytology and for inflammatory changes such as pleocytosis and oligoclonal bands to rule out MS.[4]

References

1. McKeon A, Pittock SJ, Lennon VA. CSF complements serum for evaluating paraneoplastic antibodies and NMO-IgG. *Neurology.* 2011;76:1108.
2. Graus F, Saiz A, Dalmau J. Antibodies and neuronal autoimmune disorders of the CNS. *J Neurol.* 2010;257:509.
3. Honnorat J, Antoine JC. Paraneoplastic neurological syndromes. *Orphanet J Rare Dis.* 2007;2:22.
4. Psimaras D, Carpentier AF, Rossi C; PNS Euronetwork. Cerebrospinal fluid study in paraneoplastic syndromes. *J Neurol Neurosurg Psychiatry.* 2010;81:42.

MYASTHENIA GRAVIS

❏ Definition

Myasthenia gravis results from the development of autoantibodies directed against the acetylcholine receptor (AChR) or muscle-specific tyrosine kinase (MuSK) resulting in destruction of proteins in the postsynaptic membrane of the neuromuscular junction.

❏ Clinical Presentation

The majority of patients presenting with myasthenia gravis have thymoma and occasionally SCLC, thyroid, or breast cancer.[1] Patients present with fluctuating weakness of the extraocular, bulbar, limb, and respiratory muscles. Weakness of the eyelid and extraocular muscles is present in most patients and precedes limb weakness; limb weakness alone is rare in myasthenia gravis. The differential diagnosis includes the Lambert-Eaton myasthenic syndrome, thyroid ophthalmopathy, amyotrophic lateral sclerosis, botulism, and cranial nerve or brain stem pathology.

❑ Laboratory Evaluation

Diagnosis is made by physical examination (Tensilon test), history, and serologic testing for AChR or MuSK antibodies. These tests are confirmatory in up to 94% of patients with generalized disease.[2] The most sensitive test for AChR-ab is the binding antibody test by radioimmunoassay, which is highly specific for myasthenia gravis. Antibody titers may be used to follow therapy on a particular patient but correlate poorly between patients.

References

1. Fujita J, Yamadori I, Yamaji Y, et al. Myasthenia gravis associated with small-cell carcinoma of the lung. *Chest.* 1994;105:624.
2. Meriggioli MN, Sanders DB. Myasthenia gravis: diagnosis. *Semin Neurol.* 2004;24:31.

LAMBERT-EATON MYASTHENIC SYNDROME

❑ Definition

Lambert-Eaton myasthenic syndrome (LEMS) an autoimmune disease associated with malignancy and results from the development of antibodies to the voltage-gated calcium channel (VGCC), which interfere with the normal calcium flux required for the release of acetylcholine.[1]

❑ Clinical Presentation

Patients present with symmetrical proximal muscle weakness, which starts in the lower extremities (difficulty rising from a chair), and autonomic dysfunction (dry mouth). The differential diagnosis includes myasthenia gravis, muscular dystrophy, polyneuropathies, and multiple cranial mononeuropathies. The diagnosis is made on clinical examination and confirmed by electrodiagnostic studies and the presence of antibodies to VGCC in the serum.

❑ Laboratory Evaluation

Testing for VGCC is by radioimmunoassay. Two separate antibodies can be identified. The P/Q-type VGCC is found in 85–95% of patients.[2] The N-type VGCC is found in approximately 40% of patients with LEMS and is more likely to be seen in patients with small cell lung carcinoma.[3] Higher titers of antibody are found in patients with underlying carcinoma while lower titers of antibody may be seen in patients with other neurologic paraneoplastic disorders and amyotrophic lateral sclerosis.[4]

References

1. Motomura M, Johnston I, Lang B, et al. An improved diagnostic assay for Lambert-Eaton myasthenic syndrome. *J Neurol Neurosurg Psychiatry.* 1995;58:85.
2. Pellkofer HL, Armbruster L, Krumbholz M, et al. Lambert-Eaton myasthenic syndrome differential reactivity of tumor versus non-tumor patients to subunits of the voltage-gated calcium channel. *J Neuroimmunol.* 2008;204:136.
3. Lennon VA, Kryzer TJ, Griesmann GE, et al. Calcium-channel antibodies in the Lambert-Eaton syndrome and other paraneoplastic syndromes. *N Engl J Med.* 1995;332:1467.

INFECTIONS OF THE CENTRAL NERVOUS SYSTEM*

Infections of the central nervous system (CNS) are associated with significant morbidity and mortality. Infections are caused by all types of pathogens from viruses to parasites. Organisms gain access to CNS most commonly by

- Hematogenous spread (e.g., bacterial endocarditis, nasopharyngeal colonization by *Neisseria meningitidis*)
- Direct extension from a contiguous site of infection (e.g., infected sinus)
- Direct invasion (e.g., surgery, trauma, basilar skull fracture)

Pathogenesis and signs and symptoms depend on the pathogen and site of infection, as discussed in subsequent text of this chapter and in other chapters. Primary infection may occur in the parenchyma of the CNS, as seen in encephalitis and brain abscess. Infections may also occur outside the parenchyma in locations bounded by the meninges:

- Epidural abscesses are localized in the space between the dura mater and the vertebrae.
- Meningitis occurs in the subarachnoid space (between the arachnoid and pia mater).
- Subdural abscesses are localized in the space between the dura mater and arachnoid.

Organisms may be directly visualized and isolated from CSF in patients with meningitis, as discussed later. In localized parenchymal, epidural, and subdural abscesses, organisms may not have access to the CSF, so Gram stain and culture of CSF are often negative, unless the abscess ruptures into the subarachnoid space. On the other hand, the immune response to abscesses may result in inflammatory changes detectable in the CSF, like increased WBC (usually without clear PMN predominance) and mildly elevated protein; CSF glucose is typically normal.

CENTRAL NERVOUS SYSTEM ABSCESSES

As in other tissues, CNS abscesses are localized infections with formation of pus. Disease is caused by tissue destruction and the inflammatory response to the primary infection. The forces caused by swelling of the nervous system parenchyma against the rigid structures of the skull may cause trauma (e.g., herniation) or vascular compromise. The infection may occur in the parenchyma of the brain, in the epidural or subdural space, or in other anatomic sites in the CNS. Hematogenous seeding should be suspected in patients with multiple abscesses (see eBook Figure 4-35).

A very wide variety of pathogens have been implicated in the etiology of brain abscesses. Monomicrobial and polymicrobial infections are well defined. The etiology depends on a number of factors, including age of the patient, anatomic site of infection, immune status of the patient, site of primary infection or source of organisms, and virulence of the infecting organism(s).

A broad etiology must be considered, especially in immunocompromised patients, including fungal and parasitic pathogens. *Toxoplasma gondii* reactivation

---

*Written by Michael Mitchell, MD.

should be considered in patients with defects in cell-mediated immunity, like HIV infection. Other parasitic pathogens, like *Taenia solium* or *Entamoeba histolytica*, must be considered in patients who have emigrated from endemic areas. Patients with arteriovenous malformations or other right-to-left shunts are at significantly increased risk for brain abscess.

Anaerobic organisms are frequently isolated, often as part of a polymicrobial flora. The species reflect the primary source of infection, which is commonly related to oropharyngeal, intra-abdominal, or pelvic infections. Pathogens include *Bacteroides, Prevotella, Fusobacterium, Propionibacterium*, and other species.

A wide variety of aerobic species are also implicated, including *Streptococcus* species, enteric gram-negative bacilli, and *S. aureus. Citrobacter* species have been implicated in brain abscesses and meningitis in neonates. *Klebsiella pneumoniae* has been implicated in brain abscesses associated with primary liver abscess.

❑ Clinical Presentation

Severe, sometimes localized headache unrelieved by over-the-counter analgesics is the most common symptom of brain abscess. Patients may have neck stiffness. Vomiting, change in mental status, and focal neurologic signs are signs of severe disease.

❑ Diagnosis and Laboratory Findings

Definitive diagnosis is usually made by aerobic and anaerobic culture, with Gram stain, of infected material. Patients with CNS abscesses should be carefully evaluated for increased intracranial pressure, especially prior to collection of CSF by lumbar puncture.

Typical laboratory findings include the following:

- Aspirate of infected pus should be cultured for aerobic and anaerobic bacteria, fungi, and mycobacteria, with Gram, AFB, and fungal stains.
- Histopathologic examination may provide specific diagnosis.
- CSF shows signs of inflammation, typically:
  ▼ WBC approximately 25–300/μL with increased neutrophils and lymphocytes.
  ▼ CSF protein may be normal or minimally or markedly increased (75 to >300 mg/dL).
  ▼ CSF glucose is often normal.
  ▼ Bacterial cultures of CSF may be negative, but laboratory signs of acute purulent meningitis may be seen if the abscess ruptures.
- Blood cultures are positive in approximately 10% of patients.
- Toxoplasma serology is recommended in patients with HIV infection. Other specific serologic testing is performed on the basis of epidemiologic risk.
- Laboratory findings due to associated primary disease.

ENCEPHALITIS

Encephalitis is a disease characterized by diffuse or localized inflammation of the brain parenchyma associated with neurologic dysfunction. Historically, viruses have been primary in the infectious etiology of encephalitis. Effective vaccination has reduced the incidence of several of the viruses that have been prominent causes of encephalitis, like mumps and measles viruses. The range of pathogens capable of causing encephalitis is broad. A specific diagnosis cannot be established in a significant number of patients with suspected infectious encephalitis. In patients in whom a diagnosis is established, approximately 70% are viral, approximately 20% bacterial, and approximately 10% other causes (prion, parasitic, fungal). Of note, *Mycoplasma pneumoniae* has been recognized as the cause of encephalitis in a significant proportion (approximately 30%) of children with encephalitis. Molecular testing is recommended; specific anti-*M. pneumoniae* serology was insensitive for detection. In addition, encephalitis and encephalopathy may be caused by a variety of noninfectious medical conditions.

A number of viruses are capable of causing encephalitis, either by direct infection or as an immune-mediated postinfection syndrome. Influenza; measles, mumps, and rubella; and varicella-zoster viruses have all been implicated in postinfectious encephalitis.

- *Herpes simplex virus*: HSV, usually type 1, is a common cause of sporadic encephalitis.
- *Arboviruses* (St. Louis, eastern equine, western equine, Venezuelan equine, West Nile): Arboviral encephalitis had been uncommon until the emergence of West Nile virus, which is now the most common cause of arboviral infection in the United States. These viruses show seasonal variability reflecting the distribution and activity of their mosquito vectors.
- *Rabies*: Rabies is uncommon in regions with effective vaccination programs, but low-level endemic infection is seen in host species inaccessible to vaccination, like bats and raccoons. Travel and animal exposure history are critical for timely diagnosis and treatment.
- *HIV*: HIV is neurotropic, and CNS involvement may result in a variety of types of neurologic dysfunction. In addition, severe immunosuppression associated with AIDS results in increased risk for opportunistic CNS pathogens, like CMV and JC virus.
- *Other viruses*: Encephalitis caused by other viruses is uncommon in the United States, but sporadic or epidemic encephalitis is seen in other countries caused by agents such as Arenavirus (lymphocytic choriomeningitis virus) and Nipah and Hendra viruses.

❏ Clinical Presentation
Patients present with headache, nausea, and vomiting; fever may be present. Patients usually develop changes in mental status, from subtle behavioral changes to frank obtundation. Seizures are common. Focal neurologic abnormalities may occur. Nuchal rigidity suggests a meningeal component (meningoencephalitis or isolated meningitis).

❏ Diagnosis and Laboratory Findings
Detailed history and physical examination are important in the assessment of patients. Some agents, such as rabies, may have restricted modes of transmission; other agents may show geographic restriction due to the range of the pathogen or intermediate vectors. Temporal lobe involvement suggests HSV infection. Preceding flaccid paralysis is suggestive of West Nile virus infection. Specific diagnostic testing should prioritize agents with the highest pretest probability based on presenting signs, symptoms, and epidemiology.

- CSF usually shows signs of inflammation, but these may be nonspecific. Findings overlap with aseptic meningitis and paraspinal abscesses. There is usually mild to moderate CSF pleocytosis (<250 cells/mm^3), with lymphocyte predominance. The presence of significant numbers of RBCs suggests a necrotizing encephalitis, like HSV. Protein may be mildly elevated (<150 mg/dL). CSF glucose is usually not decreased (>50% of simultaneous serum glucose concentration).
- CSF viral culture has a low diagnostic yield for CNS infections, especially for nonenteroviral and non-HSV CNS infections.
- West Nile virus should be carefully considered because of its frequency of occurrence.
- HSV should be ruled out by PCR in all patients with acute encephalitis of unknown cause because of its prominence in the differential diagnosis and the severity of sequelae in untreated infection.
- PCR is the diagnostic method of choice for most patients with acute encephalitis. The specific target pathogens are prioritized on the basis of pretest probability.
- Specific PCR for *M. pneumoniae* on CSF and throat specimens is recommended for children with acute encephalitis in whom another cause is not identified.
- Serologic testing is of limited value for patients with acute encephalitis but may be useful in patients in whom initial testing is not diagnostic. Serologic tests that may support specific diagnoses include detection of intrathecal antibody formation, production of serum or CSF IgM, or rise in antibody titer in acute and convalescent (typically >3 weeks after onset of symptoms) serum specimens. Demonstration of specific IgM in CSF provides a diagnosis of West Nile virus encephalitis.
- Brain biopsy, with routine and immunohistologic staining, may provide specific diagnosis for patients in whom initial testing by noninvasive testing is uninformative (see eBook Figure 4-36).
- In patients with postinfectious encephalitis, the virus responsible for the inflammatory response cannot be isolated from affected tissue.

MENINGITIS

Meningitis generally refers to infection in the subarachnoid space, the space between the middle (arachnoid) layer and the layer adjacent to the neural tissue (pia mater). Because the subarachnoid space is the major reservoir of CSF, CSF is usually the specimen of choice for tests to diagnose meningitis. The subarachnoid space is intrinsically "immunocompromised" outside of barrier defenses. There are relatively few phagocytic cells, and the concentrations of complement and antibodies are low. Bacteria that gain access to the subarachnoid space are able to proliferate efficiently. There is a high morbidity and mortality associated with acute bacterial meningitis, even when antibiotics are promptly administered. "Aseptic" meningitis refers generically to syndromes associated with signs and symptoms of meningeal irritation, but negative routine bacterial cultures.

Aseptic meningitis is usually caused by viruses, most commonly Enterovirus. A number of these viruses are also able to cause parenchymal infection, and distinguishing between meningitis, encephalitis, and meningoencephalitis can be challenging. Encephalitis is primarily characterized by neurologic dysfunction, whereas patients with aseptic meningitis most commonly present with photophobia, stiff neck, headache, and fever. Patients with severe aseptic meningitis, however, may develop seizures and altered mental status and progress to significant neurologic dysfunction.

A wide variety of viruses have been implicated as causing aseptic meningitis; the most common viruses are as follows:

- Enteroviruses: The incidence of enteroviral meningitis peaks in late summer and early fall, but enteroviruses cause low-level, endemic disease year-round.
- HSV-2: A significant percentage of patients with primary genital herpes simplex infection also demonstrate signs and symptoms of aseptic meningitis. HSV-2 may also cause recurrent aseptic meningitis associated with flares of genital infection.
- HIV: A subset of patients with primary HIV infection will develop signs and symptoms of aseptic meningitis or meningoencephalitis, which is usually self-limited.
- Lymphocytic choriomeningitis virus: The virus is transmitted by the urine or feces of mice and other small rodents. There is an increased rate of infection during the winter months, presumably due to increased exposure. Aseptic meningitis caused by lymphocytic choriomeningitis is unusual because CSF may show decreased glucose concentrations and WBC counts >1,000/mm^3. Diagnosis is usually established serologically.
- Mumps virus: Aseptic meningitis is a fairly frequent complication of mumps infection, but the incidence has significantly decreased due to effective vaccination programs. However, localized outbreaks continue to occur. This diagnosis may be suspected in patients with concurrent or recent parotitis.

Meningitis may be associated with CNS infection by parasitic, mycobacterial, fungal, and bacterial pathogens, as described in other sections. Other infectious agents to consider, based on clinical and laboratory findings, include

- Spirochetes (e.g., *Treponema pallidum, Borrelia burgdorferi*)
- Tick-borne agents (e.g., *Rickettsia* and *Ehrlichia* species)
- *Mycobacterium tuberculosis*
- Fungal pathogens (*Cryptococcus neoformans, Coccidioides immitis*), especially in immunocompromised patients (see eBook Figure 4-37)
- Parasites: (e.g., *Angiostrongylus*—suspect in patients with increased CSF eosinophils and risk based on epidemiology; amebas)

Aseptic meningitis may also be caused by malignancies, drugs, and other noninfectious causes.

Acute bacterial meningitis (ABM) is a medical emergency (see eBook Figure 4-38). Outcome depends on early administration of effective antibiotics and appropriate medical and neurosurgical interventions. Overall, *N. meningitidis* and *S. pneumoniae* cause a majority of cases of ABM, but the etiology of ABM depends on multiple factors. Age and route of transmission are major determinants:

- Neonates (<1 month): *Streptococcus agalactiae, E. coli, Listeria monocytogenes*, other enteric gram-negative bacteria. *Elizabethkingia meningoseptica* has been associated with outbreaks of meningitis in neonatal inpatient settings.
- Infants (1–23 months): *S. pneumoniae, N. meningitidis, S. agalactiae, Haemophilus influenzae, E. coli.*

- Older children and adults (2–50 years): *N. meningitidis, S. pneumoniae.*
- Elderly (>50 years): *N. meningitidis, S. pneumoniae, L. monocytogenes,* enteric gram-negative bacteria.
- Basilar skull fracture: *S. pneumoniae, Streptococcus pyogenes, H. influenzae.*
- Penetrating head trauma and postneurosurgical infections: staphylococci (coagulase positive and coagulase negative), aerobic gram-negative bacilli, *Propionibacterium acnes* (CSF shunts).

❑ **Clinical Presentation**

A significant proportion of adult patients with community-acquired ABM do not present with all of the classic clinical features (headache, fever, stiff neck, and altered mental status), but the majority will show at least two of the four. A significant minority of patients may be comatose on admission or show focal neurologic abnormalities. Seizures are present in approximately 5% of patients. Nonspecific symptoms are more frequent in infants and the elderly. Overall, the mortality rate is 20–25%; pneumococcal meningitis has a higher mortality rate than meningococcal (30% vs. 7%). Factors associated with increased mortality risk in patients with meningitis include:

- Age (>60 years)
- Otitis or sinusitis
- Absence of rash
- Low admission score on Glasgow Coma Scale
- Tachycardia (>120 beats/minute)
- Labs: Positive blood culture, increased ESR, decreased platelet count, low CSF WBC count (<1,000 cells/mm^3)

ABM caused by invasive medical procedures or by trauma is associated with a different etiology of infecting organisms, including *S. aureus* and enteric gram-negative bacilli. Signs and symptoms depend on the infecting organism as well as the predisposing event; those related to the trauma may overlap with those of the subsequent infection and may delay diagnosis and intervention.

The risk of meningitis is approximately 5–10% following compound skull fractures. The risk is increased when the wound is heavily contaminated with external material. Basilar skull fractures, which result in communication of the subarachnoid space with sinus cavities, are associated with a risk of meningitis up to 25%, with onset in the 2nd week after trauma. Persistent CSF leak may be associated with recurrent bacterial meningitis.

Fewer than 2% of craniotomy procedures results in bacterial meningitis. Two thirds of these infections occur within the first 2 weeks after the procedure.

Internal intraventricular catheters become infected in approximately 5–15% of cases, usually within the 1st month after placement, and usually represent intraoperative transmission. The incidence of infection of external CSF drainage catheters is <10%.

The risk of CNS infection caused by lumbar puncture is very low (approximately 1:50,000).

❑ **Diagnosis and Laboratory Findings**

When acute bacterial meningitis is suspected, appropriate laboratory testing and cultures should be collected, followed by empirical antibiotic therapy. HSV should be ruled out in patients if encephalitis is present.

- Diagnostic testing performed on CSF represents the primary approach to specific meningitis diagnosis. However, collection of CSF may be hazardous in patients with increased intracranial pressure (ICP). Cranial CT scan should be performed prior to lumbar puncture if clinical presentation suggests increased ICP. (Note: Imaging studies should not delay administration of antibiotics and dexamethasone therapy; blood cultures may be collected prior to imaging studies.) Clinical features significantly associated with increased ICP in adults include
  - ▼ Positive history of CNS disease
  - ▼ Immunocompromised state
  - ▼ Papilledema
  - ▼ Abnormal level of consciousness
  - ▼ Focal neurologic abnormalities
- Primary testing usually includes aerobic bacterial culture, Gram stain, and CSF concentration of protein and glucose. The opening pressure should be measured at the time of lumbar puncture.
- Blood cultures, CBC, and other basic metabolic tests should be undertaken for initial evaluation of all patients with suspected ABM.
  - ▼ CBC often shows changes related to acute infection (e.g., increased number of band forms, toxic granulations, Döhle bodies, vacuolization of PMNs).
  - ▼ ESR, CRP, or other tests may indicate an intense inflammatory response.
  - ▼ Infection may result in significant metabolic dysregulation.
- Gram stain is positive for the infecting organism in 25% of patients when organisms were present at 10^3 cfu/mL; sensitivity increased to 97% when organisms were present at 10^5 cfu/mL. The sensitivity of detection organisms by culture and Gram stain is improved by concentrating CSF, usually by centrifugation.
- The sensitivity of Gram stain depends on the infecting organism. Gram stain is positive in 90% of cases caused by staphylococci and pneumococci, 85% of cases caused by *H. influenzae*, 75% of cases caused by *N. meningitidis*, but only 30–50% of cases caused by gram-negative enteric bacilli. If antibiotics have been given before CSF obtained, Gram stain may be negative.
- Acridine orange staining may provide slightly greater sensitivity for detection of faintly staining organisms, but the technique requires use of a fluorescent microscope and technologist experience for smear interpretation.
- Testing for specific bacterial antigens may be used for rapid diagnosis in ABM. Kits are commercially available for detection of bacterial cell wall or capsular polysaccharide antigens of *H. influenzae* type b; *N. meningitidis* serogroups A, B, C, Y, and W135; *Streptococcus*, group B; and *S. pneumoniae*. Although tests show acceptable sensitivity and specificity, clinical studies suggest that the results of bacterial antigen testing rarely affect patient management; bacterial antigen testing is not recommended for routine evaluation of CSF in ABM.
- The most frequent and important differential diagnosis is between ABM and aseptic meningitis. The most useful test results are

▼ CSF identification of organism by stain or culture, specific nucleic acid, or antigen by PCR.

▼ Decreased CSF glucose or decreased CSF-to-serum glucose ratio if CSF glucose is normal.

▼ Increased CSF protein >1.72 mg/dL (1% of aseptic meningitis cases and 50% of ABM cases).

▼ CSF WBC >2,000/mm³ in 38% of ABM cases and PMN >1,180/mm³ but low counts do not rule out ABM.

■ Peripheral WBC count is only useful if WBC (>27,200/mm³) and total PMN (>21,000/mm³) counts are very high, which occurs in relatively few patients; leukopenia is common in infants and elderly.

■ CSF from patients with aseptic meningitis shows no organisms by Gram stain. WBC may be mildly elevated (<500 cells/mm³) with a lymphocyte predominance; protein may be moderately elevated; glucose level is usually normal.

■ CSF from patients with ABM typically demonstrates markedly increased WBC count (>1,000 cells/mm³), with a PMN predominance, increased protein (>100 mg/dL), and decreased glucose (<50% of serum glucose concentration). Opening pressure is increased (normal 100–200 mm Hg)

▼ In 50% of cases caused by *L. monocytogenes*, Gram stain may be negative; the cellular response is usually monocytic, which may cause this meningitis to be mistaken for aseptic meningitis.

■ Overall, CSF culture has a good sensitivity (70–92%) and high specificity (95%).

■ A sufficient amount of CSF must be collected to allow the testing required. Priority must be given to rule out ABM and HSV, when suspected. Repeat sampling may be needed if initial testing is not informative. A minimum of 3–5 mL of CSF should be collected for diagnostic testing for mycobacteria or fungi.

■ PCR methods have been developed for detection of some bacterial pathogens causing ABM, though FDA-approved methods are not available.

■ Gram stain of scrapings from petechial skin lesions demonstrates pathogen in approximately 70% of patients with meningococcemia; Gram stain of buffy coat of peripheral blood and, less often, peripheral blood smear may reveal this organism.

■ Laboratory findings due to preceding diseases/conditions:

▼ Pneumonia, otitis media, sinusitis, skull fracture prior to pneumococcal meningitis

▼ *Neisseria* epidemics prior to clinical cases of meningitis

▼ Bacterial endocarditis, septicemia, and so on

▼ *S. pneumoniae* in alcoholism, myeloma, sickle cell anemia, splenectomy, immunocompromised state

▼ *Cryptococcus* and *M. tuberculosis* in steroid therapy and immunocompromised state

▼ Gram-negative bacilli in immunocompromised state

▼ *H. influenzae* in splenectomy

▼ Lyme disease

- Primary diagnostic testing may also include other laboratory diagnostic tests for a patient in whom clinical presentation, epidemiologic risk factors, or signs and symptoms suggest a high prior probability of a pathogen outside the normal etiology of bacterial meningitis.
- Laboratory findings due to complications (e.g., Waterhouse-Friderichsen syndrome, subdural effusion)

Suggested Readings

Al Masalma M, Armougom F, Scheld WM, et al. The expansion of the microbiological spectrum of brain abscesses with use of multiple 16S ribosomal DNA sequencing. *Clin Infect Dis.* 2009;48:1169–1178.

Bitnun A, Ford-Jones EL, Petric M, et al. Acute childhood encephalitis and *Mycoplasma pneumoniae. Clin Infect Dis.* 2001;32:1674–1684.

Darouiche RO. Spinal epidural abscess. *N Engl J Med.* 2006;355:2012–2020.

Dumpis U, Crook D, Oksi J. Tick-borne encephalitis. *Clin Infect Dis.* 1999;28:882–890.

Glaser CA, Honarmand S, Anderson LJ, et al. Beyond viruses: clinical profiles and etiologies associated with encephalitis. *Clin Infect Dis.* 2006;43:1565–1577.

Hayden RT, Frenkel LD. More laboratory testing: greater cost but not necessarily better. *Pediatr Infect Dis J.* 2000;19:290–292.

Marciano-Cabral F, Cabral G. *Acanthamoeba* spp. as agents of disease in humans. *Clin Microbiol Rev.* 2003;16:273–307.

Matin A, Siddiqui R, Jayasekera S, et al. Increasing importance of *Balamuthia mandrillaris. Clin Microbiol Rev.* 2008;21:435–448.

Maxson S, Lewno MJ, Schutze GE. Clinical usefulness of cerebrospinal fluid bacterial antigen studies. *J Pediatr.* 1994;125:235–238.

Polage CR, Petti CA. Assessment of the utility of viral culture of cerebrospinal fluid. *Clin Infect Dis.* 2006;43:1578–1579.

Pradilla G, Ardila GP, Hsu W, et al. Epidural abscesses of the CNS. *Lancet Neurol.* 2009;8:292–300.

Tarafdar K, Rao S, Recco RA, et al. Lack of sensitivity of the latex agglutination test to detect bacterial antigen in the cerebrospinal fluid of patients with culture-negative meningitis. *Clin Infect Dis.* 2001;33:406–408.

Tattevin P, Bruneel F, Clair B, et al. Bacterial brain abscesses: a retrospective study of 94 patients admitted to an intensive care unit (1980 to 1999). *Am J Med.* 2003;115:143–146.

Tunkel AR, Glaser CA, Bloch KC, et al. The management of encephalitis: clinical practice guidelines by the Infectious Diseases Society of America. *Clin Infect Dis.* 2008;47:303–27.

van de Beek D, de Gans J, Spanjaard L, et al. Clinical features and prognostic factors in adults with bacterial meningitis. *N Engl J Med.* 2004;351:1849–1859.

van de Beek D, Drake JM, Tunkel AR. Nosocomial bacterial meningitis. *N Engl J Med.* 2010;362:146–154.

van de Beek D, de Gans J, Tunkel AR, et al. Community-acquired bacterial meningitis in adults. *N Engl J Med.* 2006;354:44–53.

CHAPTER 5

Digestive Diseases

L. Michael Snyder and Michael J. Mitchell

5

This chapter focuses on several common GI clinical presentations: abdominal pain (acute and chronic); ascites; diarrhea (acute and chronic); GI bleeding upper and lower; hepatomegaly; jaundice and associated diseases, including hepatitis. When appropriate, the discussion includes radiologic and endoscopic procedures as part of the diagnostic evaluation.

 ## DISEASE STATES ASSOCIATED WITH ABDOMINAL PAIN (ACUTE AND CHRONIC)

❑ Definition
Acute abdomen is defined as an episode of severe abdominal pain that lasts several hours or longer and requires medical attention. The acute abdomen usually, but not necessarily, has a surgical cause. However, the term "acute abdomen" should not be equated with a need for emergency surgery. The history and physical examination remain the most important aspects of diagnosis. The key feature in the evaluation of patients with acute abdomen is early diagnosis.

❑ Differential Diagnosis
- The differential diagnosis of an acute abdomen is most appropriately considered by its anatomic location (Table 5-1).
- Common gynecologic causes of lower quadrant pain include mittelschmerz, ovarian cyst, endometriosis, fibroids, ovarian torsion, pelvic inflammatory disease, ovarian tumor, ectopic pregnancy, infection of the uterus, threatened abortion, and round ligament pain secondary to pregnancy.

TABLE 5–1. Differential Diagnosis of the Acute Abdomen

Right Upper Quadrant Pain	Right Lower Quadrant Pain
Cholecystitis	Appendicitis
Choledocholithiasis	Ruptured ovarian cyst
Cholangitis	Meckel diverticulitis
Hepatitis	Cecal diverticulitis
Liver tumors	Cholecystitis
Hepatic abscess	Perforated colon
Appendicitis	Colon cancer
Peptic ulcer disease (PUD)	Urinary tract infection
Perforated ulcer	Small bowel obstruction
Pancreatitis	Inflammatory bowel disease (IBD)
Gastritis	Nephrolithiasis
Pyelonephritis	Pyelonephritis
Nephrolithiasis	Ectopic pregnancy
Pneumonia	Bowel incarceration
	Pelvic inflammatory disease (PID)

Left Upper Quadrant Pain	Lower Left Quadrant Pain
PUD	Diverticulitis
Perforated ulcer	Sigmoid volvulus
Gastritis	Perforated colon
Splenic disease (e.g., infarct, abscess, or rupture)	Colon cancer
Gastroesophageal reflux disease	Urinary tract infection
Dissecting aortic aneurysm	Small bowel obstruction
Pyelonephritis	IBD
Nephrolithiasis	Nephrolithiasis
Hiatal hernia	Pyelonephritis
Boerhaave syndrome (i.e., rupture of the esophagus)	Ectopic pregnancy
Mallory-Weiss tear	Incarceration
Diverticulitis	PID
Bowel obstruction	

Midepigastric Pain
PUD
Perforated ulcer
Pancreatitis
Abdominal aortic aneurysm
Esophageal varices
Hiatal hernia
Boerhaave syndrome (i.e., rupture of the esophagus)
Mallory-Weiss tear

■ Medical conditions that may present as acute abdomen are many. Common examples include lower lobe pneumonias, acute myocardial infarction (MI), DKA, acute hepatitis, porphyria, adrenal hemorrhage, and musculoskeletal problems. Appendicitis is a clinical diagnosis. The triad of right lower quadrant pain, anorexia, and leukocytosis is the most sensitive diagnostic tool. Nausea and vomiting usually follow the onset of pain. The patient may have a low-grade fever and mild leukocytosis. Fevers with higher temperatures or increased WBC counts suggest perforation.

- Thirty percent of patients with appendicitis have an elevated WBC count, whereas 95% have a left shift.
- The intensity of pain is somewhat in proportion to the degree of irritation to the parietal peritoneum. Therefore, a retrocecal appendix (which is the most common location) may cause only a dull ache, given the lack of contact with the parietal peritoneum.

❏ **Laboratory Findings**

- Laboratory studies are undertaken to support a clinical hypothesis. The evaluation generally includes a CBC, liver chemistries, amylase and lipase, coagulation profile, urinalysis, and urine pregnancy test.
  - ▼ Lactic acid level should be obtained for patients with suspected ischemic bowel. An elevated level is associated with tissue hypoperfusion.
  - ▼ Beta-hCG levels must be obtained for all women of childbearing age to exclude the possibility of ectopic pregnancy.
- Radiographic studies:
  - ▼ Chest radiograph should be obtained on all patients with acute abdomen to rule out free air. Pneumonia may present as an acute abdomen.
  - ▼ Abdominal radiograph is most effective in detecting either bowel obstruction or pneumoperitoneum. An upright and supine view is necessary.
    - Appendicolith can be seen in 15% of patients with appendicitis, whereas renal stones may also be visualized up to 85% of the time.
    - Other radiographic findings of acute appendicitis include right lower quadrant ileus, loss of psoas shadow, deformity of the cecal outline, free air, and soft tissue density.
- Abdominal ultrasound is the study of choice in patients with possible acute cholecystitis or ovarian cyst. A sonographic Murphy sign is more sensitive than a clinical Murphy sign for acute cholecystitis. An inflamed appendix can be visualized with compression ultrasound (sensitivity ranges from 80 to 90%).
- CT can also be used to diagnose appendicitis in patients whose clinical symptoms are ambiguous.
  - ▼ Air in the appendix or a normal-appearing contrast-filled appendix virtually rules out the diagnosis of appendicitis.
  - ▼ CT will provide an alternate diagnosis in 15% of patients when assessing for appendicitis.
- Arteriography is the test of choice for patients with suspected mesenteric ischemia.

 # DISEASE STATES ASSOCIATED WITH ABDOMINAL PAIN

DISORDERS OF THE ESOPHAGUS

MALLORY-WEISS SYNDROME

❏ **Definition**

Mallory-Weiss syndrome is characterized by spontaneous cardioesophageal laceration, usually caused by excessive retching. Laboratory findings are due to hemorrhage from cardioesophageal laceration.

PERFORATION OF THE ESOPHAGUS, SPONTANEOUS

In spontaneous perforation, gastric contents are found in thoracocentesis fluid.

PLUMMER-VINSON SYNDROME

❏ **Definition**
Plummer-Vinson syndrome is an iron deficiency anemia associated with dysphagia, atrophic gastritis, glossitis, and so on. It carries an increased risk of cancer of the esophagus and hypopharynx.

DISORDERS OF THE STOMACH

GASTRITIS, CHRONIC

- A diagnosis of chronic gastritis depends on biopsy of gastric mucosa.

❏ **Atrophic (Type A Gastritis, Autoimmune Type)**
- Gastric antrum is spared.
- Parietal cell antibodies and intrinsic factor antibodies help identify those patients prone to pernicious anemia (PA).
- Characteristics include the following:
  - ▼ Achlorhydria
  - ▼ Vitamin B_{12}–deficient megaloblastosis
  - ▼ Hypergastrinemia (due to hyperplasia of gastrin-producing cells)
  - ▼ Gastric carcinoids
  - ▼ Low serum pepsinogen I concentrations
- Laboratory findings may be due to other accompanying autoimmune diseases (e.g., Hashimoto thyroiditis, Addison disease, Graves disease, myasthenia gravis, hypoparathyroidism, type 1 DM).

❏ **Nonatrophic (Type B Gastritis)**
- Gastric antrum is involved.
- Anemia caused by iron deficiency, and malabsorption may occur.
- *Helicobacter pylori* infection is detectable in approximately 80% of patients with peptic ulcer and chronic gastritis. Diagnosis is by biopsy, culture, direct Gram staining, urease breath test, and serologic tests.
- Hypogastrinemia is caused by destruction of gastrin-producing cells in the antrum.
- Chronic antral gastritis is consistently present in patients with benign gastric ulcer.
- Gastric acid studies are of limited value. Severe hypochlorhydria or achlorhydria after maximal stimulation usually denotes mucosal atrophy.

❏ **Other Causes**
- Infections (other bacteria [syphilis], viral [e.g., CMV], parasitic [e.g., anisakiasis], fungal)
- Chemical (e.g., NSAIDs, bile reflux, other drugs)
- Lymphocytic gastritis

- Eosinophilic gastroenteritis
- Noninfectious granulomatous (e.g., sarcoidosis, Crohn disease)
- Ménétrier disease
- Radiation

CARCINOMA OF THE STOMACH

❏ Laboratory Findings
Carcinoma of the stomach should always be searched for by periodic prophylactic screening in high-risk patients, especially those with PA, gastric atrophy, or gastric polyps.

Cytology: Exfoliative cytology positive in 80% of patients; false-positive result in <2%.

Tumor markers: Increased serum CEA (>5 ng/dL) in 40–50% of patients with metastases and 10–20% of patients with surgically resectable disease. May be useful for postoperative monitoring for recurrence or to estimate metastatic tumor burden. Increased serum AFP and CA 19-9 in 30% of patients, usually incurable. Markers are not useful for early detection.

Gastric analysis: Normal in 25% of patients. Hypochlorhydria in 25% of patients. Achlorhydria following histamine or betazole in 50% of patients.

Core laboratory: Anemia due to chronic blood loss. Occult blood in stool.

DISORDERS OF THE PANCREAS

CARCINOMA OF THE PANCREAS

BODY OR TAIL
❏ Laboratory Findings
Imaging studies: Most useful tests are ultrasound or CT scanning followed by ERCP (at which time fluid is also obtained for cytologic and pancreatic function studies). This combination will correctly diagnose or rule out cancer of the pancreas in ≥90% of cases. ERCP with brush cytology has S/S = ≤25%/≤100%. Radioisotope scanning of the pancreas may be done (75Se) for lesions >2 cm.

Histology: Ultrasound-guided needle biopsy has reported sensitivity of 80–90%; false positives are rare.

Tumor markers: Serum markers for tumor (CA 19-9, CEA, and so on) are often normal. In carcinoma of the pancreas, CA 19-9 has S/S = 70%/87%, PPV = 59%, and NPV = 92%; there is no difference in sensitivity between local disease and metastatic disease. Often normal in early stages, they are *not useful for screening*. Increased values may help differentiate benign disease from cancer. Declines to normal in 3–6 months if cancer is completely removed so may be useful for prognosis and follow-up. Detects tumor recurrence 2–20 weeks before clinical evidence. Not specific for pancreas because high levels may also occur in other GI cancers, especially those affecting the colon and bile duct. CEA level in bile (obtained by percutaneous transhepatic drainage) was reported increased in 76% of a small group of cases.

Testosterone: Dihydrotestosterone ratio <5 (normal approximately 10) in >70% of men with pancreatic cancer (due to increased conversion by tumor); less sensitive but more specific than CA 19-9 and present in higher proportion of stage I tumors.

Serum amylase and lipase: May be slightly increased in early stages (<10% of cases); with later destruction of the pancreas, they are normal or decreased. They may increase following secretin–pancreozymin stimulation before destruction is extensive; therefore, the increase is less marked with a diabetic glucose tolerance curve. Serum amylase response is less reliable. See Serum Glycoprotein 2.

Glucose tolerance: Curve is of the diabetic type, with overt diabetes in 20% of patients with pancreatic cancer. Flat blood sugar curve with IV tolbutamide tolerance test indicates destruction of islet cell tissue. *Unstable, insulin-sensitive diabetes that develops in an older man should arouse suspicion of carcinoma of the pancreas.*

Serum LAP: Increased (>300 U) in 60% of patients with carcinoma of the pancreas due to liver metastases or biliary tract obstruction. *It may also be increased in chronic liver disease.*

Other: Triolein-^{131}I test demonstrates pancreatic duct obstruction with absence of lipase in the intestine, causing flat blood curves and increased stool excretion.

HEAD (SEE JAUNDICE)

■ The abnormal pancreatic function tests and increased tumor markers that occur with carcinoma of the body of the pancreas may be evident.

❑ Laboratory Findings

Core laboratory: Serum bilirubin is increased (12–25 mg/dL), mostly conjugated (increase persistent and nonfluctuating). Serum ALP is increased. Both urine and stool urobilinogen are absent. Increased serum cholesterol (usually >300 mg/dL) with esters not decreased. Other liver function tests are usually normal. See Serum Glycoprotein 2.

Hematology: Increased prothrombin time (PT); normal after IV vitamin K administration.

Other: Secretin–cholecystokinin stimulation evidences duct obstruction when duodenal intubation shows decreased volume of duodenal contents (<10 mL/10-minute collection period) with usually normal bicarbonate and enzyme levels in duodenal contents. Acinar destruction (as in pancreatitis) shows normal volume (20–30 mL/10-minute collection period), but bicarbonate and enzyme levels may be decreased. Abnormal volume, bicarbonate, or both are found in 60–80% of patients with pancreatitis or cancer. In carcinoma, the test result depends on the relative extent and combination of acinar destruction and of duct obstruction.

Histology: Cytologic examination of duodenal contents shows malignant cells in 40% of patients. Malignant cells may be found in up to 80% of patients with periampullary cancer.

CYSTIC FIBROSIS OF THE PANCREAS

Core laboratory: Hypochloremic metabolic alkalosis and hypokalemia. Serum protein electrophoresis shows increasing IgG and IgA with progressive pulmonary disease; IgM and IgD are not appreciably increased. Serum albumin is often decreased (because of hemodilution due to cor pulmonale; may be found before cardiac involvement is clinically apparent). Serum chloride, sodium, potassium, calcium, and phosphorus are normal unless complications occur (e.g., chronic pulmonary disease with accumulation of CO_2; massive salt loss due to sweating may cause hyponatremia). Urine electrolytes are normal. Excessive loss of electrolytes in sweat and stool. Impaired glucose intolerance in approximately 40% of patients with glycosuria, and hyperglycemia in 8% precedes DM. Protein–calorie malnutrition, hypoproteinemia; fat malabsorption with vitamin deficiency. Stool and duodenal fluid show lack of trypsin digestion of x-ray film gelatin; useful screening test up to age 4; decreased chymotrypsin production.

Saliva findings: Submaxillary saliva is more turbid, with increased calcium, total protein, amylase, chloride, and sodium but not potassium. These changes are not generally found in parotid saliva.

Other findings: Overt liver disease, including cirrhosis, fatty liver, bile duct strictures, and cholelithiasis, in ≤5% of cases. Meconium ileus during early infancy. Chronic or acute and recurrent pancreatitis. Pancreatic insufficiency frequency by age 1 >90%; in adults >95%. Increased incidence of GI tract cancers. GU tract abnormalities with aspermia in 98% due to obstructive changes in the vas deferens and epididymis are confirmed by testicular biopsy.

MACROAMYLASEMIA IN VIVO ARTIFACT

❏ Definition
Complex of amylase with IgA, IgG, or other high molecular weight plasma proteins that cannot filter through the glomerulus due to its large size associated with no specific symptoms or disease states.

❏ Laboratory Findings
Core laboratory: Serum lipase is normal; normal pancreatic-to-salivary amylase ratio. Urine amylase normal or low. Serum amylase *persistently* increased (often 1–4× normal) without apparent cause. Amylase–creatinine clearance ratio <1% with normal renal function is very useful for this diagnosis; should make the clinician suspect this diagnosis. Macroamylase is identified in serum by special gel filtration or ultracentrifugation technique.

❏ Limitations
- Macroamylase may be found in approximately 1% of randomly selected patients and 2.5% of persons with increased serum amylase level. Same findings may also occur in patients with normal molecular weight hyperamylasemia in which excess amylase is principally salivary gland isoamylase types 2 and 3.

PANCREATITIS

PANCREATITIS, ACUTE

❏ Laboratory Findings
Lipase: Serum lipase increases within 3–6 hours with peak at 24 hours and usually returns to normal over a period of 8–14 days; is superior to amylase; increases to a greater extent and may remain elevated for up to 14 days after amylase returns to normal. In patients with signs of acute pancreatitis, pancreatitis is highly likely (clinical specificity = 85%) when lipase ≥5× upper reference limit (URL); if values

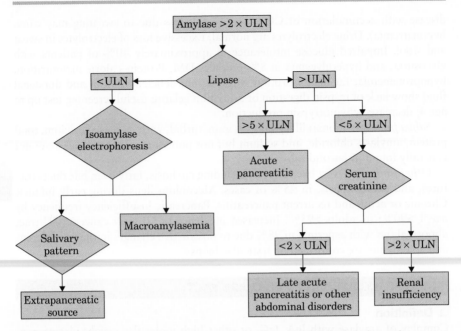

Figure 5–1 *Algorithm for increased serum amylase and lipase. ULN, upper limit of normal.*

change significantly with time, and if amylase and lipase changes are concordant. (*Lipase should always be determined whenever amylase is determined.*) Urinary lipase is not clinically useful. It has been suggested that a lipase:amylase ratio >3 (and especially >5) indicates alcoholic rather than nonalcoholic pancreatitis. If lipase ≥5x URL, acute pancreatitis or organ rejection is highly likely but unlikely if <3x URL (Figure 5-1).

Amylase: Increase begins in 3–6 hours, rises rapidly within 8 hours in 75% of patients, reaches maximum in 20–30 hours, and may persist for 48–72 hours; >95% sensitivity during the first 12–24 hours. The increase may be ≤40x normal, but the height of the increase and rate of fall do not correlate with the severity of the disease, prognosis, or rate of resolution. In patients with signs of acute pancreatitis, amylase >3x ULN or >600 Somogyi units/dL is very suggestive of acute pancreatitis. An increase >7–10 days suggests an associated cancer of the pancreas or pseudocyst, pancreatic ascites, or nonpancreatic etiology. Similar high values may occur in obstruction of the pancreatic duct; they tend to fall after several days; ≤19% of patients with acute pancreatitis (especially when seen more than 2 days after onset of symptoms) may have normal values, especially with an alcoholic etiology and longer duration of symptoms, even when dying of acute pancreatitis. May also be normal in relapsing chronic pancreatitis and patients with hypertriglyceridemia (technical interference with test). Frequently normal in acute alcoholic pancreatitis. Acute abdomen due to GI infarction or perforation rather than acute pancreatitis is suggested by only moderate increase in serum amylase and lipase (<3x URL), evidence of bacteremia. Of patients with acute alcoholic intoxication, 10–40% have elevated serum amylase (about half are salivary type); they often present with abdominal pain, but increased serum amylase is usually <3x URL.

Levels >25× URL indicate metastatic tumor rather than pancreatitis. Serum pancreatic isoamylase can distinguish elevations due to salivary amylase that may account for 25% of all elevated values. (In healthy persons, 40% of total serum amylase is pancreatic type and 60% is salivary type.) Only slight increase in serum amylase and lipase values suggests a different diagnosis than acute pancreatitis. *Many drugs increase both amylase and lipase in serum.*

Increased urinary amylase tends to reflect serum changes by a time lag of 6–10 hours, but sometimes, increased urine levels are higher and of longer duration than serum levels. The 24-hour level may be normal even when some of the 1-hour specimens show increased values. Amylase levels in hourly samples of urine may be useful. Ratio of amylase clearance to creatinine clearance is increased (>5%) and avoids the problem of timed urine specimens; also increased in any condition that decreases tubular reabsorption of amylase (e.g., severe burns, DKA, chronic renal insufficiency, multiple myeloma, acute duodenal perforation). Considered not specific and now discouraged by some but still recommended by others.

Calcium: Serum level is decreased in severe cases 1–9 days after onset (due to binding to soaps in fat necrosis). The decrease usually occurs after amylase and lipase levels have become normal. Tetany may occur. (*Rule out hyperparathyroidism if serum calcium is high or fails to fall in hyperamylasemia of acute pancreatitis.*)

Bilirubin: Serum levels may be increased when pancreatitis is of biliary tract origin but is usually normal in alcoholic pancreatitis. Serum ALP, ALT, and AST may increase and parallel serum bilirubin rather than amylase, lipase, or calcium levels. Marked amylase increase (e.g., >2,000 U/L) also favors biliary tract origin. Fluctuation >50% in 24 hours of serum bilirubin, ALP, ALT, and AST suggests intermittent biliary obstruction.

Trypsin: Serum level is increased. High sensitivity makes a normal value useful for excluding acute pancreatitis. But low specificity (increased in large proportion of patients with hepatobiliary, bowel, and other diseases and renal insufficiency; increased in 13% of patients with chronic pancreatitis, 50% with pancreatic carcinoma) and RIA technology limit utility.

CRP: Level peaks 3 days after onset of pain; at 48 hours, sensitivity = 65–100%, PPV = 37–77%. Level of 150 mg/L distinguishes mild from severe disease.

Laboratory criteria for severe disease or predictor of mortality:

- PaO_2 <60 μmol/L
- Creatinine >2 mg/dL after rehydration
- Blood glucose >250 mg/dL
- Hemoconcentration (Hct >47% or failure to decrease in 24 hours after admission), but Hct may be decreased in severe hemorrhagic pancreatitis
- GI bleed >500 mL/24 hours
- Presence, volume, and color of peritoneal fluid
- Methemalbumin may be increased in serum and ascitic fluid (AF) in hemorrhagic (severe) but not edematous (mild) pancreatitis; may distinguish these two conditions but not useful in diagnosis of acute pancreatitis.
- WBC is slightly to moderately increased (10,000–20,000/μL).
- Glycosuria appears in 25% of patients.
- Hypokalemia, metabolic alkalosis, or lactic acidosis may occur.

Laboratory findings due to predisposing conditions (may be multiple):

- Alcohol abuse accounts for approximately 36% of cases.
- Biliary tract disease accounts for 17% of cases.
- Idiopathic accounts for >36% of cases.
- Infections (especially viral such as mumps and coxsackievirus, CMV, and AIDS).
- Trauma and postoperative factors account for >8% of cases.
- Drugs (e.g., steroids, thiazides, azathioprine, estrogens, sulfonamides; children taking valproic acid) account for >5% of cases.
- Hypertriglyceridemia (hyperlipidemia—types V, I, IV) accounts for 7% of cases.
- Hypercalcemia from any cause.
- Tumors (pancreas, ampulla).
- Anatomic abnormalities of the ampullary region causing obstruction (e.g., annular pancreas, Crohn disease, duodenal diverticulum).
- Hereditary.
- Renal failure; renal transplantation.
- Miscellaneous (e.g., collagen vascular disease, pregnancy, ischemia, scorpion bites, parasites obstructing the pancreatic duct [*Ascaris*, fluke], Reye syndrome, fulminant hepatitis, severe hypotension, cholesterol embolization).

Laboratory findings due to complications:

- Pseudocysts of the pancreas.
- Pancreatic infection or abscess diagnosed by increased WBC count, Gram staining, and culture of aspirate.
- Polyserositis (peritoneal, pleural, pericardial, synovial surfaces). Ascites may develop cloudy or bloody or "prune juice" fluid, 0.5–2.0 L in volume, containing increased amylase with a level higher than that of serum amylase. No bile is evident (unlike in perforated ulcer). Gram stain shows no bacteria (unlike infarct of the intestine). Protein >3 g/dL and marked increase in amylase.
- Adult respiratory distress syndrome (with pleural effusion, alveolar exudate, or both) may occur in approximately 40% of patients; arterial hypoxemia is present.
- DIC.
- Hypovolemic shock.
- Others.

❏ **Prognostic Laboratory Findings**

- On admission
  WBC >16,000/µL
  Blood glucose >200 mg/dL
  Serum LD >350 U/L
  Serum AST >250 U/L
  Age >55 years

- Within 48 hours
  >10% decrease in Hct
  Serum calcium <8.0 mg/dL
  Increase in BUN >5 mg/dL
  Arterial pO_2 <60 mm Hg
  Metabolic acidosis with base deficit >4 mEq/L

- Mortality
  1%, if 3 signs are positive
  15%, if 3 to 4 signs are positive
  40%, if 5 to 6 signs are positive
  100%, if ≥7 signs are positive
- Degree of amylase elevation has no prognostic significance.
- CT scan, MRI, and ultrasound are useful for confirming diagnosis or identifying causes or other conditions.

Suggested Readings

Papachristou GI, Whitcomb DC. Inflammatory markers of disease severity in acute pancreatitis. *Clin Lab Med.* 2005;25:17.
Whitcomb DC. Acute pancreatitis. *N Engl J Med.* 2006;354:2142.

PANCREATITIS, CHRONIC

- See also Malabsorption.

❏ Laboratory Findings

Laboratory findings are often normal.

Imaging studies: CT, ultrasound, and ERCP are most accurate for diagnosing and staging chronic pancreatitis. Radioactive scanning of the pancreas (selenium) yields variable findings in different clinics.

Cholecystokinin–secretin test: Measures the effect of IV administration of cholecystokinin and secretin on volume, bicarbonate concentration, and amylase output of duodenal contents and increase in serum lipase and amylase. This is the most sensitive and reliable test (gold standard) for chronic pancreatitis especially in the early stages. However, it is technically difficult and is often not performed accurately; gastric contamination must be avoided. Some abnormality occurs in >85% of patients with chronic pancreatitis. Amylase output is the most frequent abnormality. When all three are abnormal, there is a greater frequency of abnormality in the tests listed below.

- Normal duodenal contents:
  - ▼ Volume: 95–235 mL/hour
  - ▼ Bicarbonate concentration: 74–121 mEq/L
  - ▼ Amylase output: 87,000–276,000 mg
- Serum amylase and lipase increase after administration of cholecystokinin and secretin in approximately 20% of patients with chronic pancreatitis. They are more often abnormal when duodenal contents are normal. Normally serum lipase and amylase do not rise above normal limits.
- Fasting serum amylase and lipase are increased in 10% of patients with chronic pancreatitis.

Serum pancreolauryl test: Fluorescein dilaurate with breakfast is acted on by a pancreas-specific cholesterol ester hydrolase–releasing fluorescein, which is absorbed from gut and measured in serum; preceded by administration of secretin and followed by metoclopramide. Reported S/S = 82%/91%.

Glucose tolerance test (GTT): In 65% of patients with chronic pancreatitis and frank diabetes in >10% of patients with chronic relapsing pancreatitis. When GTT is normal in the presence of steatorrhea, the cause should be sought elsewhere than in the pancreas.

Laboratory findings due to malabsorption: Occurs when >90% of exocrine function is lost.

- Bentiromide test is usually abnormal with moderate to severe pancreatic insufficiency but often normal in early cases.
- Schilling test may show mild malabsorption of vitamin B_{12} (no longer performed).
- Xylose tolerance test and small bowel biopsy are not usually done but are normal.
- Chemical determination of fecal fat demonstrates steatorrhea. It is more sensitive than tests using triolein-[131]I.
- Triolein-^{131}I is abnormal in one third of patients with chronic pancreatitis.
- Starch tolerance test is abnormal in 25% of patients with chronic pancreatitis.

  Laboratory findings due to chronic pancreatitis and pancreatic exocrine insufficiency:
- Alcohol in 60–70%
- Idiopathic in 30–40%
- Obstruction of pancreatic duct (e.g., trauma, pseudocyst, pancreas divisum, cancer, or obstruction of duct or ampulla)
- Others occasionally (e.g., CF, primary hyperparathyroidism, heredity, malnutrition, miscellaneous [Z-E syndrome, Shwachman syndrome, $alpha_1$-antitrypsin deficiency, trypsinogen deficiency, enterokinase deficiency, hemochromatosis, parenteral hyperalimentation])

PSEUDOCYST OF THE PANCREAS

❏ Laboratory Findings

Imaging studies: Detected by ultrasound or CT scan.

Core laboratory: Serum conjugated bilirubin is increased (>2 mg/dL) in 10% of patients. Serum ALP is increased in 10% of patients. Fasting blood sugar is increased in <10% of patients.

Secretin–pancreozymin stimulation: Duodenal contents usually show decreased bicarbonate content (<70 mEq/L) but normal volume and normal content of amylase, lipase, and trypsin.

Pancreatic cyst fluid findings: High fluid viscosity and CEA indicate mucinous differentiation and exclude pseudocyst, serous cystadenoma, other nonmucinous cysts, or cystic tumors. Pancreatic enzymes, leukocyte esterase, and NB/70K are increased in pseudocyst fluid. Increased CA 72-4, CA 15-3, and tissue polypeptide antigen are markers of malignancy; if all are low, pseudocyst or serous cystadenoma is most likely. CA 125 is increased in serous cystadenoma.

Other: Laboratory findings due to conditions preceding acute pancreatitis are noted (e.g., alcoholism, trauma, duodenal ulcer, cholelithiasis), infection, perforation, and hemorrhage by erosion of blood vessel or into a viscus.

DYSPEPSIA AND PEPTIC ULCER DISEASE

❏ **Definition**

- Dyspepsia encompasses any or all of a great variety of upper abdominal symptoms, including upper abdominal pain or discomfort, nausea, bloating, heartburn, early satiety, regurgitation, and belching.
- Nonulcerative dyspepsia is defined as persistent or recurrent abdominal pain or discomfort centered in the upper abdomen without definite structural or biochemical explanation. By definition, nonulcerative dyspepsia is a diagnosis of exclusion. Possible mechanisms include dysmotility of the stomach or small intestine, heightened visceral sensitivity, altered intestinal or gastric reflexes, and psychological distress.
- Peptic ulcer disease (PUD)
    - ▼ Epigastric abdominal pain is the most common symptom. Pain is nonradiating and is described as a "gnawing" or "hunger pain." Pain occurs 1–2 hours postprandially and is relieved characteristically by food or antacids.
    - ▼ Nocturnal pain is more specific for PUD and is due to the physiologic increase in acid secretion, which occurs in the early morning hours.
    - ▼ Asymptomatic:
        - Patients with PUD induced by NSAIDs are frequently asymptomatic.
        - As many as 60% of patients who develop bleeding as a complication of PUD are also asymptomatic.
- Dyspepsia is typically a chronic relapsing condition. Between 65% and 86% of patients with dyspepsia will experience dyspeptic symptoms, at least intermittently, 2 to 3 years after the initial presentation. Long duration of symptoms and intermittent symptoms can also occur in PUD and esophagitis; therefore, these characteristics are not reassuring as to the absence of pathology.
- Gastroesophageal reflux disease (GERD) and dyspepsia have similar symptoms. Gastroesophageal reflux is a normal physiologic process that occurs daily in all individuals. GERD (expressed clinically as heartburn).
- *Helicobacter pylori* infection is clearly implicated in the etiology of recurrent PUD, yet its role in nonulcerative dyspepsia remains unclear. Between 30% and 60% of patients with nonulcerative dyspepsia have *H. pylori*. However, the background prevalence in the general population is also high.

❏ **Recommended Tests**

- Laboratory investigation may not be necessary in young patients (<45 years of age) who have a normal examination and no indicators for organic disease. The etiology of dyspepsia is presented in Table 5-2.
- In older patients at increased risk, the minimal laboratory workup should include a CBC, electrolytes, calcium, and liver chemistries.
- Thyroid tests, hCG, amylase, and stool studies should be ordered if specific features of the history or examination are suggestive.
- *Additional studies*
    - ▼ *Upper endoscopy* (i.e., esophagogastroduodenoscopy [EGD]): In the majority of cases, this is the study of first choice when further evaluation of dyspepsia is required, including the ability to obtain biopsies. As many as two thirds of endoscopies are completely normal in younger patients

TABLE 5–2. Differential Diagnosis of Dyspepsia

Structural Disease Involving the Stomach or Esophagus

Peptic ulcer disease (15–25% of cases)
Reflux esophagitis (5–15% of cases)
Gastric or esophageal cancer (<2% of cases)
Infiltrative disease
Eosinophilic gastritis
Crohn disease
Sarcoidosis

Other gastrointestinal-related diseases

Gallstones
Chronic pancreatitis or pancreatic cancer
Celiac disease
Lactose intolerance
Hepatoma

Medications

Nonsteroidal anti-inflammatory drugs
Digitalis
Theophylline
Erythromycin
Alcohol
Caffeine
Nicotine

Other possible causes

Hypothyroidism
Hypercalcemia
Intestinal angina
Pregnancy
Nonulcerative dyspepsia*

*Nonulcerative dyspepsia occurs in up to 60% of cases, but the diagnosis requires the exclusion of other diagnostic entities.

(i.e., <45 years of age). Therefore, it is best applied to older patients and to younger patients with classic symptoms.

▼ *Upper GI radiography*: This test is less accurate than upper endoscopy and cannot provide tissue diagnosis. It is best reserved for situations where endoscopy expertise is unavailable, for patients who refuse endoscopy or have low pretest probability of disease, and in situations where endoscopy might be considered unsafe.

■ *Helicobacter pylori testing*

■ *Gastric emptying studies*: Gastric scintigraphy and gastroduodenal manometry studies generally do not influence medical management and are reserved for patients with normal laboratory tests and a normal EGD, yet who continue to have frequent or protracted vomiting suggestive of a motility disorder. Even in these cases, empiric treatment with prokinetic agents should probably be tried first. Disorders of the gallbladder (see Biliary Extrahepatic Obstruction, Complete).

Suggested Readings

Dominguez-Munoz JE, Malfertheiner P. Optimized serum pancreolauryl test for differentiating patients with and without chronic pancreatitis. *Clin Chem.* 1998;44:869.

Ferry GD. Causes of acute abdominal pain in children. www.uptodate.com, May 2009.

Khan F, Sachs H, Pechet L, et al. *Guide to Diagnostic Testing.* Philadelphia, PA: Lippincott Williams & Wilkins; 2002.

Penner RM, Majumdar SR. Diagnostic approach to abdominal pain in adults. www.uptodate.com, May 2009.

ASCITES

5

❑ Definition

- Ascites is a collection of free fluid in the peritoneal cavity.
- Etiology
  - ▼ Chronic liver disease (infectious hepatitis and alcoholism) causes 80% of cases of ascites (see Hepatomegaly, Jaundice).
  - ▼ Multiple causes, including cirrhosis, peritoneal carcinomatosis, or tuberculous peritonitis, account for 3–5% of cases.
  - ▼ Carcinomatosis causes <10% of cases of ascites.
  - ▼ Heart failure is responsible for <3–5% of cases, and nephritic syndrome is a rare cause of ascites.
  - ▼ Cryptogenic cirrhosis may account for up to 10% of cases.

❑ Classification

- Ascites is currently classified as high gradient or low gradient, depending on the serum ascites albumin gradient (SAAG). Calculation of SAAG involves the difference (not the ratio) between serum values and AF values.
- *High-gradient ascites* results from portal hypertension, whether on the basis of cirrhosis or noncirrhosis. Nephrotic syndrome is an exception and will usually cause low-gradient ascites due to marked hypoalbuminemia.
- *Low-gradient ascites* usually occurs as the result of cardiac failure, malignant carcinomatosis of the peritoneum, infections (such as TB), perforation of the bowel, connective tissues diseases, SLE, and chemical inflammation as in pancreatitis.

❑ Laboratory Findings (Figure 5-2)

- *Culture*: Bedside inoculation of AF in blood culture bottles has increased the positive bacterial yield to interpreted in concert with the cell count. A Gram stain should also be done.

  Imaging studies: Ultrasonography is useful for detecting the presence of ascites as well as for determining the etiology. It may reveal evidence of chronic liver disease, malignancy, hepatomegaly, and pancreatic disorder.

  Ascites fluid findings: AF examination is the principle diagnostic tool. Using abdominal paracentesis to obtain and study the fluid is crucial to making a diagnosis.

- *Transparent to pale fluid*: Is seen in cases of portal hypertension. Neutrophilia in excess of 1,000/mL results in opalescence. A concentration of RBCs in excess of 10,000/mL gives a faint pink tinge, and cell counts >20,000/mL

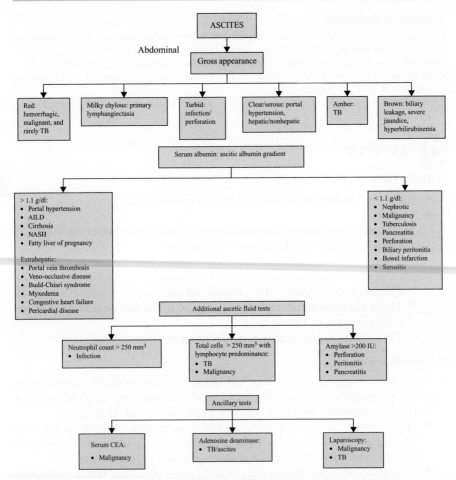

Figure 5–2 *Algorithm for the workup of patients with ascites. AILD, alcohol-induced liver disease; CEA, carcinogenic embryonic antigen; NASH, nonalcoholic steatohepatitis; TB, tuberculosis; TNC, total neutrophil count.*

color it red. A traumatic tap is evident by a streak of blood rather than homogeneously red fluid and the tendency to clot. Hepatocellular carcinoma and, rarely, metastatic disease; can cause a bloody tap. TB is only a rare cause of hemorrhagic ascites.

■ *Chylous or milky ascites:* Has a higher triglyceride concentration than serum and >200 mg/dL. It is rarely seen and is usually an indication of cirrhosis rather than lymphoma or TB as was previously thought. The triglycerides are >1,000 mg/dL in truly milky ascites. Dark-brown ascites may be seen in significant hyperbilirubinemia, biliary perforation (when ascitic bilirubin is higher than serum bilirubin), pancreatitis, and, rarely, in malignant melanoma.

■ *Bloody ascites fluid:* Once a traumatic tap has been ruled out, 50% of cases are due to hepatocellular carcinoma. TB rarely causes bloody fluid.

- *Staining*: Gram staining has low yield. Even with centrifugation, it has 10% sensitivity in spontaneous bacterial peritonitis. AFB smear for TB have very low sensitivity. In an appropriate clinical setting of low-grade fever, malaise, and weight loss, a high cell count with lymphocytic predominance and low SAAG is suggestive of TB ascites.
- *Protein concentration* of AF categorized ascites into exudative (ascitic protein >2.5 g/dL) or transudative (ascitic protein <2.5 g/dL). The significance of this has never been evaluated adequately and objectively.
- *Cell count and differential*: In uncomplicated cirrhosis, the total WBC count is <500 cells/μL with <250 neutrophils/μL. After diuresis, the total cell count may go up, but the neutrophil count remains below 250 cells/μL. In spontaneous bacterial peritonitis, the total WBC count and neutrophil count are usually, but not always, raised. In TB and carcinomatosis, the cell count rises but with a predominance of lymphocytes. In traumatic taps, for every 250 RBCs, one neutrophil is subtracted from the total WBC count.

Core laboratory: The serum and AF glucose concentrations are nearly the same in uncomplicated portal hypertension (large numbers of WBCs, bacteria, or tumor cells consume glucose and may lead to diminished levels). Amylase values may be about 3–5 times higher than the serum values. LD levels rise because of release of LD from the neutrophils. The rise occurs in cases of secondary peritonitis, TB, and pancreatitis.

Cytology: Has limitations in the diagnosis of malignant ascites and has been replaced largely laparoscopic examination of the peritoneum along with biopsy and culture.

❏ **Limitations**
- Errors may occur if serum albumin is very low or when serum and ascitic samples are not obtained within a short space of time from each other.
- A high globulin level in serum may also give a false result.

DISORDERS OF THE PERITONEUM ASSOCIATED WITH ASCITES

CHRONIC LIVER DISEASE (SEE P. 198)

- This disease differs from ascites caused by malignancy.

❏ **Laboratory Findings**
Albumin: Almost always ≥1.1 g/dL in cirrhosis (most common cause), alcoholic hepatitis, massive liver metastases, fulminant hepatic failure, portal vein thrombosis, Budd-Chiari syndrome, cardiac ascites, fatty liver, acute fatty liver of pregnancy, myxedema, mixed (e.g., cirrhosis with peritoneal TB). May be falsely low if serum albumin <1.1 g/dL or the patient in shock. May be falsely high with chylous ascites (lipid interferes with albumin assay). Albumin levels <1.1 g/dL in >90% of cases of peritoneal carcinomatosis (most common cause), TB, pancreatic or biliary ascites, nephrotic syndrome, bowel infarction or obstruction, and serositis in patients without cirrhosis.

Ascites fluid findings: AF total protein >2.5 mg/dL in cancer is only 56% accurate because of high protein content in 12–19% of these ascites as well as changes caused by albumin infusion and diuretic therapies. AF/serum albumin ratio <0.5 in cirrhosis (>90% accuracy). AF/serum ratio of LD (>0.6) or protein (>0.5) is not more accurate (approximately 56%) than only total protein for diagnosis of exudate. AF cholesterol <55 mg/dL in cirrhosis (94% accuracy). Albumin gradient (serum albumin minus AF albumin) reflects portal pressure. Total WBC count is usually <300/μL (50% of cases) and PMN <25% (50% of cases).

Core laboratory: Liver function tests are abnormal.

Other: Cirrhosis findings are similar with or without hepatocellular carcinoma. Cardiac ascites is associated with a blood–AF albumin gradient >1.1 g/dL, but malignant AF shows blood–AF albumin gradient <1.1 g/dL in 93% of cases.

INFECTED ASCITIC FLUID

❏ **Laboratory Findings**

Culture: AF in blood culture bottles has 85% sensitivity.

Ascites fluid findings:

- WBC count >250/μL: sensitivity = 85%, specificity = 93%, and neutrophils >50% are presumptive of bacterial peritonitis.
- pH <7.35 and arterial–AF pH difference >0.10; both these findings are virtually diagnostic of bacterial peritonitis and the absence of the above findings virtually excludes bacterial peritonitis.
- Lactate >25 mg/dL and arterial–AF difference >20 mg/dL are often present. LD is markedly increased. Phosphate, potassium, and gamma-glutamyltransferase may also be increased. Glucose is unreliable for diagnosis. Total protein <1.0 g/dL indicates high risk for SBP.
- Gram stain shows few bacteria in spontaneous bacterial peritonitis (SBP) but many when caused by intestinal perforation. Culture sensitivity = 50% for SBP and approximately 80% for secondary peritonitis. TB acid-fast stain sensitivity = 20–30% and TB culture sensitivity = 50–70%.

SECONDARY PERITONITIS

- This condition shows polymicrobial infection, total protein >1.0 g/dL, AF/LD greater than serum upper limit of normal, and glucose <50 mg/dL compared with spontaneous bacterial peritonitis (SPB).
- Prevalence of SBP 15%; due to *Escherichia coli* approximately 50%, *Klebsiella*, and other gram-negative bacteria; gram-positive bacteria approximately 25% (especially streptococci).

CONTINUOUS AMBULATORY PERITONEAL DIALYSIS

Monitor dialysate for the following:

- *Infection*: Peritonitis is defined as WBC count >100/μL, usually with >50% PMNs (normal is <50 WBC/μL, usually mononuclear cells), or positive

Gram stain or culture (most prevalent: coagulase-negative staphylococci, *Staphylococcus aureus*, *Streptococcus* sp.; multiple organisms, especially mixed aerobes and anaerobes occur with bowel perforation). Successful therapy causes fall in WBC count within first 2 days and a return to <100/μL in 4–5 days; differential returns to predominance of monocytes in 4–7 days with increased eosinophils in 10% of cases. Patients check outflow bags for turbidity. Turbid dialysate can occur occasionally without peritonitis during the first few months of placing catheter (due to catheter hypersensitivity) with WBC count 100–8,000/μL, 10–95% eosinophils, sometimes increased PMNs, and negative cultures. Occasional RBCs may be seen during menstruation or with ovulation at midcycle. *Because of low WBC decision level, manual hemocytometer count rather than an automated instrument must be used.*

- *Metabolic change*: Assay dialysate for creatinine and glucose; calculate ultrafiltrate volume by weighing dialysate fluid after 4-hour dwell time and subtracting it from preinfusion weight using specific gravity of 1.0.

PANCREATIC DISEASE

- AF amylase level greater than serum amylase level is specific for pancreatic disease, but both levels are normal in 10% of cases.
- Methemalbumin in serum or AF and total protein >4.5 g/dL indicate poor prognosis.

MALIGNANT ASCITES

- Increased fluid cholesterol (>45 mg/dL) and fibronectin (>10 mg/dL) have S/S 90%/82%.
- Positive cytology has S/S 70%/100%.
- Increased AF CEA (>2.5 mg/dL) has S/S 45%/100%.

ASCITES IN FETUS OR NEONATE

❑ **Causes**

- Nonimmune (occurs in 1 in 3,000 pregnancies)
  - ▼ Cardiovascular abnormalities causing CHF (e.g., structural, arrhythmias) (40% of cases)
  - ▼ Chromosomal (e.g., Turner and Down syndromes are most common; trisomy 13, 15, 16, and 18) (10–15% of cases)
  - ▼ Hematologic disorders (any severe anemia) (10% of cases)
  - ▼ Inherited (e.g., α-thalassemia, hemoglobinopathies, G6PD deficiency)
  - ▼ Acquired (e.g., fetal–maternal hemorrhage, twin-to-twin transfusion, congenital infection [parvovirus B19], methemoglobinemia)
  - ▼ Congenital defects of the chest and abdomen.
  - ▼ Structural (e.g., diaphragmatic hernia, jejunal atresia, volvulus, intestinal malrotation)

Peritonitis caused by GI tract perforation, congenital infection (e.g., syphilis, TORCH [*toxoplasmosis, other agents, rubella, CMV, and herpes simplex], hepatitis), meconium peritonitis

- ▼ Lymphatic duct obstruction
- ▼ Biliary atresia
- ▼ Nonstructural (e.g., congenital nephrotic syndrome, cirrhosis, cholestasis, hepatic necrosis, GI tract obstruction)
- ▼ Lower GU tract obstruction (e.g., posterior urethral valves, urethral atresia, and ureterocele) is most common cause
- ▼ Inherited skeletal dysplasias (enlarged liver causing extramedullary hematopoiesis)
- ▼ Fetal tumors, most often teratomas and neuroblastomas
- ▼ Vascular placental abnormalities
- ▼ Genetic metabolic disorders (e.g., Hurler syndrome, Gaucher disease, Niemann-Pick disease, G_{M1} gangliosidosis type I, I-cell disease, β-glucuronidase deficiency)
- ■ Immune (maternal antibodies reacting to fetal antigens [e.g., Rh, C, E, Kell])

PERITONITIS, ACUTE

- ■ See Figures 5-3 and 5-4.

PRIMARY PERITONITIS

Ascites fluid findings: Gram stain of direct smear and culture of peritoneal fluid usually shows streptococci in children. In adults, it is caused by *E. coli* (40–60%) or *S. pneumoniae* (15%), other gram-negative bacilli, and enterococci; usually one organism. May be caused by *Mycobacterium tuberculosis*. Marked increase in WBC (≤50,000/µL) and PMN (80–90%).

Peritoneal lavage fluid findings: Shows WBC count >200/µL in 99% of cases.

Other: Laboratory findings due to nephrotic syndrome and post–necrotic cirrhosis and occasionally bacteremia in children and cirrhosis with ascites in adults.

SECONDARY PERITONITIS

Occurs and recurs very frequently in continuous ambulatory peritoneal dialysis.

Laboratory findings due perforation of hollow viscus (e.g., appendicitis, perforated ulcer).

Dialysate findings: Turbid (indicates >300 WBC/µL); Gram stain, culture, and leukocytosis may be absent. Caused by gram-positive bacteria in approximately 70%, enteric gram-negative bacilli and *P. aeruginosa* in 20–30%, others in 10–20%, and sterile in 10–20%. *If more than one pathogen is found, rule out perforated viscus.* Usually more than one organism is found.

Suggested Readings

Cárdenas A, Gelrud A, Chopra S. Chylous, bloody, and pancreatic ascites. www.uptodate.com, May 2009.

Khan F, Sachs H, Pechet L, et al. *Guide to Diagnostic Testing*. Philadelphia, PA: Lippincott Williams & Wilkins; 2002.

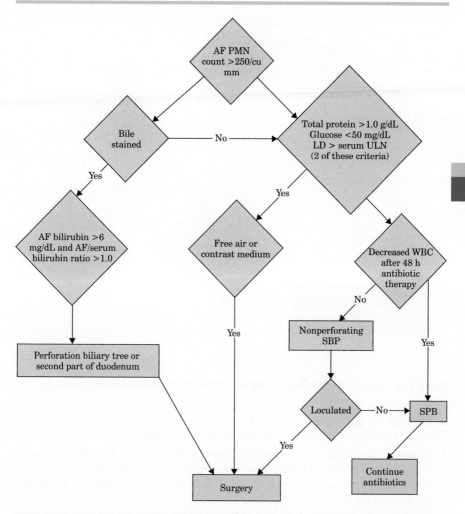

Figure 5–3 *Algorithm for differentiating secondary from spontaneous bacterial peritonitis. AF, ascitic fluid; PMN, polymorphonuclear leukocytes; LD, lactate dehydrogenase; ULN, upper limit of normal; WBC, white blood cell; SBP, spontaneous bacterial peritonitis.*

Runyon B. Diagnosis and evaluation of patients with ascites. www.uptodate.com, May 2009.
Runyon B. Diagnosis of spontaneous bacterial peritonitis. www.uptodate.com, May 2009.

 DIARRHEA

☐ **Definition**

- Diarrhea is defined as >200 g of stool or an increase in the frequency or fluidity of normal stools. It may be acute or chronic, and it is considered chronic when it lasts at least 4 weeks.

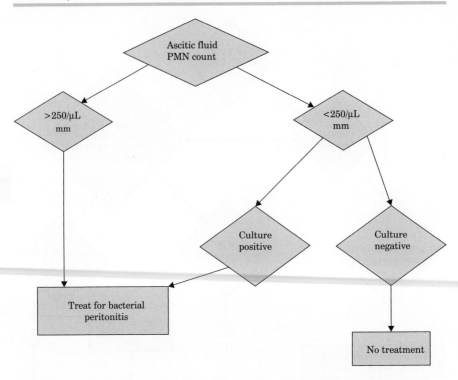

Figure 5–4 *Algorithm for spontaneous bacterial peritonitis. PMN, polymorphonuclear leukocytes.*

❏ Etiology

Diarrhea can result from any of the following mechanisms.

1. Osmosis: Molecules not normally present in the intestinal lumen increase the osmolality of chime, drawing water into the lumen (i.e., lactose)
2. Secretion: Substances can cause intestinal cells to secrete sodium and water (i.e., cholera toxin).
3. Inflammation results in denuding of the intestinal lining, which in turn disrupts normal absorption, thereby allowing compounds from the lining to leak into the lumen resulting in an increased osmosis.
4. Motility: Hypermotility leads to an increased stool volume. Hypomotility can lead to bacterial overgrowth, which causes diarrhea through several different mechanisms.
5. Anal sphincter dysfunction causes fecal incontinence, which can be interpreted by the patient as diarrhea.

❏ Differential Diagnosis

1. Laxative abuse accounts for approximately 15% of all chronic causes. It should be suspected in patients with a mental health disorder.
2. Sorbitol can cause diarrhea. In one study, approximately 17% of people had diarrhea following the ingestion of 4–5 minutes containing sorbitol.
3. Both bile salts and fatty acids cause secretion of chloride followed by water into the colon. Excess bile salts also lead to a mild degree of fat malabsorption.

4. Bacterial overgrowth can occur secondary to diabetes, blind loop syndrome, amyloidosis, diverticulitis, and scleroderma, among other causes.
5. Irritable bowel syndrome classically presents with diarrhea alternating with constipation, but it can also occur in a diarrhea-predominant form.
6. Gastric surgery syndrome results in a decreased contact time with the luminal surface and decreased digestive juices mixing with the chyme.
7. Hyperthyroidism usually has increased frequency and amount of diarrhea but not fluidity. Diarrhea is present in approximately 25% of hyperthyroid cases.
8. Inflammatory bowel disease (IBD):
   ▼ Ulcerative colitis is a relapsing and remitting disease that leads to acute inflammation of the colorectal mucosa. The rectum is involved in 55% of cases. In severe cases, bloody diarrhea often leads to weight loss, anemia, and electrolyte imbalance.
   ▼ Crohn disease is a chronic relapsing disorder characterized by transmural, asymmetric, and segmental inflammation. It typically involves the ileum, colon, or perianal region; right lower quadrant pain associated with bloody diarrhea is present in 80% of patients.
9. Neoplasia:
   ▼ Villous adenoma produces prostaglandins, which stimulate chloride and water secretion from the colon.
   ▼ Serotonin from carcinoid cells stimulates gut motility and increases intestinal secretion.
   ▼ Tumor-associated calcitonin stimulates gut motility.
   ▼ Gastrinoma leads to increased gastric acid, which directly causes fluid secretion.
10. Infection:
   ▼ Refer to p. 624, Foodborne Infectious Illnesses, and see other sections on specific agents that cause diarrheal disease.

❏ Laboratory Findings

Endoscopy: Lower endoscopy may help. One series has a 20% yield in identifying a pathologic diagnosis. In non–HIV-infected patients, the role of sigmoidoscopy versus colonoscopy is unclear. When clinically suspected, even if no gross abnormalities are noted, consider doing blind biopsies looking for lymphocytic and collagenous colitis. The yield of biopsy with no gross abnormalities ranges from 6% to 42%. Upper endoscopy is useful for making the diagnosis of sprue, Whipple disease, and other small bowel infiltrative processes.

Radiology: An upper GI series with small bowel follow-through is most commonly used when evaluating for Crohn disease. Enteroclysis is superior, with 100% sensitivity and 98% specificity for small bowel involvement with Crohn disease.

Recommended laboratory tests of stool:

- Fecal leukocytes.
- Stool for osmolality gap: The osmolality gap is calculated by the following formula: 2 (stool Na + K). The accuracy is fair in distinguishing between osmotic (if gap is 50) and secretory (if gap is >50) diarrhea.
- Stool for pH: For carbohydrate intolerance (e.g., lactose or sorbitol), one small study found the pH <5.6. For bile acid–induced diarrhea, the pH is usually over 6.8.

- Stool for fecal fat: This test is used to detect steatorrhea on the basis of malabsorption.
- Qualitative: Sensitivity is 97–100%, but the specificity varies from 56% to 86%.
- Quantitative: Based upon a 72-hour collection, the patient should be on a 75- to 100-g fat diet. A nutritional consult is advised to maximize compliance.
- Test(s) for infectious agents (e.g., stool culture, O&P examination, rotavirus detection) based on clinical presentation.

Other recommended tests:

- *Nutrition indices*: CBC, albumin, and potassium (sensitivity of hypokalemia is 100% for pancreatic cholera or [VIPoma]) are routine studies in the evaluation of chronic diarrhea.
- *Hormonal studies*: TSH, fasting serum gastrin level, calcitonin level, and 24-hour urine collection for 5-hydroxy indole acetic acid (5-HIAA) are recommended.
- *D-xylose testing*: This tests for small bowel malabsorption syndromes (e.g., sprue, Crohn disease, amyloidosis). Twenty-five grams of *D-xylose* are administered. A 5-hour urine collection and a 1-hour serum sample are obtained. A decreased amount of *D-xylose* in the urine and serum indicates small bowel malabsorption. The sensitivity of the test is decreased in the following situations: creatinine clearance of <30 mg/dL, portal hypertension, ascites, delayed gastric emptying, fiber supplements, glucose load, aspirin, and glipizide.
- *Bentiromide test* (to test for pancreatic exocrine insufficiency): N-benzoyl-L-tyrosyl para-aminobenzoic acid (NBT PABA) is administered orally. The molecule is cleaved by chymotrypsin; PABA is absorbed and then measured in a 6-hour urine collection. PABA alone is a somewhat inaccurate measure, so additional markers have been used to increase the accuracy.
- *Serum immune markers*: Several serum immune markers performed by ELISA have been found to be valuable for the diagnosis, stratification, and management of IBD (see Celiac Disease):
  - ▼ Deoxyribonuclease (DNAse)-sensitive perinuclear antineutrophil cytoplasmic antibody (P-ANCA) is positive in 60–80% of adults with ulcerative colitis (UC) and in 83% of children with UC. P-ANCA is positive in 10% of patients with Crohn disease.
  - ▼ Anti-*Saccharomyces cerevisiae* antibody (ASCA) is present in 70% of patients with Crohn disease.
  - ▼ Pancreatic antibody may be positive in 30–40% of patients with Crohn disease.
  - ▼ Outer membrane porin from *E. coli* (OmpC) antibody: An immunoglobulin A (IgA) response to OmpC is seen in 55% of patients with Crohn disease.
  - ▼ Lactoferrin, stool: A sensitive and specific marker for detecting inflammation or from irritable bowel syndrome (IBS) once infectious causes of inflammation and colorectal cancer are ruled out.
  - ▼ Calprotectin for screening of patients with diarrhea to help distinguish between active IBD and IBS.

DIARRHEA, ACUTE

OSMOTIC DIARRHEA

❑ **Definition**

Defined as diarrhea with a <3-week (upper limit 6–8 weeks) duration. Increased osmotically active solutes in the bowel; diarrhea usually stops during fasting.

Causes

- Exogenous
  - ▼ Laxatives (e.g., magnesium sulfate, milk of magnesia, sodium sulfate [Glauber salt], sodium phosphate, polyethylene glycol/saline)
  - ▼ Drugs (e.g., lactulose, colchicine, cholestyramine, neomycin, para-amino-salicylic acid [PAS])
  - ▼ Foods (e.g., mannitol, sorbitol [in diet candy, chewing gum, soda])
- Endogenous
  - ▼ Congenital malabsorption
    - ● Specific (e.g., lactase deficiency, fructose malabsorption)
    - ● General (e.g., abetalipoproteinemia and hypobetalipoproteinemia, congenital lymphangiectasia, cystic fibrosis)
  - ▼ Acquired malabsorption
    - ● Specific (e.g., pancreatic disease, celiac sprue, parasitic infestation, rotavirus enteritis, metabolic disorders [thyrotoxicosis, adrenal insufficiency], jejunoileal bypass, bacterial overgrowth, short-bowel syndrome, inflammatory disease [e.g., mastocytosis, eosinophilic enteritis])

SECRETORY (ABNORMAL ELECTROLYTE TRANSPORT) DIARRHEA

❑ **Definition**

Diarrhea caused by increased water and chloride secretion; normal water and sodium absorption may be inhibited.

Due to

- Exogenous
  - ▼ Drugs
    - ● Laxatives (e.g., aloe, anthraquinones, bisacodyl, castor oil, dioctyl sodium sulfosuccinate, phenolphthalein, senna)
    - ● Diuretics (e.g., furosemide, thiazides), asthma (theophylline), thyroid drugs
    - ● Cholinergic drugs (cholinesterase inhibitors, quinidine, clozapine, ACE inhibitors)
  - ▼ Toxins (e.g., arsenic, mushrooms, organophosphates, alcohol)
  - ▼ Infectious agents (For a discussion of infectious causes of diarrhea, see the Infectious Gastrointestinal Diseases section in this chapter and Chapter 13)
- Endogenous
  - ▼ Hormones (serotonin, calcitonin, VIP)
  - ▼ Gastric hypersecretion (Z-E syndrome, systemic mastocytosis, short-bowel syndrome)

▼ Bile salts (e.g., disease or resection of the terminal ileum)
▼ Fatty acids (e.g., disease of small intestine mucosa, pancreatic insufficiency)
▼ Congenital (e.g., congenital chloridorrhea, congenital sodium diarrhea)

❑ **Laboratory Findings**
Stool findings: Watery stool, volume >1 L/day, blood and pus are absent, stool osmolality close to plasma osmolality with no anion gap.

EXUDATIVE DIARRHEA (INFLAMMATORY CAUSES)

Due to infection, injury, ischemia, vasculitis, abscess, and/or idiopathic.
   Laboratory findings: Stool contains blood and pus.

MOTILITY DISTURBANCES

Due to

- Decreased small intestinal motility (e.g., hypothyroidism, DM, amyloidosis, scleroderma)
- Increased small intestinal motility (e.g., hyperthyroidism, carcinoid syndrome)
- Increased colonic motility (e.g., irritable bowel syndrome)

INFECTIOUS GASTROINTESTINAL DISEASES

❑ **Definition**
Ingestion of viable pathogenic microorganisms or toxins is responsible for a wide variety of gastrointestinal complaints. Ingestion of toxic nonbiologic agents, such as heavy metals, may also cause gastrointestinal symptoms, as discussed above. Disease is usually manifested by GI tract signs and symptoms but may be manifested by systemic or localized illness without significant GI symptoms (e.g., enteric fever, botulism). Fecal–oral transmission of infectious agents is commonly mediated by contamination of food but may be mediated by contaminated environmental sources. A foodborne illness is any illness related to food ingestion. Foodborne illnesses and other transmissible enteric diseases are of interest to public health authorities, and many are subjected to mandated reporting because of the possibility of widespread dissemination. Department of Public Health epidemiologists often coordinate clinical and laboratory investigations.
   A foodborne illness may be restricted to a single individual or a small group, or may represent a large outbreak with many patients linked to a common source of infection. In the United States, enteric viruses cause most infectious diarrhea cases; common bacterial pathogens associated with gastroenteritis are *Salmonella* spp., *Campylobacter* spp., *E. coli* (STEC) O157 and *Shigella* spp.

❑ **Who Should Be Suspected?**
Patients with foodborne illness usually present with a variety of symptoms including nausea, vomiting, abdominal pain, diarrhea, and anorexia. Certain foodborne illnesses, however, may be associated with minimal GI symptoms but have prominent systemic or localized symptoms.

Diarrheal illness may be noninflammatory or inflammatory. Noninflammatory diarrhea is usually caused by disease of the small intestine resulting in hypersecretion or decreased absorption. There is usually abrupt onset and resolution after a brief duration of illness. Systemic symptoms are usually absent or mild. Dehydration may be a complication, especially in the young or elderly.

Inflammatory diarrhea is characterized by mucosal invasion or cytotoxic damage by the pathogen. The large intestine is most commonly affected. The mucosal invasion typically results in bloody stools with many fecal leukocytes. Systemic symptoms are typical, including fever, abdominal pain and tenderness, nausea and vomiting, headache, and malaise.

When evaluating a patient with a likely foodborne illness, a number of issues should be pursued:

- What is the interval between likely exposure and onset of symptoms?
- What is the duration of clinical symptoms in affected patients?
- What are the prominent signs and symptoms of disease?
- Does any of the patient's recent contacts have similar illness?
- Has the patient eaten any unusual food? Eaten at any function with mass-produced meals? Eaten any raw or incompletely cooked or pasteurized food?
- Has there been new contact with animals: domesticated, farm, or wild?
- Has the patient had recent travel to regions where foodborne illness is endemic?
- Does the patient, or does a close contact, attend or reside in a day care center, long-term care facility, or other facility at which transmission of an agent may be facilitated?

The following lists provide common agents based on disease presentation. In addition to the clinical presentation, epidemiologic risk should be considered when determining diagnostic and therapeutic strategies. Additional information is provided for a number of agents in *Chapter 11. Infectious Diseases*.

- Gastroenteritis with vomiting as the prominent symptom. Suspect:
  - ▾ Anisakiasis
  - ▾ Enteric viruses (e.g., rotavirus, norovirus, enteric adenovirus)
  - ▾ Preformed toxin ingestion (*S. aureus*, *B. cereus*)
- Noninflammatory diarrhea (watery without marked fecal WBCs or RBCs). Suspect:
  - ▾ *Clostridium perfringens*
  - ▾ *Cryptosporidium* species
  - ▾ *Cyclospora cayetanensis*
  - ▾ Enteric virus (astrovirus, norovirus or other calicivirus, adenovirus, rotavirus)
  - ▾ Enterotoxigenic *E. coli*
  - ▾ *Giardia lamblia*
  - ▾ *Vibrio cholerae*
- Inflammatory diarrhea as the prominent symptom (grossly bloody stool, pus or increased fecal WBCs, fever, and systemic signs and symptoms). Suspect
  - ▾ *Campylobacter* species
  - ▾ *Entamoeba histolytica*

  ▼ *Escherichia coli*, enteroinvasive, or enterohemorrhagic
  ▼ *Salmonella* species
  ▼ *Shigella* species
  ▼ Noncholera *Vibrio* species
  ▼ *Yersinia enterocolitica*
- Persistent diarrhea as the prominent symptom (2 weeks or longer). Suspect
  ▼ *Cryptosporidium parvum*
  ▼ *Cyclospora cayetanensis*
  ▼ *Entamoeba histolytica*
  ▼ *Giardia lamblia*
- Neurologic manifestation as the prominent symptom (paraesthesia, respiratory depression, cranial nerve palsy, respiratory difficulty). Suspect
  ▼ *Clostridium botulinum* toxin
  ▼ Guillain-Barré syndrome (after *Campylobacter jejuni* gastroenteritis)
  ▼ Intoxication/poisoning (scombroid fish poisoning, ciguatera fish poisoning, *Tetraodon* [fish] poisoning, shellfish poisoning)
  ▼ Mushroom poisoning
  ▼ Organophosphate/insecticide poisoning
  ▼ Thallium poisoning
- Systemic signs and symptoms as the predominant presentation, with minimal GI symptoms. Suspect
  ▼ *Brucella* species
  ▼ *Entamoeba histolytica* liver abscess
  ▼ HAV and HEV
  ▼ *Listeria monocytogenes*
  ▼ *Salmonella* typhi or paratyphi
  ▼ *Toxoplasma gondii*
  ▼ *Trichinella spiralis*
  ▼ *Vibrio vulnificus*

❏ Diagnosis and Reporting

Most cases of diarrheal illness are mild and self-limited, and testing to establish a specific cause is rarely necessary. Diagnostic testing is recommended for patients with profuse, watery diarrhea, passage of stools with blood or mucus, persistent diarrhea (>48 hours), immunocompromised patients, and patients with severe gastrointestinal or systemic symptoms (like severe abdominal pain, fever, or hypovolemia). Testing to establish a specific diagnosis is also recommended for patients at risk for complications of gastrointestinal infections, like patients with inflammatory bowel disease, patients involved in any investigation of a possible outbreak of diarrheal illness, and patients who may be at increased risk for transmitting infection to others, like food handlers.

Because of the diverse etiology and variety of tests required to make a specific diagnosis, consultation with infectious disease experts and clinical microbiologists may improve diagnostic strategies. For many agents of foodborne diseases, reporting to the local department of public health is required; public health officials may be able to provide important information concerning ongoing outbreaks or diagnostic support.

Diagnostic testing: The type of testing will depend on the agent suspected, clinical presentation, source of specimen submitted for testing and other factors. Diagnostic techniques for microbial pathogens are discussed in other sections of this book.

- *Bacteria*: Bacterial pathogens may be isolated by culture of stool, vomitus, or other patient specimen. Stool culture is most commonly submitted. Consider submitting stool for culture in patients with
  - ▼ Immunocompromise or increased risk for complication of bacterial gastroenteritis
  - ▼ Inflammatory bowel disease, to distinguish between infection and flare
  - ▼ Severe illness, including severe vomiting or diarrhea, abdominal pain, hypovolemia, or prolonged duration
  - ▼ Signs of inflammation, like blood, mucus, or leukocytes in stool; fever; or sepsis; involvement of organ systems outside the gastrointestinal tract

Fecal culture requires use of selective, differential media optimized for isolation of specific pathogens. The pathogens routinely tested may vary from laboratory to laboratory. *Campylobacter, Salmonella,* and *Shigella* spp. are typically isolated by routine stool cultures. Antigen assays are also available for sensitive and specific direct detection of *Campylobacter* in stool specimens. Special cultures may have to be requested if another pathogen is suspected on clinical or epidemiologic grounds (e.g., *E. coli* O157:H7, other Shiga-toxigenic enteric GNB, *Vibrio* spp., *Aeromonas* spp., *Listeria monocytogenes*). Bacterial pathogens are present in high concentrations during acute symptomatic infection. Therefore, submission of a single specimen is usually sensitive for detection of bacterial causes of diarrhea; repeat cultures may be necessary for detection of *Shigella* or asymptomatic carriage of an enteric pathogen.

After isolation, additional testing may be required to detect specific pathogenic mechanisms (e.g., enteropathogenic *E. coli*, Shiga toxin production) or for epidemiologic studies (e.g., serotype analysis of *Salmonella* isolates). Culture of blood, CSF, and other specimens are recommended for patients with signs of systemic illness or localized infection outside the gastrointestinal tract.

In hospitalized patients with onset of symptoms more than 48 hours after admission, testing for *Clostridium difficile* is recommended; routine stool culture or O&P evaluation is unlikely to yield clinically significant results. Several different assays may be used to detect toxigenic *C. difficile*, including toxin A and B EIA, specific glutamate dehydrogenase, cytotoxicity, isolation by anaerobic bacterial culture and PCR.

Evaluation of food or environmental specimens for enteric pathogens is typically performed by a Public Health Laboratory, or other specialized reference laboratory, and is usually performed only as part of a formal epidemiologic investigation.

- *Enteric viruses*: Viral gastroenteritis is most commonly mild and self-limited with few systemic symptoms and may be effectively treated symptomatically without establishing a specific diagnosis. Four viral pathogens are responsible for most cases of viral gastroenteritis in the United States: norovirus, rotavirus, enteric adenoviruses, and astroviruses.
  - ▼ *Viruses may be* detected in stool by electron microscopic techniques, but this testing is not available for routine evaluation of patient specimens.

▼ *Viral culture* is also of limited utility because of long turnaround time as well as the limited availability of the specialized viral cultures required for enteric viruses that may be isolated in culture. Some clinical laboratories may provide viral culture testing to rule out enteric adenoviruses (serotypes 40 and 41).

▼ *Antigen detection* testing is available for several enteric viruses and provides reliable detection of rotavirus and enteric adenovirus in stool specimens.

▼ *Molecular diagnostic* tests now play an important role in the detection of enteric virus infection because of their high sensitivity and specificity, as well as short turnaround time for most assays. Many Public Health and Reference Laboratories offer testing for relevant viruses, and an increasing number of approved assays are becoming commercially available.

■ *Parasites:* O&P testing is not cost-effective for routine testing of patients with gastrointestinal complaints but should be considered in patients with

▼ *Persistent diarrhea*

▼ *Specific epidemiologic* risks, like travel to regions with a high endemic rate of enteric parasitic infections, exposure to infants in day care centers, diarrhea in men who have sex with men, patients with HIV infection, and patients who develop diarrhea during a waterborne or other regional outbreak of diarrhea caused by parasitic pathogens

▼ *Sensitive and specific* stool antigen testing is available for *Cryptosporidium*, *Giardia*, and *E. histolytica*. Antigen testing may serve as cost-effective initial testing for patients who require testing to rule out parasitic infection. Because ova and parasites may be shed intermittently, three specimens for O&P testing should be submitted, separated by at least 24 hours, over 3–6 days, *if needed.*

■ *Serology:* Detection of specific IgM and IgG is used for diagnosis of acute hepatitis A virus infection. Serology plays a minor role in the diagnosis of acute infection by other enteric pathogens. However, patient seroconversion may provide important diagnostic information during the convalescent phase, especially for epidemiologic investigations regarding the cause or scope of a potential epidemic of gastrointestinal disease.

■ *Toxins:* Clinical laboratories do not routinely offer testing for detection of specific toxins, like botulinum toxin, in food or patient specimens. Testing for toxins is typically performed by a Public Health Laboratory, or other specialized reference laboratory, and is usually performed only as part of a formal epidemiologic investigation.

❑ Conclusion

It is important for health care providers to

■ Consider the possibility of foodborne illness in evaluating a patient's illness.

■ Realize that many, but not all, foodborne illnesses present with prominent GI tract illness. Patients may present with predominant systemic, neurologic, or other signs and symptoms.

■ Understand the testing required for likely pathogens. When specific diagnosis is required, ensure that appropriate specimens and cultures, or other tests, are submitted for testing.

- Obtain a clinical history that may provide clues regarding the source of the illness as well as assessing the possibility of a larger outbreak.
- Report suspect cases to public health officials, as appropriate. Be aware that a patient may be a part of a larger outbreak in the community.
- Instruct patients about how to prevent further transmission of illness to contacts.

Suggested Readings

Bresee JS, Marcus R, Venezia RA, et al. The etiology of severe gastroenteritis among adults visiting emergency departments in the United States. *J Infect Dis.* 2012;205:1374–1381.

Centers for Disease Control and Prevention. Diagnosis and management of foodborne illnesses: a primer for physicians and other health care professionals. *MMWR.* 2004;53(No. RR-4):1–33.

Centers for Disease Control and Prevention. Diagnosis and management of foodborne illnesses: a primer for physicians. *MMWR.* 2001;50(No. RR-2):1–70.

Denno MD, Shaikh N, Stapp JR, et al. Diarrhea etiology in a pediatric emergency department: a case control Study. *Clin Infect Dis.* 2012;55(7):897–904.

DuPont HL. Bacterial diarrhea. *N Engl J Med.* 2009;361:1560–1569.

Payne DC, Vinjé J, Szilagyi PG, et al. Norovirus and medically attended gastroenteritis in U.S. children. *N Engl J Med.* 2013;368:1121–1130.

Scallan E, Hoekstra RM, Anguolo FJ, et al. Foodborne illness acquired in the United States— major pathogens. *Emerg Infect Dis.* 2011;17:7–15.

Steele JCH Jr, (ed). Food-borne diseases. *Clin Lab Med.* 1999;19:469–703.

Thielman NM, Guerrant RL. Acute infectious diarrhea. *N Engl J Med.* 2004;350:38–47.

DIARRHEA, CHRONIC

❑ Definition

Chronic diarrhea is diarrhea that lasts for more than 4 weeks.

❑ Causes

- Infectious agents (For a discussion of infectious causes of diarrhea, see the Infectious Gastrointestinal Diseases section in this chapter and Chapter 11)
- IBD (e.g., Crohn disease, UC, collagenous colitis)
- Carbohydrate malabsorption (e.g., lactase or sucrase deficiency)
- Foods (e.g., ethanol, caffeine, sweeteners such as sorbitol, fructose)
- Drugs (e.g., antibiotics, antihypertensive, antiarrhythmic, antineoplastic, colchicine, cholestyramine; see previous section on acute diarrhea.)
- Laxative abuse, factitious
- Endocrine (e.g., DM, adrenal insufficiency, hyperthyroidism, hypothyroidism)
- Hormone-producing tumors (e.g., gastrinoma, VIPoma, villous adenoma, medullary thyroid carcinoma, pheochromocytoma, ganglioneuroma, carcinoid tumor, mastocytosis, somatostatinoma, ectopic hormone production by lung or pancreas carcinoma)
- Injury caused by radiation, ischemia, and so on
- Infiltrations (e.g., scleroderma, amyloidosis, lymphoma)
- Colon carcinoma
- Previous surgery (e.g., gastrectomy, vagotomy, intestinal resection)
- Immune system disorders (e.g., systemic mastocytosis, eosinophilic gastroenteritis)

- Intraluminal maldigestion (bile duct obstruction, pancreatic exocrine insufficiency)
- Celiac sprue
- Whipple disease
- Abetalipoproteinemia
- Dermatitis herpetiformis
- Intestinal lymphangiectasia
- Allergy
- Idiopathic

OTHER GASTROINTESTINAL CONDITIONS ASSOCIATED WITH CHRONIC DIARRHEA

DIVERTICULOSIS, COLON

❏ Laboratory Findings
Core laboratory: Hypochromic microcytic anemia, increased WBCs. Increased ESR. Positive occult blood.

ENTEROCOLITIS, NECROTIZING, IN INFANCY

❏ Definition
Syndrome of acute intestinal necrosis of unknown cause. It is especially associated with prematurity and exchange transfusions.

❏ Laboratory Findings
There may be oliguria, neutropenia, and anemia. Persistent metabolic acidosis, severe hyponatremia, and DIC are a common triad in infants. Bloody stools feature no characteristic organisms; significant organisms are often found by frequent repeated cultures of blood, urine, and stool.

INFLAMMATORY BOWEL DISEASE

❏ Definition
IBD refers to a chronic relapsing spectrum of disorders of unknown cause with destructive mucosal immune reaction in a genetically susceptible host. It is caused by an aberrant immune response and loss of tolerance to normal intestinal flora, leading to chronic inflammation of the gut.

REGIONAL ENTERITIS (CROHN DISEASE)

❏ Definition
Systemic inflammatory disease with predominantly GI tract involvement. There are no pathognomonic findings for Crohn disease or to distinguish it from ulcerative colitis.

❑ Laboratory Findings

Histology: Endoscopic biopsy may show granulomas in >60% of cases of Crohn disease but in only 6% of cases of UC.

Serology: Atypical perinuclear-staining antineutrophil cytoplasmic antibodies (P-ANCA) are found in <15% of cases of Crohn disease but in ≤70% of ulcerative colitis patients. Anti-*S. cerevisiae* (baker's or brewers' yeast) antibodies (ASCA) are found in approximately 60% of Crohn disease cases but in only approximately 10% of cases in ulcerative colitis.

Lactoferrin and calprotectin high sensitivity and specificity distinguishing between IBD and noninflammatory IBS.

Hematology: Increased WBC, ESR, CRP, and other acute-phase reactants correlate with disease activity. Mild increase of WBC indicates activity, but a marked increase suggests suppuration (e.g., abscess). ESR tends to be higher in disease of the colon than of the ileum. Anemia due to iron deficiency or vitamin B_{12} or folate deficiency or chronic disease.

Core laboratory: Decreased serum albumin, increased γ-globulins. Hyperchloremic metabolic acidosis, dehydration, decreased sodium, potassium, magnesium. Mild liver function test changes due to pericholangitis (especially increased serum ALP). Laboratory changes due to complications or sequelae (e.g., malabsorption, perforation and fistula formation, abscess formation, arthritis, sclerosing cholangitis, iritis, uveitis).

ULCERATIVE COLITIS, CHRONIC NONSPECIFIC

❑ Definition

There are no pathognomonic findings for this disease, nor are there findings that distinguish it from Crohn disease.

❑ Laboratory Findings

Serology: P-ANCA are found in 70% of ulcerative colitis patients but only occasionally in cases of Crohn disease. Stools are negative for usual enteric pathogens and parasites.

Hematology: With diarrhea and fever, hemoglobin <7.5 g/dL, increased neutrophil count, and ESR >30 mm/hour indicate severe disease.

Core laboratory: Serum ALP often increased slightly. Other liver function tests are usually normal. Stools are positive for blood.

❑ Other Considerations

- Laboratory changes due to complications or sequelae (e.g., hemorrhage, carcinoma, electrolyte disorders, toxic megacolon with perforation).
- The lower sensitivity of combined serologic tests only modestly influences pretest and posttest probability in IBD but is very useful in distinguishing Crohn disease from UC. Serial measurements are not useful and do not correlate with disease activity; titers are stable over time.

Suggested Reading

Bossuyt X. Serologic markers in inflammatory bowel disease. *Clin Chem.* 2006;52:171–181.

MALABSORPTION

❏ **Definition**
Malabsorption is defective nutrient absorption by the small intestine.

❏ **Causes**
- Inadequate mixing of food with bile salts and lipase (e.g., pyloroplasty, subtotal or total gastrectomy, gastrojejunostomy)
- Inadequate lipolysis due to lack of lipase (e.g., CF of the pancreas, chronic pancreatitis, cancer of the pancreas or ampulla of Vater, pancreatic fistula, vagotomy)
- Inadequate emulsification of fat due to lack of bile salts (e.g., obstructive jaundice, severe liver disease, bacterial overgrowth of the small intestine, disorders of the terminal ileum)
- Primary absorptive defect in the small bowel
- Inadequate absorptive surface due to extensive mucosal disease (e.g., regional enteritis, tumors, amyloid disease, scleroderma, irradiation)
- Biochemical dysfunction of mucosal cells (e.g., celiac sprue syndrome, severe starvation, or administration of drugs such as neomycin sulfate, colchicine, or PAS)
- Obstruction of mesenteric lymphatics (e.g., by lymphoma, carcinoma, intestinal TB)
- Inadequate length of normal absorptive surface (e.g., surgical resection, fistula, shunt)
- Miscellaneous (e.g., "blind loops" of the intestine and diverticula, Z-E syndrome, agammaglobulinemia, endocrine and metabolic disorders)
- Infection (e.g., acute enteritis, tropical sprue, Whipple disease [*Tropheryma whippelii*]; in common variable hypogammaglobulinemia, 50–55% of patients have chronic diarrhea and malabsorption caused by a specific pathogen such as *G. lamblia* or overgrowth of bacteria in the small bowel.)

❏ **Laboratory Findings**
Core laboratory: Serum cholesterol may be decreased. Decreased serum carotene, albumin, and iron; increased stool weight (>300 g/24 hours) and stool fat (>7 g/24 hours).

Hematology: PT may be prolonged because of malabsorption of vitamin K. Increased ESR.

Anemia is caused by deficiency of iron, folic acid, vitamin B_{12}, or various combinations, depending on their decreased absorption.

Other: Normal D-xylose test, low serum trypsinogen, and pancreatic calcification on radiograph of the abdomen establish diagnosis of chronic pancreatitis. If calcification is absent (as occurs in 70–80% of cases), abnormal contents of pancreatic secretion after secretin–cholecystokinin stimulation or abnormal bentiromide tests establish diagnosis of chronic pancreatitis.

❏ **Recommended Tests**
Fat absorption indices (steatorrhea): Direct qualitative stool examination. ≥2 random stool samples are collected on diet of >80 g of fat daily.

Serum trypsinogen: <10 ng/mL in 75–85% of patients with severe chronic pancreatitis (those with steatorrhea) and 15–20% of those with mild to moderate disease; occasionally low in cancer of the pancreas; normal (10–75 ng/mL) in nonpancreatic causes of malabsorption.

Carotene tolerance test: Measure serum carotene following daily oral loading of carotene for 3–7 days. Low values for serum carotene levels are usually associated with steatorrhea. Increase of serum carotene by >35 µg/dL indicates previously low dietary intake of carotene and/or fat. Patients with sprue in remission with normal fecal fat excretion may still show low carotene absorption.

Vitamin A tolerance test (for screening steatorrhea): Measure plasma vitamin A level 5 hours after ingestion. Normal rise is 9× fasting level. Flat curve in liver disease. Not useful after gastrectomy. With vitamin A as ester of long-chain fatty acid, flat curve occurs in both pancreatic disease and intestinal mucosal abnormalities; when water-soluble forms of vitamin A are used, the curve becomes normal in patients with pancreatic disease but remains flat in intestinal mucosal abnormalities. An abnormal result indicates a defect in small bowel mucosal absorption function (e.g., sprue, Whipple disease, regional enteritis, TB enteritis, collagen diseases involving the small bowel, extensive resection). Abnormal pancreatic function does not affect the test.

CARBOHYDRATE ABSORPTION INDICES

- Disaccharide malabsorption
  - ▼ Causes
    - Primary malabsorption (congenital or acquired) because of absence of specific disaccharidase in brush border of small intestine mucosa
    - Isolated lactase deficiency (also called milk allergy, milk intolerance, congenital familial lactose intolerance, lactase deficiency) (is most common of these defects; occurs in approximately 10% of whites and 60% of blacks; infantile type shows diarrhea, vomiting, failure to thrive, malabsorption, and so on; often appears first in adults; become asymptomatic when lactase is removed from diet)
  - ▼ Sucrose–isomaltose malabsorption (inherited recessive defect)
    - Oral sucrose tolerance curve is flat, but glucose plus fructose tolerance test is normal. Occasionally, there is an associated malabsorption with increased stool fat and abnormal D-xylose tolerance test, although intestinal biopsy is normal.
    - Hydrogen breath test after sucrose challenge.
    - Intestinal biopsy with measurement of disaccharidase activities.
    - Sucrose-free diet causes cessation of diarrhea.
  - ▼ Glucose–galactose malabsorption (inherited autosomal recessive defect that affects the kidney and intestine)
    - Oral glucose or galactose tolerance curve is flat, but IV tolerance curves are normal.
    - Glucosuria is common. Fructose tolerance test is normal.
  - ▼ Secondary malabsorption
    - Resection of >50% of the colon disaccharidase activity. Lactose is most marked, but there may also be sucrose. Oral disaccharide tolerance

(especially lactose) is abnormal, but intestinal histology and enzyme activity are normal.

▼ Diffuse intestinal disease—especially celiac disease in which activity of all disaccharidases may be decreased, with later increase as intestine becomes normal on gluten-free diet; also cystic fibrosis of the pancreas, severe malnutrition, UC, severe *Giardia* infestation, blind loop syndrome, β-lipoprotein deficiency, effect of drugs (e.g., colchicine, neomycin, birth control pills). Oral tolerance tests (especially lactose) are frequently abnormal, with later return to normal with gluten-free diet. Tolerance tests with monosaccharides may also be abnormal because of defect in absorption as well as digestion.

▼ Small intestinal bacterial overgrowth (see Figure 5-4)

● Quantitative aerobic and anaerobic culture of aspirate of small bowel content showing >10^5 cfu/mL of anaerobic organisms is considered diagnostic. The utility of culture is limited, however, because it requires invasive collection; there may be sampling error due to limited regions of involvement within the small bowel, and culture techniques and interpretation are not standardized.

● ^{14}C-D-xylose breath test has good specificity.

● Hydrogen breath tests (glucose-H$_2$, lactulose-H$_2$)—not recommended because of limited sensitivity and specificity.

CELIAC DISEASE (GLUTEN-SENSITIVE ENTEROPATHY, NONTROPICAL SPRUE, IDIOPATHIC STEATORRHEA)

❏ **Definition**
Celiac disease is an autoimmune multisystem disorder (principally manifested in the GI tract) in genetically susceptible persons that may be caused by a mucosal injury by a complex of gliadin (a protein from dietary gluten in wheat, rye, barley, or oats) with tissue transglutaminase (tTG), a cross-linking enzyme. Findings are caused by malabsorption and autoimmunity.

❏ **Laboratory Findings**
Although there are no universally accepted tests for the diagnosis of celiac disease, specific serologic testing and small bowel biopsy are very sensitive and specific for making the diagnosis. All tests must be performed while patients are on a diet of food that contains gluten (Figure 5-5).

Histology: Biopsy of jejunum is the diagnostic gold standard; shows characteristic although not specific mucosal lesions. Establishing the diagnosis is essential; patients should not be committed to lifelong gluten-free diet without first assessing intestinal mucosal histology. False-negative results may occur because of patchy distribution of pathology.

Stool findings: Steatorrhea demonstrated by positive Sudan stain on ≥2 stool samples or quantitative determination of fat in 72-hour pooled stool sample.

Anti-human IgA tTG antibodies: (by ELISA) has S/S = >90%/>95%. False-negative results may occur in patients with IgA deficiency (present in 2.5% of patients with celiac disease for whom corresponding IgG antibody tests may be useful). More reproducible than EMA test.

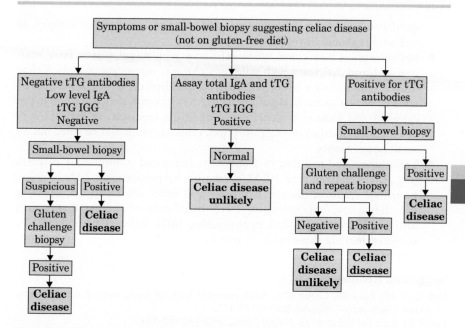

Figure 5–5 *Symptoms or small bowel biopsy suggesting celiac disease. tTG, transglutaminase.*

Anti-IgA deamidated gliadin IgG/IgA antibodies: Deamidated gliadin antibody (DGA) recognizes an antigen related to dietary gluten and is responsible for initiating inflammation in celiac disease. Antigliadin IgA antibodies (by ELISA) have been superseded by these more sensitive tests; has S/S = 80%/80–90%. IgA antigliadin antibodies become undetectable 3–6 months after gluten abstinence; may be used to monitor dietary compliance. May be most effective marker for children <3 years of age. Gliadin is a component of gluten. False-negative results may occur in patients on immunosuppressive therapy. If patient is IgA deficient, serology using IgG-tTG or IgG-EMA should be used.

Molecular tests: HLA variation DQ2 is expressed in approximately 95% of patients; HLA-DQ8 performed by DNA testing is expressed in approximately 5% of patients; absence of these virtually excludes this diagnosis.

Gluten challenge: No longer considered essential to establish the diagnosis. It is done if the diagnosis is uncertain and not documented by biopsy before gluten withdrawal, to determine if symptoms and mucosal changes occur.

Xylose tolerance test: Distinguishes malabsorption caused by impaired transport across diseased mucosa from that caused by impaired digestion in the lumen. Normal in many patients with mild to moderate disease not usually performed.

Considerations

- Firm diagnosis requires definite clinical response to gluten-free diet in 3–9 months, preferably with histologic documentation that the mucosa has reverted to normal by repeat biopsy. If the patient fails to respond to rigid dietary control, biopsy should be repeated to rule out GI lymphoma, giardiasis, hypogammaglobulinemia, and other causes of villous atrophy, as well as diet should be rechecked.

- Malabsorption may cause folate deficiency with megaloblastic bone marrow and iron deficiency with mild hypochromic macrocytic anemia. Celiac disease should always be considered in cases of iron deficiency or macrocytic anemia. May also have coagulopathy due to vitamin K deficiency and hypocalcemia and vitamin D deficiency causing osteomalacia. In patients with unexplained diarrhea or malabsorption, celiac sprue should be ruled out by small bowel biopsy.
- Laboratory findings due to frequently associated autoimmune diseases (e.g., thyroid, liver, type 1 DM, dermatitis herpetiformis [≤20% of celiac patients], Addison disease, arthritis) and other diseases (e.g., selective IgA deficiency; hyposplenism, T-cell lymphoma of the small intestine; also Down syndrome, IgA nephropathy, IBD). Patients who should be screened include those with steatorrhea, malabsorption, or autoimmune diseases.

Suggested Readings

Dukowicz AC, Lacy BE, Levine GM. Small intestinal bacterial overgrowth: a comprehensive review. *Gastroenterol Hepatol.* 2007;3:112–122.

Farrell RJ, Kelly CP. Celiac sprue. *N Engl J Med.* 2002;346:180–188.

Mäki M, Mustalahti K, Kokkonen J, et al. Prevalence of celiac disease among children in Finland. *N Engl J Med.* 2003;348:2517–2524.

ENTEROPATHY, PROTEIN LOSING

❑ Definition

This condition refers to the GI loss of plasma protein in abnormal amounts.

❑ Causes

- Secondary (i.e., disease states in which clinically significant protein-losing enteropathy may occur as a manifestation)
    - ▼ Giant hypertrophy of gastric rugae (Ménétrier disease)
    - ▼ Eosinophilic gastroenteritis
    - ▼ Gastric neoplasms
    - ▼ Infections (e.g., Whipple disease, bacterial overgrowth, enterocolitis, shigellosis, parasitic infestation, viral infections, *C. difficile* infection) (See relevant sections in Chapter 11, Infectious Diseases)
    - ▼ Nontropical sprue
    - ▼ Inflammatory and neoplastic diseases of the small and large intestines, including UC, regional enteritis
    - ▼ Constrictive pericarditis
    - ▼ Immune diseases (e.g., SLE)
    - ▼ Lymphatic obstruction (e.g., lymphoma, sarcoidosis, mesenteric TB)
- Primary (i.e., hypoproteinemia is the major clinical feature)
    - ▼ Intestinal lymphangiectasia
    - ▼ Nonspecific inflammatory or granulomatous disease of the small intestine

❑ Laboratory Findings

Core laboratory: Serum cholesterol usually normal. Serum total protein, albumin, γ-globulin, and calcium are decreased. Serum α- and β-globulins normal. Proteinuria absent.

Hematology: Mild anemia. Eosinophilia (occasionally).

Stool findings: Steatorrhea with abnormal tests of lipid absorption.

Other: Increased permeability of the GI tract to large molecular substances shown by IV iodine-131-polyvinylpyrrolidone (^{131}I-PVP) test (see Malabsorption).

COLITIS, COLLAGENOUS

5

❑ Definition

Syndrome of chronic nonbloody diarrhea. The incidence is approximately 3/1,000 in such patients. Diagnosis is established by biopsy of the colon in patients thought to have irritable bowel syndrome.

❑ Laboratory Findings

Hematology: ESR is increased, and anemia and hypoalbuminemia occur in some patients. Eosinophil count is increased in some patients.

COLITIS, PSEUDOMEMBRANOUS

- See *Clostridium difficile* in Chapter 11, Infectious Diseases.

GALLSTONE ILEUS

- Laboratory findings caused by preceding chronic cholecystitis and cholelithiasis
- Laboratory findings caused by acute obstruction of the terminal ileum (accounts for 1–2% of patients)

GASTROENTERITIS, EOSINOPHILIC

❑ Definition

Diagnosis requires histologic evidence of predominant eosinophilic (>20 eosinophils/HPF) infiltration of the GI tract in the absence of parasitic infection or extraintestinal disease.

❑ Laboratory Findings

Hematology: Eosinophilia in 80% of cases.

Other: Eosinophilic ascites with predominant disease of serosal layer. IgE may be increased, especially in children.

Suggested Readings

Bonis PAL, LaMont JT. Approach to the adult with chronic diarrhea in developed countries. www.uptodate.com, May 2009.

Khan F, Sachs H, Pechet L, et al. *Guide to Diagnostic Testing.* Philadelphia, PA: Lippincott Williams & Wilkins; 2002.

Wanke C. Approach to the adult with acute diarrhea in developed countries. www.uptodate.com, May 2009.

GASTROINTESTINAL BLEEDING

UPPER GASTROINTESTINAL BLEEDING (ADULT)

❑ Definition

Upper GI bleeding is defined as emanating from a source above the ligament of Treitz. This is the most common medical emergency for gastroenterologists. The mortality is approximately 8%, and it is not usually due to exsanguination but rather due to the adverse effect on comorbid conditions.

❑ Who Should Be Suspected?

The patient may present with stigmata of chronic blood loss (*iron deficiency* anemia and related symptoms) or acute blood loss (weakness or syncope).

Screening: Currently, screening for asymptomatic ulcerated lesions of the GI tract is generally recommended, especially for carcinoma of the colon and large adenomas.

❑ Differential Diagnosis of Upper Gastrointestinal Bleeding (Table 5-3)

- PUD (see discussion of acute abdomen under Abdominal Pain) (40–50% of patients) is associated with risk factors including *H. pylori* infection, use of NSAIDs, stress, and increase of gastric acid. It accounts for gastritis in 10% of patients, esophagitis 6% associated with gastric reflux (GERD). Risk factors for stress-related bleeding include respiratory failure and coagulopathy. Portal hypertension and varices (18% of patients) indicate the severity of a patient's underlying cirrhosis. These patients have an associated mortality of 50% even after control of the hemorrhage.
- Mallory-Weiss tears (5% of patients) occur in the distal esophagus, at the site of the gastroesophageal junction, usually following a bout of retching. Most tears heal uneventfully within 24–48 hours. The diagnosis is made by

---

TABLE 5-3. Differential Diagnosis of Upper Gastrointestinal Bleeding

- Peptic ulcer disease (40–50%; idiopathic; induced by drug, toxin, or stress; related to an infection; associated with Zollinger-Ellinger syndrome)
- Erosive esophagitis, gastritis, and duodenitis 25%
- Portal hypertension and varices (10–15%; esophageal, gastric, duodenal, and portal hypertensive gastropathy)
- Mallory-Weiss tear (5%)
- Rare causes: arteriovenous malformations, Rendu-Osler-Weber syndrome, watermelon stomach (gastric antral vascular ectasia), Dieulafoy lesion, stomal ulcer, neoplasm (benign, primary, and metastatic malignancy), connective tissue disease (scleroderma, Ehlers-Danlos syndrome), aortic enteric fistula, hemobilia, uremic gastritis, foreign body
- Carcinoma of the stomach
- Heyde syndrome (acquired von Willebrand, angiodysplasia, aortic stenosis)

endoscopic evaluation, at which time therapeutic interventions may be utilized as well as stratifying the risk of rebleeding.

- Neoplasm of the esophagus and stomach accounts for <5% of all cases of severe bleeding. It is generally a late manifestation and represents a negative prognostic feature. Uncommonly, tumors may metastasize to the gastric mucosa.
- Anticoagulant therapy: GI hemorrhage occurs in 3–4% of patients on anticoagulant therapy; it may be spontaneous or secondary to unsuspected disease (e.g., peptic ulcer, carcinoma, diverticula, hemorrhoids). Occasionally, there is hemorrhage into the wall of the intestine with secondary ileus. PT may be in the therapeutic range or, more commonly, is increased. Warfarin (Coumadin) drug action is potentiated by administration of aspirin, antibiotics, phenylbutazone, and thyroxine and by T-tube drainage of the common bile duct, especially if pancreatic disease is present.
- Occult bleeding.
- Rendu-Osler-Weber syndrome is associated with telangiectasia of the lips, oral mucosa, and fingertips. Dieulafoy lesion correlates with a dilated aberrant submucosal vessel, which erodes the overlying mucosa in the absence of an ulcer. This should be suspected in the patient with recurrent episodes of undiagnosed upper GI bleeding (GI bleeding in 10–40% of patients).

❑ **Causes**

- Mass (e.g., carcinoma, adenoma). In addition to the main cause of bleeding, 50% of patients have an additional lesion that could cause hemorrhage (especially duodenal ulcer, esophageal varices, hiatal hernia). With previously known GI tract lesions, 40% of patients bled from an altogether different lesion.
- Inflammation (e.g., IBD, Crohn disease, erosive esophagitis).
- Vascular disorders (e.g., varices, hemangioma).
- Infections (e.g., TB, amebiasis, hookworm, whipworm, strongyloidiasis, ascariasis).
- Other sites (e.g., hemoptysis, epistaxis, oropharynx).
- Others (e.g., factitious, coagulopathies, long-distance running).
- Use of fecal occult blood test (See: Occult Blood, Stool, in *Chapter 16. Laboratory Tests.*)

❑ **Laboratory Findings**

- Initial assessment: Assess magnitude of blood loss (CBC, vital signs).
  - ▼ Check coagulation (PT, PTT, platelets) and other tests to rule out either an acquired or a congenital bleeding disorder.
  - ▼ Type and cross-match number of units appropriate for severity of blood loss.
- Esophagogastroduodenoscopy (EGD) is the diagnostic procedure of choice for patients presenting with acute GI bleeding. Advantages of early EGD include the following:
  - ▼ Confirmation or modification of the working diagnosis, proposed by the history and physical examination
  - ▼ Providing therapeutic measures, which lessen transfusion requirements and the need for surgery

▼ Potentially averting the need for hospitalization

▼ In patients with iron deficiency, recommend upper and lower endoscopy plus workup for celiac disease

❑ **Limitations**

■ Adenomas <2 cm in greatest diameter are less likely to bleed. Upper GI tract bleeding is less likely than lower GI tract bleeding to cause a positive test.

■ Long-distance running is associated with positive guaiac test in ≤23% of runners.

■ Stools may appear grossly normal with GI bleeding of 100 mL/day.

■ Consistent melena requires 150–200 mL blood in the stomach.

GASTROINTESTINAL BLEEDING, SMALL INTESTINE

■ The small intestine is an uncommon site of hemorrhage, accounting for only 3–5% of GI bleeding. Patients usually present with occult blood loss and may have evidence of melena or hematochezia.

❑ **Differential Diagnosis of Gastrointestinal Bleeding from the Small Intestine (Table 5-4)**

■ Angiodysplasia accounts for the majority of cases of bleeding from the small intestine (70–80%). Bleeding can be either brisk or occult. An isolated episode of bleeding does not mandate therapy, as the lesions do not usually rebleed (approximately 50%). Angiodysplasia may be an incidental finding and needs to be documented to be considered as a source of blood loss.

■ Tumors account for 5–10% of cases of blood from the small intestine. Of these, one third are benign (leiomyoma and adenomas most commonly) and two thirds are malignant (45% adenocarcinoma, usually of the duodenum, 30% carcinoid, 14% lymphoma, and 11% leiomyosarcoma). The three

---

TABLE 5–4. Differential Diagnosis of Gastrointestinal Bleeding from the Small Intestine

• Angiodysplasia
• Small bowel tumors
• Less common causes:
  • Ulcerative diseases (most commonly Crohn disease)
  • Meckel diverticulum (the cause in two thirds of men younger than 30 years of age)
  • Zollinger-Ellison syndrome (causes ulcerations)
  • Infections (e.g., tuberculosis, syphilis, typhoid, histoplasmosis)
  • Medications (e.g., potassium, nonsteroidal anti-inflammatory drugs, 6-mercaptopurine)
  • Vasculitis
  • Radiation enteritis (injury can occur 6–24 months after exposure, secondary to the development of occlusive vasculitis)
  • Jejunal diverticula (<5% actually bleed, but bleeding is usually massive, with mortality as high as 20%)
  • Vascular lesions (varices, venous ectasias, telangiectasias, hemangiomas, arteriovenous malformations)

most common malignancies are generally associated with chronic blood loss. Metastatic disease may also occur, most commonly from melanoma and breast cancer.

❏ Laboratory Findings

- Plain abdominal films may show evidence of obstruction suggestive of stricture or tumor, but they are not likely to be diagnostic.
- Contrast radiography
  - ▼ Small bowel series have a low yield in identifying a bleeding source (i.e., a 5% detection rate). This may be increased to 10% with use of enteroclysis. If the bleeding source is a small intestine malignancy, the yield is considerably better.
  - ▼ Barium studies cannot diagnose angiodysplasias, but they may be useful in identifying mass lesions and mucosal defects.
  - ▼ Despite the low diagnostic yield, contrast radiography is the initial study in a patient where small intestinal bleeding is suspected (i.e., when the evaluation of upper and lower GI tracts are nondiagnostic).
- Endoscopic studies
  - ▼ Routine EGD reaches the junction of the second and third portions of the duodenum.
  - ▼ Conventional push enteroscopy (either a dedicated enteroscope or a pediatric colonoscope) can reach the proximal jejunum. Yield with push enteroscopy varies from 24 to 75% in detecting a bleeding source. Push enteroscopy also has therapeutic value.
  - ▼ Sonde enteroscopy is a newer procedure that is being developed to visualize the entire jejunum and ileum. It is a flexible fiberoptic instrument carried through the bowel by peristalsis. It is not a routinely available procedure, and it is best reserved for those patients with comorbid conditions that may preclude intraoperative enteroscopy (video capsule endoscopy).
- Angiography detects a bleeding rate of 0.5 mL/minute. It can localize the site of bleeding in 50–72% of cases if bleeding is massive, but in only 25–50% of cases if bleeding has slowed. It has a low yield in diagnosing angiodysplasias and tumors.
- Nuclear imaging
  - ▼ Technetium-99 bleeding scan may detect bleeding at a rate as slight as 0.1 mL/minute. Like angiography, it is only of value in the setting of active bleeding. It can define a general area of bleeding, but it cannot identify the precise source.
  - ▼ Technetium-99 Meckel scan, which is taken up by ectopic gastric mucosa in the diverticulum, is not useful if the diverticulum does not contain gastric mucosa.
- Surgical evaluation
  - ▼ Intraoperative enteroscopy is a procedure whereby the bowel is manually advanced over an endoscope. It is the most common way to examine the entire small bowel. It is successful in identifying a bleeding source 83–100% of the time.
  - ▼ Exploratory surgery is often considered in patients with recurrent GI bleeding of unclear origin. Simple exploration has a low success rate, with

5

a diagnostic yield of only 10% when unaccompanied by other evaluations (i.e., enteroscopy).

■ Stepwise approach to evaluation: In a study of 77 patients, the interval from presentation to diagnosis was >20 months, because of the relatively asymptomatic nature of the conditions and the difficulty in evaluating small bowel bleeding sources.

■ Determine the source of bleeding
  ▼ In those with a nondiagnostic evaluation of lower and upper GI tracts, small bowel evaluation will be necessary.
  ▼ Once the small bowel is assumed to be the bleeding source (i.e., standard examinations are nondiagnostic), proceed to small bowel series.

■ If the source is not identified
  ▼ Proceed to push enteroscopy, before considering repeat EGD or colonoscopy.
  ▼ Sonde enteroscopy may be considered.
  ▼ Withhold bleeding scans and angiography, unless the patient is actively bleeding.
  ▼ Exploratory surgery can be done with intraoperative endoscopy if needed.
  ▼ Video capsule endoscopy.

❑ **Neoplasms Caused by Primary Diseases of the Small Intestine**

■ Biopsy of lesions confirms the diagnosis.
■ Laboratory findings due to complications (e.g., hemorrhage, obstruction, intussusception, malabsorption).
■ Laboratory findings due to underlying conditions (e.g., Peutz-Jeghers syndrome, carcinoid syndrome).

LOWER GASTROINTESTINAL BLEEDING (ADULT), ACUTE

❑ **Overview**

■ Lower GI bleeding is usually defined by bleeding originating from below the ligament of Treitz.
■ If the initial assessment does not clearly distinguish between upper and lower sources of GI bleeding, evaluation of the upper tract should be pursued, as this is the more common site of massive GI bleeding.

❑ **Differential Diagnosis of Lower Gastrointestinal Bleeding (Table 5-5)**

■ Angiodysplasia: In elderly patients, angiodysplasia is diagnosed with proportional greater frequency. Angiodysplasia is not visualized by barium enema. The bleeding tends to be self-limited, frequently arising from the right colon.
■ Benign anorectal pathology: In younger patients (<35 years of age), benign anorectal pathology (e.g., hemorrhoidal bleeding) is the most common etiology.
■ Diverticulosis: Less than 33% of patients with diverticulosis develop significant bleeding. The bleeding is typically painless and occurs in the absence of diverticulitis. Although diverticula are more commonly located on the left side of the colon, right-sided lesions account for a significant portion of diverticular bleeding.

TABLE 5–5. Differential Diagnosis of Lower Gastrointestinal Bleeding

- Diverticulosis (~33%)
- Angiodysplasia (~28%)
- Neoplasia (benign and malignant ~19%)
- Colitis (ulcerative, Crohn, ischemic, pseudomembranous, infectious disease, radiation exposure approximately 18%)
- Hemorrhoid (approximately 3%)
- Less common causes:
  - Solitary ulcers
  - Nonsteroidal anti-inflammatory drugs
  - Venous lakes
  - Blue rubber nevus
  - Anastomotic ulcerations and suture lines
  - Mechanical trauma
  - Postbiopsy or polypectomy
  - Coagulopathy and anticoagulation therapy
  - Autoimmune disease (e.g., rheumatoid vasculitis, Henoch-Schönlein purpura)

5

- Colon cancer polyps account for 19% of patients with lower gastrointestinal blood loss in patients older than 50 years of age.
- Coagulopathy usually causes bleeding in patients with a comorbid GI condition. Therefore, a patient with coagulopathy always requires further evaluation.
- Suspect upper GI bleeding in patients presenting with hematochezia.
- Hemorrhoids and bloody diarrhea from inflammation need to be ruled out.

❑ **Diagnostic Evaluation**

- Initial assessment
  - ▼ Check coagulation studies (PT, PTT, platelets, CBC, BUN, creatinine). Bleeding in uremic patients with angiodysplasia may be a result of acquired coagulopathy. May present as iron deficiency. Perform serum ferritin.
  - ▼ Type and cross-match number of units appropriate for severity of blood loss.
- Endoscopic studies (assuming an upper GI bleed is excluded by virtue of nonbloody bilious fluid obtained via nasogastric lavage)
  - ▼ Anoscopy may be performed to rule out bleeding hemorrhoids in appropriately selected patients.
  - ▼ Colonoscopy will identify a bleeding source in approximately 80% of patients and will help control bleeding in up to 40% of patients. Other advantages include assisting in preoperative assessment.
- Neoplasms, colon: Blood in stool (occult or gross). Annual screening for occult blood detects <50% of cancers and 10% of adenomas.

Suggested Readings

Bonis PAL, Bynum TE. Angiodysplasia of the gastrointestinal tract. www.uptodate.com, May 2009.

Jutabha R. Etiology of lower gastrointestinal bleeding in adults. www.uptodate.com, May 2009.

Jutabha R. Approach to the adult patient with lower gastrointestinal bleeding. www.uptodate.com, May 2009.

Jutabha R, Jensen D. Approach to the adult patient with upper gastrointestinal bleeding. www.uptodate.com, May 2009.

Khan F, Sachs H, Pechet L, et al. *Guide to Diagnostic Testing.* Philadelphia, PA: Lippincott Williams & Wilkins; 2002.

Travis A, Saltzman J. Evaluation of occult gastrointestinal bleeding. www.uptodate.com, May 2009.

Villa X. Approach to upper gastrointestinal bleeding in children. www.uptodate.com, 1–27, May 2009.

HEPATOMEGALY

❏ **Definition**

■ Hepatomegaly refers to an enlarged liver with a vertical span >12 cm as percussed in the midclavicular line. Studies have suggested that by ultrasound, a midhepatic (sagittal) diameter >15.5 cm indicates hepatomegaly in 75% of the cases. By radioisotope scanning, a span of >15–17 cm in the midclavicular line indicates hepatomegaly.

■ Hepatomegaly may occur in the absence of pathology (i.e., normal variant) or as a result of a depressed right hemidiaphragm, Riedel lobe, or subdiaphragmatic space occupying lesions.

❏ **Differential Diagnosis and Workup (Figure 5-6)**

■ The causes of hepatomegaly can be subdivided into processes involving the following:

▼ Hypertrophy or hyperplasia of cells intrinsic to the normal liver parenchyma

▼ Hepatomegaly secondary to infiltration of the liver by cells or organisms not normally present

▼ Vascular causes resulting in congestion of the liver

■ Common causes: Fatty liver (nonalcoholic steatohepatitis) is a common cause of hepatomegaly. The most common cause of fatty liver in the United States is chronic alcoholism. Other causes of fatty liver include diabetes, obesity, hyperlipidemia (metabolic syndrome), protein malnutrition, and prolonged TPN.

▼ Other causes: In addition to infectious and drug-related causes, clinically important causes of hepatomegaly include hemochromatosis, α_1-antitrypsin deficiency, Wilson disease, autoimmune hepatitis, SLE, and RA.

▼ Cholangiohepatitis is a rare disorder in which intrahepatic and extrahepatic bile ducts become obstructed with bile stones, leading to secondary inflammation of the liver.

▼ Congestion from heart failure includes all causes of elevated right heart pressures (e.g., cor pulmonale, tricuspid regurgitation, constrictive pericarditis, ventricular dysfunction).

▼ Hepatocellular carcinoma represents approximately 2.5% of all carcinomas in the United States and approximately 30–50% of all carcinomas in Asians living in Asia, where chronic active hepatitis due to hepatitis B virus is common. Other risk factors include chronic hepatitis C or chronic liver disease of any type.

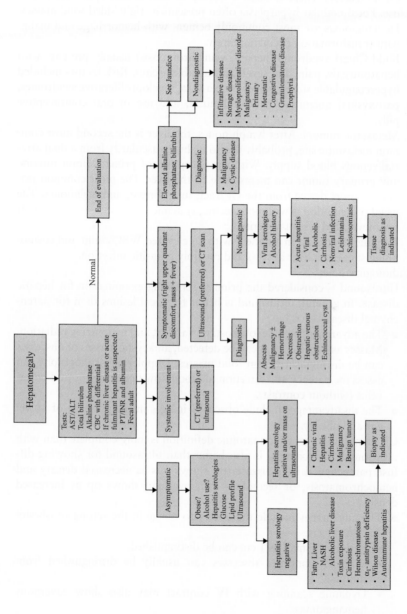

Figure 5–6 *Algorithm for the workup of hepatomegaly, if the vertical span is >12 cm by physical examination or imaging. ALT, alanine aminotransferase; AST, aspartate aminotransferase; CBC, complete blood count; CT, computed tomography; FOBT, fecal occult blood test; GI, gastrointestinal; INR, international normalized ratio; NASH, nonalcoholic steatohepatitis; PT, prothrombin time.*

▼ Benign tumors include adenomas, focal nodular hyperplasia, and hemangiomas. Adenomas are more commonly seen in women 30–40 years of age, mostly in the right lobe and can be as large as 10 cm in greatest dimension. There is often a history of oral contraceptive (estrogen) use. Focal nodular hyperplasia often presents as right-sided solid masses. Hemangiomas are most commonly benign, with hemorrhage and malignant transformation occurring rarely.

▼ Budd-Chiari syndrome (hepatic vein thrombosis) usually presents with hepatomegaly, pain, and severe, intractable ascites. Risk factors included hypercoagulable states, polycythemia vera, myeloproliferative syndromes, paroxysmal nocturnal, hemoglobinuria, and use of oral contraceptive pills.

▼ Metastatic tumors: After lymph nodes, the liver is the second most common metastatic site, probably due to its high vascularity from a dual arterial/venous blood supply. With the exception of primary brain tumors, any primary tumor can metastasize to the liver. The most common primary tumors derive from the GI tract, lung, breast, and melanoma. The usual presentation is with nonspecific, systemic symptoms such as weight loss, fever, and loss of appetite.

▼ A tender liver mass in a patient with an elevated WBC count and eosinophilia suggests a liver abscess and possibly parasitic infection.

■ Radiologic studies

 ▼ Ultrasound is considered the primary screening examination for hepatic disease. In general, ultrasound is better for focal lesions than for parenchymal disease.

 ● The advantages include low cost, portability, and no ionizing radiation. Masses as small as 1 cm can be detected, and cystic masses or abscesses can be distinguished from solid masses. Doppler ultrasonography can assess the patency and direction of blood flow in the hepatic and portal veins (without contrast).

 ● The disadvantages include obscured images in the presence of bowel gas and obesity.

 ▼ CT scanning: In general, anatomic definition is more complete than with ultrasound. CT scanning is also better than ultrasound for showing diffuse parenchymal liver disease (fat shows ups as decreased density and hemochromatosis, or secondary iron overload shows up as increased density).

 ● The advantages include the ability to image in the setting of obesity and bowel gas.

 • Lesions as small as 1 cm can be distinguished.

 • With IV contrast, abscesses can usually be distinguished from tumors.

 • Dynamic scanning with IV contrast may also show cavernous hemangiomas.

 • Mass lesions can be biopsied under either ultrasound or CT guidance.

 ● The disadvantages include cost, radiation, and possible exposure to IV contrast.

▼ Magnetic resonance imaging (MRI): Sensitivity is superior to CT scanning for mass lesions.
  ● The advantages include lack of ionizing radiation and different planes of imaging.
    • It is the technique of choice to look for hemangiomas.
    • It is useful in distinguishing between a regenerating nodule and a tumor in the cirrhotic liver.
    • MRI can be used to monitor the liver for iron and copper deposition and, with some modification, can identify fatty liver and can produce an estimated quantification of fat content.
    • It can sometimes detect Budd-Chiari syndrome (hepatic vein thrombosis) without the need for IV iodinated contrast media (gadolinium is required).
  ● The disadvantages include cost; slow time to acquire images, leading to more artifact; and limitations for patients with metal implants due to the use of a large magnet. MRI cannot distinguish a primary versus metastatic tumor.
▼ Radioisotope scanning has been largely replaced by ultrasound and CT scanning.
  ● Technetium-99m–labeled sulfur colloid scanning depends on uptake of phagocytic cells (Kupffer) and can help assess size and shape of the liver. Any disease where Kupffer cells are replaced by tumors, cysts, and abscesses produces a cold spot (adenomas); whereas with focal nodular hyperplasias, the liver will light up. Resolution for mass lesions is approximately 2 cm. Scintigraphy using radioactively labeled antibodies to tumor antigens is being developed as a diagnostic tool.
  ● Gallium scanning uses gallium that is preferentially taken up in tissues synthesizing proteins (tumors or abscesses), and such areas show up as hot spots.
▼ Imaging of the biliary tract
  ● ERCP allows for therapy (e.g., stone removal or stenting) as well as diagnosis.
  ● Percutaneous transhepatic cholangiography (PTC) allows for imaging of the proximal biliary ducts and some therapy (e.g., stent placement or percutaneous drainage) of the ducts.
  ● More recently, magnetic resonance cholangiopancreatography (MRCP) has demonstrated diagnostic accuracy similar to ERCP. The principal disadvantages include spatial resolution, which may not be as good as that achieved with ERCP; lack of therapeutic benefit; and decreased ability to visualize the ampulla.

FATTY LIVER

■ Nonalcoholic steatohepatitis in most cases may have a history of metabolic syndrome. Nutritional (e.g., alcoholism, malnutrition, starvation, rapid weight loss)

❏ Causes

- Drugs (e.g., aspirin,[†] glucocorticoids,[*] synthetic estrogens,[*] some antiviral agents,[*,†] calcium channel blockers,[†] cocaine,[†] methotrexate,[*] valproic acid[†])
- Metabolic/genetic (e.g., acute fatty liver of pregnancy, dysbetalipoproteinemia, Weber-Christian disease, cholesterol ester storage,[‡] Wolman disease[‡])
- Other (e.g., HIV infection, *B. cereus* toxins, liver toxins [e.g., organic solvents, phosphorus], small bowel disease [inflammatory, bacterial overgrowth], fatty liver of pregnancy)

❏ Laboratory Findings

- *Histology*: Biopsy of the liver establishes the diagnosis. Fatty liver may be the only postmortem finding in cases of sudden, unexpected death.
- *Core laboratory*: Most commonly, serum AST and ALT are increased 2–3×; usually ALT > AST in NAFL. Serum ALP is normal or slightly increased in <50% of patients. Other liver function tests are usually normal. Increased serum ferritin (≤5×) and transferrin saturation occur in approximately 60% of cases.
- *Serology*: Tests for viral hepatitis are negative.

Considerations

- Laboratory findings are due to underlying conditions (most commonly alcoholism; nonalcoholic fatty liver [NAFL] is commonly associated with type 2 DM [≤75%], obesity [69–100%], hyperlipidemia [20–81%]; hypertension malnutrition, toxic chemicals). NAFL is distinguished by negligible history of alcohol consumption and negative random blood alcohol assays. Cirrhosis occurs in ≤50% of alcoholic and ≤17% of nonalcoholic cases.

FATTY LIVER OF PREGNANCY, ACUTE

- The incidence is ≤1 per 15,000 deliveries; usually occurs >35th week of pregnancy.
- This is a medical emergency because of high maternal and fetal mortality that is markedly improved by termination of pregnancy.
- Often associated with preeclampsia (see Chapter 8, Renal and Urinary Tract Diseases).

❏ Laboratory Findings

- *Histology*: Biopsy of the liver confirms the diagnosis.
- *Core laboratory*: Increased AST and ALT to approximately 300 U (rarely >500 U) is used for early screening in suspicious cases; ratio is not helpful in differential diagnosis. Serum bilirubin may be normal early but will rise unless pregnancy terminates. Serum uric acid is increased disproportionately to BUN and creatinine, which may also be increased. Blood glucose is often decreased, sometimes markedly. Blood ammonia is usually increased. Neonatal liver function tests are usually normal but hypoglycemia may occur.
- *Hematology*: Increased WBC in >80% of cases (often >15,000/µL). Evidence of DIC in >75% of patients.

---

[*]May principally cause macrovesicular steatosis due to imbalance in hepatic synthesis and export of lipids.
[†]May principally cause microvesicular steatosis due to defective mitochondrial function.
[‡]May principally cause accumulation of phospholipids in lysosomes.

NEOPLASMS OF THE LIVER: HEPATOCELLULAR CARCINOMA (HEPATOMA)

❏ **Laboratory Findings**

- *Core laboratory*: Serum AFP may be increased for up to 18 months before symptoms; is a sensitive indicator of recurrence in treated patients, but a normal postoperative level does not ensure the absence of metastases. Levels >500 ng/dL in adults strongly suggest hepatoma. Levels >100× URL have S/S = 60%/100%. In ≤30% of hepatoma cases, AFP <4× URL; such increases are common in chronic HBC and HCV. Serum GGT hepatoma–specific band (HSBs I′, II, II′) by electrophoresis activity >5.5 U/L has S/S = 85%/97%, accuracy = 92%. Does not correlate with AFP or tumor size.
- *Hematology*: ESR and WBC sometimes increased. Anemia is common; polycythemia occurs occasionally. Hemochromatosis (≤20% of patients die of hepatoma).
- *Serology*: Markers of viral hepatitis are frequently present.
- *Tumor markers*: Serum CEA is usually normal. CEA in bile is increased in patients with cholangiocarcinoma and intrahepatic stones but not in patients with benign stricture, choledochal cysts, and sclerosing cholangitis. Increases with progression of disease and declines with tumor resection.

Considerations

- Sudden progressive worsening of laboratory findings of underlying disease (e.g., increased serum ALP, LD, AST, bilirubin).
- Relative absence of hepatoma associated with cirrhosis of Wilson disease.
- Laboratory findings due to obstruction of hepatic (Budd-Chiari syndrome) or portal veins or the inferior vena cava may occur.

Suggested Readings

Friedman LS. Congestive hepatopathy. www.uptodate.com, May 2009.

Khan F, Sachs H, Pechet L, et al. *Guide to Diagnostic Testing.* Philadelphia, PA: Lippincott Williams & Wilkins; 2002.

Yao DF, Yao DB, Wu XH, et al. Diagnosis of hepatocellular carcinoma by quantitative detection of hepatoma-specific bands of serum γ-glutamyltransferase. *Am J Clin Pathol.* 1998; 110:743.

 JAUNDICE (SEE HEPATOMEGALY)

❏ **Overview**

- Jaundice is a yellowish staining of the integument, sclerae, and deeper tissues and is associated with conditions that have increased excretions of bile pigments, which are increased in the plasma.
- Physiology
  - ▼ Serum bilirubin accumulates when its production from heme exceeds its metabolism and excretion.
  - ▼ An imbalance between the production and clearance of serum bilirubin results either from excess release of bilirubin into the bloodstream or

from physiologic processes that impair the hepatic uptake, metabolism, or excretion of this metabolite.

▼ Jaundice is clinically detectable when the serum bilirubin exceeds 2.0–2.5 mg/dL. Because elastin has a high affinity for bilirubin, and scleral tissue is rich in elastin, scleral icterus is usually a more sensitive sign than generalized jaundice.

■ Bilirubin metabolism

▼ Unconjugated bilirubin: More than 90% of serum bilirubin in normal individuals is in an unconjugated form, circulating as an albumin-bound complex. This is not filtered by the kidneys.

▼ Conjugated bilirubin: The remainder is conjugated (primarily as a glucuronide), rendering it water soluble, and thus capable of being filtered and excreted by the kidney.

▼ Hepatic phase: Hepatic metabolism has three phases: uptake, conjugation, and excretion.

● Uptake phase: Unconjugated bilirubin is bound to albumin and is presented to the hepatocyte, where the complex dissociates and bilirubin enters the cell either by diffusion or by transport across the membrane.

● Conjugation phase: Bilirubin is then conjugated in a two-step process. This occurs in the endoplasmic reticulum and is catalyzed by glucuronyl transferase. Bilirubin glucuronide is generated.

● Excretion phase: In an energy-dependent process occurring in the biliary canaliculi, conjugated bilirubin is excreted into the bile. It is important to remember that this is the rate-limiting step. When this phase is impaired, either through obstruction or through excretory defects, the conjugated bilirubin is presumed to reflux through the hepatic sinusoids into the bloodstream.

▼ Intestinal phase: After excretion into the bile, conjugated bile is transported into the duodenum. It is not reabsorbed by intestinal mucosa. In the intestine, it is either excreted in the feces unchanged or metabolized by intestinal bacteria to urobilinogen. Urobilinogen is then reabsorbed, where a small portion is metabolized in the liver, and the remainder bypasses the liver and is excreted by the kidney.

❏ **Differential Diagnosis of Jaundice (Table 5-6)**

■ Extrahepatic biliary obstruction

▼ The history, physical examination, and initial laboratory assessment have a sensitivity of 90–95%. The specificity, however, is only 76%. When radiologic imaging is factored in, the specificity rises to 98%.

▼ Approximately 40% of patients with this diagnosis present with jaundice.

▼ In the setting of complete obstruction, alcoholic stools are seen and no urobilinogen is detected in the urine (see Cancer Head of the Pancreas, Acute Abdomen).

▼ In patients with extrahepatic biliary obstruction, ALP would be expected to rise to levels 2–3 times normal. A normal level would be uncommon. Serum transaminases would generally be <300 U/L.

TABLE 5–6. Differential Diagnosis of Jaundice

Conjugated Hyperbilirubinemia

- Hepatocellular jaundice
  - Hepatitis virus
  - Toxin or drugs (alcohol)
  - Cirrhosis
  - Ischemia
- Extrahepatic biliary obstruction
  - Choledocholithiasis
  - Ascending cholangitis
  - Pancreatitis—see Abdominal Pain
  - Sclerosing cholangitis
  - HIV cholangiopathy
  - Biliary stricture or cyst
  - Malignancy
    - Pancreas—see Abdominal Pain
    - Ampullary carcinoma
    - Cholangiocarcinoma
    - Metastatic
- Intrahepatic cholestasis
  - Abscess
  - Tumor
  - Primary biliary cirrhosis
  - Cholestatic jaundice of pregnancy
  - Dubin-Johnson syndrome
  - Rotor syndrome
  - Benign recurrent intrahepatic cholestasis
  - Sepsis
  - Infiltrative disease
    - Sarcoid
    - Amyloid

Unconjugated Hyperbilirubinemia

- Hemolysis
- Gilbert syndrome
- Ineffective erythropoiesis
- Hematoma resorption

- Intrahepatic cholestasis: Consider intrahepatic etiologies in the differential diagnosis because high levels may be seen in patients with primary biliary cirrhosis and granulomatous hepatitis.
  - This group of disorders is defined by the lack of evidence of mechanical obstruction and cannot be explained on the basis of hepatocellular injury alone. Among these disorders are those characterized by disordered enzyme function (intrinsic/acquired), infiltrative disorders, and drugs.
  - A diagnosis of intrahepatic cholestasis made by clinical assessment and supported by negative findings from ultrasound or CT scan offers 95% specificity. In a patient in whom extrahepatic obstruction is not strongly suspected, no further investigation of the extrahepatic biliary tree is indicated.

HYPERBILIRUBINEMIA

UNCONJUGATED HYPERBILIRUBINEMIA

❏ **Causes**

- Increased destruction of RBCs
  - ▼ Isoimmunization (e.g., incompatibility of Rh, ABO, other blood groups)
  - ▼ Biochemical defects of RBCs (e.g., G6PD deficiency, pyruvate deficiency, hexokinase deficiency, congenital erythropoietic porphyria, and α- and γ-thalassemias)
  - ▼ Structural defects of RBCs (e.g., hereditary spherocytosis, hereditary elliptocytosis, infantile pyknocytosis, hereditary xerocytosis)
  - ▼ Physiologic hemolysis of the newborn
    - Infection (viral, bacterial, and protozoal)
    - Congenital causes
    - Extravascular blood (e.g., subdural hematoma, ecchymoses, hemangiomas)
    - Erythrocytosis (e.g., maternal-to-fetal or twin-to-twin transfusion, delayed clamping of the umbilical cord)

❏ **Recommended Laboratory Evaluation**

These studies are of proven benefit in determining the proximate etiologies in the patient presenting with jaundice. With this approach, the clinician can confidently assign probabilities to the major categories that most frequently account for jaundice.

- The first step is to determine the total bilirubin and the bilirubin fractions. This allows the clinician to determine whether the problem is due to an excess production or impaired conjugation (indirect/unconjugated predominant) versus impaired excretion (direct/conjugated predominant).
- ALP elevations out of proportion to the hepatic transaminases would favor extrahepatic or intrahepatic cholestasis.
- Hepatic transaminase elevations out of proportion to the alkaline phosphatase favor hepatocellular etiologies.
- The CBC can be extremely useful. The most important points include the interpretation of or for
  - ▼ Anemia (hemolysis, bleeding) (see Chapter 10, Hematologic Disorders)
  - ▼ Mean corpuscular volume (microcytosis suggests iron deficiency; round macrocytosis suggests chronic liver disease or ineffective erythropoiesis; GI malignancy)
  - ▼ Thrombocytopenia (sequestration in portal hypertension, sepsis, autoimmune disease, bone marrow suppression [alcohol])
  - ▼ Reticulocytosis (hemolysis) (see Chapter 10, Hematologic Disorders)
- Urinalysis provides information about bilirubinuria and urobilinogen. In reality, data from urinalysis add little incremental benefit to the decision-making process.
  - ▼ The presence of urobilinogen eliminates the possibility of complete biliary tract obstruction. That is, bile has entered the intestine, where it undergoes enterohepatic metabolism.
  - ▼ The presence of bilirubinuria, on the other hand, suggests that conjugation is taking place.

- Coagulation studies are useful in two areas.
  - ▼ If an invasive intervention is considered, coagulation studies can be used to assess bleeding risk.
  - ▼ If the prothrombin time is prolonged and other causes of coagulopathy are unlikely, chronic liver disease or hepatocellular etiologies become increasingly likely.
- Serum amylase would be obtained in cases where extrahepatic obstruction is suspected on the basis of history and physical examination.

❑ Diagnostic Imaging

- It is estimated that 25–40% of common bile duct obstructions are missed by both ultrasound and CT scanning. However, when intrahepatic cholestasis or hepatocellular etiologies are suspected, either of these noninvasive strategies is acceptable.
- *Ultrasound*: This is the least invasive and most inexpensive of the imaging procedures available to assess obstructive jaundice. Ultrasound determines the presence of obstructive jaundice by detecting dilated bile ducts.
  - ▼ The sensitivity is 55–93%, and the specificity is 73–96%.
  - ▼ False negatives are generally due to two factors:
    - Inability to visualize the biliary tree (often secondary to interposed bowel gas)
    - Absence of biliary dilation in the presence of obstruction
  - ▼ It may be preferable, given its lower cost and radiation exposure.
- CT scanning is slightly more sensitive (74–96%) and specific (90–94%) than ultrasound in detecting the presence of biliary obstruction.
  - ▼ A CT scan is more likely to show the site and cause of obstruction when compared with ultrasound.
  - ▼ CT scan also gives information in instances where staging a suspected neoplasm has clinical significance (see Cancer Head of the Pancreas).
  - ▼ In patients for whom mass lesions (i.e., malignancy, abscess) are suspected or where technical limitations make ultrasound difficulty to interpret, CT is preferred.
- *Percutaneous transhepatic cholangiography (PTC)*: The technical success rate of this procedure is approximately 90–99%. Its use is limited by a major complication rate of 3–5% and has been largely supplanted by endoscopic retrograde cholangiopancreatography (ERCP). ERCP offers a lower complication rate than PTC and provides a greater number of therapeutic options (stone extraction, stent placement).
  - ▼ This test could reasonably be used in patients with a high likelihood of extrahepatic obstruction (e.g., those who have had recent biliary surgery, symptoms of cholangitis, palpable gallbladder, pain or fever, pancreatitis).
  - ▼ When palliation is the primary intent, ERCP is an appropriate initial procedure.
- *Magnetic resonance cholangiopancreatography (MRCP)* is a radiologic technique that produces images of the pancreaticobiliary tree, which are similar in appearance to those obtained by invasive methods. It appears to have diagnostic accuracy similar to that of ERCP.

5

▼ MRCP is indicated for patients with allergies to iodinated contrast media and patients with altered anatomy (i.e., secondary to surgical procedures or congenital abnormalities).

▼ ERCP has advantages over MRCP, which include the ability to perform therapeutic interventions, perform manometry or endoscopic ultrasound, directly visualize the ampulla, and biopsy lesions.

DISEASES ASSOCIATED WITH JAUNDICE

CONJUGATED HYPERBILIRUBINEMIA/HEPATOCELLULAR JAUNDICE

CIRRHOSIS OF THE LIVER

❑ **Laboratory Findings**

▪ *Bilirubin*: Serum levels are often increased; may be present for years. Fluctuations may reflect liver status due to insults to the liver (e.g., alcoholic debauches). Most bilirubin is of the unconjugated type unless cirrhosis is of the cholangiolitic type. Higher and more stable levels occur in post–necrotic cirrhosis; lower and more fluctuating levels occur in Laennec cirrhosis. Terminal icterus may be constant and severe. Urine bilirubin is increased; urobilinogen is normal or increased.

▪ *AST*: Serum levels are increased (<300 U) in 65–75% of patients. Serum ALT is increased (<200 U) in 50% of patients. Transaminases vary widely and reflect activity or progression of the process (i.e., hepatic parenchymal cell necrosis).

▪ *ALP*: Serum levels are increased in 40–50% of patients.

▪ *Total protein*: Usually normal or decreased. Serum albumin parallels functional status of parenchymal cells and may be useful for following progress of liver disease, but it may be normal in the presence of considerable liver cell damage. Decreasing serum albumin may reflect development of ascites or hemorrhage. Serum globulin level is usually increased; it reflects inflammation and parallels the severity of the inflammation. Increased serum globulin (is usually gamma) may cause increased total protein, especially in chronic viral hepatitis and post–hepatitic cirrhosis.

▪ *Total cholesterol*: Normal or decreased. Progressive decrease in cholesterol, HDL, LDL with increasing severity. Decrease is more marked than in chronic active hepatitis. LDL may be useful for prognosis and selecting patients for transplantation. Decreased esters reflect more severe parenchymal cell damage.

▪ *Other core laboratory findings*: BUN is often decreased (<10 mg/dL); increased with GI hemorrhage. Serum uric acid is often increased. Electrolytes and acid–base balance are often abnormal and reflect various combinations of circumstances at the time, such as malnutrition, dehydration, hemorrhage, metabolic acidosis, respiratory alkalosis. In cirrhosis with ascites, the kidney retains increased sodium and excessive water, causing dilutional hyponatremia. Increased blood ammonia in liver coma and cirrhosis and with portacaval shunting of blood.

- *Hematology*: WBC is usually normal with active cirrhosis; increased (<50,000/μL) with massive necrosis, hemorrhage, and so on; decreased with hypersplenism. Anemia reflects increased plasma volume and some increased destruction of RBCs. If more severe, rule out hemorrhage in the GI tract, folic acid deficiency, and excessive hemolysis.

  CSF findings: CSF is normal except for increased glutamine levels, which reflect brain ammonia levels (due to conversion from ammonia). Glutamine >35 mg/dL is always associated with hepatic encephalopathy (normal = 20 mg/dL); correlates with depth of coma and is more sensitive than arterial ammonia.

Considerations

- See Tables 5-7 and 5-8.
- Laboratory findings due to complications or sequelae, often in combination.
- Abnormalities of coagulation mechanisms (see Chapter 10, Hematologic Disorders) such as prolonged PT (does not respond to parenteral vitamin K as frequently as in patients with obstructive jaundice). Prolonged bleeding time in 40% of cases due to decreased platelets and/or fibrinogen.
- Hepatic encephalopathy (neurologic and mental abnormalities in some patients with liver failure or portosystemic shunt). Diagnosis is clinical; characteristic laboratory findings are supportive but not specific.
- See Table 5-9.
- Markers that may indicate progression to cirrhosis include decreased albumin; increased globulins; AST/ALT ratio >1; increased bilirubin, mainly unconjugated; increased PT; and decreased platelet count.

TABLE 5–7. Causes of Liver Disease with Associated Conditions

Laboratory Findings Due to Causative/Associated Diseases or Conditions	Frequency in the United States
Alcoholism	60–70%
Biliary disease (e.g., primary biliary cirrhosis and sclerosing cholangitis)	5–10%
Cryptogenic	10–15%
Chronic viral hepatitis (HBV with or without HDV; HCV)	10%
Hemochromatosis	5%
Wilson disease	Rare
Alpha$_1$-antitrypsin deficiency	Rare
Autoimmune chronic active hepatitis	
Cystic Fibrosis	
Glycogen storage diseases	
Galactosemia	
Porphyria	
Fructose intolerance	
Tyrosinosis	
Infections (e.g., congenital syphilis, schistosomiasis)	
Gaucher disease	
Ulcerative colitis	
Osler-Weber-Rendu disease	
Venous outflow obstruction (e.g., Budd-Chiari syndrome, venoocclusive disease, congestive heart failure)	

TABLE 5–8. Comparison of Different Mechanisms of Jaundice

	Cholestasis	Hepatocellular	Infiltration
Disease Example	Common Duct Stone	Acute Viral Hepatitis	Metastatic Tumor, Granulomas, Amyloid
	Drugs		
Serum bilirubin	6–20 mg/dL*	4–8 mg/dL	Usually <4 mg/dL, often normal
AST, ALT (U/mL)	May be slightly I, <200	Markedly I, often 500–1,000	May be slightly I, <100
Serum ALP	3–5 times N	1–2 times N	2–4 times N
Prothrombin time	I in chronic cases	I in severe disease	N
Response to parenteral vitamin K	Yes	No	

N, normal; I, increase.

*Serum bilirubin >10 mg/dL is rarely seen with common duct stone and usually indicates carcinoma.

Increased serum ALP <3× normal in 15% of patients with extrahepatic biliary obstruction, especially if obstruction is incomplete or due to benign conditions. Occasionally, AST and LD are markedly increased in biliary obstruction or liver cancer.

TABLE 5–9. Comparison of Three Main Types of Liver Disease Due to Drugs

	Predominantly Cholestatic	Predominantly Hepatocellular	Mixed Biochemical Pattern
Example of drugs	Anabolic steroids,* estrogens*	Cinchophen	Phenylbutazone
		Isonicotinic acid hydrazide	Phenytoin
	Organic arsenicals, antithyroid drugs (e.g., methimazole), chlorpromazine, PAS, erythromycin, sulfonylurea derivatives (including sulfonamides, phenothiazine tranquilizers, oral diuretics, antidiabetic drugs)	Monamine oxidase inhibitors (particularly iproniazid)	PAS and other antituberculosis agents
Serum bilirubin	May be ≥30 mg/dL		
AST, ALT, LD (U/mL)	Mild to moderate increase	More markedly increased	
Serum ALP, LAP	More markedly increased; may remain increased for years after jaundice has disappeared	Less markedly increased	

*ALP, AST, and ALT are not increased as much compared with other drugs.

INFECTIOUS DISEASE: VIRAL HEPATITIS

❏ Definition

Five hepatitis viruses cause the majority of clinically important viral infections of the liver: HAV, HBV, HCV, HDV, and HEV. They are all RNA viruses except for HBV, which is a DNA virus. All of these viruses can cause acute hepatitis; only HBV, HCV, and HDV are able to cause chronic hepatitis infections in immunologically normal patients. Coinfection with two hepatitis viruses or hepatitis virus infection in patients with preexisting liver disease is frequently associated with greater disease severity (Table 5-10). Other viruses or infectious agents may cause liver infection associated with systemic or localized infections. Agents include herpes viruses—like HSV, CMV, and EBV—rubella, *M. tuberculosis*, ameba, and leishmania. See the discussions for these agents in Chapter 11. *Infectious Diseases*. A variety of hepatotoxins, autoimmune diseases, and other diseases may also cause hepatitis that is clinically similar to diseases caused by the hepatitis viruses.

Viral hepatitis may be suspected in patients with nonspecific symptoms (see Prodromal Phase) or specific symptoms, like jaundice or RUQ pain (see Acute Phase). Viral hepatitis may also be considered in asymptomatic patients in whom liver function abnormality, like hyperbilirubinemia or elevated levels of AST or ALT, is detected by screening tests. For these patients, evaluation with an acute hepatitis panel is recommended; the different viral agents cannot be reliably distinguished by clinical signs and symptoms. The acute hepatitis panel includes hepatitis A IgM antibody, hepatitis B core IgM antibody, hepatitis B surface antigen, and hepatitis C antibody. Further testing, as described below, is recommended on the basis of results of the tests in the acute hepatitis panel.

❏ Laboratory Overview

- The results for acute hepatitis panel, and additional virus-specific tests, are discussed with the agents below.
- Because the signs and symptoms of infection with other infectious agents and hepatotoxins may be indistinguishable from those caused by the hepatitis viruses, specific testing to rule out other causes of liver damage is recommended, based on clinical history, epidemiology, laboratory, and other relevant information.
- In addition to testing for specific viral markers of infection, the patient's hematologic, coagulation, and hepatic function should be evaluated over the course of illness.
- The earliest laboratory signs of acute viral hepatitis include elevations in ALT and AST, which typically precede elevation of bilirubin levels. In acute illness, the degree of ALT elevation typically exceeds AST elevation. Peak aminotransferase levels >1,000 U/L are common. The level of aminotransferase elevation does not reliably predict the severity or prognosis of disease. Total bilirubin may increase to 5–20 mg/dL at peak. ALP is normal or mildly elevated in most cases.
- CBC may show mild neutropenia with a relative lymphocytosis, often with atypical lymphocytes. Serum globulins are normal or mildly elevated. In severe liver disease, synthesis of albumin and coagulation factors may be compromised, resulting in increased PT.

TABLE 5–10. Comparison of Different Types of Viral Hepatitis

	A	B	C	D	E
Genome	ssRNA	dsDNA	ssRNA	ssRNA	ssRNA
Classification	Picornaviridae	Hepadnaviridae	Flaviviridae	Unclassified	Caliciviridae
New cases in the United States, 2007 (www.cdc.gov)	25,000	43,000	17,000	Uncommon. Always associated with HBV; 4% of acute HBV cases have HDV coinfection	Rare; occurs in travelers to endemic areas
Incubation period (days)	15–60	45–160	14–180	42–180	15–64
Transmission					
Enteric	Yes	No	No	No	Yes
Sexual	No	Yes	Possible	Possible	No
Perinatal	No	Yes	Possible	Possible	No
Parenteral	Rare	Yes	Yes	Yes	No
Posttransfusion incidence (%)	None	1 case per 137,000 units transfused	1 case per 2 million units transfused	Virtually eliminated by HBV screening	None
Viremia	Transient	Prolonged	Prolonged	Prolonged	Transient
Fecal excretion of virus	+	–	–	–	+
Onset	Abrupt	Insidious	Insidious	Abrupt	Abrupt
Course	Mild, often subclinical, self-limited	Acute* and chronic infection	Acute infection typically mild; high incidence of chronic infection	Increases severity of underlying HBV infection	Usually mild, self-limited†
Asymptomatic	Most children	Most children; 50% adults	<75%	Rare	Often
Jaundice	Child: 10% Adult: 70–80%	15–40%‡	10–25%	Varies	25–50%
Chronic hepatitis after acute infection (%)	0%	1–10% (90% of neonates)	70–85%	Common; high in superinfection	0%
Hepatocellular carcinoma association	No	Yes	Yes	Yes	Unlikely
Acute liver failure	1–2%	0.1–1%	Very rare	5%	1–2%; 20% in pregnancy

*≤20% have serum sickness-like prodroma.

†Resembles hepatitis A. Case fatality 1–2% except ≤20% in pregnancy; usually milder infection and biochemical abnormalities than HBV or HAV infection. One percent of icteric cases become fulminant (<8 weeks) and 90% die within 2–4 weeks; associated with encephalopathy; renal, electrolyte, acid–base imbalances; hypoglycemia; coagulation derangements.

‡A nonicteric patient is more likely to progress to chronic hepatitis.

❏ Disease Manifestations

Viral hepatitis infections may show many and varied clinical features, but most patients with acute viral hepatitis are asymptomatic or experience minimal constitutional symptoms. On the other hand, any of the hepatitis viruses may cause fulminant disease with extensive liver damage and hepatic failure. One cannot distinguish different types of viral hepatitis by clinical features or routine chemistries; specific serologic tests are needed. Hepatitis virus infections demonstrate the following clinical phases.

❏ Prodromal Phase

- After a variable, virus-specific incubation period, patients may develop non-specific symptoms, including low-grade fever, headache, fatigue and malaise, and arthralgias. Anorexia, nausea, and vomiting are common and may be associated with abdominal pain (epigastric or right upper quadrant).
- Prodromal symptoms typically last 1–2 weeks before the onset of signs and symptoms of acute liver disease. Dark urine may precede the onset of jaundice. Acholic stools may be seen in HAV and HEV infections.
  - ▼ During the prodrome:
    - Specific serologic markers appear in serum (see Figure 5-7).
    - ESR is normal.
    - Leukopenia (lymphopenia and neutropenia) is noted with onset of fever, followed by relative lymphocytosis and monocytosis. Plasma cells and <10% atypical lymphocytes may be seen.
    - Urinary urobilinogen and total serum bilirubin increase just before the onset of jaundice.
    - Serum AST and ALT levels increase during the prodromal phase and show very high peaks (>500 U) during the acute phase.

❏ Acute Hepatitis Phase

- Signs and symptoms of the prodromal phase usually abate with the onset of jaundice and the acute phase of hepatitis.
- Acute hepatitis may be icteric or anicteric. The majority of cases of acute HCV infections and HAV and HBV infections in children are anicteric.
  - ▼ Asymptomatic: Many patients infected with hepatitis viruses may remain clinically asymptomatic or show only mild or transient symptoms. The diagnosis of viral hepatitis may be suspected by finding abnormal LFT or other tests collected for other reasons.
  - ▼ Symptomatic, icteric:
    - Patients develop jaundice; examination of the sclerae may provide the most sensitive site for detection. LFT and other laboratory testing demonstrates liver cell damage and the extent of hepatic function compromise. The levels of conjugated and unconjugated bilirubin are typically comparable. In acute hepatitis, there is usually marked elevation of aminotransferases, with ALT > AST; the degree of elevation does not correlate with the extent of hepatic cellular damage. LD may be mildly elevated. Serum AST and ALT fall rapidly in the several days after jaundice appears and become normal 2–5 weeks later with resolution of infection.

5

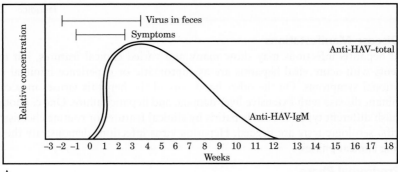

A

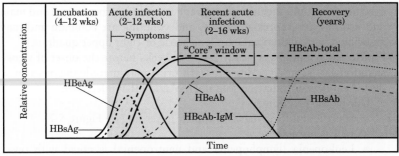

B

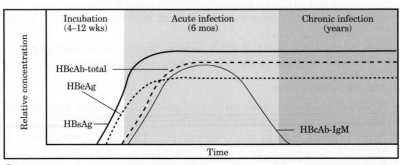

C

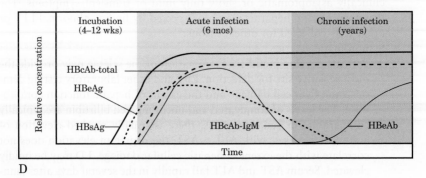

D

Figure 5–7 *Hepatitis serologic profiles.* **A.** *Antibody response to hepatitis A.* **B.** *Hepatitis B core window identification.* **C, D.** *Hepatitis B chronic carrier profiles: no seroconversion* **(C)**; *late seroconversion* **(D)**. *(Reproduced with permission of Hepatitis Information Center, Abbott Laboratories, Abbott Park, IL).*

- Other laboratory tests may be abnormal, depending on severity of the disease. ALP and albumin levels are usually normal. Serum protein electrophoresis may show mild elevation of the γ-globulin fraction. Serum cholesterol-to-ester ratio is usually depressed early; total serum cholesterol is decreased only in severe disease. Serum phospholipids are increased in mild but decreased in severe hepatitis. Urine urobilinogen is increased in the early icteric period; at peak of the disease, it disappears for days or weeks; urobilinogen simultaneously disappears from stool.
  - ▼ Severe hepatocellular damage is predicted by prolonged PT, markedly elevated bilirubin, hypoglycemia, or decreased serum albumin concentration. A prolonged and complicated course is more common in the elderly, in patients with significant underlying medical (especially hepatic) conditions, and in patients presenting with severe symptoms, like peripheral edema or encephalopathy during the acute phase.
  - ▼ Symptomatic, anicteric: Laboratory abnormalities are usually mild compared to patients with icteric hepatitis; there is slight or no increase in serum bilirubin.
- Nonspecific laboratory abnormalities may be associated with the acute phase of viral hepatitis. ESR is increased but decreases during convalescence. Serum iron is often increased. Urine examination may show cylinduria, and albuminuria occurs occasionally. The renal concentrating ability is sometimes decreased.
- Acute Fulminant Hepatitis/Acute Liver Failure (ALF)
  - ▼ Acute fulminant hepatitis may be recognized by triad of prolonged PT, increased PMNs, and nonpalpable liver. A prolonged PT, especially >20 seconds, indicates the likely development of acute hepatic insufficiency; therefore, the PT should be performed with the initial patient evaluation.
  - ▼ Acute fulminant hepatitis is associated with failure of liver function. Patients present with hepatic encephalopathy and hepatic synthetic dysfunction. The manifestations of encephalopathy may range from drowsiness and confusion to stupor and coma. Synthetic dysfunction is usually manifested by coagulopathy. Multiorgan failure may ensue. Ascites is typical. Bacterial superinfection, especially with streptococci and *S. aureus*, may occur.
  - ▼ ALF is more common with coinfection with two hepatitis viruses, like HBV and HDV, or with hepatitis infections in patients with preexisting liver disease. HBV infection is the most common cause of ALF (approximately 1–3% of adults). HAV is associated with ALF only in adults and occurs in 1.8% of patients >60 years of age. ALF after HEV is rare, except for pregnant women, where up to 20% of patients may develop ALF. ALF is an extremely rare complication of acute HCV infection. ALF may occur as a complication of systemic HSV infection. There is a high mortality associated with ALF, but if the patient survives, complete biochemical and histologic recovery are the rule.
  - ▼ In addition to clinical signs of hepatic failure, significant metabolic derangement and laboratory abnormalities are common:
    - As the patient's condition deteriorates, titers of HBsAg and HBeAg often fall and disappear.
    - Serum bilirubin progressively increases and may reach very high levels.

- Increased serum AST and ALT levels are seen, but levels may fall abruptly terminally; serum ALP and GGT may be increased.
- Serum cholesterol and cholesterol esters are markedly decreased.
- Albumin and total protein levels are decreased.
- Increased ammonia level in blood.
- Hematologic abnormalities.
- Evidence of DIC is common.
  - Decreased factors II, V, VII, IX, and X cause prolonged PT and aPTT.
  - Decreased antithrombin III.
  - Platelet count <100,000 in two thirds of patients.
  - Hemorrhage, especially in the GI tract.
- Metabolic markers are typically abnormal, including
  - Hypokalemia (early), with metabolic alkalosis
  - Respiratory alkalosis
  - Lactic acidosis
  - Hyponatremia, hypophosphatemia
  - Hypoglycemia in approximately 5% of patients
- Renal function tests may be abnormal. Hepatorenal syndrome may develop.

❏ Postacute Hepatitis Phase

In uncomplicated viral hepatitis, symptoms of the acute phase should resolve within 1 to 6 months, depending on the virus, with correction of the biochemical abnormalities in the subsequent months. Persistence of clinical or biochemical abnormalities suggests progression to chronic hepatitis in hepatitis B, C, or D infections.

- Resolution: During recovery, systemic symptoms abate. Liver tenderness and biochemical abnormalities may persist. Complete clinical and biochemical recovery occurs 1–2 months after HAV and HEV infections and 3–6 months after uncomplicated HBV. HAV and HEV infections are not associated with progression to chronic infection. HBV, HCV, and HDV may progress to chronic infection. Recovery from acute HBV infection is more likely after clinically apparent (icteric) versus subclinical infection
- Chronic infection
  - ▼ The persistence of clinical and laboratory abnormalities for >6 months after acute hepatitis is characteristic of chronic infection. Chronic liver infection may develop with HCV, HBV, or HBV plus HDV infections. The clinical presentation varies from asymptomatic disease through progression to end-stage liver failure. Signs and symptoms may be fairly constant or marked by flares in severity, increasing the progression of liver injury. Cirrhosis may develop. Liver damage is influenced by virus factors, as discussed later, and host factors. Host factors include coexisting diseases, especially liver disease, the host immune response, and alcohol consumption or exposure to other hepatotoxins.
  - ▼ The degree of laboratory abnormalities may not accurately reflect the degree of histologic changes. Aminotransferase elevation may be variable. In mild disease, ALT elevation is typically greater than the degree of AST elevation. Marked elevation of bilirubin levels is associated with

advanced liver damage and cirrhosis. In advanced cirrhosis, the pattern of aminotransferase elevation is usually reversed, with the degree of AST elevation exceeding that of ALT elevation. The synthetic function of the liver decreases with advanced chronic disease and cirrhosis, with resulting clinical manifestations of coagulopathy, metabolic derangements, and so on.

- *Hepatocellular carcinoma*: Hepatocellular carcinoma (HCC) may occur as a complication of chronic viral hepatitis. In HBV infection, HCC may occur in patients with or without cirrhosis. Risk factors for the development of HCC in HBV-infected patients include infection early in life, coexisting immunocompromising diseases, and HDV coinfection. HCC may also complicate HCV infection but occurs only in patients with cirrhosis.

HEPATITIS VIRUSES

Most cases of acute viral hepatitis in the United States are caused by HAV, HBV, and HCV. In a CDC surveillance survey in 2012, there were an estimated 69,000 new cases of acute hepatitis caused by these agents (50% HBV; 25% HAV; 25% HCV).

- The acute hepatitis panel (HBsAg, total anti-HBc, IgM anti-HBc, IgM anti-HAV, and total anti-HVC) is recommended for evaluation of patients with suspected acute infectious hepatitis. Repeat testing to confirm negative results may be considered in patients at high risk for viral hepatitis. In addition, testing for rheumatoid factor may be considered if false-positive antibody tests are suspected. Further testing is determined by results of the initial screening tests. Repeat screening after negative results should be considered for patients with a high clinical suspicion or prior risk in order to rule out false-negative results due to a window period. Window periods represent intervals prior to immune response or during a transition from phases of antigen predominance to antibody predominance (e.g., HBsAg positive → anti-HBs positive). There are no FDA-approved diagnostic tests for HDV or HEV; diagnostic testing, when indicated, may be pursued through the CDC/Public Health Laboratory or Reference Laboratories. Specific testing for HDV is not necessary if HBV infection has been ruled out. Testing for HEV is usually unneeded unless a patient has recently traveled to an area where HEV infection is endemic. Specific hepatitis viruses and diagnostic testing are presented in subsequent text of this chapter.

❑ **Hepatitis Viruses Transmitted by Enteric Routes (HAV and HEV)**

- *HAV*
  - ▼ HAV infections, caused by a nonenveloped, single-stranded RNA picornavirus, occur worldwide.
  - ▼ Only approximately 25% of patients with acute HAV infection report risk factors in the 2–6 weeks prior to onset of symptoms. Risk factors include close contact with a patient with documented HAV infection or person at increased risk for HAV infection, employment or attendance at a nursery, day care center or preschool, exposure to a foodborne or waterborne outbreak, or high-risk sexual practices.

▼ Overall, 68% of patients develop jaundice. Childhood infections are most commonly anicteric (>90%), whereas infections in adults are often severe, with icteric infection occurring in approximately 80% of patients. Most symptomatic infections resolve in 1–2 months. Rare cholestatic variants may remain symptomatic for months but eventually resolve completely. The fatality rate for HAV infection is <1% (0.02/100,000 population), most commonly in patients >75 years of age.

▼ The prodromal period after exposure is approximately 4 weeks (range 2 to 7 weeks). Fecal excretion of virus begins late in the prodromal phase. IgM appears in the late prodrome; IgM may remain detectable for 6–12 months. After 3 months, IgM levels usually begin to drop, whereas rising IgG levels are detected. IgG levels persist indefinitely. Acute liver failure is uncommon in HAV infection (0.1%). Chronic infection does not occur in HAV infections.

■ *HAV diagnosis*:
  ▼ Anti-HAV-IgM positive: Acute infection
    ● Anti-HAV-IgM appears at the same time as symptoms in >99% of cases and peaks within the 1st month. IgM becomes undetectable within 12 (usually 6) months.
    ● The presence of anti-HAV-IgM confirms diagnosis of recent acute infection. Serial testing is usually not needed for diagnosis.
    ● Serum bilirubin is usually 5–10 times the normal level. Jaundice lasts a few days to 12 weeks. Patients are usually not infectious after the onset of jaundice.
    ● Serum AST and ALT are increased for 1–3 weeks.
    ● Relative lymphocytosis is frequent.
  ▼ Anti-HAV-IgG positive: Remote infection/immune
    ● Anti-HAV-IgG is usually detectable for life after resolution of acute HAV infection and indicates immunity to HAV infection.
  ▼ Anti-HAV-total may be predominantly IgG or IgM, depending on infection status. A negative anti-HAV-total effectively excludes acute HAV but does not distinguish recent from past infection, for which anti-HAV-IgM test is needed. Tests for anti-HAV-total (minimum detection approximately 100 mU/mL) may be insensitive for detection of protective antibody after HAV vaccine (minimum protective antibody concentration is <10 mU/mL).
  ▼ Nonspecific elevation of IgM is common in acute HAV infection.

■ *HEV*
  ▼ HEV infections are caused by an unenveloped, single-stranded RNA virus of the Caliciviridae family and are clinically similar to HAV infections.
  ▼ HEV infection is most common in developing countries with inadequate sanitation and limited access to clean water supplies, including countries in Asia, Africa, and Central America; symptomatic infection is rare in the United States and usually occurs in persons with recent travel to an endemic region.
  ▼ HEV infections are transmitted by the fecal–oral route. The symptoms of acute HEV infection are similar to those of acute hepatitis caused by other viruses; specific testing is needed to establish HEV infection.

▼ Asymptomatic infection occurs in approximately 60–90% of patients during outbreaks. Symptomatic infections are most common in young adults (20–40 years); acute liver failure may occur in 1–2% of patients overall but in 10–20% of pregnant women with HEV infection. A cholestatic presentation (duration of infection >3 months), with prolonged jaundice, fatigue, and pruritus, occurs more frequently in HEV infections compared to HAV, but infection eventually resolves completely.

■ *HEV diagnosis*
  ▼ Diagnostic testing is performed by special reference laboratories, like the CDC.
  ▼ Anti-HEV-IgM positive: Acute infection.
  ▼ Anti-HEV-IgG positive: Remote infection.
  ▼ Recent travel to an endemic area should be documented (e.g., Mexico, India, Africa, or Russia).

❑ **Hepatitis Viruses Transmitted by Blood-Borne Routes (HBV, HCV, and HDV)**

HBV, HCV, and HDV are most commonly transmitted by exposure to blood, semen, or infected body fluids. Infection may also be transmitted by perinatal/vertical (especially in HBV in areas with high endemic rate) and sexual routes (now the most common exposure for HBV infection). Transmission by transfusion or transplantation has fallen as a result of screening.

■ *HBV* (see Figure 5-7)
  ▼ HBV is a double-stranded DNA *Hepadnavirus*. HBV infection occurs worldwide.
  ▼ In a 2010 CDC survey, only 36% of patients with acute HBV infection reported any high-risk behavior or known exposure in the 6 months prior to illness. Specific high-risk behaviors or exposure risks include employment in health care settings involving contact with blood or potential needle-stick injury, dialysis or kidney transplant, transfusion of blood products, recent surgery, injection drug use, high-risk sexual practices, or close contact with any person at high risk for HBV infection. The case fatality rate for acute HBV infection is approximately 1.5% (1.1 case/100,000 population). It is highest in patients 30–39 years of age.
  ▼ Symptoms and disease: Symptomatic disease occurs in a minority of patients with acute HBV infection (<1 year old: <1%; 1–5 years old: 5–15%; >5 years old: 30–50%). Symptoms and evidence of active infection occurs approximately 2–3 months (range 2 to 5 months) after exposure. HBsAg, anti-HBc IgM, and HBeAg appear late in the prodromal phase. In patients who recover without progression to chronic infection, the titer of these markers, as well as the ALT, begin to fall during the phase of active disease, usually returning to normal within 4 to 6 months. Most patients with acute HBV infection recover completely. The risk of chronic infection depends on the age of acquisition of HBV infection (>90% of infants; 25–50% of children aged 1 to 5 years; 6–10% of older children and adults).

■ *HBV Diagnosis and Laboratory Testing*

A number of laboratory tests are used to different stages of HBV infection:

▼ Hepatitis B surface antigen (*HBsAg*) is the earliest indicator of active HBV infection. HBsAg is usually detectable within 27–41 days (as early as 14 days) of the onset of infection. HBsAg appears 7–26 days before transaminase abnormalities and peaks as ALT rises. HBsAg detection persists during the acute illness. HBsAg usually disappears 12–20 weeks after onset of symptoms in uncomplicated HBV infection.

▼ Detection of HBsAg for >6 months defines chronic infection or a chronic carrier state. Hepatitis B vaccination does not cause a positive HBsAg. HBsAg titers are not of clinical value and may never be detected in some patients; diagnosis of acute HBV infection is based on detection of HBc-IgM.

▼ Antibody to HBsAg (*anti-HBs*), without detectable HBsAg, indicates recovery from HBV infection, absence of infectivity, and immunity from future HBV infection. Anti-HBs may be seen after transfusion due to passive transfer. Anti-HBs is found in 80% of patients after clinical cure. The appearance of anti-HBs may take several weeks or months after HBsAg has disappeared and ALT has returned to normal, causing a 2- to 6-week "window" period.

▼ Anti-HBs is the only antibody produced in response to vaccine. Its presence indicates immunity. Antibody develops in approximately 95% of healthy adults after a three-dose immunization series. Seroreactivity may wane in vaccinated individuals, but immunity to infection is typically preserved. Escape mutants, which lack the "a" determinant of the vaccine, may cause infection in vaccinated patients who demonstrate anti-HBs.

▼ Antibodies to hepatitis B core antigens (anti-HBc) are the first antibodies to appear after HBV infection. Total and IgM antibodies typically appear 4–10 weeks after appearance of HBsAg. *Anti-HBc-total* remains detectable for years or for lifetime. In chronic HBV infection, total anti-HBc and HBsAg are always present, and anti-HBs is absent.

▼ *Anti-HBc-IgM* is the earliest specific antibody to develop in response to HBV infection. It is found in high titer for a short time during the acute disease stage and is the sole marker of HBV infection during the window between HBsAg and anti-HBs detection. Anti-HBc-IgM declines to low levels during recovery. Because this is the only test unique to recent infection, it may be used to differentiate acute from chronic HBV. However, because some patients with chronic Hepatitis B infection become positive for anti-HBc-IgM during flares, it is not an absolutely reliable marker of acute illness. Before anti-HBc-IgM disappears, anti-HBc-IgG appears and lasts indefinitely.

▼ Hepatitis B e-antigen (*HBeAg*) indicates virus replication and a highly infectious state. HBeAg appears within 1 week after HBsAg. HBeAg disappears prior to the disappearance of HBsAg during resolution of acute infection. HBeAg is detected only when HBsAg and HBV DNA are detectable in the circulation. HBeAg occurs early in disease, before biochemical changes, and disappears after the serum ALT peaks. Levels are usually detectable for 3–6 weeks in uncomplicated HBV infection. It is a marker of active HBV replication in the liver. HBeAg at the time of delivery is an accurate predictor of risk (approximately 90%) of vertical transmission to neonates.

▼ HBeAg may be used to determine resolution of HBV infection. Persistence >20 weeks suggests progression to chronic carrier state and possible chronic hepatitis. Antibody to HBe (*anti-HBe*) appears after HBeAg disappears and remains detectable for years. Detection of anti-HBe is associated with decreasing infectivity and suggests a good prognosis for resolution of acute infection. A positive reaction for anti-HBe and anti-HBc, in the absence of HBsAg and anti-HBs, confirms recent acute infection (2–16 weeks).

▼ Detection of *HBV DNA* by PCR indicates active infection. It is the most sensitive and specific assay for early diagnosis of HBV infection and may be detected when all other markers are negative (e.g., in immunocompromised patients). Detection of HBV DNA indicates active viral replication, even if HBeAg is not detectable. HBV DNA viral load may be used to assess disease status and prognosis or to monitor the response to therapy. A level of 100,000 copies per mL has been proposed for initiation of therapy in HBeAg-positive patients. DNA levels decrease in patients who respond to therapy. An increased risk for the development of HCC and cirrhosis is seen in chronically infected patients with persistently elevated HBV DNA levels ($>10^5$ copies/mL).

▼ HBV genotype analysis may be useful for management of patients with chronic HBV infection who are treated with antiviral agents. The replication of the HBV genome is prone to misreading, resulting in a pool of "quasispecies" in the patient's circulating pool of HBV. A quasispecies resistant to the antiviral agent may become the predominant circulating form of virus in the presence of antiviral selection, resulting in failure of therapy. Genotype analysis may identify quasispecies with specific mutations of the HBV polymerase gene that confer resistance to the antiviral agents used to treat chronic HBV. If identified early, therapy may be changed before hepatitis reactivation occurs.

Correlation of HBV Serologic Test Results and Disease Status

Typical patterns of HBV serologic tests for different disease status are given below. Atypical patterns may be due to testing during transitions between disease phases but may also be caused by false-positive or false-negative test results. Unexpected test results should be confirmed and, if confirmed, repeated after several months to see if the pattern resolves. Additional testing, like genetic analysis, may be performed, if relevant, for resolution.

▼ *No HBV infection*: Negative reactions for HBsAg and anti-HBc IgM rule out acute HBV infection.

▼ *HBV immune status*: Anti-HBs may be added to assess a patient's immune status. Patients with immunity due to natural infection show positive reactions for anti-HBs and anti-HBc and a negative reaction for HBsAg. Patients with immunity due to hepatitis B vaccination are positive for anti-HBs and negative for HBsAg and anti-HBc.

▼ *Acute HBV infection*: HBsAg and anti-HBc antibodies (total and IgM) are positive, and anti-HBs is negative. HBV DNA is detectable.

▼ Acute HBV infection usually lasts for 1–6 months with mild or no symptoms. Aminotransferases are increased >10-fold. HBsAg gradually arises to high titers during the active phase; HBeAg also appears. Serum bilirubin is usually normal or only slightly increased in acute disease. Immune complex–mediated diseases may be seen in 10–20% of patients (e.g., serum sickness, arthritis, dermatitis, glomerulonephritis, vasculitis). Immune complex–mediated glomerulonephritis or nephrotic syndrome may progress to chronic renal failure. Acute HBV usually resolves in 3–6 months in uncomplicated infection. In patients who recover from acute HBV infection, titers of HBsAg fall to undetectable levels, followed by the emergence of anti-HBs after 4 to 8 weeks. During this "window," anti-HBc total and IgM antibodies are detectable; HBV DNA is also usually detectable.

▼ *Acute HBV infection with recovery*: After complete resolution of HBV infection, patient testing shows HBsAg negative, anti-HBs positive, HBeAg negative, anti-HBe positive, anti-HBc-IgG positive, and HBV DNA falls to undetectable levels. Full recovery is more common after clinically apparent acute HBV infection. Acute liver failure is uncommon, occurring in 0.1–1% of patients.

▼ *Chronic HBV infection*: Chronic infection is uncommon, occurring in 1–10% of patients overall, but approximately 90% perinatal infections. The typical pattern of HBV markers shows that HBsAg and total anti-HBc are positive, while anti-HBc-IgM and anti-HBs are negative.

▼ *Laboratory Evaluations for Patients with Chronic HBV Infection*:
   ● Tests for HBV active replication (e.g., HBeAg/anti-HBe, HBV viral load) are used for initial assessment and ongoing monitoring of patients.
   ● Laboratory tests to assess impact of infection (e.g., CBC, PT, hepatic function panel) are used for initial assessment and ongoing monitoring of patients.
   ● Laboratory tests to rule out coinfection with other viruses (e.g., HCV, HDV, HIV).
   ● Consider liver biopsy to stage liver disease histologically.
   ● Consider screening for hepatocellular carcinoma (e.g., AFP, ultrasound).

Continued transaminase elevation for >6 months is seen in chronic hepatitis. Chronic HBV infection may last for only 1 year or for several decades with mild or severe symptoms. Most patients resolve spontaneously, but some develop progressive liver failure and cirrhosis. AST and ALT fall to 2–10 times normal range. Detection of HBeAg indicates continuing active viral replication, but patients with active HBV replication, as demonstrated by HBV DNA, may be HBeAg negative. A chronic carrier state with nonreplicating virus may also develop. Patients are usually asymptomatic. AST and ALT fall to normal or <2 times normal levels. Anti-HBe is detectable; HBeAg is negative. HBsAg is present but at decreasing titers. HBV viral load may be negative or low positive. Total anti-HBc is usually present in high titer (>1:512). HBV carrier patients may experience flares of active, symptomatic hepatitis accompanied by a change in their serologic markers: HBsAg positive, anti-HBc-IgM positive, anti-HBs negative, anti-HBe negative, and HBeAg may be detected. The development of anti-HBs marks the end of the carrier stage. Chronic replicative infection may be caused by hepatitis B viruses with mutations that affect normal HBeAg expression, resulting in an atypical pattern of HBV markers. Patients infected with precore or core promoter mutants tend to have more severe disease, more flares, and more rapid progression to cirrhosis. Patients are HBsAg positive, anti-HBs negative, anti-HBc-IgG positive, anti-HBc-IgM negative, HBeAg negative, and anti-HBe positive. Effective treatment of chronic HBV hepatitis causes ALT, HBeAg, and HBV DNA to become normal.

- *HDV*
  - ▼ HDV, delta agent, is a small defective single-stranded RNA virus enveloped by hepatitis B surface antigens. HDV requires simultaneous HBV infection but relies on HBV only for envelope protein (HBs). The epidemiology of HDV infection is similar to HBV except that sexual and perinatal infection is less efficient. Although uncommon in the United States, HDV is distributed worldwide, with perhaps 5% of HBV-infected patients coinfected with HDV.
  - ▼ HDV infection may be transmitted simultaneously with HBV infection. In these patients, clinical manifestations may be similar to patients with HBV infection alone, but coinfection is often more severe in terms of clinical signs and symptoms. In HBV/HDV coinfection, the risk for progression to chronic hepatitis is no greater than is seen in HBV infection alone.
  - ▼ HDV may also be transmitted to patients with preexisting chronic HBV infection. Such HDV superinfections usually lead to clinical deterioration, increased chronicity, and may lead to ALF.
  - ▼ HDV infection may be suspected on the basis of exposure in regions of high endemicity, history of injection drug abuse, unusually severe HBV disease, or deterioration in chronic HBV infections.
    - Antigen detection is the most reliable laboratory test for diagnosis, but levels may be variable. Serum HDVAg and HDV-RNA appear during the incubation period after the appearance of HBsAg and before a rise in ALT, which often shows a biphasic elevation. HBsAg and HDVAg are transient; HDVAg resolves with clearance of HBsAg. Total anti-HDV supports a diagnosis; anti-HDV-IgM is not reliable for distinguishing between acute and chronic infection but is detectable more often than anti-HDV-IgG. In HBV/HDV coinfections, detectable anti-HDV elevations are not clearly predictable, may be of low titer, and often disappear with resolution of acute infection. In superinfection, however, high anti-HDV levels are seen, and these last indefinitely. Determination of the class of anti-HBc, IgG versus IgM, can help distinguish between HDV coinfection and superinfection. Chronic HDV infection is more severe and has higher mortality than other types of viral hepatitis. The risk of HCC is threefold greater in patients with chronic HBV infection in whom anti-HDV is detected compared to patients who are negative.
- *HDV diagnosis* (see Tables 5-11 and 5-12)

Commercial assays for detection of HDV antigen, antibody, and RNA are commercially available but not FDA approved in the United States.

  - ▼ Anti-HDV positive: HDV infection
    - Anti-HDV positive, HBsAg positive, anti-HBc-IgM positive: HBV/HDV coinfection. HDAg, anti-HDV-IgM, and HDV RNA may be detected. Low titer anti-HDV-total appears late.

TABLE 5–11. Comparison of Types of Hepatitis D Virus (HDV) Infections

	Coinfection	Superinfection	Chronic HDV
HBV infection	Acute	Chronic	Chronic
HDV infection	Acute	Acute to chronic	Chronic
Chronicity rate	<5%	>75%	Cirrhosis in >70%
Serology			
HBsAg	+	Usually persistent	Persistent
HBcAb-IgM	+	Negative	Negative
Anti-HDV-total	Negative or low titer	+	+
Anti-HDV-IgM*	Transient+	Transient	High titer
HDV-RNA (HDAg)	Transient+	Usually persistent	Persistent
Liver HDAg	Transient+	Usually persistent	Persistent

+, Positive.
*Decrease in anti-HDV-IgM usually predicts resolution of acute HDV. Persistent anti-HDV-IgM typically predicts progression to chronic HDV infection. High titer correlates with active liver inflammation.

- Anti-HDV-total positive, anti-HBc-IgM negative, HBsAg positive, anti-HBc-IgG positive, HDV RNA positive, total, and IgM anti-HDV rapidly increase: Acute HDV superinfection. HDAg may be missed. HDAg can be demonstrated on liver biopsy by immunohistochemical staining. HDAg is not detected in chronic HDV infection.

■ HCV

▼ HCV is an enveloped, single-stranded RNA Flavivirus. HCV infections occur worldwide but with geographic variation in prevalence of infection.

TABLE 5–12. Serologic Diagnosis of Hepatitis B Virus (HBV) and Hepatitis D Virus (HDV)

Test				
HBsAg	HBcAb-IgM	Anti-HDV-IgM	Anti-HDV-IgG	Interpretation
Transient+	+High titer	Transient+	Transient low titer	Acute HBV and acute HDV*
Transient decrease due to inhibitory effect of HDV on HBV synthesis	Negative or low titers	High titer first, low titer later	Increasing titers	Acute HDV and chronic HBV†
May remain + in chronic HBV	Replaced by anti-HBc-IgG in chronic HBV	+Correlates with HDAg in hepatocytes	High titers correlate with active infection; may remain + for years after infection resolves	Chronic HDV and chronic HBV‡

+, Positive.
*Clinically resembles acute viral hepatitis; fulminant hepatitis is rare, and progression to chronic hepatitis is unlikely. If HBV does not resolve, HDV can continue to replicate indefinitely.
†Clinically resembles exacerbation of chronic liver disease or of fulminant hepatitis with liver failure.
‡Clinically resembles chronic liver disease progressing to cirrhosis.

Transmission is almost exclusively by percutaneous exposure. Transmission by sexual and perinatal exposure is rare.

▼ In 2011, a CDC study showed the rate of newly diagnosed HCV infection of 85 per 100,000 population. Among newly diagnosed patients, only 50% had testing for active infection (i.e., HCV RNA detection). The highest prevalence and percentage of deaths were seen in patients born during the period 1945–1965.

▼ In 2012, the CDC published revised recommendations for HCV testing, as described below. The new recommendations were issued (1) to reflect changes in diagnostic tests, like improved immunoassays and unavailability of RIBA HCV confirmatory testing; (2) to expand one-time screening of everyone born between 1945 and 1965, regardless of specific risk factors; (3) to include initial evaluation for active infection (HCV viremia detection) in all patients with positive HCV serology to facilitate optimal treatment. The recommendations stress the impact of new direct-acting antivirals for improved outcome in patients with chronic HCV infection and likely decreased transmission of infection.

▼ Specific risk factors are well described for HCV acquisition, but 38% of patients report no known risk for exposure. Significant risk factors for HCV infection include the following:
- Any person born from 1945 through 1965
- HIV infection
- History of IV drug abuse
- History of blood product transfusion or organ transplantation before July 1992 or clotting factor concentrate before 1987
- History of long-term hemodialysis
- Known exposure to HCV, like health care workers exposed to HCV-positive blood by needle-stick injury or the recipient of blood or organ transplant from a patient subsequently shown to be HCV positive
- Children born to HCV-positive mothers
- Persistently elevated serum ALT

HCV risk may also be increased in noninjection illicit drug use, like intranasal cocaine use, patients with tattoos or body piercing, patients with a history of STD or multiple sex partners, patients with a long-term sexual relationship with an HCV-positive partner.

▼ The acute phase of HCV infection usually occurs 2 months after exposure (range: 2–26 weeks) and is typically mild; 70–80% of patients remain anicteric and asymptomatic. ALF is very rarely seen as a complication of acute HCV infection.

▼ The reported rate of spontaneous recovery after acute HCV infection has varied between 14% and 50%; the variability is likely due to the patient population studied and mode of acquisition of infection. Reinfection after spontaneous clearance, in some patient populations, may also be misinterpreted as chronic infection. Patients with symptomatic infection during the acute phase are more likely to spontaneously recover; most patients who recover after acute HCV infection do so within 3 months after the onset of acute infection. Because the HBV RNA viral load may vary over time, even to undetectable levels, a single negative value should not be relied on as a marker of recovery; several repeat laboratory evaluations to confirm recovery should be performed at 3-month intervals.

▼ Chronic HCV infection develops in 75–85% of infected patients, but in most patients, it is associated with relatively mild clinical disease, in spite of progressive hepatic damage. Risk factors for more severe disease and rapid progression include alcohol abuse (or other hepatotoxin exposure); coexisting liver disease; immunocompromised status, especially HIV infection; and genetic and other factors. The risk of progression to cirrhosis is markedly increased in patients with hypogammaglobulinemia. Transaminase elevations are typically lower than in HBV infection; episodic fluctuations are common. Occult HBV infection is present in about one third of patients with chronic HCV liver disease.

■ *Initial HCV Diagnostic Tests*
  ▼ *Serology*: Patients with suspected HCV infection should first be tested for HCV antibody. Current "second-generation" EIA assays are very sensitive; tests are positive at presentation in half of patients and within 1 month of presentation in approximately 95% of patients. False-negative results may be seen in dialysis, transplant, or immunocompromised patients (e.g., HIV-infected patients) in spite of circulating HVC RNA. The specificity of HCV serology tests is also very high (>99%), but false-positive reactions must be ruled out in asymptomatic patients with a low prior probability of infection, as in blood donor screening.

  ▼ The FDA has approved several waived, rapid diagnostic tests for HCV antibody detection. These tests have sensitivities comparable to laboratory-based EIA tests. These assays may improve care by providing direct testing with immediate results at the point of patient encounter, like a physician's office, clinic, or emergency room.

  ▼ A negative result for HCV antibody rules out infection in immunologically intact patients. In patients who might not mount a solid antibody response, testing for HCV RNA should be performed.

  ▼ A positive result for HCV serology testing indicates HCV infection or a false-positive result. In antibody-positive patients with a low prior probability of HCV infection, like healthy blood donors, unexpectedly positive HCV serology screens should be followed by repeat HCV antibody testing using a different test method from the one used for initial testing.

  ▼ Positive HCV serology tests cannot distinguish between resolved versus active infection, which requires testing for HCV RNA.

  ▼ *Molecular diagnostic testing*: Molecular testing for HCV RNA should be performed on all patients with positive HCV serology to determine the presence of active HCV replication. The recombinant immunoblot assay (RIBA HCV) is no longer available for routine diagnostic testing.

  ▼ HCV RNA detection tests may be qualitative or quantitative. The most sensitive method available should be used to rule out active infection. Real-time (RT) PCR and other quantitative assays may now provide reliable quantification to levels as low as those provided by qualitative assays. An advantage of the use of quantitative HCV (viral load) assays to confirm HCV infection is that they can provide information to predict likely response to antiviral therapy and to determine response to antiviral therapy. Even though HCV RNA assays are calibrated to an international standard, results may vary across different assays. Therefore, the use of a single assay is recommended for serial testing of a patient's HCV viral load.

- ● Anti-HCV positive (confirmed), HCV RNA negative: Resolved HCV infection.
- ● Anti-HCV positive (confirmed), HCV RNA positive: Active HCV infection.
- ▼ *HCV genotype analysis*: HCV genotype should be determined for patients with acute or chronic HCV infection. There are six different HCV genotypes and many subtypes. The prevalence of different genotypes shows geographic variability; genotype 1 is most common in the United States.
- ▼ There are genotype-specific differences in response to therapy; the HCV genotype is a factor used to determine the dose and duration of antiviral treatment for chronic HCV infection. Genotypes 2 and 3 have better response rates than genotypes 1 and 4.
- ■ *Laboratory testing in chronic HCV infection*: A number of medical conditions may impact the severity of chronic HCV infection and affect response to treatment. In addition, chronic HCV infection may have disease manifestations outside the liver. In addition to *HCV viral load* testing, tests to evaluate patients for treatment and to monitor response to therapy include the following:
  - ▼ Testing to rule out other chronic diseases, including *infection* (like HIV, hepatitis A, and hepatitis B), *genetic condition* (like hemochromatosis, Wilson disease, α_1-antitrypsin deficiency), or *autoimmune disease* (like positive reactions for ANA, AMA, or antiactin antibody).
  - ▼ A patient *IL28B genotype* predicts a more favorable response to therapy.
  - ▼ *Hepatic function panel*: Serum aminotransferase levels typically increase within 2–8 weeks after infection but commonly show significant variability and may return to almost-normal levels (formerly called *acute "relapsing" hepatitis*). The degree of ALT elevation is an unreliable predictor of histology in HCV infection; biopsy is needed to define the severity of liver damage. Abnormal bilirubin and alkaline phosphatase levels suggest a cholestatic process.
  - ▼ *CBC and PT.*
  - ▼ Metabolic assessment: including *renal* and *thyroid function panels* and *25-hydroxy-vitamin D3 level.*
  - ▼ Assess the patient for alcohol and drug abuse; consider *drug screen.*
  - ▼ Abdominal ultrasound and *AFP* to assess the patient for liver tumor and ascites.
  - ▼ Liver biopsy to assess fibrosis, inflammation, iron overload, steatosis, or other histologic abnormality.
- ■ *Assessment of response to HCV antiviral therapy*: The goal of antiviral treatment is a sustained virologic response (SVR), which is defined as undetectable HCV RNA 6 months after the end of therapy.
  - ▼ *Patient factors*: Pretreatment factors associated with a lower rate of SVR include inability to comply with the treatment regimen, diabetes or insulin resistance, increased body weight, older age, increased portal hypertension

or abnormal liver histopathology (fibrosis, cirrhosis, steatosis), statin use, increased triglyceride or HDL, and decreased LDL.

▼ *Baseline*: Patients with pretreatment HCV viral loads >800,000 IU/mL are less likely to achieve SVR, compared to patients with lower baseline viral loads.

▼ *Rapid virologic response (RVR)*: Monitoring HCV viral load should begin as early as 2–4 weeks after initiation of antiviral therapy with pegylated interferon/ribavirin or triple therapy (e.g., pegIFN/RBV plus telaprevir or boceprevir). The rate of fall of the HCV viral load is an important predictor of SVR, especially for genotype 1 virus. Patients with negative HCV RNA at 4 weeks have high (>90%) rates of SVR and may be eligible for a shortened duration of therapy.

▼ Early virologic response (EVR): HCV viral load should be assessed at 12 weeks in patients who did not achieve RVR. SVR is seen in 65% of patients overall in whom the HCV viral load shows a >2 $\log_{10}$ reduction compared to baseline; SVR >70% is seen in patients with undetectable HCV RNA at 12 weeks.

● Patients who do not show a >2 $\log_{10}$ reduction in HCV viral load, compared to their baseline, are unlikely to achieve an SVR (<2%).

Suggested Readings

Beinhardt S, Rutter K, Stättermayer AF, et al. Revisiting the predictors of a sustained virologic response in the era of direct-acting antiviral therapy for hepatitis C virus. *Clin Infect Dis.* 2013;56:118–122.

Bräu N. Evaluation of the hepatitis C virus-infected patient: the initial encounter. *Clin Infect Dis.* 2013;56(6):853–860.

Center for Disease Control and Prevention. *Viral Hepatitis.* www.cdc.gov/hepatitis/index.htm. Accessed June 18, 2013.

Centers for Disease Control and Prevention. Vital Signs: Evaluation of Hepatitis C Virus Infection Testing and Reporting—Eight U.S. Sites, 2005–2011. *MMWR.* 2013;62(No. 18):357–361.

Ferenci P. Response guided therapy in patients with chronic hepatitis C—yesterday, today and tomorrow. *Best Pract Res Clin Gastroenterol.* 2012;26:463–469.

Hoofnagle JH, Nelson KE, Purcell RH. Hepatitis E. *N Engl J Med.* 2012;367:1237–1244.

Niesters HGM, Zoulim F, Pichoud C, et al. Validation of the INNO-LiPA HBV DR assay (version 2) in monitoring hepatitis B virus-infected patients receiving nucleoside analog treatment. *Antimicrob Agents Chemother.* 2010;54:1283–1289.

Rotman Y, Liang TJ. Hepatitis C virus. In: Richman DD, Whitley RJ, Hayden FG. *Clinical Virology,* 3rd ed. Washington, DC: ASM Press; 2009.

Sherman KE. Therapeutic approach to the treatment-naïve patient with hepatitis C virus genotype 1 infection: a step-by-step approach. *Clin Infect Dis.* 2012;55:1236–1241.

Sonneveld MJ, Zoutendijk R, Flink HJ, et al. Close monitoring of hepatitis B surface antigen levels helps classify flares during peginterferon therapy and predicts treatment response. *Clin Infect Dis.* 2013;56:100–105.

Strader DB, Wright T, Thomas DL, et al. Diagnosis, management, and treatment of hepatitis C. *Hepatology.* 2004;39:1147–1171.

VASCULAR AND ISCHEMIC DISORDERS OF THE LIVER

BUDD-CHIARI SYNDROME

❑ **Definition**

Heterogeneous group of disorders due to obstruction of hepatic venous outflow

❏ Causes

- Thrombosis due to hypercoagulable states (e.g., polycythemia vera [10–40% of cases], essential thrombocythemia, myelofibrosis; antiphospholipid syndrome; and deficiencies of protein C, protein S, and antithrombin III) (See Chapter 10, Hematologic Disorders, Paroxysmal Nocturnal Hemoglobinuria)
- Membranes and webs
- Others (e.g., neoplasms, collagen vascular diseases, cirrhosis, and polycystic liver disease)

❏ Laboratory Findings

- *Core laboratory*: Due to parenchymal cell necrosis and malfunction (e.g., increased serum AST), ALT may be increased >5 times in acute and fulminant forms. ALP and bilirubin may be increased and serum albumin decreased. Ascitic fluid total protein is usually >2.5 g/dL.
- Radiologic visualization (e.g., ultrasound, CT scan, MRI, hepatic angiography).
- Liver biopsy.

Suggested Reading

Menon KVN, Shah N, Kamath PS, et al. The Budd-Chiari syndrome. *N Engl J Med*. 2004;350:578.

CONGESTIVE HEART FAILURE

❏ Laboratory Findings Related to Altered Liver Function

- *Core laboratory*: Pattern of abnormal liver function tests is variable depending on severity of heart failure; the mildest show only slightly increased ALP and slightly decreased serum albumin; moderately severe also show slightly increased serum bilirubin and GGT; one fourth to three fourths of the most severe will also show increased AST and ALT (≤200 U/L) and LD (≤400 U/L). All return to normal when heart failure responds to treatment. Serum ALP is usually the last to become normal, and this may be weeks to months later. AST and ALT may be increased 2–3× normal in less than one third of cases but much higher in severe acute heart failure. Serum albumin is slightly decreased in <50% of patients but is rarely. Serum bilirubin is increased in ≤70% of cases (unconjugated more than conjugated); usually <3 mg/dL but may be >20 mg/dL. It usually represents combined right- and left-sided failure with hepatic engorgement and pulmonary infarcts. Serum bilirubin may suddenly rise rapidly if superimposed myocardial infarction occurs. Serum cholesterol and esters may be decreased. Serum ammonia may be increased. Urine urobilinogen is increased. Urine bilirubin is increased in the presence of jaundice.
- *Hematology*: PT may be slightly increased in 80% of cases, with increased sensitivity to anticoagulant drugs. Fails to correct with vitamin K.

PORTAL HYPERTENSION

- This condition may be
  - ▼ Prehepatic (e.g., portal vein thrombosis, splenic arteriovenous fistula)
  - ▼ Intrahepatic

- Presinusoidal (e.g., metastatic tumor, granulomas such as sarcoid, schistosomiasis)
- Sinusoidal (e.g., cirrhosis)
- Postsinusoidal (e.g., hepatic vein thrombosis, alcoholic hepatitis)
▼ Posthepatic (e.g., pericarditis, tricuspid insufficiency, inferior vena cava web)

BILIARY EXTRAHEPATIC OBSTRUCTION, COMPLETE

DISEASES OF THE GALLBLADDER AND BILIARY TREE (INTRAHEPATIC OR EXTRAHEPATIC) (SEE ABDOMINAL PAIN)

❑ **Laboratory Findings**

- *Liver enzymes*: AST is increased (≤300 U/L), and ALT is increased (≤200 U/L); they usually return to normal within 1 week after relief of obstruction. In *acute* biliary duct obstruction (e.g., due to common bile duct stones or acute pancreatitis), AST and ALT are increased >300 U/L (and often >2,000 U/L) and decline 58–76% in 72 hours without treatment; simultaneous serum total bilirubin shows less marked elevation and decline, and ALP changes are inconsistent and unpredictable. Typical pattern of extrahepatic obstruction includes increased serum ALP (>2–3× normal), AST <300 U/L, and conjugated serum bilirubin. In extrahepatic type, the increased ALP is related to the completeness of obstruction. Normal ALP is extremely rare in extrahepatic obstruction. Very high levels may also occur in cases of intrahepatic cholestasis.
- Conjugated serum bilirubin is increased; unconjugated serum bilirubin is normal or slightly increased. Urine bilirubin is increased; urine urobilinogen decreased. There is decreased stool bilirubin and urobilinogen (clay-colored stools).
- *Lipids*: Serum phospholipids are increased. Serum cholesterol is increased (acute, 300–400 mg/dL; chronic, ≤1,000 mg/dL).
- *Hematology*: PT is prolonged, with response to parenteral vitamin K more frequent than in hepatic parenchymal cell disease.

Considerations

- Laboratory findings due to underlying causative disease are noted (e.g., stone, carcinoma of duct, metastatic carcinoma to periductal lymph nodes).
- Bile duct obstruction (one): Characteristic pattern is serum bilirubin that remains normal in the presence of markedly increased serum ALP.

CANCER OF THE GALLBLADDER AND BILE DUCTS

❑ **Laboratory Findings**

- Laboratory findings of duct obstruction are of progressively increasing severity in contrast to the intermittent or fluctuating changes due to duct obstruction caused by stones. A papillary intraluminal duct carcinoma may undergo periods of sloughing, producing the findings of intermittent duct obstruction.

These reflect varying location and extent of tumor infiltration that may cause partial intrahepatic duct obstruction or obstruction of the hepatic or common bile duct, metastases in the liver, or associated cholangitis; 50% of patients have jaundice at the time of hospitalization.

- *Hematology*: Anemia is present.
- *Cytology*: Examination of aspirated duodenal fluid may demonstrate malignant cells.
- *Stool findings*: Silver-colored stool due to jaundice combined with GI bleeding may be seen in carcinoma of the duct or ampulla of Vater.

CHOLANGITIS, ACUTE

5

❑ **Laboratory Findings**

- *Culture*: Blood culture positive in approximately 30% of cases; 25% of these are polymicrobial. Infection of bile ducts usually due to gram-negative (e.g., *E. coli*, *Klebsiella* sp., gram-positive, and anaerobic [*Streptococcus faecalis*, enterococcus, *Bacteroides fragilis*]) organisms usually associated with obstruction
- *Hematology*: Marked increase in WBC (≤30,000/μL) with increase in granulocytes
- Core laboratory: Increased serum AST and ALT. Increased urine urobilinogen

Considerations

- Laboratory findings of incomplete duct obstruction due to inflammation or of preceding complete duct obstruction (e.g., stone, tumor, scar). See Choledocholithiasis
- Laboratory findings of parenchymal cell necrosis and malfunction

CHOLANGITIS, PRIMARY SCLEROSING

- Chronic fibrosing cholestatic inflammation of intra- and extrahepatic bile ducts predominantly in men younger than age 45; rare in pediatric patients; ≤75% are associated with IBD, especially UC. Slow, relentless, progressive course of chronic cholestasis to death (usually from liver failure). Twenty-five percent of patients are asymptomatic at the time of diagnosis.

❑ **Diagnostic Criteria**

1. Cholestatic biochemical profile for >6 months
   - ▼ Serum ALP may fluctuate but is always increased (usually ≥3 times upper limit of normal).
   - ▼ Serum GGT is increased.
   - ▼ Serum AST is mildly increased in >90%. ALT > AST in three fourths of cases.
   - ▼ Serum bilirubin is increased in 50% of patients; occasionally is very high; may fluctuate markedly; gradually increases as disease progresses. Persistent value >1.5 mg/dL is a poor prognostic sign that may indicate irreversible medically untreatable disease.

2. Compatible clinical history (e.g., IBD) and exclusion of other causes of sclerosing cholangitis (e.g., previous bile duct surgery, gallstones, suppurative cholangitis, bile duct tumor or damage due to floxuridine, AIDS, congenital duct anomalies)
3. Characteristic cholangiogram to distinguish from primary biliary cirrhosis
   ▼ Increased γ-globulin in 30% and increased IgM in 40–50% of cases
   ▼ Antineutrophil cytoplasmic antibody (ANCA) is present in approximately 65% of cases, and antinuclear antibodies are noted in <35% of cases and are present at higher levels than in other liver diseases, but diagnostic significance is not yet known.
   ▼ In contrast to primary biliary cirrhosis, antimitochondrial antibody, smooth muscle antibody, rheumatoid factor, and ANA are negative in >90% of patients.
   ▼ HBsAg is negative.
   ▼ Liver biopsy provides only confirmatory evidence in patients with compatible history, laboratory, and x-ray findings. Liver copper is usually increased, but serum ceruloplasmin is also increased.

Other Considerations
   ■ Laboratory findings due to sequelae.
   ■ Cholangiocarcinoma in 10–15% of patients may cause increased serum CA 19-9.
   ■ Portal hypertension, biliary cirrhosis, secondary bacterial cholangitis, steatorrhea and malabsorption, cholelithiasis, and liver failure.
   ■ Laboratory findings due to underlying disease (e.g., ≤7.5% of UC patients have this disease; much less often with Crohn disease). Associated with syndrome of retroperitoneal and mediastinal fibrosis.

CHOLECYSTITIS, ACUTE

❑ **Laboratory Findings**
   ■ *Hematology*: Increased ESR, WBC (average 12,000/μL; if >15,000, suspect empyema or perforation), and other evidence of acute inflammatory process.
   ■ *Core laboratory*: Serum AST is increased in 75% of patients. Increased serum bilirubin in 20% of patients (usually >4 mg/dL; if higher, suspect associated choledocholithiasis). Increased serum ALP (some patients) even if serum bilirubin is normal. Increased serum amylase and lipase in some patients

Considerations
   ■ Laboratory findings of associated biliary obstruction if such obstruction is present
   ■ Laboratory findings of preexisting cholelithiasis (some patients)
   ■ Laboratory findings of complications (e.g., empyema of the gallbladder, perforation, cholangitis, liver abscess, pyelophlebitis, pancreatitis, gallstone ileus)

CHOLECYSTITIS, CHRONIC

   ■ May be mild laboratory findings of acute cholecystitis or no abnormal laboratory findings

- May be laboratory findings of associated cholelithiasis
- Laboratory findings of sequelae (e.g., carcinoma of the gallbladder)

CHOLEDOCHOLITHIASIS

- Gallstones in bile ducts due to passage from the gallbladder or anatomic defects (e.g., cysts, strictures)

❏ **Laboratory Findings**

- *Core laboratory*: Increased serum and urine amylase. Increased serum bilirubin in about one third of patients. Increased urine bilirubin in about one third of patients. Increased serum ALP
- *Hematology*: Increased WBC
- Considerations
  - ▾ Laboratory evidence of fluctuating or transient cholestasis. Persistent increase of WBC, AST, and ALT suggests cholangitis.
  - ▾ Laboratory findings due to secondary cholangitis, acute pancreatitis, obstructive jaundice, stricture formation, and so on.
  - ▾ In duodenal drainage, crystals of both calcium bilirubinate and cholesterol (some patients); 50% accurate (only useful in nonicteric patients).

❏ **Cholelithiasis**

- Laboratory findings of underlying conditions causing
  - ▾ Hypercholesterolemia (e.g., DM, malabsorption)
  - ▾ Chronic hemolytic disease (e.g., hereditary spherocytosis)
- Laboratory findings due to complications (e.g., cholecystitis, choledocholithiasis, gallstone ileus)

ATRESIA, EXTRAHEPATIC BILIARY, CONGENITAL

- Conjugated serum bilirubin increased in early days of life in some infants but not until 2nd week in others. Level is often <12 mg/dL during the first few months, with subsequent rise later in life.
- Laboratory findings as in complete biliary obstruction.
- Liver biopsy to differentiate from neonatal hepatitis.
- Laboratory findings due to sequelae (e.g., biliary cirrhosis, portal hypertension, frequent infections, rickets, hepatic failure).
- ^{131}I-rose bengal excretion test.

OTHER CONSIDERATIONS

- Most important to differentiate this condition from neonatal hepatitis, for which surgery may be harmful.
- More than 90% of cases of extrahepatic biliary obstruction in newborns are due to biliary atresia; occasional cases may be due to choledochal cyst (causes intermittent jaundice in infancy), bile plug syndrome, or bile ascites (associated with spontaneous perforation of the common bile duct).

INTRAHEPATIC OBSTRUCTION CHOLESTASIS

- Causes of intrahepatic cholestasis:
  - ▼ Intrahepatic obstruction
    - Space-occupying lesions (e.g., amyloidosis, sarcoidosis, metastases; non-Hodgkin lymphoma more often than Hodgkin disease)
    - Drugs (e.g., estrogens, anabolic steroids)—most common cause (Table 5-13)
    - Normal pregnancy
    - Alcoholic hepatitis
    - Infections (e.g., acute viral hepatitis, gram-negative sepsis, toxic shock syndrome, AIDS, parasitic, fungal)
    - Sickle cell crisis
    - Postoperative state following long procedure and multiple transfusions
    - Benign recurrent familial intrahepatic cholestasis—rare condition
- Autosomal recessive condition; attacks begin after age 8, last weeks to months, complete resolution between episodes, may recur after months or years; exacerbated by estrogens

❑ **Laboratory Findings**

- *Core laboratory*: Increased serum ALP, but GGT is usually normal. Serum direct bilirubin may be normal or ≤10 mg/dL. Transaminase usually <100 U.
- *Histology*: Liver biopsy shows centrolobular cholestasis without inflammation, bile pigment in hepatocytes and canaliculi; little or no fibrosis.

CIRRHOSIS, PRIMARY BILIARY (CHOLANGIOLITIC CIRRHOSIS, HANOT HYPERTROPHIC CIRRHOSIS, CHRONIC NONSUPPURATIVE DESTRUCTIVE CHOLANGITIS, ETC.)

- Slow progressive multisystem autoimmune disease; chronic nonsuppurative inflammation and asymmetric destruction of small intrahepatic bile ducts producing chronic cholestasis, cirrhosis, and ultimately liver failure

TABLE 5–13. Comparison of Various Types of Cholestatic Disease

Disorder	Bilirubin (mg/dL)	ALP	AST	ALT	Albumin
CBD obstruction N					
Stone	0–10	N–10	N–10	N–10	N
Cancer	5–20	2–10	N	N	N
Intrahepatic					
Drug-induced	5–10	2–10	N–5	10–50	
Acute viral hepatitis	0–20	N–3	10–50	10–50	N
Alcoholic liver disease	0–20	5	<10	<50% of AST	N/sl D

CBD, common bile duct; N, normal; sl D, slightly decreased.
*Serum value, times normal.

❑ **Diagnostic Criteria**

- Definitive diagnosis requires all three criteria; probable diagnosis requires two criteria.
  - ▼ Antimitochondrial autoantibodies present
  - ▼ Cholestatic pattern (increased ALP) of long duration (>6 months) not due to known cause (e.g., drugs)
  - ▼ Compatible histologic findings on liver biopsy
- Serum ALP is markedly increased; is of liver origin. Reaches a plateau early in the course and then fluctuates within 20% thereafter; changes in serum level have no prognostic value. 5′-N and GGT parallel the ALP. *This is one of the few conditions that will elevate both serum ALP and GGT to striking levels.*
- Serum mitochondrial antibody titer is strongly positive in approximately 95% of patients (1:40–1:80) and is hallmark of disease (98% specificity); titer >1:160 is highly predictive of primary biliary cirrhosis (PBC), even in the absence of other findings. Does not correlate with severity or rate of progression. Titers differ greatly in patients. Similar titers occur in 5% of patients with chronic hepatitis; low titers occur in 10% of patients with other liver disease; rarely found in normal persons. Titer may decrease after liver transplantation but usually remains detectable.
- Serum bilirubin is normal in early phase but increases in 60% of patients with progression of disease and is a reliable prognostic indicator; an elevated level is a poor prognostic sign. Conjugated serum bilirubin is increased in 80% of patients; levels >5 mg/dL in only 20% of patients; levels >10 mg/dL in only 6% of patients. Unconjugated bilirubin is normal or slightly increased.
- Laboratory findings show relatively little evidence of parenchymal damage.
  - ▼ AST and ALT may be normal or slightly increased (≤1–5 times normal), fluctuate within a narrow range, and have no prognostic significance.
  - ▼ Serum albumin, globulin, and PT normal early; abnormal values indicate advanced disease and poor prognosis; not corrected by therapy.
- Marked increase in total cholesterol and phospholipids with normal triglycerides; serum is not lipemic; serum triglycerides become elevated in late stages. Associated with xanthomas and xanthelasmas. In early stages, LDL and VLDL are mildly elevated and HDL is markedly elevated (thus atherosclerosis is rare). In advanced stage, LDL is markedly elevated with decreased HDL and presence of lipoprotein-X (nonspecific abnormal lipoprotein seen in other cholestatic liver disease).
- Serum IgM is increased in approximately 75% of patients; levels may be very high (four to five times normal). Other serum immunoglobulins are also increased.
- Hypocomplementemia.
- Polyclonal hypergammaglobulinemia. Serum IgM is increased in approximately 75% of patients with failure to convert to IgG antibodies; levels may be very high (four to five times normal). Other serum immunoglobulins are also increased.
- Biopsy of the liver categorizes the four stages and helps assess prognosis, but needle biopsy is subject to sampling error because the lesions may be spotty; findings consistent with all four stages may be found in one specimen.
- Serum ceruloplasmin is characteristically elevated (in contrast to Wilson disease).

5

- Liver copper may be increased 10–100 times normal; correlates with serum bilirubin and advancing stages of disease.
- ESR is increased one to five times normal in 80% of patients.
- Urine contains urobilinogen and bilirubin.
- Laboratory findings of steatorrhea:
  ▼ Serum 25-hydroxyvitamin D and vitamin A are usually low.
  ▼ PT is normal or restored to normal by parenteral vitamin K.
- Laboratory findings due to associated diseases:
  ▼ More than 80% have one, and >40% have at least two, other circulating antibodies to autoimmune disease (e.g., RA, autoimmune thyroiditis [hypothyroidism in 20% of patients], Sjögren syndrome, scleroderma) although not useful diagnostically.

CONGENITAL CONJUGATED HYPERBILIRUBINEMIA

DUBIN-JOHNSON SYNDROME (SPRINZ-NELSON DISEASE)

- An autosomal recessive disease (gene located on chromosome 10q24) due to inability to transport bilirubin–glucuronide through hepatocytes into canaliculi, but conjugation of bilirubin–glucuronide is normal. Characterized by mild chronic, recurrent jaundice. May have hepatomegaly and right upper quadrant abdominal pain. Usually is compensated except in periods of stress. Jaundice (innocuous and reversible) may be produced by estrogens, birth control pills, or last trimester of pregnancy; may resemble mild viral hepatitis.

❏ **Laboratory Findings**

- See Table 5-14.
- *Histology*: Liver biopsy shows large amounts of yellow-brown or slate-black pigment in centrolobular hepatic cells (lysosomes) and small amounts in Kupffer cells.
- *Core laboratory*: Serum total bilirubin is increased (1.5–6.0 mg/dL); rarely ≤25 mg/dL during intercurrent illness; significant amount is conjugated. Normal in heterozygotes. Other liver function tests are normal. No evidence of hemolysis. Urine contains bile and urobilinogen.
- *Other*: Urine total coproporphyrin is usually normal, but approximately 80% is coproporphyrin I (normally 25% is coproporphyrin I and 75% is coproporphyrin III); diagnostic of Dubin-Johnson syndrome. Not useful to detect individual heterozygotes. Fecal coproporphyrins are normal. BSP excretion is impaired with late (normal at 45 minutes; increased at 90 and 120 minutes); virtually pathognomonic but is no longer performed.

ROTOR SYNDROME

- Autosomal recessive, familial, asymptomatic, benign defective uptake, and storage of conjugated bilirubin and possibly in transfer of bilirubin from the liver to bile or in intrahepatic binding; usually detected in adolescents or adults. Jaundice may be produced or accentuated by pregnancy, birth control pills, alcohol, infection, or surgery.
- See Table 5-14.

TABLE 5–14. Differential Diagnosis of Hereditary Jaundice with Normal Liver Chemistries and No Signs or Symptoms of Liver Disease

| | | | | Unconjugated Hyperbilirubinemias | |
| | | | | Crigler-Najjar Syndrome | |
	Dubin-Johnson Syndrome	Rotor Syndrome	Gilbert Disease	Type I	Type II
Incidence	Uncommon	Rare	≤7% of population	Very rare	Uncommon
Inheritance mode	AR	AR	AD	AR	AD
Serum bilirubin usual total (mg/dL)	2–7; ≤25	2–7; ≤20	<3; ≤6	>20	<20
Defect in bilirubin metabolism	Direct ~60%; Impaired biliary excretion of conjugated organic anions and bilirubin	Direct ~60%	Mostly indirect; increases with fasting; Hepatic UDP-glucuronyl transferase activity Decreased	All indirect; Absent	All indirect; Marked decrease
Impaired excretion of dyes requiring conjugation (e.g., BSP)	Yes; initial rapid fall, then rise in 45–90 minutes	Yes; slow clearance; no later increase	May be slightly impaired in ≤40% of patients		
Effect of phenobarbital		Decrease to normal	None	Marked decrease	
Urine coproporphyrin Total	Normal	Increased			
I/III*	>80%	<80%			
Age at onset of jaundice	Childhood, adolescence	Adolescence, early adulthood	Adolescence	Infancy	Childhood, adolescence
Usual clinical features	Asymptomatic jaundice in young adults	Asymptomatic jaundice	Appear in early adulthood; often first recognized with fasting; very mild hemolysis in ≤40% of patients	Jaundice, kernicterus in infants, young adults	Asymptomatic jaundice; kernicterus rare
Oral cholecystogram	GB usually not visualized	Normal	Normal	Normal	Normal
Liver biopsy	Characteristic pigment	No pigment	Normal	Normal	Normal
Treatment	Not needed		Not needed	Liver transplant; no response to phenobarbital	Phenobarbital
Animal model	Corriedale sheep	None		Gunn rat	

AD, autosomal dominant; AR, autosomal recessive; BSP, sulfobromophthalein; GB, gallbladder; UDP-glucuronyl transferase, uridine diphosphate–glucuronosyl transferase.

*Normally coproporphyrin III, 75% of total.

CAUSES OF UNCONJUGATED HYPERBILIRUBINEMIA

UNCONJUGATED BILIRUBINEMIA

❑ **Causes**
- Increased destruction of RBCs
  - ▼ Isoimmunization (e.g., incompatibility of Rh, ABO, other blood groups)
  - ▼ Biochemical defects of RBCs (e.g., G6PD deficiency, pyruvate deficiency, hexokinase deficiency, congenital erythropoietic porphyria, α- and γ-thalassemias)
  - ▼ Structural defects of RBCs (e.g., hereditary spherocytosis, hereditary elliptocytosis, infantile pyknocytosis, *xerocytosis*)
  - ▼ Physiologic hemolysis of the newborn
  - ▼ Infection

PHYSIOLOGIC JAUNDICE

❑ **Definition**
Transient unconjugated hyperbilirubinemia (physiologic jaundice) that occurs in almost all newborns resulting from physiologic hemolysis

❑ **Laboratory Findings**
- In a normal full-term neonate, average maximum serum bilirubin is 6 mg/dL (≤12 mg/dL is in physiologic range) that occurs during the 2nd to 4th day and then rapidly falls to approximately 2.0 mg/dL by 5th day (phase I physiologic jaundice). Declines slowly to <1.0 mg/dL during the 5th to 10th day but may take 1 month to fall to <2 mg/dL (phase II physiologic jaundice). Phase I due to deficiency of hepatic bilirubin glucuronyl transferase activity, and sixfold increase in bilirubin load presented to the liver. In Asian and Native American newborns, the average maximum serum levels are approximately double (10–14 mg/dL) the levels in non-Asians, and kernicterus is more frequent. Serum bilirubin >5 mg/dL during the first 24 hours of life is indication for further workup because of risk of kernicterus.
- In older children (and adults), icterus is apparent clinically when serum bilirubin is >2 mg/dL, but in newborns, clinical icterus is not apparent until serum bilirubin is >5–7 mg/dL; therefore, only half of the full-term newborns show clinical jaundice during the first 3 days of life.
- In premature infants—average maximum serum bilirubin is 10–12 mg/dL and occurs during the 5th to 7th day. Serum bilirubin may not fall to normal until 30th day. Further workup is indicated in all premature infants with clinical jaundice because of risk of kernicterus in some low birth weight infants with serum levels of 10–12 mg/dL.
- In postmature infants and half of small-for-date infants—serum bilirubin is <2.5 mg/dL, and physiologic jaundice is not seen. When mothers have received phenobarbital or used heroin, physiologic jaundice is also less severe.
- When a pregnant woman has unconjugated hyperbilirubinemia, similar levels occur in cord blood, but when the mother has conjugated hyperbilirubinemia (e.g., hepatitis), similar levels are *not* present in cord blood.

NONPHYSIOLOGIC JAUNDICE

Cause should be sought for underlying pathologic jaundice if
- Total serum bilirubin >7 mg/dL during the first 24 hours or increases >5 mg/dL/day or visible jaundice
- Peak total serum bilirubin >12.5 mg/dL in white or black full-term infants or >15 mg/dL in Hispanic or premature infants
- Conjugated serum bilirubin >1.5 mg/dL

HEREDITARY AND/OR CONGENITAL CAUSES OF UNCONJUGATED HYPERBILIRUBINEMIA

5

CRIGLER-NAJJAR SYNDROME (HEREDITARY GLUCURONYL TRANSFERASE DEFICIENCY)

- A rare familial autosomal recessive disease due to marked congenital deficiency or absence of glucuronyl transferase, which conjugates bilirubin to bilirubin glucuronide in hepatic cells (counterpart is the homozygous Gunn rat)

❑ **Laboratory Findings**
- See Table 5-14.

Type I
Histology: Liver biopsy is normal.
Core laboratory: Unconjugated serum bilirubin is increased; it appears on the 1st or 2nd day of life, rises in 1 week to peak of 12–45 mg/dL and persists for life. No conjugated bilirubin in serum or urine. Liver function tests are normal; BSP is normal. Fecal urobilinogen is very low.

❑ **Other Considerations**
- Untreated patients often die of kernicterus by age 18 months.
- Nonjaundiced parents have diminished capacity to form glucuronide conjugates with menthol, salicylates, and tetrahydrocortisone.
- Type I should always be ruled out when there are persistent unconjugated bilirubin levels of 20 mg/dL after 1 week of age without obvious hemolysis and especially after breast milk jaundice has been ruled out.

GILBERT DISEASE

- Chronic, benign, intermittent, familial (autosomal dominant with incomplete penetrance), nonhemolytic unconjugated hyperbilirubinemia with evanescent increases of unconjugated serum bilirubin, which is usually discovered on routine laboratory examinations; due to defective transport and conjugation of unconjugated bilirubin.
- Jaundice is usually accentuated by pregnancy, fever, exercise, and various drugs, including alcohol and birth control pills.
- Rarely identified before puberty.
- May be mildly symptomatic; 3–7% prevalence in total population.

NEONATAL JAUNDICE: BREAST MILK JAUNDICE

- Due to the presence in mother's milk of pregnanediol, which inhibits glucuronyl transferase activity

❑ **Laboratory Findings**
- Severe unconjugated hyperbilirubinemia. Develops in 1% of breast-fed infants by the 4th to 7th day. May reach peak of 15–25 mg/dL by the 2nd to 3rd week; then gradually disappears in 3–10 weeks in all cases. If nursing is interrupted, serum bilirubin falls rapidly by 2–6 mg/dL in 2–6 days and may rise again if breast-feeding is resumed; if interrupted for 6–9 days, serum bilirubin becomes normal.
- No other abnormalities are present.
- Kernicterus does not occur.

LUCEY-DRISCOLL SYNDROME (NEONATAL TRANSIENT FAMILIAL HYPERBILIRUBINEMIA)

- Syndrome is due to some factor in mother's serum only during the last trimester of pregnancy that inhibits glucuronyl transferase activity; disappears about 2 weeks postpartum.
- Newborn infants have severe nonhemolytic unconjugated hyperbilirubinemia usually ≤20 mg/dL during the first 48 hours and a high risk of kernicterus.

WILSON DISEASE

- Autosomal recessive defect that impairs copper excretion by the liver, which may cause copper accumulation in the liver and brain resulting in cirrhosis, neuropsychiatric disease, and corneal pigmentation.
- Heterozygous gene for Wilson disease occurs in 1 of 200 in the general population; 10% of these have decreased serum ceruloplasmin; liver copper is not increased (<250 µg/g of dry liver). Serum copper and ceruloplasmin and urine copper are inadequate to detect heterozygous state.
- Homozygous gene (clinical Wilson disease) occurs in 1 of 200,000 in the general population.
- Liver biopsy may show no abnormalities, moderate to marked fatty changes with or without fibrosis, or active or inactive mixed micronodular–macronodular cirrhosis.

❑ **Laboratory Findings**
- Findings of liver function tests may not be abnormal, depending on the type and severity of the disease. In patients presenting with acute fulminant hepatitis, Wilson disease is suggested if there is a disproportionately low serum ALP and relatively mild increase in AST and ALT. ALP is frequently decreased; ALP/bilirubin ratio <2.0 is said to distinguish Wilson disease as cause of fulminant liver failure with S/S = 100%/100%.

- *Radiocopper incorporation* into ceruloplasmin is reduced significantly compared with heterozygotes or normal persons. ^{64}Cu is administered IV or PO and serum concentration is plotted against time. Serum ^{64}Cu disappears within 4–6 hours and then reappears in persons without Wilson disease; secondary reappearance is absent in Wilson disease because incorporation of ^{64}Cu into ceruloplasmin is decreased. Useful when liver biopsy is contraindicated but rarely used since advent of transjugular liver biopsy. Can use mass spectroscopy rather than radioactive Cu.
- Chelating agent (e.g., d-penicillamine) produces urine Cu excretion of 2–4 mg/day.

❑ **Other Considerations**

- Diagnosis should be ruled out in any patient with hepatitis with negative serology for viral hepatitis, Coombs-negative hemolysis (due to copper released from necrotic liver cells), or neurologic symptoms to allow for early diagnosis and treatment of Wilson disease.

Suggested Reading

Ferenci P. Diagnosis and current therapy of Wilson disease. *Aliment Pharmacol Ther.* 2004;19:157.

TRAUMA

- May be laceration, hematoma, or vascular

❑ **Laboratory Findings**

- Core laboratory: Serum LD is frequently increased (>1,400 units) 8–12 hours after major injury. Shock due to any injury may also increase LD. Other serum enzymes and liver function tests are not generally helpful.

Endocrine Diseases

Hongbo Yu

This chapter focuses on six common groups of endocrine disorders based on organ systems: diabetes mellitus, disorders of the thyroid gland, disorders of the adrenal gland, gonadal disorders, disorders of the pituitary gland, and disorders of the parathyroid gland and mineral metabolism. For each organ system, the diseases are further discussed according to clinical presentations and/or laboratory findings. The differential diagnosis, laboratory workup, and radiologic studies for each disease are also considered. Of note, male hypogonadism is covered in the Genitourinary Diseases, Chapter 7.

General principles in the diagnosis of endocrine diseases include the following:

- Stimulatory tests should be performed if hypofunction is suspected and suppression tests if hyperfunction is suspected.
- Suppression tests suppress normal glands but not autonomous secretion.
- Patient preparation is particularly important for hormone studies, results of which may be markedly affected by many factors such as stress, position, fasting state, time of day, preceding diet, and drug therapy. These all should be recorded on the laboratory test requisition form and discussed with the laboratory prior to test ordering.
- Appropriate and timely transportation to the laboratory and preparation of specimen are essential.

- No single test adequately reflects the endocrine status in all conditions.
- Multiple gland hypofunction should evaluate the pituitary gland.

DIABETES MELLITUS

❑ Definition

The term "diabetes mellitus" (DM) refers to a group of disorders of abnormal carbohydrate metabolism sharing in common the clinical finding of hyperglycemia. DM is associated with a relative or absolute impairment in insulin secretion, along with varying degrees of peripheral resistance to the action of insulin.

❑ Overview

DM affects approximately 5% of the world population and 8% of the US population. It is the fourth leading cause of death in the United States. Of the estimated 18 million people with primary DM in the United States, 90–95% have type 2 DM.

❑ Types and Classification

The recent classification focuses on the underlying pathophysiologic process, rather than descriptions based upon age at onset or type of treatment.

1. Type 1: immune mediated, results in an absolute insulin deficiency.
2. Type 2: relative insulin deficiency due to abnormalities of both insulin secretion and insulin action. Insulin levels are sufficient to prevent lipid mobilization and ketosis.
3. Gestational diabetes: diagnosed during pregnancy. Only 2% of patients with gestational diabetes remain diabetic after delivery. Forty percent of the patients will develop overt diabetes within 15 years, mostly type 2, but occasionally type 1.
4. Specific types of diabetes:
   a. Genetic defects of beta cell function
   b. Genetic defects in insulin action
   c. Diseases of the exocrine pancreas, such as pancreatitis, trauma, pancreatectomy, neoplasia, cystic fibrosis (CF), hemochromatosis, and fibrocalculous pancreatopathy
5. Associated with endocrinopathies (i.e., Cushing syndrome), drugs (i.e., corticosteroids), or chemicals.

❑ Who Should Be Suspected?

The clinical onset of diabetes can be acute or insidious, depending both on the degree of insulin deficiency as well as on the intercurrent level of physiologic stress. Patients with the following symptoms and signs should be tested:

1. Classic symptoms of hyperglycemia, such as thirst, polyuria, weight loss, visual blurring
2. Serendipitous finding of hyperglycemia or known impaired glucose tolerance
3. Complications of diabetes, such as proteinuria, neuropathy, cardiovascular complications, and retinopathy
4. Evidence of dehydration, orthostatic hypotension, confusion, or coma

❑ Screening for Diabetes Mellitus

A. In the absence of specific symptoms

   Routine screening for type 1 DM is not recommended, since there is no accepted treatment for the asymptomatic phase of type 1 DM.

However, for type 2 DM, the American Diabetes Association (ADA) recommends screening for diabetes or prediabetes in all adults with body mass index (BMI) ≥25 kg/m² and one or more additional risk factors for diabetes (see subsequent text of this chapter). In individuals without risk factors, testing should begin at age 45 years. Fasting plasma glucose is the recommended screening test, since it is faster, easier to perform, more convenient, acceptable to patients, and less expensive.

B. Risk factors for diabetes
1. Age ≥45 years
2. Overweight (body mass index ≥25 kg/m²)
3. Family history diabetes mellitus in a first-degree relative
4. Habitual physical inactivity
5. Belonging to a high-risk ethnic or racial group (e.g., African American, Hispanic, Native American, Asian American, and Pacific Islander)
6. History of delivering a baby weighing >4.1 kg (9 lb) or of gestational DM
7. Hypertension (blood pressure ≥140/90 mm Hg)
8. Dyslipidemia defined as a serum high-density lipoprotein cholesterol concentration ≤35 mg/dL (0.9 mM) and/or a serum triglyceride concentration ≥250 mg/dL (2.8 mM)
9. Previously identified impaired glucose tolerance (IGT) or impaired fasting glucose (IFG)
10. Polycystic ovary syndrome
11. History of vascular disease

❏ How to Confirm the Diagnosis
ADA Criteria for the diagnosis of diabetes mellitus:

a. Symptoms of diabetes and a casual plasma glucose ≥200 mg/dL (11.1 mM). Casual is defined as any time of day without regard to time since the last meal. The classic symptoms of diabetes include polyuria, polydipsia, and unexplained weight loss.

Or

b. Fasting plasma glucose ≥126 mg/dL (7.0 mM). Fasting is defined as no caloric intake for at least 8 hours.

Or

c. Two-hour plasma glucose ≥200 mg/dL (11.1 mM) during an oral glucose tolerance test (OGTT). The test should be performed using a glucose load containing the equivalent of 75 g anhydrous glucose dissolved in water.

Or

d. Glycosylated hemoglobin A1c (HbA$_{1c}$) ≥6.5%. In 2010, the ADA added this as another criterion for the diagnosis of DM. The diagnostic test should be performed using a method that is certified by the National Glycohemoglobin Standardization Program (NGSP) and standardized or traceable to the Diabetes Control and Complications Trial reference assay. Point-of-care HbA$_{1c}$ assays are not sufficiently accurate at this time to use for diagnostic purposes. HbA$_{1c}$ is an extremely valuable clinical tool useful both in the diagnosis and in management of diabetic patients. HbA$_{1c}$ has a circulating life span of about 90 days, and thus the measurement of HbA$_{1c}$ provides information about the level of glycemic control over a 3-month period. However, if the patient's red blood cells have abnormal survival time, the value of HbA$_{1c}$ may not be reliable. It will be falsely low in patients with hemolytic anemias, and it may be falsely elevated in patients with polycythemia vera or postsplenectomy. It cannot be used as a reliable index for glycemic control in patients with chronic liver diseases due to increased erythrocyte turnover.

In the absence of unequivocal hyperglycemia, the diagnosis of DM must be confirmed on a subsequent day by measuring any one of the three criteria (b, c, and d). However, in symptomatic patients with blood glucose ≥200 mg/dL (11.1 mM) or patients with ketonuria and clear manifestations of type 1 DM, the diagnosis is established and further evaluation is not needed.

Patients with prediabetic conditions (Table 6-1) should be counseled on issues related to lowering their risk for macrovascular diseases (smoking cessation, use of aspirin, diet, and exercise), should have measurements of blood pressure and serum lipids, and should also be encouraged to modify their lifestyle and reduce their weight.

❑ Complications

Evaluation for complications of diabetes should be done routinely in diabetic patients.

A. Routine eye examination
B. Routine foot examination
C. Screening for microalbuminuria
D. Screening for coronary heart disease

Acute Complications

Excessive and prolonged hyperglycemia associated with uncontrolled diabetes can cause fluid and electrolyte imbalance, which may be life-threatening.

A. *Diabetic ketoacidosis* (mostly in type 1 DM, may also be seen in type 2 DM): Absolute insulin deficiency leads to the unopposed action of the counterregulatory hormones, including glucagon on the liver, adipose tissue, and muscle, leading to unchecked gluconeogenesis and lipolysis.
   a. *Signs and symptoms*
      1. Dehydration, fruity breath smell, orthostatic hypotension, tachypnea, tachycardia, abdominal pain, nausea, vomiting, and confusion
      2. Antecedent history of viral or bacterial illness, trauma, or emotional stress

TABLE 6–1. Diagnostic Thresholds for Diabetes and Prediabetic Conditions

Category	Fasting Plasma Glucose	Two-Hour Plasma Glucose	Glycosylated Hemoglobin A_{1c}
Normal	<100 mg/dL (5.6 mM)	<140 mg/dL (7.8 mM)	<5.7%
Impaired fasting glucose	100–125 mg/dL (5.6–5.9 mM)		
Impaired glucose tolerance		140–199 mg/dL (7.8–11.0 mM)	
Increased risk			5.7–6.4%
Diabetes mellitus	≥126 mg/dL (7.0 mM)	≥200 mg/dL (11.1 mM)	≥6.5%

b. *Laboratory findings*
1. Hyperglycemia (generally ≥300 mg/dL), glucosuria, ketonemia and keto-nuria, low bicarbonate, elevated blood urea nitrogen, elevated creatinine, pH usually <7.3.
2. Decreased total body potassium and phosphorus. Serum levels may be normal due to acidosis and shifts to the extracellular space.

B. *Hyperosmolar hyperglycemic nonketotic coma:* Hyperglycemia in patients with type 2 DM can lead to hyperosmolar coma. The degree of hyperglycemia and dehydration that develop is often far more severe than in patients with type 1 DM.

a. *Signs and symptoms*
1. Usually occurs in elderly patients with decreased ability to obtain free water; precipitated by illness or drugs
2. Deceased mentation, coma
3. Dehydration

b. *Laboratory findings*
1. Hyperglycemia (glucose often ≥600 mg/dL)
2. Serum osmolarity often ≥320 mOsm/kg
3. Bicarbonate remains ≥15 mEq/L
4. pH remains ≥7.3

Chronic Complications

A. Microvasculopathy
a. Diabetic nephropathy
1. Diabetes is now the most common cause of end-stage renal disease in Western countries.
2. Twenty to thirty percent of patients with diabetes will develop evidence of nephropathy.
3. The earliest evidence of nephropathy is the appearance of low levels of albumin (30 mg/day or 20 µg/minute) in the urine, termed microalbuminuria.
4. Eighty percent of type 1 DM and 20–40% of type 2 DM patients who develop microalbuminuria will progress to overt nephropathy (≥300 mg/day or 200 µg/minute) over a period of 10–15 years if not treated.
5. Of those patients who develop overt nephropathy, end-stage renal disease can be expected to develop in 75% of patients with type 1 DM and 20% of patients with type 2 DM over 20 years.
b. Retinopathy and neuropathy
B. Macrovasculopathy and vascular atherosclerosis are also major complications of DM.

Suggested Readings

Khan F, Sachs H, Pechet L. *Guide to Diagnostic Testing*. Philadelphia, PA: Lippincott Williams & Wilkins; 2002.

Kronenberg HM, Melmed S, Polonsky KS, et al. *Williams Textbook of Endocrinology*, 11th ed. Philadelphia, PA: Saunders, Elsevier Inc.; 2008.

Laffel L, Svoren B. Epidemiology, presentation, and diagnosis of type 2 diabetes mellitus in children and adolescents. In: Rose B, (ed). *UpToDate*, Waltham, MA: UpToDate, Inc.; 2009.

Levitsky LL, Misra M. Epidemiology, presentation, and diagnosis of type 1 diabetes mellitus in children and adolescents. In: Rose B, (ed). *UpToDate*, Waltham, MA: UpToDate, Inc.; 2009.

McCulloch DK. Diagnosis of diabetes mellitus. In: Rose B, (ed). *UpToDate*, Waltham, MA: UpToDate, Inc.; 2009.

McCulloch DK. Overview of medical care in adults with diabetes mellitus. In: Rose B, (ed). *UpToDate*, Waltham, MA: UpToDate, Inc.; 2009.

McCulloch DK. Screening for diabetes mellitus. In: Rose B, (ed). *UpToDate*, Waltham, MA: UpToDate, Inc.; 2009.

DISORDERS OF THE THYROID GLAND

THYROTOXICOSIS/HYPERTHYROIDISM

❑ Definition

Thyrotoxicosis refers to the classic physiologic manifestations of excessive quantities of the circulating thyroid hormones. The term hyperthyroidism is reserved for disorders that result from sustained overproduction of the hormone by the thyroid itself. Thyrotoxicosis can be caused by hyperthyroidism, or by exogenous thyroid hormone, iatrogenic, or self-administered.

❑ Overview

The clinical manifestations of thyrotoxicosis are largely independent of its cause. However, the disorder that causes thyrotoxicosis may have other effects. The most common form is Graves disease, comprising 70–80% of the cases.

❑ Common Causes

1. Graves disease (diffuse toxic goiter) is the prototypic autoimmune hyperthyroid condition. Prevalence is approximately 1–2% in women; in men, the prevalence is about one tenth of that. Patients commonly have a family history of thyroid dysfunction (hyperthyroidism or hypothyroidism). It may be accompanied by an infiltrative orbitopathy and ophthalmopathy. In patients and their relatives, there is an increased frequency of other autoimmune disorders, such as DM, pernicious anemia, and myasthenia gravis. The radioactive iodine uptake (RAIU) is typically elevated unless the patient has been exposed to excess iodine or acutely to large dose of glucocorticoids. The circulating autoantibodies specific to Graves disease are directed against the thyroid-stimulating hormone (TSH) receptor and can be measured directly.

2. Toxic multinodular goiter (MNG) is a disorder in which hyperthyroidism arises in a multinodular goiter, usually of long standing. The overproduction of thyroid hormone is usually less than in Graves disease and is almost never accompanied by infiltrative ophthalmopathy. All patients with MNG should be screened annually with a serum TSH.

3. Toxic adenoma is usually caused by a single adenoma sometimes referred to as hyperfunctioning solitary nodule or toxic nodule. It often shows a suppressed TSH, which appears in a radioiodine thyroid scan as a localized area of increased radioiodine accumulation.

4. Chorionic gonadotropin–induced hyperthyroidism can be physiologic during pregnancy (transient gestational thyrotoxicosis) or associated with trophoblastic tumors.

5. Iodide-induced hyperthyroidism. Administration of supplemental iodine to subjects with endemic iodine deficiency goiter can result in iodide-induced hyperthyroidism. Amiodarone, an antiarrhythmic medication, is the most common drug that has been reported to be associated with iodine-induced thyrotoxicosis.

6. Autoimmune (Hashimoto's) thyroiditis can be associated with transient thyrotoxicosis, which is caused by thyroid cell breakdown, and the hyperthyroid symptoms are of abrupt onset and short duration.

7. Subacute thyroiditis is an acute inflammatory disorder of the thyroid gland, which is caused directly or indirectly by a viral infection. The symptoms of fever, malaise, and neck soreness frequently overshadow the symptoms of hyperthyroidism. Characteristic findings are of a tender thyroid gland, an elevated erythrocyte sedimentation rate (ESR), and a low RAIU.

8. Excess thyroid hormone ingestion can be either iatrogenic or factitious. The presence of a low, rather than elevated, serum thyroglobulin level in a patient with thyrotoxic manifestations and a low RAIU is very suspicious for exogenous hormone ingestion rather than thyroid hyperfunction.

9. Thyroid storm (accelerated hyperthyroidism) represents an extreme accentuation of thyrotoxicosis. It is an uncommon but serious complication, with a mortality of 10–75%. Manifestations include severe fever, marked tachycardia, cardiac arrhythmias, tremulousness, and altered mental status.

10. Subclinical (mild) hyperthyroidism refers to the situation that there are no signs or symptoms of thyrotoxicosis, but the serum TSH is subnormal despite normal serum free thyroid hormone concentrations. The diagnosis requires several subnormal TSH concentration results spaced months apart.

11. Ectopic thyroid hormone excretion from the ovary (struma ovarii).

❏ **Who Should Be Suspected?**

Signs and symptoms of thyrotoxicosis include

1. Anxiety, emotional lability, nervousness, and irritability
2. Heat intolerance and increased perspiration
3. Weight loss despite a normal or increased appetite
4. Tremor, palpitations, tachycardia, proximal muscle weakness, and exophthalmos
5. Oligomenorrhea in women; gynecomastia and erectile dysfunction in men

❏ **Laboratory Findings**

The availability of sensitive and reliable assays for serum TSH and free thyroxine (T_4) has made the laboratory diagnosis of hyperthyroidism rather straightforward (Figure 6-1).

■ Serum TSH is the most cost-effective screening test. If the value is normal, the patient is very unlikely to have hyperthyroidism. In hyperthyroidism, serum TSH is below normal and frequently <0.1 µIU/mL. TSH may remain decreased for many months in treated formerly hyperthyroid patients; therefore, thyroid hormone levels more accurately reflect the clinical situation.

■ Serum free T_4 is important to confirm and determine the degree of hyperthyroidism in a patient with a low TSH.

■ Serum T_3 is usually elevated with hyperthyroidism. Assessment of T_3 levels is important to determine the severity of the hyperthyroidism and to monitor the response to treatment.

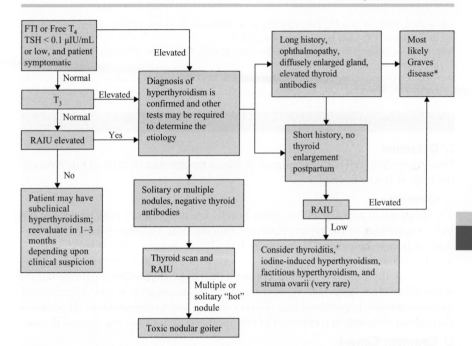

Figure 6–1 *Algorithm for the diagnosis of hyperthyroidism. *Graves disease can be confirmed by measuring thyroid antibodies. ⁺Suspect postpartum thyroiditis if within 6 months of delivery, subacute thyroid if associated with tender gland and constitutional symptoms, and silent thyroiditis if neither. T_4, thyroxine; FTI, free thyroxine index; RAIU, radioactive iodine uptake; T_3, triiodothyronine; TSH, thyroid-stimulating hormone.*

- RAIU is often elevated in Graves disease. However, the diagnostic accuracy of RAIU in hyperthyroidism does not approach that of the serum TSH plus free T_4 measurement. Therefore, determining RAIU is not useful in the diagnosis of straightforward Graves disease but is useful in excluding thyrotoxicosis not caused by hyperthyroidism. Very low values of RAIU in association with thyrotoxicosis signal the presence of factitious thyrotoxicosis, ectopic thyroid tissue, subacute thyroiditis, or the thyrotoxic phase of autoimmune thyroiditis.
- Thyrotropin receptor autoantibodies are present in 70–100% of the patients with Graves disease, and their measurement is not usually necessary for diagnosis, but it may be helpful in prognosis because patients who have high titers that do not decrease with antithyroid drug treatment are unlikely to go into remission. Measurement of thyrotropin receptor autoantibodies is important in pregnancy, because a high titer at the end of pregnancy correlates with an increased risk of neonatal hyperthyroidism.
- Abnormal TSH can also been seen in various nonthyroidal diseases. Simultaneous measurement of TSH with free T_4 is useful in evaluating the differential diagnoses.

Suggested Readings

Khan F, Sachs H, Pechet L, et al. *Guide to Diagnostic Testing*. Philadelphia, PA: Lippincott Williams & Wilkins; 2002.

Kronenberg HM, Melmed S, Polonsky KS, et al. *Williams Textbook of Endocrinology*, 11th ed. Philadelphia, PA: Saunders, Elsevier Inc., 2008.

Ross DS. Diagnosis of hyperthyroidism. In: Rose B, (ed). *UpToDate*, Waltham, MA: UpToDate, Inc.; 2009.

Ross DS. Overview of the clinical manifestations of hyperthyroidism in adults. In: Rose B, (ed). *UpToDate*, Waltham, MA: UpToDate, Inc.; 2009.

HYPOTHYROIDISM

❑ Definition

Hypothyroidism refers to a condition in which the amount of thyroid hormones in the body is below normal.

❑ Overview

The diagnosis of hypothyroidism relies heavily upon laboratory tests because of the lack of specificity of the typical clinical manifestations. The prevalence of hypothyroidism is approximately 5% in adults and 15% in women older than 65 years of age. Hypothyroidism is less common in men, with a five to eight times lower incidence. Hypothyroidism is far more common than hyperthyroidism. Hypothyroidism is usually easily treated with thyroid hormone replacement. It is now hypothesized that autoimmune hyperthyroidism (Graves disease) and hypothyroidism (Hashimoto thyroiditis) represent two extremes of one spectrum of autoimmune thyroid disease.

❑ Common Causes

I. Primary hypothyroidism
  A. Hashimoto thyroiditis is the most common cause of hypothyroidism in areas of the world in which dietary iodine is sufficient. It usually presents with goiter, hypothyroidism, or both. Goiter usually develops gradually. The diagnosis of Hashimoto thyroiditis is confirmed by the presence of thyroid autoantibodies, including thyroid peroxidase (TPO) antibody and thyroglobulin antibody.
  B. Iatrogenic: Thyroidectomy and radioiodine therapy or external irradiation for the treatment of carcinoma, hyperthyroidism, or goiter can lead to hypothyroidism.
  C. Iodine deficiency (endemic goiter) almost always occurs in areas of environmental iodine deficiency. The incidence of endemic goiter has been greatly reduced by the introduction of iodized salt.
  D. Drugs: thioamides, lithium, amiodarone, interferon, and interleukin-2
  E. Infiltrative diseases such as fibrous thyroiditis, hemochromatosis, and sarcoidosis
  F. Transient hypothyroidism is defined as a period of reduced free T_4 with suppressed, normal, or elevated TSH levels that are eventually followed by an euthyroid state. This form of hypothyroidism usually occurs in the clinical context of subacute (postviral) thyroiditis, lymphocytic (painless) thyroiditis, or postpartum thyroiditis
  G. Congenital thyroid agenesis, dysgenesis, or defect in hormone synthesis
  H. Subclinical hypothyroidism is defined as a normal serum free T_4 concentration and a slightly high serum TSH concentration. These patients usually have nonspecific symptoms and a substantial proportion of them eventually develop overt hypothyroidism

II. Secondary and tertiary (central) hypothyroidism refers to hypothyroidism induced by deficiency of either TSH or thyrotropin-releasing hormone (TRH). This type of hypothyroidism is much less common than primary hypothyroidism, and the symptoms are usually milder than in primary hypothyroidism.

III. Generalized thyroid hormone resistance

❏ Who Should Be Suspected?

Signs and symptoms of hypothyroidism include:

1. Fatigue, weight gain, depression, and cold intolerance
2. Dry skin, brittle hair, constipation, and muscle cramps
3. Hypermenorrhea in women
4. Thyroid enlargement (goiter), puffy face and hands (myxedema), and delayed ankle reflex relaxation phase
5. Hypothyroidism in infants and children leads to retardation of mental development and of growth. Severe hypothyroidism in infancy is termed cretinism.
6. Myxedema coma refers to severe prolonged hypothyroidism, which is manifested by bradycardia, congestive heart failure, hypothermia, hypoventilation, and paralytic ileus. It is an uncommon but life-threatening condition if not detected and treated promptly.
7. Secondary and tertiary hypothyroidism should be suspected in patients with known hypothalamic or pituitary disease, patients with a pituitary mass, or in patients with other hormonal deficiencies.

❏ Laboratory Findings (Figure 6-2)

■ Laboratory confirmation of the diagnosis of hypothyroidism consists of measuring serum TSH and free T_4. Primary hypothyroidism is characterized by a high serum TSH concentration and a low serum free T_4 concentration. Secondary hypothyroidism is characterized by a low serum TSH concentration as well as a low serum T_4 concentration.

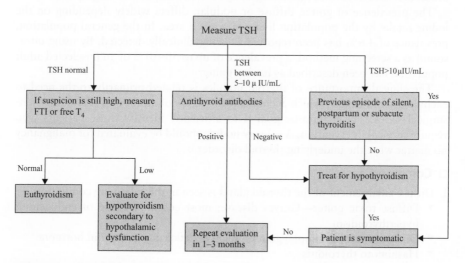

Figure 6–2 *Algorithm for the diagnosis of hypothyroidism. T_4, thyroxine; FTI, free thyroxine index; TSH, thyroid-stimulating hormone.*

- Total T_4, RAIU, and free T_4 index are usually decreased in hypothyroidism, but they are less sensitive than TSH and free T_4 measurement.
- Antithyroid peroxidase (TPO) antibodies are detected in almost all patients with Hashimoto disease and its variants, in 70% of patients with Graves disease, and in a smaller number of patients with various other thyroid disorders such as MNG, nontoxic goiter, and thyroid carcinoma.

Suggested Readings

Khan F, Sachs H, Pechet L, et al. *Guide to Diagnostic Testing*. Philadelphia, PA: Lippincott Williams & Wilkins, 2002.
Kronenberg HM, Melmed S, Polonsky KS, et al. *Williams Textbook of Endocrinology*, 11th ed. Philadelphia, PA: Saunders, Elsevier Inc., 2008.
Ross DS. Diagnosis of and screening for hypothyroidism. In: Rose B, (ed). *UpToDate*, Waltham, MA: UpToDate, Inc.; 2009.
Ross DS. Subclinical hypothyroidism. In: Rose B, (ed). *UpToDate*, Waltham, MA: UpToDate, Inc.; 2009.

GOITER AND THYROID NODULES

❑ Definition

Goiter refers to an enlargement of the thyroid gland. It can be classified in different ways. Toxic goiter refers to goiter with hyperthyroidism. Nontoxic goiter refers to an enlarged thyroid gland with normal or low thyroid hormone levels.

A thyroid nodule is defined as a discrete lesion within the thyroid gland that is due to an abnormal focal growth of thyroid cells.

❑ Overview

Thyroid enlargement or nodules come to clinical attention when noted by the patient, or as an incidental finding during routine physical examination, or during a radiologic procedure, such as carotid ultrasonography or neck computed tomography (CT).

The prevalence of goiter, diffuse or nodular, differs widely depending on the iodine intake by the population living in a given area. In the general population, prevalence of 4.6% has been reported as being clinically detected. By using ultrasound as a screening method, a prevalence of up to 30–50% of an unselected adult population has been described as having goiter.

The clinical importance of thyroid nodules is related primarily to the need to exclude thyroid cancer, which accounts for 4–6.5% of all thyroid nodules in nonsurgical series. The diagnostic goal is to efficiently identify those patients who require surgical intervention. A solitary nodule should be evaluated for malignancy no matter what the underlying thyroid disorder is.

❑ Common Causes

I. Diffuse enlargement of the thyroid gland is seen in the following conditions:
   ▼ Diffuse toxic goiter—Graves disease; most common cause of endogenous hyperthyroidism
   ▼ Diffuse nontoxic (simple) goiter—relative deficiency of thyroid hormone
   ▼ Hashimoto thyroiditis
   ▼ Organification defect (abnormality in the incorporation of iodine into thyroid hormone precursors)

II. Nodular enlargement of the thyroid gland is seen in the following situations:
   A. Benign solid nodule.
      - Hyperplastic (or colloid) nodule
      - Follicular adenoma
   B. Malignant tumors.
      - Thyroid carcinomas, including papillary, follicular, anaplastic, and medullary carcinomas

   Papillary/follicular/anaplastic carcinomas arise from thyroid follicular epithelial cells. Papillary and follicular cancers are considered differentiated cancers, and patients with these tumors are often treated similarly despite numerous biologic differences. Most anaplastic (undifferentiated) cancers appear to arise from differentiated cancers.

   Medullary carcinoma arises from calcitonin-secreting C cells and can occur in both sporadic and hereditary forms. The sporadic (noninherited) form accounts for 80% of cases and is usually unilateral. The hereditary form makes up 20% of the cases, is usually multicentric, and can be transmitted as a single entity and part of multiple endocrine neoplasia (MEN) types 2A and 2B, and familial non-MEN.

      - Lymphomas. Most primary thyroid lymphomas arise in patients who have chronic autoimmune thyroiditis.
   C. Multinodular goiter can present with or without thyrotoxicosis. A retrospective study showed that the risk of malignancy was similar in patients with multinodular goiter and one or more dominant nodules to the patients with solitary nodule. Therefore, a dominant nodule in a multinodular goiter should be evaluated as if it were a single nodule.
   D. Simple cyst.

❑ Who Should Be Suspected?

As mentioned earlier, thyroid nodules can be noted by the patient on self-examinations or by the physician on routine physical examinations. In addition, the presence of goiter or thyroid nodules should be suspected in patients with the following symptoms or signs.

1. Pain, pressure, or fullness in the neck
2. Hoarseness or change in voice
3. Trouble swallowing

❑ Laboratory Findings (Figure 6-3)

1. Serum TSH should be measured in any patient with a goiter or nodules. It may be used as a first-line screening test. In multinodular goiter, TSH usually is in normal or low-normal range; it is rarely increased.
2. Calcitonin level is increased in virtually all patients with clinical medullary carcinoma. However, it is not cost-effective or necessary in patients without clinical suspicion due to rarity of the disease and high frequency of false-positive results.
3. Measurement of serum antithyroid peroxidase antibody and antithyroglobulin antibody levels may be helpful in the diagnosis of chronic autoimmune thyroiditis, especially if the serum TSH level is elevated.
4. Fine needle aspiration (FNA) biopsy of the nodule is the most time- and cost-efficient evaluation. The reported overall rates of sensitivity and specificity exceed

90% in iodine-sufficient geographic areas. FNA biopsy should be performed in any patient with a solitary or predominant nodule in a multinodular gland, unless the TSH is suppressed, implying autonomous function and, therefore, a low likelihood of malignancy.

❑ **Imaging Studies (see Figure 6-3)**

1. Ultrasonography should be used to assess both morphology and size of the goiter and assist in screening and follow-up of thyroid nodules that are difficult to palpate. It may also be useful in directing a FNA biopsy in selected patients. However, this technique cannot distinguish between benign and malignant nodules.

2. Thyroid scintigraphy. Radionuclide scans can be performed with either iodine-123 or technetium-99m pertechnetate. Most thyroid carcinomas are inefficient in

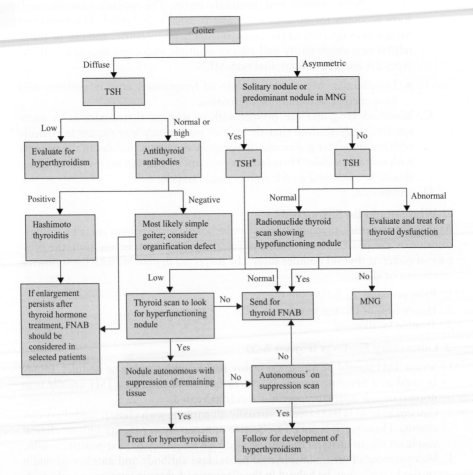

Figure 6-3   *Algorithm for the diagnosis of goiter and thyroid nodules. *Include measurement of serum calcitonin if there is a family history of medullary cancer or multiple endocrine neoplasm, type 2 (MEN2). †Autonomy is defined as the ability to concentrate radioactive iodine despite TSH suppression. FNAB, fine needle aspiration biopsy; MNG, multinodular goiter; TSH, thyroid-stimulating hormone.*

trapping and organifying iodine and appear as cold nodules. Unfortunately, most benign nodules also do not concentrate iodine and, therefore, are cold nodules. The only situation in which an iodine scan can exclude malignancy with reasonable certainty is in the case of a toxic adenoma, which is characterized by significantly increased uptake within the nodule, so-called "hot" nodule, and markedly suppressed or absent uptake in the remainder of the gland.

Suggested Readings

Khan F, Sachs H, Pechet L, et al. *Guide to Diagnostic Testing*. Philadelphia, PA: Lippincott Williams & Wilkins; 2002.

Kronenberg HM, Melmed S, Polonsky KS, et al. *Williams Textbook of Endocrinology*, 11th ed. Philadelphia, PA: Saunders, Elsevier Inc.; 2008.

Ross DS. Clinical manifestations and evaluation of obstructive or substernal goiter. Rose B, (ed). *UpToDate*, Waltham, MA: UpToDate, Inc.; 2009.

Ross DS. Diagnostic approach to and treatment of thyroid nodules. In: Rose B, (ed). *UpToDate*, Waltham, MA: UpToDate, Inc.; 2009.

6

 # DISORDERS OF THE ADRENAL GLAND

CUSHING SYNDROME

❏ Definition
Cushing syndrome refers to hypercortisolism of any cause. Whereas, Cushing disease refers to hypercortisolism due to an adrenocorticotropic hormone (ACTH)-producing pituitary adenoma.

❏ Overview
The incidence of Cushing disease is 5–25 cases per 1,000,000 people per year. Other causes of Cushing syndrome are much less common.

❏ Common Causes
Cushing syndrome may be either ACTH dependent or ACTH independent.

I. ACTH-dependent Cushing syndrome
   A. Cushing disease is the most common cause of Cushing syndrome and comprises 65–70% of the cases. Almost all patients with Cushing disease have a pituitary adenoma. The adenomas are frequently small, and even a gadolinium-enhanced, high-resolution magnetic resonance imaging (MRI) of the sella identifies only 50% of them. Pituitary adenoma cells have a higher than normal set point for cortisol feedback inhibition. This feature is clinically important because it permits the use of dexamethasone suppression to distinguish between pituitary and ectopic ACTH secretion; the latter is usually very resistant to glucocorticoid negative feedback.
   B. Ectopic ACTH secretion by nonpituitary tumors accounts for 10–15% of the cases of Cushing syndrome. A wide variety of tumors, usually carcinomas rather than sarcomas or lymphomas, have been associated with ectopic ACTH secretion. The most common causes are small cell carcinomas of the lung, bronchial or pulmonary carcinoid tumors, and pancreatic islet cell tumors and thymic tumors. Ectopic secretion of ACTH causes bilateral adrenocortical hyperplasia and hyperfunction.

   C. Ectopic corticotropin-releasing hormone (CRH) syndrome constitutes <1% of Cushing syndrome. CRH secretion by nonhypothalamic tumors causes pituitary hyperplasia, hypersecretion of ACTH, and bilateral adrenal hyperplasia.

II. ACTH-independent Cushing syndrome
   A. Adrenal tumors account for 18–20% of the cases of Cushing syndrome. It is important to be sure of the biochemical diagnosis prior to performing any adrenal imaging, since 4% of patients have an adrenal incidentaloma.
   B. Iatrogenic or factitious Cushing syndrome is usually caused by the use of prednisone, or potent inhaled, injected, and topical glucocorticoids, such as beclomethasone and fluocinolone. Exogenous glucocorticoids inhibit CRH and ACTH secretion, leading to bilateral adrenocortical atrophy. Plasma ACTH, serum cortisol, and urinary cortisol excretion are all low.

❏ Who Should Be Suspected?

Symptoms and signs of Cushing syndrome include hypertension, type 2 DM, and menstrual and psychiatric disorders. Physical examination findings include central obesity, proximal muscle weakness, wide purple striae, spontaneous ecchymoses, and facial plethora (moon face).

❏ Laboratory Findings

I. Diagnosis of Cushing syndrome involves three steps (Figure 6-4). The first step is to suspect Cushing syndrome based on the symptoms and signs. The second step is to confirm the presence of excess cortisol production by biochemical testing. The third step is to determine if the hypercortisolism is ACTH dependent, and, if so, the source of the ACTH.

II. Tests used to establish the diagnosis of Cushing syndrome are listed in Table 6-2. Urinary cortisol, late night salivary cortisol, and low-dose dexamethasone suppression tests are now recommended as first-line tests. At least two first-line tests should be unequivocally abnormal to establish the diagnosis of Cushing syndrome. Urinary and salivary cortisol measurements should be obtained at least twice.

   A. Twenty-four–hour urinary cortisol excretion provides a direct and reliable practical index of cortisol secretion. It is an integrated measurement of plasma free cortisol; as cortisol secretion increases, the binding capacity of cortisol-binding globulin is exceeded and results in a disproportionate rise in urinary free cortisol. The two most important factors in obtaining a valid result are collection of a complete 24-hour specimen and a reliable reference laboratory.

   B. Late-night or midnight salivary cortisol concentration can also be used. Saliva is easily collected, and cortisol is stable in saliva for several days even at room temperature. The criteria used to interpret salivary cortisol results vary among different studies. Midnight salivary cortisol is an accurate diagnostic test. A cortisol value >2.0 ng/mL has 100% sensitivity and 96% specificity for diagnosing Cushing syndrome.

   C. Low-dose dexamethasone suppression tests include an overnight 1-mg test and a standard 2-day test. In normal patients, the administration of

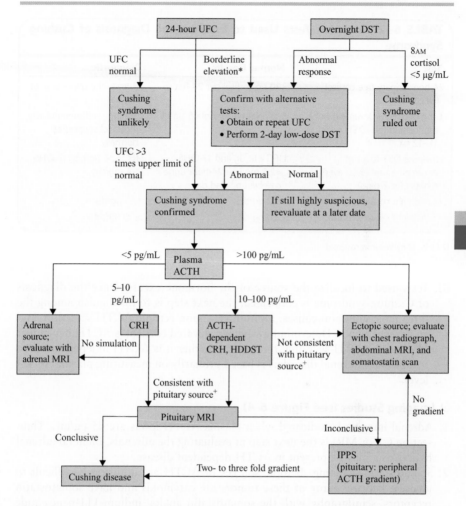

Figure 6–4 *Algorithm for the evaluation of Cushing syndrome. *Patients with alcoholism or depression may have pseudo-Cushing syndrome and require a CRH test for further evaluation. ⁺With a pituitary source, ACTH should increase with CRH, and cortisol production should decrease with HDDST. ACTH, adrenocorticotropic hormone; CRH, corticotropin-releasing hormone; DST, dexamethasone suppression test; HDDST, high-dose dexamethasone suppression test; MRI, magnetic resonance imaging; IPPS, inferior petrosal sinus sampling; UFC, urinary free cortisol.*

glucocorticoid results in suppression of ACTH and cortisol secretion. Whereas in Cushing syndrome of whatever cause, there is a failure of this suppression and the cortisol concentration remains elevated.

D. Midnight serum cortisol is based on the fact that the normal evening or night nadir in serum cortisol is preserved in obese and depressed patients (pseudo-Cushing syndrome) but not in those with Cushing syndrome. The test needs to be repeated on at least two nights. Accuracy of midnight cortisol requires an indwelling catheter, and it is clearly not convenient in an outpatient setting.

TABLE 6–2. Common Tests Used to Establish the Diagnosis of Cushing Syndrome

Test	Normal Results	Diagnostic
24-hour urinary free cortisol (UFC)	<90 µg cortisol per 24-hour period	>3 times the upper limit of normal
1 mg overnight dexamethasone suppression test (DST) given at 11–12 PM	8 AM plasma cortisol <5 µg/dL	Cushing syndrome unlikely if cortisol suppresses normally
Low-dose DST (0.5 mg dexamethasone given every 6 hours for 2 days)	UFC <10 µg and 17-OHS <2.5 mg in a 24-hour urine collected on 2nd day	UFC >36 µg/day 17-OHS >4 mg/day
12 midnight cortisol	<5.0 µg/dL	>7.5 µg/dL
12 midnight salivary cortisol	<2.0 ng/mL	>2.0 ng/mL

17-OHS, 17-hydroxycorticosteroid.

III. Tests used to localize the source of the hormone excess: Once the diagnosis of Cushing syndrome is confirmed, the next step is to distinguish among the three most common causes: a pituitary tumor, ectopic ACTH secretion, and an adrenal tumor. Determining whether elevated cortisol is ACTH dependent (due to an ACTH-secreting tumor) or whether it is ACTH independent (due to a primary adrenal disorder) is based primarily on measuring plasma ACTH level.

❑ Imaging Studies (see Figure 6-4)

1. Adrenal imaging is indicated when plasma ACTH levels are <5 pg/mL. Thin-section CT or MRI is the next step in evaluating the adrenals. Bilateral adrenal hyperplasia may be present in ACTH-dependent disease.
2. Somatostatin scanning. Ectopic sources of ACTH are notoriously difficult to identify. Because many of these tumors are carcinoids and have somatostatin receptors, scintigraphy with the somatostatin analog indium-111-pentreotide can sometimes localize tumors not found by conventional techniques.
3. Because both incidental pituitary and adrenal tumors are common, biochemical evaluation should be completed before any imaging studies.

❑ Additional Study

Petrosal sinus sampling is used when the anatomic localization fails to identify an unequivocal lesion as suggested by the biochemical testing. This test allows confirmation of the pituitary source of ACTH and identifies the side of the ACTH-secreting lesion. ACTH is measured simultaneously in samples from catheters placed in the left and right inferior petrosal sinuses and compared to peripheral levels. A gradient of two- to threefold is consistent with a pituitary source of ACTH. CRH can also be given during the procedure to enhance its accuracy.

Suggested Readings

Khan F, Sachs H, Pechet L, et al. Guide to Diagnostic Testing. Philadelphia, PA: Lippincott Williams & Wilkins; 2002.

Kronenberg HM, Melmed S, Polonsky KS, et al. *Williams Textbook of Endocrinology*, 11th ed. Philadelphia, PA: Saunders, Elsevier Inc.; 2008.

Nieman LK. Causes and pathophysiology of Cushing's syndrome. In: Rose B, (ed). *UpToDate*, Waltham, MA: UpToDate, Inc.; 2009.

Nieman LK. Clinical manifestations of Cushing's syndrome. In: Rose B, (ed). *UpToDate*, Waltham, MA: UpToDate, Inc.; 2009.

Nieman LK. Establishing the cause of Cushing's syndrome. In: Rose B, (ed). *UpToDate*, Waltham, MA: UpToDate, Inc.; 2009.

Nieman LK. Establishing the diagnosis of Cushing's syndrome. In: Rose B, (ed). *UpToDate*, Waltham, MA: UpToDate, Inc.; 2009.

ADRENAL INSUFFICIENCY

❏ Definition

Adrenal insufficiency is defined as a deficiency of hormones synthesized by the adrenal cortex.

6

❏ Common Causes

I. Primary adrenal insufficiency (Addison disease): due to intrinsic diseases of the adrenal glands
   A. Autoimmune adrenalitis. It is the most common cause of primary adrenal insufficiency and comprises approximately 70–80% of the cases. Some of the patients also have other autoimmune disorders, such as hypoparathyroidism, type 1 DM, Hashimoto thyroiditis, Graves disease, or pernicious anemia.
   B. Infections. Common infectious etiologies include tuberculosis, fungi (histoplasmosis, paracoccidioidomycosis), bacteria (meningococcemia, *Pseudomonas aeruginosa*), and viruses (HIV, CMV).
   C. Adrenal hemorrhage or infarction. Adrenal hemorrhage has been associated with meningococcemia (Waterhouse-Friderichsen syndrome) or *Pseudomonas aeruginosa*. Anticoagulants are a major risk factor for adrenal hemorrhage.
   D. Metastatic disease. Infiltration of the adrenal glands by metastatic cancers is common. The primary site includes the lung, breast, stomach, and colon. Similar findings can be seen with melanomas or lymphomas.
   E. Drugs. Several drugs may cause adrenal insufficiency by inhibiting cortisol biosynthesis. They include etomidate, ketoconazole, metyrapone, and suramin.
   F. Other risk factors include antiphospholipid syndrome, thromboembolic disease, trauma, stress, adrenoleukodystrophy, and abetalipoproteinemia.
II. Secondary adrenal insufficiency: due to inadequate ACTH secretion by the pituitary
   A. Panhypopituitarism. Symptoms are due to a decrease in all pituitary hormones, resulting in hypoadrenalism.
   B. Isolated ACTH deficiency.
   C. Megestrol acetate. Megestrol is used as an appetite stimulant in patients with metastatic breast cancer or AIDS. It suppresses the hypothalamic–pituitary–adrenal axis.
III. Tertiary adrenal insufficiency: due to inadequate CRH secretion by the hypothalamus
   A. Following abrupt cessation of high-dose glucocorticoid therapy
   B. Following correction of Cushing syndrome

❑ Who Should Be Suspected?

Clinical symptoms and signs of adrenal insufficiency vary depending on the rate and extent of loss of adrenal function, whether mineralocorticoid production is preserved, and the degree of stress.

1. Adrenal crisis. It refers to acute adrenal insufficiency, and the predominant manifestation is shock. Other symptoms include anorexia, nausea, vomiting, abdominal pain, weakness, fatigue, lethargy, confusion, or coma. Adrenal crisis may occur in patients with gradual onset who have been stressed by infection, trauma, or surgery.
2. The most common symptoms of chronic adrenal insufficiency are chronic malaise, anorexia, nausea, vomiting, and generalized weakness.
3. Patients with long-standing primary adrenal insufficiency may present with hyperpigmentation. Other frequent signs are hypotension or orthostatic hypotension. Calcification of the auricular cartilage occurs exclusively in men.
4. Patients with secondary and tertiary adrenal insufficiency usually have intact mineralocorticoid function and do not develop hyponatremia and/or hyperkalemia.

❑ Laboratory Findings (Figure 6-5)

1. Serum cortisol concentration. Cortisol is secreted in a diurnal pattern with highest levels in the morning. Levels measured later in the day are unreliable. Healthy people have early morning serum cortisol concentration of >15 µg/dL. Values <15 µg/dL are suggestive of adrenal insufficiency and require further testing.

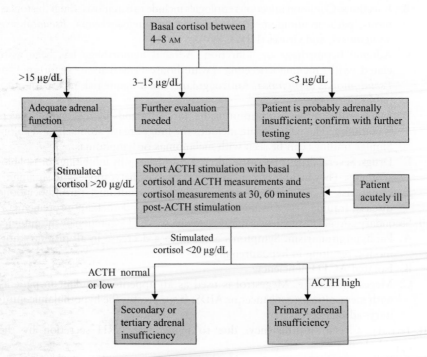

Figure 6–5 *Algorithm for the diagnosis of adrenal insufficiency. ACTH, adrenocorticotropic hormone.*

2. Basal plasma ACTH concentration. An elevated morning ACTH plasma level in the presence of low cortisol is diagnostic of primary adrenal insufficiency. In contrast, plasma ACTH concentrations are low or low normal in secondary or tertiary adrenal insufficiency.

3. ACTH stimulation tests. If the diagnosis of adrenal insufficiency is being considered and the patients have early morning serum cortisol concentration <15 μg/dL, a short ACTH stimulation test should be performed. A subnormal response confirms the diagnosis of adrenal insufficiency.

4. Corticotropin-releasing hormone test. Differentiation between secondary and tertiary adrenal insufficiency can be done by a corticotropin-releasing hormone test. Patients with secondary adrenal insufficiency show little or no ACTH response, whereas patients with tertiary disease usually have an exaggerated and prolonged ACTH response.

5. Antiadrenal antibodies. Antibodies against 21-hydroxylase (P450c21) are identified in 60–70% of patients with autoimmune adrenal insufficiency. They frequently precede the onset of disease. They are also present in 20% of patients with hypoparathyroidism.

6. Patients with suspected adrenal crisis should be treated with dexamethasone, which does not cross-react in the cortisol assay, and confirmatory tests should be performed within 1–2 days.

❏ Imaging Studies

In patients with primary adrenal insufficiency, abdominal CT or MRI with specific attention to adrenals should be obtained to identify the etiology. Enlarged adrenals suggest infectious, hemorrhagic, or metastatic diseases. Pituitary CT or MRI should be performed to look for masses in patients with secondary or tertiary adrenal insufficiency.

Suggested Readings

Khan F, Sachs H, Pechet L, et al. *Guide to Diagnostic Testing*. Philadelphia, PA: Lippincott Williams & Wilkins; 2002.

Kronenberg HM, Melmed S, Polonsky KS, et al. *Williams Textbook of Endocrinology*, 11th ed. Philadelphia, PA: Saunders, Elsevier Inc.; 2008.

Nieman LK. Causes of primary adrenal insufficiency (Addison's disease). In: Rose B, (ed). *UpToDate*, Waltham, MA: UpToDate, Inc.; 2009.

Nieman LK. Causes of secondary and tertiary adrenal insufficiency in adults. In: Rose B, (ed). *UpToDate*, Waltham, MA: UpToDate, Inc.; 2009.

Nieman LK. Clinical manifestations of adrenal insufficiency in adults. In: Rose B, (ed). *UpToDate*, Waltham, MA: UpToDate, Inc.; 2009.

Nieman LK. Diagnosis of adrenal insufficiency in adults. In: Rose B, (ed). *UpToDate*, Waltham, MA: UpToDate, Inc.; 2009.

Nieman LK. Evaluation of the response to ACTH in adrenal insufficiency. In: Rose B, (ed). *UpToDate*, Waltham, MA: UpToDate, Inc.; 2009.

PRIMARY HYPERALDOSTERONISM

❏ Definition

Primary hyperaldosteronism is a syndrome characterized by hypertension, hypokalemia, and suppressed plasma renin activity associated with increased aldosterone excretion.

❑ Common Causes

1. Aldosterone-producing adenoma accounts for 65% of the cases. Patients tend to have more severe hypertension, lower potassium levels, higher aldosterone secretion, and are of younger age than patients with idiopathic hyperaldosteronism. Unilateral adrenalectomy is curative.
2. Bilateral idiopathic hyperaldosteronism comprises approximately 20–30% of the cases. Bilateral hyperplasia is present.
3. Primary adrenal hyperplasia refers to unilateral aldosterone secretion in patients with physiologic changes similar to those of bilateral idiopathic hyperaldosteronism.
4. Aldosterone-producing adrenocortical carcinoma
5. Ectopic aldosterone-secreting tumors can be of ovarian or renal origin.

❑ Who Should Be Suspected?

The classic presenting signs of primary aldosteronism are hypertension, hypokalemia, and edema.

1. Hypertension. The blood pressure in primary aldosteronism is often substantially elevated with mean values of 184/112 and 161/105 mm Hg in patients with adrenal adenoma and adrenal hyperplasia, respectively. However, malignant hypertension rarely occurs.
2. Hypokalemia. Potassium level is low with inappropriate potassium wasting. Plasma potassium tends to be relatively stable at least over the short-term as the potassium-wasting effect of excess aldosterone is counterbalanced by the potassium-retaining effect of hypokalemia itself. Progressive hypokalemia does not occur unless some other factor is added. Hypokalemia may not be the initial presentation, but it is a common finding after administration of diuretics such as furosemide.
3. Metabolic alkalosis
4. Peripheral edema
5. Hypomagnesemia
6. Muscle weakness

❑ Laboratory Findings (Figure 6-6)

1. Plasma aldosterone. High plasma aldosterone concentration (PAC) more than 30 ng/dL is suggestive of hyperaldosteronism. Plasma aldosterone concentrations show diurnal variation with highest concentrations at the time of awakening and lowest in the evening. Aldosterone concentrations are related to extracellular fluid volume, being increased by dietary sodium restriction or diuresis and decreased by sodium loading. A rise of plasma aldosterone can occur right after the assumption of upright position. In practice, most centers draw a morning ambulatory upright sample for the assessment of aldosterone and renin levels.
2. Urine aldosterone excretion. Elevated 24-hour urinary aldosterone excretion >15 μg/day is suggestive of hyperaldosteronism.
3. Plasma renin activity (PRA). Plasma renin activity relies on endogenous angiotensinogen in the plasma without addition of angiotensinogen. Renin cleaves angiotensinogen to produce angiotensin I, which can be measured by radioimmunoassay. Plasma renin activity is expressed as the amount of angiotensin I generated per unit of time. Plasma renin activity is low in primary

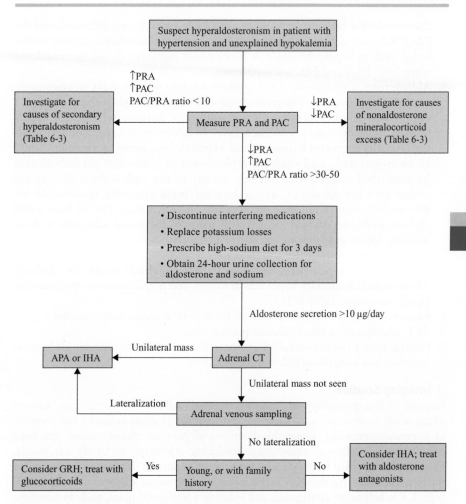

Figure 6–6 *Algorithm for the diagnosis of hyperaldosteronism. APA, aldosterone-producing adenoma; CT, computed tomography; GRH, glucocorticoid remediable hyperaldosteronism; IHA, idiopathic hyperaldosteronism; PAC, plasma aldosterone concentration; PRA, plasma renin activity.*

hyperaldosteronism. Conversely, high plasma renin activity can be seen with renovascular or malignant hypertension or secondary to diuretic usage.

4. Plasma aldosterone-to-plasma renin ratio (PAC/PRA ratio). The 2008 Endocrine Society guidelines recommend that the PAC/PRA ratio be used for case detection of primary aldosteronism. Because 30% of the patients with essential hypertension will have low upright renin levels, an elevated plasma aldosterone is required for diagnosis. Hypokalemia must be corrected, and the patient must be off diuretics, angiotensin-converting enzyme (ACE) inhibitors, and high-dose beta-blockers. Primary aldosteronism should be suspected when PRA is suppressed and PAC is increased. Secondary hyperaldosteronism (e.g., renovascular

disease) should be considered when both PRA and PAC are increased and the PAC/PRA ratio is <10. An alternate source of mineralocorticoid receptor stimulation such as hypercortisolism or licorice root ingestion should be considered when both PRA and PAC are suppressed.

5. Aldosterone suppression. Oral sodium loading over 3 days is commonly used in many centers. The patients should receive a high-sodium diet for 3 days. The risk of increasing dietary sodium in patients with severe hypertension must be assessed in each case. In addition, because sodium loading typically increases kaliuresis and hypokalemia, serum potassium should be measured daily and vigorous replacement of potassium chloride should be prescribed as indicated. On the 3rd day of the high-sodium diet, serum electrolytes are measured, and a 24-hour urine specimen is collected for the measurement of aldosterone, sodium, and creatinine. The 24-hour urine sodium excretion should exceed 200 meq to document adequate sodium loading. Urine aldosterone excretion 14 µg/day in this setting is consistent with hyperaldosteronism.

6. Other causes of hypertension with associated hypokalemia need to be ruled out. These include secondary hyperaldosteronism and nonaldosterone mineralocorticoid excess (see Table 6-3).

7. Patients should be off spironolactone for at least 6 weeks before testing.

8. ACE inhibitors can falsely elevate plasma renin.

9. Patients need to be normokalemic prior to the evaluation of aldosterone because hypokalemia suppresses aldosterone secretion.

❏ Imaging Studies

Because of the possibility of "nonfunctioning" adrenal incidentaloma, adrenal image study is recommended after the biochemical analysis indicates the presence of hyperaldosteronism. Once the diagnosis of primary aldosteronism has been established, a unilateral aldosterone-producing adenoma, or rarely carcinoma, must be distinguished from bilateral hyperplasia, since the treatment is different for the two disorders. Adrenal CT is the recommended initial study to determine subtype. CT is helpful in confirming and locating a unilateral mass, such as adenoma or carcinoma. The diagnosis of carcinoma should be suspected when a unilateral adrenal mass is >4 cm in diameter. An abnormality in both glands such as adrenal thickening suggests adrenal hyperplasia. However, patients with hyperplasia may also have normal-appearing adrenal glands on CT.

TABLE 6–3. Other Causes of Hypertension Associated with Hypokalemia

Secondary Hyperaldosteronism (High Renin and High Aldosterone)	Nonaldosterone Mineralocorticoid Excess (Low Renin and Low Aldosterone)
Diuretic usage	Congenital adrenal hyperplasia
Renovascular hypertension	Exogenous mineralocorticoids
Renin-secreting tumors	Deoxycorticosterone (DOC)-producing tumor
Coarctation of the aorta	Cushing syndrome
Malignant hypertension	Liddle syndrome
Bartter syndrome	Chronic licorice ingestion

❏ Additional Study

Adrenal vein sampling can also provide additional information. Measurement of aldosterone in samples of adrenal venous blood, obtained by an experienced radiologist, is the criterion standard test to distinguish between unilateral adenoma and bilateral hyperplasia. Unilateral disease is associated with a marked increase in PAC on the side of the tumor, usually fourfold greater, whereas in patients with bilateral hyperplasia, there is little difference between the two sides.

Suggested Readings

Khan F, Sachs H, Pechet L, et al. *Guide to Diagnostic Testing*. Philadelphia, PA: Lippincott Williams & Wilkins; 2002.

Kronenberg HM, Melmed S, Polonsky KS, et al. *Williams Textbook of Endocrinology*, 11th ed. Philadelphia, PA: Saunders, Elsevier Inc.; 2008.

Stowasser M. Assays of the renin-angiotensin-aldosterone system in adrenal disease. In: Rose B, (ed). *UpToDate*, Waltham, MA: UpToDate, Inc.; 2009.

Young WF, Jr, Kaplan NM, Rose BD. Approach to the patient with hypertension and hypokalemia. In: Rose B, (ed). *UpToDate*, Waltham, MA: UpToDate, Inc.; 2009.

Young WF, Jr, Kaplan NM, Rose BD. Clinical features of primary aldosteronism. In: Rose B, (ed). *UpToDate*, Waltham, MA: UpToDate, Inc.; 2009.

6

ADRENAL MASSES

❏ Definition

Adrenal masses refer to any enlargement of the adrenal glands.

❏ Overview

Adrenal masses can be found in up to 4% of abdominal CT scans done on patients without suspected adrenal problems. The majority of adrenal masses are benign, nonfunctioning adenomas discovered incidentally on abdominal imaging studies (adrenal incidentalomas).

❏ Classification

I. Based on hormonal activity
  A. Hormonally active (functional, hypersecretory)
  - Hypersecreting adrenal adenoma or carcinoma
  - Pheochromocytoma
  - ACTH-dependent Cushing's syndrome with nodular hyperplasia
  - Congenital adrenal hyperplasia
  - Primary aldosteronism
  B. Hormonally inactive (nonfunctional, nonhypersecretory)
II. Based on the tumor's biologic behavior
  A. Malignant
  - Adrenal carcinoma
  - Metastatic carcinoma, lymphoma, leukemia
  B. Benign
  - Adrenal adenoma
  - Granulomatous infection
  - Hemorrhage or hematoma
  - Amyloidosis

- Cysts
- Other benign tumors such as angiomyolipoma, ganglioneuroma, lipoma, hamartoma, and teratoma

❏ Who Should Be Suspected?

The presence of symptoms or signs suggestive of hormonal activity warrants further evaluation with appropriate biochemical screening tests (Figure 6-7; Table 6-4).

❏ Laboratory Findings

1. The goal of evaluation is to determine which masses are functional and which ones have the likelihood of being malignant. Benign tumors without hormonal activity need only to be followed, whereas most hormonally active and primary

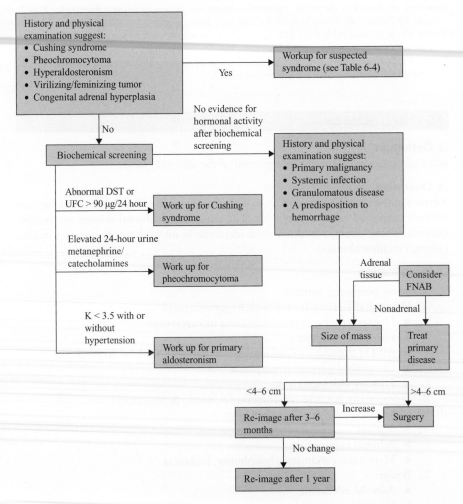

Figure 6–7 *Algorithm for the diagnosis of adrenal masses. Consider both clinical presentation and appearance on imaging in deciding cutoff size. DST, dexamethasone suppression test; FNAB, fine needle aspiration biopsy; UFC, urinary free cortisol.*

TABLE 6–4. Clinical Presentations of Hormonal Hypersecretion and Recommended Screening Tests

Disease	Suggestive Clinical Findings	Screening Recommendations
Pheochromocytoma	Hypertension, paroxysms of headaches, sweating, palpitations, tachycardia, orthostasis, flushing, pallor, glucose intolerance	24-hour urine for fractionated metanephrines and catecholamines*
Cushing syndrome	Cushingoid habitus, hypertension, thin skin, muscle weakness, facial plethora purplish striae	Overnight 1 mg dexamethasone suppression test, midnight salivary cortisol, or 24-hour urinary free cortisol*
Primary aldosteronism	Hypertension with hypokalemia, metabolic alkalosis	Blood pressure and serum potassium (in salt-replete state)* Upright plasma rennin activity and plasma aldosterone concentration 24-hour urine aldosterone
Sex hormone–secreting tumor	Virilization: hirsutism, amenorrhea, frontal balding, acne, clitoromegaly Feminization (very rare): gynecomastia, penile or testicular atrophy	DHEAS, testosterone, urinary 17-ketosteroid for virilizing tumors, estradiol for feminizing tumors
Congenital adrenal hyperplasia (especially late-onset 21-hydroxylase deficiency)	In women acne, hirsutism, amenorrhea, infertility may have suggestive family history	Serum 17α-OHP. If not significantly elevated, perform ACTH stimulation test for 17-OHP (to be considered in patients 21 years of age or younger in the presence of suspicious clinical features)

*Screen in all patients with an incidental adrenal mass.
ACTH, adrenocorticotropic hormone; DHEAS, dehydroepiandrosterone sulfate; 17α-OHP, 17-hydroxyprogesterone.

malignant tumors need to be removed. Appropriate biochemical screening tests are listed in the table and algorithm. In patients with no apparent signs or symptoms, a basic biochemical screening is necessary because up to 11% of the cases will have unsuspected abnormal adrenal function.

2. CT and MRI are helpful in determining the likelihood of the adrenal masses being malignant. Size is the most important predictor. Masses >4–6 cm are recommended for surgical removal. Close follow-up is recommended for smaller masses for any change in size.

3. FNA biopsy can differentiate adrenal from nonadrenal masses, but not benign from malignant adrenal tissue. Therefore, it is most useful for evaluation of metastatic disease in patients with a known or suspected cancer outside the adrenal gland.

Suggested Readings

Khan F, Sachs H, Pechet L, et al. *Guide to Diagnostic Testing*. Philadelphia, PA: Lippincott Williams & Wilkins; 2002.

Kronenberg HM, Melmed S, Polonsky KS, et al. *Williams Textbook of Endocrinology*, 11th ed. Philadelphia, PA: Saunders, Elsevier Inc.; 2008.

Lacroix A. Clinical presentation and evaluation of adrenocortical tumors. In: Rose B, (ed). *UpToDate*, Waltham, MA: UpToDate, Inc.; 2009.

Young WF Jr, Kaplan NM. The adrenal incidentaloma. In: Rose B, (ed). *UpToDate*, Waltham, MA: UpToDate, Inc.; 2009.

PHEOCHROMOCYTOMA

❏ Definition
Pheochromocytoma refers to catecholamine-secreting tumors arising from the chromaffin cells of the adrenal medulla or the sympathetic ganglia (extra-adrenal).

❏ Overview
Pheochromocytomas are rare neoplasms with an annual incidence of 2–8 cases per 1,000,000 people. This entity constitutes <0.2% of patients with hypertension. These tumors are curable when diagnosed and treated properly, but they are potentially fatal if missed.

❏ Classification
The 10% rules refers to the following: 10% pheochromocytomas are extra-adrenal, 10% are seen in children, 10% are bilateral, 10% represents recurrence, 10% are malignant, and 10% are familial.

Familial syndromes include

A. Familial pheochromocytomas
B. Multiple endocrine neoplasia (MEN) type 2
   ▼ MEN type 2A: pheochromocytoma, medullary carcinoma of the thyroid, and hyperparathyroidism
   ▼ MEN type 2B: pheochromocytoma, medullary carcinoma of thyroid, mucosal neuromas, marfanoid body habitus
C. Neurofibromatosis 1 (NF1). The main features of NF1 are neurofibromas and dermal café-au-lait spots. NF1 has been associated with a variety of endocrine neoplasms including pheochromocytoma, somatostatin-producing carcinoid tumors of duodenal wall, medullary carcinoma of thyroid, and hypothalamic or optic nerve tumors.
D. von Hippel-Lindau disease (VHL). It is an autosomal dominant neoplastic syndrome characterized by hemangioblastomas of central nervous system, retinal angiomas, renal cell carcinomas, visceral cysts, pheochromocytoma, and islet cell tumors.

❏ Who Should Be Suspected?
The classic triad of symptoms includes episodic headache, sweating, and tachycardia. However, not all patients have the three classic symptoms, and patients with essential hypertension may have the same symptoms. Therefore, pheochromocytoma should be suspected in patients who have one or more of the following:

1. Sustained or paroxysmal hypertension
2. Generalized sweating, palpitations, headache, tremor, and panic attack–type symptoms
3. Familial syndrome of MEN2, NF1, or VHL

4. Family history of pheochromocytoma
5. An adrenal mass incidentally discovered by imaging studies
6. Hypertension and diabetes
7. Onset of hypertension at young age (<20 years)
8. History of gastric stromal tumor or pulmonary chondroma (Carney triad)

❏ Laboratory Findings (Figure 6-8)

Evaluation includes analysis of plasma or urinary catecholamine and their metabolites. The diagnosis is typically confirmed by measurements of urinary and plasma fractionated metanephrines and catecholamines.

1. Twenty-four–hour urine catecholamines and metanephrines. It is traditionally relied upon by many institutions for the diagnosis of pheochromocytomas. Sensitivity and specificity of this test are approximately 98%. Measurement of urinary creatine should also be included to verify an adequate urine collection. A positive test is considered to be twofold elevation above the upper limit of normal in urine catecholamines or metanephrines.
2. Fractionated plasma free metanephrines. Some groups have advocated that fractionated plasma free metanephrines should be a first-line test for pheochromocytoma. The sensitivity of this test is 96–100%, and the specificity is approximately 85–89%. Therefore, the predictive value of a negative test is extremely high.
3. Patients must be off all interfering medications before urine or plasma catecholamines can be measured. Levels can be increased by tricyclic antidepressants, labetalol, levodopa, decongestants, amphetamines, ethanol, and benzodiazepines. Levels can be decreased by metyrosine and methylglucamine, which are

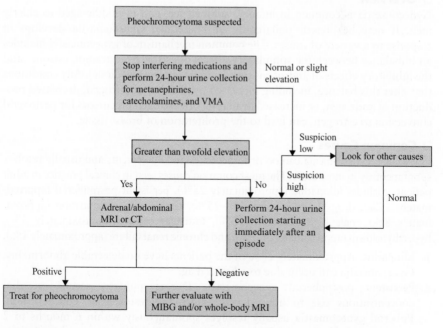

Figure 6–8 *Algorithm for the diagnosis of pheochromocytoma. CT, computed tomography; MIBG, [123I]–metaiodobenzylguanidine; MRI, magnetic resonance imaging; VMA, vanillylmandelic acid.*

present in contrast media. Patients should avoid acetaminophen (Tylenol) during the sample collection.

❑ Imaging Studies

1. CT and MRI will detect most sporadic tumors because they are usually larger than 3 cm in greatest dimension. MRI has some advantage, since pheochromocytomas have a typical hyperintense appearance on T2-weighted images.
2. [^{123}I]-metaiodobenzylguanidine (MIBG) scintigraphy is useful in patients with negative CT or MRI.

Suggested Readings

Khan F, Sachs H, Pechet L, et al. *Guide to Diagnostic Testing.* Philadelphia, PA: Lippincott Williams & Wilkins; 2002.

Kronenberg HM, Melmed S, Polonsky KS, et al. *Williams Textbook of Endocrinology,* 11th ed. Philadelphia, PA: Saunders, Elsevier Inc.; 2008.

Young WF, Jr, Kaplan NM. Clinical presentation and diagnosis of pheochromocytoma. In: Rose B, (ed). *UpToDate,* Waltham, MA: UpToDate, Inc.; 2009.

GONADAL DISORDERS

GYNECOMASTIA

❑ Definition

Gynecomastia is defined as excess development of male mammary tissue.

❑ Overview

Gynecomastia is common in infancy, adolescence, and in middle-aged to elderly men. It may be present unilaterally or bilaterally. Gynecomastia develops in response to a variety of causes. The common mechanism of gynecomastia includes an imbalance between the stimulatory effects of estrogens (estradiol, estrone) and the inhibitory effects of androgens (testosterone, androstenedione). Any conditions that alter this balance, including increased production of estrogen, decreased production of androgen, or increased availability of estrogen precursors for peripheral conversion to estrogen, can lead to the proliferation of breast tissue.

❑ Common Causes

Physiologic gynecomastia can occur in neonates and adolescents and usually resolves spontaneously in most cases. The most common causes seen in clinical practice in adult patients includes idiopathic (approximately 25%), persistent postpubertal (approximately 25%), drugs (approximately 10–25%), cirrhosis or malnutrition (approximately 8%), male hypogonadism (10%), testicular tumors (approximately 3%), hyperthyroidism (approximately 1.5%), and chronic renal failure (approximately 1%).

1. Idiopathic. Approximately 25% of the patients have no detectable abnormality. Gynecomastia can occur due to advanced age.
2. Persistent postpubertal gynecomastia. During puberty, serum estradiol concentrations rise to adult levels before the testosterone concentration. Pubertal gynecomastia usually resolves spontaneously within 6 months to 2 years of onset but in some instances may persist, leading to postpubertal gynecomastia. It is likely due to estrogen–androgen imbalance.

3. Drugs.
   a. Androgen antagonists and inhibitors. For example, spironolactone, cimetidine, marijuana, flutamide, leuprolide, ketoconazole, finasteride, diazepam, tricyclic antidepressants, phenothiazines, alcohol, and chemotherapeutic agents
   b. Estrogenic effects. For example, digitalis, diethylstilbestrol, marijuana, heroin, isoniazid, and alcohol
   c. Increased availability of substrate or activity of aromatase. For example, exogenous administration of gonadotropins, testosterone, or phenytoin
   d. Unknown mechanisms. For example, methyldopa, antihypertensives (ACE inhibitors, calcium channel blockers), narcotics, metronidazole, amiodarone, and omeprazole
4. Cirrhosis or malnutrition.
   a. Gynecomastia can occur in up to 67% of cirrhotic patients. There are two mechanisms for this. First, the damaged hepatocytes have an impaired ability to clear androstenedione, which is then available for peripheral aromatase activity and subsequent conversion to estrogens. The second mechanism is through induction of sex hormone–binding globulin (SHBG). Because SHBG binds testosterone with greater affinity than estrogen, any condition that increases SHBG will alter the estrogen–androgen ratio in favor of estrogen.
   b. Malnutrition. During starvation, gynecomastia can occur due to decreased gonadotropin and testosterone levels and normal estrogen production from adrenal precursors. Refeeding is associated with rising gonadotropin, resulting in increased testosterone secretion and marked elevated estrogen production. Therefore, patients during refeeding can develop gynecomastia.
5. Male hypogonadism. Gynecomastia occurs due to androgen deficiency.
   a. Primary hypogonadism. It accounts for approximately 8% of gynecomastia cases. It can be due to a congenital abnormality such as Klinefelter syndrome, testosterone synthesis defects, or testicular defects (trauma, torsion, or infection)
   b. Secondary hypogonadism. It accounts for approximately 2% gynecomastia cases. It is usually due to a hypothalamic or pituitary abnormality. Pituitary abnormality includes infarction and adenoma. Men with hyperprolactinemia show erectile dysfunction and loss of libido but can also develop galactorrhea and gynecomastia. Prolactin levels >200 ng/mL are almost always indicative of a pituitary tumor. The principal mechanism is through prolactin's indirect effects on reducing the secretion of gonadotropins, thereby resulting in a shift in the estrogen–testosterone balance favoring estrogen.
6. Testicular neoplasms. The mechanism is related to elevation of the estrogen level either by direct production from the tumor cells or through stimulation of interstitial cells by beta-HCG. Approximately 20% of Leydig cell tumors and 33% of Sertoli cell tumors are associated with gynecomastia. These non–germ cell tumors cause gynecomastia through increased production of estrogen by the tumor cells. Germ cell tumors, on the other hand, under the influence of beta-human chorionic gonadotropin (HCG), cause a disproportionate increase in the production of estrogen over testosterone.
7. Hyperthyroidism. Gynecomastia has been reported in 10–40% of men with Graves disease.

8. Chronic renal failure. Gynecomastia occurs in approximately 50% of patients treated with maintenance hemodialysis. The mechanism of gynecomastia in renal failure is multifactorial.

   a. Renal failure is associated with an increased luteinizing hormone (LH) level, which stimulates the production of estradiol by the Leydig cells.

   b. Other etiologies include low testosterone levels related to primary testicular dysfunction and hyperprolactinemia related to deceased clearance.

   c. Increased prolactin levels, linked to secondary hyperthyroidism, may also contribute.

9. Other rare causes include feminizing adrenocortical tumors, ectopic HCG production by tumors of the lung, liver, and gastrointestinal tract, true hermaphroditism, androgen insensitivity syndromes, and aromatase excess syndrome.

❏ Who Should Be Suspected?

Combination of a careful history and physical examination and a few diagnostic tests can result in the identification of the cause of gynecomastia in the majority of patients.

  I. History:

    A. Pain. Gynecomastia tends to present with discomfort, as opposed to breast cancer, which is more typically painless.

    B. Symmetry. Gynecomastia is often bilateral, albeit asymmetrically, whereas breast cancer is often unilateral.

    C. Medication history

    D. Assess for other historical features of family history of cancer, rapid onset, older age, and breast discharge (which suggests breast cancer).

    E. Assess for loss of libido and erectile dysfunction (which suggests hypogonadism).

    F. Check for a history of liver disease or for risk factors associated with liver disease, chronic renal insufficiency, a pituitary mass, thyroid dysfunction, or Cushing syndrome.

    G. Check for symptoms of an underlying malignancy, specifically focusing on testicular, lung, and gastrointestinal sources.

    H. Assess weight changes and refeeding.

 II. Physical examination:

    1. Breast examination.

        a. Breast cancer usually manifests as a hard nodule that is fixed to the underlying soft tissue. Other characteristics include a unilateral presence, nipple discharge, eccentric positioning, skin ulceration, and axillary adenopathy.

        b. Gynecomastia is usually characterized by firm, rubbery, well-defined masses, discoid in shape, mobile, concentric with origination beneath the nipple or areolar region, frequently bilateral, and tender to palpation. Unilateral gynecomastia may be seen as a stage in the development of bilateral gynecomastia. Asymmetry is a frequent finding in patients with gynecomastia.

    2. Testicular examination. Assess for signs of hypogonadism or neoplasm.

    3. Neurologic examination. Assess the visual fields and cranial nerves.

    4. Palpate the thyroid gland for size and nodularity.

    5. Assess for stigmata of Cushing syndrome (strength, striae, fat pad distribution, hirsutism).

❏ Laboratory Findings (Figure 6-9)
1. Initial evaluation should include:
   A. Beta-HCG level, obtained for the evaluation of ectopic production.
   B. Serum total and free testosterone, LH, follicle-stimulating hormone (FSH), and estradiol concentrations.
   C. Chest radiograph can be used to rule out pulmonary malignancy.
2. Supplemental hormonal evaluation is performed as determined by clinical judgment.
   A. Prolactin levels should be obtained in any patients with suspicion of a mass lesion or erectile dysfunction, or when secondary hypogonadism is identified (i.e., low testosterone or low to normal LH).
   B. Dehydroepiandrosterone sulfate (DHEAS) assesses for adrenocortical tumor in the setting of elevated estradiol.
   C. TSH and overnight dexamethasone suppression test (or 24-hour urinary free cortisol).

❏ Imaging Studies (see Figure 6-9)
Neuroimaging should be reserved for those cases in which a mass lesion is suspected (e.g., headache, visual field defect, cranial nerve palsy) or the hormonal evaluation leads one to suspect a pituitary tumor (i.e., elevated prolactin level or Cushing disease).

Suggested Readings
Braunstein GD. Causes and evaluation of gynecomastia. In: Rose B, (ed). *UpToDate*, Waltham, MA: UpToDate, Inc.; 2009.

Braunstein GD. Epidemiology and pathogenesis of gynecomastia. In: Rose B, (ed). *UpToDate*, Waltham, MA: UpToDate, Inc.; 2009.

Khan F, Sachs H, Pechet L, et al. *Guide to Diagnostic Testing*. Philadelphia, PA: Lippincott Williams & Wilkins; 2002.

HIRSUTISM

❏ Definition
Hirsutism refers to the presence of excess terminal hair in androgen-dependent areas in women, including face, chest, areola, linea alba, lower back, buttock, inner thigh, and external genitalia.

❏ Overview
Hirsutism may affect 5–10% of women of reproductive age. There are two conditions characterized by generalized hair growth that do not represent true hirsutism.

1. Hypertrichosis. It refers to excess terminal hair throughout the body. This is a rare condition that is usually caused by a drug, such as phenytoin, penicillamine, diazoxide, minoxidil, or cyclosporine. It can also occur in patients with systemic diseases, such as hypothyroidism, anorexia nervosa, malnutrition, porphyria, and dermatomyositis.
2. Increased vellus hair. It is the soft, unpigmented hair that covers the whole body, and it is androgen-independent hair.

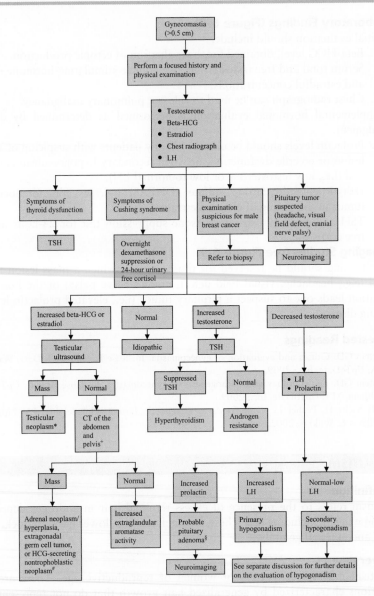

Figure 6–9 *Algorithm for the workup of gynecomastia. CT, computed tomography; HCG, human chorionic gonadotropin; LH, luteinizing hormone; TSH, thyroid-stimulating hormone. *The neoplasm is likely a germ cell tumor if the HCG is elevated, or a non–germ cell tumor if the estradiol is elevated. ⁺Abdomen and pelvic images are obtained to identify either an extragonadal germ cell tumor or an HCG-secreting nontrophoblastic neoplasm. An adrenal mass or hyperplasia is sought if the estradiol is elevated. ‡Common nontrophoblastic neoplasms include lung and gastrointestinal sources. §An elevated prolactin level may be seen secondary to hypothyroidism, resulting from an elevated TSH. A number of medications can elevate the prolactin level. Before proceeding with neuroimaging, be certain to exclude these possibilities. A prolactin level >200 ng/mL is usually indicative of an adenoma.*

❑ Common Causes

Hirsutism is a result of the interaction between circulating serum androgens and the sensitivity of hair follicle to androgens. The most common causes of hirsutism are polycystic ovary syndrome and idiopathic hirsutism (Table 6-5).

❑ Who Should Be Suspected?

The clinical approach to a patient with hirsutism includes the degree of androgen excess and its cause. The goal is to identify the small number of women who have potentially serious disorders such as androgen-secreting tumors or women with polycystic ovary syndrome.

I. History:
   A. Menstrual history. Women with consistently regular menstrual cycles and symptoms of ovulation are unlikely to have severe hyperandrogenemia.
   B. Time course of symptoms. Hirsutism occurring at a later age, with rapid onset, associated with the abrupt cessation of menses, or the presence of other features of virilization, is more often associated with potentially serious disorders, such as adrenal or ovarian tumors.
   C. Weight history
   D. Medication history
   E. Family history
   F. The presence of hirsutism alone is usually a benign condition.

TABLE 6–5. Differential Diagnosis of Conditions Accompanied by Hirsutism and Their Specific Features

Differential Diagnosis	Specific Features
Idiopathic hirsutism	Hirsutism accompanied by no other clinical or biochemical abnormalities
Polycystic ovary syndrome (PCOS)	Onset of hirsutism around the time of puberty, gradual increase in hair growth, menstrual irregularity, obesity, glucose intolerance
Hyperprolactinemia	Galactorrhea, amenorrhea, or both may be present
Drugs	Danazol, androgenic progestins, phenothiazines, phenytoin, diazoxide, minoxidil; cyclosporine can cause hypertrichosis
Late-onset congenital adrenal hyperplasia	Usually present at birth or in infancy, but the nonclassical form of 21α-hydroxylase deficiency can present prepubertally; 17α-hydroxyprogesterone >1,000 ng/dL after administration of adrenocorticotropic hormone; less common from is 11β-hydroxylase deficiency
Hyperthecosis	Increased ovarian testosterone production by luteinized stromal theca cells
Ovarian tumors	Usually occur later in life, serum testosterone usually >150–200 ng/dL
Adrenal tumors	More often carcinomas can be with or without evidence of Cushing syndrome, DHEAS usually 800 µg/dL
Insulin-resistant syndromes	Frequently associated with acanthosis nigricans
Menopause	Secondary to altered estrogen–androgen ratios

DHEAS, dehydroepiandrosterone sulfate.

II. Physical examination:
 A. Look for and quantify increased hair in androgen-dependent regions.
 B. Look for evidence of virilization, such as clitoral enlargement, deepening of voice, frontal balding, increased musculature, and loss of female body contour.
 C. Look for evidence of Cushing syndrome, such as skin striae, thin skin, or bruising.
 D. Body habitus. Height, weight, and a calculation of body mass index (BMI) should be obtained. Many women with polycystic ovary syndrome are obese.
 E. Galactorrhea. The presence of any breast discharge is suggestive of hyperprolactinemia, and a serum prolactin level should be measured.
 F. Abdominal and pelvic examinations. These examinations may reveal mass lesions producing androgen.

❑ Laboratory Findings (Figure 6-10)

1. Serum androgens. Almost all women with hirsutism have an increased production rate of androgens, usually testosterone. Total serum testosterone is adequate to exclude testosterone-secreting tumors, but free testosterone may be necessary to identify smaller increases in testosterone, especially since the carrier protein for testosterone, sex hormone–binding globulin, is suppressed by hyperandrogenism and hyperinsulinemia (in patients with polycystic ovary disease). Free testosterone may be elevated, even with a normal total testosterone due to deceased serum binding. Serum DHEAS should be obtained if there is a suspicion of an adrenal androgen-secreting tumor.
2. Serum prolactin. If the patient also has irregular menses, serum prolactin should be measured for evaluation of possibility of hyperprolactinemia.
3. Serum LH. Women with polycystic ovary syndrome tend to have elevated serum LH concentrations and normal or low serum FSH concentrations.

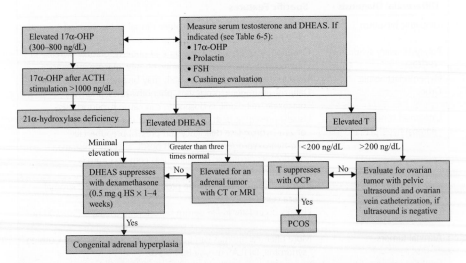

Figure 6–10 *Diagnostic algorithm for hirsutism. 17α-OHP, 17α-hydroxyprogesterone; ACTH, adrenocorticotropic hormone; CT, computer tomography; DHEAS, dehydroepiandrosterone sulfate; FSH, follicle-stimulating hormone; MRI, magnetic resonance imaging; OCP, oral contraceptive pill; PCOS, polycystic ovary syndrome; T, testosterone.*

4. 17α-hydroprogesterone (17α-OHP). Testing for nonclassic 21-hydroxylase deficiency should be considered in women with an early onset of hirsutism, hyperkalemia, or a family history of congenital adrenal hyperplasia. Basal serum 17α-hydroprogesterone concentrations may be only slightly high, especially late in the day. 17α-hydroprogesterone varies with menstrual cycle and increases with ovulation. A morning value of >300 ng/mL in the early follicular phase strongly suggests the diagnosis of 21-hydroxylase deficiency, which may be confirmed by an ACTH stimulation test. The response to ACTH is usually exaggerated.

5. Dexamethasone suppression testing. Circulating testosterone is derived from both ovarian and adrenal sources and precursors (androstenedione, DHEA, DHEAS). The administration of dexamethasone will suppress the production of adrenal androgens to a greater extent than it will suppress the production of ovarian androgens. Normal adrenal suppression indicates adrenal production of androgens such as congenital adrenal hyperplasia. Failure of suppression of DHEAS level strongly suggests the presence of an androgen-secreting adrenal tumor.

❏ Imaging Studies (see Figure 6-10)

An adrenal CT scan is recommended to look for an adrenal androgen-secreting tumor when serum DHEAS is markedly elevated. Pelvic ultrasonography with a transvaginal probe is an effective way to look for polycystic ovary or ovarian androgen-secreting tumors.

Suggested Readings

Barbieri RL, Ehrmann DA. Evaluation of women with hirsutism. In: Rose B, (ed). *UpToDate*, Waltham, MA: UpToDate, Inc.; 2009.

Barbieri RL, Ehrmann DA. Pathogenesis and cause of hirsutism. In: Rose B, (ed). *UpToDate*, Waltham, MA: UpToDate, Inc.; 2009.

Khan F, Sachs H, Pechet L, et al. *Guide to Diagnostic Testing*. Philadelphia, PA: Lippincott Williams & Wilkins; 2002.

GALACTORRHEA

❏ Definition

Galactorrhea refers to any persistent discharge of milk or milk-like secretion from the breasts in the absence of a gestational event or beyond 6 months postpartum in a woman who is not nursing.

❏ Overview

Galactorrhea needs to be distinguished from other forms of nipple discharge. Galactorrhea is usually manifested by bilateral milky nipple discharge involving multiple ducts. Green, yellow, bloody, or multicolored fluid should lead the clinicians to look for other causes of nipple discharge. When gross inspection does not permit the identification of the nipple discharge, microscopic examination can be helpful. Milk is rich in lipid content, and thus a fat stain is highly sensitive in confirming the diagnosis of galactorrhea.

❏ Common Causes (Table 6-6)

I. Physiologic causes

A. Galactorrhea from perpetuation or reactivation of lactation. This accounts for the vast majority of galactorrhea cases. In general, prolactin levels,

TABLE 6–6. Causes of Galactorrhea

Physiologic causes
- Excessive breast stimulation or tight garments
- Perpetuation or reactivation of postpartum lactation
- Stress, surgery, venipuncture
- Coitus
- Pseudocyesis

Pathologic causes

Pituitary disorders
- Prolactinomas
- Pituitary angiosarcoma
- Acromegaly
- Cushing disease
- Empty sella syndrome
- Stalk transection or compression (postsurgical, head trauma, tumor)

CNS and hypothalamic disorders
- Craniopharyngioma
- Rathke pouch cyst
- Ectopic pinealomas
- Encephalitis
- Pseudotumor cerebri
- Infiltrative hypothalamic processes (e.g., glioma, histiocytosis, sarcoidosis, tuberculosis)
- Irradiation

Metabolic and endocrinologic disorders
- Adrenal hyperplasia or carcinoma
- Hypothyroidism or hyperthyroidism
- Liver disease
- Chronic renal failure
- Sheehan syndrome
- Anovulatory disorders (e.g., polycystic ovarian disease, Chiari-Frommel syndrome)
- Idiopathic galactorrhea and amenorrhea

Chest wall lesions

Ectopic prolactin production
- Bronchogenic carcinoma
- Renal cell carcinoma

Pharmacologic causes
- Antidepressants (e.g., tricyclics, monoamine oxidase inhibitors, selective serotonin reuptake inhibitors)
- Neuroleptics (e.g., phenothiazines and butyrophenones)
- Opiates and narcotics
- H_2-blockers (e.g., cimetidine)
- Oral contraceptive pills
- Calcium channel blockers (e.g., verapamil)
- Benzamines (e.g., metoclopramide)
- Alpha-receptor blockers (e.g., reserpine, methyldopa)
- Cocaine
- Amphetamines

Functional/idiopathic

menses, and fertility are normal. Reactivation of pregnancy-related lactation may occur after a spontaneous first-trimester pregnancy loss, therapeutic abortion, or ectopic pregnancy.

B. Disorders of the chest wall. Although rare, chest wall injury from surgery such as mastectomy, trauma, infiltrating tumors, and herpes zoster eruptions can produce galactorrhea. Hyperprolactinemia may or may not be present. The mechanism for this milk formation is uncertain, but it may result from chronic neuronal stimulation from the breast to the hypothalamus. Other causes must be ruled out prior to attributing galactorrhea to this cause.

II. Pathologic causes

A. Pituitary tumors. The most important evaluation in a patient with galactorrhea is the consideration of a pituitary tumor.

B. Idiopathic galactorrhea with amenorrhea. Generally, the patients in this group have elevated prolactin levels and normal imaging. Possible mechanisms for this disorder include interference of luteinizing hormone–releasing hormone (LHRH), release in the hypothalamus by prolactin, alternation of pituitary sensitivity to LHRH, or interference with steroidogenic action of gonadotropins at the level of the ovary.

C. Anovulatory syndromes.

1. Chiari-Frommel syndrome. It is characterized by galactorrhea and amenorrhea that occurs more than 6 months postpartum in the absence of nursing and in the absence of a pituitary tumor. Approximately 50% of these women will resume normal menses over the next few months. A small minority may have occult microadenomas of pituitary, which may become clinically apparent with time.

2. Polycystic ovary syndrome (PCOS). It is characterized by obesity, oligomenorrhea, infertility, and hirsutism. Elevated prolactin levels may accompany this syndrome, thereby leading to galactorrhea.

D. Endocrinopathies

1. Hypothyroidism is a rare cause of galactorrhea. Prolactin levels may be normal or slightly elevated. Galactorrhea is corrected with restoration of euthyroidism.

2. Galactorrhea is a frequent finding in women with thyrotoxicosis. Serum prolactin is normal, and the mechanism of galactorrhea is unknown.

3. Cushing syndrome and acromegaly can be associated with galactorrhea. Workup for these conditions should be undertaken only if specific signs and symptoms are present.

E. Ectopic prolactin production. It is a very rare cause of galactorrhea, and other causes should be excluded first. Tumors that have been associated with ectopic prolactin production include renal cell carcinoma and bronchogenic carcinoma.

III. Pharmacologic causes

A. Galactorrhea associated with elevated prolactin levels. Most pharmacologic agents that cause prolactin release either block dopamine receptors (e.g., neuroleptics) or deplete dopamine in the tuberoinfundibular neurons (e.g., centrally acting alpha-blockers). All types of antidepressants can cause galactorrhea, but selective serotonin reuptake inhibitors (SSRIs) do so more commonly than other antidepressants.

B. Galactorrhea associated with oral contraceptive pills (OCPs). Both usage and discontinuation of OCPs can cause galactorrhea. The exact mechanisms are unknown. The abrupt cessation of estrogen and progesterone mimics withdrawal at the time of delivery and can trigger milk production. Estrogen at postmenopausal replacement dose is not associated with galactorrhea.

❑ Who Should Be Suspected?

Differential diagnosis of galactorrhea is broad. The goal is to identify the small number of women with pituitary adenoma or other space-occupying lesions as the cause of galactorrhea.

I. History:
   A. Menstrual and reproductive history: Galactorrhea can be seen during pregnancy, including ectopic pregnancy, and in the immediate postpartum period. Hyperprolactinemia can lead to hypoestrogenemia, with amenorrhea and infertility. Higher levels of prolactin are associated with more significant menstrual derangements. Galactorrhea in men suggests a pathologic process and should always have an aggressive workup assessing for a pituitary adenoma and hypogonadism.
   B. Medication history.
   C. History of chest wall surgery, trauma, or herpes zoster eruption.

II. Physical examination (Figure 6-11):
   A. Eye examination: Check visual acuity and visual fields and examine the cranial nerves. Assess for symptoms of pituitary diseases such as cranial neuropathies (nerves III, IV, or VI), visual field deficits (bitemporal hemianopsia, optic chiasm, or optic nerve compression), or headache.
   B. Breast and chest wall examination: Confirm galactorrhea; palpate for masses, scars, and eruption. Endocrine laboratory testing should be ordered without performing either breast examination or nipple stimulation.
   C. Skin examination: Note abnormal skin texture (e.g., myxedema), striae, pigmentation, or hirsutism.
   D. Endocrine examination: Assess for thyroid dysfunction, stigmata of Cushing syndrome (striae, buffalo hump, and central obesity), and acromegaly. Abnormalities of temperature, thirst, and appetite regulation suggest hypothalamic disease.
   E. Pelvic examination: Check ovarian and uterine sizes for causes of amenorrhea and anovulation.

❑ Laboratory Findings

1. Serum prolactin: The concentrations may increase slightly during sleep, strenuous exercise, occasionally emotional or physical stress, intense breast stimulation, and high-protein meals. Therefore, a slightly high value should be confirmed before the patient is considered to have hyperprolactinemia. Mildly elevated prolactin levels should prompt investigation for a tumor, even if no other clear cause for the hyperprolactinemia is identified or if symptoms and signs of pituitary and central nervous system (CNS) processes are present.

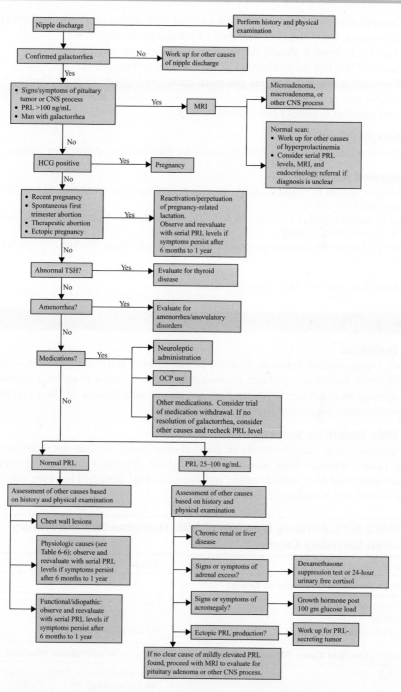

Figure 6–11 *Algorithm for the workup of galactorrhea. CNS, central nervous system; HCG, human chorionic gonadotropin; MRI, magnetic resonance imaging; OCP, oral contraceptive pill; PRL, prolactin; TSH, thyroid-stimulating hormone.*

Sample dilutions may be needed in patients with strong suspicion for hyperprolactinemia, but normal or low level of plasma prolactin levels.
2. Beta-HCG level: It should be obtained to exclude pregnancy.
3. Serum TSH: For the evaluation of hyper- or hypothyroidism.
4. Consider a workup for less common endocrinopathies such as Cushing syndrome and acromegaly after excluding more common causes and only if history and physical findings raise clinical suspicion.

❏ **Imaging Studies**
High-resolution CT scan or MRI is useful for localization of pituitary tumors.

Suggested Readings

Golshan M, Iglehart D. Nipple discharge. In: Rose B, (ed). *UpToDate*, Waltham, MA: UpToDate, Inc.; 2009.

Khan F, Sachs H, Pechet L, et al. *Guide to Diagnostic Testing*. Philadelphia, PA: Lippincott Williams & Wilkins; 2002.

Snyder PJ. Causes of hyperprolactinemia. In: Rose B, (ed). *UpToDate*, Waltham, MA: UpToDate, Inc.; 2009.

Snyder PJ. Clinical manifestations and diagnosis of hyperprolactinemia. In: Rose B, (ed). *UpToDate*, Waltham, MA: UpToDate, Inc.; 2009.

MALE HYPOGONADISM* (TABLE 6-7)

❏ **Definition**
Male hypogonadism refers to decrease in one or both testicular functions—sperm production and/or testosterone production. The root cause is either a disease of or damage to the testes (primary hypogonadism) or a disease of the pituitary or hypothalamus (secondary hypogonadism).

❏ **Who Should be Suspected?**
In general, early manifestations in postpubertal males include decreased energy and libido, whereas later manifestations include decreased androgen-dependent development of hair, muscle mass, and bone mineral density. However, there are age-related or physiologic considerations.

TABLE 6-7 Laboratory Diagnosis of Male Hypogonadism and Primary versus Secondary Causes

Test	Result	Cause
Hypogonadism (Products of Testes)		
Serum total testosterone	Low	Low
And/or		
Sperm concentration	Decreased	Decreased
Hypogonadism Cause (Testicular Damage vs. Pituitary or Hypothalamic Disease)		
LH & FSH	Elevated	Testicular disease or damage (primary hypogonadism)
	Not elevated	Pituitary or hypothalamic disease (secondary hypogonadism)

*Submitted by Charles R. Kiefer, PhD.

- Manifestations in infants may include ambiguous genitalia or cryptorchidism (bearing in mind that a retractile testis usually descends into the scrotum within the first year of life). A micropenis at birth may indicate deficient gonadotropin-releasing hormone during the third trimester of pregnancy.
- Manifestations in teenage boys may be signaled by failure to develop pubertal changes at the normal rate, resulting from low serum testosterone and normal or subnormal concentrations of LH (luteinizing hormone) and/or FSH (follicle stimulating hormone). If just delayed puberty, it will correct spontaneously. However, it may be the result of secondary hypogonadism, which becomes a more likely possibility the longer the delay.
- In the severely obese (BMI > 40), there may be secondary hypogonadism as well as decreasing the serum concentration of sex hormone–binding protein.
- In older men undergoing male senescence, although serum total testosterone falls slightly, free testosterone falls more significantly, so that levels after age 80 are one half to one third of those at age 20.
- Within each of the two classes of male hypogonadism (primary or secondary), there exist both congenital and acquired causes. Primary congenital causes include Klinefelter syndrome (47XXY) and androgen synthesis disorders; whereas primary acquired causes include infection (e.g., mumps, orchitis), trauma, and chemotherapy or radiation therapy. Secondary congenital causes include Kallmann syndrome, hypopituitarism, and idiopathic hypogonadotropic hypogonadism; whereas secondary acquired causes include mass lesions in the pituitary or hypothalamus, hyperprolactinemia, and trauma to the base of the skull.

❑ Laboratory Findings

- The salient diagnostic test for male hypogonadism is measurement of serum testosterone concentration—a low value being indicative of the condition. Serum total testosterone (free plus protein bound) accurately reflects secretion of testosterone in most cases. Measurement of free testosterone concentration could be considered in cases of obesity (reduces testosterone protein binding) or male senescence (slightly increases protein binding). Time of serum collection from young men should take into account diurnal variation of testosterone levels, which are maximal at about 8 AM and minimal at about 8 PM (about 70% of maximum). Measurement should be repeated if the first 8 am value is low or borderline, or at variance with the clinical picture. If testosterone levels are normal, and infertility is a problem, then a semen analysis should be obtained for further workup.
- With a normal testosterone level but a low sperm count, the gonadotropins should be measured. If the LH level is normal and the FSH level is high, then the indication is seminiferous tubule damage (leaving testosterone production by the Leydig cells intact).
- With a low or borderline testosterone level and a low sperm count, then LH and FSH levels can distinguish primary from secondary causes of hypogonadism. If the gonadotropins are above normal, the indication is primary hypogonadism. If they are normal or low, then the indication is secondary hypogonadism.
- Table 6-7 summarizes the diagnosis of hypogonadism, and the laboratory differentiation of primary vs secondary causes.

Suggested Readings

Nachtigall LB, Boepple PA, Pralong FP, et al. Adult-onset idiopathic hypogonadotropic hypogonadism—a treatable form of male infertility. *N Engl J Med.* 1997;336:410–415.

Smyth CM, Bremner WJ. Klinefelter syndrome. *Arch Intern Med.* 1998;158:1309–1314.

Bremner WJ, Vitiello MV, Prinz PN. Loss of circadian rhythmicity in blood testosterone levels with aging in normal men. *J Clin Endocrinol Metab.* 1983;56:1278–1281.

Giagulli VA, Kaufman JM, Vermeulen A. Pathogenesis of the decreased androgen levels in obese men. *J Clin Endocrinal Metab.* 1994;79:997–1000.

Mingrone G, Greco AV, Giancaterini A, et al. Sex hormone-binding globulin levels and cardiovascular risk factors in morbidly obese subjects before and after weight reduction induced by diet or malabsorptive surgery. *Atherosclerosis.* 2002:161:455–462.

Deslypere JP, Vermeulen A. Leydig cell function in normal men: effect of age, life-style, residence, diet, and activity. *J Clin Endocrinol Metab.* 1984;59:955–962.

 # DISORDERS OF THE PITUITARY GLAND

HYPOPITUITARISM

❑ Definition

Hypopituitarism is the deficiency of one or more pituitary hormones resulting from either pituitary or hypothalamic dysfunction. The term panhypopituitarism is used when all the anterior pituitary hormones are absent. When hypothalamic disease is also present, vasopressin deficiency may occur.

❑ Overview

The prevalence of hypopituitarism is 46 cases per 100,000 individuals. The incidence is approximately 4 cases per 100,000 per year.

❑ Causes

Pituitary tumors and other neoplastic processes are the most common causes of acquired hypopituitarism.

I. Pituitary diseases
  1. Mass lesions. They include pituitary adenomas, cysts, lymphocytic hypophysitis, metastatic cancers, and other lesions.
  2. Following surgical or radiation treatment of the pituitary
  3. Infiltrative diseases
     a. Hereditary hemochromatosis in the pituitary is characterized by ion deposition in pituitary cells, which leads to hormonal deficiencies.
     b. Lymphocytic hypophysitis often associates with pregnancy and occurs in the postpartum period. It is initially characterized by lymphocytic infiltration and enlargement of the pituitary and then followed by destruction of the pituitary cells. Affected patients typically present with headaches of an intensity out of proportion to the size of the lesion and hypopituitarism.
  4. Pituitary infarction (Sheehan syndrome). Typically, the patients have a history of severe postpartum hemorrhage to cause hypotension and require blood transfusions. Severe hypopituitarism can be recognized during the first days or weeks after delivery by the development of lethargy, anorexia, weight loss, and inability to lactate.
  5. Pituitary apoplexy. Sudden hemorrhage into pituitary gland is called pituitary apoplexy. Hemorrhage often occurs into a pituitary adenoma. It is

manifested by sudden onset of headache, cranial nerve defects, visual defects, and hypopituitarism.
  6. Empty sella syndrome. An empty sella refers to an enlarged sella turcica that is not entirely filled with pituitary tissue.
    a. Primary empty sella is due to a congenital defect in the sellar diaphragm.
    b. Secondary empty sella is due to surgery, radiation treatment, or tumor infarction.
  7. Genetic defects. Mutations in genes encoding transcription factors necessary for differentiation of anterior pituitary cells have been identified, and they lead to congenital deficiency of one or more pituitary hormones.
II. Hypothalamic diseases
  A. Mass lesions. These include primary benign tumors, such as craniopharyngiomas, and metastatic malignant tumors, such as lung and breast carcinomas.
  B. Hypothalamic radiation. It is often associated with radiation treatment for brain tumors and nasopharyngeal carcinomas.
  C. Infiltrative diseases. Sarcoidosis and Langerhans cell histiocytosis can cause deficiencies of anterior pituitary hormones.
  D. Infections. The most common etiology is tuberculous meningitis.
  E. Basal skull fracture or head trauma

❏ Who Should Be Suspected?

Hypopituitarism should be suspected in any patient with midline defects or pituitary and/or hypothalamic masses. Symptoms are mainly secondary to target gland dysfunction (i.e., thyroid, adrenal, gonads) due to deficiency of TSH, ACTH, growth hormone, or gonadotropin but can also be related to local symptoms if a mass is present (i.e., headache, visual disturbances). In pituitary apoplexy, symptoms can be dramatic.

❏ Laboratory Findings

I. ACTH and cortisol
  1. Basal ACTH secretion. Serum cortisol should be measured between 8 and 9 AM. Serum cortisol value ≤3 µg/dL is strongly suggestive of cortisol deficiency and in a patient with pituitary or hypothalamic disease indicates ACTH deficiency. Cortisol values ≥18 µg/dL indicate sufficient basal ACTH secretion. Values between 3 and 18 µg/dL, which persist on repeat determination, are an indication for the evaluation of ACTH reserve.
  2. ACTH reserve.
    a. Metyrapone test. Metyrapone blocks the conversion of 11-deoxycortisol to cortisol by CYP11B1 (11β-hydroxylase, P450c11), the last step in the synthesis of cortisol, and induces a rapid fall of cortisol and an increase of 11-deoxycortisol in serum. The metyrapone test can be performed as an overnight single-dose test or as a 2- or 3-day test. Cortisol and 11-deoxycortisol should be measured at 8 AM. A normal response is 8 AM serum 11-deoxycortisol concentration of 7–22 µg/dL. A serum cortisol concentration at 8 AM of <5 µg/dL confirms adequate metyrapone blockade and thereby documents compliance and normal metabolism of metyrapone. Serum 11-deoxycortisol concentrations <7 µg/dL with concomitantly suppressed cortisol values indicate adrenal insufficiency.

   b. Insulin tolerance test (insulin-induced hypoglycemia test). Patients should be administered regular insulin 0.1 U/kg intravenously, and glucose and cortisol should be measured at 15, 30, 60, 90, and 120 minutes after injection. If glucose level falls to 35–40 mg/dL, cortisol should increase to >18 μg/dL. Decreased cortisol levels indicate adrenocortical insufficiency secondary to hypopituitarism. The test requires close observation for hypoglycemia and is risky in patients with cardiac or neurologic dysfunction.

   c. ACTH stimulation test. Cosyntropin is synthetic ACTH, which has the full biologic potency of native ACTH. It is a rapid stimulator of cortisol and aldosterone secretion. The response to ACTH varies with the underlying disorder. If the patient has hypopituitarism with deficient ACTH secretion and secondary adrenal insufficiency, then the intrinsically normal adrenal gland should respond to maximally stimulating concentrations of exogenous ACTH if given for a sufficient length of time. The response may be less than in normal subjects and initially sluggish due to adrenal atrophy resulting from chronically low stimulation by endogenous ACTH. If, on the other hand, the patient has primary adrenal insufficiency, endogenous ACTH secretion is already elevated and there should be little or no adrenal response to exogenous ACTH.

II. TSH
   A. Basal function. Low FTI or free T_4 in the absence of appropriately elevated TSH is suggestive of secondary hypothyroidism. Medications that decrease thyroid hormone binding such as phenytoin, salsalate, or high-dose aspirin should be ruled out. Patient should also be taken off glucocorticoid treatment.
   B. TRH test. TRH is administrated intravenously (200–500 μg). Three blood specimens are collected for serum TSH testing, one immediately prior to TRH injection, and one 15 minutes and one 30 minutes after TRH injection. A significant rise in serum TSH from a basal level of 2–3 μU/mL is normal. Secondary (pituitary) hypothyroidism shows no rise in the decreased TSH level. A delayed peak is suggestive of hypothalamic rather than pituitary dysfunction, but is relatively nonspecific.

III. Gonadotropins
   A. Low levels of FSH and LH in postmenopausal women or in men with low testosterone are suggestive of gonadotropin deficiency.
   B. Gonadotropin-releasing hormone (GnRH) test. Patients should be given GnRH (100 μg intravenously), and LH and FSH should be measured at 0, 30, and 60 minutes. LH should increase by 10 IU/L and FSH by 2 IU/L.

IV. Growth hormone (GH)
   A. Basal GH and insulin-like growth factor-I (IGF-I) levels are nonspecific.
   B. Provocative tests with insulin, L-arginine, vasopressin, glucagon, or L-dopa should not be used. Peak GH should be >5–10 ng/mL.

V. Vasopressin
   A. Basal serum sodium, osmolality, and urine osmolality. Hypotonic urine in the presence of increased serum sodium and serum osmolality is suggestive of diabetes insipidus. Twenty-four–hour urine should be collected for volume and specific gravity measurement.
   B. Water deprivation test. The inability to concentrate urine with a response to exogenous vasopressin is diagnostic of central diabetes insipidus.

❏ Imaging Studies

A. An MRI scan (T1, T2 +/− gadolinium) is the first choice to evaluate the pituitary gland, hypothalamus, and pituitary stalk.

B. A high-resolution CT with thin sections through the pituitary fossa is a reasonable alternative.

Suggested Readings

Khan F, Sachs H, Pechet L, et al. *Guide to Diagnostic Testing.* Philadelphia, PA: Lippincott Williams & Wilkins; 2002.

Snyder PJ. Causes of hypopituitarism. In: Rose B, (ed). *UpToDate*, Waltham, MA: UpToDate, Inc.; 2009.

Snyder PJ. Clinical manifestations of hypopituitarism. In: Rose B, (ed). *UpToDate*, Waltham, MA: UpToDate, Inc.; 2009.

Snyder PJ. Diagnosis of hypopituitarism. In: Rose B, (ed). *UpToDate*, Waltham, MA: UpToDate, Inc.; 2009.

6

PITUITARY TUMORS

❏ Definition

Pituitary tumors are represented by any new growth of the pituitary gland, independent of size or symptoms.

❏ Overview

Pituitary adenomas are the most common cause of sellar masses. Most tumors are considered benign.

❏ Classification

1. Hormonally active tumors
    A. Growth hormone–secreting tumors
    B. Prolactin-secreting tumors
    C. ACTH-secreting tumors
2. Hormonally inactive tumors
    A. Nonsecreting pituitary adenoma
    B. Metastatic tumor (breast and lung are the most common primary sites)
    C. Other brain tumors such as craniopharyngioma, meningioma, and glioma

❏ Who Should Be Suspected?

Pituitary masses can present with neurologic symptoms, abnormalities related to undersecretion or oversecretion of pituitary hormones, or as an incidental finding on radiologic examination performed for some other reason.

I. Symptoms
    A. Hormonally active tumors can be associated with symptoms of secretion or deficiency.
        a. Growth hormone–secreting tumors present with symptoms of acromegaly.
        b. Prolactin-secreting tumors present with symptoms of galactorrhea.
        c. ACTH-secreting tumors present with symptoms of Cushing syndrome.
    B. Nonsecreting tumors do not become symptomatic until their size becomes sufficient to cause with pituitary hormone insufficiency (e.g., gonadal dysfunction, secondary hypothyroidism, adrenal insufficiency, growth failure, delayed puberty in children).

C. Neurologic symptoms.
  a. Visual defects. Impaired vision is the most common symptom that leads a patient with a nonfunctioning adenoma to seek medical attention. Visual impairment is caused by suprasellar extension of the adenoma, leading to compression of the optic chiasm. The most common complaint is diminished vision in the temporal fields (bitemporal hemianopsia).
  b. Headaches
  c. Diplopia
II. Signs
  A. Pituitary apoplexy. Sudden hemorrhage into the adenoma can cause excruciating headache and diplopia. It usually occurs spontaneously but occasionally is precipitated by administration of an anticoagulant.
  B. Pituitary incidentaloma. Pituitary masses discovered incidentally on imaging studies are further evaluated based on their sizes. Incidental microadenomas refer to masses <10 mm in diameter. Patients with microadenomas should be evaluated clinically for hormonal hypersecretion and chemically for any hypersecretion suspected clinically. Serum prolactin level should be measured if there is no clinical suspicion of hormonal hypersecretion. When a macroadenoma (≥10 mm in diameter) is identified, evidence for hormonal excess should be sought and assessment of overall pituitary function and formal visual fields is required.

❏ Laboratory Findings (Figure 6-12)

1. A serum prolactin of >200 ng/mL almost always indicates a prolactinoma, although other causes should be considered, such as pregnancy, lactation, stress, dopamine receptor antagonists (e.g., neuroleptics, metoclopramide), primary hypothyroidism, and renal failure. Concentrations between 20 and 200 ng/mL could be due to a lactotroph adenoma or to any other sellar mass. The finding of a large tumor with only minimally elevated prolactin indicates that the tumor is not a prolactinoma but is causing pituitary stalk compression and loss of dopamine inhibition of prolactin secretion.

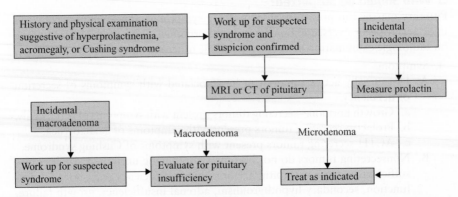

Figure 6-12 *Pituitary tumor algorithm. CT, computed tomography; MRI, magnetic resonance imaging.*

2. The best test for the diagnosis of acromegaly and growth hormone–secreting tumors is measurement of serum insulin-like growth factor I (IGF-I). IGF-I levels need to be corrected for age and sex. Among patients with equivocal values, serum growth hormone secretion after oral glucose administration can be obtained. Random growth hormone measurements are not reliable, since growth hormone is secreted episodically and may be elevated with anxiety, exercise, acute illness, chronic renal failure, and diabetes.
3. Twenty-four–hour urine free cortisol quantification or midnight salivary cortisol test for Cushing disease
4. LH, FSH, with testosterone in male patients or estradiol in female patients
5. TSH and free T_4 for thyroid function assessment

Suggested Readings

Khan F, Sachs H, Pechet L, et al. *Guide to Diagnostic Testing*. Philadelphia, PA: Lippincott Williams & Wilkins; 2002.

Kronenberg HM, Melmed S, Polonsky KS, et al. *Williams Textbook of Endocrinology*, 11th ed. Philadelphia, PA: Saunders, Elsevier Inc.; 2008.

Snyder PJ. Causes, presentation and evaluation of sellar masses. In: Rose B, (ed). *UpToDate*, Waltham, MA: UpToDate, Inc.; 2009.

Snyder PJ. Clinical manifestations and diagnosis of gonadotroph and other clinically nonfunctioning adenomas. In: Rose B, (ed). *UpToDate*, Waltham, MA: UpToDate, Inc.; 2009.

Snyder PJ. Pituitary incidentaloma. In: Rose B, (ed). *UpToDate*, Waltham, MA: UpToDate, Inc.; 2009.

6

DIABETES INSIPIDUS

❏ Definition

Diabetes insipidus (DI) is a disorder characterized by excretion of a large volume of dilute hypotonic urine.

❏ Common Causes

1. Central DI is caused by inability to synthesize or secrete vasopressin [antidiuretic hormone (ADH)] in the neurohypophyseal system. In complete central DI, ADH levels are undetectable and polyuria is severe. In partial central DI, ADH levels are subnormal but detectable, and polyuria is less extreme. The most common causes of central DI include the following:
   a. Idiopathic disease. It has been suggested that autoimmune destruction to the ADH-producing cells is involved in many patients.
   b. Familial and congenital disorders
   c. Primary or secondary tumors. Most often due to primary suprasellar and intrasellar tumors including craniopharyngiomas and germinomas, metastatic carcinomas (lung, breast), leukemias, and lymphomas.
   d. Infiltrative disorders. Patients with Langerhans cell histiocytosis are at particularly high risk for central DI. Other infiltrative disorders include granulomatous lesions such as sarcoidosis, tuberculosis, syphilis, and Wegener granulomatosis.
   e. Neurosurgery or trauma
   f. Hypoxic encephalopathy
   g. Post–supraventricular tachycardia
   h. Anorexia nervosa

2. Nephrogenic DI is characterized by renal resistance to the action of ADH, leading to a decrease in urinary concentrating ability. The most common causes of nephrogenic DI include
   a. Chronic renal failure seen in chronic pyelonephritis, analgesic nephropathy, or nephrosclerosis
   b. Other tubulointerstitial diseases such as polycystic kidney disease, medullary cystic kidney disease, sickle cell disease or trait, renal amyloidosis, and Sjögren syndrome
   c. Release of bilateral urinary tract obstruction
   d. Drugs such as lithium, cidofovir, foscarnet, vasopressin V2 receptor antagonists, amphotericin B, demeclocycline, ifosfamide, ofloxacin, orlistat, and didanosine
   e. Pregnancy
   f. Hereditary renal tubular unresponsiveness to vasopressin due to genetic mutations in the vasopressin V2 receptor gene or aquaporin-2 gene
   g. Prolonged potassium depletion and hypokalemia (condition is reversed by restoring potassium level to normal)
   h. Prolonged hypercalciuria, usually with hypercalcemia (condition is reversed by restoring calcium level to normal)
3. Primary polydipsia is characterized by a primary increase in water intake. It can be due to
   a. Psychogenic illnesses
   b. Hypothalamic lesions affecting thirst center
   c. Drugs (such as thioridazine, chlorpromazine, anticholinergic agents) causing dry mouth and leading to increased thirst

❑ **Who Should Be Suspected?**

The main clinical manifestation of DI is polyuria. Polyuria is defined as urine volume exceeding 3 L/day in adults and 2 L/m^2 in children. It must be differentiated from other similar urinary complaints such as urinary frequency, nocturia, urgency, and urinary incontinence, which are not associated with an increase in the total urine output.

The cause of polyuria is often suggested from the history such as age of onset. In the majority of hereditary nephrogenic DI, severe polyuria manifests during the first week of life. In familial central DI, polyuria may present after the first year of life, sometimes in young adulthood. In adults, the onset of polyuria is usually abrupt in central DI and almost always gradual in acquired nephrogenic DI or primary polydipsia. The new onset of nocturia in the absence of other causes of nocturia (e.g., prostatic enlargement in men over 50 years of age or urinary tract infection in children) is often a first clue to DI. Family history of polyuria suggests the familial forms of both central and nephrogenic DI.

❑ **Laboratory Findings**

1. Measurement of urine output. To confirm the presence of polyuria, one can collect a 24-hour urine specimen or the patient can keep a diary for 24 hours, recording the volume and the time of each voided urine.
2. Serum sodium and urine osmolality. A low serum sodium concentration (<137 mEq/L) with a low urine osmolality (e.g., less than one-half the plasma

osmolality) is usually indicative of water overload due to primary polydipsia. A high-normal serum sodium concentration (>142 mEq/L) points toward DI, particularly if the urine osmolality is less than the plasma osmolality. A normal serum sodium concentration is not helpful in diagnosis but, if associated with a urine osmolality more than 600 mOsm/kg, excludes a diagnosis of DI. Hypernatremia during the first year of life is a common feature in children with hereditary nephrogenic DI.

3. Water deprivation test (also known as water restriction test). This test is important to differentiate the major forms of DI. Each of the causes of DI produces a distinct pattern to water deprivation and desmopressin (dDAVP) administration. Complete central DI is associated with urine osmolality <200 mOsm/kg after deprivation and marked increase (more than 100%) in urine osmolality after dDAVP administration. Partial central DI shows urine osmolality between 200 and 800 mOsm/kg after deprivation and variable increase (15–50%) in urine osmolality after dDAVP administration. Nephrogenic DI demonstrates submaximal rise in urine osmolality (usually below 300 mOsm/kg) after deprivation and little or no elevation in urine osmolality after dDAVP administration. Primary polydipsia is associated with a rise in urine osmolality (usually above 500 mOsm/kg) after water deprivation and no response to dDAVP administration.

Water deprivation tests for older infants and children should be performed in the hospital under close medical supervision. The patient should not be allowed to lose more than 5% of his or her body weight.

Water deprivation is not performed in newborns or very young infants suspected to have hereditary nephrogenic DI. The preferred diagnostic test in this setting is the administration of dDAVP with the measurement of the urine osmolality at baseline and at 30 minutes over the next 2 hours. If the urine osmolality does not increase by more than 100 mOsm/kg over baseline, the diagnosis of nephrogenic DI is made and DNA should be obtained for mutation analysis.

4. Plasma ADH measurement. When results of water deprivation test are ambiguous, plasma ADH assay is a useful adjunct. Plasma samples collected at baseline and following water deprivation (prior to the administration of ADH) should be sent for the measurement of ADH. Baseline plasma ADH should be low in patients with central DI and high in patients with nephrogenic DI. Primary polydipsia can associate with normal or low plasma ADH. If there is an increase in plasma ADH in response to the rising urine osmolality, central DI is excluded. If there is an appropriate elevation in urine osmolality and plasma ADH rises, nephrogenic DI is excluded.

5. Solute diuresis needs to be differentiated from DI. Solute diuresis is a form of polyuria in which large amount of filtered, nonreabsorbable solute gain entry to the renal tubules. The most common clinical example of solute diuresis is glycosuric diuresis seen in diabetic hyperglycemia. The urine osmolality in a solute diuresis is usually above 300 mOsm/kg, in contrast to the dilute urine typically found with a water diuresis seen in DI. Total solute excretion (calculated on a 24-hour urine collection from the product of the urine osmolality and the urine volume) is normal with a water diuresis (600–900 mOsm/day) but markedly increased with a solute diuresis.

Suggested Readings

Bichet DG. Clinical manifestations and causes of central diabetes insipidus. In: Rose B, (ed). *UpToDate*, Waltham, MA: UpToDate, Inc.; 2009.

Bichet DG. Clinical manifestations and causes of nephrogenic diabetes insipidus. In: Rose B, (ed). *UpToDate*, Waltham, MA: UpToDate, Inc.; 2009.

Bichet DG. Diagnosis of polyuria and diabetes insipidus. In: Rose B, (ed). *UpToDate*, Waltham, MA: UpToDate, Inc.; 2009.

Khan F, Sachs H, Pechet L, et al. *Guide to Diagnostic Testing*. Philadelphia, PA: Lippincott Williams & Wilkins; 2002.

Kronenberg HM, Melmed S, Polonsky KS, et al. *Williams Textbook of Endocrinology*, 11th ed. Philadelphia, PA: Saunders, Elsevier Inc.; 2008.

SYNDROME OF INAPPROPRIATE ANTIDIURETIC HORMONE SECRETION

❑ Definition

The syndrome of inappropriate antidiuretic hormone secretion (SIADH) is a disorder in which ADH release is either autonomous or poorly regulated. SIADH results when plasma levels of ADH are elevated and when the physiologic secretion of ADH from the posterior pituitary would normally be suppressed.

❑ Overview

SIADH is the most common cause of euvolemic hypoosmolality, and it is also the single most common cause of hypoosmolality encountered in clinical practice. It accounts for 20–40% among all hypoosmolar patients.

❑ Common Causes

1. Tumors. Ectopic production of ADH by a tumor is most often due to a small cell carcinoma of the lung but is also occasionally seen with other lung tumors. Less common causes include carcinomas of the pancreas, duodenum, prostate, and head and neck.
2. CNS disorders. A large number of different CNS disorders including stroke, hemorrhage, infection, trauma, and psychosis can enhance ADH release.
3. Drugs. Various drugs can lead to SIADH, and they include antineoplastic agents (vincristine, cyclophosphamide), antidepressant drugs (amitriptyline, phenothiazines), serotonin reuptake inhibitors (fluoxetine, sertraline), chlorpropamide, carbamazepine, oxcarbazepine, and clofibrate.
4. Pulmonary diseases. Infectious diseases such as tuberculosis, bacterial and viral pneumonia, aspergillosis, and empyema can lead to the SIADH. A similar response may occasionally be seen with asthma, atelectasis, acute respiratory failure, and pneumothorax.
5. HIV infection
6. Major surgery. Major abdominal or thoracic surgery is often associated with transient hypersecretion of ADH.
7. Hormone deficiency. Both adrenal insufficiency and hypothyroidism may be associated with hyponatremia and SIADH, which can be corrected by hormone replacement.
8. Idiopathic. Some patients appear to have idiopathic SIADH, with a higher rate in the elderly.

❏ Who Should Be Suspected?

The hallmark of SIADH is hypoosmolality. Clinical manifestations of hypoosmolality are mainly a broad spectrum of neurologic symptoms, ranging from mild nonspecific symptoms (e.g., headache, nausea) to more significant disorders (e.g., disorientation, confusion, obtundation, focal neurologic deficits, and seizures). This neurologic symptom complex has been known as hyponatremic encephalopathy. Nonneurologic symptoms are relatively uncommon.

Clinical euvolemia is usually present, and it is defined by the absence of signs of hypovolemia (orthostasis, tachycardia, decreased skin turgor, dry mucous membranes) or hypovolemia (subcutaneous edema, ascites).

❏ Laboratory Findings

1. Decreased plasma osmolality
2. Hyponatremia
3. Inappropriately elevated urine osmolality (above 100 mOsm/kg and usually above 300 mOsm/kg)
4. Elevated urine sodium concentration (usually above 40 mEq/L)
5. Low blood urea nitrogen (BUN) and serum uric acid concentration
6. Relatively normal serum creatinine concentration
7. Normal acid–base and potassium balance
8. Causes such as adrenal insufficiency and hypothyroidism need to be identified since the associated SIADH can be corrected by hormone replacement.
9. Currently, measurement of plasma ADH levels has very limited role in the diagnosis of SIADH. There are several reasons for this. First, the elevated plasma ADH levels seen in SIADH generally remain within normal reference range and are abnormal only in relation to plasma osmolality. Second, the current assays for ADH cannot detect elevations in 10–20% of patients with SIADH. Third, most disorders of volume depletion are associated with elevation of plasma ADH levels and thus cannot be distinguished.

Suggested Readings

Kronenberg HM, Melmed S, Polonsky KS, et al. *Williams Textbook of Endocrinology*, 11th ed. Philadelphia, PA: Saunders, Elsevier Inc.; 2008.

Rose BD. Pathophysiology and etiology of the syndrome of inappropriate antidiuretic hormone secretion (SIADH). In: Rose B, (ed). *UpToDate*, Waltham, MA: UpToDate, Inc.; 2009.

Sterns RH. Evaluation of the patient with hyponatremia. In: Rose B, (ed). *UpToDate*, Waltham, MA: UpToDate, Inc.; 2009.

DISORDERS OF THE PARATHYROID GLAND AND MINERAL METABOLISM

HYPERPARATHYROIDISM

❏ Definition

Primary hyperparathyroidism is autonomous hypersecretion of parathyroid hormone (PTH) from the parathyroid glands. Secondary hyperparathyroidism occurs in patients with chronic advanced renal disease that causes retention of phosphate, inadequate vitamin D activation, chronic low serum calcium, and therefore compensatory hyperplasia of the parathyroid glands with compensatory secretion of PTH. This chapter focuses solely on primary hyperparathyroidism.

❑ Overview
Primary hyperparathyroidism is frequently identified in asymptomatic patients with an elevated serum calcium concentration. It is estimated to have a prevalence of 1 case per 1,000 people. Primary hyperparathyroidism can occur at any age, but the majority of cases occur in patients >45 years of age.

❑ Common Causes
Primary hyperparathyroidism can usually be differentiated from other causes of hypercalcemia by the demonstration of an elevated serum PTH concentration.

1. Parathyroid adenoma is the most common cause of hyperparathyroidism and accounts for approximately 90% of the cases. Most patients have a single enlarged gland with a single adenoma. The remaining glands are usually normal.
2. Parathyroid hyperplasia accounts for approximately 6% of the cases. It involves all four glands and can occur either as isolated or as part of a syndrome such as MEN type 1 or 2 or familial hyperparathyroidism.
3. Parathyroid carcinoma is a rare cause of hyperparathyroidism and constitutes 1–2% of the cases. The diagnosis of carcinoma requires demonstration of local invasion of contiguous structure, metastases to lymph node, or distant metastases.
4. Familial hypocalciuric hypercalcemia is caused by an inactivating mutation in the calcium-sensing receptor in the parathyroid glands and the kidneys. It is characterized by a family history of hypercalcemia, a young age of onset, lack of symptoms or complications, and specifically by a low urine calcium excretion with calcium/creatinine (Ca/Cr) clearance ratio <0.01 in 90% of patients. These patients have normal or only very slightly elevated PTH concentrations.

❑ Who Should Be Suspected?
Primary hyperparathyroidism should be suspected in patients with

1. Elevated serum calcium levels, especially when it persists for years
2. Nephrolithiasis
3. Metabolic acidosis
4. Unexplained osteoporosis, bone pain, and pathologic fractures
5. Osteitis fibrosa cystica, which is characterized by subperiosteal bone resorption on the radial aspect of middle phalanges, tapering of distal clavicles, "salt and pepper" appearance of the skull, bone cysts, and brown tumors of the long bones

❑ Laboratory Findings
The diagnosis of primary hyperparathyroidism depends on demonstrating elevated serum calcium in the presence of increased PTH (Figure 6-13).

1. Measurement of serum calcium. A single elevated serum calcium concentration should be repeated to confirm the presence of hypercalcemia. Both total and ionized calcium concentrations should be obtained. The patient's oral calcium and vitamin D supplements should be withheld before the workup.

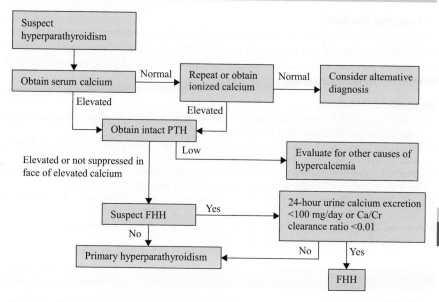

Figure 6–13 *Algorithm for the workup of hyperparathyroidism. Ca/Cr, calcium/creatinine; FHH, familial hypocalciuric calcemia; PTH, parathyroid hormone.*

2. Measurement of PTH. Approximately 80–90% of patients with primary hyperparathyroidism have elevated PTH. In the remaining patients, normal or only minimally elevated PTH is detected, but these values are inappropriately high in the setting of an elevated serum calcium level. In patients with non–PTH-mediated hypercalcemia, intact PTH is <25 pg/mL. Parathyroid hormone–related protein (PTHrP), which is the humoral cause of cancer-related hypercalcemia, is not detected in the intact PTH assay.

3. Urinary calcium excretion. A 24-hour urine calcium quantitation should be measured if familial hypocalciuric hypercalcemia is suspected. The finding of 24-hour urine calcium excretion <100 mg and Ca/Cr clearance ratio <0.01 confirms the diagnosis.

4. Patients who have a familial history of hyperparathyroidism or those suspected of having hyperparathyroidism in the context of MEN syndromes should also be evaluated for associated disorders, particularly for pheochromocytoma and thyroid medullary carcinoma.

5. Vitamin D metabolites. Patients with primary hyperparathyroidism convert more calcidiol to calcitriol than normal individuals. Therefore, serum concentrations of *1,25-dihydroxyvitamin D_3* (calcitriol) may be at upper limits of normal or elevated. However, an elevated value is not specific, and thus the measurement of *1,25-dihydroxyvitamin D_3* (calcitriol) is not generally needed to confirm the diagnosis. However, it is helpful to differentiate from the cases with an isolated PTH increase in the absence of hypercalcemia due to vitamin D deficiency.

❏ Imaging Studies

Localization studies such as ultrasonography, technetium-99m sestamibi, CT, or MRI scanning should not be used to establish the diagnosis of primary hyperparathyroidism but are commonly used to facilitate unilateral neck exploration and minimally invasive surgeries.

Suggested Readings

Fuleihan GE, Arnold A. Pathogenesis and etiology of primary hyperparathyroidism. In: Rose B, (ed). *UpToDate*, Waltham, MA: UpToDate, Inc.; 2009.

Fuleihan GE, Silverberg SJ. Clinical manifestations of primary hyperparathyroidism. In: Rose B, (ed). *UpToDate*, Waltham, MA: UpToDate, Inc.; 2009.

Fuleihan GE, Silverberg SJ. Diagnosis and differential diagnosis of primary hyperparathyroidism. In: Rose B, (ed). *UpToDate*, Waltham, MA: UpToDate, Inc.; 2009.

Khan F, Sachs H, Pechet L, et al. *Guide to Diagnostic Testing*. Philadelphia, PA: Lippincott Williams & Wilkins; 2002.

Kronenberg HM, Melmed S, Polonsky KS, et al. *Williams Textbook of Endocrinology*, 11th ed. Philadelphia, PA: Saunders, Elsevier Inc.; 2008.

HYPERCALCEMIA

❏ Definition

Hypercalcemia refers an abnormally high concentration of calcium compounds in the circulating blood.

❏ Overview

Hypercalcemia is a relatively common clinical problem. It results when the entry of calcium into circulation exceeds the excretion of calcium into urine or deposition in bone. Hypercalcemia occurs when there is accelerated bone resorption, excessive gastrointestinal absorption, or deceased renal excretion of calcium. There are many causes of hypercalcemia, but hyperparathyroidism and malignancy are the most common, accounting for >90% of the cases.

❏ Common Causes

Hypercalcemia can be divided into major categories based on the mechanisms of increased bone resorption and increased calcium absorption.

1. Disorders with increased bone resorption
   a. Primary hyperparathyroidism
   b. Secondary and tertiary hyperparathyroidism
   c. Malignancy. The most common etiology with nonmetastatic solid tumor is secretion of PTHrP. Rarely, it is due to a result of ectopic production of PTH.
   d. Thyrotoxicosis
   e. Immobilization
   f. Paget disease of bone
   g. Tamoxifen used in patients with breast cancer and skeletal metastases
   h. Hypervitaminosis A
2. Disorders with increased calcium absorption
   a. Increased calcium intake. A high calcium intake alone rarely causes hypercalcemia, but it can lead to hypercalcemia when combined with decreased urinary excretion.

b. Chronic renal failure. It occurs in patients who are treated with calcium carbonate or calcium acetate to bind dietary phosphate.

c. Milk-alkali syndrome. Excess intake of calcium- and alkali-containing antacids (such as calcium carbonate or sodium bicarbonate) leads to hypercalcemia, metabolic alkalosis, and renal failure. It typically occurs in the situation of taking excess calcium carbonate supplementation to treat osteoporosis or dyspepsia.

3. Hypervitaminosis D can cause hypercalcemia by increasing calcium absorption and bone resorption. High concentration of either 25-hydroxyvitamin D (calcidiol) or 1, 25-dihydroxvitamin D (calcitriol) can lead to hypercalcemia. High serum concentration of 1, 25-dihydroxvitamin D is usually caused by ingestion of calcitriol as treatment for hypoparathyroidism or for the hypocalcemia and secondary hyperparathyroidism of renal failure, but it also can be due to increased endogenous production in patients with granulomatous disease and lymphoma.

4. Miscellaneous causes:
   a. Lithium
   b. Thiazide diuretics
   c. Pheochromocytoma
   d. Adrenal insufficiency
   e. Rhabdomyolysis and acute renal failure
   f. Theophylline toxicity
   g. Familial hypocalciuric hypercalcemia
   h. Metaphyseal chondrodysplasia
   i. Congenital lactase deficiency

❏ Who Should Be Suspected?

- Patients with mildly elevated serum calcium (<12 mg/dL) may be asymptomatic, particularly if the elevation is chronic, or they may report nonspecific symptoms, such as constipation, fatigue, and depression.
- Patients with moderately elevated serum calcium (12–14 mg/dL) may have symptoms of polyuria, polydipsia, nausea, anorexia, vomiting, constipation, muscle weakness, and change in sensorium. Acute hypercalcemia leads to a shortened QT interval, which reflects the shortened myocardial action potential.
- Severe hypercalcemia (>14 mg/dL) can lead to progression of above symptoms and confusion, lethargy, stupor, and even coma and death.

❏ Laboratory Findings (Table 6-8; Figure 6-14)

The main goal of hypercalcemia workup is to differentiate PTH-mediated hypercalcemia from non–PTH-mediated hypercalcemia.

- Interpretation of serum calcium. Approximately 40–50% protein bound (predominantly to albumin), but only the ionized or free of the circulating calcium concentration is physiologically important. Hypercalcemia is caused by an elevation in the ionized or free calcium concentration. In patients with hypo- or hyperalbuminemia, the measured calcium concentration should be corrected for abnormality in albumin. Pseudohypercalcemia

TABLE 6–8. Laboratory Results in Common Causes of Hypercalcemia

Disorder	Serum Phosphate	Intact PTH	Urine Calcium Excretion	Miscellaneous
Primary hyperparathyroidism	↓	↑	NL or ↑	Metabolic acidosis
Familial hypocalciuric hypercalcemia	Variable	NL or SL ↑	↓	
Humoral hypercalcemia of malignancy	↓	↓	NL or ↑	↑ PTHrP
Granulomatous disease	NL or ↑	↓	↑↑	↑ 1,25-OH vitamin D, ↑ angiotensin-converting enzyme
Vitamin D toxicity	NL or ↑	↓	↑↑	↑ 1,25-OH vitamin D
Milk-alkali syndrome	NL or ↑	↓	↓	Metabolic alkalosis and decreased GFR
Metastatic bone disease	NL or ↑	↓	↑	
Thiazide diuretics	NL	↓	↓	
Lithium	NL	↑	↓	

NL, normal level; PTHrP, parathyroid hormone–related protein; SL, slightly.
Normal values: urine calcium: 100–250 mg/24 h (females) and 100–300 mg/24 h (males); serum phosphate: 2.5–4.5 mg/dL; PTH (intact): 12–72 pg/mL; 1,25-OH Vitamin D: 14–78 pg/mL; angiotensin-converting enzyme: 17–70 units; PTHrP: <2.8 pmol/L.

should be excluded; it is related to increased protein binding due to either severe dehydration and hyperalbuminemia or production of calcium-binding paraprotein in patients with multiple myeloma. On the contrary, in patients with hypoalbuminemia due to chronic illness or malnutrition, total serum calcium concentration may be normal when serum ionized calcium is elevated.

■ Calcium results need to be repeated if abnormal. A single elevated serum calcium concentration should be repeated to confirm the diagnosis.

■ Serum calcium should not be measured after a recent high-calcium meal.

■ A 24-hour urine calcium quantification is useful in differentiating primary hyperparathyroidism from familial hypocalciuric hypercalcemia (FHH).

■ PTH. Measurement of intact PTH via immunoradiometric assays is the current standard for the diagnosis of hyperparathyroidism. PTH will be elevated in 80–90% of patients with primary hyperparathyroidism.

■ Parathyroid hormone–related protein (PTHrP). In the presence of hypercalcemia, if PTH level is appropriately suppressed, then evaluation for other causes should include the measurement of PTHrP. PTHrP is the most common tumor product implicated in the hypercalcemia of malignancy.

■ Vitamin D metabolites. Serum concentrations of the vitamin D metabolites, 25-hydroxyvitamin D, and 1, 25-dihydroxvitamin D should be measured if there is no obvious malignancy and neither PTH nor PTHrP levels are elevated. An elevated serum concentration of calcidiol is indicative of vitamin D intoxication. However, an increased level of calcitriol may be due to direct intake, extrarenal production in granulomatous disease or lymphoma, or increased renal production.

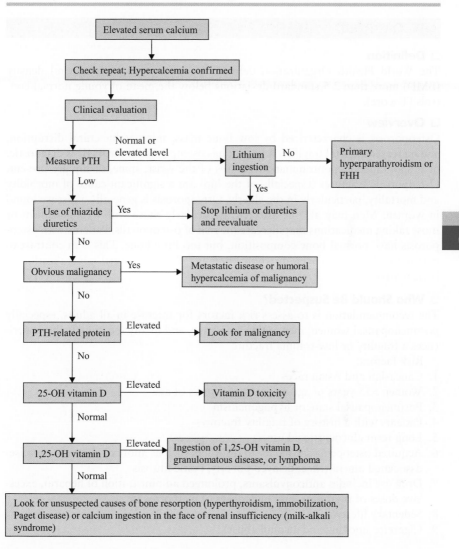

Figure 6–14 *Algorithm for the workup of hypercalcemia. FHH, familial hypocalciuric hypercalcemia; PTH, parathyroid hormone.*

Suggested Readings

Agus ZS. Clinical manifestations of hypercalcemia. In: Rose B, (ed). *UpToDate*, Waltham, MA: UpToDate, Inc.; 2009.

Agus ZS. Diagnostic approach to hypercalcemia. In: Rose B, (ed). *UpToDate*, Waltham, MA: UpToDate, Inc.; 2009.

Agus ZS. Etiology of hypercalcemia. In: Rose B, (ed). *UpToDate*, Waltham, MA: UpToDate, Inc.; 2009.

Khan F, Sachs H, Pechet L, et al. *Guide to Diagnostic Testing*. Philadelphia, PA: Lippincott Williams & Wilkins; 2002.

OSTEOPOROSIS

❑ Definition
The World Health Organization defines osteoporosis as bone mineral density (BMD) more than 2.5 standard deviations below the mean of young normal controls (T-score).

❑ Overview
Osteoporosis is characterized by low bone mass, microarchitectural disruption, and increased skeletal fragility. A patient has osteoporosis if the BMD is diagnostic, or if spontaneous, nontraumatic fractures of the wrist, spine, or hip are present. Osteoporotic fractures (especially of the hip) are a significant cause of morbidity and mortality, particularly in the elderly. Osteoporosis is generally a disease found in women. Men may also be affected, particularly those with hypogonadism or those taking medications that increase the risk of osteoporosis. Patients with osteoporosis have normal bone composition, but too little bone. This is in contrast to patients with osteomalacia, in whom there is failure of normal mineralization of bone matrix.

❑ Who Should Be Suspected?
The recommendation is to assess risk factors for fracture in all adults, especially postmenopausal women, men >60 years of age, and in any individual who experiences a fragility or low-trauma fracture

Risk factors:
1. Caucasian and Asian races
2. Women >55 years of age and men >65 years of age
3. Postmenopausal state or hypogonadism
4. Patients with a history of fragility fractures
5. Long-term glucocorticoid use
6. Acquired osteopenia secondary to disorders such as anorexia nervosa, exercise-associated amenorrhea, delayed puberty, cystic fibrosis
7. Drug use includes anticonvulsants, prolonged administration of heparin, excessive doses of thyroxine, and high doses of methotrexate
8. Sedentary lifestyle
9. Cigarette smoking and alcohol abuse

❑ Laboratory Findings (Figure 6-15; Table 6-9)
Bone densitometry: Bone density measurements are used in conjunction with fracture risk assessment for osteoporosis screening. Multiple techniques have been developed for the measurement of bone mass, and usage depends mainly on local availability. Dual-energy x-ray absorptiometry (DXA) is the most widely used method. Because BMD varies between sites, evaluation at more than one site is recommended.

Laboratory evaluation in a patient with suspected osteoporosis is listed in Table 6-9. It is also important to test for plasma albumin and 25-hydroxycholesterol levels.

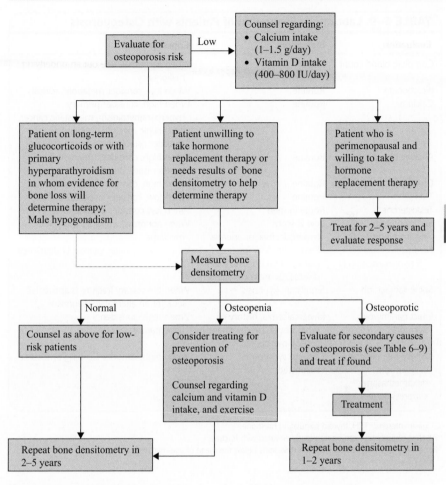

6

Figure 6-15 *Algorithm for the evaluation of a patient with suspected osteoporosis.*

TABLE 6–9. Laboratory Evaluation of Patients with Osteoporosis

Evaluation	Indication	Consideration
Complete blood count	Routine	When abnormal, rule out an underlying malignancy
Bicarbonate	Routine	When low, consider metabolic acidosis
Calcium	Routine	When high, consider primary hyperparathyroidism, metastatic cancer, or multiple myeloma. When low, consider osteomalacia or renal failure
Alkaline phosphatase	Routine	When high, consider osteomalacia or another bone disease*
Creatinine	Routine	When high, consider renal failure
TSH	Routine	When low, consider hyperthyroidism
Testosterone	Route in men	When low consider hypogonadism
Serum protein electrophoresis	Low Z-score[†], hypercalcemia, or anemia	When abnormal, consider multiple myeloma
Serum 25-hydroxyvitamin D	Elderly with poor intake, history of GI disease, liver disease, or anticonvulsants	When low, consider vitamin D deficiency
Spine radiograph	Significant kyphosis	When the solitary fracture is above T-7, look for an alternative diagnosis
Intact parathyroid hormone	Hypercalcemia, history of renal stones, predominantly cortical osteopenia	When high, consider hyperparathyroidism
Urinary free cortical or overnight dexamethasone suppression test	Cushing syndrome suspected	When high, consider Cushing syndrome

GI, gastrointestinal; TSH, thyroid-stimulating hormone.
*Alkaline phosphatase can be transiently elevated with fracture.
[†]Bone mineral density is >2.5 standard deviations below the mean of age-matched controls.

Suggested Readings

Khan F, Sachs H, Pechet L, et al. *Guide to Diagnostic Testing.* Philadelphia, PA: Lippincott Williams & Wilkins; 2002.

Raisz LG. Pathogenesis of osteoporosis. In: Rose B, (ed). *UpToDate*, Waltham, MA: UpToDate, Inc.; 2009.

Raisz LG. Screening for osteoporosis. In: Rose B, (ed). *UpToDate*, Waltham, MA: UpToDate, Inc.; 2009.

CHAPTER 7

Genitourinary System Disorders

Charles R. Kiefer

This chapter reorganizes the diseases and disorders of the genitourinary (GU) tracts and includes the latest information for the diagnosis of prostate and urinary tract diseases. Each entry is organized with a brief definition of the disorder and information regarding clinical presentation, laboratory findings, and limitations, if appropriate.

 NEOPLASTIC DISEASES

BLADDER CANCER

❏ **Definition**

- Cancer arising in the urinary bladder is a carcinoma of urothelial (transitional cell) origin in the United States and Europe (90% of cases). Less frequently, urothelial carcinomas may originate in the renal pelvis, ureter, or urethra. In other parts of the world, bladder carcinomas of nonurothelial origin are more common.

❏ Who Should Be Suspected?

- Suspected patients are older than age 40 years, more commonly males with a history of cigarette smoking, who present with hematuria (painless, intermittent, grossly visible, and present throughout micturition), or irritative voiding symptoms (frequency, urgency, dysuria) that suggest carcinoma in situ (CIS) of the bladder.
- The association of pain with bladder cancer (located to the flank; suprapubic, hypogastric, and perineal; abdominal or right upper quadrant areas; bone pain; or headache/disordered cognitive function) can be signs of locally advanced or metastatic disease. Constitutional symptoms (fatigue, weight loss, anorexia, failure to thrive) are usually signs of advanced or metastatic disease and carry a poor prognosis.
- The definitive diagnosis and staging of bladder cancer are by cystoscopy, beginning with a baseline evaluation of the bladder and uninvolved mucosa to record the number, size, location, appearance, and growth type (papillary or solid) of all lesions observed. Visible lesions can be biopsied or resected for histologic analysis.

❏ Laboratory Findings

- Urinalysis: A positive dipstick test (detecting one to two red cells per high-power field [HPF]) should be confirmed by microscopic analysis (below). Infection should be ruled out by a urine culture prior to further workup of hematuria.
- Urine sediment: Hematuria is significant if there are greater than three red cells per HPF, present throughout micturition. The presence of dysmorphic red cells or casts suggests a glomerular origin, whereas normally formed red cells likely originate from infections, tumors, or obstructions/calculi. The specimen should be maintained at room temperature and examined within 30 minutes of collection.
- Urine cytology: Urine cytologic analysis by fluorescence in situ hybridization (e.g., UroVysion™ FISH) can be a useful noninvasive aid both in the primary diagnosis of urothelial carcinoma and in monitoring tumor recurrence (occurring in about 70% of cases after initial treatments). UroVysion™ FISH is designed to detect certain numerical chromosomal abnormalities commonly associated with urothelial carcinoma (either amplifications of chromosomes 3, 7, and 17 or deletions of the 9p21 locus).
- Urine biomarkers: Several urine-based biomarkers have been approved for diagnosis or surveillance of patients with a history of the disease. However, their sensitivity is low, and their use is not recommended for an initial workup of a suspected case.

❏ Limitations on Interpretation of the UroVysion™ FISH Test for Bladder Cancer

- A positive result in the absence of clinical evidence of urothelial bladder cancer may indicate urothelial malignancies of other organs along the GU tract (kidney, ureter, prostate, or urethra).
- A negative result in the presence of other signs or symptoms of urothelial carcinoma may suggest a false-negative test.

Suggested Readings

Getzenberg RH. Urine-based assays for bladder cancer. *Lab Med.* 2003;34:613–617.

Lotan Y, Roehrborn CG. Sensitivity and specificity of commonly available bladder tumor markers versus cytology: results of a comprehensive literature review and meta-analyses. *Urology.* 2003;61:109–118.

PROSTATE CANCER

❑ Definition

- Prostate cancer is an adenocarcinoma of the prostate gland, most commonly occurring in the peripheral zone. There is a close association of the cancer with small clumps of cancer cells—carcinoma in situ or prostatic intraepithelial neoplasia (PIN)—although it has not been proven that PIN is the cancer precursor.
- Prostate cancer is generally so indolent that most men die of other causes before the disease becomes clinically advanced. However, globally it is the sixth leading cause of cancer deaths in men (second leading cause in the United States and first in the United Kingdom).

❑ Who Should Be Suspected?

- Prostate cancer tends to develop in men over age 50. In the early stage of the disease, most men have no symptoms directly linked to the cancer, but because the gland surrounds the prostatic urethra, changes in urinary function can occur with disease progression.
- As a presenting symptom, a change in urinary function (frequency, urgency, nocturia, hesitancy) is the most common, but benign prostatic hyperplasia (BPH) figures into the differential diagnosis and is usually the cause.
- Hematuria and hematospermia are uncommon symptoms but, if present, also are more likely to be caused by BPH. However, if occurring in older men, prostate cancer should be included in the differential diagnosis.
- Bone pain, often in the vertebrae, pelvis, or ribs, if present, would indicate metastatic disease.

❑ Early Detection

- The two methods for early detection of *suspected* prostate cancer are the digital rectal examination for asymmetric areas of induration or nodules on the posterior and lateral aspects of the prostate gland and measurement of serum prostate-specific antigen (PSA). About 20% of early detections occur through a suspicious digital rectal examination and the remaining 80% through a suspicious PSA test. A definitive diagnosis of prostate cancer by either method of early detection is established by a positive biopsy.
- Screening of *unsuspected* cases for prostate cancer via the PSA test is controversial. Because of the low specificity of elevated PSA levels for prostate cancer versus BPH or prostatitis, the benefits of screening are outweighed by the harms of unnecessary treatment. Screening is not recommended by the U.S. Preventive Services Task Force (Grade "D," 2012) and the Centers for

Disease Control and Prevention. The American Society of Clinical Oncology and the American College of Physicians discourage screening in those expected to live less than another 10–15 years. The American Urological Association recommends shared decision making in those from age 55 to 69 and no more often than every 2 years.

❏ **Laboratory Findings**

■ PSA testing: PSA levels normally correlate with age and prostate size, averaging 1 ng/mL for men under age 50 and 3 ng/mL for men over age 60. A value of 4.0 ng/mL is widely used as a cutoff for prostate cancer. There are two effective methods of enhancing the specificity of the PSA test—use of an age-based reference range and calculation of the free versus total PSA ratio.

▼ Age-based reference range: A PSA reference range based on age should be calculated for each laboratory performing PSA testing.

▼ PSA free versus total ratio: The risk of prostate cancer is increased if the ratio of free to total PSA is <25%.

▼ PSA velocity: An annual rate of change in the PSA level >2.0 ng/mL, while not an effective screening test, offers value in assessing preoperative mortality risk.

Suggested Readings

Berger AP, Cheli C, Levine R, et al. Impact of age on complexed PSA levels in men with total PSA levels of up to 20 ng/mL. *Urology.* 2003;62:840–844.

Catalona WJ, Partin AW, Slawin KM, et al. Use of the percentage of free prostate-specific antigen to enhance differentiation of prostate cancer from benign prostatic disease: a prospective multicenter clinical trial. *JAMA.* 1998;279:1542–1547.

Crawford ED, DeAntoni EP, Etzioni R, et al. Serum prostate-specific antigen and digital rectal examination for early detection of prostate cancer in a national community-based program. The Prostate Cancer Education Council. *Urology.* 1996;47:863–869.

D'Amico A, Chen M, Roehl K, Catalona W. Preoperative PSA velocity and the risk of death from prostate cancer after radical prostatectomy. *N Engl J Med.* 2004;351:125–135.

CARCINOMA OF THE RENAL PELVIS AND URETER

❏ **Definition**

■ Carcinomas of the renal pelvis and ureter are primary tumors of urothelial (transitional cell) origin. Primary tumors arising in the renal pelvis include urothelial carcinomas (>90% of cases), squamous cell carcinomas (8%), and adenocarcinomas (rare).

❏ **Who Should Be Suspected?**

■ Individuals with carcinoma of the renal pelvis or ureter are most likely to have hematuria (70–95% of cases) or flank pain (8–40%) stemming from obstruction of the ureter or ureteropelvic junction by a tumor mass. Other types of urinary tract symptoms (bladder irritation, constitutional symptoms) are less likely to be seen at diagnosis (<10%). Calculi or chronic infection may precede the squamous cell carcinomas.

❑ Laboratory Findings

- Urine cytology: Examination of urinary sediment for malignant cells is a less reliable method for diagnosis of these cases than for bladder cancers because of the poor yield of low-grade tumors and the likelihood of synchronous bladder cancer (40–50% of cases).

Suggested Readings

Olgac S, Mazumdar M, Dalbagni G, et al. Urothelial carcinoma of the renal pelvis: a clinicopathologic study of 130 cases. *Am J Surg Pathol.* 2004;28:1545–1552.

Paonessa J, Beck H, Cook S. Squamous cell carcinoma of the renal pelvis associated with kidney stones: a case report. *Med Oncol.* 2011;28(Suppl 1):S392–S394.

LEUKOPLAKIA OF THE RENAL PELVIS

❑ Definition

- Leukoplakia of the renal pelvis is a visualized grayish patch observed on the mucosal surface epithelium of the renal pelvis (part of the kidney urothelium) and represents metaplastic squamous plaque (squamous metaplasia and keratinization).

❑ Who Should Be Suspected?

- Candidates are typically middle-aged individuals with recurrent episodes of renal or ureteric colic. In 90% of cases, the lesion is unilateral.

❑ Laboratory Findings

- Urine cytology (cell block or Pap smear): The finding of sheets of desquamated keratinized epithelial cells in urine during an attack of renal colic is pathognomonic.
- Flow cytometry (DNA): High-grade (aneuploid) tumors can be detected in >90% of cases.

Suggested Readings

Hertle L, Androulakakis P. Keratinizing desquamative squamous metaplasia of the upper urinary tract: leukoplakia—cholesteatoma. *J Urol.* 1982;127:631–635.

Smith BA Jr, Webb EA, Price WE. Renal leukoplakia: observations of behavior. *J Urol.* 1962;87:279–287.

Terry TR, Shearer RJ. Conservative surgical management of leukoplakia of upper urinary tract. *J R Soc Med.* 1986;79:544–545.

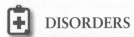 DISORDERS

BENIGN PROSTATIC HYPERPLASIA (BPH)

❑ Definition

- BPH is enlargement of the prostate resulting from hyperplasia of prostatic stromal and epithelial cells, compressing the periurethral region of the prostate and causing partial or complete obstruction of the urethra.

❑ Who Should Be Suspected?

- Candidates are men, generally older than 30 years, with moderate to severe lower urinary tract symptoms (frequency, nocturia, hesitancy, urgency, weak stream) that gradually progress with time.
- A history and physical examination should include a digital rectal examination of the prostate. A urine culture and urinalysis for hematuria should be undertaken to rule out other or more serious disorders that could cause symptoms similar to those of BPH (urinary tract infection, bladder calculi, prostatitis, prostate cancer, or bladder cancer). On digital rectal examination, symmetric enlargement and firmness of the prostate are typical of BPH, whereas asymmetric areas are suggestive of prostate cancer.

❑ Laboratory Findings

- Serum prostate-specific antigen (PSA): In 20% of BPH patients, serum PSA may be increased from the widely used prostate cancer cutoff value of 4.0–10 ng/mL. In fact, BPH is a more common cause of elevated PSA levels than is prostate cancer.
- Serum creatinine: While not recommended by the American Urological Association in the management of patients with BPH, a high serum creatinine value may suggest a bladder outlet obstruction or underlying renal or prerenal disease and an increased risk for post–prostate surgery complications and mortality.

Suggested Readings

Barry MJ, Fowler FJ Jr, O'Leary MP, et al. The American Urological Association symptom index for benign prostatic hyperplasia. The Measurement Committee of the American Urological Association. *J Urol.* 1992;148:1549–1557.
Jacobsen SJ, Girman CJ, Lieber MM. Natural history of benign prostatic hyperplasia. *Urology.* 2001;58:5–16.
Madersbacher S, Alivizatos G, Nordling J, et al. EAU 2004 guidelines on assessment, therapy and follow-up of men with lower urinary tract symptoms suggestive of benign prostatic obstruction (BPH guidelines). *Eur Urol.* 2004;46:547–554.

CALCULI

❑ Definition

- A renal calculus (kidney stone) is a solid concretion/crystalline aggregate formed in the kidneys by supersaturation of dietary minerals in the urine, one or more of which nucleate seed crystals. Both the supersaturation and the crystalline aggregation processes are pH dependent.
- Calculi can be classified by their location and chemical composition.
  - ▼ Locations include the kidney (nephrolithiasis), ureter (ureterolithiasis), or bladder (cystolithiasis).
  - ▼ Varieties of chemical composition include calcium containing (primarily calcium oxalate but also calcium phosphate); struvite (magnesium ammonium phosphate); uric acid; and cystine.

- Calcium oxalate or calcium phosphate calculi occur in 85% of male and 70% of female patients. Calcium oxalate crystals require an acid environment. Calcium phosphate crystals occur with hypercalciuria, hypocitraturia, and an alkaline environment (Figure 7-1). A comparison of idiopathic causes of hypercalciuria is presented in Table 7-1.
- Struvite stones (staghorn calculi), occurring in 10–15% of patients, are generated by UTI urea-splitting bacteria, including *Proteus* species (>50% of cases; after ruling out *Klebsiella*, *Pseudomonas*, *Serratia*, and *Enterobacter*), and in patients with persistently alkaline urine. Although not producing symptoms unless inducing urinary tract obstruction or infection, this type of calculus can lead to renal failure over years if present bilaterally. Staghorn calculi should be cultured.
- Cystine stones are rare, occurring in patients with homozygous congenital familial cystinuria, and characterized by bilateral obstructive staghorn calculi with associated renal failure.

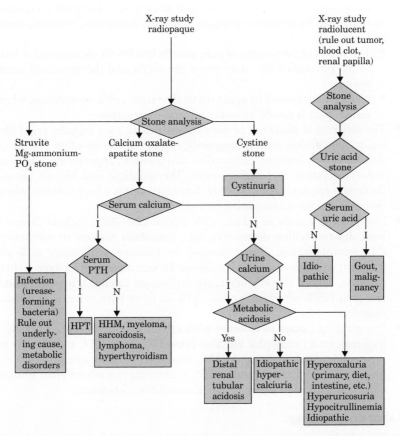

Figure 7–1 *Algorithm for diagnosis of renal calculi, as revealed by flank pain, renal colic, hematuria, fever, and urinalysis findings. I, increased; N, normal; PTH, parathyroid hormone; HPT, hyperparathyroidism; HHM, humeral hypercalcemia of malignancy.*

TABLE 7-1 Comparison of Types of Idiopathic Hypercalciuria

	Resorptive	Absorptive	Renal
Due to	Primary hyperparathyroidism	Primary increase in intestinal absorption; reabsorption autosomal	Abnormal renal tubular dominant
Frequency	Least common	Most common	1/10 as common as absorptive type
2-hour urine after fasting			
Calcium	30 mg	<20 mg	Increased
Calcium/creatinine ratio	>0.15	<0.15	>0.15

❑ **Who Should Be Suspected?**

■ In adults, the most common symptom of calculi that obstruct the ureter or renal pelvis is excruciating, intermittent pain that radiates from the flank to the groin or to the genital area and inner thigh. The pain is commonly accompanied by urinary urgency, restlessness, hematuria, sweating, nausea, and vomiting.

▼ The waves or paroxysms of pain usually last 20–60 minutes and is related to the passage of the stone down the ureter and the associated ureteral spasm.

▼ Flank pain is caused by upper ureteral or renal pelvic obstruction, whereas genital pain is caused by lower ureteral obstruction.

■ The differential diagnosis of patients with flank pain includes renal bleeding, pyelonephritis, ectopic pregnancy, rupture or torsion of an ovarian cyst, dysmenorrhea, intestinal obstruction, diverticulitis, appendicitis, biliary colic and cholecystitis, and herpes zoster. The intestinal and hepatic causes of flank pain are not accompanied by hematuria nor is a herpes zoster infection (which is usually accompanied by a rash).

■ Precipitating causes in adults with calculi (20–30%) include destructive bone diseases (either destructive, e.g., metastatic tumors; or osteoporotic, e.g., immobilization, Paget disease, or Cushing syndrome); milk-alkali (Burnett) syndrome; hypervitaminosis D; sarcoidosis; RTA-type I (hypercalciuria, highly alkaline urine, normal serum calcium); hyperthyroidism; and gout (25% of primary cases, 40% of cases with marrow-proliferative disorders).

■ Precipitating causes in children with calculi include infections (13–40%); hypercalciuria (idiopathic but also caused by distal RTA and therapy with furosemide, prednisone, or ACTH); oxaluria (3–13%); uric acid (4%); cystinuria (5–7%); hypocitraturia (10%); xanthine (an inborn error of metabolism); and adenine phosphoribosyltransferase deficiency.

❑ **Laboratory Findings**

■ Two 24-hour urine specimens should be collected and tested for daily volume and levels of magnesium, sodium, uric acid, calcium, citrate, and oxalate.

▼ A urine culture should be performed to detect infecting microorganisms.

▼ Urine microscopy should be performed to detect the presence and level of red cells, white cells, urinary casts, and crystals.

▼ Calculi should be collected by urination through a stone screen, for chemical analysis.

■ Hematuria: Gross or microscopic, occurs in 80% of symptomatic patients and is the single most definitive predictor of a calculus in patients with unilateral flank pain. However, hematuria is not detected in 10–30% of patients with documented nephrolithiasis.

■ Renal function tests: Useful for interpretation of hypercalcemia.

■ Crystalluria: Diagnostically useful for cystine crystals (in familial cystinuria) or struvite crystals.

■ Cyanide-nitroprusside test: Positive (false positive may occur with sulfur-containing drugs). Calcium oxalate, phosphate, and uric acid should arouse suspicion about possible causes, but they may occur in normal urine.

■ Neutrophilia: Suggestive of infection, for example, in the finding of struvite crystals.

Suggested Readings

Coe FL, Parks JH, Asplin JR. The pathogenesis and treatment of kidney stones. *N Engl J Med.* 1992;327:1141–1152.

Elton TJ, Roth CS, Berquist TH, et al. A clinical prediction rule for the diagnosis of ureteral calculi in emergency departments. *J Gen Intern Med.* 1993;8:57–62.

Teichman JM, Long RD, Hulbert JC. Long-term renal fate and prognosis after staghorn calculus management. *J Urol.* 1995;153:1403–1407.

7

HEMATURIA

❏ Definition

■ The term *hematuria* refers to the microscopic detection in urine of >2 RBCs per high-power field. It should not to be confused with hemoglobinuria, a term reserved for the presence of free hemoglobin in urine.

■ Hematuria may be macroscopic (grossly visible as red or brown urine) or microscopic (detectable only by microscopy). It can be classified as glomerular or nonglomerular in origin. Centrifugation allows one to differentiate hematuria (RBCs in sediment) from hemoglobinuria (normal sediment, heme-pigmented supernatant), which can be tested for heme with a urine dipstick.

❏ Who Should Be Suspected?

■ Hematuria is common and, in many patients, particularly young adults, is transient and inconsequential. With increasing age, common causes can include inflammation or infection of the prostate or bladder and calculi. In patients over age 35, hematuria is associated with a higher risk of benign prostatic hyperplasia and renal or GU malignancies.

■ Patients on oral anticoagulants and those with a high international normalized ratio (INR) are at higher risk of hematuria. Even if present in such patients, it is necessary to investigate for alternative source(s) of the condition.

■ Isolated hematuria occurs in patients with calculi, trauma, prostatitis, sickle cell trait or disease, tuberculosis, and *Schistosoma haematobium* infection. Acute cystitis or urethritis in women can cause gross hematuria. Hypercalciuria and hyperuricosuria are also risk factors for unexplained isolated hematuria.

■ *Benign familial* or *recurrent hematuria* refers to asymptomatic, recurrent hematuria without proteinuria or other laboratory abnormalities. Persistent or recurrent hematuria, even if only microscopic, should be investigated, especially in patients over age 50. Other family members may be affected. The condition may clear spontaneously.

❑ **Laboratory Findings**

■ The single most important test in the evaluation of hematuria is the microscopic analysis of urine sediment, which can often distinguish glomerular from nonglomerular bleeding.

■ Microscopy of centrifuged urinary sediment should be examined under high dry magnification. Note that <3% of normal persons have ≥3 RBC per HPF. RBCs or casts indicate that the blood is of glomerular origin. The most common causes of isolated glomerular hematuria are IgA nephropathy, hereditary nephritis (Alport syndrome), and thin basement membrane disease. The presence of clots rules out a glomerular origin—large thick clots suggest a bladder origin, whereas small stringy clots indicate upper urinary tract disease. The presence of WBCs suggests inflammation or infection.

■ The urine dipstick can detect RBCs at a level equivalent to one to two RBCs per HPF, but results in more false-positive tests owing to a number of interfering factors (listed below), and so a positive dipstick test must be confirmed by microscopic examination of the urine. Proteinuria is also detected by dipstick, and a 2+ proteinuria in the presence of microscopic hematuria indicates glomerular disease.

■ Immunocytochemical staining for human Tamm-Horsfall protein is positive with >80% of RBCs of renal origin and <13.1% of RBCs of nonrenal origin.

■ Imaging studies, urinary cytology, cystoscopy, or occasionally renal biopsy may be indicated in cases of persistent hematuria with no obvious etiology.

❑ **Limitations on the Urine Dipstick Test**

■ Causes of false-positive results
  ▼ Vaginal bleeding (menstruation)
  ▼ Viral illness
  ▼ Bacteriuria
  ▼ Certain foods (beets, blackberries, rhubarb)
  ▼ Pigmenturia (myoglobin, porphyrin, hemoglobin)
  ▼ Drugs (rifampin, phenolphthalein, iodides, bromides, copper, oxidizing agents, permanganate)
  ▼ Postejaculate semen
  ▼ Red diaper syndrome
  ▼ Trauma
  ▼ Vigorous exercise prior to collection

- ▼ pH > 9
- ▼ Factitious
- Causes of false-negative results
  - ▼ Reducing agents (high doses of vitamin C)
  - ▼ pH < 5.1

Suggested Readings

Cohen RA, Brown RS. Clinical practice. Microscopic hematuria. *N Engl J Med.* 2003;348:2330–2338.

Grossfeld GD, Litwin MS, Wolf JS, et al. Evaluation of asymptomatic microscopic hematuria in adults: the American Urological Association best practice policy—part I: definition, detection, prevalence, and etiology. *Urology.* 2001;57:599–603.

HEMOGLOBINURIA

❑ Definition

- Hemoglobinuria refers to the presence of free hemoglobin (Hb) in urine. The condition is often associated with hemolytic anemia, wherein intravascular red cell destruction increases levels of free plasma Hb. The excess Hb is filtered by the kidneys and excreted into the urine where it is visibly detected. The renal threshold for hemoglobinuria is 100–140 mg Hb/dL plasma.
- Although free Hb directly passing the glomeruli in the ultrafiltrate is relatively uncommon (usually, RBCs enter the urinary tract and undergo various amounts of lysis), nevertheless, conditions resulting in intravascular hemolysis have the potential of producing hemoglobinuria once all available plasma haptoglobin is bound by Hb. Hb is readily absorbed by the renal proximal tubules as dissociated dimers and catabolized to ferritin. In turn, ferritin is denatured to hemosiderin that can be found in urine in cases of severe, prolonged hemoglobinuria.

❑ Who Should Be Suspected?

- Candidates include patients with red urine but no red cells in urinary sediment, especially if there is a history suggesting intravascular hemolysis. The classic patient with hemolysis may have many of the following findings: rapid onset of pallor, anemia, jaundice, a history of pigmented (bilirubin) gallstones, splenomegaly, the presence of circulating spherocytic or fragmented red cells on the peripheral blood smear, and/or a positive direct antiglobulin test (Coombs test).
- Inciting causes of hemoglobinuria fall into several categories:
  - ▼ Hemolytic anemias with intravascular hemolysis
    - Paroxysmal nocturnal hemoglobinuria
    - Paroxysmal cold hemoglobinuria
    - Microangiopathic hemolytic anemias (thrombotic thrombocytopenic purpura/hemolytic uremic syndrome), prosthetic heart valves, severely damaged natural valves (especially aortic)
    - Severe autoimmune hemolytic anemias
    - Fava bean sensitivity, G6PD deficiency, and other hemoglobinopathies
    - Severe hereditary spherocytosis
  - ▼ Other hematologic crises (e.g., disseminated intravascular coagulation [DIC], incompatible transfusion reactions).

▼ Infections (e.g., *Clostridium perfringens* [previously known as *Clostridium welchii*]; *E. coli* bacteremia from transfused blood; *Bartonella bacilliformis*, the agent of Oroya fever or Carrion disease).

▼ Parasitemias (e.g., malaria).

▼ Organ damage (e.g., kidney infarction, diabetic acidosis).

▼ Physical or chemical trauma (e.g., strenuous exercise, march hemoglobinuria, thermal burns, infusion or bladder irrigation with hypotonic solutions, naphthalene, sulfa drugs).

❏ **Laboratory Findings**

▪ The diagnosis of intravascular hemolysis is usually based on the medical history and analysis of blood and urine specimens. A positive dipstick test and the microscopic absence of urine RBCs and RBC casts suggest hemoglobinuria or myoglobinuria.

▪ Serum LDH and haptoglobin: The combination of an increased level of serum LDH and a reduced level of haptoglobin has been shown to be 90% specific for the diagnosis of hemolysis, whereas the combination of a normal serum LDH and a serum haptoglobin >25 mg/dL has been shown to be 92% sensitive for ruling out hemolysis.

▪ Free Hb: In correlation with hemosiderin in the urine sediment, the finding of free Hb in the plasma and/or urine is highly specific for the presence of intravascular hemolysis.

▪ Spectrophotometry: Presence of Hb in both urine and plasma (deoxy Hb highest absorption peak is at 420 nm, with a secondary peak at 580 nm) is indicative of intravascular hemolysis.

▪ Serum conjugated bilirubin and urine urobilinogen: Both are elevated with hemolysis.

❏ **Limitations**

▪ Causes of false-positive dipstick results
  ▼ Delayed processing of hematuria specimen, resulting in hemolysis of RBCs
  ▼ Non-Hb urine pigments that may mimic hemoglobinuria (myoglobin, porphyrin)
  ▼ Presence of pus, iodides, or bromides

Suggested Readings

Marchand A, Galen RS, Van Lente F. The predictive value of serum haptoglobin in hemolytic disease. *JAMA.* 1980;243:1909–1911.

Prahl S. Optical absorption of hemoglobin. http:omlc.ogi.edu/spectra/hemoglobin. December 15, 1999.

HYPEROXALURIAS

❏ **Definitions**

▪ Primary hyperoxalurias (PHs) are rare inborn errors of glyoxylate metabolism, characterized by the overproduction of oxalate, which is deposited as calcium oxalate in various organs, primarily the kidneys. End-stage renal disease results in a significant number of cases. PH types 1–3 stem from autosomal recessive enzymatic defects in

- ▼ (PH type 1) the hepatic peroxisomal enzyme alanine:glyoxylate aminotransferase, which is involved in the conversion of glyoxylate to glycine (80% of PH cases)
- ▼ (PH type 2) the cytosolic glyoxylate reductase/hydroxypyruvate reductase, which is involved in the conversion of glyoxylate to glycolate (10% of PH cases)
- ▼ (PH type 3) the mitochondrial 4-hydroxy-2-oxoglutarate aldolase (5% of PH cases)
- ■ Secondary hyperoxaluria results from increased enteric absorption of oxalate, most commonly caused by fat malabsorption via the binding of calcium by free fatty acids in the colon. This decreases the amount of calcium available to bind to oxalate for the formation of insoluble calcium oxalate, leaving the free oxalate to be more easily absorbed.
  - ▼ Specific disorders of fat malabsorption result from pancreatic insufficiency, inflammatory bowel disease, bowel resection or jejunoileal or gastric bypass, use of the weight reduction drug orlistat (which causes fat malabsorption by inhibiting gastric and pancreatic lipases), and cystic fibrosis (which causes pancreatic insufficiency and promotes calcium deposition via hypercalciuria).
  - ▼ Secondary hyperoxaluria may also be precipitated by the chronic ingestion of oxalate precursors (e.g., ascorbic acid) or of foods rich in oxalic acid (e.g., rhubarb, parsley, cocoa, nuts, or star fruit [carambola]).

❑ Who Should Be Suspected?

- ■ PH type 1: The age range at diagnosis varies from <1 to >50.
  - ▼ Infants (26% of PH type 1 cases) are generally diagnosed younger than 6 months of age with nephrocalcinosis (91%), failure to thrive (22%), urinary tract infection (21%), and end-stage renal disease (ERSD, 14%).
  - ▼ Those diagnosed in childhood generally present with symptoms of recurrent urolithiasis and rapidly declining renal function (30%), that is, renal colic, hematuria, and urinary tract infection, although a few will have bilateral obstruction and acute renal failure.
  - ▼ Adults are diagnosed either by the occasional calculus formation (30%) or only after failed isolated renal transplant (10%).

❑ Laboratory Findings

- ■ Urinary oxalate: PH type 1 or 2, usually >100 mg/24 hours unless renal function is diminished; secondary disease, usually 50–100 mg/24 hours.
- ■ Molecular genetic testing (PH type 1): Demonstrates the mutation of the alanine:glyoxylate aminotransferase (AGXT) gene.

Suggested Readings

Hoppe B. An update on primary hyperoxaluria. *Nat Rev Nephrol.* 2012;8:467–475.
Hoppe B, Leumann E, von Unruh G, et al. Diagnostic and therapeutic approaches in patients with secondary hyperoxaluria. *Front Biosci.* 2003;8:e437–e443.

PRIAPISM

❑ **Definition**

■ Priapism is a persistent erection of the penis (or clitoris), lasting at least 4 hours, that is not associated with sexual stimulation or desire. This relatively rare condition can occur in all age groups (although it exhibits a bimodal peak distribution of incidence at ages 5–10 and 20–50) and is especially common in those with sickle cell disease. Classified as either ischemic or non-ischemic, ischemic priapism is a urologic emergency, whereas nonischemic priapism is usually self-limited.

■ Ischemic (low flow, anoxic, or venoocclusive) priapism is the most common form of the condition. The prolonged nitric oxide–mediated relaxation and paralysis of cavernosal smooth muscle results in a compartment syndrome with increasing hypoxia and acidosis in the cavernous tissue. Structural damage to the erectile tissue is believed to occur at the microscopic level as early as 4–6 hours after the onset of the erection, with significant structural changes in the cavernous smooth muscle after 12 hours and irreversible damage as early as 24 hours after onset.

■ Nonischemic (high flow, arterial, or congenital) priapism usually results from a fistula between the cavernosal artery and the corpus cavernosum. It commonly follows penile or perineal trauma, or blunt trauma (such as from bicycling). It may also stem from a congenital arterial malformation. In any event, nonischemic priapism is not an emergency condition because the cavernous blood is well oxygenated.

■ Recurrent (stuttering) priapism is a form of the ischemic condition (usually occurring in men with sickle cell anemia), which begins with erections of short duration (usually during sleep), then persisting on waking, becoming of longer duration, and increasing frequency until transforming into the classical ischemic form.

❑ **Who Should Be Suspected?**

■ Patients typically present with an erection of 2–4 hours in the absence of sexual excitation. The duration may be shorter for patients with recurrent priapism.

■ Causes can be classified into seven categories:
  ▼ Thromboembolic disease (sickle cell disease or trait, polycythemia, pelvic thrombophlebitis)
  ▼ Infiltrative diseases (e.g., leukemia, bladder or prostate carcinoma)
  ▼ Penile trauma
  ▼ CNS infection (e.g., syphilis, TB) or spinal cord injury or anesthesia
  ▼ Intracavernous injectables for treatment of erectile dysfunction (papaverine, alprostadil, phentolamine)
  ▼ Other medications: Antihypertensives, antipsychotics (e.g., chlorpromazine, clozapine), antidepressants (especially trazodone), anticoagulants, testosterone, heparin, and recreational drugs (alcohol, cocaine, marijuana, cantharides)
  ▼ Other causes: Prostatitis and retroperitoneal bleeding. Phosphodiesterase type 5 (PDE5) inhibitors (sildenafil, tadalafil, vardenafil) have only rarely been implicated.

❑ **Laboratory Findings**

- Cavernous blood gas analysis and/or Doppler ultrasonography can be used to distinguish immediately ischemic from nonischemic priapism persisting longer than 4 hours.
- A volume of 3–5 mL is aspirated with a 19- to 21-gauge needle from one side of the corpus cavernosum.
  - ▼ The color of ischemic blood will be black, and blood gas analysis will reveal hypoxia, hypercarbia, and acidemia.
  - ▼ The color of nonischemic blood will be red, and blood gas analysis will reveal normal levels of oxygen, carbon dioxide, and pH.

Suggested Readings

Burnett AL, Bivalacqua TJ. Priapism: current principles and practice. *Urol Clin North Am.* 2007;34:631–642.

Cherian J, Rao AR, Thwaini A, et al. Medical and surgical management of priapism. *Postgrad Med J.* 2006;82:89–94.

7

RETROPERITONEAL FIBROSIS

❑ **Definition**

- Retroperitoneal fibrosis (formerly Ormond disease) is a rare condition (incidence of 0.1–1.3 per 100,000 for the idiopathic form) characterized by the proliferation of inflammatory and fibrous tissue in the retroperitoneum, often encasing the ureters or abdominal organs and resulting in ureteral blockage.
- The disorder occurs primarily (70% of cases) in idiopathic form among individuals at age 40–60 (70%). There are also secondary forms of the disorder with a variety of identified causes (certain drugs, malignancies, infections, radiation therapy, retroperitoneal hemorrhage, and surgical sequelae).
- The pathogenesis of the disorder is unclear, but two leading theories suggest (each with some evidence) either an exaggerated local inflammatory reaction to aortic atherosclerosis (incited by oxidized low-density lipoprotein) or a manifestation of systemic autoimmune disease.

❑ **Who Should Be Suspected?**

- Compiling the data from four studies, the most common presenting symptoms are pain in the lower back, abdomen, and/or flank (28–90%); testicular pain (50–64%); fatigue (60%); substantial weight loss (54%); and new-onset hypertension (33–57%). Urinary symptoms (urgency, frequency, and dysuria) are also common. Most patients have renal impairment by the time they are seen for medical attention.

❑ **Laboratory Findings**

- The diagnostic method of choice is a contrast-enhanced CT scan to visualize the extent of fibrosis, to assess the presence of lymphadenopathy and tumors, and to enable guided biopsy for tissue analysis.

- Although there are no biochemical or hematologic markers of the disorder, ureteral obstruction is assessed by measurements of BUN and serum creatinine concentration. Both are usually elevated in correlation with the presence and extent of obstruction.
- The inflammatory level of the disorder is assessed by measurement of the erythrocyte sedimentation rate and C-reactive protein, both of which are elevated in the majority of patients at presentation.
- Antinuclear antibodies may be found in up to 60% of cases.
- Anemia is found in up to 38% of cases.

Suggested Readings

Vaglio A, Salvarani C, Buzio C. Retroperitoneal fibrosis. *Lancet.* 2006;367:241–251.
van Bommel EF, Jansen I, Hendriksz TR, et al. Idiopathic retroperitoneal fibrosis: prospective evaluation of incidence and clinicoradiologic presentation. *Medicine* (Baltimore). 2009;88:193–201.

 INFECTIONS

URINARY TRACT INFECTIONS*

Urinary tract infections (UTIs) are among the most common infections encountered in both outpatient and inpatient settings.

❑ Definitions and Key Concepts

- Most UTIs are restricted to infection of the bladder (cystitis), though infection may occur in any area of the urinary tract, from the kidney to urethra.
- Most UTIs are caused by uropathogenic organisms from the gastrointestinal or vaginal florae that colonize the periurethral mucosa. Organisms are able to ascend through the urethra to the bladder by various mechanisms.
- Acute cystitis that occurs in healthy (including no history suggestive of urinary tract abnormality), premenopausal, nonpregnant women is classified as *uncomplicated*. All other UTIs are classified as *complicated*.
- Uncomplicated cystitis rarely progresses to severe infection. The goal of antibiotic therapy of uncomplicated cystitis is for amelioration of symptoms.
- Most UTIs are caused by a single uropathogenic species. Polymicrobial infections may occur in patients with anatomical abnormalities or foreign bodies, but suspect colonization or culture contamination for cultures that yield growth of more than two different species.
- Etiology: *E. coli* causes >75% of all uncomplicated UTIs. Most other UTIs are caused by other enteric gram-negative bacilli (e.g., *K. pneumoniae* and *P. mirabilis*) and gram-positive cocci (e.g., *Enterococcus* species, *S. saprophyticus*, Group B streptococcus). Resistant organisms (e.g., *C. albicans*, *P. aeruginosa*) are usually associated with nosocomial and health care–related UTIs.
- Renal tissues may be infected by ascending infection through the ureters or by hematogenous seeding during bacteremia.

---

*Written by Michael Mitchell, MD.

- *Asymptomatic bacteriuria* is defined by a urine culture, submitted by a patient without dysuria or other symptoms of UTI, that yields growth of $>10^5$ cfu/mL of a single uropathogen. Pregnant women with asymptomatic bacteriuria are at increased risk for developing UTI, including pyelonephritis, and low birth weight infants. Screening for asymptomatic bacteriuria with a routine urine culture at 12–16 weeks of gestation is recommended. Antibiotic treatment significantly reduces the risks associated with asymptomatic bacteriuria in pregnant women. The clinical value of treating asymptomatic bacteriuria in men or in nonpregnant women has not been established. Screening for asymptomatic bacteriuria in these groups is not recommended.
- *Renal abscess*: Most renal abscesses occur in the setting of obstructive pyelonephritis, caused by ascending infection. Predisposing factors include diabetes, renal stones, tumor, neurogenic bladder, and vesicoureteral reflux. Enteric bacilli are implicated most frequently, but polymicrobial infections occur commonly. Renal abscess and perinephric abscess may also occur as a result of hematologic seeding of the renal parenchyma or perirenal fat and are usually caused by *S. aureus*. Signs and symptoms of renal or perinephric abscess are similar to those of severe pyelonephritis.
- *Sterile pyuria*: Conditions other than acute bacterial UTI should be considered for patients with pyuria (≥ 10 WBC/HPF) and negative urine culture. Potential causes include infectious conditions (e.g., renal tuberculosis, urethritis/STI, prostatitis, and viral cystitis or genital infection) and noninfectious conditions (e.g., inflammation by exposure to allergen or chemical agent, mechanical irritation due to stone or instrumentation, renal diseases associated with inflammation).

❏ Who Should Be Suspected/Who Should Be Tested?

- Risk factors for complicated UTI:
  - ▼ *Pregnancy*
  - ▼ *Urinary tract abnormality*, including anatomical obstruction, indwelling foreign body, recent surgery, or instrumentation
  - ▼ *Medical conditions*, including diabetes, underlying renal disease, immunosuppression, history of complicated UTI, or recent hospitalization
- Clinical signs and symptoms
  - ▼ *Cystitis*: Dysuria, urgency, frequency, suprapubic pain, hematuria.
  - ▼ *Pyelonephritis*: Fever (>38°C), flank pain, costovertebral angle tenderness, nausea, vomiting, malaise. Signs and symptoms of cystitis are common. Patients may present with signs of sepsis and multiple organ failure.
  - ▼ Nonspecific symptoms (like failure to thrive or feeding difficulties) may be the only symptoms of UTI in infants and elderly patients.
- In uncomplicated UTI, patients respond rapidly to effective antibiotic therapy. Further evaluation, including urinalysis and culture, is recommended for patients with persistent symptoms or early recurrence to rule out pathogen resistant to initial therapy or to rule out other factors associated with complicated UTI.

❑ **Diagnostic and Laboratory Findings**

■ Uncomplicated UTI can be reliably diagnosed on the basis of typical symptoms. Urinalysis and urine culture are not routinely needed; patients may be treated empirically.

■ Uninalysis and urine culture should be performed for patients if complicated UTI is suspected, and for patients with symptoms of pyelonephritis.

■ Diagnostic Tests

▼ **Urinalysis** (dipstick or microscopic): Dipstick urinalysis performs best when urine culture yields growth >10^5 cfu/mL and dipstick shows positive leukocyte esterase and nitrite reactions (sensitivity 84%; specificity 98%). Sensitivity was significantly lower when the urine culture yielded growth <10^5 cfu/mL. The urine dipstick is not a reliable screen to rule out UTI.

However, urinalysis has good specificity and may provide evidence to support a diagnosis of UTI. Most patients with UTI have pyuria (WBCs by microscopy or dipstick leukocyte esterase); WBC casts suggest pyelonephritis. Proteinuria and hematuria are also frequent findings. A positive dipstick nitrite reaction is typical for UTI caused by *E. coli* and other *Enterobacteriaceae*, but may be negative for other uropathogens, like *Enterococcus* species, *Pseudomonas* species and *S. saprophyticus*.

Algorithms using dipstick urinalysis have been proposed to reduce unnecessary antibiotic use while awaiting culture results. In patients at low risk for complicated UTI, three variables were used: dysuria, leukocytes greater than trace, and any positive nitrite reaction, including trace. Patients positive for two or three variables were treated without culture; culture was collected for patients with no or one positive variable and antibiotics withheld pending culture results. Using the algorithm, 80% of significant UTIs were detected; unnecessary antibiotic prescriptions were reduced by 23.5% and urine cultures by 59% compared with usual physician care.

▼ **Gram stain:** Gram stain of an unconcentrated urine may be useful for detecting urine specimens that yield growth >10^5 cfu/mL, but are not reliable for detecting specimens that yield lower level, but significant growth. Because of the limited sensitivity for detecting significant cultures, and because of the labor intensity to perform, Gram staining is not recommended for urine specimens.

▼ **Routine culture:** Quantitative culture is performed by inoculation of 1 microliter of urine onto SBA and selective (e.g., MacConkey or CNA) agar. The lower level of detection, therefore, is 10^3 cfu/mL. The extent of workup (identification and susceptibility testing) depends on several factors, including: type of specimen (clean catch versus invasively collected), number of species isolated (pure culture versus mixed), pathogenic potential of isolate (typical uropathogen versus common contaminant) and quantity of growth.

Laboratory workup is usually limited (descriptive ID only; no susceptibility testing) for cultures that yield mixed growth (3 or more species in comparable quantities), organisms with low uropathogenic potential (like *Lactobacillus* and diphtheroids), or isolates growing in quantities <10^4 cfu/mL.

▼ **Culture for possible complicated UTI:** For symptomatic patients at risk for complicated UTI, bacteriuria at quantities <10^{3-4} cfu/mL may predict significant UTI. For such patients, culture methods using a 10-microliter inoculum allow detection of growth at a lower detection limit of 10^2 cfu/mL. The extent of workup follows similar guidelines used for routine cultures, except that full ID and appropriate susceptibility testing is performed when one or two uropathogens are isolated in quantities >10^3 cfu/mL (versus the 10^4 cfu/mL cutoff used for routine cultures).

Urine culture may be normal in patients with renal or perinephric abscess if the infected tissue does not communicate with the collecting system. Drainage of such localized infections is performed for therapeutic reasons, as well as to collect material for culture, Gram stain and any other laboratory evaluation.

- Other Laboratory Testing:
  - ▼ Pregnancy testing may be appropriate for women presenting with otherwise uncomplicated UTI.
  - ▼ In patients with complicated UTI, blood cultures are recommended for patients with fever, hypotension, or other signs of sepsis. Other laboratory testing appropriate for the clinical presentation is recommended.

Suggested Readings

Cai T, Mazzoli S, Mondaini N, et al. The role of asymptomatic bacteriuria in young women with recurrent urinary tract infections: to treat or not to treat. *Clin Infect Dis.* 2012;55:771–777.

Gorgon LB, Waxman MJ, Ragsdale L, et al. Overtreatment of presumed urinary tract infection in older women presenting to the emergency department. *J Am Geriatr Soc.* 2013;61:788–792.

Hooton TM. Uncomplicated urinary tract infection. *N Engl J Med.* 2012;366:1028–1037.

McIsaac WJ, Moineddin R, Ross S. Validation of a decision aid to assist physicians in reducing unnecessary antibiotic drug use for acute cystis. *Arch Intern Med.* 2007;167:2201–2206.

Nicolle LE, Bradley S, Colgan R, et al. Infectious diseases society of America guidelines for the diagnosis and treatment of asymptomatic bacteriuria in adults. *Clin Infect Dis.* 2005;40:643–654.

Semeniuk H, Church D. Evaluation of the leukocyte esterase and nitrite urine dipstick screening tests for detection of bacteriuria in women with suspected uncomplicated urinary tract infections. *J Clin Microbiol.* 1999;37:3051–3052.

U.S. Preventive Services Task Force. Recommendation statement: screening for asymptomatic bacteriuria in adults. *Ann Intern Med.* 2008;149:43–47. See: www.uspreventiveservicestaskforce.org/uspstf08/asymptbact/asbactsum.htm

Wilson ML, Gaido L. Laboratory diagnosis of urinary tract infections in adult patients. *Clin Infect Dis.* 2004;38:1150–1158.

TUBERCULOSIS, RENAL[‡]

❑ Definitions and Key Concepts

- Renal tuberculosis is a common form of extrapulmonary tuberculosis. The disease is caused by hematogenous seeding of the kidney during mycobacteremia that may occur during primary infection or late reactivation with miliary dissemination.

❑ Who Should Be Suspected/Who Should Be Tested?

- The clinical manifestations of renal TB are variable; many patients show minimal symptoms and may be identified after workup for pyuria or microscopic hema-

---

[‡]Written by Michael J. Mitchell, MD.

turia, which are almost universally seen. Systemic symptoms are uncommon. Patients may complain of dysuria; gross hematuria may occur.

- Diagnosis should be suspected in a patient with a history or increased risk of mycobacterial disease, especially TB, and signs (e.g., microhematuria or pyuria) or symptoms (e.g., dysuria) of UTI. Routine urine culture is negative, although contaminated urine or coincidental UTI may confound the diagnosis.

❑ **Diagnostic and Laboratory Findings**

- Patients with possible renal tuberculosis should be evaluated for pulmonary tuberculosis and infection at other extrapulmonary sites, as appropriate. Testing should include screening (e.g., TST), culture and imaging studies, as well as detailed physical examination and history.
- Mycobacteria are shed intermittently, so four to six first-morning samples should be submitted for mycobacterial culture. Mycobacterial culture of samples from other potentially infected sites is also recommended, as well as skin (or comparable) testing for TB. False-positive AFB smears may be seen due to nonpathogenic mycobacteria.
- Urinalysis typically shows WBCs; WBC casts are unusual. Some degree of hematuria is demonstrated in most patients.
- Renal function tests are usually normal; heavy proteinuria is uncommon.

EPIDIDYMITIS

❑ **Definition**

- Epididymitis is inflammation of the epididymis. The epididymis stores sperm cells received from the tubules of the rete testis, facilitates their maturation, and ultimately delivers them to the vas deferens.

❑ **Who Should Be Suspected?**

- Epididymitis most commonly has an infectious etiology, presenting as either an acute condition (<6 weeks) or, more typically, chronic (≥6 weeks). The acute presentation is characterized by severe scrotal swelling and exquisite pain, often accompanied by high fever, rigors, and irritative voiding symptoms (frequency, urgency, and dysuria). The chronic presentation includes scrotal pain but usually lacks irritative voiding symptoms. Asymptomatic urethritis often accompanies epididymitis originating with sexually transmitted agents.
- Noninfectious epididymitis (precipitated by, e.g., trauma, autoimmune disease, or vasculitis) generally presents as a chronic condition, with less pain and swelling (less epididymal inflammation).
- The differential diagnosis of epididymitis should consider a range of other sources of scrotal pain and swelling, e.g., testicular torsion, Fournier gangrene (necrotizing fasciitis of the perineum with mixed aerobic/ anaerobic bacteria), trauma/surgery, testicular cancer, inguinal hernia, Henoch-Schönlein purpura (IgA vasculitis), or epididymo-orchitis (e.g., post-mumps).

❏ Laboratory Findings (Infectious Epididymitis)

- A urinalysis and urine culture should be performed on all patients suspected of urethritis. A urethral swab should be obtained in patients with urethral discharge and sent for culture and nucleic acid amplification testing for chlamydia and gonorrhea.
- In sexually active men under age 35, *Chlamydia trachomatis* and *Neisseria gonorrhoeae* are the most frequent causative agents. Combined infections by both agents are more frequently found than infections by *N. gonorrhoeae* alone.
- In men over age 35, *Escherichia coli*, other coliforms, and *Pseudomonas* species are more common. Less common pathogens include *Ureaplasma* species, *Mycobacterium tuberculosis*, and *Brucella* species, cytomegalovirus or *Cryptococcus* (patients with HIV infection).
- In boys before puberty, *E. coli* is a common cause.
- In children, epididymitis may be a response following infection by enterovirus, adenovirus, or *Mycoplasma pneumoniae*.

Suggested Readings

Doble A, Taylor-Robinson D, Thomas BJ, et al. Acute epididymitis: a microbiological and ultrasonographic study. *Br J Urol.* 1989;63:90–94.
Hawkins DA, Taylor-Robinson D, Thomas BJ, et al. Microbiological survey of acute epididymitis. *Genitourin Med.* 1986;62:342–344.
Wampler SM, Llanes M. Common scrotal and testicular problems. *Prim Care.* 2010;37: 613–626.

7

PROSTATITIS

❏ Definition

- Prostatitis refers to histologic inflammation of the prostate gland, although the term is used loosely to describe several different conditions. The 1999 classification system of the National Institutes of Health Prostatitis Collaborative Network comprises four classes of prostatitis:
  - ▼ I. Acute bacterial prostatitis: Acute urogenital symptoms, with evidence of bacterial infection of the prostate. Route of entry is nearly always via the urethra or bladder through the prostatic duct, with intraprostatic reflux of urine and, sometimes, concomitant infection of the bladder or epididymis.
  - ▼ II. Chronic bacterial prostatitis: Chronic or recurrent urogenital symptoms with evidence of bacterial infection of the prostate. The route of entry is the same as for acute bacterial prostatitis.
  - ▼ IIIA. Chronic prostatitis/chronic pelvic pain syndrome, inflammatory: Chronic or recurrent urogenital symptoms with evidence of inflammation but not bacterial infection of the prostate.
  - ▼ IIIB. Chronic prostatitis/chronic pelvic pain syndrome, noninflammatory: Chronic or recurrent urogenital symptoms without evidence of inflammation or bacterial infection of the prostate.
  - ▼ IV. Asymptomatic inflammatory prostatitis: Absence of urogenital symptoms; evidence of inflammation of the prostate is found incidentally.

❑ Who Should Be Suspected?

- Acute bacterial prostatitis (WHO class I) is manifested by a spiking fever, chills, malaise, myalgia, dysuria, irritative urinary symptoms (frequency, urgency, urge incontinence), pelvic or perineal pain, and cloudy urine. On exam, the prostate is often warm, firm, edematous, and exquisitely tender.
- Chronic bacterial prostatitis (WHO class II) is manifested (in a minority of patients) by symptoms of recurrent urinary tract infection (frequency, dysuria, urgency) with repeated isolation of the same organism from urine, perineal discomfort, and occasionally a low-grade fever.

  However, other patients may be asymptomatic, with persistent or recurrent bacteria in urine found incidentally during a workup for lower abdominal/perineal/genital pain or bladder irritation/obstruction.
- Chronic prostatitis/chronic pelvic pain syndrome (CP/CPPS) is manifested by chronic pelvic pain for at least three of the preceding 6 months in the absence of other identifiable causes. Despite the name, it is uncertain that the symptoms can be traced to the prostate. WHO class IIIA CP/CPPS includes patients with inflammatory cells in expressed prostatic secretions, post–prostate massage urine, or seminal fluid. WHO class IIIB includes the balance of patients with chronic prostatitis or pelvic pain.
- Asymptomatic inflammatory prostatitis (WHO class IV) is usually diagnosed incidentally, during prostate biopsy or during a workup for infertility or cancer. The natural history of the syndrome is not well understood.

❑ Laboratory Findings

- Acute bacterial prostatitis (WHO class I)
  - ▼ Blood: leukocytosis and an elevated serum prostate-specific antigen (PSA) support the diagnosis and should be followed by a digital rectal exam.
  - ▼ Urine: A Gram stain and culture should be obtained in all suspected cases. Bacteria causing acute prostatitis are easily recoverable from urine (prostate massage is contraindicated in suspected acute prostatitis, because it may induce sepsis). Culture usually reveals the causative organism (unless antibiotics were used recently).
  - ▼ Recovered organisms are generally those that induce UTI and urethritis: *Escherichia coli, Klebsiella, Proteus, Pseudomonas, Enterobacter, Enterococcus, Serratia,* and *Staphylococcus aureus.*
  - ▼ WBCs are found in the centrifuged urine sediment of the last portion of the voided urine specimen.
- Chronic bacterial prostatitis (WHO class II)
  - ▼ A presumptive diagnosis relies on chronic (>3 months) or recurrent urogenital symptoms, especially if bacteriuria is present. The standard diagnostic confirmation test is the Meares-Stamey four-glass test, which compares cultured bacterial colony counts in the first 5–10 mL (urethral) and midstream (bladder) urine specimens, a prostatic secretion (expressed by a 1-minute gentle prostate massage), and the first 5–10 mL of post–prostatic massage voided urine. If the bacteriuria baseline is

$<10^3$/mL, chronic bacterial prostatitis is suspected if the leukocyte count in the prostatic secretion is >12 per high-power field and confirmed if >20 per high-power field (unless leukocytes were also present in the bladder urine specimen). A simpler "two-glass" method compares cultured bacterial colony counts collected from the midstream urine specimen (followed by the prostate massage) with the post–prostatic massage voided urine. This simpler method has a 100% positive and 96% negative predictive value.

▼ Cultures of the post–prostatic massage urine or expressed prostatic secretions are nearly always positive for bacteria. Repeated isolations of the same organism over time confirm the agent.

▼ Limitation: *Chlamydia trachomatis* will not grow in culture, so negative results by urine and prostatic secretion cultures should be followed by nucleic acid testing for this organism.

■ Chronic prostatitis/chronic pelvic pain syndrome (WHO classes IIIA and IIIB)

▼ A urinalysis should be performed on any patient suspected of prostatitis. The presence of hematuria should be followed up by urine cytology (for carcinoma in situ of the bladder), cystoscopy, and potentially upper tract imaging.

▼ A urine culture should also be performed to rule out a UTI. A recurrent UTI should be evaluated for chronic bacterial prostatitis (class II syndrome).

▼ Although bacterial infection has been implicated (especially in class IIIA), no agent has been consistently identified by culture or found by polymerase chain reaction (PCR) testing. Moreover, there is little correlation between histologic evidence of inflammation and the presence or absence of symptoms. The differential diagnosis is one of exclusion:

  ● There is no low-grade fever (which can occur in the class II syndrome)
  ● There is no prostatic hypertrophy, tenderness, or edema by rectal examination (as in the class II syndrome)
  ● There are no systemic or neurologic symptoms (as in urethritis, urogenital cancer, urinary tract disease, urethral stricture, or neurologic disease affecting the bladder)

Suggested Readings

Gamé X, Vincendeau S, Palascak R, et al. Total and free serum prostate specific antigen levels during the first month of acute prostatitis. *Eur Urol.* 2003;43:702–705.

Krieger JN, Nyberg L Jr, Nickel JC. NIH consensus definition and classification of prostatitis. *JAMA.* 1999;282:236–237.

Nickel JC, Nyberg LM, Hennenfent M. Research guidelines for chronic prostatitis: consensus report from the first National Institutes of Health International Prostatitis Collaborative Network. *Urology.* 1999;54:229–234.

Nickel JC, Shoskes D, Wang Y, et al. How does the pre-massage and post-massage 2-glass test compare to the Meares-Stamey 4-glass test in men with chronic prostatitis/chronic pelvic pain syndrome? *J Urol.* 2006;176:119–124.

Schaeffer AJ. Clinical practice. Chronic prostatitis and the chronic pelvic pain syndrome. *N Engl J Med.* 2006;355:1690–1698.

INFERTILITY

OVERVIEW

❑ **Definition**

- Infertility is defined as the inability to conceive after 12 or more months of regular intercourse without contraception.
- For a couple of normal fertility, the likelihood of pregnancy not occurring by 12 months is only 7%, which is close to the 5% figure often used as a threshold for a type 1 statistical error (here, falsely rejecting the null hypothesis of normal fertility). The likelihood of normal fertility decreases to 1% if pregnancy has not occurred after 3 years of intercourse without contraception. In a meta-analysis of 25 population surveys from 1991 to 2006, sampling 172,413 women, the 12-month prevalence rate of infertility ranged from 3.5 to 16.7% in more developed nations and 6.9 to 9.3% in developing nations.
- For those couples who have not been able to conceive despite 12 months of intercourse without contraception, a standard infertility evaluation is warranted for both partners. A two-part algorithm for the systematic assessment of the male partner is presented in Figure 7-2.
- Although there is an uncertain relationship between abnormalities found on tests of infertility versus actual causes of infertility, one population-based study reported the following results for all factors of infertility (male and female combined):
  - ▼ Male factors: 23%
  - ▼ Ovulatory disorders: 18%
  - ▼ Tubal damage: 14%
  - ▼ Endometriosis: 9%
  - ▼ Coital problems (e.g., impotence): 5%
  - ▼ Cervical factors: 3%
  - ▼ Unexplained: 28%
- Male factors of infertility can be divided into four general categories, of which the first three are amenable to laboratory diagnosis:
  - ▼ Testicular disease (primary defects, including Y chromosome deletions) (30–40%)
  - ▼ Posttesticular defects (disorders of sperm transport) (10–20%)
  - ▼ Secondary hypogonadism (1–2%)
  - ▼ Idiopathic (normal semen analysis, no other apparent cause) (40–50%)
- Female factors of infertility can also be divided into four general categories, of which the first category and hyperprolactinemia are amenable to laboratory diagnosis:
  - ▼ Ovulatory disorders (25%)
  - ▼ Tubal blockages or abnormalities (22%)
  - ▼ Endometriosis (15%)
  - ▼ Pelvic adhesions, hyperprolactinemia, and idiopathic (38%)

Approach to diagnosis of male infertility

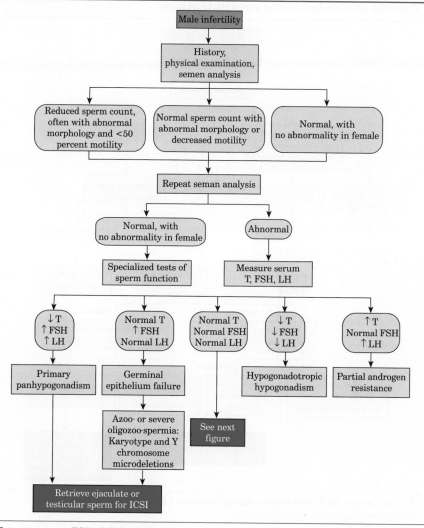

T: testosterone; FSH: follicle-stimulating hormone; LH: luteinizing hormone; ICSI: intracytoplasmic sperm injection.

A

Figure 7–2   *(From Swerdloff RS, Wang C. Evaluation of male infertility. In: Basow DS, ed. UpToDate. Waltham, MA: UpToDate, 2013.)*

Approach to diagnosis of male infertility in patients with normal serum hormone concentrations

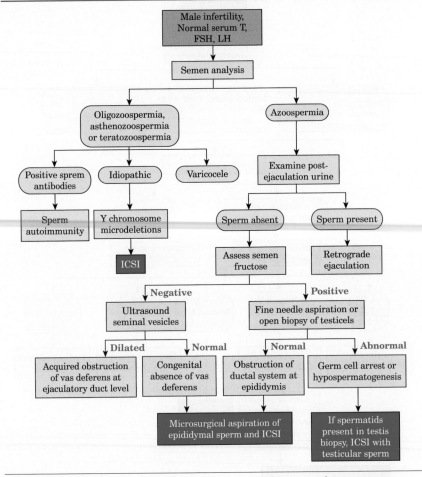

T: testosterone; FSH: follicle-stimulating hormone; LH: luteinizing hormone; ICSI: intracytoplasmic sperm injection.

B

Figure 7–2 (*Continued*)

Suggested Readings

Hull MG, Glazner CM, Kelly NJ, et al. Population study of causes, treatment and outcome of infertility. *Br Med J.* 1985;91:1693–1697.

Swerdloff RS, Wang C. Evaluation of male infertility. In: Basow DS ed. *UpToDate*, Waltham, MA: UpToDate Inc., 2013.

TESTICULAR DISEASE

❏ **Definition**

- Testicular disease refers to primary testicular defects, including congenital and developmental disorders and acquired diseases. Testicular disease accounts for 30–40% of all causes of male infertility.

❏ **Who Should Be Suspected?**

- For a couple experiencing infertility, the workup of the male begins with a history, physical examination, and standard semen analysis. Under certain circumstances, more specialized tests could help determine the cause. The presence of agglutination in the initial semen analysis suggests sperm autoimmunity, which should be confirmed by testing for antisperm autoantibodies. Azoospermia in the initial analysis, and the absence of sperm in concentrated postejaculation urine suggest a blockage, and assessing semen fructose is warranted.
- Chromosomal disorders affecting male fertility include Klinefelter syndrome (XXY and variants XXY/XY; XXXY), autosomal and X chromosome defects, and especially Y chromosome microdeletions and substitutions. Congenital disorders at the gene level include androgen receptor or postreceptor abnormalities, defective estrogen receptor or synthesis, inactivating receptor in the follicle-stimulating hormone (FSH) receptor gene, and myotonic dystrophy. Developmental disorders include cryptorchidism and varicoceles.
- Acquired diseases affecting male fertility include testicular cancer (with increasing frequency), debilitating illnesses (such as chronic renal insufficiency, cirrhosis, malnutrition, and sickle cell anemia), celiac disease, and a range of infections causing orchitis (mumps, echovirus, arbovirus, tuberculosis, leprosy, gonorrhea, and chlamydia).
- Other causes include certain drugs—alkylating agents (such as cyclophosphamide and chlorambucil), antiandrogens (such as flutamide, cyproterone, bicalutamide, spironolactone), ketoconazole, and cimetidine; ionizing radiation (doses as low as 0.015 Gy [15 rads] transiently suppressing spermatogenesis, doses above 6 Gy [600 rads] usually causing irreversible azoospermia and infertility); environmental toxins (such as lead, cadmium, mercury, and certain "endocrine disruptors" such as certain insecticides and fungicides); and smoking.

❏ **Laboratory Findings**

- A positive test for antisperm autoantibodies suggests sperm autoimmunity, which could be clinically significant if >50% of the cells are coated and when such sperm fail to penetrate preovulatory human cervical mucus or demonstrate impaired fertilizing capacity.
- Low or nondetectable semen fructose is associated with ejaculatory duct obstruction or with congenital absence of the vas deferens.

Suggested Readings

Adamopoulos DA, Lawrence DM, Vassilopoulos P, et al. Pituitary-testicular interrelationships in mumps orchitis and other viral infections. *Br Med J.* 1978;1:1177–1180.

Bronson R, Cooper G, Rosenfeld D. Sperm antibodies: their role in infertility. *Fertil Steril.* 1984;42:171–183.

Carlson HE, Ippoliti AF, Swerdloff RS. Endocrine effects of acute and chronic cimetidine administration. *Dig Dis Sci.* 1981;26:428–432.

Rowley MJ, Leach DR, Warner GA, et al. Effect of graded doses of ionizing radiation on the human testis. *Radiat Res.* 1974;59:665–678.

Vine MF, Margolin BH, Morrison HI, et al. Cigarette smoking and sperm density: a meta-analysis. *Fertil Steril.* 1994;61:35–43.

DISORDERS OF SPERM TRANSPORT

❑ Definition

- Disorders of sperm transport involve abnormalities at either of the critical sites along the male genital tract (the epididymis and the vas deferens) or ejaculatory dysfunction.

❑ Who Should Be Suspected?

- For a couple experiencing infertility, in the workup of the male, the findings of azoospermia in the initial standard semen analysis, normal-sized testes, and normal serum levels of testosterone, FSH, and luteinizing hormone (LH) warrant checking for retrograde ejaculation with a postejaculatory urine specimen. If sperm are not present in the urine specimen, then the patient has obstructive azoospermia or impaired spermatogenesis. Assessing semen fructose is the next step in distinguishing an obstruction at the epididymis from an obstruction or absence of the vas deferens.

❑ Laboratory Findings

- If semen fructose is present, epididymal obstruction is likely, but fine needle aspiration or open biopsy of the testis should be considered to confirm normal testicular histology. If the histologic analysis is abnormal, the conclusion is a germ cell arrest or hypospermatogenesis.
- If semen fructose is absent, obstruction or absence of the vas deferens is likely, and ultrasound analysis of the seminal vesicles will allow one to distinguish an acquired obstruction (dilated seminal vesicles) from congenital absence (normal seminal vesicles).

Causes of acquired vas deferens obstructions include infection (gonorrhea, chlamydia, tuberculosis) and ligation (i.e., vasectomy). Only 2% of infertile men have congenital absence of the vas deferens, most stemming from mutations of the cystic fibrosis transmembrane conductance regulator (CFTR) gene, although other findings typical of CF are absent. Primary ciliary dyskinesias (affecting cilia function and transport) are a genetically diverse group of congenital defects that lead to abnormal transport of sperm within the vas deferens.

Suggested Readings

Munro NC, Currie DC, Lindsay KS, et al. Fertility in men with primary ciliary dyskinesia presenting with respiratory infection. *Thorax.* 1994;49:684–687.

Patrizio P, Asch RH, Handelin B, et al. Aetiology of congenital absence of vas deferens: genetic study of three generations. *Hum Reprod.* 1993;8:215–220.

Wilton LJ, Teichtahl H, Temple-Smith PD, et al. Young's syndrome (obstructive azoospermia and chronic sinobronchial infection): a quantitative study of axonemal ultrastructure and function. *Fertil Steril.* 1991;55:144–151.

POSTVASECTOMY STATUS

❑ **Definition**

- Following a vasectomy, a series of semen analyses are performed for a defined period to determine the success or failure of the procedure. Azoospermia in a semen specimen is definitive evidence of a successful vasectomy.

❑ **Who Should Be Evaluated?**

- About four of five postvasectomy patients will be azoospermic after 3 months and 20 ejaculations. However, this period of time will be shorter if ejaculations are more frequent or if the patient is older.
- In a low percentage of cases, postvasectomy patients will consistently evidence nonmotile sperm, possibly reflecting an undue delay between ejaculation and laboratory analysis. Repeat testing after 1 and 2 months may confirm azoospermia, but the continued presence of rare, nonmotile sperm at this point is probably clinically insignificant.

❑ **Laboratory Findings**

- A fresh specimen should be examined using direct phase-contrast microscopy (25–50 high-power fields). If sperm are not seen on the initial slide, a centrifuged specimen should be evaluated.
- If motile sperm are present 3 months after the procedure and there have been more than 20 ejaculates, then the vasectomy is considered a failure.

Suggested Readings

Barone MA, Nazerali H, Cortes M, et al. A prospective study of time and number of ejaculations to azoospermia after vasectomy by ligation and excision. *J Urol.* 2003;170:892–896.

Griffin T, Tooher R, Nowakowski K, et al. How little is enough? The evidence for post-vasectomy testing. *J Urol.* 2005;174:29–36.

Sharlip ID, Belker AM, Honig S, et al. Vasectomy: AUA guideline. www.auanet.org/education/guidelines/vasectomy.cfm

OVULATORY DISORDERS

❑ **Definition**

- As a group, ovulatory disorders are characterized as either infrequent (oligoovulation) or absent (anovulation). In both disorders, the number of oocytes available for fertilization is reduced. Ovulatory disorders account for 25% of all causes of female infertility.

❑ **Who Should Be Suspected?**

- Candidates are women aged 16–40 years who report irregular or absent menses (amenorrhea) and irregular or absent molimina (breast tenderness, dysmenorrheal, bloating). Likely causes are pregnancy, oligoovulation (>36 days between menstrual cycles), or anovulation (>3–6 months without menses). Anovulation patients are classified by the WHO as:
  - ▼ WHO1: hypogonadotropic hypoestrogenic (15%)
  - ▼ WHO2: normogonadotropic normoestrogenic (80%)
  - ▼ WHO3: hypergonadotropic hypoestrogenic (5%)

❑ Laboratory Findings

- WHO class 1: FSH is low or low-normal, and serum estradiol is low because of decreased hypothalamic secretion of gonadotropin-releasing hormone (GnRH) or pituitary unresponsiveness to GnRH.

- WHO class 2: FSH and estradiol are normal. The majority of anovulation patients belong to this group, with heterogeneous additional symptoms that include obesity, biochemical or clinical hyperandrogenism, and insulin resistance. Follow-up testing would include prolactin (covered in the next section), thyroid-stimulating hormone (TSH), and T_4. Thyroid abnormalities occur in up to 4% of patients with infertility. In patients with signs of hirsutism, testing should include testosterone and dehydroepiandrosterone (DHEA-sulfate). This group includes patients with polycystic ovary syndrome (PCOS), of whom 70% demonstrate elevated free testosterone. An additional test for PCOS is the 2-hour glucose tolerance test, which examines insulin and glucose levels following administration of a 75 g glucose bolus.

- WHO class 3: FSH is elevated. In patients with elevated FSH and a normal karyotype, the diagnosis should consider ovarian resistance (follicular form) or premature ovarian insufficiency (absence of ovarian follicles through early menopause). In patients under age 30 with elevated FSH, a karyotype analysis should be performed to check for Turner syndrome (XO) or XY females with gonadal dysgenesis.

Suggested Reading

Davis J, Segars J. Menstruation and menstrual disorders: anovulation. *Glob Libr Women's Med.* (ISSN: 1756–2228); 2009; doi: 10.3843/GLOWM.10296

HYPERPROLACTINEMIA

❑ Definition

- Hyperprolactinemia is an abnormally high serum prolactin concentration in women of reproductive age. Excluding pregnancy, it accounts for 10–20% of cases of amenorrhea.

❑ Who Should Be Suspected?

- In premenopausal women, hyperprolactinemia causes hypogonadism, manifested by infertility, oligomenorrhea, or amenorrhea, and less often by galactorrhea. The mechanism involves inhibition of LH, and possibly FSH as well, through inhibition of the release of GnRH. The symptoms of hyperprolactinemic hypogonadism in these patients directly correlate with serum prolactin concentration. In most laboratories, a serum prolactin concentration above 15–20 ng/mL (15–20 µg/L) is considered abnormally high for women of reproductive age.

❑ Laboratory Findings (Premenopausal Women)

- 20–50 ng/mL (20–50 µg/L): Mild hyperprolactinemia, causing insufficient progesterone secretion and a short luteal phase of the menstrual cycle.

Infertility may be present despite no abnormality of the menstrual cycle. These patients account for about 20% of those evaluated for infertility.

- 50–100 ng/mL (50–100 µg/L): Moderate hyperprolactinemia, causing either amenorrhea or oligomenorrhea.
- 100 ng/mL (>100 µg/L): Associated with overt hypogonadism, subnormal estradiol secretion, and its consequences, including amenorrhea, hot flashes, and vaginal dryness.

Suggested Reading

Corenblum B, Pairaudeau N, Shewchuk AB. Prolactin hypersecretion and short luteal phase defects. *Obstet Gynecol.* 1976;47:486–488.

CHAPTER 8

Gynecologic and Obstetric Disorders

Juliana G. Szakacs

The 10th edition is updated to include the latest recommendations for cervical cancer screening and diagnostic testing for diseases of the female genital tract, including abnormalities related to menstruation. New genetic tests for the prenatal screening of heritable disorders are becoming available (see also Chapter 10). Please see the e-book version for the figures referenced in this chapter.

GYNECOLOGIC DISORDERS

CANCER OF THE BREAST

❑ Definition
Cancer of the breast is a malignancy arising from the breast epithelium (carcinoma) and/or stroma (sarcoma).

❑ Clinical Presentation
Breast cancer is the most common malignancy in women and a leading cause of cancer death. Risk factors include increased age and female gender, race, preexisting benign breast disease, family history of breast or ovarian cancer, exposure to ionizing radiation, and environmental factors.

❏ Laboratory Findings

The diagnosis of breast cancer is made on mammographic and/or ultrasound findings followed by biopsy and histologic evaluation. Patients with a familial history of breast cancer may be screened for BRCA1 and BRCA2; however, <10% of all breast cancers are associated with genetic mutations (see Chapter 10).

The histologic types of breast carcinoma include infiltrating ductal carcinoma (see eBook Figure 8-1C), infiltrating lobular (see eBook Figure 8-2D) carcinoma, and mixed ductal/lobular carcinoma. In addition, there are sarcomas and mixed tumors, phyllodes tumor (see eBook Figure 8-3C).

Molecular subtypes include luminal subtypes A and B (the majority of ER-positive breast cancers), and HER2-enriched (often negative for ER and PR), basal subtypes (triple negative) (see eBook Figures 8-1 to 8-3).

At the time of diagnosis, immunohistochemical staining is performed on the tumor to determine estrogen (ER) and progesterone (PR) receptor expression for prognosis and human epidermal growth factor 2 (HER2) receptors to determine if the patient will respond to Herceptin. Grading is based on architecture, nuclear morphology, and the number of mitoses using a system such as the Scarff-Bloom-Richardson grading system. Staging is based on the TNM system from the American Joint Committee on Cancer and the International Union for Cancer Control.

CANCER OF THE CERVIX

❏ Definition

Squamous cell carcinoma of the cervix is one of the most frequent neoplasms that affect a woman's reproductive system[1] (see eBook Figure 8-4A). Cervical squamous cell carcinoma is the result of infection with various strains of the human papilloma virus (HPV), especially (but not exclusively) the oncogenic types 16 and 18. Persistent viral infection transforms the epithelial cells that undergo a progression of changes in the cervix particularly at the squamocolumnar junction, which can be identified on Pap testing and on biopsy. The progression from acute infection to dysplasia to invasive carcinoma may take 3–7 years. Regular screening for high-risk HPV and by Pap testing has decreased the incidence of this cancer worldwide. HPV vaccination should decrease the incidence further in coming years. Adenocarcinoma of the cervix is also caused by HPV transformation of the endocervical cells but is less common than SCC and is not easily detected by Pap testing (see eBook Figure 8-4B).

❏ Clinical Presentation

Cervical carcinoma is usually seen in women in their 40s and 50s but may occur as early as the mid-20s if there is a history of early sexual activity and multiple partners. It is more likely in patients who have never been screened or who have not had a Pap test in the previous 5 years. Patients may be asymptomatic or present with abnormal or postcoital bleeding or vaginal discharge that may be watery, mucoid, or purulent and malodorous. The presence of pelvic or lower back pain suggests advanced disease. Suspicion should be high in the presence of an abnormal Pap test.

❏ Laboratory Findings

Pap testing may be performed by conventional smear or liquid methodology (SurePath Liquid-Based Pap Test and ThinPrep Pap Test). Cytology is reported in the Bethesda system as negative, atypical squamous cells (ASCUS), low-grade squamous intraepithelial lesion (LSIL), high-grade squamous intraepithelial lesion (HSIL), squamous cell carcinoma, and atypical glandular cells (AGUS) (see eBook Figure 8-5A–E). A statement on the adequacy of the cellularity for testing is also made.[2]

ACOG recommends screening for cervical cancer with cytology (smear or liquid based) and high-risk HPV DNA testing as follows[3]:

- No screening for women younger than 21 years.
- Cytology alone should be performed for women aged 21–29 years.
- HPV and cytology cotesting performed every 5 years for women aged 30–65 years.
- For women with three negative cytology tests or two negative cotesting screens, no further screening is necessary after age 65 years.
- Women with a history of treated CIN 2, CIN 3, or adenocarcinoma in situ should continue routine age-based screening for at least 20 years.
- For women who have undergone total hysterectomy and who have not had a history of CIN 2, CIN 3, or adenocarcinoma in situ in the previous 20 years, no screening is necessary.
- For women vaccinated against HPV, follow age-specific recommendations similar to unvaccinated women.

Follow-up of screening tests as follows:

- Negative cytology and negative HPV rescreen in 5 years
- ASCUS Pap and negative HPV rescreen in 3 years
- Negative cytology and positive HPV repeat cotesting in 12 months or test for HPV 16/18
  - ▼ If HPV 16/18 positive refer to colposcopy
  - ▼ If HPV 16/18 negative repeat cotesting in 12 months

Referral of patients for colposcopic examination and biopsy should be performed for patients with positive HPV 16 or 18 and any cytology results higher than LSIL or any patient with atypical glandular cells. Patients should undergo biopsy of any visualized cervical lesions and endocervical curettage if no lesions are apparent (see eBook Figures 8-6 and 8-7). For patients with abnormal Pap tests (ASCUS and HSIL), positive high-risk HPV DNA test and negative biopsy additional tissue diagnosis should be attempted with conization (loop electrocautery excision).

For women diagnosed with invasive squamous cell carcinoma of the cervix, imaging studies (CT or MRI) are recommended to evaluate possible involvement of adjacent organs or metastases.

Testing options:

Many laboratories now offer reflex testing for HPV from the liquid pap vial based on the ACOG recommendations, making it easier for the clinician. In addition, PCR testing for GC, *Chlamydia*, and *Trichomonas* may also be performed on the same liquid pap vial.

Limitations of the Pap test:

- False-negative results in approximately 5–10% of cases.
- Unsatisfactory cellularity occurs with fewer than 5,000 well-visualized, well-preserved squamous cells in a liquid-based Pap, and 8,000 cells on a conventional smear are obtained.
- Sampling problems occur in up to 10% of samples collected; these have integrity issues and are considered unsatisfactory due to the presence of blood or mucous, inflammation, insufficient cells, or problems with the slide preparation. Malignant cells may not be present if the smear is repeated too soon after a previous abnormal smear.
- The Pap test was designed to screen for squamous tumors. Other tumor types are less readily diagnosed (e.g., adenocarcinoma, lymphoma, and sarcoma).
- Human error in interpreting difficult cells; <3% of preventable cervical cancers are due to misread smears.

References

1. Saraiya M, Ahmed F, Krishnan S, et al. Cervical cancer incidence in a prevaccine era in the United States, 1998–2002. *Obstet Gynecol.* 2007;109:360–370.
2. Solomon D, Nayar R (eds). *The Bethesda System for Reporting Cervical Cytology,* 2nd ed. New York: Springer Science and Business Media, LLC; 2004.
3. Committee on Practice Bulletins—Gynecology. American College of Obstetricians and Gynecologists Practice Bulletin No. 131: screening for cervical cancer. *Obstet Genecol.* 2012;120:1222–1238.

CANCER OF THE ENDOMETRIUM

❑ Definition
Endometrial carcinoma is the most common invasive gynecologic cancer in North America (cervical carcinoma is most common worldwide). There are two types recognized. Type 1 is estrogen or tamoxifen related, is usually a low-grade endometrioid type, and is preceded by endometrial intraepithelial neoplasia.

❑ Clinical Presentation
Cancer of the endometrium is associated with PTEN mutations, obesity, and hereditary nonpolyposis colonic cancer syndrome. Concurrent ovarian carcinoma may occur in 10–20%. Type 2 is unrelated to estrogen or tamoxifen, is usually a higher-grade papillary serous or mixed type, and is associated with p53 mutations without a preceding in situ component. The progression of type 2 disease is usually rapid, and the prognosis is poor[1]. Patients with endometrial carcinoma present with a history of abnormal vaginal bleeding, especially if postmenopausal.

❑ Laboratory Findings
The diagnosis of endometrial carcinoma is made on endometrial biopsy or curettage (positive in 95% of patients) and rarely is identified on Pap test (see eBook Figure 8-8). A negative Pap test does not rule out carcinoma. Blood tests may show anemia if bleeding is chronic or severe, but otherwise are noncontributory.

Reference

1. Crum CP, Lee KR (eds). *Diagnostic Gynecologic and Obstetric Pathology.* Philadelphia, PA: Elsevier Saunders; 2006.

EPITHELIAL OVARIAN CARCINOMA

❑ Definition

Cancer of the ovary may derive from the epithelium (95% of cases) or from the stromal supporting cells or germ cells. This section will deal with the epithelial carcinomas arising from the surface of the ovary that are contiguous with the peritoneum and include low-grade serous carcinomas, serous tumors of low malignant potential, high-grade serous carcinomas, mucinous carcinoma, endometrioid carcinomas, clear cell tumors, Brenner (transitional cell) tumors, and undifferentiated carcinomas.

❑ Clinical Presentation

Patients may present with either acute symptoms such as bowel obstruction or pleural effusion or subacute symptoms such as adnexal mass, pain, bloating, urinary frequency, or early satiety. Patients with a positive family history of breast or ovarian cancer or who have BRCA1 or BRCA2 mutations or Lynch syndrome may be at increased risk (see Hereditary and Genetic Diseases, Chapter 10).

❑ Laboratory Findings

The diagnosis of ovarian cancer is made on histologic examination of tissue or cytology of peritoneal or pleural fluid if present (see eBook Figure 8-9). Rarely abnormal glandular cells may be seen on Pap test, which on further workup are found to originate from the ovary.

Imaging is the most important tool for identifying an adnexal mass. Surgical excision of the intact mass with intraoperative frozen-section diagnosis is performed whenever possible as transabdominal FNA or biopsy of ovarian tumors has been shown to increase the risk of seeding the malignant cells into the peritoneum by rupture or incision of the mass.

Screening tests for ovarian carcinoma have been sought to aid in finding these patients before symptoms occur. These include the following:

- *CA-125* is elevated in approximately 50% of patients with early-stage disease and in >80% of patients with advanced disease. It may also be elevated in normal women and in patients with endometriosis, leiomyoma, cirrhosis, PID, or other malignancies. Following serial CA-125 levels over time may be more beneficial as a screening tool.
- *Human epididymis protein 4* (HE4) is helpful in diagnosing recurrent or progressive disease or in the evaluation of a suspicious adnexal mass.
- *Carcinoembryonic antigen* (CEA) is nonspecific. Levels may be elevated in malignancies (particularly mucinous carcinomas) of the ovary, GI tract, breast, pancreas, thyroid, and lung. It is also elevated in patients who smoke, or who have mucinous cystadenoma, cholecystitis, cirrhosis, pancreatitis, pneumonia, and diverticulitis and IFD.
- *CA 19-9* is a mucin protein that may be elevated in ovarian cancer but is also positive in gastric cancers. It may be used to follow recurrence in a patient with known CA19-9–positive ovarian cancer.
- *OVA1* is a panel that includes five serum biomarkers to assess the likelihood of malignancy in patients with an adnexal mass. Two markers are

up-regulated (CA 125 II, beta-2 microglobulin) and three down-regulated (transferrin, transthyretin, apolipoprotein A1). An algorithm determines the patient's risk for ovarian cancer. OVA1 is commercially available through Quest Diagnostics.

■ *Pathologic diagnosis* of tumor type and grade forms the basis for treatment and prognosis. These tumors are staged according to the International Federation of Gynecology and Obstetrics (FIGO)/TNM system. For a complete review of the pathology of epithelial ovarian carcinomas, (see Crum and Lee).[1] *Diagnostic Gynecologic and Obstetric Pathology.* Philadelphia, PA: W B Saunders Co, 2005.

OVARIAN GERM CELL TUMORS

❑ Definition
Ovarian germ cell neoplasms originate from the germ cells of the ovary and comprise 5% of the malignant ovarian neoplasms. These tumors may be malignant or benign and include teratomas (mature, dermoid, and immature), dysgerminomas, endodermal sinus (yolk sac) tumors, embryonal carcinomas, and nongestational choriocarcinoma (see eBook Figure 8-10).

❑ Clinical Presentation
Patients presenting with ovarian germ cell neoplasms are usually between 10 and 30 years of age. They are more frequent in Asian/Pacific Islander and Hispanic women than in Caucasians. Presenting symptoms include effects of hCG production by the tumor (precocious puberty, abnormal vaginal bleeding), abdominal enlargement, ascites, or abdominal pain (including acute abdomen due to torsion).

❑ Laboratory Findings
The definitive diagnosis requires histologic evaluation at the time of surgical excision. A presumptive diagnosis may be made with an adnexal mass on pelvic imaging (CT, MRI, or ultrasound) and elevation of an associated tumor marker. Tumor markers are also used to monitor patients post–surgical resection for recurrence. These include the following:

■ *hCG* is increased in embryonal cell carcinomas, ovarian choriocarcinomas, mixed germ cell tumors, and some dysgerminomas.
■ *AFP* is increased in endodermal sinus tumors, embryonal cell carcinomas, mixed germ cell tumors, and some immature teratomas.
■ *Lactate dehydrogenase (LDH)* is increased in dysgerminomas.
■ *Pathologic diagnosis* of tumor type and grade forms the basis for treatment and prognosis. Malignant germ cell neoplasms are staged according to the FIGO/TNM system. For a complete review of the pathology of ovarian germ cell tumors (see Crum and Lee).[1] *Diagnostic Gynecologic and Obstetric Pathology.* Philadelphia, PA: W B Saunders Co, 2005.

Reference
1. Crum CP, Lee KR (eds). *Diagnostic Gynecologic and Obstetric Pathology.* Philadelphia, PA: WB Saunders Co,; 2005.

OVARIAN SEX CORD-STROMAL NEOPLASMS

❏ Definition

Ovarian sex cord-stromal neoplasms are benign or malignant tumors that arise from the cells supporting the oocytes, including ovarian hormone–producing cells. These are rare tumors comprising <2% of all ovarian cancers. These include fibromas, thecomas, granulosa cell tumors, Sertoli or Sertoli–Leydig cell tumors, and gynandroblastoma.

❏ Clinical Presentation

Patients with sex cord tumors present with abdominal distention, bloating, pain or pelvic symptoms, and a finding of adnexal mass on imaging. They also may exhibit hormonal manifestations including signs of estrogen excess (precocious puberty, abnormal uterine bleeding) or androgen excess (virilization). The risk for sex cord tumors may be decreased in current or past smokers, in women who have taken oral contraceptive pills, and in multiparous women.

❏ Laboratory Findings

The diagnosis of sex cord-stromal tumor is made on tissue evaluation at the time of surgery (see eBook Figure 8-11). For any suspected ovarian malignancy, a complete oophorectomy must be performed to prevent potential spread of neoplastic cells. Presumptive diagnosis may be made in a patient with hormonal changes, an adnexal mass on imaging (transpelvic ultrasound), or bimanual exam and elevation of an associated tumor marker. These include the following:

- *AFP* is seen in embryonal carcinoma and polyembryoma and may be seen in immature teratoma, endodermal sinus tumors, mixed germ cell tumors, and Sertoli–Leydig cell tumors.
- *hCG* is seen in embryonal carcinoma, choriocarcinoma, and polyembryoma and may be seen in mixed germ cell tumors and dysgerminoma.
- *LDH* is seen in dysgerminoma and endodermal sinus tumors and may be seen in embryonal carcinoma, choriocarcinoma, immature teratoma, and mixed germ cell tumors.
- *Inhibin* is seen in granulosa cell tumors where both inhibin A and inhibin B should be ordered, and it may be seen in Sertoli–Leydig cell tumors and gonadoblastoma.
- *Estradiol* may be seen in granulosa cell tumors, Sertoli–Leydig cell tumors, gynandroblastoma, immature teratoma, embryonal carcinoma, and dysgerminoma.
- *Testosterone* is elevated when virilization is present in Sertoli–Leydig cell tumors and may also be seen in granulosa cell tumors and gynandroblastoma.
- *Androstenedione* may be seen in gynandroblastoma and Sertoli–Leydig cell tumors.
- *DHEA* may be seen in immature teratoma, gonadoblastoma, and Sertoli–Leydig cell tumors.
- *Müllerian inhibiting substance (MIS)* appears to be a more specific tumor marker for granulosa cell tumors but is not yet available for clinical use.
- *Genetic testing* is not helpful at this time. Sex cord-stromal neoplasms have no known association with BRCA1 or BRCA2. Studies have shown a somatic mutation in *FOXL2*, a gene that encodes a transcription factor, may be associated with granulosa cell tumors, and somatic mutations affecting

the RNase IIIb domain of *DICER1* may be associated with Sertoli–Leydig cell tumors.

- *Pathologic diagnosis* of tumor type and grade forms the basis for treatment and prognosis. Sex cord–stromal neoplasms are staged according to the FIGO/TNM system. For a complete review of the pathology of ovarian germ cell tumors (see Crum and Lee).[1]

URINARY TRACT INFECTIONS

See Chapter 7

PELVIC INFLAMMATORY DISEASE*

CHORIOAMNIONITIS

❑ Definition
Pelvic inflammatory disease (PID) refers to infection of the upper genital tract of women. It may include the endometrium, myometrium, parametrium, uterine tubes, and ovaries. Other pelvic and abdominal organs may be secondarily infected (e.g., peritonitis, perihepatitis).

❑ Who Should Be Suspected?
PID is most commonly caused as a complication of STIs (85%); 15% of cases arise postoperatively or as a complication of childbirth. Factors for increased risk for PID include risk factors associated with STI: Age <25 years and young age at onset of sexual activity; new or multiple sex partners, especially partners with STI symptoms; unprotected sexual activity; and history of STI. Additional factors may include IUD use, douching, and bacterial vaginosis.

Clinical features:

- PID describes infection in any of various organs, including the uterus, ovaries, and adjacent abdominal organs. Clinical presentation depends on the primary sites and severity of infection.
- Diagnosis should be strongly considered in women presenting with abdominal pain if physical examination reveals cervical or adnexal tenderness. Diffuse, subacute abdominal pain is typical. Abdominal tenderness, sometimes with subtle peritoneal signs, and onset during menses are commonly described. Abnormal uterine bleeding is reported frequently. Nonspecific symptoms, like fever and lower genital tract symptoms, may be reported; other causes should be investigated if symptoms related to the GI or urinary tract are predominant.

❑ Laboratory Findings
- There is no gold standard for the diagnosis of PID. Evaluation must consider findings on physical examination and laboratory testing. Additional testing may be required, including imaging studies, laparoscopy, and histopathology.
- Serum pregnancy test should be performed to rule out ectopic pregnancy or other complication of pregnancy.

---

*This section contributed by Michael J. Mitchell, MD.

- A positive result of NAAT for *Neisseria gonorrhoeae* or *Chlamydia trachomatis*, with compatible clinical presentation, confirms a diagnosis of PID.
- The quality and wet mount/Gram stain of cervical/vaginal fluid should be examined for increased WBCs or other abnormality. Abnormal secretions or increased WBCs ($\geq$3 WBC per high-power field) support a diagnosis of PID.
- Positive results for peripheral blood WBC, ESR, or CRP support a diagnosis of PID.
- Supplemental tests: Inflammation of upper genital or adjacent organs, detected by laparoscopy, biopsy, peritoneal fluid analysis, or positive culture from normally sterile upper genital sites, confirms a clinical diagnosis of PID.
- Other tests: HIV and syphilis testing should be requested. Additional testing and microbiologic testing are performed on the basis of signs and symptoms in specific patients.

Suggested Reading

Peipert JF, Boardman L, Hogan JW, et al. Laboratory evaluation of acute upper genital tract infection. *Obstet Gynecol*. 1996;87:730–736.

VAGINOSIS AND VAGINITIS (BACTERIAL VAGINOSIS, TRICHOMONIASIS, VULVOVAGINAL CANDIDIASIS)*

Definition

- Vaginitis is used to describe conditions associated with significant inflammation, whereas vaginosis is used when vaginal secretions do not show a marked increase in inflammatory cells. Symptoms attributed to vaginitis may also be due to primary cervicitis, urethritis, or inflammation to other related tissues.
- Changes in the amount or character of vaginal discharge are common presenting complaints of women seeking medical attention. Although there is normal variability in vaginal secretions, infectious and other pathologic causes are common and should be carefully evaluated.

❑ Causes

- Complaints associated with noninfectious causes may be indistinguishable from those caused by genital tract infections. Common noninfectious causes include the following:
  - ▼ Allergy and irritants. Many products, such as detergents, soaps, bubble bath, latex (e.g., condoms), and topical medications, may cause inflammation of the vaginal mucosa and changes in the character and volume of secretions. Clinical management requires elimination of the allergen or irritant.
  - ▼ Atrophic vaginitis. This type of vaginitis is caused by estrogen deficiency and is usually associated with menopause but may be seen in the postpartum period or as a result of medication. Symptoms of estrogen deficiency

*This section contributed by Michael J. Mitchell, MD.

lead to vaginal dryness and itching rather than an increase in vaginal secretions. Here, there are mixed nonspecific gram-negative rods with decreased lactobacilli; vaginal cytology shows an atrophic pattern.

▼ Physiologic leukorrhea. Vaginal secretions may vary significantly in normal women, especially related to the menstrual cycle. The volume of vaginal secretion is typically greatest in mid-cycle. Significant symptoms and inflammation are not seen with physiologic leukorrhea; the odor, color, and viscosity of secretions are similar to the characteristics in the absence of leukorrhea.

■ Bacterial vaginosis, trichomoniasis, and vulvovaginal candidiasis are the most common causes of clinically significant vaginosis/vaginitis and are described in detail below. Other infectious causes of vaginitis include the following:

▼ Condyloma acuminata. Increased vaginal discharge, pruritus, and pain are common symptoms caused by anogenital warts.

▼ Foreign body or traumatic vaginitis. Foreign bodies, like a retained tampon, may cause a change in the normal vaginal flora and mild signs and symptoms of infection. Removal of the foreign body is usually all that is required for clinical management.

▼ Group A *Streptococcus*, *Staphylococcus aureus*, and other pathogens may cause acute vaginal infection with pain, edema, erythema, and purulent vaginal discharge. Gram staining and culture confirm the diagnosis.

❏ Diagnosis: General Aspects of Vaginosis

The initial diagnostic evaluation should include a detailed history and laboratory testing. (Note that symptoms may be caused by more than one infectious condition.) A detailed clinical history may provide information that is useful in distinguishing infectious vaginitis from other conditions that may cause changes in the character of vaginal discharge (e.g., urethritis, cervicitis, noninfectious inflammatory conditions). Important factors include the following:

■ Menstrual history: Vaginal secretions may vary with pregnancy and menstrual cycle. Vulvovaginal candidiasis often occurs in the premenstrual period; trichomoniasis often occurs in the postmenstrual period.

■ Sexual history: Factors associated with an increased risk of STDs, including BV and trichomoniasis, include new sexual partner, exposure to multiple sexual partners, and history of STD.

■ Recent and current medications: Antibiotics, estrogen and progestin drugs, and other medications may predispose to vaginitis through changes in the vaginal environment or flora.

■ Personal hygiene and potential irritants: Hygienic products and practices, frequent or recent douching, soaps and detergents, topical medications, and panty liners and other products may cause vaginal irritation, resulting in symptoms indistinguishable from infectious causes.

■ In addition to history and physical examination, the following tests are recommended: vaginal pH, microscopic examination of vaginal secretions (wet mount, Gram stain), and amine test. Additional testing, including testing for specific microorganisms, is recommended for patients in whom testing does not provide a diagnosis.

❏ Laboratory Tests

Specific diagnosis requires laboratory testing (see Table 8-1).

- Vaginal pH: Secretions are collected, using a dry swab, from the vaginal side-wall halfway between the cervix and introitus. A narrow-range paper (pH 4.0–5.5) should be used.
- Microscopic examination: Saline wet mount preparations are used for direct detection of yeast-like cells and pseudohyphae, trichomonads, and host cells. Vaginal secretions collected by swab are suspended in a drop of normal saline on a microscopic slide. Normal vaginal secretions show a predominance of SECs with a minimal number of PMNs. Note that although *Candida* species are common components of the normal vaginal microflora, visualization of many yeast-like cells or pseudohyphae is abnormal and characteristic of candidiasis. (Detection of yeast may be facilitated by addition of 10% KOH to the saline wet mount preparation.) "Clue" cells are squamous epithelial cells covered by coccobacillary organisms, resulting in fuzzy or indistinct cell borders.
- Gram stain: Gram stains are used for direct detection of bacteria, yeast, and host cells. Normal vaginal secretions show a predominance of SECs with a minimal number of PMNs. There is a predominance of gram-positive bacilli consistent with *Lactobacillus* species.
- Amine "whiff" test: A drop of 10% KOH may be added to vaginal secretions on a microscopic slide. The immediate release of a "fishy" (volatile amine) odor is typical of BV.
- Culture: Culture of vaginal secretions may improve the sensitivity of detection for trichomoniasis, but special techniques are required for isolation of *T. vaginalis*. Culture is not recommended for routine evaluation of vulvovaginal candidiasis. Positive cultures for yeast must be interpreted with caution because *C. albicans* and other yeast may represent normal endogenous flora. Culture may be useful for patients with recurrent vulvovaginal candidiasis, or candidiasis resistant to standard therapy. Bacterial culture, including culture for *G. vaginalis*, is not reliable for the diagnosis of BV because no single organism can be specifically implicated in the pathogenesis of BV.
- Serology: Serologic testing does not play a significant role in the diagnosis of vaginitis.
- Molecular tests: Molecular diagnostic tests are increasingly available for the diagnosis of infectious vaginitis. For example, nucleic acid hybridization provided greater sensitivity for detection of agents associated with BV, trichomoniasis, and vulvovaginal candidiasis compared with standard methods.
- HIV and syphilis serology and testing related to other STIs should be considered.

❏ Diagnosis

- Common presenting symptoms of vaginitis include change in the volume, character or odor of vaginal secretions; irritation of the genital mucosa, including erythema, burning, and itching; dysuria; and spotting.
- In premenopausal women, the volume of vaginal secretions is <5 mL/day. Secretions are typically odorless, transparent, and viscous and white to

8

TABLE 8–1. Comparison of Various Causes of Vaginitis

Condition	pH	Gram Stain/Saline Mount	10% KOH Mount	Culture	Amine Test
Normal	4.0–4.5	PMN/EC <1; gram-positive rods dominant; 3+ SECs	–		–
Bacterial vaginosis	>4.5	Clue cells; PMN/EC <1; ↓ gram-positive rods, ↑ gram-negative coccobacilli	–	No value	>70% positive
Vulvovaginal candidiasis		PMN/EC ~40%; gram-positive rods dominant; 3+ SECs	Hyphae in 70%	If wet mount is negative	–
Trichomoniasis	>4.5	Motile trichomonads in ~60%, 4+ PMNs; mixed flora	–	Use if wet mount is negative	Often positive

↓, decreased; ↑, increased; PMN/EC, ratio of polymorphonuclear cells to epithelial cells.

yellowish. Normal vaginal pH is 4.0–4.5. Microscopic examination demonstrates a predominance of normal squamous epithelial cells (SECs) and few PMNs; there is a predominance of gram-positive bacilli consistent with lactobacilli (long, slender, may form chains).

▪ Douching within 24 hours decreases the sensitivity of tests. Do not test during first few days of menstrual cycle.

Bacterial Vaginosis

▪ Bacterial vaginosis (BV) is a common cause of infectious vaginitis, accounting for approximately 50% of cases. BV is associated with sexual transmission. BV is caused by a disruption of the normal microbial flora of the vagina. Gram stain shows a loss of the predominant *Lactobacillus* species, which produce peroxide and acidify the vaginal secretions. Loss of the lactobacilli allows overgrowth of anaerobes and other microorganisms, including *Gardnerella* and *Mobiluncus*, *Atopobium vaginae*, and other species.

▪ Patients with BV may be asymptomatic or present with minimal symptoms. Typical symptoms include an increase in the volume of thin, homogeneous, often malodorous vaginal secretions. Signs of inflammation are minimal.

▪ Diagnosis of BV is based on ≥3 of the following (Amsel criteria):
  ▼ Homogeneous, thin, whitish adherent vaginal secretions
  ▼ Positive "whiff" test
  ▼ Presence of clue cells on wet mount (>20% of vaginal squamous cells coated with small coccobacilli) in 90% of cases
  ▼ Vaginal pH >4.5

▪ Gram stain, using standardized interpretive criteria, is considered the gold standard for the diagnosis of BV. BV is characterized by a loss of gram-positive rods, with overgrowth of small, curved gram-negative bacilli and gram-variable coccobacilli. Gram stain of vaginal secretions has been demonstrated to have high positive and negative predictive values (90% and 94%, respectively) compared to diagnosis using the Amsel criteria. Interpretation is based on the number of clue cells (≥2 clue cells per 20 fields) and the proportion of bacterial morphotypes (non-*Lactobacillus* > *Lactobacillus*). See Table 8-1.

Trichomoniasis

▪ This sexually transmitted protozoal infection is caused by *Trichomonas vaginalis*; it is the most common nonviral STI.

▪ Women typically present with acute, inflammatory vaginitis. Most patients (approximately 70%) present with vaginal and urethral inflammation resulting in burning, itching, dysuria, and other symptoms associated with increased vaginal secretions. Secretions are described as greenish, frothy, and foul smelling in a minority of patients.

▪ Direct detection: Rapid diagnosis may be possible by microscopic examination. Vaginal secretions typically show increased pH (>4.5) and increased numbers of PMNs. Motile trichomonads, with typical twitching or "falling leaf" motility, are diagnostic but seen in only 50–70% of cases. Organisms may lose motility as early as 10 minutes after collection.

▪ Specific diagnosis requires laboratory testing (see Table 8-1).

▼ Molecular tests:
- FDA-approved NAATs (e.g., *Trichomonas vaginalis* assay) have become the gold standard for diagnosis, providing the highest sensitivity and specificity with decreased turnaround time compared to culture.
- An FDA-approved nonamplified molecular probe assay (Affirm VP III Microbial Identification System, Becton Dickinson) showed good specificity with sensitivity (approximately 65%) compared to NAAT.

▼ Antigen testing (e.g., Trichomonas Rapid Test) provides rapid results with good sensitivity (approximately 90%) and specificity (>95%).

▼ Culture: Commercially available culture shows good sensitivity (approximately 80%), but cultures must be incubated for 3–7 days before final results are available.

▼ Urinalysis: *T. vaginalis* may be an incidental finding in routine urinalysis.

Vulvovaginal Candidiasis

■ *Candida albicans* is responsible for 80–90% of cases of vulvovaginal candidiasis, but *Candida glabrata* and other *Candida* species are capable of causing clinically significant candidiasis. Vulvar inflammation, edema, pain, and pruritus are common symptoms. Thick, adherent, curd-like vaginal secretions are well described, but thin secretions may be seen and are indistinguishable from other causes of vaginal infection. Vulvovaginal candidiasis is not significantly associated with sexual transmission.

■ Factors associated with an increased risk of vulvovaginal candidiasis include the following:

▼ Contraceptive use (especially vaginal sponges and intrauterine devices)

▼ Current or recent antimicrobial therapy

▼ DM, especially when poorly controlled

▼ Increased estrogen levels caused by pregnancy or therapeutic estrogen administration

▼ Intrinsic or acquired immunodeficiency or immunosuppressive therapy

Suggested Readings

Anderson MR, Klink K, Cohrssen A. Evaluation of vaginal complaints. *JAMA*. 2004;291:1368–1379.

Eckert LO. Acute vulvovaginitis. *N Engl J Med*. 2006;355:1244–1252.

Goonan K. Chapter 34: Vaginitis. In: Khan F, Sachs HJ, Pechet L, et al., (eds). *Guide to Diagnostic Testing*. Philadelphia, PA: Lippincott Williams & Wilkins; 2002.

Hilmarsdáttir I, Hauksdáttir GS, Jáhannesdáttir JD, et al. Evaluation of a rapid gram stain interpretation method for diagnosis of bacterial vaginosis. *J Clin Microbiol*. 2006;44:1139–1140.

Lowe NK, Neal JL, Ryan-Wenger NA. Accuracy of the clinical diagnosis of vaginitis compared with a DNA probe laboratory standard. *Obstet Gynecol*. 2009;113:89–95.

Mazzulli T, Simor AE, Low DE. Reproducibility of interpretation of gram-stained vaginal smears for the diagnosis of bacterial vaginosis. *J Clin Microbiol*. 1990;28:1506–1508.

Nugent RP, Krohn MA, Hillier SL. Reliability of diagnosing bacterial vaginosis is improved by a standardized method of gram stain interpretation. *J Clin Microbiol*. 1991;29:297–301.

Nygren P, Fr R, Freemzan M, et al. Evidence on the benefits and harms of screening and treating pregnant women who are asymptomatic for bacterial vaginosis: an update review for the U.S. preventive services task force. *Ann Intern Med*. 2008;148:220–233.

U.S. Preventive Services Task Force. Screening for bacterial vaginosis in pregnancy to prevent preterm delivery: U.S. preventive services task force recommendation statement. *Ann Intern Med*. 2008;148:214–219.

PREGNANCY AND OBSTETRIC MONITORING OF THE FETUS AND PLACENTA

PREGNANCY

❑ **Normal Laboratory Values Altered by Pregnancy***

- *Hematology*: RBC mass increases 20%, but plasma volume increases approximately 40% causing RBC, Hb, and Hct to decrease approximately 15%. WBC increases 66%. Platelet count decreased by average 20%. ESR increases markedly during pregnancy, making this a useless diagnostic test during pregnancy. Occasionally cold agglutinins may be positive and osmotic fragility increased.

- *Renal function tests*: Respiratory alkalosis with renal compensation. Normal pCO_2 = approximately 30 mEq/L, normal HCO_3^- = 19–20 mEq/L. Serum osmolality decreases 10 mOsm/kg during first trimester. Increased GFR 30–50% early until approximately 20 weeks postpartum. Renal plasma flow increases 25–50% by midpregnancy. BUN and creatinine decrease 25%, especially during first half of pregnancy. BUN of 18 mg/dL and creatinine of 1.2 mg/dL are definitely increased (abnormal) in pregnancy, although normal in nonpregnant women. *Beware of BUN >13 mg/dL and creatinine >0.8 mg/dL.* Serum uric acid decreases 35% in first trimester (normal = 2.8–3.0 mg/dL); returns to normal by term. Serum aldosterone, angiotensins I and II, and renin are increased although secondary hyperaldosteronism may also be seen with toxemia of pregnancy.

- *Urinalysis*: Urine volume is not increased. Glycosuria occurs in >50% of patients due to impaired tubular resorption. Lactosuria should not be confused with glucose in urine. Proteinuria (200–300 mg/24 hour) is common (approximately 20% of patients); worsens with underlying glomerular disease. Urine porphyrins may be increased. Urinary gonadotropins (human chorionic gonadotropin, hCG) are increased. Urine estrogens increase from 6 months to term (≤100 µg/24 hours). Urine 17-ketosteroids rise to upper limit of normal at term.

- *Serum protein findings*: Serum total protein decreases 1 g/dL during first trimester; remains at that level. Serum albumin decreases 0.5 g/dL during first trimester and 0.75 g/dL by term.
  - ▼ Serum α-1 globulin increases 0.1 g/dL. Serum α-2 globulin increases 0.1 g/dL. Serum β-globulin increases 0.3 g/dL.

- *Chemistry*: Fasting blood glucose decreases 5–10 mg/dL by end of first trimester. Serum calcium decreases 10%. Serum magnesium decreases 10%. No changes are found in serum levels of sodium (normal = approximately 135 mEq/L), potassium, chloride, or phosphorus. Serum T_3 uptake is decreased and T_4 is increased. T_7 ($T_3 \times T_4$) is normal. TBG is increased. (Check tests for thyroid function.) Serum progesterone is increased.

- *Enzyme studies*: No changes are found in serum levels of amylase, AST, ALT, LD, ICDH, acid phosphatase, and α-hydroxybutyrate dehydrogenase. Serum CK decreases 15% by 20 weeks of gestation; increases at beginning of labor to peak 24 hours postpartum; and then gradually returns to normal. CK-MB is detected at onset of labor in approximately 75% of patients with peak 24 hours

---

*Contributed by Mary Williamson.

postpartum and then returns to normal. Serum LD and AST levels remain low. Serum ALP increases (200–300%) progressively during the last trimester of normal pregnancy caused by an increase of heat-stable isoenzyme from the placenta. Serum LAP may be increased moderately throughout pregnancy. Serum lipase decreases 50%. Serum pseudocholinesterase decreases 30%.

- *Lipid studies*: Serum phospholipid increases 40–60%. Serum triglycerides increase 100–200%. Serum cholesterol increases 30–50%.
- *Iron studies*: Serum iron decreases 40% in women not on iron therapy. Serum vitamin B_{12} level decreases 20%. Serum folate decreases $\geq$50%. Overlap of decreased and normal range of values often makes this test useless in diagnosis of megaloblastic anemia of pregnancy. Serum transferrin increases 40% and percent saturation decreases $\leq$70%. Serum ceruloplasmin increases 70%.

❏ Laboratory Monitoring of Pregnancy

At the first prenatal visit, all pregnant women should receive the following:

- Pap test if not done in preceding year to rule out dysplasia.
- CBC to rule out hematologic abnormalities (may be suggestive of genetic disorders such as thalassemia or iron deficiency or B_{12}/folate deficiency anemia).
- Blood type, Rh type, and antibody screen.
- Rubella screen, rapid plasma reagin (RPR) test, or syphilis antibody EIA test; HBsAg and HIV test should be offered.
- For high-risk women, test for *N. gonorrhoeae, C. trachomatis*, and HBsAg; repeat at 28 weeks.
- For women with diabetes during pregnancy, obtain a hemoglobin A1c.

First trimester (10w3d and 13w6d) testing may include the following:

- Maternal triple screen (pregnancy-associated placental protein A (PAPP-A), total hCG, and ultrasound for nuchal translucency and genetic diseases; optimally drawn between 11 and 13 weeks 6 days) *OR*
- Serial sequential testing with combined sonography and maternal serum testing for PAPP-A in first trimester followed with testing for PAPP-A, AFP, hCG, unconjugated estriol, and dimeric inhibin A in the second trimester. The first trimester specimen must be drawn between 11 and 18 weeks' gestation and the second specimen drawn between 15 and 22 weeks' gestation.
- Genetic testing for CF and other familial diseases should be offered (see Chapter 10).
- Cell-free DNA testing (noninvasive prenatal testing, NIPT) for trisomies 21, 18, and 13 and monosomy X may be considered for high-risk patients and may be drawn as early as 9 weeks of gestation.
- For patients with positive screening tests, amniotic fluid and chromosome analysis on chorionic villus sampling (CVS) may be performed and is diagnostic. Rapid detection of aneuploidy for chromosomes 13, 18, 21, X, and Y is available by CVS or amniotic fluid FISH.

Second trimester (15w0d and 22w6d):

- Maternal Quad Screen (pregnancy-associated placental protein A, total hCG, nuchal translucency and inhibin A) and sonogram for genetic diseases should be offered if first-trimester screening or serial sequential screening was not performed (test between 16 and 18 weeks is optimal) (see Chapter 11).

▪ For women who have had first-trimester screening, a repeat alpha-fetoprotein (AFP) at 16–18 weeks should be considered.

▪ Testing to rule out open neural tube defects may be performed on amniotic fluid by AFP testing.

▪ For women with diabetes in pregnancy, obtain a glucose tolerance test at 24–28 weeks.

At 36 weeks:

▪ Optional screen for group B streptococcus

❑ **Laboratory Monitoring of the Neonate**

The healthy term newborn requires minimal testing and only rarely develops hypoglycemia or hyperbilirubinemia. Preterm infants may require additional testing for hypoglycemia, and failure to grow in the neonatal intensive care unit with serum calcium and alkaline phosphatase. Preterm infants also have an increased rate of thrombocytopenia that may be alloimmune mediated due to maternal antibody or due to increased peripheral consumption. Platelets should be monitored and may drop as low as 10,000/µL.

Glucose monitoring should be performed in infants who are large for gestational age, have a diabetic mother, who require intensive care or are premature, have polycythemia or express tremors, hypotonia, irritability, lethargy, stupor, apnea, seizures, or hypothermia.

Infants should be monitored for jaundice at regular intervals of at least 8 hours and at discharge from the hospital. Bilirubin monitoring should be performed if jaundice is present within the first 24 hours. Transcutaneous bilirubin monitoring may be used to screen; however, elevated levels must be documented with serum.

Cord blood may be sent for blood typing and Coombs tests if the mother is Rh negative or if jaundice develops prior to 24 hours.

Microbiology and infectious disease studies for syphilis, HBV, and/or toxoplasma may be performed as clinically indicated.

Newborn screening for metabolic diseases is performed on the day of discharge or follow-up at age 4 days as mandated by state law (e.g., PKU, thyroid function tests, others).

INFANTS AT INCREASED RISK

Low birth weight infants are at increased risk for infection, necrotizing enterocolitis, respiratory distress syndrome, thrombocytopenia, intracranial bleed, and a number of other disorders. Infants with low birth weight ≤2,500 g, very low birth weight 1,500 g, or extremely low birth weight 1,000 g may be seen due to prematurity or intrauterine growth restriction. At the opposite extreme, infants with high birth weight (>4,000 g), and postmature infants are at risk for hypoglycemia, and increased perinatal mortality. Infants of high-risk mothers (toxemia, diabetes, drug addiction, cardiac or pulmonary disease) and those with polyhydramnios, oligohydramnios, and cesarean delivery are also at increased risk.

❑ Laboratory Monitoring for Infants at Increased Risk

During Labor and Delivery

- Monitoring fetal pH with a scalp monitor will indicate hypoxia during extended labor; pH <7.2 increases risk.
- Pulmonary immaturity may be recognized at the time of rupture of membranes by testing amniotic fluid for the lecithin/sphingomyelin ratio, lamellar body count, or phosphatidylglycerol.
- Amnionitis may be recognized by meconium-stained amniotic fluid at the time of rupture.

During the Neonatal Period

- Respiratory distress syndrome (RDS) is diagnosed by clinical findings, increased work of breathing, increased oxygen requirement, and chest radiograph showing diffuse reticular ground glass appearance and air bronchial grams. Arterial blood gas measurements will reveal hypoxia and elevated CO_2. Chemistry may reveal hyponatremia due to water retention.
- Hypoglycemia and hypocalcemia may be monitored with serum chemistry.
- Anemia of prematurity due to insufficient erythropoietin production and shorter RBC life span of approximately 35–50 days (term infant = 60–70 days) may be detected on hemogram. Hematocrit at term is usually 60%; this drops rapidly over the first 2 weeks and by 4 weeks reaches 35% on average with a nadir at 8–10 weeks of 30%. Preterm infants' HCT averages 41% at 26–30 weeks, 45% at 28 weeks, and 47% at 32 weeks.[1]
- Hemolytic disease of the newborn (erythroblastosis fetalis) due to Rh/ABO immunization may result in anemia with extramedullary hematopoiesis and ultimately organ failure and death. Maternal and fetal ABO and Rh testing should be performed. In addition, a direct antiglobulin (Coombs) test will be positive.
- Infections are more common in preterm than in term newborns (e.g., late-onset nosocomial infection by coagulase-negative staphylococci and fungi with central venous catheters; sepsis or pneumonia due to amnionitis); appropriate culture should be performed.
- Neonatal hyperbilirubinemia (see Chapter 5).

Reference

1. Gilbert-Barness E, Barness LA. *Clinical Use of Pediatric Diagnostic Tests*. Philadelphia, PA: Lippincott Williams & Wilkins; 2003.

OBSTETRIC DISORDERS

AMNIOTIC FLUID EMBOLISM

Amniotic fluid embolism is an emergency occurring during labor or shortly after delivery with cardiogenic shock, respiratory failure, and frequently death. The diagnosis is made on physical examination with rapidly progressive hypotension progressing to shock. Blood tests will show a consumptive coagulopathy (DIC), hypoxemia, and acidosis. Unfortunately, many cases are confirmed only at autopsy. Amniotic debris consisting of squamous cells, mucin, and lanugo from the fetus can be found in the peripheral blood or on autopsy sections of the lung in the mother (see eBook Figure 8-12).

CHORIOAMNIONITIS*

❑ **Definition and Etiology**

- Intra-amniotic infections (IAI) include infections of amniotic fluid, membranes, or placenta. IAIs are a significant cause of fetal demise, premature delivery, neonatal sepsis and pneumonia, and maternal bacteremia and sepsis (see eBook Figure 8-13).
- Most IAIs are caused by vaginal microorganisms that gain access to the uterine cavity. These ascending infections are most common as a result of premature rupture of the fetal membranes. Fetal infection may also be caused by hematogenous transmission from the maternal circulation. This route is most common for viral pathogens.
- The etiology is broad. Mixed infections are common. Pathogens associated with IAI include the following: Anaerobes, including *Bacteroides* spp., *Fusobacterium* spp., and anaerobic gram-positive cocci; *E. coli*, *Proteus mirabilis*, and other enteric gram-negative rods; *Enterococcus* spp.; *Listeria monocytogenes*; group B *Streptococcus*, and group A *Streptococcus*; *Ureaplasma urealyticum* and *Mycoplasma hominis*. Nonbacterial pathogens include *Toxoplasma gondii* and viruses (e.g., CMV, HSV, rubella).

❑ **Who Should Be Suspected?**

- Risk factors for IAIs include prolonged labor and premature rupture of membranes, especially with fetal distress, and when fetal scalp monitors are used; nulliparity; IAI in previous pregnancy; and concurrent STI.
- Almost all women with IAI present with fever. Other signs and symptoms include abdominal pain and uterine tenderness, leukocytosis, maternal or fetal tachycardia, and foul-smelling amniotic fluid.

❑ **Laboratory Findings**

- Laboratory tests must be interpreted in the context of the clinical presentation. Individual tests have moderate negative predictive values but reasonably good positive predictive values. Increasing numbers of supportive laboratory test findings are associated with improved positive predictive value.
- Culture: Amniotic fluid cultures are the gold standard for diagnosis. Gram stain may demonstrate organisms.
- Two or three sets of blood cultures should be collected from the mother and baby after delivery, to evaluate the possibility of bacteremia or fungemia.
- Amniotic fluid findings: Analysis of fluid glucose concentration and WBC count is recommended. An elevated WBC, or positive leukocyte esterase reaction, supports diagnosis.
- Amniotic fluid glucose concentration is usually decreased. An amniotic fluid glucose concentration <5 mg/dL has a positive predictive value approximately

---

*This section contributed by Michael J. Mitchell, MD.

90%; a glucose concentration ≥20 mg/dL has a negative predictive value approximately 90%.

- Maternal CRP is not useful for predicting IAI.
- Histology: Fetal membranes and tissue and placenta should be submitted for histologic examination, as appropriate.

Suggested Readings

Broekhuizen FF, Gilman M, Hamilton PR. Amniocentesis for gram stain and culture in preterm premature rupture of the membranes. *Obstet Gynecol.* 1985;66:316–321.

Gauthier DW, Meyer WJ. Comparison of gram stain, leukocyte esterase activity, and amniotic fluid glucose concentration in predicting amniotic fluid culture results in preterm premature rupture of membranes. *Am J Obstet Gynecol.* 1992;1:1092–1095.

Goldenberg RL, Hauth JC, Andrews WW. Intrauterine infection and preterm delivery. *NEJM.* 2000;342:1500–1507.

Hussey M, Levy E, Pombar X, et al. Evaluating rapid diagnostic tests of intra-amniotic infection: Gram stain, amniotic fluid glucose level, and amniotic fluid to serum glucose level ratio. *Am J Obstet Gynecol.* 1998;179:650–656.

Kiltz RJ, Burke S, Porreco RP. Amniotic fluid glucose concentration as a marker for intra-amniotic infection. *Obstet Gynecol.* 1991;78:619–622.

Romero R, Gomez R, Chaiworapongsa T, et al. The role of infection in preterm labour and delivery. *Paediat Perinat Epidemiol.* 2001;15:41–56.

Sperling RS, Newton E, Gibbs RS. Intraamniotic infection in low-birth-weight infants. *J Infect Dis.* 1988;157:113–117.

8

ECTOPIC (TUBAL) PREGNANCY

❑ Definition
Ectopic pregnancy is the implantation of the conceptus outside of the endometrial cavity, in the Fallopian tube or cornu of the uterus.

❑ Clinical Presentation
Tubal pregnancy has increased in frequency and constitutes up to 2% of all pregnancies now[1]. Patients present with abdominal pain, amenorrhea, and vaginal bleeding. With rupture, there is rapid onset of hypotension from intraperitoneal bleeding and if not immediately treated may result in death. Diagnosis is made by ultrasound and hCG in the serum or urine (see eBook Figure 8-14).

❑ Laboratory Findings
- *Human chorionic gonadotropin* (hCG): Tests for hCG should recognize the following three important forms. Intact hCG, H-hCG (hyperglycosylated hCG produced by invasive cytotrophoblasts; key component in early pregnancy), and free β-hCG that many kits and point-of-care (POC) tests do not recognize.
  - ▼ hCG titer doubles about every 1.4–2.1 days during first 40 days of normal pregnancy (at least two measurements 48–72 hours apart are needed to calculate this); an abnormally slow increase in hCG (<66% in 48 hours during first 40 days of pregnancy) indicates ectopic pregnancy (S/S = 80%/91%) or abnormal intrauterine pregnancy in approximately 75% of cases[2].
  - ▼ The discrimination zone for normal versus ectopic pregnancy is reached when hCG reaches 6,500 mIU/mL (equivalent to approximately 6 weeks of gestation) without an intrauterine gestational sac seen by transabdominal

US or at 1,500–2,000 mIU/mL hCG when visualizing by transvaginal ultrasound[3]. There is no proven discriminatory level for multiple gestations.

▼ The lack of visualization of a gestational sac may also occur with spontaneous abortion.

▼ Decrease of hCG of ≥15% 12 hours after curettage is diagnostic of completed abortion, but hCG that rises or remains the same indicates ectopic pregnancy.

▼ hCG level >50,000 mIU/mL in ectopic pregnancy is rare.

▼ Serum hCG is used to monitor methotrexate treatment of ectopic pregnancy (performed weekly until undetectable).

▼ Urine pregnancy test is more variable.

■ *Progesterone*: Serum progesterone may be used to help identify ectopic pregnancy in patients with bleeding and abdominal pain with an hCG lower than expected for gestational age. A level of ≥25 ng/mL is said to indicate normal intrauterine pregnancy (sensitivity = 98%) and ≤5 ng/mL confirms nonviable fetus (100% sensitivity)[4,5].

■ *Hematology:* WBC may be increased. It usually returns to normal in 24 hours, and persistent increase may indicate recurrent bleeding. Fifty percent of patients have normal WBC; 75% of the patients have WBC <15,000/μL. Persistent WBC >20,000/μL may indicate PID. Anemia depends on degree of blood loss; it often precedes the tubal pregnancy in impoverished populations. Progressive anemia may indicate continuing bleeding into the peritoneal cavity. Absorption of blood from peritoneal hematoma may cause increased serum bilirubin.

■ *Uterine curettage* is needed to distinguish ectopic pregnancy from spontaneous intrauterine abortion by the identification of chorionic villi and implantation site in the specimen.

References

Rajkowa M, Glass MR, Rutherford AJ, et al. Trends in the incidence of ectopic pregnancy in England and Wales from 1966 to 1996. *Br J Obstet Gynaecol.* 2000;107(3):369–374.

Silva C, Sammel MD, Zhou L, et al. Human chorionic gonadotropin profile for women with ectopic pregnancy. *Obstet Gynecol.* 2006;107:605.

Barnhart KT, Simhan H, Kamelle SA. Diagnostic accuracy of ultrasound above and below the beta-hCG discriminatory zone. *Obstet Gynecol.* 1999;94:583.

Rausch ME, Barnhart KT. Serum biomarkers for detecting ectopic pregnancy. *Clin Obstet Gynecol.* 2012;55:418.

Verhaegen J, Gallos ID, van Mello NM, et al. Accuracy of single progesterone test to predict early pregnancy outcome in women with pain or bleeding: meta-analysis of cohort studies. *BMJ.* 2012;345:e6077.

FETAL DEATH IN UTERO

❑ Definition
Stillbirth is distinguished from miscarriage by a fetal weight varying from >350 to >500 g or >20 weeks of gestation.

❑ Clinical Presentation
The rate of fetal loss varies by race, maternal diabetes, and hypertension.

The most common causes are[1]:

- Obstetric complications 29.3%
- Placental disease 23.6%
- Fetal genetic/structural abnormalities 13.7%
- Maternal or fetal infection 12.9%
- Umbilical cord abnormalities 10.4%
- Hypertensive disorders 9.2%
- Other maternal medical conditions 7.8%

❑ **Laboratory Findings**

No laboratory tests are available to predict fetal loss. Screens for genetic abnormalities may be helpful to predict poor outcome. Other risks include advanced maternal age, obesity, smoking, multiple gestations, maternal hypertension, diabetes and collagen vascular disease, and a past history of fetal loss.

The diagnosis of fetal death is usually made by the mother noting decreased fetal movements and uterine bleeding or contractions. The diagnosis is confirmed by ultrasound examination.

Reference

1. Stillbirth Collaborative Research Network Writing Group. Causes of death among stillbirths. *JAMA*. 2011;306:2459.

POSTTERM PREGNANCY

❑ **Definition**

A prolonged or postterm pregnancy is defined as one lasting >294 days or 42 weeks of gestation. The etiology is unknown for most cases and rarely may be due to abnormal fetal production of hormones that are involved in parturition.

❑ **Clinical Presentation**

Patients at risk include patients with previous postterm pregnancy, nulliparity, male fetus, maternal obesity, advanced maternal age, and race (Caucasians are at a greater risk).

❑ **Laboratory Findings**

- A progressively falling rather than a rising serum estriol (E3) is usually found.
- Amniotic fluid L/S ratio is not useful.

MULTIPLE GESTATION PREGNANCY

❑ **Definition**

Pregnancy with more than one fetus.

❑ **Clinical Presentation**

Multiple gestations are increasing due to increased maternal age at childbirth and the increased use of fertility drugs such as clomiphene citrate and gonadotropins and in vitro fertilization. Thirty-one percent of the cases are monozygotic (see eBook Figure 8-15)[1]. Risks posed by multiple gestations include preterm birth, fetal growth restriction, and increased mortality due to obstetric complications and congenital anomalies. Preeclampsia is also increased.

❑ Laboratory Findings

In women with multiple gestations, estradiol, FSH, and luteinizing hormone may be elevated. The hCG may be increased, with increased maternal serum AFP.

Reference

1. Cameron AH, Edwards JH, Derom R, et al. The value of twin surveys in the study of malformations. *Eur J Obstet Gynecol Reprod Biol.* 1983;14:347.

PLACENTAE ABRUPTIO AND PREVIA

Placenta abruptio is the premature separation of normally implanted placenta after the 20th week of gestation. It causes hemorrhage and 15% of third-trimester stillbirths. There are no diagnostic laboratory findings. Laboratory findings are hypovolemic shock, acute renal failure, and DIC (it is the most common cause of DIC in pregnancy).

Placenta previa is the abnormal implantation of the placenta into the lower uterine segment. It may cover part (partial) or all (complete) of the internal os resulting in painless vaginal bleeding and increases risk for fetal demise. Laboratory findings are due to blood loss. Maternal HCT should be maintained at ≥35%.

PRETERM DELIVERY

❑ Definition

Preterm delivery is defined as a gestational age <37 weeks from the LMP; however, birth prior to 38 weeks also has increased morbidity and mortality. Prematurity may also be defined as low birth weight infants (<2,500 g), very low birth weight (<1,500 g), and extremely low birth weight (<1,000 g). Preterm birth may be due to infection, placental abruption or hemorrhage, pathologic uterine distention, or stress in the mother or fetus. It is more likely to occur in women under 20 years of age or over 35 years of age. Patients present with uterine contractions and vaginal discharge (mucus or bloody show). The diagnosis is made on physical examination with cervical dilation or defacement, regular contractions, bleeding, and ruptured membranes.

❑ Laboratory Findings

- *Fetal fibronectin* in cervical secretions >50 ng/mL (immunoassay) or rapid test identifies women who deliver before term with S/S = 60–93%/52–85%, PPV = 25%. With high-risk patients, S/S = 70/75%. NPV = 96% rules out labor within 7 days[1,2]. Normally present in early pregnancy and within 1–2 weeks of onset of labor at term but normally absent from cervicovaginal fluid after 20 weeks. It is also present in AF so testing after rupture of membranes is not helpful. If present between 24 and 36 weeks, it precedes preterm labor/birth by ≥3 weeks.
- Laboratory findings are due to associated conditions (e.g., hyaline membrane disease, intraventricular hemorrhage).

References

1. Sanchez-Ramos L, Delke I, Zamora J, et al. Fetal fibronectin as a short-term predictor of preterm birth in symptomatic patients: a meta-analysis. *Obstet Gynecol* 2009;114:631.
2. Honest H, Bachmann LM, Gupta JK, et al. Accuracy of cervicovaginal fetal fibronectin test in predicting risk of spontaneous preterm birth: systematic review. *BMJ.* 2002;325:301.

RUPTURED MEMBRANES

❑ **Definition**

The diagnosis of rupture of membranes is best made on direct observation of fluid leaking from the cervical os. Laboratory diagnosis of fluid from the posterior fornix as amniotic fluid (AF) rather than urine may be necessary.

❑ **Laboratory Findings**

Laboratory methods for detecting AF in the vagina:

- The "Fern" test is the most reliable test (>96% accuracy). AF air-dried on glass slide shows a characteristic fern-like pattern microscopically. Results are false positive in the presence of cervical mucus or semen and false negative in the presence of blood, dry swab, or insufficient drying time; they are not affected by meconium or pH.
- Amniotic fluid pH is 7.0–7.3 while normal vaginal pH is 3.8–4.2. The nitrazine paper test changes from blue to yellow if the pH is >6.5, with accuracy approximately 93%[1]. Results are false positive due to blood, semen, alkaline urine, trichomoniasis, and bacterial vaginosis. A reagent strip test pH ≥7 and protein ≥100 mg/dL indicate the presence of AF (Table 8-2).
- Placental alpha microglobulin-1 protein assay point of care test using immunochromatography to detect trace amounts of placental alpha microglobulin-1 protein in vaginal fluid[2]. Compared to fern testing or nitrazine paper testing, the cost of this test is significantly higher and should be limited to use when the diagnosis remains uncertain following the previous tests.
- Measurement of AFP in vaginal secretions is unreliable; same concentration in AF and maternal plasma in the third trimester.

References

1. Abe T. The detection of rupture of fetal membranes with the nitrazine indicator. *Am J Obstet Gynecol.* 1940;39:400.
2. Abdelazim IA, Makhlouf HH. Placental alpha microglobulin-1 (AmniSure(®) test) for detection of premature rupture of fetal membranes. *Arch Gynecol Obstet.* 2012;285:985.

TOXEMIA OF PREGNANCY (PREECLAMPSIA/ECLAMPSIA)

❑ **Definition**

Preeclampsia is characterized by hypertension, proteinuria, and edema (of the face, hands, and legs) after the 20th week of pregnancy. It is a multisystem disorder and when severe will show signs of end-organ injury. Eclampsia refers to the new onset of seizures in a patient with preeclampsia. The incidence of preeclampsia is ≤7.5% of pregnancies worldwide.[1] The etiology is unknown and likely involves maternal and fetal/placental factors. There is abnormal placental vasculature early in pregnancy, which may result in underperfusion, hypoxia, and ischemia. This may lead to circulating antiangiogenic factors that cause maternal endothelial dysfunction resulting in hypertension and proteinuria.[2]

❑ **Laboratory Findings**

The diagnosis of mild preeclampsia is made in a previously normotensive woman with new onset of hypertension and proteinuria after 20 weeks of gestation (BP ≥140/90 and proteinuria ≥0.3 g in 24 hours or a protein: creatinine ratio

≥0.3 mg/mg). (Collect urine by catheter if membranes have ruptured or in presence of vaginitis.)

- Alternate tests: >1+ on dipstick on two occasions >6 hours but <1 week apart *or* two specimens ≥1+ by dipstick 6 hours but <1 week apart *or* a single specimen ≤2+ by dipstick
- Increased serum inhibin A (at 15–20 weeks) and activin A (at approximately 30 weeks) may indicate preeclampsia and preterm labor[3].

The diagnosis of severe preeclampsia is made with a blood pressure >160/110 on two occasions at least 6 hours apart, proteinuria of >5 g/day, and persistent visual or mental abnormalities.

Additional tests:

- Proteinuria >3+ on dipstick on two occasions >6 hours apart or significant new-onset proteinuria ≥3.0–5.0 g/24 hours or >3+ by dipstick on two occasions.
- Oliguria—urine output ≤500 mL/24 hours.
- AST or ALT abnormal with persistent right upper quadrant or epigastric pain.
- CBC may show a platelet count <100,000/μL and increased HCT.
- Blood smear may show schistocytes if microangiopathic hemolysis is present.
- Serum uric acid is increased in virtually all cases of preeclampsia; correlates with disease severity.
- Serum creatinine >1.2 mg/dL. Creatinine clearance is decreased, causing increased BUN and creatinine.
- BUN may be normal unless the disease is severe or there is a prior renal lesion. (BUN usually decreases during normal pregnancy because of the increase in the GFR.)
- Urinalysis: RBCs and RBC casts are not abundant; hyaline and granular casts are present.
- Histology: Biopsy of kidney is pathognomonic (swelling of glomerular and mesangial endothelial cells) and also rules out primary renal disease or hypertensive vascular disease.

References

1. Wallis AB, Saftlas AF, Hsia J, et al. Secular trends in the rates of preeclampsia, eclampsia, and gestational hypertension, United States, 1987–2004. *Am J Hypertens.* 2008;21:521.
2. Maynard SE, Karumanchi SA. Angiogenic factors and preeclampsia. *Semin Nephrol.* 2011;31:33.
3. Cukle H, Sehmi I, Jones R. Maternal serum Inhibin A can predict preeclampsia. *Br J Obstet Gynaecol.* 1998;105:1101.

ECLAMPSIA

❏ Definition

Eclampsia is the new onset of seizures or coma without other neurologic condition occurring in a woman who meets the criteria for preeclampsia. Approximately 20% of women who develop eclampsia have only mild hypertension and may have no evidence of proteinuria or edema[1]. Eclampsia is a severe form of the preeclampsia eclampsia continuum and remains a common cause of maternal death. Seizures are believed to result from severe hypertension resulting in hypertensive encephalopathy[2]. Stroke with cerebral hemorrhages is the cause of death in up to 20% of patients with eclampsia[3].

❑ **Laboratory Findings**

- Laboratory findings due to complications (e.g., cerebral hemorrhage, pulmonary edema, renal cortical necrosis).
- $MgSO_4$ treatment requires urine output ≥100 mL/4 hours. Monitoring serum magnesium levels is not required.
- Beware of associated or underlying conditions (e.g., hydatidiform mole, twin pregnancy, prior renal disease, DM, or nonimmune hydrops fetalis).

References

1. Sibai BM. Eclampsia. VI. Maternal-perinatal outcome in 254 consecutive cases. *Am J Obstet Gynecol.* 1990;163:1049
2. Zeeman GG, Fleckenstein JL, Twickler DM, et al. Cerebral infarction in eclampsia. *Am J Obstet Gynecol.* 2004;190:714.
3. Lewington S, Clarke R, Qizilbash N, et al. Age-specific relevance of usual blood pressure to vascular mortality: a meta-analysis of individual data for one million adults in 61 prospective studies. *Lancet.* 2002;360:1903.

TROPHOBLASTIC NEOPLASMS

8

❑ **Definition**

Gestational trophoblastic disease is due to a group of abnormal gestations and neoplasms arising from the trophoblast associated with pregnancy. Most common is the partial hydatidiform mole (PHM) followed by complete hydatidiform mole (CHM), placental site trophoblast tumor, and choriocarcinoma. Risk factors include advanced maternal age, Asian ethnicity, lower social–economic status, and a prior molar pregnancy.

❑ **Clinical Presentation**

PHM occurs in one in 100 pregnancies. It develops when a normal egg is fertilized by two spermatozoa or one spermatozoon that has undergone nondisjunction in meiosis resulting in triploidy (see eBook Figure 8-16A–C).

❑ **Laboratory Findings**

- HCG levels are variable and spontaneously regress in >95% of cases requiring chemotherapy.
- Endometrial curettings reveal hydropic and normal villi, amniotic membranes with or without fetal parts. A fetus if present may express syndactyly.
- Histologically, there is focal mild syncytial trophoblastic hyperplasia. A p57 immunostain will be positive.
- Flow cytometry will demonstrate triploidy.
- A karyotype will demonstrate 69 XXY in most cases, 69 XXX, and rarely 69 XYY.

❑ **Clinical Presentation**

CHM occurs in 1:1,000 pregnancies. It develops when an anucleate ovum is fertilized by one or two spermatozoa resulting in a diploid cell with two sets of paternal chromosomes (see eBook Figure 8-16D–F). Ninety percent are homozygous 46 XX; the rest are heterozygous, mostly 46 XY with few 46 XX.[1]

❑ **Laboratory Findings**

- HCG levels are increased, usually >100,000 mIU/mL.
- Endometrial curettings reveal grape-like transparent villi. A fetus is not present.
- Histology reveals villi with prominent cisterns, trophoblastic hyperplasia, and atypia particularly of the implantation site. A p57 immunostain is negative.
- Flow cytometry reveals diploid cells.

Following treatment by evacuation of the molar pregnancy, the following laboratory studies should be performed to determine whether residual neoplastic trophoblasts persist. Risk for persistence includes increased maternal age, a longer interval from a previous pregnancy, and higher hCG levels.

- Serum hCG is used for diagnosis and management of both benign and malignant types. A persistently elevated or slowly declining level by the end of first trimester indicates persistent trophoblastic disease and the need for systemic therapy for invasive mole or choriocarcinoma (see below). An hCG level >500,000 mIU/L is virtually diagnostic.
- After evacuation of the uterus, hCG is negative by 40 days in 75% of cases. If the test is positive at 56 days, 50% have trophoblastic disease.
- Repeat hCG test every 1–2 weeks with clinical examination for 6 months. Disease remits in 80% without further treatment. Plateau or rise of titer indicates persistent disease. Chemotherapy is indicated if disease persists or metastasizes.
- A negative hCG test should be rechecked every 3 months for 1–2 years.
- High-risk patients are indicated by initial serum titer >40,000 mIU/L. Frequent follow-up titers are indicated after radiation therapy with lifelong titers every 6 months.
- Measurement of hCG in the CSF (ratio of serum to CSF <60:1) is used in the diagnosis of brain metastases.

❑ **Limitations of hCG Testing**

- Beware of false low results due to artifactual "hook effect" of immunoassays due to large antigen excess (>1 × 10⁶ mIU/L); this is eliminated by a two-stage immunoassay.
- Clinical and biochemical evidence of hyperthyroxemia may occur because α subunits of TSH and hCG are identical.

❑ **Clinical Presentation**
Persistent gestational trophoblastic disease or invasive mole occurs when the villi are present within the myometrium or its vascular spaces (invasion) and may occur with either PHM or CHM. Following invasion, trophoblasts may embolize to distant sites (metastatic). This type of mole requires surgical resection and usually responds to chemotherapy.

❑ **Laboratory Findings**

- HCG may plateau or rise following evacuation of the uterus.
- Endometrial curettings reveal minimal residual villous tissue.

❏ Clinical Presentation

Placental site trophoblastic tumor, previously known as trophoblastic pseudotumor, presents as a mass in the endometrium that can be identified on sonogram. These tumors are not well understood and are primarily seen in reproductive age women with rare cases in postmenopausal women. It may follow a normal term delivery, abortion, or a molar pregnancy. Women present with irregular bleeding months to years following the preceding pregnancy. The tumor is composed of cytotrophoblasts, which invade in a pattern similar to normal placental implantation. Immunohistochemistry may help differentiate this tumor from choriocarcinoma. Prognosis for poor outcome is suggested by the length of time from the previous pregnancy. Diagnosis >2 years following the pregnancy has a worse outcome.[2,3]

❏ Laboratory Findings

- HCG measurement reveals persistent low levels (<50 mIU/L).
- Endometrial curettings demonstrate a fleshy mass in the endomyometrium.
- Histology reveals sheets of mononuclear atypical trophoblasts that dissected between the muscle fibers.
- Immunostaining is positive for human placental lactogen, keratin, and p63, and MIB-1 fraction is usually >15%.

❏ Choriocarcinoma

May occur following molar pregnancy, abortion, ectopic pregnancy, or normal pregnancy. The diagnosis is usually made several months following the pregnancy. Patients present with abnormal uterine bleeding or may have symptoms of metastatic disease. Prognosis is better if diagnosed following a molar pregnancy most likely due to closer patient surveillance and earlier diagnosis.[4]

❏ Laboratory Findings

- HCG rises 2 weeks after delivery.
- Endometrial curettage demonstrates hemorrhagic tumor nodules, no villi are present.
- Histologic evaluation reveals atypical syncytial trophoblasts and cytotrophoblasts.
- Immunostaining reveals strongly positive β-hCG.

References

1. Hemming JD, Quirke P, Womack C, et al. Diagnosis of molar pregnancy and persistent trophoblastic disease by flow cytometry. *J Clin Pathol.* 1987;40(60):615–620.
2. Feltmate CM, Genest DR, Goldstein DP, et al. Advance as in the understanding of placental site trophoblastic tumor. *J Reprod Med.* 2002;47:337–341.
3. Papadopolous AJ, Foskett M, Seckl MJ, et al. Twenty-five years' clinical experience with placental site trophoblastic tumors. *J Reprod Med.* 2002;47(6):460–464.
4. Soper JT. Gestational trophoblastic neoplasia. *Curr Opin Obstet Gynecol.* 1990;2(1):92–97.

CHAPTER 9

Hematologic Disorders

Liberto Pechet

9

This chapter covers blood diseases encompassing pathology of the formed elements of blood (red cells, white cells, and platelets), monoclonal plasmatic dyscrasias, hemorrhagic and thrombotic diseases, and lastly metabolic disorders that have a major impact on hematologic parameters.

 RED BLOOD CELL DISORDERS

ANEMIAS

❏ **Definition**
Anemia is a reduction in Hb leading to decrease in oxygen supply to peripheral tissues. Normal hemoglobin (Hb) range is established by population studies, but range should be adjusted for different age groups, especially for children, and levels are lower in women and in African Americans. There is some debate whether people of older ages have *physiologically* lower Hg levels. Most likely lower values reflect underlying pathology. Hb values are more accurate than hematocrit (Hct) values, because Hb is measured directly by automated analyzers, whereas the Hct is a calculated value.

❏ **Diagnosis**
- There are many ways to classify anemias, but the differential diagnosis of anemia can be narrowed by using the RBC size, as reflected in the MCV and the reticulocyte count. See Figure 9-1.

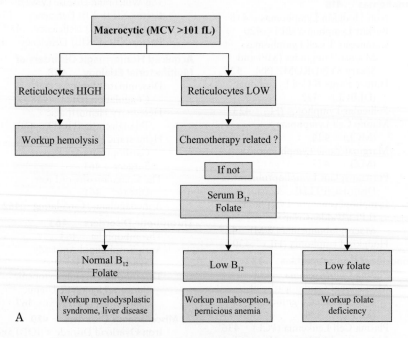

Figure 9–1 *Workup of anemias based on the mean corpuscular volume (MCV).*

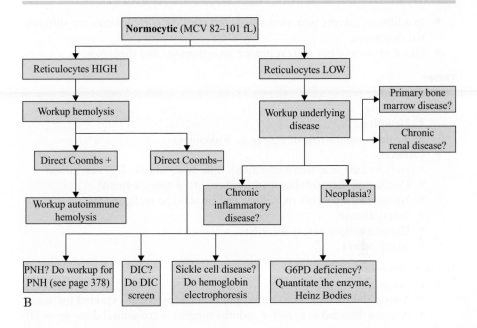

B

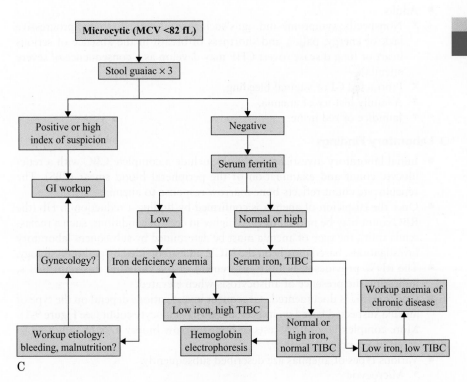

C

Figure 9–1 *(Continued)*

■ In addition, insight into mechanism and etiology complements the differential diagnosis.

■ Onset of anemia has a great impact on symptoms and diagnosis.

Onset

■ Acute
  ▼ Bleeding
  ▼ Hemolysis
  ▼ Acute bone marrow disease (e.g., leukemias)
■ Chronic
  ▼ Deficiencies: iron (most common), folic acid, vitamin B_{12}, nutritional
  ▼ Congenital (hemoglobinopathies, hereditary spherocytosis)
  ▼ Neoplasia, especially metastatic or hematologic malignancies
  ▼ Renal disease
  ▼ Chronic inflammatory disorders
  ▼ Many others

When to Suspect Anemia

■ Children
  ▼ Young child who fails to thrive and is not as active as expected for age.
  ▼ Anemia detected at ages 3–6 months suggests a congenital disorder of Hb synthesis or structure.
■ Adults.
  ▼ Nonspecific symptoms and signs such as weakness, dizziness, progressive lack of energy, pallor, and shortness of breath in the absence of serious heart or lung disease (overt CHF may develop as a consequence of severe anemia).
  ▼ Protracted GI or vaginal bleeding.
  ▼ A family history of anemia.
  ▼ Jaundice or red urine.

❑ Laboratory Findings

■ Initial laboratory investigation should include a complete CBC with a reticulocyte count and examination of the peripheral blood smear (PBS). The reticulocyte count reflects bone marrow response to anemia.

■ Once the suspicion of anemia is confirmed by finding a reduction in Hb (the RBC count may be normal or even higher in certain conditions, such a thalassemia trait), the type of anemia must be determined by subsequent laboratory investigations, based mostly on the MCV, and subdivided by pathophysiology.

■ The RDW provides a useful measurement of the variation in size of RBCs, indicating the presence of anisocytosis when elevated.

■ Once anemia is documented, subsequent investigations depend on the type of anemia suspected based on indices and the reticulocyte count (see Figure 9-1). More complex laboratory tests or bone marrow biopsy may be indicated to ascertain its precise etiology.

■ Various types of anemias are described subsequently.
  ▼ Microcytic
  ▼ Macrocytic
  ▼ Normocytic

▼ Aplastic
▼ Hemoglobinopathies
▼ Hemolytic anemias
▼ Sickle cell
▼ HbC, HbD, HbE diseases
▼ Thalassemias

Suggested Readings

Beutler E, Waalen J. The definition of anemia: what is the lower limit of normal of the blood hemoglobin concentration? *Blood.* 2006;107:1747–1750.

Tefferi A. Anemia in adults: a contemporary approach to diagnosis. *Mayo Clin Proc.* 2003; 78:1274–1280.

MACROCYTIC ANEMIAS

❑ Definition

Anemias in which the RBCs are oval macrocytes, with an MCV larger than normal (>101 fL).

❑ Who Should Be Suspected?

A patient with macrocytic anemia, hypersegmented neutrophils on peripheral blood smear, and symptoms of malabsorption, poor diet, chronic hemolysis without folate supplementation, chemotherapy, or hypothyroidism. Folate deficiency is seen with alcoholism; in third-world countries, it may be associated with sprue-like syndromes. Vitamin B_{12} (cobalamin) deficiency increases in incidence with aging, and should be searched for, even in the absence of anemia in the elderly with neurologic deficits. Cobalamin and folic acid deficiencies often coexist. Other causes of macrocytic anemias are liver cirrhosis, myelodysplastic syndrome (MDS), azidothymidine (AZT) therapy for AIDS, Down syndrome, and normal newborns.

9

❑ Laboratory Findings

Laboratory investigation of macrocytic anemias must differentiate between macrocytic anemias without megaloblastosis and true megaloblastic anemias resulting from vitamin B_{12} and/or folate deficiency. Megaloblastic anemia is a morphologic definition based on bone marrow examination. B_{12} deficiency may be the result of pernicious anemia (PA) (lack of intrinsic factor) or may have other etiologies.

- CBC:
  ▼ Anemia with oval macrocytes, poikilocytosis and anisocytosis, small teardrop cells
  ▼ High RDW
  ▼ Thrombocytopenia and leukopenia in severe cases
  ▼ Hypersegmented polymorphonuclear cells and giant metamyelocytes in megaloblastic anemias
  ▼ Reticulocyte count: inadequate for the degree of anemia.
- Serum or RBC folate and serum cobalamin are obtained if another etiology is not obvious. The specific metabolites methylmalonic acid and homocysteine accumulate in these deficiencies; they are additional assays and may help discriminate between cobalamin and folate deficiencies and other etiologies for macrocytic anemias. These assays, as well as RBC folate, are more expensive

and should be reserved for patients with borderline folate or cobalamin values but strong suspicion of one or the other.

- Serum cobalamin if <200 pg/mL is consistent with vitamin B_{12} deficiency.
- Serum folate if <2 ng/mL is consistent with folate deficiency.
- Serum or urine methylmalonic acid if increased confirms vitamin B_{12} deficiency. It may be normal in folate deficiency.
- Homocysteine (total) if elevated is compatible with either cobalamin or folate deficiency. If normal, both can be excluded.
- Documentation of cobalamin deficiency does not establish the diagnosis of PA, an autoimmune disease characterized by deficiency of intrinsic factor (IF) and lack of HCl gastric secretion. PA was traditionally diagnosed by the absorption of orally administered radiolabeled cobalamin, the Schilling test (no longer available in the United States). In its absence, the assays mentioned above are helpful, but not specific for PA. Fifty percent to 70% of PA patients will have positive serum anti-IF antibodies, thus documenting PA (100% specificity). The patients who are negative for IF antibodies cannot be distinguished from non-PA cases of cobalamin malabsorption but will respond to oral vitamin B_{12} if not PA. Antiparietal antibodies are less sensitive or specific. Recently, chronic *Helicobacter pylori* infection has been implicated in the etiology of PA and the lack of IF.
  - ▼ Bone marrow aspirate (indicated in very selected cases) may reveal marked red cell hyperplasia and megaloblastic maturation in both vitamin B_{12} and folate deficiencies. Otherwise, it may uncover other reasons for macrocytosis, such as myelodysplastic syndrome MDS.
  - ▼ Serum LDH and indirect bilirubin are elevated in folate and vitamin B_{12} deficiency.

❑ **Limitations**

- In the presence of coexisting iron deficiency, MCV may not be elevated, even in cases of overt folate or cobalamin deficiency.
- Low cobalamin levels develop during pregnancy.
- One hospital meal may normalize serum folate level (but not RBC).

Methylmalonic acid increases in renal insufficiency.

MICROCYTIC ANEMIAS

❑ **Definition**

Anemias characterized by low MCV (<82 fL) and hypochromia. Most common: iron deficiency anemia, to be differentiated from the thalassemias and occasionally from anemia of chronic diseases. Despite the high frequency of iron deficiency anemia, patients should not be treated automatically with iron without determining the cause of the anemia.

❑ **Who Should Be Suspected?**

Suspect iron deficiency if the following are present:

- History of GI, vaginal, or massive, repeated urinary bleeding
- Microcytosis, hypochromic
- Poor diet

❏ **Laboratory Findings**

■ First line of investigation: serum ferritin has a specificity of 98% but a sensitivity of only 25% for a 12 µg/L threshold. Because ferritin is an acute-phase reactant, it may be normal or even increased despite iron deficiency when the patients have serious medical problems, such as chronic inflammatory conditions and active liver disease. As a consequence, a normal ferritin value does not exclude iron deficiency. Very low values are definitely diagnostic, iron deficiency is confirmed, and there is no need to obtain serum iron and total iron-binding capacity (TIBC). Investigation of etiology (history, stool examination for occult blood, GI investigation, pelvic and rectal examinations) is mandatory.

■ If serum ferritin is normal or borderline, serum iron and transferrin (usually reported as TIBC) are the next assay to be ordered.

■ If the serum iron is very low and TIBC elevated (with the ratio of serum iron divided by TIBC <16%), diagnosis is confirmed.

■ Normal serum iron and TIBC: iron deficiency is excluded in most cases.

■ Low serum iron, low TIBC: most likely anemia of chronic disease; workup underlying etiology.

■ High serum iron, normal TIBC: the most likely diagnosis is thalassemia.

■ Two additional blood tests: the soluble transferrin receptor and the reticulocyte Hb content are optional. When used in conjunction with ferritin, these tests improve further our ability to accurately diagnose iron deficiency. Not widely used.

■ As a last resort, if the diagnosis is still in doubt: bone marrow aspirate/biopsy for Prussian blue stain. If it is negative, iron deficiency is definitely present.

9

NORMOCYTIC ANEMIAS

❏ **Definition**
Anemias with normal MCV.

❏ **Who Should Be Suspected?**
Patients with anemias secondary to an underlying nonhematologic disease (also known as "anemias of chronic disease" [ACD]). The term "anemia of chronic inflammation" may be used too, but it does not cover all situations (see the following paragraph). The most common conditions leading to ACD:

■ Anemia of chronic inflammation (infections, rheumatologic diseases) is the prototype of normocytic anemias; the red cell may occasionally be borderline microcytic.

■ The etiology of anemia of chronic renal failure is in part the reduced production of erythropoietin; additional factors are a shortened red cell survival and frequent bleeding.

■ Anemia in cancer patients is a common, multifactorial finding. Microangiopathic hemolytic anemia and myelophthisic anemia may be an additional feature resulting from disseminated carcinoma.

■ Aplastic anemias (AAs) can be congenital or acquired. In AA, hematopoiesis fails. All blood lineages are decreased (pancytopenia), with the possible exception of lymphocytes. Pure red cell anemia is a variant of AA in which only, or mostly, the red cell line is affected.

❏ **Laboratory Findings**

- CBC: Moderate anemia, normal to slightly reduced MCV in inflammatory conditions; normal red cell morphology, with only mild variation in RDW. In anemia of chronic renal failure, burr cells can be seen on the peripheral blood smear (PBS).
- Inadequate reticulocyte response.
- Increased serum ferritin; reduced serum iron and TIBC.
- Serum erythropoietin is inadequate for the level of anemia, especially in renal failure.

APLASTIC ANEMIA (AA)

❏ **Definition**

Although the name refers only to anemia, AA is characterized by peripheral blood pancytopenia. It is the paradigm of bone marrow failure. The diagnosis of AA is one of exclusion. There is variable bone marrow hypocellularity due to diminished or absent hematopoietic precursors, the result of injury to the pluripotent stem cell. The absence of a myeloproliferative neoplasm or an MDS is a prerequisite for the diagnosis.

❏ **Etiology**

- AA may be acquired or congenital (Fanconi anemia; see below). More than 50% of the acquired cases are idiopathic, most likely due to an autoimmune mechanism that destroys or suppresses the hematopoietic stem cell via cytotoxic T lymphocytes and the cytokines they produce.
- Other cases may result from drugs, such as chemotherapy, anticonvulsants, and many more. It is essential to obtain a history of drug or toxin exposure.
  - ▼ Immunologic disorders such as graft versus host disease.
  - ▼ Thymomas.
  - ▼ Exposure to ionizing radiation.
  - ▼ Viral infections: EBV and the putative agent of seronegative hepatitis.
  - ▼ Severe malnutrition: kwashiorkor, anorexia nervosa.
  - ▼ Leukemia may be the underlying disease in 1–5% of patients who present with AA.
  - ▼ PNH (see p. 378) develops in 5–10% of patients with AA; conversely, AA develops in 25% of patients with PNH.

❏ **Who Should Be Suspected?**

An individual who presents with a clinical picture of increasing symptoms of anemia, mucosal bleeding, or fever, mucosal ulcerations, and bacterial infections due to neutropenia, in whom an initial CBC demonstrates pancytopenia. Pancytopenia from other causes, such as chemotherapy, should be ruled out (see below). The disease is frequent in East Asia.

❏ **Laboratory Findings**

- RBC: anemia is normocytic, normochromic. Hg may be <7 g/L. RDW is normal. MCV is frequently elevated at presentation.
- Reticulocytes are invariably decreased to absent.

- WBC: neutropenia (absolute neutrophil count <1,500/µL) is always present, often accompanied by monocytosis. Abnormal WBCs are not seen. Lymphocyte count is normal (false lymphocytosis if one observes the percent of WBC rather than the absolute count).
- Platelets are decreased, but severity varies.
- Bone marrow (BM) is hypocellular, with an "empty" marrow in severe cases. Less than 30% of residual cells are hematopoietic. Hematopoiesis is not megaloblastic. The appearance of the BM in inherited or acquired AA is identical. Aspiration and biopsy are both necessary to rule out MDS, leukemias, granulomatous disease, or tumors. The BM examination must also exclude the viral hemophagocytic syndrome.
- *Cytogenetics*: normal karyotype.
- *Flow cytometry* phenotyping shows virtual absence of CD34 hematopoietic stem cells in blood and marrow. AA and PNH overlap in approximately 40–50% of cases.
- Serum iron studies are normal.

Suggested Reading
Sheinberg P, Young N. How I treat acquired aplastic anemia. *Blood.* 2012;120:1185–1196.

PANCYTOPENIA

❑ **Definition**

Pancytopenia is a disorder in which all three blood lines, red cells, white cells, and platelets, are reduced. It is not a disease entity, but a triad of findings that may result from a number of disease processes, most of which involve the bone marrow. Occasionally early on, only two of the three blood lines may be decreased: *bycytopenia*. Eventually, all three lineages become affected.

❑ **Etiology**

Pancytopenia may be the result of a congenital anomaly, neoplasia, or autoimmunity or may be iatrogenic (Figure 9-1). The following mechanisms may account for pancytopenia:

- Decreased production of hematopoietic cells by the bone marrow resulting in a hypocellular marrow;
- Ineffective hematopoiesis with a cellular (or even hypercellular) marrow;
- Infiltration of the bone marrow by extraneous elements;
- Systemic conditions.

A *bone marrow aspirate and biopsy* are mandatory in most cases without a clear etiology. Deciding the bone marrow cellularity may at times be difficult, because of imprecise quantitation of cellularity or sample error due to unequal distribution of bone marrow tissue. In some cases, biopsies from multiple sites may be necessary. Moreover, hypocellular marrow due to aplastic anemia may evolve over time into a hypercellular marrow. This happens for instance when acute leukemia or PNH develops.

A *thorough history and physical examination* also play a prominent role in establishing the etiology of pancytopenia, with important clues, such as a history of any drug or toxin exposure or splenomegaly, directing the clinician to possible etiologic causes.

When to suspect pancytopenia:

- Finding a persistent decrease in all three hematopoietic lines on a routine CBC
- Clinical symptoms suggestive of anemia, bleeding, or prolonged fever
- Repeated infections

Tests recommended:

- CBC with differential.
- Chemistry, immunology, or infectious investigations as suggested by systemic manifestations.
- Flow cytometry to rule out paroxysmal nocturnal hemoglobinuria (PNH) or hematologic malignancies.
- Bone marrow aspiration and biopsy (see above).
- Cytogenetic and FISH analysis may establish the precise diagnosis in myelodysplastic syndromes or other hematologic malignancies. Newer whole-genome scanning technologies such as single nucleotide polymorphism (SNP) array–based karyotyping may be an additional diagnostic technology.
- Histochemistry for infiltrative congenital disorders.

Suggested Readings

Nester CM, Thomas CP. Atypical hemolytic uyremic syndrome: what it is, how is it diagnosed, and how is it treated. *Hematology Am Soc Hematol Educ Program*. 2012;2012: 617–625.
Scheinberg P, Young NS. How I treat acquired aplastic anemia. *Blood*. 2012;120:1185–1196.

PURE RED CELL APLASIA (PRCA)

❑ Definition

Chronic condition of profound anemia, characterized by severe reduction or absence of reticulocytes, and absent bone marrow erythroid precursors. (The congenital pure red cell aplasia is described below under Diamond-Blackfan anemia.) All other cell lines are normal. Most cases are mediated by IgG autoantibodies. PRCA may be associated with certain drugs, thymomas, collagen vascular syndromes, or CLL, or follow parvovirus B19 infection. It may also be part of the 5q⁻myelodysplastic syndrome. PRCA may also develop following administration of recombinant erythropoietin due to the development of antierythropoietin antibodies.

❑ Laboratory Findings

- CBC: severe reduction but normal-appearing RBCs; normal WBC and platelet counts.
- Reticulocytes are severely decreased or absent.
- Bone marrow is normocellular, but erythroid precursors cells are absent (giant normoblasts may be seen if the etiology is a parvovirus infection). White cell precursors and megakaryocytes (except in the 5q⁻ syndrome) are normal.
  ▼ Serum iron and transferrin saturation are increased.

FANCONI ANEMIA (FA)

❏ **Definition**
The most common inherited AA. Autosomal recessive syndrome in childhood, associated with congenital anomalies of short stature, rudimentary thumbs, hypoplastic radii, renal anomalies, and skin spots. There is an increased incidence of myelodysplastic syndrome, acute myelogenous leukemia, and squamous cell carcinomas. The diagnosis is usually made between the ages of 6 and 9 years, but in rare cases, it may not been made until adulthood.

❏ **Laboratory Findings**
The hematologic findings evolve over months or years: macrocytic anemia, leukopenia due to neutropenia, and mild to moderate thrombocytopenia.

- *Cytogenetics*: Normal chromosome numbers but structural instability causing breaks, gaps, constrictions, and rearrangements. The diagnosis is made by the presence of increased chromosomal breakage in lymphocytes cultured in the presence of DNA cross-linking agents.
- *Genetics*: Multiple genes appear to be responsible for Fanconi anemia. The genes are dispersed through the genome.
- Fetal Hb is increased (>28%).
- i antigen may be observed.
  - ▾ Serum alpha-protein levels are frequently elevated.

DIAMOND-BLACKFAN ANEMIA (DBA)

❏ **Definition**
DBA is a congenital pure red cell aplasia. It is usually sporadic but may be inherited in an autosomal dominant manner. Onset is before 12 months. DBA is associated with congenital anomalies of the kidneys, eyes, skeleton, and heart. Spontaneous remissions have been observed in 20–30% of cases after months or years.

❏ **Laboratory Findings**
- RBC: severe macrocytic, anemia that is refractory to conventional therapies.
- Reticulocytes are <1%.
- WBC, differential white cell count, and platelet count are normal.
- Bone marrow is normocellular but presents with a marked decrease in erythroid precursors. All other cell lines are normal.
- Fetal Hb is increased.
- Adenosine deaminase is increased in RBCs.
- Serum iron and all other hematologic parameters are normal.
- Serum erythropoietin is elevated.

 HEMOGLOBINOPATHIES

Hemoglobinopathies constitute the most common inherited disorders in humans as a result of selective pressure of endemic falciparum malaria. Human hemoglobins (Hb) are proteins containing a heme moiety and two pairs of globin genes. Normal adult Hb is composed of two alpha and two β-chains, which together add up to

97% of total Hb in red cells (RBC). The balance globins are composed of Hb A2 (approximately 2.5%) and fetal Hg (HbF) usually 0.8–2%. More than 1,000 mutations involving the globin genes have been described; they result from amino acid substitution or from abnormalities of synthesis. The majority of these variants do not cause clinical or hematologic problems. Several variants, such as sickle cell disease and β-thalassemias (described below), are protective and asymptomatic in the heterozygous; however, they result in severe morbidity in the homozygous. Initial screening and definitive diagnosis for Hb variants are described in Chapter 16. Table 9-1 describes the most common hemoglobinopathies encountered in North America: sickle cell syndromes, HbC disease, and β- and α-thalassemias. Genetic analysis may be necessary for uncommon or unknown variants. In North America, it is done in a few specialized laboratories.

SICKLE CELL ANEMIA

❑ Definition
The term sickle cell disease (SCD) describes all the conditions associated with sickling of RBC. SCD encompasses a group of conditions with autosomal inheritance of abnormal Hb β chain resulting from a substitution of valine for glutamic acid in the beta globin chain. This substitution results in polymerization of poorly soluble deoxy-HbS, leading to a marked decrease in red cells' deformability and irreversible distortion of red cells into the sickle cell shape, with their removal by the spleen (prior to the occurrence of autosplenectomy) and macrophages. SCD is encountered mostly in populations of African or Arab ancestry, as well as in some Indian groups.

- Sickle cell anemia (SCA) is the homozygous state where the majority of Hb is S. This results in the precipitation and polymerization of Hb, causing rigid crystals that deform red cells (sickling), leading to microvascular occlusions and hemolysis.
- Sickle cell trait (SCT) is the heterozygous form, in which the CBC is normal. Although generally asymptomatic, its diagnosis is important for genetic counseling.
- Sickle cell syndromes (diseases) represent combinations of sickle cell trait with other hemoglobinopathies, most commonly with β-thalassemia or Hb C.

❑ Who Should Be Suspected?
- SCA should be suspected in a child with a family history of sickle cell disease, failure to thrive, progressive hemolytic anemia, and vasoocclusive crises (repeated painful episodes that lead to organ damage).
- Clinical manifestations are not present at birth, but become apparent after 3–6 months of life, as the concentration of HbF declines, and that of HbS increases. By 2 years of age, 61% of children have already had painful vasoocclusive episodes.
- *Aplastic crises* are self-limited episodes of erythroid aplasia lasting 5–10 days. They are due to infections (most commonly parvovirus B19) and may require emergency transfusions.
- Bilirubin gallstones are present in 30% of patients by age 18 and 70% by age 30.
- Organ damage develops by the time SCA patients are in their teens, with the lungs, kidneys, heart, and liver involvement. Cerebrovascular accidents are also common.

TABLE 9–1. Hemoglobinopathies

Condition	HbA (%)	HbA$_2$ (%)	HbF (%)	HbS (%)	HbC (%)	Other (%)
Normal	≥94	2–3.5	0.5–1	0	0	0
Sickle cell trait	50–70	2–4.5	0.5–1	30–45	0	0
Sickle cell anemia	0	2–4	1–25	75–95	0	0
HbC trait	50–60	sl ↑	0.5–1	0	30–40	0
HbCC (homozygous)	0	<3.5	sl ↑	0	95	0
HbS/HbC disease	Trace	0	<1	50–55	45–50	0
β-Thalassemia minor	90–95	3.5–7	1–5	0	0	0
β-Thalassemia major	β+: Trace β–: 0	2–sl ↑	60–95 95–98	0	0	0
α-Thalassemia with 1–2 abnormal genes	Varies with genetic type	2–3.5	0.5–1	0	0	0
α-Thalassemia: 3-gene defect (HbH disease)	<60	<2	<1–1	0	0	HbH: 5–40
α-Thalassemia: 4-gene defect (hydrops fetalis)	0 or trace	<2	0 or trace	0	0	Hb Bart's 70–80
HbS/β-thalassemia	10–30	4–6	<1–10	70–90	0	0
Hereditary persistence of fetal Hb (HPFH)	Heterozygous: 70–85 Homozygous: 0	1–2.1 0	15–30 100	0	0	0

9

❏ Laboratory Findings

- A "sickle cell screen" can be obtained for a rapid preliminary diagnosis. It is positive in SCA, SCT, in some *non-S sickling* hemoglobinopathies, and in combined SCD with other hemoglobinopathies.

- Hb variant analysis (HPLC or electrophoresis) is used to identify different hemoglobins. Newborns have predominantly HbF with a small amount of HbS and no HbA1. Because other sickle cell syndromes may have similar patterns, it is recommended to study the parents, or repeat the test after 1 year of age, when the adult pattern of SCA is established: very high HbS. HbF may be slightly elevated (1–4%) and especially in patients treated successfully with hydroxyurea where it may reach 15% or more, resulting in marked diminution in morbidity.

- The newborn with SCT will have HbA, HbF, and HbS. Adults have >50% HbA1 and 35–45% HbS.

- Prenatal testing: gene analysis of fetal DNA may be performed on chorionic villi (7–10 weeks of gestation) or amniocytes (15–20 weeks of gestation). DNA testing may be also useful in newborns or children in cases with high levels of HbF if hereditary persistence of fetal hemoglobin is suspected.

- Patients with HbSC disease (see below) have equal amount of HbS and C.

- Patients with sickle cell trait–β-thalassemia (+) have HbA1, elevated HbA2, and HbS.

  - ▼ *CBC* in patients with SCA.
  - ▼ RBC: mild to moderate chronic hemolytic anemia (Hct 15–30%, Hb 5–10 g/dL), punctuated by aplastic crises (sudden, life-threatening episodes of very severe anemia) (see above).
  - ▼ Reticulocytes 3–15% (they may account for an elevated MCV).
  - ▼ MCV is in general normal (except as noted above); MCHC is elevated. Microcytosis and hypochromia may be present, however, if there is coexisting α- or β-thalassemia, or iron deficiency in nontransfused patients.
  - ▼ Peripheral blood smear (PBS): visible sickle cells, polychromasia, and Howell-Jolly bodies in older children, reflecting hyposplenism due to autosplenectomy. Nucleated red cells, basophilic stippling, and Pappenheimer bodies are usually found.
  - ▼ WBCs may be higher than normal. A persistent leukocytosis augurs a poor prognosis.
  - ▼ Platelets may be elevated, in part the result of loss of splenic function.
  - ▼ Bone marrow aspirate (not necessary for diagnosis) is hyperplastic.
  - ▼ Serum erythropoietin may be inappropriately low in some patients, possibly as the result of progressive renal disease.
  - ▼ Serum iron and ferritin may be low, and transferrin elevated, due to iron loss in urine.
  - ▼ Serum folate is low due to overutilization, if not replaced therapeutically.
  - ▼ Serum LDH is elevated.
  - ▼ Serum bilirubin is commonly elevated.
  - ▼ Serum haptoglobin is decreased.
  - ▼ Serum aminotransferase is often elevated.
  - ▼ Ferritin becomes very elevated in multiply transfused patients.
  - ▼ Urine hemosiderin and urobilinogen are present (not necessary for diagnosis).

HEMOGLOBIN S–HEMOGLOBIN C DISEASE

❑ **Definition**

A moderately severe sickling disease, clinically intermediate between sickle cell anemia and sickle cell trait. Occurs in 1 of 833 people of African ancestry.

❑ **Laboratory Findings**

- Hb electrophoresis: HbA is absent; HbS and HbC are present in approximately equal amounts. HbF is ≤6%.
- CBC.
  ▼ Anemia: mild to moderate normochromic, normocytic.
  ▼ Peripheral blood smear (PBS): tetragonal crystals within the RBC in 70% of patients. Target cells and plump/angulated sickle cells, rather than typical sickle cells, are identified.
  ▼ MCV is low, or low normal; MCHC is high.

SICKLE CELL–α-THALASSEMIA DISEASE

α-Thalassemia modifies the severity of sickle cell anemia. Otherwise, it is usually clinically insignificant.

SICKLE CELL–β-THALASSEMIA DISEASE

❑ **Definition**

Condition of mild to moderate severity found in 1 of every 1,667 people of African ancestry.

❑ **Laboratory Findings**

- Hb electrophoresis: HbS varies between 20% and 90%; HbF between 2% and 20%. If the HbS is very high and HbA1 is suppressed, the disease is severe. In milder cases, HbA1 is 25–50%. HbA2 is increased (due to the presence of β-thalassemia), but it has to be differentiated from HbC, which has a similar migration pattern.
- CBC
  ▼ RBC: hypochromic, microcytic anemia with decreased MCV (iron deficiency must be ruled out).
  ▼ Peripheral blood smear (PBS): target cells are prominent; other findings resemble those of sickle cell anemia.

SICKLE CELL–PERSISTENT HIGH FETAL HEMOGLOBIN

❑ **Definition**

Condition seen in 1 in 25,000 African Americans but also frequent in Arab populations. May be mimicked in patients with sickle cell anemia responding to hydroxyurea therapy. Clinical picture and findings intermediate between sickle cell anemia and trait.

❏ **Laboratory Findings**

- Hb electrophoresis: HbF is 20–40%; HbA1 and A2 are absent; HgS is approximately 65%.
- RBC: HbF is unevenly distributed among RBC.

SICKLE CELL–HEMOGLOBIN D DISEASE

❏ **Definition**
Condition resembling HbS/HbC disease; less severe than sickle cell anemia. Found in 1 in 20,000 individuals of African ancestry. Clinically a mild syndrome.

❏ **Laboratory Findings**

- Intermediate between those of sickle cell anemia and sickle cell trait.
- Hb electrophoresis cannot distinguish HbS from HbD at alkaline pH but can be separated at pH 6.2.

Suggested Readings

Vichinsky EP, Mahoney DH Jr. Diagnosis of sickle cell syndromes. UpToDate. In: Basow DS (ed). Waltham, MA: UpToDate, Inc.; 2013.
Ware RE. How I use hydroxyurea to treat young patients with sickle cell anemia. *Blood.* 2010;115:5300–5311.

HEMOGLOBIN C DISEASE

❏ **Definition**
A hemoglobinopathy prevalent in individuals with ancestral roots in West Africa.
Autosomal transmission.

- HbC trait: found in 2% of African Americans, less frequently in other groups; asymptomatic, no anemia.
- Homozygous HbC disease: mild hemolytic anemia.

❏ **Laboratory Findings**

- HbC trait: Hb variant analysis shows 50% HbA1 and 30–40% HbC.
- Homozygous condition: There is no HbA1, and HbC forms the majority variant Hb; HgF is slightly increased. Peripheral blood smear (PBS) shows a variable number of target cells (≤40%), a variable number of microsphero-cytes, occasionally nucleated RBCs, and a few tetragonal crystals within RBCs.

HEMOGLOBIN C–β-THALASSEMIA

HbC-β-thalassemia is a form of β-thalassemia (see below). Affected individuals are commonly asymptomatic, although moderate hemolysis may be present. These individuals have a moderate microcytic, hypochromic, hemolytic anemia, and splenomegaly. Their red cells may show Hb C crystals.

HEMOGLOBIN D DISEASE

❏ **Definition**
Autosomal inherited hemoglobinopathy prevalent in Southeast Asia and in parts of India (HbD Punjab). The heterozygous form is asymptomatic with no anemia.

❏ **Laboratory Findings**
- Hb variant analysis demonstrates the abnormal Hb at acid pH (it has the same mobility as HbS at alkaline pH). There are no other laboratory abnormalities in the *heterozygous* individual.
- RBC: mild hemolytic, microcytic anemia in *homozygous* individuals; their peripheral blood smear (PBS) shows target cells and spherocytes.

HEMOGLOBIN E DISEASE

❏ **Definition**
The most common structural hemoglobinopathy in the United States after HbS and HbC. Autosomal inherited hemoglobinopathy, prevalent in Southeast Asia (15–30% of the population in Cambodia, Thailand, parts of China, Burma, and Vietnam). Heterozygous individuals have similar findings as patients with β-thalassemia trait (see below). Homozygotes exhibit more microcytosis but are asymptomatic.

❏ **Laboratory Findings**
- Hb variant analysis shows 95–97% HbE in the homozygous (the rest is HbF); 30–35% in individuals carrying HbE trait. Electrophoretic mobility is the same as for HbA2, but it is present in much higher concentrations. It separates from HbC and O on citrate agar electrophoresis at acid pH.
- CBC.
  - ▼ Mild hemolytic, microcytic (MCV 55–70 fL) anemia or no anemia in the homozygous.
  - ▼ Erythrocytosis may be present (RBC approximately 5,500/μL) in both the trait and in the homozygous.
  - ▼ Peripheral blood smear (PBS) shows 25–60% target cells and microcytes in the homozygous individuals.

HEMOGLOBIN E–β-THALASSEMIA

❏ **Definition**
The most common symptomatic thalassemia in Southeast Asia. A severe condition that resembles β-thalassemia intermedia or β-thalassemia major (see below).

❏ **Laboratory Findings**
- Hemolytic anemia varies from moderate to severe, similar to β-thalassemias (see below).
- Peripheral blood smear (PBS) shows severe hypochromia and macrocytosis and marked anisopoikilocytosis with many teardrop and target red cells. Nucleated RBC and basophilic stippling may be present.

HEMOGLOBIN E–ALPHA-THALASSEMIA

A mild hemolytic anemia encountered in Southeast Asia. It causes microcytosis. The severity depends on the number of α genes deleted (see α-thalassemia below).

 # THE THALASSEMIAS

Thalassemias are chronic, microcytic, hemolytic anemias. They result from defective synthesis of either β- or α-globin subunits of the Hb A molecule. Thalassemias are classified into β- or α-thalassemia according to which of the globin chain is affected. The thalassemias are among the most common genetic disorders worldwide. They have an autosomal recessive inheritance resulting in either homozygous (thalassemia major) or subtle (thalassemia minor) clinical abnormalities. The β-thalassemia syndromes are extremely heterogenous. In addition to β-thalassemia trait and β-thalassemia major described below, there are combinations with other hemoglobinopathies and variants described above.

β-THALASSEMIA MAJOR

❑ Definition and Who Should Be Suspected

A severe condition resulting from impaired or absent production of the β globin chains of Hb. The resulting excess α chains precipitate inside the red cells with dire consequences: severe hemolysis, skeletal changes, liver abnormalities, premature gallbladder bilirubin stones, splenomegaly, aplastic crises, impaired growth, endocrine and cardiopulmonary complications, and hemosiderosis resulting from RBC transfusions. The clinical expression of the severe phenotype is extremely heterogenous. A milder form of β-thalassemia, *β-thalassemia intermedia*, is seen in patients with one β (–) allele mutation that produce no β globin chains and with a β (+) mutation from the second allele. It produces a small amount of β chains, thus these patients are less severely affected.

- β-thalassemia is most common in individuals of Mediterranean ancestry (mutations result from protection against endemic malaria in the Mediterranean basin); it is also found in African Americans and in some groups in India.
- Infants are well at birth, depending on high levels of HbF (no β chains, just α and fetal globins), for tissue oxygenation. The diagnosis is usually established at 6–12 months of age due to increasing symptoms: pallor, irritability, growth retardation abdominal swelling due to hepatosplenomegaly, followed by abnormal skeletal development, the result of an expanding extramedullary hematopoiesis.
- Coinheritance of an α-thalassemia trait may ameliorate the morbidity of β-thalassemia major.

❑ Laboratory Findings

- CBC.
  - ▼ RBC: profound anemia, microcytosis, reduced MCV and MCHC, very elevated RDW. Hb levels may be as low as 3–4 g/dL. The anemia may become acutely life threatening during *aplastic crises*, mostly provoked by infection with parvovirus B19, which infects precursor erythroid cells.

- ● Red cell morphology shows extreme hypochromia and poikilocytosis, tear drop cells, and many target cells. Heinz bodies are readily identified when the smears are stained with supravital stains.
  - ▼ WBC is elevated (in part falsely so, due to enumeration of nucleated RBCs as WBCs by some automated counters), but true leukocytosis is usually present.
  - ▼ Platelets may be reduced due to hypersplenism but become elevated in splenectomized patients.
  - ▼ Peripheral blood smear (PBS): marked poikilocytosis with many target cells, tear drop cells, nucleated RBCs, and basophilic stippling of RBCs.
  - ▼ Reticulocyte count is inappropriately low, in part the result of ineffective erythropoiesis. It may become 0 during aplastic crises.
- ■ Bone marrow aspirate shows red cell hyperplasia with marked shift to early red cell progenitors due to intramedullary hemolysis, in turn the result of accelerated apoptosis. Megaloblastic morphology may be observed in the absence of folate supplements. Extramedullary hematopoiesis develops in the skeletal bones, liver, and spleen.
- ■ Hb variant analysis shows absence of HbA1 in $\beta(0)$ thalassemia, where only HbA2 and HbF are present. HbA2 may increase to 3–6% (unless iron deficiency is also present). HbA1 is present after RBC transfusions.
- ■ Serum iron and ferritin increase progressively throughout life due to RBC transfusions.
- ■ Serum bilirubin is elevated.
- ■ Liver function tests are abnormal, in part the result of transfusional viral hepatitis. This problem is becoming rare with present-day transfusion practice.
- ■ LDH and uric acid are elevated.
- ■ Haptoglobin is decreased.
- ■ Endocrine abnormalities are related to extensive iron deposits, with laboratory evidence of hypogonadism and diabetes.
- ■ Hypercoagulability: abnormalities in the level of clotting factors and their inhibitors have been reported in some cases.

β-THALASSEMIA MINOR (TRAIT)

❏ **Definition**

Heterozygotes who carry one normal β-globin allele and one β-thalassemic allele are clinically normal but have an abnormal hematologic picture that may mislead for a diagnosis of iron deficiency.

❏ **Laboratory Findings**

- ■ CBC shows microcytic anemia. The anemia is milder (Hg 10–13 g/dL), but the microcytosis is more profound (MCV 60–70 fL) than seen in iron deficiency. RBC count may be higher than normal (another contrast to iron deficiency anemia). RDW is normal, since the RBCs are uniformly microcytic and hypochromic. On peripheral blood smear (PBS), basophilic stippling of RBCs and target cells may be observed. During pregnancy, carriers may develop a more profound anemia, than attributable to the physiologic anemia of pregnancy.
- ■ Hb variant analysis: HbA2 is elevated, sometimes as high as 7–8% with the ratio HbA2/HbA1 being 1:20 instead of the normal 1:40; HgF is slightly

elevated in 50% of cases. Some forms of β-thalassemia trait may have a normal concentration of HbA2. Definitive diagnosis can only made by molecular genetic techniques.

ALPHA-THALASSEMIA SYNDROMES

❏ Definition
Normal subjects have four α globin genes, two on each chromosome. The α-thalassemias are caused by mutations or deletions affecting the production of one or more of the four α globin genes. This defect results in a relative excess of β globin chains, which may lead to hemolysis.

❏ Who Should Be Suspected?
α-Thalassemia should be suspected based on a family history of anemia and geographic and ethnic background. The condition is prevalent in populations of African, Middle East, or Southeast Asian ancestry. The diagnosis is further suspected in cases of microcytic, hypochromic anemia not due to iron deficiency, with normal levels of HbA_2 on hemoglobin variant analysis.

❏ Diagnosis
The severity of the syndrome depends on the number of α genes affected.

- Loss of all four α globin loci results in *hydrops fetalis with Hb Bart*, condition incompatible with extrauterine life. This condition is not seen in populations of African ancestry, but it is encountered in Asian populations. Hb Bart is composed of four γ globin chains, which fails to deliver oxygen to tissues. It is fast moving on Hb electrophoresis.
- Loss of three α loci results in *Hemoglobin H disease*. These patients have a moderate microcytic, hypochromic anemia with inclusion bodies present on the peripheral blood smear (PBS). Hb levels are usually 8–10 g/dL. Hb electrophoresis or chromatographic techniques show 5–30% HbH, which is the result of tetrameric β-chains. HbH disease can be acquired in hematologic malignancies, especially in myelodysplastic syndromes.
- Loss of two loci results in α-thalassemia-1 trait (*α-thalassemia minor*). There are two variants, depending if the two affected genes are on the same chromosome, or one per chromosome. Adult patients may have a mild microcytic, hypochromic anemia. In these cases, the red cells are microcytic, hypochromic, and target cells are present. Hb electrophoresis is normal. Definitive diagnosis can only made by molecular genetic techniques.
- Loss of only one locus results in α-thalassemia-2 trait (*α-thalassemia minima* or silent carrier of α-thalassemia). There are no hematologic abnormalities, and Hb electrophoresis is normal. The diagnosis can only be made by DNA analysis.
- Hemoglobin Constant Spring is a common structural variant associated with α-thalassemia in Asia. It is associated with a normal α chain, but the Constant Spring allele functions as a severe α-thalassemia gene. Patients show a minor, very slowly migrating abnormal Hg component of Hg electrophoresis. Homozygosity results in a mild form of HbH disease.
- Couples at risk for having offsprings with homozygous thalassemia may choose *antenatal diagnosis* by direct gene analysis of the fetus.

Suggested Readings

Benz EJ. Newborn screening for α-thalassemia-keeping up with globalization. *N Engl J Med.* 2011;364:770–771.
Forget BG. Thalassemia. *Hematol Clin North Am.* 2010;24:1–140.
Rachmilewitz EA, Giardina PJ. How I treat thalassemia. *Blood.* 2011;118:3479–3488.

 # HEMOLYTIC INTRINSIC RED BLOOD CELL DEFECTS

ENZYMOPATHIES

The most common enzymopathies are glucose-6-phosphate dehydrogenase (G6PD) and pyruvate kinase (PK) deficiencies. Other rare deficiencies of RBC enzymes do occur but will not be discussed here.

GLUCOSE-6-PHOSPHATE DEHYDROGENASE (G6PD) DEFICIENCY

❏ Definition

G6PD deficiency is an X-linked inherited RBC enzyme deficiency. Incidence is high in regions where malaria is or was prevalent. More than 300 variants have been described. G6PD deficiency can be divided into three classes, with the normal genotype being designated G6PD type B.

- Class 1 (Mediterranean variant, also designated G6PD type B–): <5% of normal RBC enzyme activity. It results in a *chronic* hemolytic anemia exacerbated by oxidant drugs or febrile illnesses. Very severe hemolytic attacks develop after the ingestion of fava beans (*favism*).
- Class 2 (African variant, G6PD type A–): <10% of normal RBC enzyme activity; patients have *episodic* hemolytic attacks produced by certain infections, oxidant drugs, or diabetic ketoacidosis. It is not triggered by ingestion of fava beans.
- Class 3: 10–60% of the normal enzyme activity. There is no hemolysis except for limited episodes (2–3 days) after ingestion of oxidant drugs or following infections. Similar G6PD levels are found in female carriers.

❏ Who Should Be Suspected?

G6PD deficiency should be considered in the differential diagnosis of a patient with nonimmune (Coombs negative) hemolytic anemia.

❏ Laboratory Findings

Basis of diagnosis:

- Generation of NADPH from NADP as detected by either quantitative spectrophotometric analysis or, more rapidly, by screening tests, such as a fluorescent spot test.
- G6PD levels may be normal during and shortly following a hemolytic episode in type A– cases, because very young RBCs contain sufficient enzyme. *Assays for G6PD should be postponed for at least 6 weeks after an acute episode.*

CBC: Hemolytic anemia: chronic in class 1 and intermittent in classes 2 and 3. It is seen 2–4 days after ingestion of an oxidant drug (primaquine and sulfa drugs are the most common offending agents) or after fava beans consumption. Female carriers: possible mild hemolytic episodes that are difficult to diagnose with conventional methodology; they can be diagnosed by genetic methods.

- Peripheral blood smear (PBS): Heinz bodies in RBCs (require brilliant cresyl blue supravital special stain), nucleated RBCs, spherocytes, poikilocytes, fragmented RBCs, and bite cells.
- Reticulocytosis.
  - ▼ MCV may be elevated in type A– patients if not supplemented with folic acid.
  - ▼ Bilirubin is elevated correlating to the degree of hemolysis. Neonatal jaundice develops in 5% of affected newborns of African or Mediterranean ancestry after the first 24 hours of life. Serum indirect bilirubin reaches a peak (often >20 mg/dL) at 3rd to 5th day with resulting kernicterus if not treated promptly.

PYRUVATE KINASE (PK) DEFICIENCY

❑ **Definition**

PK deficiency is an autosomal recessive, nonspherocytic *chronic* hemolytic anemia. Affected individuals are either homozygous for a single mutation or heterozygous for two different PK mutations. The mechanism of hemolysis has not been elucidated.

❑ **Who Should Be Suspected?**

A patient with chronic, sometimes severe, nonimmune (Coombs negative) hemolytic anemia.

There is a wide range of clinical and laboratory findings. The severity of anemia varies from severe neonatal anemia requiring transfusions to a fully compensated hemolytic process in adults who have 10–20% of the normal enzyme in their RBCs. The severely affected patients may require frequent red cell transfusions and as a consequence develop iron storage overload. The severe cases present with jaundice, pallor, and splenomegaly. Such patients may also develop gallstones. The anemia may worsen after certain infections (aplastic crises). PK deficiency is more common in persons of northern European extraction and possibly in Chinese. The disease is particularly severe among the Amish of Pennsylvania.

❑ **Laboratory Findings**

- Peripheral blood smear (PBS) shows no characteristic changes, particularly no spherocytes.
- The laboratory diagnosis is based on demonstrating low erythrocytic PK enzymatic levels. A screening test using crude hemolysate detects heterozygous carriers in persons who are hematologically normal. This assay may miss some variants. Quantitation of the enzyme can be performed in specialized laboratories.
- Genetic tests are the most definitive approach to diagnosis.
- Elevated levels of LDH and decreased haptoglobin can be seen.

HEREDITARY SPHEROCYTOSIS (HS)

❏ Definition

HS is a congenital red cell membrane abnormality resulting from defects in one of six genes encoding proteins involved in vertical linkages that tie the membrane skeletal network of the RBCs with the lipid bilayer. The ankyrin gene is the one most commonly involved. HS is inherited as autosomal dominant transmission in 75% of affected individuals. The condition is recessive or presents as a new mutation in the remaining 25%. HS is seen mostly in patients of northern European origin.

❏ Who Should Be Suspected

- Patients with mild to severe anemia, jaundice, splenomegaly, and cholelithiasis early in life, and a family history of a hereditary hemolytic anemia.
- Exacerbations of anemia may occur in aplastic (infections with parvovirus B19 or other viruses), hemolytic crises (with some viral infections), or due to the development of megaloblastic anemia, usually the result of folate deficiency.

❏ Laboratory Findings

- CBC: Anemia of varying severity, but with acute exacerbations (see above). Moderately severe anemia occurs in approximately 70% of cases. Approximately 20% have mild, compensated hemolysis. Approximately 10% of HS patients have severe, debilitating anemia and are transfusion dependent, unless splenectomized (splenectomy ameliorates the anemia, but spherocytosis persists). Indices: normal or slightly low MCV (except elevated when the reticulocyte count is very high or if the patient is folate deficient), elevated MCHC (the most helpful red cell index in HS), and RDW.
- Reticulocytosis (5–20%).
- Peripheral blood smear (PBS): Spherocytosis of various degrees is invariably present. Howell-Jolly bodies indicate previous splenectomy. The presence of spherocytes on peripheral blood smear (PBS) is not pathognomonic: it may be due to acquired hemolytic anemias rather than HS.
- Osmotic fragility reveals increased RBC fragility, but it may be abnormal (increased) also in patients with acquired hemolytic anemias.
- Ektacytometry, acidified glycerol lysis test, cryohemolysis test, and especially the flow cytometric eosin-5-maleimide tests have *surpassed the osmotic fragility test in sensitivity and specificity* but may only be available in specialized laboratories.
- Haptoglobin: decreased.
- Coombs test: negative.
- Hemoglobin: usually normal at birth but decreases sharply during the subsequent 20 days of life.
- Bilirubin is slightly elevated, except in neonatal cases with severe hemolysis, when it may be elevated at birth, resulting in kernicterus if not treated promptly.
- Genetic tests: offered in some research laboratories, usually unnecessary.

❏ Other Considerations

- Laboratory findings may reflect cholelithiasis or aplastic crises.
- Falsely elevated potassium (hyperkalemia) is due to potassium leaking from RBCs.

HEREDITARY ELLIPTOCYTOSIS (HE)

❏ **Definition**

HE is a congenital heterogeneous disorder of the membrane skeleton of RBCs, most commonly a defect in spectrin. It is transmitted in an autosomal dominant mode of inheritance. Occasionally, the transmission is recessive. Individuals who are heterozygous for HE are asymptomatic. Individuals who are homozygous or compound heterozygous (10% of patients) exhibit mild to severe anemia. The disorder is more frequent in African Americans and in patients of Mediterranean origin (previous areas of endemic malaria). Affected neonates may have transient overt hemolytic anemia until adult Hb supervenes.

❏ **Laboratory Findings**

- Peripheral blood smear (PBS): more than 50% of RBCs are ellipsoidal or rod shaped. Other markers of hemolysis are uncommon, except in the approximately 10% of severely affected patients. In severe cases of HE, severe poikilocytosis is common.
- Indices: decreased MCV, MCH, MCHC; increased RDW.
- Variant Hb studies and osmotic fragility (see above under HS) are normal.

❏ **Other Considerations**

- Some degree of elliptocytosis may be seen in peripheral blood smear (PBS) of other types of anemia.

HEREDITARY PYROPOIKILOCYTOSIS (HP)

❏ **Definition**

HP is considered a subtype of HE. In homozygous individuals, it results in a severe congenital hemolytic anemia. It occurs primarily in people of African ancestry.

❏ **Laboratory Findings**

Peripheral blood smear (PBS): RBCs are markedly misshapen (fragments, microspherocytes, elliptocytes, pyknotic forms). The RBCs *fragment* when heated at 45–46°C (normal RBCs show budding and fragmentation only when heated at 49°C). Severe microcytosis and micropoikilocytosis are present.

HEREDITARY OVALOCYTOSIS (HO)

❏ **Definition**

HO is a condition of altered membrane deformability. It is very common in Southeast Asia, where its prevalence is 5–25% in malaria endemic areas. Transmission is autosomal dominant, but so far only heterozygous individuals have been identified. Most affected people express minimal hemolysis.

❏ **Laboratory Findings**

Peripheral blood smear (PBS): oval-shaped RBCs with one or two transverse ridges or a longitudinal slit.

❏ **Other Considerations**

Hereditary ovalocytosis can be confused with hereditary elliptocytosis.

HEREDITARY STOMATOCYTOSIS

❑ Definition
Hereditary stomatocytosis is an uncommon autosomal dominant disease resulting from defective RBC permeability to sodium and potassium ions.

❑ Laboratory Findings
Peripheral blood smear (PBS):

- Homozygous individuals: >35% of RBCs show slit-like areas of central pallor, producing a mouth-like appearance.
- Heterozygous individuals: 1–25% stomatocytes.
- Anemia: similar to that of hereditary ovalocytosis.
- Homozygous individuals: varying degrees of hemolysis.
- Heterozygous individuals: no anemia.

❑ Other Considerations

- Stomatocytes may be seen on the peripheral blood smear (PBS) of many acquired disorders, such as alcoholism, liver disease, and drug-induced hemolytic anemias.

 # HEMOLYTIC EXTRINSIC RED BLOOD CELL DEFECTS

AUTOIMMUNE HEMOLYTIC ANEMIAS (AIHAS)

AIHAs anemias may be classified on the basis of the type of antibody present: warm (binding optimally at 37°C), cold (binding optimally at 4°C), or occasionally combined warm and cold antibodies. Each of these AIHAs may be idiopathic or secondary to other diseases.

❑ Definition
Warm-Reactive AIHAs
Warm-reactive AIHAs are due to the presence of IgG antibodies that react with RBC antigens at body temperature. About 60% are idiopathic, and the remaining 40% are the result of lymphomas, leukemias, other neoplasms, or autoimmune disorders such as SLE. They may also accompany HIV or other viral infections.

Cold-Reactive AIHAs and Cold Agglutinin Disease
These AIHAs result from the presence of IgM antibodies that react to polysaccharide antigens on the RBC surface at temperatures below that of the body's. The antibodies fix complement.

Most of the chronic cases, for which the term *cold agglutinin disease* is commonly used, have an underlying B-cell neoplasm (CLL/small lymphocytic lymphoma [SLL], lymphomas, macroglobulinemia) as their etiology. Some cases are idiopathic. Acute cases either are the result of viral infections such as mycoplasma pneumonia and infectious mononucleosis or belong to a group known as paroxysmal cold hemoglobinuria. There are variable degrees of hemolysis; the disease can be intravascular or extravascular. The symptoms are exacerbated in cold weather; Raynaud phenomena are common, with vascular obstruction due to RBC clumps, cyanosis of exposed parts, and pallor. Splenomegaly is uncommon; the liver is the site for sequestering the coated RBCs.

❏ Laboratory Findings
Warm-Reactive AIHA
- Hb moderate to severe decrease, in the range of 7–10 g/dL.
- Reticulocytes: elevated in most cases.
- Indices: increased MCV due to reticulocytosis; increased MCHC reflects the presence of spherocytes.
- Peripheral blood smear (PBS): microspherocytes, polychromasia, and occasionally nucleated RBCs.
- Coombs test: direct IgG and C3d are positive. The warm antibodies are in most cases directed against IgG1 and less frequently against IgG3.
- Unconjugated bilirubin, LDH, urine, and fecal urobilinogen: elevated.
- Haptoglobin: decreased.

Cold-Reactive AIHA and Cold Agglutinin Disease
- Anemia (severity depends on cold agglutinin titer) with anomalous high MCV and MCHC (artifacts due to RBC clumping at room temperature).
- Peripheral blood smear (PBS): RBC clumping.
- Reticulocyte count: high.
- Anticomplement (C3) Coombs test (positive). Anti-I antibodies are best detected using cord blood red cells.
- Cold agglutinin titers: elevated.

PAROXYSMAL NOCTURNAL HEMOGLOBINURIA (PNH)

❏ Definition
PNH is an acquired disorder of hematopoietic stem cells, characterized by intravascular hemolysis and hemoglobinuria. Only 25% of cases present with classical nocturnal and paroxysmal hemolysis. The clinical triad of intravascular hemolysis, venous thrombosis (the leading cause of death), and bone marrow failure is typical. The chronic intravascular hemolysis results in iron deficiency. There is a high risk of evolution into aplastic anemia, myelodysplastic syndrome, or AML. Clinically, the polymorphism of PNH can be roughly divided into two presentations:
- Classic PNH: hemolysis without bone marrow failure
- Aplastic anemia–PNH syndrome (AA-PNH): hemolysis with bone marrow failure

❏ When To Suspect Paroxysmal Nocturnal Hemoglobinuria
- Patients with Coombs-negative intravascular hemolysis, especially if concurrently iron deficient.
- Patients with hemoglobinuria.
- Patients with venous thrombosis involving unusual sites (mesenteric, hepatic, portal, cerebral, or dermal veins) and especially patients with otherwise unexplained Budd-Chiari syndrome. Such patients should also be investigated for the JAK2 V617F (see p. 1021) mutation if the etiology remains unclear.
- Patients with unexplained refractory anemia.

❏ Laboratory Findings

Highly Recommended

- Flow cytometry (high sensitivity and specificity).
  - ▼ At least two different monoclonal antibodies, directed against two different glycosylphosphatidylinositol (GPI) anchored proteins, either absent or greatly diminished in PNH, on at least two different cell lineages, should be used to diagnose a patient with PNH. In fact, the preferred approach includes the detailed evaluation of leukocytes, because some red blood cells may be lost secondary to hemolysis or diluted from their true frequency by repeated transfusions.
  - ▼ CD59 and CD55 are the most commonly assessed. Other monoclonal antibodies directed against determinants on leukocytes such as CD14, CD16, and CD24, can be used.
- Fluorescently labeled aerolysin (FLAER): This reagent is more sensitive and specific than the available monoclonal antibodies. This allows the simultaneous detection of PNH clones in monocyte and neutrophil lineages in a single-tube, multiparameter flow cytometric assay.
- Direct Coombs test: negative.

Recommended

- CBC: RBC indices: macrocytic anemia evolving into a microcytic picture. Reticulocytes are increased, but not commensurate with the degree of anemia. Mild leukopenia and thrombocytopenia may be present; if severe, a combination with aplastic anemia or another bone marrow failure syndrome should be considered.
- Bone marrow: normoblastic hyperplasia; indicated if an additional underlying hematologic disease is suspected.
- Haptoglobin: reduced.
- Serum iron and ferritin: decreased.
- Karyotype: normal.
- LDH: increased.
- Leukocyte alkaline phosphatase (LAP): absent or reduced.
- Liver function studies: unconjugated bilirubin: increased; AST/ALT: normal; ALP: normal.
- Methemalbumin: reduced.
- Hemoglobin, plasma: increased (hemoglobinemia).
- Urinalysis: hemoglobinuria, hemosiderinuria, and no intact RBCs in urine sediment.

Suggested Readings

Hill A, Kelly RJ, Hillmen P. Thrombosis in paroxysmal nocturnal hemoglobinuria. *Blood.* 2013;121:4985–4996.

Parker CJ. Management of paroxysmal nocturnal hemoglobinuria in the era of complement inhibitory therapy. *Hematology Am Soc Hematol Educ Program.* 2011;2011:21–29.

PAROXYSMAL COLD HEMOGLOBINURIA (PCH)

❏ Definition

PCH is an acute hemolytic anemia that results from characteristic antibodies (Donath-Landsteiner) that cross-react with P blood group on RBC membrane

TABLE 9–2. Drugs Most Commonly Implicated in Hemolytic Anemias

Mechanisms	Offending Drugs
Acute intravascular: positive direct Coombs test in the presence of the drug	Sulfonamides, quinidine, quinine, stibophen
Chronic extravascular: positive direct and indirect Coombs test without the drug present	α-Methyldopa, mefenamic acid, levodopa
Unknown mechanism	Ribavirin
Intravascular and extravascular: positive Coombs test in the presence of the drug	High-dose penicillin and analogs, cephalothin, streptomycin

causing osmotic lysis. This transient hemolysis occurs following exposure to a cold environment, with sudden hemoglobinuria. PCH may be associated with the convalescence phase of an acute viral illness (mumps, measles, infectious mononucleosis) or seen in patients with syphilis. PCH may also be idiopathic.

❏ **Laboratory Findings**

- Plasma appears scarlet and becomes maroon or brown after a few hours (free Hb is oxidized to metHb, as well as due to the formation of methemalbumin).
- Peripheral blood smear (PBS): spherocytes, nucleated RBCs, anisocytosis, and poikilocytosis.
- Donath-Landsteiner test: when the blood is cooled, then brought to 37°C, hemolysis develops.
- Complement-directed Coombs test: may be positive but the IgG Coombs is negative.

Drug-Induced Hemolytic Anemias

This hemolytic anemia is due to anti-RBC antibodies that develop as the result of drug effects. The drugs most commonly implicated and the mechanisms involved are described in Table 9-2.

HEMOLYTIC DISEASE OF THE NEWBORN

❏ **Definition**

Hemolysis occurs when fetal RBCs cross the placenta and the mother is immunized with a fetal RBC antigen that is not present on her RBCs. Some women may be immunized with more than one type of RBC antigen. The resulting immune response triggers the production of IgG antibodies that are then transferred to the fetus and cause hemolysis of the fetal RBCs. The most frequent cases are due to immunization against the D antigen of the Rh blood group. Next most common are due to immunization against the Kell antigen.

❏ **Laboratory Findings**

- Laboratory findings are those of hemolysis in the newborn.
- After birth, the by-products of RBC destruction occur, especially increased unconjugated bilirubin, with attended complications (bilirubin encephalopathy and kernicterus).

MECHANICAL HEMOLYSIS

❏ **Definition**

Physical trauma to RBCs damages them, resulting in RBC fragmentation and intra-vascular hemolysis. Mechanical hemolytic anemias can be divided into two groups:

- Microangiopathic: endothelial cell injury in small blood vessels due to fibrin strands in vessel lumens, as seen in DIC, TTP, HUS, disseminated malignancy; malignant hypertension; vasculitis; HELLP syndrome; scleroderma insertion of foreign bodies into the circulation; Kasabach-Merritt syndrome (giant hemangioma); chemotherapy; and the "catastrophic" antiphospholipid antibody syndrome.
- Macroangiopathic: RBC injury from malfunctioning valvular prosthesis, severe cardiac valve deformities, or aortic atheromata (Waring blender syndrome).

Mechanical hemolysis may also occur in hypersplenism, march hemoglobinuria (runner's hemoglobinuria), and freshwater drowning or inadvertent infusion of water.

❏ **Laboratory Findings**

- Laboratory diagnosis: directed to the causative disease.
- Anemia: commensurate with the severity of underlying process.
- Peripheral blood smear (PBS): >5 of 500 RBCs are deformed (schistocytes) or helmet cells (a subtype of schistocytes) or are microspherocytes.
- Platelets: varying degrees of thrombocytopenia, occasionally without anemia.
- D-dimer and fibrinogen degradation products (FDPs): elevated if DIC is present.
- Plasma Hb and urine hemosiderin: elevated.
- Plasma haptoglobin: decreased.

Suggested Reading

Mohandas N, Gallagher PG. Red cell membrane: past, present, and future. *Blood.* 2008;112:3939–3948.

EVANS SYNDROME

❏ **Definition**

Evans syndrome is characterized by the simultaneous (or sequential) development of autoimmune hemolytic anemia and immune thrombocytopenia (ITP) and/or immune neutropenia, without a demonstrable underlying etiology. Evans syndrome may be associated occasionally with SLE lymphoproliferative neoplasms or primary immune deficiencies.

❏ **Laboratory Findings**

As described for autoimmune hemolytic anemias (see p. 377 under Anemia, hemolytic) and immune thrombocytopenias (see p. 442 under Platelets, thrombocytopenias). When neutropenia is present, studies for antileukocyte antibodies should be undertaken.

Suggested Reading

Michel M, Chanet V, Dechartres A, et al. The spectrum of Evans syndrome in adults: new insight into the disease based on the analysis of 68 cases. *Blood.* 2009;114:3167–3172.

ERYTHROCYTOSIS

- Increased red cell mass (>25% above predicted hemoglobin, or >18.4 g/dL in males, or >16.4 in females)
- Causes of erythrocytosis (see algorithm on Figure 9-2)
- Clonal: polycythemia vera
- Nonclonal:
  - ▼ Relative erythrocytosis (hemoconcentration)
  - ▼ Hypoxia, high altitude, pulmonary disease, right to left shift, sleep apnea, high affinity hemoglobin, carbon monoxide poisoning
  - ▼ Renal disease
  - ▼ Certain tumors (hypernephroma, hepatoma, cerebellar hemangioblastoma, adrenal tumors, pheochromocytoma, uterine fibromyoma)
  - ▼ Androgen therapy, testosterone or erythropoietin abuse
  - ▼ Familiar erythrocytosis

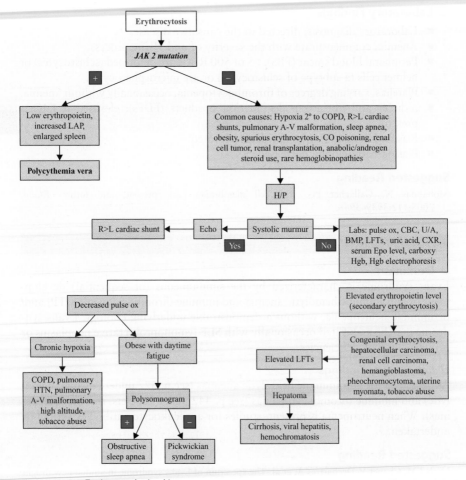

Figure 9–2 *Erythrocytosis algorithm.*

WHITE BLOOD CELL DISORDERS

LEUKOCYTOSIS AND LEUKOPENIAS

Leukocytosis refers to a total white cell count >10,300/µL (in our laboratory). Counts up to 11,000 may be considered physiologic by allowing two standard deviations above the upper limit. Leukocytosis may reflect an absolute increase of neutrophils, lymphocytes, eosinophils, monocytes, basophils, or combinations. Leukopenia is defined as a total white cell count <4,300/µL.

❑ Causes of Neutrophilia (Neutrophilic Leukocytosis)

In adults, neutrophilia is defined as an increase in the absolute neutrophil count >7,500/µL (or >72%). A *relative* neutrophilia is seen when the other cellular elements (mostly the lymphocytes) are decreased. The *absolute* neutrophil count, as reported by automated counters, is a more reliable parameter than the percent count. Spurious neutrophilia may be reported by automated counters in the presence of clumped platelets or cryoglobulins. The counters will flag such results as not acceptable. Causes of neutrophilia can be divided into primary (clonal) and secondary.

Primary Neutrophilia
- Myeloproliferative neoplasms
- Neutrophilic leukemia (see p. 405)
- Hereditary, giant neutrophilia (occasional large neutrophils with multiple nuclear lobes)
- Hereditary neutrophilia, a rare autosomal dominant condition without medical problems
- Chronic idiopathic neutrophilia, condition not associated with medical problems

Secondary Neutrophilia
- Acute infections
  - ▼ Localized (e.g., pneumonia, meningitis, tonsillitis, abscess, acute otitis media in children)
  - ▼ Systemic (e.g., septicemia). Certain bacteria, such as pneumococcal, *staphylococcal*, and clostridial species, may cause very elevated neutrophil and band counts.
- Inflammation, especially during chronic diseases' flare-ups
- Vasculitis
- Acute rheumatic fever
- Crohn disease and ulcerative colitis
- Rheumatoid arthritis
- Chronic hepatitis
- Metabolic (uremia, acidosis, eclampsia, acute gout)
- Poisoning by chemicals (mercury), venoms (e.g., black widow spider)
- Parenteral (foreign proteins, vaccines)

9

- Drugs: epinephrine, steroids, lithium, retinoic acid therapy for acute promyelocytic leukemia, therapeutic cytokines, especially granulocyte (or granulocyte–monocyte) colony–stimulating factors
- Acute hemorrhage
- Acute hemolysis
- Tissue or tumor necrosis
- Acute myocardial infarction
- Tumor necrosis
- Burns
- Gangrene
- Bacterial necrosis
- Physiologic conditions
  - ▼ Strenuous exercise
  - ▼ Emotional stress
- Labor
- Smoking
- Leukoerythroblastic reaction (myelophthisis): neutrophilia associated with immature granulocytes, nucleated red cells, and teardrop red cells; it is associated with tumor invasion of the bone marrow, TB, and other granulomatous diseases.

NEUTROPENIA

❑ **Definition**

Less than 43% of leukocytes, or an absolute neutrophil and band count <1,600/µL (or <1,000/µL in people of African ancestry). Absence of granulocytes: agranulocytosis. A greatly reduced number of neutrophils: granulocytopenia. Absolute neutrophil counts below 500/µL increase susceptibility of bacterial or fungal infections.

❑ **Causes of Neutropenia**

- *Decreased bone marrow production*
  - ▼ Myelodysplastic syndromes
  - ▼ Aplastic anemia
  - ▼ Chemotherapy
  - ▼ Acute leukemia
  - ▼ Radiation therapy or accident
  - ▼ Folic acid or vitamin B_{12} deficiency
- *Increased bone marrow production but decreased survival of neutrophils*
  - ▼ Autoimmune and isoimmune neutropenia
  - ▼ SLE and RA
  - ▼ Felty syndrome
  - ▼ Hypersplenism
  - ▼ Large granular lymphocytosis
- *Viral infections* (various mechanisms)
  - ▼ Infectious mononucleosis
  - ▼ HIV infection
  - ▼ Hepatitis

- ▼ Influenza
- ▼ Measles
- ▼ Rubella
- ▼ Psittacosis
- ■ *Bacterial infections*
  - ▼ Overwhelming sepsis
  - ▼ Miliary TB
  - ▼ Typhoid and paratyphoid
  - ▼ Brucellosis
  - ▼ Tularemia
- ■ *Rickettsial infections*
  - ▼ Scrub typhus (tsutsugamushi disease)
  - ▼ Sandfly fever (caused by Sicilian or Naples virus)
- ■ *Other infections*
  - ▼ Malaria
  - ▼ Kala-azar
- ■ *Drugs*
  - ▼ Sulfa drugs (TMP/SMX)
  - ▼ Antibiotics (chloramphenicol, vancomycin, cephalosporin, macrolides)
  - ▼ Antimalarials (chloroquine, quinine, amodiaquine)
  - ▼ Antifungal agents (amphotericin B, flucytosine)
  - ▼ Antidiabetics (chlorpropamide, tolbutamide)
  - ▼ Anti-inflammatory (sulfasalazine, gold salts, phenacetin, phenylbutazone)
  - ▼ Anticonvulsants (carbamazepine, phenytoin, valproate, ethosuximide)
  - ▼ Psychotropic drugs (clozapine, phenothiazines, tricyclic and tetracyclic antidepressants, meprobamate)
  - ▼ Cardiovascular (procainamide, ticlopidine, ACE inhibitors, propranolol, dipyridamole, digoxin)
  - ▼ Diuretics (thiazides, furosemide, spironolactone, acetazolamide)
  - ▼ Antithyroid drugs (thioamides)
  - ▼ Dermatologic drugs (dapsone, isotretinoin)
- ■ *Chronic idiopathic neutropenia*
- ■ *Neonatal and infantile neutropenia*
  - ▼ Maternal immune neutropenia
  - ▼ Maternal isoimmunization to fetal leukocytes
- ■ *Congenital neutropenia* as seen with certain inborn errors of metabolism and other congenital syndromes

Suggested Reading
Boxer LA. How to approach neutropenia. *Hematology Am Soc Hematol Educ Program.* 2012;2012:174–182.

AGRANULOCYTOSIS

❏ Definition
The term agranulocytosis literally means total absence of granulocytes in the peripheral blood. When the neutrophils and bands are <500/µL, the term severe

granulocytopenia is used. A count <500/μL confers a high risk for sepsis; a count of <200 is certain to lead to overwhelming bacterial infection.

Agranulocytosis may be the result of

- Peripheral destruction of PMNs (often drug related)
- Bone marrow failure

❑ Who Should Be Suspected?

Agranulocytosis should be suspected in anyone started recently or restarted on any drug, who suddenly develops fever, chills, and signs of infection. Sore throat is a common presenting symptom. Patients may develop overwhelming sepsis.

❑ Laboratory Findings

- CBC: normal Hb and platelets (except under special circumstances, such as postchemotherapy); absent or extremely decreased neutrophils and bands. The granulocytes may show pyknosis or vacuolization. Normal lymphocytes and monocytes (but relative lymphocytosis and monocytosis).
- Bone marrow shows an absence of cells in the granulocytic series but normal erythroid and megakaryocytic series.
- ESR is increased.
- Other laboratory findings reflect the infection.
- Hb, RBC count and morphology, platelet count, and coagulation tests are normal.

LYMPHOCYTOSIS

❑ Definition

Lymphocytosis is defined as an absolute lymphocyte count >3,400/μL (or >43%) in adults, >7,200 in adolescents, and >9,000 in young children and infants. Spurious lymphocytosis: neutropenia with relative lymphocytosis, but normal absolute lymphocyte count.

❑ Primary (Clonal) Lymphocytosis

- Chronic lymphocytic leukemia (CLL)
- Monoclonal B-cell lymphocytosis (>4,000 but <5,000 clonal lymphocytes)
- Acute lymphocytic leukemia (ALL)
- Prolymphocytic leukemia
- Hairy cell leukemia
- Follicular, mantle cell, and splenic marginal zone lymphomas in leukemic phase
- Large granular lymphocytic leukemia (see p. 404)

❑ Secondary (Reactive) Lymphocytosis

- Infections (e.g., pertussis, infectious mononucleosis [EBV], infectious lymphocytosis [especially in children], infectious hepatitis, CMV, mumps, German measles, chickenpox, toxoplasmosis, babesiosis, chronic TB, cat scratch disease)
- Noninfectious causes (e.g., hypersensitivity reactions, stress)
- Drugs: efalizumab (Raptiva)

LYMPHOCYTOPENIA

❑ **Definition**
Lymphocytes are <1,600/μL (or <18%) in adults and <3,000/μL in children

❑ **Causes**

- Corticosteroid therapy or Cushing syndrome; epinephrine injection
- Certain infections (e.g., acute and chronic retroviral infections, TB)
- Sarcoidosis
- Congenital immunoglobulin disorders
- Chemotherapy and radiation therapy
- Neoplastic diseases, especially Hodgkin lymphoma
- ARDS
- Autoimmune disorders
- Idiopathic CD4+ lymphocytopenia
- CHF
- Increase loss via the GI tract (e.g., intestinal lymphectasia, thoracic duct drainage, obstruction to intestinal lymphatic drainage)

MONOCYTOSIS

❑ **Definition**
Absolute monocyte count of >1,200/μL or >12% of a differential count

❑ **Causes**

- Acute monocytic or myelomonocytic leukemia, chronic myelomonocytic leukemia (as part of myelodysplastic syndromes, or myeloproliferative neoplasms)
- Hodgkin lymphoma, non-Hodgkin lymphomas, multiple myelomas
- Carcinomas of the ovary, stomach, and breast
- Lipid storage diseases (e.g., Gaucher disease)
- Postsplenectomy
- Recovery from agranulocytosis, chemotherapy, or subsidence of acute infection
- Protozoan infections (e.g., malaria, kala-azar, trypanosomiasis)
- Some rickettsial infections (e.g., Rocky Mountain spotted fever, typhus)
- Certain bacterial infections (e.g., bacterial endocarditis, TB, syphilis, brucellosis)
- Ulcerative colitis, regional enteritis, sprue
- Sarcoidosis and other connective tissue diseases (e.g., SLE, RA)
- Tetrachloroethane poisoning
- Chronic corticosteroid therapy
- Acute minor viral infections (counts should be rechecked in 1 month)
- Diurnal variations

EOSINOPHILIA

❑ **Definition**
Eosinophil count of >600/μL or >8% of the differential count. Eosinophilia may be primary (clonal), reactive, or idiopathic.

❑ **Associated Conditions**

▪ *Primary*
  ▼ Hematologic: hypereosinophilic syndrome
  ▼ Neoplastic disorders: chronic eosinophilic leukemia, myelomonocytic leukemia with inversion 16 mastocytosis, and T-cell lymphomas that secrete interleukin-5
▪ *Secondary*
  ▼ Allergic diseases: atopic and related diseases, medication related
  ▼ Infectious diseases: parasitic infections, mostly helminths, some fungal infections, infrequently other infections
  ▼ Collagen vascular disorders
  ▼ Autoimmune disorders such as the vasculitis of the Churg-Strauss syndrome
  ▼ Tumors with secondary eosinophilia: T-cell lymphomas (e.g., mycosis fungoides, Sézary syndrome), Hodgkin lymphoma
  ▼ Pulmonary diseases: (hypersensitivity pneumonia, Loeffler pneumonia)
  ▼ Endocrine: adrenal insufficiency
  ▼ Immunologic reactions, transplant rejection
  ▼ Cholesterol embolism syndrome

PERSISTENT EOSINOPENIA

❑ **Definition**
No lower limit can be determined because the eosinophil count may be 0% in some normal patients.

❑ **Associated Conditions**
  ▪ Drugs: corticosteroids or epinephrine administration
  ▪ Cushing syndrome
  ▪ Infections in conjunction with neutrophilia
  ▪ Inflammation: acute

BASOPHILIA

❑ **Definition**
Basophilia is defined as >300/μL or >2% of leukocytes. (The basophil is the rarest of leukocytes.)

❑ **Associated Conditions**
  ▪ Basophilia frequently accompanies myeloproliferative neoplasms, and its progression may herald a blast crisis in chronic myelogenous leukemia. The existence of basophilic leukemia is controversial. One case was recently described by our group.
  ▪ Other causes of basophilia are
    ▼ Hypersensitivity states (drugs, foods, foreign protein injection)
    ▼ Myxedema
    ▼ Anemias, chronic hemolytic, iron deficiency (in some patients)

▼ Ulcerative colitis
▼ Postsplenectomy
▼ Hodgkin lymphoma
▼ Chronic sinusitis
▼ Chickenpox
▼ Smallpox
▼ Nephrotic syndrome (in some patients)

❑ **Basophilopenia (No Lower Limit Can Be Determined Because Some Normal Subjects Have 0% Basophils)**

▪ Hyperthyroidism
▪ Irradiation or chemotherapy
▪ Drugs: corticosteroids
▪ Ovulation and pregnancy
▪ Stress

LEUKEMOID REACTIONS

❑ **Definition**

A count >50,000/µL white cells in nonleukemic conditions defines a leukemoid reaction. The peripheral blood smear (PBS) shows increase in and shift to the left of myeloid cells (bands, metamyelocytes, myelocytes, some promyelocytes, and rare myeloblasts); increased primary granules in the myeloid cells (toxic granulation) and Döhle bodies, cytoplasmic vacuolization. If the left shift consists of an elevation of bands only (>700/µL), the term bandemia is applied. Frequently it signals the onset of a septic episode such as acute appendicitis.

❑ **Causes of Leukemoid Reactions**

▪ Severe sepsis (osteomyelitis, empyema, disseminated TB)
▪ Burns
▪ Tissue necrosis (gangrene, mesenteric vein thrombosis)
▪ Therapy with granulocyte colony–stimulating factor (G-CSF) or granulocyte monocyte colony–stimulating factor (GM-CSF)
▪ Metastatic infiltration of the marrow

 ACUTE LEUKEMIAS*

B LYMPHOBLASTIC LEUKEMIA/LYMPHOMA (B-ALL)

❑ **Definition**

B-ALL is a clonal disease affecting the lymphocytic B line, with heavy infiltration of bone marrow and peripheral blood. If the neoplasm is confined to a mass with no or minimal evidence of peripheral blood or bone marrow involvement, the term B lymphoblastic lymphoma is appropriate. With modern therapy, B-ALL has a good prognosis in children, but not in adults. To what this difference is attributable is not yet clear.

---

*Co-authored by Patricia Minehart Miron, PhD & Hongbo Yu, MD, PhD.

❏ Who Should Be Suspected?

- B-ALL is the most common form of cancer in childhood, comprising >85% of leukemias in children. The disease can however occur at any age. Children (peak incidence at age 2–3 years) or adults older than 65, presenting with acute onset of fever, infection, bleeding, fatigue, musculoskeletal pain (particularly in adolescents), and characteristic findings on the CBC. Lymphadenopathy and hepatosplenomegaly are present in the majority of patients but are not massive.
- Predisposing factors: children with certain genetic disorders such as Down syndrome, neurofibromatosis type 1, Bloom syndrome, and ataxia telangiectasia.
- Poor prognostic signs at presentation: WBC count >100,000/μL, platelet count <50,000/μL, CD10 negativity, certain karyotypic abnormalities, occurrence of the disease before age 1 (probably having occurred before birth) or after age 10, and induction failure. Mature B leukemic phenotype rather than the precursor B cell is associated with poorer prognosis.

❏ Laboratory Findings

Laboratory diagnosis is based on morphology, immunophenotype, and cytogenetic/genetic analysis.

Morphology

- Blood: CBC
  - ▼ Anemia, moderate to severe.
  - ▼ Thrombocytopenia.
  - ▼ WBC is usually elevated, with lymphocytosis and neutropenia, but approximately 50% of children have WBC counts <10,000 at presentation.
  - ▼ Lymphoblasts are usually identified on the peripheral blood smear (PBS).
  - ▼ Bone marrow generally shows >50% lymphoblasts. It should be obtained before starting therapy to determine immunophenotype, cytogenetics, and overall cellularity. Peripheral blood may be sufficient for these studies in cases with high peripheral blood blast count. Once the diagnosis of leukemia is confirmed, definitive assignment to the subtype of B-ALL, as provided by immunophenotyping and cytogenetic studies, is mandatory before deciding on therapeutic protocol.

Immunophenotype

- Seventy percent to 80% of childhood ALL are of the B-precursor lineage. The expression of markers on the leukemic lymphoblasts does not correlate strictly with normal lymphoid maturation. B-ALL lymphoblasts are positive for CD19; cytoplasmic CD79a; and cytoplasmic and surface CD22, CD24, PAX5, and TdT. The expression of CD34, CD10 (CALLA antigen), and CD20 is variable. Myeloid markers CD13 and CD33 may also be present. The aberrant immunophenotype serves to identify minimum residual disease in the bone marrow following therapy.

  A simple classification is offered below:

- Mature B-cell phenotype (1–2% of cases in children and 5% in adults). Surface monoclonal immunoglobulins. Indistinguishable from Burkitt lymphoma.

- B-progenitor ALL present in 80–85% of childhood B-ALL. Eighty to 90% express CD10. The majority have an immunoglobulin gene rearrangement, predominantly involving the IgH gene. Different subsets are based on various cell markers: pro-B ALL (CD10–, no cytoplasmic Ig [cIg]), early pre-B ALL (CD10+, but no cIg), and pre-B ALL (CD10+, cIg positive). The prognosis among these various forms of immature B-ALL depends mostly on their genetic etiology as reflected in karyotypes or by interphase FISH (see below).

Cytogenetic/Genetic Analysis

- In addition to immunophenotype, cytogenetic and molecular genetic abnormalities are used in the prognostic evaluation and therapy of B-ALL. Both numerical and structural abnormalities of the chromosomes are associated with prognosis and influence treatment.
  - ▼ t(9;22)(q34;q11.2); BCR-ABL (the Ph chromosome) is present in ≤25% of adults and 3% of children. Its presence denotes poor prognosis in B-ALL patients, but patients may respond to tyrosine kinase inhibitors.
  - ▼ t(12;21)(p13;q22); tETV6-RUNX1: favorable prognosis.
  - ▼ t(1;19)(q23;p13.3); E2A-PBX1 intermediate to poor prognosis.
  - ▼ MLL (11q23) rearrangements, most commonly t(4;11)(q21;q23) with AFF1(AF4)/MLL and t(11;19)(q23;p13.3) with (MLL; MLLT1(ENL); poor prognosis.
  - ▼ IGH (14q32) rearrangements; most commonly t(8;14)(q24;q32) with MYC-IGH.
  - ▼ Deletion/rearrangement of 9p (CDKN2A deletion); favorable prognosis in adults; possibly poor prognosis in children.
  - ▼ Hyperdiploidy (54–58 chromosomes especially if associated with the combined trisomies of chromosomes 4 and 10 have the best prognosis).
  - ▼ Hypodiploidy (the blasts contain <45 chromosomes, poor prognosis). Note that hyperdiploidy may represent doubling of a hypodiploid clone. This doubled clone still confers poor prognosis. High hyperdiploidy may also be seen in combination with BCR-ABL1 and with t(1;9) and also carries a poor prognosis.
- In addition to the genetic abnormalities demonstrated by chromosome and FISH studies, high-density single nucleotide polymorphism (SNP) arrays and gene expression profiles are being increasingly used to stratify patients and determine prognosis and therapeutic protocols.
- Once the initial profile of the leukemic cells had been established, the information is used to establish the effect of therapy as revealed by the presence of minimal residual disease (MRD), which correlates well with clinical outcome.

Additional Information

- CSF may show increased protein and cells, some recognizable as lymphoblasts. Because of high incidence of meningeal involvement, examination of CSF is part of all protocols.
- Serum LDH and sedimentation rate are elevated.
- Hypercalcemia, hyperpotassemia, hyperphosphatemia, and hyperuricemia may be present at diagnosis or develop as the result of therapy.
- Acute lysis syndrome may develop as the result of therapy.

9

Suggested Readings

Borowitz MJ, Chan JKC. B lymphoblastic leukaemia/lymphoma not otherwise specified. In: *WHO Classification of Tumours of Haematopoietic and Lymphoid Tissues*, 4th ed. Lyon, France: International Agency for Research on Cancer; 2008:168–170.

Mulligan CG. The molecular genetic makeup of acute lymphoblastic leukemia. *Hematology Am Soc Hematol Educ Program*. 2012;2012:389–396.

ACUTE MYELOID LEUKEMIA (AML)

❏ **Definition**

AML is a hematopoietic neoplasm involving a clonal proliferation of the myeloid line, involving granulocytic, or erythroid, or megakaryocytic hematopoietic stem cells. It is characterized by acquisition of somatic mutations that confer proliferative or survival advantage to the clonal cells and impair normal hematopoiesis. AML is a markedly heterogeneous disease with numerous genetic aberrations.

❏ **Classification**

- The 2008 WHO classification will guide the description of AML variants in this section. AML is divided into six major groups:
  1. AML with recurrent genetic abnormalities: these abnormalities impact prognosis. The most common ones are balanced abnormalities that create a fusion gene encoding a chimeric protein. Best examples: acute promyelocytic leukemia (APL); AML with inv(16)(p13.1q22); AML with t(8;21)(q22;q22).
  2. AML with myelodysplasia-related changes comprises three subgroups: AML arising from previous MDS or MDS/MPN; AML with an MDS-related cytogenetic abnormality; AML with multilineage dysplasia. This group has a poor prognosis.
  3. Therapy-related myeloid neoplasms: the leukemia occurs as a late complication of cytotoxic chemotherapy or radiation therapy.
  4. AML not otherwise specified: cases that do not fulfill criteria for the other groups. These cases of AML are classified basically by morphology, and follow closely the FAB[†] classification, except for having eliminated acute promyelocytic leukemia (formerly M3).
  5. Myeloid sarcoma: extramedullary myeloid tumor. It may precede or coincide with overt AML.
  6. Myeloid proliferations related to Down syndrome (DS): DS individuals have a 50- to 150-fold increase in the incidence of AML in the first 5 years of life. In some cases, the leukemia is acute megakaryocytic. In addition, 10% of DS newborns have *a transient* episode of abnormal myelopoiesis expressed mainly as thrombocytopenia and marked leukocytosis.

❏ **Who Should Be Suspected?**

- AML is the most common acute leukemia in adults. It should be suspected during the 1st months of life (initiating events are in utero), in middle age, or in the elderly, in a patient who is acutely ill, and with nonspecific presenting

---

[†]French-American-British classification, as previously used, was based on morphologic criteria.

signs and symptoms that reflect profound disturbances in hematopoiesis: fatigue, malaise, infections, ulcerations of mucous membranes, bleeding, diffuse bone tenderness, joint pain, and swelling.

- Other findings:
  - ▼ Modest splenic enlargement is present in 50% of cases.
  - ▼ Lymphadenopathy is not present. Isolated masses (myeloid sarcoma [chloroma]), which are collection of blasts in extramedullary sites, may precede systemic AML.

❏ Laboratory Findings

Morphologic, cytochemical or immunophenotypic, cytogenetic, and molecular studies, if available, should be performed in every case to maximize the precise diagnosis and prognosis classification.

- CBC
  - ▼ Anemia, normochromic, normocytic, is universally present. Nucleated red cells may be identified on the peripheral blood smear (PBS).
  - ▼ Thrombocytopenia is severe in most cases.
  - ▼ WBC: Leukocytosis with neutropenia is present in more than half the cases; some patients may present with leukopenia, especially if AML follows MDS. Greater than 20% of white cells are blasts. There are few or no intermediate granulocytic cells (myelocytes, metamyelocytes, bands). Auer rods are present in certain subtypes with granulocytic differentiation and help to establish the diagnosis, especially by determining myelogenous rather than lymphoid etiology at the first inspection of the patient's peripheral blood smear (PBS).
- *Bone marrow aspirate and biopsy* are mandatory for cytochemical, immunophenotypic, cytogenetic, and genetic studies. The WHO classification defines AML as with either >20% blasts in bone marrow or PBS or with specific cytogenetic findings: t(8;21)(q22;q22) RUNX1-RUNX1T1; inv(16)p;(13.1q22); 6(16:16)(p13.1;q22 CBFB-MYH11; t(15;17)(q24.1;q21.1) PML-RARA. The bone marrow is hypercellular in most cases, with a predominance of early progenitor cells (myeloblasts and promyelocytes or monoblasts and promonocytes) depending on the leukemic subtype. Initial assessment is based on counting 500 cells on the aspirate. AML–erythroleukemia is established when >50% of precursor cells are erythroid, and myeloblasts comprise >20% of nonerythroid cells. Careful assessment of megakaryocytes and the degree of marrow fibrosis are also part of the initial studies.
- *Coagulation studies.* Bleeding, a severe complication of AML, is usually due to the severe thrombocytopenia, compounded by platelet functional defects. In addition, patients with the t(15;17) and hypergranular promyelocytes frequently develop a proteolytic state akin to DIC either spontaneously or following the initial chemotherapy. The mechanism is thought to be release of tissue factor from the promyelocytes' granules. PT and PTT are elongated, FDP and latex D-dimers are elevated, and fibrinogen, initially elevated, decreases dramatically.
- Metabolic and electrolyte abnormalities are common; the patients must be monitored carefully, especially during induction chemotherapy. Renal failure from multifactorial causes is common.

▼ Hyperuricemia is the most frequent biochemical abnormality. Hyperuricuria may also be present.

▼ Tumor lysis syndrome may develop during induction chemotherapy. It is characterized by rapid development of hyperuricemia, hyperkalemia, hyperphosphatemia, and hypocalcemia.

▼ Acute promyelocytic leukemia (APL) differentiation syndrome (previously the retinoic acid syndrome) develops in 2–27% of patients in the 1st to 3rd week after initiating all-trans retinoic acid (ATRA) therapy for this type of AML. The most susceptible patients are those with hyperleukocytosis and abnormal serum creatinine. Lactic acidosis has been described in patients with AML.

▼ Hypokalemia is common and may be profound.

▼ Lysozyme is released from the leukemic cells and may induce renal tubular damage.

▼ Hypercalcemia and hypocalcemia have been reported.

▼ Spuriously high potassium and decreased serum glucose may be the result of circulating metabolically active white cells.

■ CNS involvement is infrequent in AML (5–7% of patients). It is more common in patients with a monocytic predominant clone, with hyperleukocytosis, and patients under 2 years of age. MLL rearrangements, inv(16) and complex karyotypes may also predispose to CNS involvement.

■ Cytochemistry, although extremely useful in the past, is taking a secondary role in the era of cytogenetic/genetic and immunophenotyping diagnosis and classification. It plays a role when a rapid result is beneficial, such as rapidly differentiating AML from ALL. The most commonly used stains are as follows:

▼ Myeloperoxidase or Sudan Black B: positive in AML with maturation, in myelomonocytic leukemia, and in erythroleukemia; strongly positive in APL, negative in ALL, minimally differentiated AML, monoblastic leukemia without differentiation and in megakaryocytic leukemia.

▼ Chloroacetate esterase: positive in AML with differentiation and in acute myelomonocytic leukemia; negative in ALL, AML without differentiation, and in acute monoblastic and erythroleukemia.

▼ Nonspecific esterase: positive (and inhibited by sodium fluoride) in acute myelomonocytic or monoblastic leukemia with or without differentiation; negative in ALL, and AML with granulocytic line as the main component.

▼ Periodic acid–Schiff (PAS): the pattern of granules staining with PAS may differentiate lymphoid from myeloid precursors (e.g., very coarse granules in ALL lymphoblasts).

▼ Lysozyme is positive in AML with monocytic differentiation.

■ *Immunophenotype*: Most cases of AML are characterized by their complex immunophenotypes. There is great variation in immunophenotype depending on the leukemic subtype. Blasts are positive for CD34 (except for APL and some cases with monocytic differentiation, where CD34 may be weakly expressed or absent), and in some cases HLA-DR (except for APL) and CD117. The AML variants with differentiation toward the granulocytic phenotype express CD13, CD33, CD15, and CD65. Those with monocytic characteristics are positive for CD14, CD4, CD11b, CD11c, CD64, and CD36. The megakaryoblastic leukemias express platelet antigens, such as CD41 and/or CD61. CD2 is expressed in subsets of APL, more often in microgranular variant. CD19 is expressed in AML with RUNX1-RUNX1T1. Other T- or B-cell antigens are expressed in acute leukemia of ambiguous lineage (mixed phenotype acute leukemia). Because of this possibility and its impact on prognosis (poor), their panel of antigens used at the time of diagnosis must contain multiple myeloid, B- and T-cell markers.

- *Cytogenetic/molecular genetic* investigations determine to a great extent prognosis and therapeutic protocols and have become the major criteria the WHO uses for subclassification of AML. Cytogenetics is also critical in distinguishing AML from chronic myeloid leukemia in blast crisis. There are specific cytogenetic abnormalities seen only in AML, example t(1;22)(p13;q13). Complex karyotype has consistently been associated with poor outcome. Although cytogenetic studies are essential for diagnosis and classification, many of the variant translocations can be detected by real-time polymerase chain reaction (RT-PCR) that has higher sensitivity and as such is useful for residual disease monitoring. Abnormalities in certain genes, such as mutations in FLT3, nucleophosphin (NMP1), KIT of CEBPA, as well as gene expression profiles confer prognostic significance. Gene expression profiling leads to further subclassifications of AML, with prognostic and therapeutic implications. Ultimately, it is expected that a proteomic-based classification will emerge.

  ▼ AML with t(8;21)(q22;q22) with RUNX1-RUNX1T1 fusion is found in approximately 5% of AML cases. Generally shows maturation in the neutrophilic lineage, occurs in a younger population, and may present as myeloid sarcomas. Good response to chemotherapy.

  ▼ AML with inv(16)(p13.1q22) or t(16;16)(p13.1;q22) with fusion of the CBFB, and MYH11 genes shows monocytic and granulocytic differentiation and abnormal eosinophils in the bone marrow. This rearrangement may be difficult to detect without FISH or PCR. It is important to alert the cytogenetics laboratory if this variant is suspected. Myeloid sarcomas may be present at diagnosis or at relapse. This variant constitutes 5–8% of AML cases. Patients respond well to chemotherapy.

  ▼ Acute promyelocytic leukemia (APL) with t(15;17)(q24;q21), with the PML–RARA retinoic acid receptor-α translocation. Five percent to 8% of acute leukemias. Use of FISH analysis for *rapid diagnosis* may be useful for early initiation of ATRA therapy together with an anthracycline.

  There are two varieties of APL: the majority (considered typical APL) have hypergranular promyelocytes, many containing large Auer rods and high incidence of acute DIC; the microgranular (variant) PML, presents with bilobed nuclei and very high WBC. APL provided the first paradigm of molecularly targeted therapy, ATRA. Variant RARA translocations can be detected by classical cytogenetics and by FISH and are important to distinguish, as not all variants respond to ATRA. Prognosis is most favorable among all AML subtypes when treated promptly with ATRA and an anthracycline.

- AML with t(9;11)(p22;q23); the MLL gene on chromosome 11q23 is involved in numerous translocations with different partner genes, most commonly in association with MLLT3 at 9p22. Most frequently, the morphology is monocytic or myelomonocytic. Detected in 9–12% of pediatric and 2% of adult AML. Intermediate prognosis; other MLL rearrangements tend to have poorer prognosis.
- AML with t(6;9)(p23;q34) fuses DEK on chromosome 6, with NUP214 (CAN) on chromosome 9. May have monocytic, basophilic, and multi-lineage dysplastic features. Incidence: 0.7–1.8% of AML. Presents with lower WBC than other AML and pancytopenia. Poor prognosis.
- AML with inv(3)(q21q26.2) or t(3;3)(q21;q26.2) with rearrangement of EVII, and RPN1 genes may present de novo or evolve from MDS with normal or increased platelet counts and atypical megakaryocytes in the bone marrow. Comprises 1–2% of all AML. Trilineage dysplastic morphology is common; aggressive disease with short survival.
- AML (megakaryoblastic) with t(1;22)(p13;q13). Fusion of RBM15-MKL1 genes. Very rare leukemia that occurs in infants and young children. Marked hepatosplenomegaly.
- AML with MDS-related changes may have complex karyotypes, unbalanced abnormalities, such as −7/7q− or −5/5q−, or balanced abnormalities.
- Therapy-related myeloid neoplasms have abnormal karyotypes in >90% of cases. Approximately 70% of patients have unbalanced chromosomal aberrations, mainly whole or partial loss of chromosomes 5 and/or 7, frequently associated with other chromosomal abnormalities.

■ *Molecular genetics*: In addition to the genetic mutations with cytogenetic abnormalities described above, specific gene mutations are also common and may be present in cases with or without detectable cytogenetic abnormalities. Mutations in FLT3 (fms-related tyrosine kinase 3) and NPM1 (nucleophosmin) are of particular prognostic import. In normal karyotype cases, FLT3-ITD (internal tandem duplication) carries an unfavorable prognosis, whereas NPM1 mutation is considered favorable. Similarly, CEBPA (CCAAT/enhancer-binding protein α) mutation in a normal karyotype background is considered favorable.

■ Monitoring of minimal residual disease (MRD) remains an active field of investigation. MRD is defined as any measurable disease or leukemic cells detectable above a certain threshold level. Finding of MRD after intensive therapy affects survival negatively. As of now, half of AML patients lack a molecular target suitable for MRD monitoring. For those patients with a suitable target, multiparameter flow cytometry can be applied to peripheral blood investigations. Protocols are in place for pediatric AML, but not for adults with the disease.

Suggested Readings

Arber DA, Brunning RD, LeBeau MM, et al. Acute myeloid leukaemia with recurrent genetic abnormalities. In: *WHO Classification of Tumours of Haematopoietic and Lymphoid Tissues*, 4th ed. Lyon, France: International Agency for Research on Cancer; 2008:110–123. (See also pp. 124–144.)

Grossmann V, Schnittger S, Kohlmann A, et al. A novel hierarchical prognostic model of AML solely based on molecular mutations. *Blood.* 2012;120:2963–2972.

Paietta E. Minimal residual disease in acute myeloid leukemia: coming of age. *Hematology Am Soc Hematol Educ Program.* 2012;2012:35–42.

Walter RB, Othus M, Burnett AK, et al. Significance of FAB subclassification of "acute myeloid leukemia, NOS" in the 2008 WHO classification: analysis of 5848 newly diagnosed patients. *Blood.* 2013;121:2424–2431.

T LYMPHOBLASTIC LEUKEMIA/LYMPHOMA (T-ALL)

❑ Definition

T-ALL is a neoplasm of lymphoblasts committed to the T-cell lineage. The term lymphoma is preferred to leukemia when the presenting manifestation is a tumor, rather than peripheral blood involvement. The incidence of T-ALL in children with ALL ranges between 10% and 15% and in adults between 20% and 25%.

❑ Who Should Be Suspected?

Presentation is similar as for B-ALL (see p. 389), but there is more predominant extramedullary involvement, including frequent CNS and anterior mediastinal thymic masses.

❑ Laboratory Findings

- CBC: (see B-ALL at p. 389, but note higher leukocytosis at presentation).
- Immunophenotype: CD3 is T-lineage specific. The lymphoblasts are TdT positive and express CD1a, CD2, CD4, CD5, CD7, and CD8 to variable degrees. CD10 may also be positive.
- Molecular genetics: Clonal rearrangement of the T-cell receptor gene (TCR) is almost always present.
- Cytogenetics: Abnormal karyotypes are present in 50–70% of cases. The most common recurrent abnormality involves the α and Δ TCR loci at 14q11.2.

Suggested Reading

Borowitz MJ, Chan JKC. T lymphoblastic leukaemia/lymphoma. In: *WHO Classification of Tumours of Haematopoietic and Lymphoid Tissues*, 4th ed. Lyon, France: International Agency for Research on Cancer; 2008:176–178.

 CHRONIC LEUKEMIAS‡

CHRONIC MYELOGENOUS LEUKEMIA

[See Myeloproliferative Neoplasms]

CHRONIC EOSINOPHILIC LEUKEMIA (CEL) AND HYPEREOSINOPHILIC (HES) SYNDROME*

❑ Definition

CEL is a rare clonal myeloproliferative disease characterized by the overproduction of eosinophils. It must be distinguished from the HES, reactive eosinophilia, or other leukemias with predominant eosinophilia. It may undergo blastic transformation.

‡Co-authored by Patricia Minehart Miron, PhD & Hongbo Yu, MD, PhD.

HES is defined as persistent (>6 months' duration) eosinophilia of >1,500 eosino-phils/mL with no demonstrable disease that could cause eosinophilia, no abnormal T-cell population, and no evidence of another clonal myeloid disorder. It leads to end-organ damage because of the proinflammatory role of eosinophils; any organ may be involved. If untreated, HES may be fatal.

- Persistent peripheral blood eosinophilia (≥1,500/μL).
- Myeloblasts <20% in peripheral blood or bone marrow, and there are no cytogenetic features diagnostic of AML.
- No evidence of other myeloproliferative neoplasms or MDS/MPN.
- No BCR-ABL1 gene rearrangement.
- No PDGFRA, PDGFRB, or FGFR1 gene rearrangements.
- Evidence of clonality by either cytogenetic or molecular studies, or blast cells are >2% in the peripheral blood or >5% in the bone marrow.

❑ Neoplasms With Eosinophilia and Abnormalities of PDGFRA, PDGFRB, or FGFR2

Involve rearrangement of tyrosine kinase gene. PDGFRA and PDGFRB rearrange-ments common in CEL; PDGFRB rearrangements can be detected with routine cytogenetic analysis, PDGFRA is typically cryptic and require FISH for detection.

❑ Who Should Be Suspected?

Patients with eosinophilia for longer than 6 months. Presumptive signs and symp-toms of organ involvement, especially cardiac or neurologic.

❑ Laboratory Findings

- CBC in CEL:
  - ▼ Eosinophilia with mostly mature eosinophils; the WBC count is usually <25,000/μL but may be >90,000, with rare immature forms.
  - ▼ Mild anemia in half the patients; thrombocytopenia in one third of cases; thrombocytosis may also be present.
  - ▼ Increase in dysplastic-appearing or immature eosinophils.
- Bone marrow:
  - ▼ Hypercellular marrow with 25–75% of eosinophils and increase in eosin-ophil precursors; no reticulin fibrosis.
  - ▼ Hyperplasia with increase in abnormal eosinophils and eosinophilic precursors.
  - ▼ The most common mutation associated with the myeloproliferative vari-ant of the *HES* is that presenting with the fusion tyrosine kinase FIPIL1/ PDGFRA (F/P).
  - ▼ F/P is cytogenetically cryptic and requires FISH analysis for detection. Patients with these genetic markers respond to tyrosine kinase inhibitors such as ima-tinib mesylate and are considered and classified as separate entities.
  - ▼ *CEL:* Certain clonal abnormalities may be demonstrated, most frequently involving chromosomes 5, 7, 8 (the 8p11 syndrome), 10, 15, or 17. The best defined entity in CEL is t(5;12)(q33;p13) involving PDGFRB. In the absence of clonal abnormalities, the diagnosis is more difficult, and the hypereosinophilic syndrome may be considered.
- Interleukin 5: overproduction in some patients.
- Elevated troponin levels suggest cardiac involvement by HES.

Suggested Readings

Klion AD. How I treat hypereosinophilic syndrome. *Blood*. 2009;114:3736–3741.

Oliver JW, Deol I, Morgan DL, et al. Chronic eosinophilic leukemia and hypereosinophilic syndromes. *Cancer Genet Cytogenet*. 1998;107:111–117.

Tefferi A. Blood eosinophilia: a new paradigm in disease classification, diagnosis, and treatment. *Mayo Clin Proc*. 2005;80:75–83.

CHRONIC LYMPHOCYTIC LEUKEMIA (CLL)/SMALL LYMPHOCYTIC LYMPHOMA (SLL)

❑ Definition

CLL/SLL is an indolent clonal proliferation of mature B lymphocytes, leading to an accumulation of these cells in the peripheral blood, bone marrow, spleen, and lymph nodes. B-cell CLL is considered identical (one disease at different stages) with the mature B-cell neoplasm small lymphocytic lymphoma (SLL), an indolent non-Hodgkin lymphoma. SLL by itself refers to the nonleukemic cases. This section will present CLL/SLL as one entity.

❑ Who Should Be Suspected?

Individuals who present with persistent (at least 3 months) absolute lymphocytosis of ≥5,000/µL, frequently with lymphadenopathy and splenomegaly. The patient may be asymptomatic or present with symptoms related to anemia, neutropenia, or immune deficiency, but rarely bleeding.

In the absence of extramedullary tissue involvement, there must be ≥5,000/µL monoclonal lymphocytes with CLL phenotype in the peripheral blood for the diagnosis of CLL. CLL/SLL is more common in patients >55 years of age, but it may be encountered in young individuals.

❑ Diagnosis

The simplest way to diagnose CLL is by flow cytometry, where the presence of a clone of mature B lymphocytes with characteristic immunophenotype confirms the diagnosis (see below for details).

❑ Laboratory Findings

- CBC
  - ▼ Anemia, when present, is normochromic, normocytic and connotes advanced disease. In some cases, it is autoimmune, with a positive direct Coombs test. If the etiology of anemia is autoimmune, the anemia by itself does not categorize the disease as being in an advanced stage. Autoimmune hemolytic anemia may also develop as a complication of purine analog therapy.
  - ▼ Platelet count is decreased in advanced disease. Occasionally, there is an autoimmune component to thrombocytopenia (ITP). In these cases, the bone marrow reveals a normal number of megakaryocytes. If thrombocytopenia is solely immune in etiology, it does not indicate advanced disease.
  - ▼ WBC count is increased, usually 50,000–250,000/µL, with >90% lymphocytes. Neutropenia indicates progressive disease, unless it is the result of therapy. Recently, an entity of monoclonal B lymphocytosis has been described, and it refers to monoclonal B lymphocytes in patients with absolute lymphocyte counts <5,000/µL. MBL is best detected by flow cytometric

analysis of peripheral blood in the absence of a history of B-cell leukemia or another related lymphoproliferative disease. Some of these patients may eventually evolve into typical CLL and need to be followed closely.

▼ In stable CLL/SLL, the lymphocytes are small, with clumped chromatin, indistinct nucleoli, and scanty cytoplasm. Smudge cells are numerous; their presence suggests CLL/SLL even if the WBC count is not greatly elevated. Increasing numbers of lymphocytes (lymphocyte doubling time in <1 year) or increased percentage of prolymphocytes indicate progressive disease.

■ *Bone marrow*: Bone marrow aspiration and biopsy are seldom required for diagnosis. Bone marrow biopsy may show a pattern of nodular, interstitial, combined nodular and interstitial, or diffuse infiltration by lymphocytes. Progressive replacement of erythroid, myeloid, and megakaryocytic series by lymphocytes takes place over time.

■ *Lymph node biopsy*: The histopathologic findings in CLL and SLL are identical. The lymph nodes show diffusely effaced nodal architecture with pale areas corresponding to proliferation centers in a dark background of small cells. The cells in the proliferation are mostly small, noncleaved lymphocytes with condensed chromatin, round nuclei, and occasionally single small nucleoli. There is an admixture of prolymphocytes and paraimmunoblasts usually clustered in proliferation centers. The proliferation index is low.

■ *Immunophenotype analysis, usually by flow cytometry, is a key component to the diagnosis of CLL.* A major criterion for the diagnosis of CLL is the demonstration of clonality of circulating B lymphocytes. Flow cytometry reveals the expression of B-cell–associated antigens CD19, CD20 (weak), CD22, CD23, CD43, CD79a, and CD11c (weak). Cyclin D1, CD10, FMC7, CD79b, and CD103 are negative; CD5, a T-cell–associated antigen, is *uniformly present on CLL/SLL cells.* Mantle cell lymphoma cells (Table 9-3) are also positive for CD5. Staining for surface IgM/κ or IgM/λ (whichever represents the abnormal clone) is dim. Minimal residual disease assessment in posttherapy hematologic remission is determined by multicolor flow cytometry and compared with the initial pattern.

■ *Cytogenetics*: Chromosomal abnormalities can be detected in most cases of CLL, particularly with the recent use of CpG-rich oligonucleotides as a

TABLE 9–3. Differential Immunophenotypic Markers for Four Chronic Lymphoproliferative Diseases

Marker	CLL/SLL	B-PLL	HCL	Mantle Cell Lymphoma
Surface immunoglobulin	Dim	Bright	Positive	Bright
CD5	+	+/−	−	+
CD11c	Weakly +	−	+	−
CD22	+	−	+	+
CD103	−	−	+	−
CD23	+	−	−	−
CD25	−	−	+	+
TRAP	−	−	+	−

B-PLL, prolymphocytic leukemia; CLL, chronic lymphocytic leukemia; HCL, hairy cell leukemia; SLL, small lymphocytic lymphoma; TRAP, tartrate-resistant acid phosphatase.

mitogen in cell culture. Common abnormalities include trisomy 12, 11q22-23 (ATM) deletion, 13q14.3 deletion, 17p13 (TP53) deletion, and 6q21 deletion. Deletion of 13q is often cytogenetically cryptic and requires detection by FISH. The other deletions may also be cryptic and are typically included in a CLL FISH panel.

- *Prognostic markers*
  - ▼ The expression on leukemic cells of ZAP-70, CD38, and unmutated immunoglobulin heavy chain variable region is associated with aggressive disease. Because of lack of methodologic standardization, immunoglobulin mutation status assays are not recommended at this time.
  - ▼ Cytogenetic studies segregate prognosis as follows (in order of decreasing survival): isolated deletion 13q14.3 (best survival), normal karyotypes, trisomy 12 (the prognostic value of trisomy 12 is not clear, but so far considered as being intermediate), 11q/ATM deletion, and 17p/p53 deletion (shortest survival).
- *Genomic studies* may emerge in the future as the best tools for determining the clinical course of CLL/SLL. Genetic complexity is associated with aggressive disease. Loss or mutation of TP53 (a tumor suppressing gene) places patients in the highest risk prognostic group. Down-regulation of miR-29c and miR-223, and possibly other microRNAs, has been associated with adverse prognosis. MiR-34a indicates resistance to chemotherapy. This is an area that is developing rapidly. The integration of genomic mutations and cytogenetic lesions improves the accuracy of survival prediction in CLL.
- *Serum immunoglobulins*: Hypogammaglobulinemia develops and progresses as the disease becomes more advanced. A monoclonal protein, usually of the same class as the surface membrane immunoglobulin, is found in 5% of patients.
- LDH, β-2 microglobulin, and thymidine kinase are elevated in more than half the patients. Their increase parallels a worsening prognosis.

❏ Transformation

- The most common transformation is reflected by a progressive increase in prolymphocytes. When $\geq 55\%$ of the leukemic lymphocytes acquire characteristics of prolymphocytes, the disease becomes known as prolymphocytic leukemia (see below). It connotes a grave prognosis.
- Richter syndrome is an aggressive transformation from CLL/SLL seen in 2–8% of patients. Diffuse large B-cell lymphoma is the most common histology. This lymphoma may arise from the CLL clone, but occasionally it represents an independent clone. It is considered a very aggressive lymphoma, but a large recent study demonstrated genetic heterogeneity and that survival can vary from a few weeks to 15 years.

Suggested Readings

Gribben JG. How I treat chronic lymphocytic leukemia. *Blood.* 2010;115:187–197.

Rawstron AC, Bennett FL, O'Connor SJM, et al. Monoclonal B-cell lymphocytosis and chronic lymphocytic leukemia. *N Engl J Med.* 2008;359:575–583.

Rossi D, Rasi S, Spina V, et al. Integrated mutational and cytogenetic analysis identifies new prognostic subgroups in chronic lymphocytic leukemia. *Blood.* 2013;121:1403–1412.

Rossi D, Spina V, Deambrogy C, et al. The genetics of Richter syndrome reveals disease heterogeneity and predicts survival after transformation. *Blood.* 2011;117:3391–3401.

PROLYMPHOCYTIC (PLL) LEUKEMIA OF B- AND T-CELL SUBTYPE

❑ **Definition**
B-cell PLL is a rare, aggressive, clonal lymphoproliferative disease composed mainly of B-cell prolymphocytes. It involves peripheral blood, bone marrow, and spleen. T-cell PLL is still rarer and will not be discussed further.

❑ **Who Should Be Suspected?**
Patients who present with prominent splenomegaly but no lymphadenopathy, B symptoms and WBC counts of >100,000 comprised nearly exclusively of abnormal appearing lymphocytes and frequently with anemia and thrombocytopenia. Some have a history of CLL/PLL, which occasionally transforms into B-cell PLL (see p. 402).

❑ **Laboratory Findings**
- *CBC:* 50% of patients present with anemia and thrombocytopenia.
- *Peripheral blood smear (PBS)* is heavily populated by medium/large-sized "prolymphocytes," with moderately condensed chromatin and a single, prominent, vesicular nucleolus. The prolymphocytes must exceed 55% of lymphocytes but are frequently >90%.
- *Bone marrow* is infiltrated in an interstitial pattern by prolymphocytes.
- *Lymph nodes* may show vague nodularity, but proliferation centers are absent.
- *Immunophenotype*
  - ▼ The prolymphocytes express bright surface IgM and IgD and bright CD20 (see Table 9-3) as well as CD19, CD20, CD22, CD79a and b, and FMC7.
  - ▼ Expression of CD5 and CD23 is weak or absent. CD25, CD11c, and CD103 are negative.
  - ▼ ZAP 70 and CD38 are expressed in half the cases.
- *Cytogenetics.* There are few studies available. Cases with t(11;14)(13;q32) should be considered leukemic variants of mantle cell lymphoma. Similarly, abnormalities common in CLL including deletions in 6q 11q (ATM), 13q, and 17p (TP53) are considered evidence of progression, from CLL. Molecular studies of p53 detect mutations in more than half the cases.

Suggested Reading
Campo E, Catovsky D, Montserrat E, et al. B-cell prolymphocytic leukaemia. In: *WHO Classification of Tumours of Haematopoietic and Lymphoid Tissues*, 4th ed. Lyon, France: International Agency for Research on Cancer; 2008:183–184.

HAIRY CELL LEUKEMIA

❑ **Definition**
Hairy cell leukemia (HCL) is a rare indolent B-cell lymphoproliferative neoplasm, characterized by the accumulation of small mature B lymphocytes with abundant cytoplasm and hairy projections. The disease has a 4:1 to 3:1 male-to-female ratio.

❏ Who Should Be Suspected?

Individuals who present with abdominal fullness due to splenomegaly and fatigue, weakness, and weight loss. Because of severe cytopenias, some patients may present with infections or excessive bleeding.

❏ Laboratory Findings

- *CBC*:
  - ▼ Anemia and thrombocytopenia are common, in part due to bone marrow infiltration and in part to hypersplenism.
  - ▼ WBC is usually decreased at presentation, but it may also be increased if the abnormal lymphocytes are elevated. Neutropenia and monocytopenia may be present.
  - ▼ Usually from 10% to 90% of lymphocytes in the peripheral blood smear reveal lymphocytes with cytoplasmic projections (hairy). Nucleoli are not visible. Ten percent of patients present with marked leukocytosis and the HCL cells predominate.
- *Bone marrow*:
  - ▼ Aspirate is difficult to obtain because of reticulin fibrosis.
  - ▼ Biopsy shows a hypercellular marrow, with diffuse or interstitial infiltration by hairy cells in a characteristic loose, widely spaced, fashion, with a well-defined rim of cytoplasm leaving a clear zone around the cells, producing a "fried egg" appearance. The hairy projections are not clearly seen on the biopsy specimen. No nucleoli are seen. There is no paratrabecular involvement. In some patients, there may be a hypocellular marrow that may resemble aplastic anemia. Reticulin stain shows moderate to marked increase in reticulin fibers.
- *Spleen and lymph nodes*: The leukemic cells are found in the red pulp with infiltration of the cords and sinuses, whereas the white pulp is atrophic. Angiomatous lakes are formed.
- *Cytochemistry*: Tartrate-resistant acid phosphatase (TRAP) is invariably positive (see Table 9-3) on involved white cells. It requires peripheral blood smear or bone marrow aspirate. Positivity appears as cytoplasmic granularity. It is rarely performed nowadays, having been replaced with the more specific flow cytometric studies.
- *Flow cytometry*
  - ▼ Flow cytometry (see Table 9-3) is positive for CD19, CD20 (bright), CD22, CD25, CD11c, CD103, and often annexin A1, and CD123. Cyclin D1 is weakly positive. Hairy cells lack expression of CD10, CD5, CD21, and CD23. Surface immunoglobulin is positive.
  - ▼ The hairy cell variant is negative for CD25 and CD123. This distinction is important therapeutically.
- *Molecular genetics*: Analysis of the immunoglobulin variable region genes shows somatic mutations in the majority of cases. Recent studies suggest that most cases demonstrate BRAF mutations. However, genetic studies have not been incorporated yet in the diagnostic criteria for HCL.
- *Karyotype*: No consistent karyotypic abnormalities are found. Abnormalities of 5q may be detected.

- *Hairy cell leukemia variant* is no longer considered a subtype of HCL, but a distinct lymphoproliferative entity. It is associated with extreme leukocytosis, with morphologic features between HCL and prolymphocytic leukemia.

Suggested Reading

Grever MR. How I treat hairy cell leukemia. *Blood.* 2010;115:21–28.

T-CELL LARGE GRANULAR LYMPHOCYTIC LEUKEMIA (T-LGL)

❑ Definition

T-LGL is a clonal disease of large granular natural killer (NK) cells. It is characterized by a persistent (>6 months) increase in the number of clonal peripheral blood large granular lymphocytes (LGLs), usually between 2,000 and 20,000/µL (the absolute number of LGLs in normal subjects is 2–400), without a clearly identified cause, splenomegaly, and cytopenias. T-LGLs may be associated with other diseases, such as RA or other hematologic disorders.

❑ Who Should Be Suspected?

A middle age or elderly patient with neutropenia and/or anemia, together with peripheral blood lymphocytosis, and moderate splenomegaly. The patient may be asymptomatic for long periods of time or may suffer from repeated bacterial infections. If the total lymphocyte count is not elevated, the disease may be suspected if an increased number of LGLs are present on examination of the peripheral blood.

❑ Laboratory Findings

- *CBC*
  - ▼ RBC: Anemia is present in half the patients, occasionally with oval macrocytosis.
  - ▼ WBC: Neutropenia is present in the majority of patients. LGLs are increased; they are large with abundant cytoplasm containing fine or coarse azurophilic granules and a reniform or round nucleus.
  - ▼ Thrombocytopenia is present in approximately 20% of patients.
- *Bone marrow* may show diffuse infiltration with LGL, but the extent of bone marrow involvement is variable.
- *Immunophenotype*: Most T-LGL leukemias show a profile of cytotoxic T cells, with positive CD3, CD8, CD16, CD57, and the alpha/beta T-cell receptor (TCR). Diminished or lost expression of CD5 and/or CD7 is common. T-LGL cells can also express CD2, CD45RA, and IL-2 receptor beta (CD122).
- *Molecular studies* help define the disease by finding TCR gene rearrangement. Developing technology found a number of genes whose expression was active in LGL T cells, but silent in normal T cells.
- *Cytogenetics* reveals no consistent karyotypic abnormalities, deletion of 6q may be the most common.
- *Serum protein electrophoresis* shows hypergammaglobulinemia in half the patients, rarely a monoclonal IgG gammopathy.
- *Serologic findings*: A positive RF is common, and antinuclear antibodies and circulating immune complexes are present in half the cases.

Suggested Reading
Zhang D, Loughran TP. Large granular lymphocytic leukemia: molecular pathogenesis, clinical manifestations, and treatment. *Hematology Am Soc Hematol Educ Program.* 2012;2012:652–659.

CHRONIC NEUTROPHILIC LEUKEMIA

❑ Definition
A rare myeloproliferative disease in which the predominant blood peripheral cells are mature granulocytes.

❑ Who Should Be Suspected?
Patients with persistent neutrophilia in whom a chronic infection, neoplasm, or inflammatory process is excluded. Clinical picture of splenomegaly and hepatomegaly of unknown etiology. Twenty-five to 30% of patients present with mucocutaneous bleeding. Polycythemia vera, primary myelofibrosis, and essential thrombocythemia should be excluded.

❑ Laboratory Findings
- *CBC*: Characterized by persistent leukocytosis (WBC $\geq 2,500 \times 10^9/\mu L$) due to neutrophilia (segmented neutrophils and bands are >80% of WBC). Immature granulocytes are <10% on the peripheral blood smear (PBS). Hb and platelets are normal early in the disease, but anemia and thrombocytopenia develop as the disease progresses.
- *Bone marrow*: Hypercellular with increase in mature neutrophils, but <5% myeloblasts.
- *Cytogenetics and genetic studies*: No rearrangement of BCR-ABL1, PDGFRA, PDGRFB, or FGFR1.

Suggested Reading
Bain BJ, Brunning RD, Vardiman JW, et al. Chronic neutrophilic leukaemia. In: *WHO Classification of Tumours of Haematopoietic and Lymphoid Tissues*, 4th ed. Lyon, France: International Agency for Research on Cancer; 2008.

 # MULTILINEAGE DISEASES**

MYELOPROLIFERATIVE NEOPLASMS (MPNS)

❑ Definition
Chronic MPNs are a heterogeneous group of clonal malignant disorders that arise from mutations in hematopoietic stem cells/progenitors. Clonal overexpansion leads to terminal myeloid expansion, reflected by various combinations of erythrocytosis, leukocytosis, thrombocytosis, bone marrow hypercellularity/fibrosis, and splenomegaly. There is a predisposition of the progenitor cells to undergo terminal transformation into leukemic blast cells. The three most common nonleukemic MPNs are polycythemia vera, essential thrombocythemia, and primary myelofibrosis. They are characterized by clonal dominance and unregulated increase in

---

**Co-authored by Patricia Miron, PhD

the circulation of erythrocytes, leukocytes, or platelets, each lineage alone, or in combination. Diagnostic challenges ensue because of the overlap of clinical and laboratory manifestations among these three disorders (phenotypic mimicry). This mimicry has been enhanced by the discovery of a common mutation *(V617F)* in *JAK2*, which belongs to the Janus family of tyrosine kinases.

■ *Bone marrow biopsies* are valuable for distinguishing among the various MPNs and for monitoring disease progression or effect of therapy. Following the discovery of mutations in crucial genes, the diagnosis of MPNs is becoming both morphologic and cytogenetic/molecular.

❑ **Classification**

■ Below is the revised (2008) WHO classification of MPNs, which includes the classic MPNs, and the atypical ones:
  ▼ Chronic myelogenous leukemia, BCR-ABL + [t(9:22)]
  ▼ Chronic neutrophilic leukemia
  ▼ Polycythemia vera
  ▼ Primary myelofibrosis
  ▼ Essential thrombocythemia
  ▼ Chronic eosinophilic leukemia, not otherwise classified
  ▼ Mastocytosis (not discussed further because of its rarity)
  ▼ *Atypical MPNs*: Myeloproliferative neoplasm, unclassifiable. These conditions include chronic myeloid disorders that are currently unclassifiable as belonging to either classical MPNs or myelodysplastic syndromes.
■ The diagnostic approach of these entities will be presented under separate headings.

Suggested Reading

Spivak JL. Narrative review: thrombocytosis, polycythemia vera, and JAK2 mutations: the phenotypic mimicry of chronic myeloproliferation. *Ann Intern Med.* 2010;152:300–306.

CHRONIC MYELOGENOUS LEUKEMIA (CML)

❑ **Definition**

CML is a myeloproliferative neoplasm characterized by the dysregulated production and uncontrolled proliferation originating in an abnormal pluripotential bone marrow stem cell. It is consistently associated with the BCR-ABL1 fusion gene. It results in an increase of myeloid cells, and, to a lesser extent, erythroid and platelets in the peripheral blood, and marked hyperplasia in the bone marrow. CML is induced by a chimeric gene that results from the fusion of the ABL1 gene on chromosome 9 with the BCR gene on chromosome 22, leading to the formation of a new leukemia-specific fusion gene that codes for a constitutionally activated protein tyrosine kinase. The Philadelphia (Ph) chromosome is the abnormal chromosome 22, reflecting the 95% of cases where the translocation between chromosomes 9 and 22 is balanced.

If untreated, CML progresses from the chronic phase to acute leukemia (blastic transformation) within 3–5 years, frequently with an intermediate "accelerated" phase. It may also present in the accelerated or blastic phase when first diagnosed.

❑ Who Should Be Suspected?

Patients found to have persistent, and not otherwise explained, myeloid leukocytosis. Patients with fatigue, anorexia, weight loss, excessive sweating, early satiety, abdominal fullness due to splenomegaly, and bleeding episodes.

❑ Laboratory Findings

Chronic Phase

- **CBC:**
  - ▼ WBC count is markedly elevated, usually 50,000–300,000/μL, predominantly neutrophils, bands, metamyelocytes, and myelocytes. The presence of a greater percentage of myelocytes than metamyelocytes (leukemic hiatus or myelocyte bulge) is a classic finding. Blasts account for <2% of cells. Basophilia is nearly always present. Eosinophilia may also be present. Absolute monocytosis is usually present but absolute lymphocytes are normal.
  - ▼ Hct/Hb may be normal or slightly decreased or increased; if anemia is present, it is normochromic, normocytic. Normoblasts are usually seen on the peripheral blood smear (PBS). Reticulocyte count is <3%.
  - ▼ Platelets may be normal, but in approximately 50% of cases, they are elevated. Occasionally, the platelets may be decreased, especially as the disease progresses. Large platelets (megathrombocytes) may be conspicuous.
- **Bone marrow**
  - ▼ Hyperplastic, with increase mainly in the myelocytic line, increased myeloid-to-erythroid ratio.
  - ▼ Myeloblasts are <5%. Increase in basophils and eosinophils, including immature forms. Megakaryocytes may be increased. Small megakaryocytes with hypolobulated nuclei are commonly found. Increases in reticulin fibrosis and vascularity are frequently found.
- **Cytogenetics**

  Demonstration of t(9,22)(q34;q11) involving BCR-ABL1 genes is the gold standard for diagnosis. Approximately 5% of CML patients do not demonstrate the t(9;22) by karyotyping but demonstrate the BCR-ABL1 gene fusion by FISH or real-time PCR techniques.[††] Patients may have variant complex translocations involving other chromosome or other cryptic translocations, but all result in the formation of the Ph chromosome with the BCR-ABL1 rearrangement. Patients whose cells lack evidence of BCR-ABL1 gene fusion by FISH or RT-PCR do not have CML. The V617F JAK2 mutation is absent.

- **Immunostains:** Leukocyte (neutrophil) alkaline phosphatase (LAP) (NAP): Low or absent LAP is not necessary for diagnosis in Philadelphia chromosome–positive patients. Nevertheless, it may be helpful for the rapid differentiation of CML from leukemoid reactions or other myeloproliferative neoplasms, while results of cytogenetic studies are pending.

- **Uric acid:** elevated

[††]Atypical CML is referred by some hematologists to cases mimicking CML, but without evidence of BCR-ABL gene fusion. These cases are classified by WHO in the group of myeloproliferative/myelodysplastic disorders. Another variant is the rare chronic neutrophilic leukemia, characterized by mature granulocytic hyperplasia and elevated LAP, but absent Philadelphia chromosome.

Accelerated Phase

- Progression to accelerated phase (or blast crisis) requires the acquisition of other chromosomal or molecular changes.

  The most common chromosomal abnormalities are trisomy 8, trisomy 19, an additional copy of the Ph chromosome, and isochromosome 17q.

- For diagnosis, 10–19% blasts of peripheral blood cells or nucleated bone marrow cells are required.
- ≥20% peripheral blood basophiles
- Persistent thrombocytopenia (<100,000/µL) unrelated to therapy
- Increasing spleen size and increasing WBC count unresponsive to therapy

  Blast Crisis

- ≥20% blasts of peripheral blood cells or of nucleated bone marrow cells.
- Extramedullary blast proliferation
- Large foci or clusters of blasts in the bone marrow biopsy
- Some patients present with Ph-positive acute leukemia; Some of these patients represent CML presenting in blast crisis, whereas others have de novo acute leukemia.

❏ Laboratory Criteria for Monitoring Response in Treated Patients

- Disease monitoring is one of the key management strategies of CML to assess the response to therapy and to detect early relapse. The most sensitive approach to detect CML is the quantitative real-time PCR (RT-PCR) of the BCR-ABL messenger RNA. By this methodology, one CML cell can be detected in 100,000 to 1 million cells. Another advantage of this methodology is the use of peripheral blood rather than bone marrow tissue. In cases of complete cytogenetic response, present guidelines suggest molecular testing starting 3 months.
- In patients treated with tyrosine kinase inhibitors, monitoring for new mutation in ABL is recommended, because such mutations predict the development of resistance to therapy. Certain mutations, such as those harboring BCR-ABL T315I, are resistant to therapy (a new tyrosine kinase inhibitor is presently being investigated for its effectiveness in patients with this mutation).

Complete Hematologic Response

- Complete normalization of peripheral blood counts with leukocytes <10,000/µL
- Platelet count <450,000/µL
- No immature cells in peripheral blood

Cytogenetic Response

- Complete: no translocation detected in a minimum of 20 metaphases
- Major: 0–30% positive metaphases
- Minor: 35–90% positive metaphases

Molecular Response

- Defined by the magnitude of reduction in BCR-ABL transcripts from a standard value.
- *Complete* molecular response: *BCR-ABL1* mRNA undetectable by RT-PCR.

- *Major* molecular response: >3-log reduction of *BCR-ABL1* mRNA; it correlates well with survival. No patient who achieved complete cytogenetic response and a major molecular response at 18 months progressed to accelerated or blast phase at 60 months.

Suggested Readings

Luatti S, Castagnetti F, Marzocchi G, et al. Additional chromosomal abnormalities in Philadelphia-positive clone: adverse prognostic influence on frontline imtinib therapy: a GIMEMA Working Party on CML analysis. *Blood.* 2012;120:761–767.
Branford S. Monitoring after successful therapy for chronic myeloid leukemia. *Hematology Am Soc Hematol Educ Program.* 2012;2012:105–110.

POLYCYTHEMIA VERA (PV)

❑ Definition
PV is the most common chronic myeloproliferative neoplasm (MPN). It is characterized by overproduction of morphologically normal erythroid cells, leading to an elevated red cell mass (RCM), as reflected by high hemoglobin and hematocrit. An increased RCM alone is insufficient to establish the diagnosis, because the RCM may be increased in secondary polycythemias, such as conditions associated with hypoxia, or with tumors secreting erythropoietin, or in congenital conditions.

❑ Classification
- The revised 2008 WHO criteria for the diagnosis of PV are presented:
- Major criteria
  - ▼ Hemoglobin >18.5 in men, >16.5 in women, or other evidence of increased red cell mass.
  - ▼ Presence of V617F JAK2 mutation in exon 14, or other functionally similar mutation such as JAK2 exon 12 mutation.
- Minor criteria
  - ▼ Bone marrow biopsy showing hypercellularity for age with trilineage growth (panmyelosis) and with prominent erythroid, granulocytic, and megakaryocytic proliferation.
  - ▼ Serum erythropoietin level below the reference range of normal.
  - ▼ Endogenous erythroid colony formation in vitro (not generally available in clinical laboratories).

The diagnosis requires the presence of *both* major criteria and *one* minor criterion or the presence of the first major criterion with two minor criteria. The first major criterion (high RCM) may be missed in patients with gastrointestinal bleeding.

❑ Who Should Be Suspected?
- Patients found to have an elevated Hb and Hct (the disease may be asymptomatic for long time) that cannot be explained otherwise.
- Mostly middle aged to elderly patients (median age at presentation is sixth decade).
- Patients with a history of familial polycythemic disorders and elevated Hb/Hct.
- Patients with otherwise unexplained thrombotic or bleeding events. The course of PV is characterized by thrombotic events, frequently in splanchnic vessels.

9

- Patients with splenomegaly of unknown etiology.
- Patients with pruritus, erythromelalgia, transient visual disturbances, headaches, weakness, dizziness, gastrointestinal symptoms, and excessive sweating.

❏ Laboratory Findings

- *CBC*: elevated Hb, Hct, and red cell count; platelets and granulocytes, but neither monocytes nor lymphocytes are frequently elevated.
- *Red cell mass (RCM)*: elevated (requires isotope study availability); plasma volume is normal or elevated.
- *Blood gases*: O_2 >92%.
- *Bone marrow*: Hyperplasia of erythroid, granulocytic, and megakaryocytic lines, without increase in immature cells; decreased iron stores; increased reticulin, especially as the disease progresses. Absence of stainable iron is a nearly universal finding.
- *Molecular genetics*: V617F JACK2 mutation in the exon 14 is present in 95–97% of PV patients, but it is not specific for PV as it may also be present in essential thrombocythemia and primary myelofibrosis. Increasing amounts of V617F allele correspond to a more pronounced myeloproliferative phenotype, favoring higher Hb levels and leukocyte counts. Other mutations seen in a minority of patients include mutations, insertions, or deletions in exon 12 of the JACK2 gene.
- *Cytogenetics or FISH*: Absence of BCR-ABL1 (t(9;22)). Other abnormalities that may be found but are not specific for PV include 20q⁻, +8, +9, and gain of 9p.
- *Serum erythropoietin*: low or immeasurable.
- *Other*: Leukocyte alkaline phosphatase and serum vitamin B_{12} are elevated, but not necessary for diagnosis.

Suggested Reading
Passamonti F. How I treat polycythemia vera. *Blood.* 2012;120:275–284.

ESSENTIAL THROMBOCYTHEMIA (ET)

❏ Definition
ET is a chronic myeloproliferative neoplasm (MPN) involving mainly the megakaryocytic lineage, characterized by persistent thrombocytosis. It is a diagnosis of exclusion.

❏ Who Should Be Suspected?

- Patients, especially females, with persistent thrombocytosis without an underlying cause, not meeting criteria for polycythemia vera, primary myelofibrosis, chronic myelogenous leukemia, myelodysplastic syndromes, or other myeloid neoplasms.
- Patients with unexplained splenomegaly.
- Patients with unexplained thrombosis or hemorrhages.
- No evidence of reactive thrombocytosis.

❏ Laboratory Findings

- *CBC*: sustained platelet count >450,000 (some recommend persistent elevated counts for ≥8 months).
- *Bone marrow biopsy* shows proliferation of the megakaryocytic lineage with increased numbers of enlarged, mature megakaryocytes; no increase and no left shift of granulopoiesis or erythropoiesis. Iron stores are normal.
- *Genetic test*: V617F JAK2 mutation can be demonstrated in about half the cases of ET; in its absence, reactive thrombocytosis should be ruled out, especially by demonstrating normal serum ferritin to exclude iron deficiency.

Cytogenetics: No cytogenetic abnormalities are specific for ET. The incidence of clonal cytogenetic abnormalities is approximately 5–10%. Abnormalities include +8, +9, and 20q–. The absence of BCR-ABL1 (t[9;22]) must be documented to exclude CML.

Suggested Reading

Passamonti F, Thiele J, Girodon F, et al. A prognostic model to predict survival in 867 World Health Organization-defined essential thrombocythemia at diagnosis: a study by the International Working Group on Myelofibrosis Research and Treatment. *Blood*. 2012;120:1197–1201.

PRIMARY MYELOFIBROSIS (PMF)

❏ Definition

PMF is a Philadelphia (Ph) chromosome–negative chronic myeloproliferative neoplasm (MPN) characterized by progressive bone marrow fibrosis, clonal proliferation of myeloid cells, and ineffective hematopoiesis. All patients have marked splenomegaly. It may follow transformation of PV or ET into myelofibrosis (no longer "primary"). PMF has a prefibrotic (initial) and a fibrotic stage. The prefibrotic stage is frequently difficult to diagnose. PMF is characterized by a leukoerythroblastic blood picture, teardrop poikilocytosis of red cells, and extramedullary hematopoiesis, with progressive hepatosplenomegaly. Other causes of marrow fibrosis must be excluded.

❏ Classification

- The WHO-proposed revision requires the presence of major and minor criteria:
  - ▼ *Major criteria*
    - Presence in the bone marrow biopsy of megakaryocytic proliferation and atypia, usually accompanied by either reticulin and/or collagen fibrosis; in the absence of significant reticulin fibrosis, the megakaryocyte changes must be accompanied by an increased bone marrow cellularity characterized by granulocytic proliferation and often decreased erythropoiesis (the prefibrotic cellular-phase disease).
    - Not meeting WHO criteria for PV, CML, MDS, or other myeloid neoplasms.
    - Demonstration of JAK2 V617F or other clonal markers such as MPL, or in the absence of a clonal marker, no evidence that the bone marrow fibrosis is due to an underlying inflammatory or other neoplastic diseases.

▼ *Minor criteria*
- Leukoerythroblastosis
- Increased serum LDH
- Anemia
- Palpable splenomegaly

❑ Who Should Be Suspected of PMF?

■ Patients with progressive splenomegaly reaching enormous size and resulting in hypersplenism as manifested by pancytopenia. Hepatomegaly may also be present.

■ Patients aged >65 with constitutional symptoms: severe fatigue, symptoms due to enlarged spleen, weight loss, signs of a hypermetabolic state, pruritus, and pulmonary hypertension.

■ Patients with progressive unexplained anemia with bizarre peripheral blood smear (PBS) morphology, and leukocytosis.

■ Patients with thrombosis of splanchnic veins.

❑ Laboratory Findings

■ *CBC*

▼ RBCs: Normochromic, normocytic progressive anemia caused by hemolysis, ineffective hematopoiesis, splenic sequestration, bleeding, and a variety of other cases. Peripheral blood smear (PBS) shows marked anisocytosis and poikilocytosis with teardrop RBCs (dacrocytes), polychromasia, and nucleated red cells (part of a leukoerythroblastic picture). Reticulocyte count is increased.

▼ WBCs may be decreased, normal, or increased; abnormal or immature forms may be present and increase with time. The blasts are initially <5%, but as the disease progresses, the WBCs and blasts in the peripheral blood may increase and may reflect transformation into blast crisis/acute myeloid leukemia. Basophils and eosinophils may be increased.

▼ Platelets may be decreased, normal, or increased. Thrombocytopenia becomes more profound with disease progression. Abnormal or large forms are present. Deficient aggregation with collagen or epinephrine is common.

■ *Bone marrow* shows progressive fibrosis that can be visualized with silver stain for reticulin and trichrome stain for mature collagen. Bone marrow sinusoids are expanded, and there is intravascular hematopoiesis. Early on the bone marrow may be hypercellular with minimal fibrosis (prefibrotic or cellular phase of PMF). Frequently, the bone marrow aspirate results in a dry tape. The biopsy shows a progressively hypocellular marrow replaced by fibrosis. Megakaryocytes are the last remaining hematopoietic elements, most of which have abnormal morphology.

■ *Lymph node biopsy* (usually not necessary) shows extramedullary hematopoiesis involving all three cell lines. Foci of extramedullary hematopoiesis may occur in almost any organ.

■ *Genetics and flow cytometry*

▼ The JAK2 V617F gene mutation is present in approximately 50–60% of cases.

▼ MPL (W515K/L): Activating mutations affecting MPL thrombopoietin receptors are present in 5–7% of cases.

▼ Elevated CD34+ hematopoietic precursors can be detected in peripheral blood and distinguishes PMF from PV and ET in which they are absent in the chronic phases.

■ Chromosome abnormalities occur in 35–50% of patients at diagnosis. Favorable abnormalities include sole deletions in 13q or 20q or trisomy 9. Deletion of 5q, 7q, or 12p, trisomy 8, or >3 aberrations predict a poor survival. Patients with abnormalities 17p– have the poorest survival. Additional karyotypic abnormalities that may develop during the course of the disease may further affect prognosis.

Cytogenetic studies are recommended not only to determine prognosis but most importantly to rule out CML through the absence of BCR-ABL translocation.

■ *Coagulation*: PT or PTT may be prolonged and laboratory evidence of DIC is occasionally found.

■ *Leukocyte alkaline phosphatase* (LAP) is increased (not routinely recommended).

■ *Other*: LDH, serum uric acid, and vitamin B_{12} are often increased.

Suggested Readings

Levine RL, Gilliland DG. Myeloproliferative disorders. *Blood*. 2008;112:2190–2198.

Mascarenhas J, Hoffman R. A comprehensive review and analysis of the effect of ruxolitinib therapy on the survival of patients with myelofibrosis. *Blood*. 2013;121:4832–4837.

Tam CS, Abruzzo LV, Lin KI, et al. The role of cytogenetic abnormalities as a prognostic marker in primary myelofibrosis: applicability at time of diagnosis and later during disease course. *Blood*. 2009;113:4171–4178.

MYELODYSPLASTIC SYNDROME (MDS)

❏ Definition

MDS is a group of clonal disorders of the hematopoietic system, characterized by ineffective hematopoiesis. Dysplasia (abnormal morphology) involving at least 10% of a specific myeloid lineage, peripheral blood cytopenias, and increased risk of transformation into acute myeloid leukemia. Approximately two thirds of patients present initially with low-risk disease. Higher grade disease categories tend to progress to acute myeloid leukemia. Refractory cytopenias are the principal cause of mortality and morbidity. The differential diagnosis of MDS includes various causes of macrocytic or refractory anemias, alcohol consumption, and thyroid disease.

❏ Who Should Be Suspected?

An elderly patient, presenting with cytopenia(s) discovered by routine CBC, or with symptoms resulting from anemia (fatigue, weakness, exercise intolerance, new angina), less frequently infections, bruising, or bleeding. Splenomegaly and lymphadenopathy are absent. The presence of monocytosis is suggestive of chronic myelomonocytic leukemia (CMML). Previous exposure to environmental toxins such as benzene, radiation therapy, or treatment with alkylating agents or topoisomerase II inhibitors may result in secondary MDS. Alternatively, young patients with an inherited hematologic disorder are predisposed to develop MDS.

❑ Classification

- The WHO classification has proved helpful for prognosis and in selection of therapy and is updated periodically. The 2008 WHO classification of MDS contains eight entities:
  1. Refractory cytopenias with unilineage dysplasia (RCUD).
  2. Refractory anemia (RA): <5% bone marrow blasts, ≤1% blasts in the peripheral blood; <15% of erythroid precursors are ringed sideroblasts (characterized by at least five granules of iron that encircle the nucleus of erythroid precursors).
     - Refractory neutropenia (RN)
     - Refractory thrombocytopenia (RT)
  3. Refractory anemia with ringed sideroblasts (RARS): similar to RA, but with ≥15% ringed sideroblasts in the bone marrow. Erythroid dysplasia only.
  4. Refractory cytopenias with multilineage dysplasia (RCMD): dysplasia in ≥10% of cells in two or three lineages and <5% bone marrow blasts; ±15% ringed sideroblasts.
  5. Refractory anemia with excess blasts-1 (RAEB-1): 5–9% blasts in the bone marrow but no Auer rods. Cytopenia(s) but <5% blasts in peripheral blood.
  6. Refractory anemia with excess blasts-2 (RAEB-2): 10–19% blasts in bone marrow, Auer rods ±; 5–19% blasts in peripheral blood, cytopenia(s).
  7. Myelodysplastic syndrome unclassified (MDS-U): <5% blasts in bone marrow; dysplasia in <10% of cells when accompanied by a cytogenetic abnormality is considered presumptive evidence for a diagnosis of MDS; cytopenias and ≤1% blasts in peripheral blood.
  8. MDS associated with isolated del (5q) (the 5q⁻ syndrome). Bone marrow: normal or increased mononuclear megakaryocytes with spherical nuclei; <5% blasts; no Auer rods; del(5q) as the only cytogenetic abnormality. Peripheral blood: anemia, normal or increased platelet count, and no or rare blasts (<1%).
- Syndromes with mixed features of myelodysplastic–myeloproliferative disorders are classified separately as MDS/MPS. The prototype is CMML.

❑ Laboratory Findings

- Findings vary with subtype of MDS (see above). Common findings will be described, as well as those distinguishing ones for various subtypes.
  - ▼ *CBC.* Unilineage, bilineage, or trilineage cytopenias are common, but in the absence of dysplastic features, they are insufficient for the diagnosis of MDS.
    - Red cells: commonly macrocytic anemia (high MCV); hypochromic, microcytic cells in RARS; ovalomacrocytosis; basophilic stippling; Howell-Jolly bodies; and megaloblastoid nucleated red cells may be present on peripheral blood smear (PBS).
    - WBC: Leukopenia resulting from neutropenia is present at diagnosis in half the patients. Granulocytes have reduced or absent granulation, reduced segmentation of nuclei (pseudo-Pelger-Huet nuclei), clumped chromatin pattern, ring-shaped nuclei, and nuclear sticks. The granulocytes may be dysfunctional, leading to infections. Lymphopenia due

to a reduction of T4 lymphocytes is seen in hypertransfused patients. Mild monocytosis is common, but if the monocytes are markedly elevated, consider CMML.

- Platelets: Varying degrees of thrombocytopenia are present at the time of diagnosis in about 25% of patients. Giant or agranular platelets can be seen on peripheral blood smear (PBS). Platelets may be functionally defective, and platelet aggregation is often abnormal. Thrombocytosis may be present in some patients with RARS; thrombocytosis is also part of the 5q⁻ syndrome or in patients with translocations involving chromosome 3.

▼ *Bone marrow examination* is mandatory for diagnosis and classification of the MDS subtype. Marrow fibrosis can be seen in approximately 10% of the MDS cases, and it is usually associated with excess blasts and aggressive clinical course. In most cases, the bone marrow is hyperplastic, and erythroid hyperplasia, in association with ineffective erythropoiesis. The erythroid precursors show alterations in their nuclei. Approximately 10–15% of patients have a hypocellular marrow that is difficult to distinguish from aplastic anemia.

- Defective maturation in the myeloid series is common, and counting the number of blasts is essential to determine subtype and prognosis.
- Megakaryocytes are normal or increased in number; they sometimes occur in clusters. Abnormal morphology of megakaryocytes is common.
- Cytochemical stains of the bone marrow (especially iron stains of erythroblasts) are helpful in the diagnosis of the various subtypes of MDS.
- Immunophenotyping of the bone marrow is useful in determining percentage of CD34+ cells, which usually parallels the number of blasts on the aspirate smear. Assessment of maturation patterns of myeloid and monocytic elements can also provide supporting evidence for the diagnosis of MDS.

▼ *Cytogenetic studies* are helpful for diagnosis, may provide prognostic information, and are useful for monitoring response to therapy. Patients with the 5q⁻ anomaly (isolated or in combination with other abnormalities) may be treated differently, as they often respond to immunomodulatory therapy. Clonal cytogenetic abnormalities are seen in approximately 50–75% of cases and are not specific to subtypes, although certain cytogenetic abnormalities may be associated with characteristic morphology, for instance the association of *EVI1* rearrangements at 3q26 with abnormal megakaryocytes. Recurrent abnormalities include ⁻5/5q⁻, ⁻7/7q⁻, trisomy 8, and 20q⁻. In the International Prognostic Scoring System (IPSS) for MDS, normal chromosomes, ⁻Y, 5q⁻, and 20q⁻ are considered good prognosis; ⁻7/7q⁻ or complex karyotype (≥3 abnormalities) are considered poor prognosis, and other findings are considered intermediate. Del(17p) is associated with the presence of pseudo-Huët granulocytes containing small vacuoles, a deletion of TP53, and a relatively high risk of leukemic transformation. Abnormalities of *MLL* at 11q23 often represent therapy-related MDS and are associated with poor prognosis. Certain clonal cytogenetic abnormalities, for example, ⁻Y and 20q⁻, are not diagnostic of MDS in the absence of positive morphologic findings.

▼ *Molecular genetic studies* reveal 30% higher abnormalities than classic karyotyping. The finding of recurrent molecular genetic alterations with prognostic and diagnostic impact indicates that in the near future, implementing comprehensive genetic studies will play an important role in clinical practice.

▼ *Serum B_{12} and folate* should be obtained to exclude deficiencies that may mimic MDS morphologically. The karyotype is normal in these deficiencies.

▼ *Hb electrophoresis* may reveal acquired Hb H disease, or rarely acquired thalassemic syndrome, but it is not necessary for the diagnosis of MDS.

▼ *Serum immunoglobulins* are variably abnormal, with hypogammaglobulinemia, polyclonal hypergammaglobulinemia, and even monoclonal gammopathies reported.

▼ Studies for PNH help differentiate the two diseases or reveal various combinations of PNH with aplastic anemia or refractory anemias as part of a MDS picture.

▼ *Serology for HIV infection* may be indicated in some cases, since AIDS may be associated with dysplastic hematopoiesis and cytopenias.

❑ **Prognosis**

■ The International Prognosis Scoring System (IPSS) classifies MDS patients into four prognostic categories based on the number of cytopenias, cytogenetics, and percent of blasts in the bone marrow.

Suggested Readings

Abdel-Wahab O, Figueroa ME. Interpreting new molecular genetics in myelodysplastic syndromes. *Hematology Am Soc Hematol Educ Program.* 2012;2012:56–64.

Brunning RD, Orazi A, Germing U, et al. Myelodysplastic syndromes/neoplasms, overview. In: *WHO Classification of Tumours of Haematopoietic and Lymphoid Tissues*, 4th ed. Lyon, France: International Agency for Research on Cancer; 2008:88–93.

Nimer SD. Myelodysplastic syndromes. *Blood.* 2008;111:4841–4851.

Stone RM. How I treat patients with myelodysplastic syndromes. *Blood.* 2009;113:6296–6303.

Tefferi A, Vardiman JW. Mechanisms of disease: myelodysplastic syndromes. *N Engl J Med.* 2009;361:1872–1885.

CHRONIC MYELOMONOCYTIC LEUKEMIA (CMML)

❑ **Definition**

According to the 2008 WHO classification, CMML belongs to the group of myelodysplastic/myeloproliferative neoplasms. CMML is subdivided into two subcategories:

■ CMML-1: blasts (including promonocytes) <5% in the peripheral blood and <10% in the bone marrow

■ CMML-2: blasts (including promonocytes) 5–19% in the peripheral blood or 10–19% in the bone marrow or the presence of Auer rods

❑ **Who Should Be Suspected?**

An elderly patient with persistent monocytosis of >3 months' duration and massive splenomegaly in 25% of cases. Hepatomegaly, lymphadenopathy, tissue infiltrations, or serous effusions may also be presenting findings.

❑ **Laboratory Findings**

- *CBC*: One, two, or all three lineages present dysplastic features.
  - ▼ RBC: Severe anemia is common.
  - ▼ WBC: Persistent absolute monocyte count of >1,000/μL (>10% of leukocytes) in the peripheral blood. The monocytes may be morphologically normal or may have dysplastic features. In cases without dysplasia, other causes of monocytosis must be excluded. Neutropenia or neutrophilia may also be present, but neutrophil precursors account for <10% of the leukocytes. They may have dysplastic features. In some cases, eosinophilia is present (CMML with eosinophilia).
- *Platelets*: Moderate thrombocytopenia with atypical, large platelets may be present.
- *Bone marrow* is hypercellular with striking granulocytic and to a less extent monocytic proliferation. Esterase stains distinguish the monocytic line. There are <20% blasts. An increase in erythroid precursors with dyserythropoietic features may also be present. Abnormal megakaryocytes complete the morphologic picture. Lysozyme (muramidase) activity may be elevated in blood and urine.
- *Immunophenotype*: Myeloid antigens CD33 and CD13 are positive; monocytic antigens CD14, CD68, and CD64 are variably expressed. Aberrant features are frequently present. An increasing CD34 population forecasts transformation into acute leukemia.
- *Immunostain* for lysozyme on tissue sections is positive for the monocytic cells.
- *Cytogenetics*: Nonspecific clonal cytogenetic abnormalities are found in 20–40% of patients. The most frequent abnormalities are +8, –7/del(7q), and structural abnormalities of 12p. Some patients with t(5;12)(q33;p13) may have eosinophilia and may respond to therapy with tyrosine kinase inhibitors. This group of patients is no longer included in the CMML category, since they result from fusions of PDGFRB with other genes (see above).
- *Genetic studies*: PDGFRA or PDGFRB are not rearranged. Rearrangements must be excluded in cases with eosinophilia. The BCR-ABL 1 fusion gene must be excluded.

Suggested Reading

Itzykson R, Kosmider O, Renneville A, et al. Clonal architecture of chronic myelomonocytic leukemias. *Blood*. 2013;121:2186–2198.

SPLENOMEGALY

❑ **Definition**

Enlargement of the spleen that can be demonstrated either by physical examination or by imaging studies. Splenomegaly reflects an underlying disease. Finding splenomegaly should trigger systemic investigation of its etiology.

❑ **Who Should Be Suspected?**

Patients with abdominal fullness, early satiety, or chronic or acute left upper abdominal pain.

- Common causes of splenomegaly are as follows:
  - ▼ Infections
    - Infectious endocarditis
    - Infectious mononucleosis
    - Brucellosis
    - Miliary tuberculosis
    - Parasitic infections: malaria, schistosomiasis, kala-azar
    - Fungal diseases
  - ▼ Vascular (systemic or portal) congestion (congestive splenomegaly)
  - ▼ Immune disorders
    - RA (Felty syndrome)
    - SLE
    - Sarcoidosis
  - ▼ Hematologic conditions
    - Hemolytic anemias
    - Thalassemia major
    - Hereditary (spherocytosis), ovalocytosis
    - Polycythemia vera
    - Essential thrombocythemia
    - Chronic lymphocytic leukemia
    - Non-Hodgkin lymphomas
    - Hodgkin lymphoma
    - Chronic myeloid leukemia (massive)
    - Primary myelofibrosis (massive)
    - Systemic mastocytosis
    - Infiltrative splenomegaly
    - Lipid storage diseases—Gaucher disease, Niemann-Pick disease, and many more
    - Amyloidosis
    - Sarcoidosis
    - Metastatic disease
  - ▼ Developmental anomalies
  - ▼ Multitransfused patients
- In many cases of splenomegaly, the spleen's ability to engulf blood cells is increased (hypersplenism), resulting in mono-, bi-, or pancytopenias.

LYMPHOMAS[‡‡]

NON-HODGKIN LYMPHOMAS

❑ **Definition**

- Non-Hodgkin lymphomas are neoplasms of lymphoid tissues comprising numerous variants. They are a heterogeneous group of distinct disorders, mostly unrelated to one another, with a spectrum of histologic grades and clinical behavior. The present classification, as updated by the WHO in 2008, recognizes three categories of lymphoid neoplasms: B-cell, T-cell,

[‡‡]Co-authored by Patricia Minehart Miron, PhD & Hongbo Yu, MD, PhD.

and NK cell lymphomas, and separately Hodgkin lymphoma and plasma cell disorders. Among the non-Hodgkin lymphomas, most are derived from B cells. The present classification is based on currently available morphologic, immunophenotypic, and genetic techniques, with an attempt to correlate the various types with their clinical behavior. The latter is utilized as a guide for predicting prognosis and therapy in the International Prognostic Index.

- Many issues remain unresolved, and the 2008 WHO classification represents evolving concepts. Rapidly evolving genomic technologies, which include gene rearrangement and microarray techniques, reveal multiple subtypes of different molecular etiologies, clinical evolution, and response to therapy, all within the presently accepted types of lymphomas.

- In addition, studies of microRNA (miRNA) (small noncoding RNAs that orchestrate many aspects of cell physiology and their deregulation is often linked to distinct neoplasms) have demonstrated clusters, such as 17–92 overexpressed in a variety of B-cell lymphomas.

- Because of the extreme rarity of some lymphomas (B- or T-cell lymphoblastic leukemia/lymphoma, primary cutaneous follicle center lymphoma, aggressive NK cell leukemia, angioimmunoblastic T-cell lymphoma, peripheral T-cell lymphoma [unspecified], hepatosplenic T-cell lymphoma, T-cell lymphoma, nasal type, adult T-cell leukemia/lymphoma, anaplastic large cell lymphoma, ALK positive or negative, enteropathy-associated intestinal T-cell lymphoma, subcutaneous panniculitis-like T-cell lymphoma, primary cutaneous gamma-delta T-cell lymphoma, primary cutaneous CD30⁺ T-cell lymphoproliferative disease, lymphomatoid papulosis, and primary cutaneous anaplastic large cell lymphoma) and space constraints, these entities will not be included. The reader is referred to the WHO classification manual or specialty hematopathology textbooks.

- The following types of non-Hodgkin lymphoma and diagnostic approaches are described in subsequent sections:
  - Diffuse large cell (see p. 422)
  - Follicular (see p. 423)
  - Mantle zone (see p. 424)
  - Marginal zone (see p. 425)
  - Burkitt (see p. 420)
  - Cutaneous (see p. 421)
  - Lymphoplasmacytic (see p. 427)
  - Posttransplantation (see p. 427)

❏ Common Laboratory Findings (Type-Specific Findings Will Be Presented With Each Lymphoma Chapter)

- Abnormalities of humoral immunity: hypogammaglobulinemia and occasionally monoclonal gammopathies
- Autoimmune hemolytic anemia and/or thrombocytopenia
- Laboratory findings due to involvement of other organs (CNS, liver, kidneys, GI tract, testes)
- Laboratory and clinical findings related to therapy:
  - Cytopenias
  - Peripheral neuropathies

▼ As the result of infections
▼ Gonadal dysfunction
■ History of AIDS

Suggested Readings

Jaffe ES, Harris LN, Stein H, et al. Classification of lymphoid neoplasms: the microscope as a tool for disease discovery. *Blood*. 2008;112:4384–4399.

Swedlow SH, Campo E, Harris NL, et al. *WHO Classification of Tumours of Haematopoietic and Lymphoid Tissues*, 4th ed. Lyon, France: International Agency for Research on Cancer; 2008:158–166.

BURKITT LYMPHOMA (BL)

❏ Definition

BL is a highly aggressive, B-cell lymphoma with distinctive morphologic, genetic, and cytogenetic alterations. Translocations involving the MYC oncogene are the molecular hallmark of BL, being present in 100% of cases. There are three distinctive forms of BL: endemic (in Equatorial Africa), sporadic (in Western countries), and associated with immunodeficiency.

❏ Who Should Be Suspected?

1. For the endemic form is the most common childhood cancer in equatorial Africa. It is manifested as tumors of the jaw or facial bones. Nearly all endemic cases are associated with EBV infection.

2. The sporadic forms involve mostly nonhematopoietic organs, with a predication to invade the bone marrow and CNS. The peak incidence is in the second and third decades. BL has a propensity to invade. Only 20% of cases are associated with EBV infection.

3. Immunodeficiency-associated BL occurs most commonly in patients infected with HIV (HIV-BL), but rarely in other immunocompromised patients.

❏ Laboratory Findings

■ *For diagnosis, a biopsy with studies of morphologic, genetic, and cytogenetic analysis and immunophenotyping is necessary.*

▼ *Morphology*: Medium-sized uniform-appearing cells with round nuclei and 2–5 basophilic nucleoli. The cytoplasm of BL cells is deeply basophilic, with numerous lipid vacuoles. A "starry sky" pattern is characteristic for BL-positive biopsies.

▼ *CBC*: A leukemic, ALL-like phase can be seen in patients with bulky disease (Burkitt leukemia variant).

▼ *Immunophenotype*: BL has a mature B-cell phenotype. The cells have monotypic surface IgM and are positive for CD10, CD19, CD20, CD22, CD38, CD43, and CD79a. CD5 and TdT are negative. Bcl-2 is typically absent. Proliferation fraction by Ki-67 is nearly 100%.

▼ *Cytogenetics*: Translocation *(8;14) (q24;q32)* is found in 80% of cases; in the rest, *t(8;22)(q24;q11)* or *t(2;8)(p11;q24)*. These translocations are readily detected by metaphase analysis. FISH analysis may also be used but can miss some rearrangements because the break points are widely heterogeneous.

▼ *Genetic studies*: C-MYC dysregulation with BCL-6⁺ has long been associated with BL. The MYC translocation is considered a primary event. However, deregulation of MYC has been shown to occur in other B-cell lymphomas, most often as a secondary event, the so-called "double-hit," indicating an aggressive course. Gene profile studies help differentiate atypical BL from diffuse large cell lymphoma, but no uniform criteria have yet been established.

Suggested Readings

Jaffe ES, Pittaluga S. Aggressive B-Cell lymphomas: a review of new and old entities in the WHO classification. *Hematology Am Soc Hematol Educ Program.* 2011;2011:506–514.

Piccaluga PP, De Falco G, Kustagi M, et al. Gene expression analysis uncovers similarity and differences among Burkitt lymphoma subtypes. *Blood.* 2011;117:3596–3608.

CUTANEOUS T-CELL LYMPHOMAS: MYCOSIS FUNGOIDES (MF) AND SÉZARY SYNDROME (SS)

❑ Definition
Cutaneous T-cell lymphomas (CTCL) are a heterogeneous group of T-cell lymphomas. MF and SS are tumors of the CD4$^+$ helper T cells. MF is the more common; it is an indolent, extranodal non-Hodgkin lymphoma. SS is a leukemic variant in which typical malignant Sézary cells circulate in the peripheral blood; they can also be found in skin and lymph nodes.

❑ Who Should Be Suspected?
An elderly patient with persistent and progressive pruritic patches, plaques, or subcutaneous tumors (MF). An elderly patient with a high number of atypical (cerebriform) T-cell lymphocytes in the peripheral blood; erythroderma and extracutaneous infiltrates, with marked lymphadenopathy (SS).

❑ Laboratory Findings
Diagnosis is established by the typical morphology of skin biopsy for MF and SS, as well as by the study of peripheral blood for SS.

- *Bone marrow and liver biopsies* are usually normal.
- *CBC* is normal in MF. Total WBC count is often increased in SS. More than 1,000/μL cells are atypical, easily identifiable lymphocytes.
- *Skin biopsy* in MF demonstrates atypical mononuclear cells with cerebriform nuclei, infiltrating the upper dermis.
- *ESR, Hb, and platelet counts* are usually normal in both conditions.
- *Immunophenotyping* may be technically difficult. Both conditions have CD4$^+$, CD3$^+$, CD45RO$^+$ CLA$^+$ phenotype. In MF, the cells are positive for CD4, CD2, CD3, CD5, and CLA, but, in most cases, MF cells are negative for CD8. In addition to CD4, SS cells express CD27, CCR7, L-selectin, and CCR4. Alterations in the expression of T-cell antigens are commonly seen, with loss of expression of CD7 and CD26 being the most common, but not distinctive for malignant T cells. Immunophenotyping helps to distinguish CTCL from reactive or inflammatory lymphoid infiltrates in the skin, which usually express all mature T-cell antigens. An epidermal/dermal discordance for CD2, CD3, CD5, and CD7 suggests the diagnosis of CTCL. In SS, the neoplastic lymphocytes are markedly expanded in the peripheral blood with a CD4/CD8 ratio of >10.

- *Molecular genetic studies*: T-cell receptor gene rearrangement may help establish the diagnosis of MF when the skin biopsy and immunophenotyping results are ambiguous. Gene expression profiles and microRNA profiling suggest that MF and SS may be separate entities with differing pathogenesis.
- *Cytogenetics*: In many patients, the tumor cells have complex karyotypes.

Suggested Reading

Van Doorn R, van Kester MS, Dijkman R, et al. Oncogenomic analysis of mycoides fungoides reveals major differences with Sezary syndrome. *Blood.* 2009;113:127–136.

DIFFUSE LARGE B-CELL LYMPHOMA (DLBCL)

❑ Definition

DLBCL is characterized by clinical, morphologic, cytogenetic, and molecular heterogeneity and can be divided in many subgroups that are biologically distinct, with different responses to therapy. One of the most consistent predictors of outcome is the Rituxan-International Prognostic Index.

❑ Who Should Be Suspected?

Patients in their 60s who present with rapidly enlarging lymphadenopathy and/or with tumors at extranodal sites, the most common being the GI tract. The bone marrow may also be involved, and in many of these cases, lymphoma cells may be detected in the peripheral blood.

❑ Laboratory Findings

- *Diagnosis is best established by biopsy of an enlarged lymph node or another affected organ. The morphologic pattern and immunophenotype establish the diagnosis and its variants.*
  - ▼ *Immunophenotype*: In most cases, the tumor cells are positive for the B-cell markers CD19, CD20, CD22, CD79a, and CD45. Monoclonal cell surface membrane IgM is usually positive. Occasionally, DLBCL cells may be CD5 or CD10 positive. It has recently been reported that expression of CD30 by the lymphoma cells is associated with better outcome in patients treated with R-CHOP chemoimmunetherapy.
  - ▼ *Cytogenetics*: There are no karyotypic abnormalities specific for DLBCL. Up to 30% of cases show rearrangement of 3q27, involving the BCL6 gene; 30% carry a t(14;18)(q32;q21) causing a *BCL2-IGH* rearrangement, more typically found in follicular lymphomas, and 10–20% carry a *C-MYC* rearrangement (see below).
  - ▼ *Genetics*: Increasingly, genomic studies offer better differentiation and prognostication. Gene expression profiling—not universally available for clinical use—has identified three distinct molecular subgroups: germinal center B-cell like, activated B-cell like, and primary mediastinal B-cell lymphoma. They have different survival patterns and respond differently to therapy. C-MYC expression or amplification is associated with resistance to therapy and a poor prognosis, especially if associated with BCL2 and BCL6 translocations or overexpressions.
  - ▼ *Other*: Elevated serum LDH indicates aggressive disease.

Suggested Readings

Horn H, Ziepert M, Becher C, et al. MYC status in concert with BCL2 and BCL6 expression predicts outcome in diffuse large B-cell lymphoma. *Blood.* 2013;121:2253–2263.

Perry AM, Cardesa-Salzmann TM, Meyer PM, et al. A new biologic prognostic model on immunohistochemistry predicts survival in patients with diffuse large B-cell lymphoma. *Blood.* 2012;120:2290–2296.

FOLLICULAR LYMPHOMA (FL)

❏ Definition

FL is defined primarily by its morphologic pattern, and by the translocation t(14;18), that leads to deregulated expression of the antiapoptotic BCL-2 protooncogene. FL is the second most common lymphoma in Western countries comprising approximately 20% of all lymphomas. It is considered an indolent lymphoma because in general, the disease shows a slow rate of progression, in spite of its clinical presentation with advanced disease in the majority of patients. It is an incurable disease since most cases eventually transform into aggressive lymphomas. The prognosis can be determined by criteria known as The Follicular Lymphoma International Prognostic Index (FLIPI).

❏ Who Should Be Suspected?

Patients in their 50s or 60s, complaining of generalized, progressive lymphadenopathy and splenomegaly, but otherwise asymptomatic, despite the high incidence of bone marrow involvement and generalized disease.

❏ Laboratory Findings

The diagnosis is established by biopsy of an involved lymph node. According to the number of centroblasts present in the neoplastic infiltrate, FL is subdivided into grades 1 to 3A that constitute a biologic continuum. Grade 3B is composed exclusively of centroblasts and is usually negative for t(14;18), as is pediatric FL.

- *Bone marrow biopsy and peripheral blood*: Whenever the bone marrow is involved, paratrabecular lymphoid aggregates are seen. With leukemic involvement of the peripheral blood, notched or clefted lymphocytes are identified.
- *Immunohistochemistry* for BCL2 is valuable for the diagnosis of FL (see below).
- *Immunophenotype*: FL cells (obtained from lymph node, bone marrow biopsy, or peripheral blood) are positive for CD19, CD20, CD22, and CD79a. In most cases, the cells are also CD10 positive. Some cases especially in grade 3 (advanced) disease may lack CD10 expression. The cells also express BCL-2 and BCL-6 and lack expression of CD5 and CD43. Immunoglobulins heavy and light chains are rearranged. About half of the affected cells express IgM and 40% IgG.
- *Cytogenetics and molecular genetics*: One of the earliest events in the developing of FL is thought to occur in the B-cell precursors in the bone marrow, giving rise to the t(14;18) (q32;q21) translocation that juxtaposes the BCL2 gene on chromosome 18, to the immunoglobulin heavy chain gene locus, resulting in overproduction of the BCL2 protein. This translocation is observed in 85% of cases of FL, but it is not specific for FL, since 30%

of DLBCL are also positive. Moreover, it was found that many healthy persons have this translocation in their circulating lymphocytes, without any evidence of FL.

▪ *CBC*: Hemoglobin below 12 g/dL is associated with advanced disease.
▪ *Other*: Serum LDH is usually normal, but a high LDH connotes a poor prognosis.

Suggested Readings

Solai-Celigny P, Roy P, Colombat P, et al. Follicular lymphoma international prognostic index. *Blood.* 2004;104:1258–1265.

Stevenson FK, Stevenson GT. Follicular lymphoma and the immune system: from pathogenesis to antibody therapy. *Blood.* 2012;119:3659–3667.

MANTLE CELL LYMPHOMA (MCL)

❑ Definition

MCL is a CD-5–positive mature B-cell lymphoma. MCL is considered one of the most aggressive lymphomas. Recently, a subgroup of patients with an indolent course has been identified through gene expression profile studies. MCL comprises about 7% of non-Hodgkin lymphomas. The t(11;14)(q13;q32), which involves CCND1 and IGH, is usually present. The translocation determines the ectopic and deregulated expression of cyclin D1, which is considered the primary molecular event in the pathogenesis of MCL. Less common are the variant CCND1 rearrangements with IGK or IGL genes. Rarely (approximately 5%), mantle cell lymphoma can results from dysregulation of CCND2 (12p13) and CCND3 (6p12) genes. These genes can be seen rearranged with IGH, IGK, or IGL. The MCL-affected cells are usually positive for CD5, creating difficulties in the differentiation from CLL/SLL.

❑ Who Should Be Suspected?

Elderly patients with generalized disease: constitutional symptoms, nonbulky lymphadenopathy, possibly hepatosplenomegaly, lymphocytosis, bone marrow invasion, some with multiple lymphomatous polyposis of the intestine, and constitutional symptoms.

❑ Laboratory Findings

Laboratory diagnosis of MCL is based mainly on lymph node morphology, flow cytometry, and cytogenetics.

▪ *CBC*: Anemia and thrombocytopenia are commensurate with the clinical stage, the degree of bone marrow infiltration, or may reflect chemotherapy. Increasing lymphocyte count, characterized by a leukemic phase, denotes a poor prognosis.
▪ *Lymph node biopsy* shows lymphoid proliferation with vaguely nodular, diffuse, or mantle zone pattern. Lymphocytes are homogenous, small to medium in size with irregular or "cleaved" nuclei, and inconspicuous nucleoli.
▪ *Immunophenotype*: Cells express intense surface IgM/IgD and show lambda light chain restriction in up to 80% of cases. The cells are positive for CD5, CD19, CD20, and FMC-7. They are negative for CD10, BCL6, and in contrast to CLL/SLL, CD23 is negative or weakly positive. All cases are BCL2 positive. Nuclear staining for cyclin D1 (BCL-1) is positive in 95% of cases.

- *Molecular genetics*: Immunoglobulin heavy and light chain genes are rearranged. The IgV region genes lack somatic mutations in most cases, indicating a pregerminal center stage of differentiation, consistent with an origin from immunologically naive mantle zone B cells. The neural transcription factor SOX11 is overexpressed in most MCL but is not detected in other mature B-cell lymphomas nor in normal lymphoid cells. Gene expression profiles may play a future role in subclassifying MCL.
- *Cytogenetics*: The *t(11;14)(q13;q32)* is present in most cases of MCL. (See above.)
- *Other*: LDH elevation is associated with poor prognosis.

❑ **Transformation**

- Transformation is characterized morphologically by increase in cell size (blastic variant), frequent mitoses, and an aggressive clinical course.
- Additional karyotypic abnormalities are associated with a poor prognosis.

Suggested Readings

Ghielmini M, Zucca E. How I treat mantle cell lymphoma. *Blood*. 2009;114:1469–1476.

Hoster E, Dreyling M, Klapper W, et al. A new prognostic index (MIPI) for patients with advanced-stage mantle cell lymphoma. *Blood*. 2008;111:558–565.

Perez-Galan P, Dreyling M, Wiestner A. Mantle cell lymphoma: biology, pathogenesis, and the molecular basis of treatment in the genomic era. *Blood*. 2011;117:26–38.

MARGINAL ZONE LYMPHOMA (MZL)

❑ **Definition**

MZL includes three distinct entities that originate from memory B lymphocytes, normally present in the marginal zone of secondary lymphoid follicles: splenic MZL (±villous lymphocytes); extranodal MZL of mucosa-associated lymphoid tissue (MALT); and nodal MZL. These three lymphoma subtypes account for 5–17% of all non-Hodgkin lymphomas. They are clinically distinct.

- The first two types will be presented in this section.
  A. Splenic marginal B-cell lymphoma is an indolent lymphoma composed of small lymphocytes that surround and replace the splenic white pulp germinal centers. The condition may be associated with villous lymphocytes in the peripheral blood. Splenic hilar lymph nodes and the bone marrow are often involved.
  B. MALT lymphoma is a low-grade lymphoma originating in sites normally devoid of lymphoid tissues, such as stomach (the most prevalent), salivary glands, small bowel, lung, and thyroid. It is often preceded by chronic inflammation of the affected site or is associated with autoimmune diseases such as Sjögren syndrome and Hashimoto thyroiditis. Bacterial infection with *Helicobacter pylori* is associated with 92% of gastric MALT lymphomas. Usually, MALT presents as a localized disease.

❑ **Who Should Be Suspected?**

Splenic marginal B-cell lymphoma: Elderly patients with abdominal discomfort due to splenomegaly, lymphocytosis, and cytopenias. Peripheral lymphadenopathy and involvement of extralymphatic organs–except bone marrow—are uncommon.

The course is extremely indolent, but it has the potential to transform into a high-grade lymphoma.

MALT lymphoma: A patient (median age 60) with GI symptoms not otherwise diagnosed or with demonstrated *H. pylori* infection of the stomach and a gastric lesion. The majority of patients present with stage I or II disease.

❏ Laboratory Findings

Splenic B-Cell Marginal Zone Lymphoma

- *CBC*: Anemia, thrombocytopenia (both may have an autoimmune etiology), and neutropenia are commonly present; lymphocytosis is frequently present, but not essential for diagnosis. The lymphocytes have a round nucleus, condensed chromatin, and abundant basophilic cytoplasm with small surface "villous" projections. A combination of hemoglobin <12 g/dL, elevated LDH, and serum albumin <3.5 g/dL is predictive of short survival.
- *Coagulation*: PTT may be prolonged due to an acquired inhibitor, such as the lupus anticoagulant.
- *Bone marrow or lymph node biopsy* is indicated in the absence of diagnostic peripheral blood findings or available spleen histology. Bone marrow involvement may be mild and difficult to identify.
- *Immunophenotype*: The neoplastic lymphocytes express surface immunoglobulins (IgM or IgD), B-cell antigens (CD19, CD20, CD22), and BCL-2. They are CD5, CD10, CD43, CD23, CD25, and CD103 negative. Negative CD10 and BCL6 help exclude follicular lymphoma.
- *Cytogenetics and molecular genetics*: The majority of the patients show an abnormal karyotype; recurrent aberrations include gain of 3q and deletion of 7q22-36. Deletion of 17p is associated with an aggressive clinical course. A gene expression profile, different from other B-cell lymphomas, has been described.

MALT Lymphoma

For patients presenting with gastric MALT lymphoma, the diagnosis is established by endoscopic biopsy.

- *Microbiology*: Studies for *H. pylori* are positive for gastric MALT lymphoma, but other microbes, as well as chronic stimulation due to autoimmune diseases, have been implicated in pathogenesis.
- *Immunophenotype*: The tumor cells express B-cell–associated antigens: CD19, CD20, CD22, CD79a, and complement receptors CD21 and CD35. They are negative for CD5, CD10, and CD23. This immunophenotype is helpful in the differential diagnosis of other lymphomas.
- *Cytogenetics*: Four recurrent chromosomal translocations have been described: t(11;18) (q21;q21) BIRC3-MALT1; t(14;18)(q32;q21) IGH-MALT1; and less commonly, t(1;14)(p22;q32) BCL10-IGH; and t(3;14) (p13;q32) FOXP-IGH. Trisomy 3 is present in 60% of cases.
- *Immunohistochemistry*: Nuclear expression of BCL-10 or NF-kappa B is associated with resistance to antibiotic therapy.

Suggested Reading

Zinzani PL. The many faces of marginal zone lymphoma. *Hematology Am Soc Hematol Educ Program*. 2012;2012:426–432.

POSTTRANSPLANT LYMPHOPROLIFERATIVE DISORDER (PTLD)

❑ **Definition**

Lymphoma is the most common malignancy following stem cell or solid organ transplantation. PTLD comprises a spectrum of lymphomas classified by the WHO as early lesions, polymorphic PTLD, monomorphic PTLD (classified according to B-/T-cell lymphomas they resemble), and classic Hodgkin lymphoma-like PTLD. More than 90% of early cases (<1 year after transplantation) are EBV positive. Later cases (>2 years posttransplantation) are less often associated with EBV positivity, and their etiology is uncertain.

❑ **Who Should Be Suspected?**

Posttransplant patients who present with fever, generalized lymphadenopathy, hepatosplenomegaly not due to a documented infection. The GI tract, lungs, and liver may also be involved, occasionally as initial localizations. The incidence of PTLD correlates with the intensity of immunosuppression. It is seen sometimes following unrelated donor allogeneic stem cell transplantation or umbilical cord blood transplants after intensive immunosuppression.

❑ **Laboratory Findings**

- Peripheral blood may show very atypical plasmacytic lymphocytes.
- Lymph node biopsy or fine needle aspiration is essential for diagnosis and classification. It reveals atypical plasmacytoid lymphoid cells.
- Bone marrow biopsy should be done if no other tissue source is readily obtained.
- Flow cytometry of lymph nodes or bone marrow biopsy reveals κ/λ ratio of 5:1.
- EBV clonality and load help define the etiology.

Suggested Reading

Swerdlow SH, Webber SA, Chadburn A, et al. Post-transplant lymphoproliferative disorders. In: *WHO Classification of Tumours of Haematopoietic and Lymphoid Tissues*, 4th ed. Lyon, France: International Agency for Research on Cancer; 2008:343–349.

LYMPHOPLASMACYTIC LYMPHOMA (LPL)/WALDENSTRÖM MACROGLOBULINEMIA (WM)

❑ **Definition**

LPL/WM results from the accumulation, predominantly in the bone marrow, of clonally lymphoplasmacytic cells that secrete a monoclonal IgM protein, resulting in elevated serum IgM paraprotein. Most cases of LPL are IgM associated, a few secrete IgA or IgG, and some are nonsecretory, hence falling outside the classical denomination of WM. Clinically, classical WM can be distinguished from lymphoplasmacytic lymphoma on the basis of symptoms of hyperviscosity. However, there seems no rationale for separating these entities. We will use the terms interchangeably, as LPL/WM. The term LPL/WM should be reserved for a distinct neoplasm of small lymphoid cells that are CD5⁻, CD10⁻, CD23⁻, and have a pan-B-cell marker–positive phenotype. There is variable involvement of bone marrow, lymph nodes, and spleen. Monoclonal gammopathy of undetermined significance (MGUS) of

IgM class (defined as <10% marrow infiltration and <3 g/dL of serum monoclonal IgM) and smoldering WM (defined by the presence of ≥3 g/dL IgM and/or ≥10% lymphoplasmacytic infiltration, but no evidence of end-organ damage) have been associated with an increased risk of developing LPL/WM.

❑ Who Should Be Suspected?

Patients with lymphadenopathy, hepatosplenomegaly, oronasal bleeding, and constitutional symptoms (weakness, fatigue, weight loss, fever, night sweats, recurrent infections—especially pneumonias with pleural effusion). The presentation may be characteristic of the hyperviscosity syndrome: blurring or loss of vision, headache, vertigo, dizziness, diplopia retinal vein engorgement and flame-shaped hemorrhages, and papilledema. *Severe hyperviscosity is a medical emergency.* Patients with type I or II cryoglobulinemia and cold agglutinin hemolytic anemia should also be investigated for LPL/WM. The disease may also present with pulmonary symptomatology or with CNS infiltration (Bing-Neel syndrome).

❑ Laboratory Findings

- **CBC**
  - ▼ Red cells: Moderate to severe normochromic, normocytic anemia with rouleaux formation on the peripheral blood smear (PBS). The anemia is multifactorial, in part due to bone marrow infiltration, but to a large extent being the result of red cell dilution by increased plasma volume. Autoimmune hemolytic anemia may develop on the basis of cold or warm antibodies.
  - ▼ WBC: Lymphocytosis or monocytosis is common. Occasionally, leukopenia is present.
  - ▼ Platelets: Thrombocytopenia may be present; it is occasionally immune in etiology. Platelet function is impaired secondary to coating of the platelet surface receptors by IgM paraproteins, resulting in impaired platelet adhesiveness. Platelet aggregation may show a thrombocytopathy.
- *Immunoglobulins*
  - ▼ Serum protein electrophoresis reveals a homogenous spike (M component), almost always of γ mobility.
  - ▼ Total serum protein and globulin are markedly increased.
  - ▼ Quantitation of immunoglobulins reveals increased IgM (>30 g/L in most cases, but no specific cutoff is required for the diagnosis). There is reciprocal decrease of IgG and of IgA. Serial quantitation of serum IgM is used to monitor the effect of therapy or disease progression.
  - ▼ Immunofixation is a more definitive diagnostic assay because it identifies the M spike as a monoclonal IgM protein.
  - ▼ Serum light chains: A preponderance of κ over λ light chains, with a reported 4.5:1 incidence ratio. Serum free light chain determination could be used as a surrogate tumor marker.
  - ▼ A serum monoclonal IgM is not pathognomonic for WM. It may be seen in rare cases of multiple myeloma (WM can be excluded if such patients have osteolytic lesions) and splenic marginal zone lymphoma. In asymptomatic patients, a diagnosis of smoldering LPL/WM may be entertained. If the bone marrow is infiltrated with <10% clonal cells and the patient is asymptomatic, the diagnosis of IgM-MGUS should be considered.

- *Serum viscosity*: Clinical symptoms of hyperviscosity begin when serum viscosity is >4 centipoise. At a viscosity of >6 centipoise the symptoms become more severe. The frequency of hyperviscosity ranges from 6% to 20% of cases. There may be great variability in the serum viscosity level at which patients become symptomatic.

- *Bone marrow biopsy* is recommended for all patients. Bone marrow *aspirate* appears often to be hypocellular. The *biopsy* specimen, however, demonstrates hypercellularity with ≥10% infiltration by small lymphocytic and plasmacytoid or plasma cells. The intratrabecular pattern of infiltration may be nodular, interstitial, or diffuse. The abnormal cells have a nuclear spoke-wheel pattern of plasma cells but have high nuclear/cytoplasmic ratio more typical of small lymphocytes. Nevertheless, typical plasma cells with Russell and Dutcher bodies may be seen. Mast cells are frequently increased.

- *Lymph node biopsy* shows lymphoplasmacytic infiltration, but the normal architecture is preserved. Distinguishing LPL/WM from other B-cell lymphomas, especially marginal zone B-cell lymphoma, may be difficult.

- *Histologic transformation*: LPL can transform in a more aggressive form of lymphoma, similar to Richter transformation in CLL. Transformation can be demonstrated by lymph node or bone marrow biopsy. It connotes an aggressive clinical picture resistant to therapy. Occasionally, the disease may evolve into AL amyloidosis.

- *CNS infiltration* with plasma cells and lymphocytes (the Bing-Neel syndrome) has been described. Peripheral neuropathy is seen in up to 20–25% of patients. The evaluation of anti–myelin-associated glycoprotein antiganglioside MI and antisulfatide IgM antibodies may be appropriate.

- *Flow cytometry* demonstrates an earlier stage of B-cell differentiation in addition to the plasmacytic cells. The clonal cells are surface IgM^+, $CD19^+$ $CD20^+$, $CD22^+$, $CD25^+$, $CD38^+$, $CD79a^+$, $FMC7^+$, $BCL2^+$, $PAX5^+$; $CD3^-$, $CD103^-$. A small subset of patients may express CD5 in their lymphocytic component.

  - ▼ *Cytogenetics*: Cytogenetic examination may be useful in differentiating LPL/WM from IgM myeloma. Eighty-three percent of patients have chromosomal abnormalities. The most common reported recurrent abnormality is 6q deletion (encompassing 6q21-25).

- *Molecular genetics*: MYD88 L265P is a commonly recurring mutation that can be useful in differentiating LPL/WM and non-IgM LPL from B-cell disorders that have some of the same features. miRNA expression profiling reveals a specific signature, but the technology is available only in some research laboratories.

- *Coagulation*: Thrombin time is prolonged due to inhibition of fibrin polymerization by the paraprotein (impaired coagulation may play a role in the bleeding diathesis).

- *Serum β-2 microglobulin* is elevated in half the patients.

- *Sedimentation rate* and *C-reactive protein* may be very elevated.

- *LDH and alkaline phosphatase* when elevated correlate with an unfavorable course.

- *Hyperuricemia and hypercalcemia* have been reported.

- *Azotemia* may be present on the basis of light chain or amyloid depositions, as well as parenchymal renal involvement by lymphoplasmacytic cells.
- *Tests no longer recommended*
  - ▼ Immunoelectrophoresis (replaced by immunofixation).
  - ▼ BJ protein may be replaced by measuring serum light chains because the amount of IgM excreted in urine may be below detection level and does not correlate well with tumor burden. In addition, obtaining serum light chain analysis obviates the need to collect 24-hour urine.

❑ Limitations

- Spurious results: The high-level IgM may interfere with automated analyzer results, especially producing an artificially low HDL cholesterol or falsely elevated Hgb.
- Serum IgM may occasionally be artifactually low because of the polymerization of IgM. A warm bath collection should be obtained for blood specimens in patients suspected of having cryoglobulinemia to avoid underestimation of serum IgM.
  - ▼ Low serum ferritin levels may be the result of interference of the IgM paraprotein with ferritin measurements.
- Difficulty in cross-matching blood may be encountered.

Suggested Readings

Ghobrial IM. Are you sure this is Waldenstrom macroglobulinemia? *Hematology Am Soc Hematol Educ Program.* 2012;2012:586–594.
Vijay A, Gertz MA. Waldenstrom macroglobulinemia. *Blood.* 2007;109:5096–5103.

HODGKIN LYMPHOMA (HL)

❑ Definition

HL is a neoplasm of transformed B-lymphocytes, characterized morphologically by the presence of Hodgkin or Reed-Sternberg HRS cells. In many ways, HL remains an enigmatic neoplasm.

HL is comprised of two major subgroups based on morphologic appearance and immunophenotype of the tumor cells: nodular lymphocyte predominant HL (NLPHL) and classical HL (cHL). The tumor cells of NLPHL retain the phenotypic feature of germinal center B cells, whereas they are inconspicuous in cHL. cHL is in turn subdivided into four subtypes with distinct morphology, epidemiology, and prognosis: nodular sclerosis (NSHL), mixed cellularity (MCHL), lymphocyte rich (LRHL), and lymphocyte depleted (LDHL), the latter having the worst prognosis.

❑ Who Should Be Suspected?

In North America and Western countries, HL has a bimodal age distribution: one peak in young adults and one in an older age group (approximately 65 years of age). Commonly, an adult with indolent lymphadenopathy, often in the cervical area. Occasionally, the patient may present with B symptoms (fever, night sweats, weight loss, and pruritus) or dyspnea in cases with advanced mediastinal involvement. Risk factors: a history of infectious mononucleosis, autoimmune disorders, immunosuppression (organ or stem cell transplantation), therapy with immuno-suppressive drugs, and HIV infection.

❏ Laboratory Findings

- *The diagnosis of HL is based on the morphology found on excisional tissue biopsy of an involved lymph node. RS cells are large cells with slightly basophilic cytoplasm; they have bilobed or multiple nuclei, surrounded by T lymphocytes. Hodgkin cells represent the mononuclear variant.*

  In addition to the laboratory tests described below, *imaging studies* have a very important role in establishing the extent of disease and differentiating HL from other conditions, especially when involving the mediastinum. Among them, *sarcoidosis*, an inflammatory disease characterized by non-caseating granulomas, involves the lungs in >90% of patients. In stage 1, sarcoidosis presents with hilar adenopathy alone, which radiologically may be very similar to HL radiographic image.

- *Bone marrow biopsy* is positive for malignant cells in up to 6.5% of advanced cases. It affects therapy only marginally.

- *CBC*
  - ▼ Normochromic, normocytic anemia in advanced cases. Anemia or leukopenia at presentation denotes a poor prognosis. Eosinophilia occurs in ≈20% of patients. Lymphopenia or monocytosis may also occur.
  - ▼ Platelets may be decreased (in some cases, immune thrombocytopenia is present) or increased.

- *Elevated ESR, elevated LDH*, and low serum albumin are associated with advanced disease.

- *Liver function* tests may be abnormal.

- *Serum calcium* may be elevated due to bony involvement or overproduction of calcitriol.

- *Immunophenotype*: The neoplastic cells in *cHL* express CD30, and CD15, but *lack* pan-B antigens (CD19, CD20, CD79a), pan-T antigens (CD3, CD7), and CD45. The expression of epithelial membrane antigen (EMA) is mostly negative. Ninety-five percent of cases are weakly positive for PAX-5/BSAP. The HRS cells of cHL also express MUM1. By contrast, in NLPHL, the neoplastic cells stain positively for CD20, CD79a, CD45, OCT-2, BOB.1, and EMA. They lack CD15 and CD30.

- *Cytogenetics*: Cytogenetic abnormalities are found in the majority of cases of cHL; however, there are no typical cytogenetic abnormalities, and cytogenetic analysis is not considered to be clinically important.

- *Molecular genetic studies* have not reached the clinical practice yet. Genomic analysis detects EBV positivity in 40% of LRHL, 70% of MCHL, and nearly 100% of LDHL, but not in NSHL or NLPHL. Activation of NF-κB pathway is a central event in HL pathogenesis.

Suggested Readings

Aster JC. Epidemiology, pathologic features, and diagnosis of classical Hodgkin lymphoma. In: Basow DS (ed). *UpToDate*, Waltham, MA: UpToDate Inc.; 2013.

Greaves P, Gribben JG. Laser-capturing the essence of Hodgkin lymphoma. *Blood*. 2012;120:4451–4452.

MONOCLONAL GAMMOPATHIES[§§]

This section describes disorders of plasma cells and of plasma proteins. These neoplasms result from the expansion of a clone of Ig-secreting, terminally differentiated B lymphocytes. These neoplasms are known as monoclonal gammopathies because they express monoclonal products of homogenous immunoglobulins (or fragments) produced by the neoplastic abnormal B cells. The monoclonal proteins may be present in serum, urine, and CSF. The section will follow the fourth edition of the *WHO Classification of Tumours of Haematopoietic and Lymphoid Tissues*. It includes plasma cell myeloma, plasmacytoma, the benign precursor monoclonal gammopathy of undetermined significance (MGUS), and the syndromes defined by the consequence of tissue immunoglobulin deposition, primary amyloidosis (AL), and light and heavy chain deposition disease. Lymphoplasmacytic lymphoma and the heavy chain diseases are described separately.

Suggested Reading
Swerdlow SH, Campo E, Harris NL, et al. *WHO Classification of Tumours of Haematopoietic and Lymphoid Tissues*, 4th ed. Lyon, France: International Agency for Research on Cancer; 2008:200–213.

PLASMA CELL MYELOMA (PCM)

❑ Definition
Plasma cell myeloma (multiple myeloma, MM) is a B-cell neoplasm consisting of neoplastic proliferation of plasma cells primarily occurring in the bone marrow. The current WHO classification stratifies this disorder into two distinct categories based on specific criteria: (1) symptomatic plasma cell myeloma and (2) asymptomatic (smoldering) myeloma (see below).

Clinically, plasma cell myeloma is manifested by osteolytic lesions, renal failure, hypercalcemia, anemia, hyperviscosity, and serum/urine M (monoclonal) protein.

❑ Who Should Be Suspected?
Patients in their 60s and 70s who present with anemia, bone pain, unexplained fractures, frequent infections, bleeding, symptoms of hypercalcemia (excessive thirst and urination, constipation, nausea, loss of appetite and mental confusion), and neurologic symptoms arising from compression fractures of vertebrae. There is a wide clinical spectrum ranging from an asymptomatic state to aggressive forms and disorders due to deposition of immunoglobulin chains in tissues.

❑ Diagnosis and Laboratory Findings
The diagnosis is based on established criteria (WHO) for plasma cell myeloma:

- Symptomatic plasma cell myeloma
  - ▼ M protein in serum or urine: >30 g/L IgG, or >20 g/L IgA, or >1 g/24 hour urine light chain; some patients with symptomatic myeloma may have lower levels.
  - ▼ Bone marrow clonal plasma cells (usually >10% of nucleated cells) or extramedullary plasmacytoma(s).

[§§]Co-authored by Patricia Minehart Miron, PhD.

▾ Related organ or tissue impairment (hypercalcemia, renal insufficiency, anemia, bone lesions, amyloidosis, hyperviscosity or recurrent infections).

■ Asymptomatic (smoldering) myeloma: patients progress into symptomatic myeloma or amyloidosis at a rate of 10% per year in the first 5 years.

▾ M protein in serum or urine (>30 g/L IgG, >20 g/L IgA, or >1g/24 hour or urine light chain)

and/or

▾ 10% or more clonal plasma cells in bone marrow

▾ No related organ or tissue impairment

❏ Laboratory Findings

Laboratory studies are essential for initial diagnosis and prognosis upfront and for determining the presence of a complete remission (CR) following therapy. The current definition of CR is based on serologic and cytologic results, rather than molecular studies.

■ *Bone marrow biopsy and aspirate*: Aspirate and biopsy are recommended for identification and quantitation of plasma cells morphologically and by immunophenotype (CD138⁺). Plasma cells are seen in sheets or abnormal clusters. Morphology may vary from normal-appearing plasma cells to primitive plasmablasts that may be difficult to identify morphologically.

■ *CBC*: Normochromic, normocytic anemia with or without leukopenia, thrombocytopenia, and presence of normoblasts in cases with extensive marrow replacement. Rouleaux formation (due to paraproteinemia) is present on peripheral blood smear (PBS).

■ *Serum protein* is markedly elevated with increased globulins and hypoalbuminemia. Decrease in polyclonal gamma globulins is also present and is one of the reasons for repeated infections. Hypogammaglobulinemia in light chain myelomas that produce only light chains.

■ *Serum protein electrophoresis and immunofixation* reveal a monoclonal protein (κ or λ) and identify a specific heavy chain (IgG 50%, IgA 20%, IgD, IgE, IgM, and biclonal in <10% of cases). Light chain only is found in 20% of cases (light chain disease).

■ *Urine protein electrophoresis and immunofixation* reveal M protein (Bence Jones protein) reflecting urine light chain. With extensive renal damage, albumin and whole immunoglobulin molecules can be found in urine.

■ *Serum free light chain immunoassay*: Normal κ:/λ is 0.26–1.65. The ratio is altered in nonsecretory myeloma, oligosecretory myeloma, and light chain myeloma. This assay is useful for diagnosis, monitoring during and after treatment, and perhaps prognosis of patients with multiple myeloma and an intact immunoglobulin.

■ Cold agglutinins or cryoglobulins may be present.

■ Serum calcium may be elevated due to osteolytic lesions.

■ Hypercalciuria results from dehydration and renal tubular dysfunction.

■ Serum uric acid is elevated in 50% of cases.

■ ESR (is usually [90% cases]) markedly elevated.

■ Serum β2 microglobulin can be elevated. A level >6 μg/mL portends poor prognosis.

- Renal function tests may be abnormal in the presence of monoclonal light chain proteinuria.
- *Immunophenotype*: The neoplastic plasma cells classically are CD138$^+$, CD38^{high}, CD19$^-$, CD56$^+$ (60–80%), and CD79a$^+$ and express monotypic cytoplasmic κ or λ. In addition, plasma cells may also aberrantly express CD117, CD20, CD52, CD10, and occasionally myeloid and monocytic antigens. Cyclin D1 expression may be seen in cases with t(11,14) translocation.
- *Genetics and cytogenetics*: New genetic technology now allows insight into the genetic aberrations in MM at a genome-wide scale and across different developmental stages in the course of an individual's disease. Risk scores based on gene expression profiling have been recently presented as powerful prognostic predictors. While not yet applicable clinically, these advances will also lead to improved targeted therapies. At the cytogenetic level, the MM genome is recognized as being extremely complex. Nevertheless, *cytogenetic evaluation is mandatory* in all patients with newly diagnosed MM. Genetic abnormalities can be detected by interphase FISH in nearly 100% of cases. Cytogenetic abnormalities can be classified into two groups: *structural (translocations)*, involving the IGH locus, and *genomic imbalances, including gains and losses*. The most common IGH translocations are t(11;14)(q13;q32) CCND1-IGH (15–18%), t(14;16)(q32;q23) MAF-IGH (5%), t(4;14)(p16.3;q32) FGFR3-IGH (15%), and t(14;20)(q32;q12) MAB-IGH (2%). CCND1-IGH is considered a favorable finding with associated therapy; the other IGH partners are considered to be poor prognostic findings. Hyperdiploidy, typically with trisomy of chromosomes 3, 5, 7, 9, 11, 15, 19, and 21, is a favorable finding, while hypodiploidy is unfavorable. Hypodiploid clones often double and must be distinguished from hyperdiploid clones. Deletion of 13q or loss of 13 is common, and its prognostic impact, particularly as a sole abnormality, is unclear. Deletion of 17p (TP53) and MYC rearrangements represent progression of disease as do the molecular genetic findings of K or NRAS mutations (30–40%), FGFR3 mutation, and inactivation of RB1 or p18^{INK4c}.
- *Microbiology*: Repeated bacterial infections caused by *Diplococcus pneumoniae*, *Staphylococcus aureus*, and *Escherichia coli*.
- Test no longer recommended: serum immunoelectrophoresis.

Suggested Readings

Bergsagel PL, Mateos M-V, Gutierres NC, et al. Improving overall survival and overcoming adverse prognosis in the treatment of cytogenetically high-risk multiple myeloma. *Blood*. 2013;121:884–892.

Kyle RA, Rajkumar SV. Multiple myeloma. *Blood*. 2008;111:2962–2972.

MONOCLONAL GAMMOPATHY OF UNDETERMINED SIGNIFICANCE (MGUS)

❑ Definition

MGUS is an asymptomatic preneoplastic condition characterized by the presence in the serum of

- Monoclonal (M)-protein, but <3 g/dL
- Bone marrow clonal plasma cells <10%

- No lytic lesions, anemia, hypercalcemia, or renal insufficiency (see below), that is, no end-organ damage that can be attributed to the plasma cell proliferative disorder. A special situation was recently discussed: monoclonal gammopathies associated with kidney disease and the term "monoclonal gammopathy of renal significance" was proposed.
- No clinical manifestations or evidence of another B-cell proliferative disorder.

In most cases, neoplastic plasma cells are present in the bone marrow; however, clonal IgM-producing cells may be seen originating in the spleen and lymph nodes. The risk of progression to an overt plasma cell myeloma, amyloidosis (), lymphoplasmacytic lymphoma , or other lymphoproliferative disorder is 1% per year. MGUS patients with abnormal free light chain ratio are at high risk of developing amyloidosis. MGUS has been divided into three subtypes with different modes of progression: non-IgM MGUS, the most prevalent, IgM-MGUS, and light chain MGUS.

❑ Who Should Be Suspected?

MGUS is more common in men (1.5:1) and African American subjects; its incidence is 4.2% in individuals older than 50 years and 5% in those older than 70. There are no distinctive symptoms or physical findings associated with this disorder. Seventy-nine percent to 82% of patients with the systemic capillary leak syndrome have MGUS.

❑ Laboratory Findings

- Bone marrow biopsy and aspirate. Plasma cells are increased, but <10; interstitial and in small cluster distribution.
- CBC is usually normal. Rouleaux formation (due to paraproteinemia) may be seen.
- Serum proteins may be elevated with increased globulins (decreased A:G ratio) and hypoalbuminemia.
- Hypogammaglobulinemia may be present in light chain MGUS where only light chains are produced.
- Serum protein electrophoresis and immunofixation reveal a monoclonal protein (κ or λ) and identify preponderance of a specific immunoglobulin chain (IgG 70% of cases, IgA 12%, light chain 20%, IgM 15%, and biclonal 3%).
- Urine protein electrophoresis and immunofixation reveal M protein (Bence Jones protein) in one third of cases, reflecting urine light chains.
- Serum free light chain immunoassay. Normal κ-to-λ ratio is 0.26:1.65. Abnormal ratio in MGUS is a significant risk factor for progression to myeloma.
- Renal function tests may be abnormal in MGUS. Light chains and proteinuria may be present.
- Immunophenotype: Flow cytometry analysis frequently shows two populations of plasma cells: one with normal immunophenotype (CD38 bright+, CD19+, and CD56⁻) with polytypic cytoplasmic light chain expression and another with an aberrant phenotype (CD38+, CD19–, CD56+) with monotypic cytoplasmic light chain expression.
- Cytogenetics: The primary cytogenetic abnormalities can be divided into two, partially overlapping, entities: (1) hyperdiploidy in half the cases, with

trisomies of chromosomes 3, 5, 7, 9, 11, 15, 19, and 21 and (2) nonhyper-diploid in the remaining 50% of cases, often associated with a translocation event at the IgH locus (on chromosome 14) with recurrent chromosomal patterns and oncogene deregulation. Dysregulation of a Cyclin D gene is found in all MGUS and plasma cell myeloma clones. Additional genomic events represent progression of MGUS to plasma cell myeloma.

Suggested Readings

Leung N, Bridoux F, Hutchinson CA, et al. Monoclonal gammopathy of renal significance: when MGUS is no longer undetermined or insignificant. *Blood*. 2012;120:4292–4295.

Merlini G, Palladini G. Differential diagnosis of monoclonal gammopathy of undetermined significance. *Hematology Am Soc Hematol Educ Program*. 2012;2012:595–603.

PLASMA CELL LEUKEMIA (PCL)

❑ Definition

PCL is an aggressive form of plasma cell myeloma consisting of clonal plasma cells circulating in the peripheral blood. PCL can occur de novo (primary PCL) or evolve as a late feature in the course of plasma cell myeloma (secondary PCL). It has a poor prognosis with a median survival of 7–11 months in treated cases.

❑ Who Should Be Suspected?

PCL is more common in men and in African Americans. The incidence is 0.02–0.03 cases/100,000 population. Secondary PCL occurs in 1–4% of plasma cell myeloma cases. Patients with PCL present with clinical features similar to those of plasma cell myeloma (PCM). Patients with primary PCL have smaller M-protein peak in serum, higher platelet count, younger age (55 vs. 65 for secondary PCL), and longer survival. In addition to peripheral blood and bone marrow, clonal plasma cells are found frequently in the spleen, liver, pleural effusions, ascites, and CNS.

❑ Laboratory Findings

- *CBC*: Leukocytosis with clonal plasma cells exceeding 2,000/µL or 20% of differential count. Mild anemia and/or thrombocytopenia can also be observed. The plasma cells have relatively scant cytoplasm and may resemble plasmacytoid lymphocytes. They may also have the morphology of plasmablasts.
- *Bone marrow* biopsy and aspirate are similar to that for PCM (see p. 432).
- *Serum protein electrophoresis and immunofixation* reveal a monoclonal protein (κ or λ) and identify a specific heavy chain.
- *Urine protein electrophoresis and immunofixation* reveal M protein.
- *Serum free light chain immunoassay*. Abnormal κ-to-λ ratio may be seen.
- *Renal function tests* may be abnormal in cases with monoclonal light chain proteinuria.
- *Immunophenotype*: Bright CD38 and/or CD138 with monoclonal cytoplasmic κ or λ is usually observed. Contrary to PCM, CD56 staining is rarely observed. CD19 and/or CD20 is frequently absent.
- *Cytogenetics*: Abnormal karyotypes (similar to PCM) are frequently found, and there is a higher incidence of unfavorable cytogenetics—del 13q14, t(4;14)(p16.3;q32), t(14;16)(q32;q23), and del 17p13.

Suggested Reading
Swerdlow SH, Campo E, Harris NL, et al. *WHO Classification of Tumours of Haematopoietic and Lymphoid Tissues*, 4th ed. Lyon, France: International Agency for Research on Cancer; 2008:203.

MONOCLONAL LIGHT AND HEAVY CHAIN DEPOSITION DISEASES

❑ Definition
These disorders include light chain deposition disease (LCDD), heavy chain deposition disease (HCDD), and light and heavy chain deposition disease (LHCDD). They are seen in the context of plasma cell disorders or of lymphomas with plasmacytic differentiation. There is abnormal deposition of light chain, heavy chain, or both light and heavy chains in tissues, but in contrast to amyloidosis, they do not form β sheets and do not stain with Congo red. Median survival is 4 years.

❑ Who Should Be Suspected?
Middle-aged (median age 56 years) male patients with symptoms of Ig deposition in various organs: the kidney (nephrotic syndrome and renal failure), heart, liver, peripheral nerves, lungs, blood vessels, and joints.

❑ Laboratory Findings
- *Bone marrow biopsy and aspirate*: Evidence of plasmacytosis, overt PCM, lymphoplasmacytic lymphoma, or marginal zone lymphoma may be present.
- *Tissue biopsy of involved organs* (e.g., heart, kidneys, liver) shows evidence of nonamyloid, nonfibrillary, amorphous eosinophilic material. LCCD is diagnosed by renal biopsy, showing nodular sclerosing glomerulopathy by light microscopy, diffuse linear staining of glomerular and tubular basement membrane κ or λ light chains by immunofluorescence, and nonfibrillar electron-dense deposits by electron microscopy. The deposits must be Congo red negative.
- *CBC* is usually normal. Rouleaux formation (due to paraproteinemia) may be seen.
- *Serum protein* may be elevated, and hypogammaglobulinemia may be present.
- *Serum complement* levels may be decreased in HCDD.
- *Serum protein electrophoresis and immunofixation* reveal a monoclonal light chain (κ in 80% cases), heavy chain protein or both.
- *Urine protein electrophoresis and immunofixation* demonstrate M protein that is composed of urine light chain.
- *Serum free light chain immunoassay* altered κ:λ ratio.
- *Renal function tests* may be abnormal in cases with monoclonal light chain proteinuria. Increased serum creatinine is associated with poor prognosis.
- *Immunophenotype*: Plasma cells have immunophenotype similar to that described for plasma cell myeloma and MGUS.

Suggested Reading
Swerdlow SH, Campo E, Harris NL, et al. *WHO Classification of Tumours of Haematopoietic and Lymphoid Tissues*, 4th ed. Lyon, France: International Agency for Research on Cancer; 2008:209.

PLASMACYTOMA

❑ Definition
Plasmacytoma(s) refers to single (or multiple) monoclonal plasma cell tumors with no involvement of bone marrow or blood. There are no typical clinical features associated with plasmacytoma.

- Plasmacytomas are classified as either
  1. Solitary plasmacytoma of bone (SPB), a localized bone lesion
  or
  2. Extraosseous plasmacytoma (EP), localized plasma cell neoplasm that arise in tissues other than bone (upper respiratory tract, sinuses, larynx, GI system, lymph nodes, bladder, breast, thyroid, testis, parotid, CNS, and skin)
- SPB and EP constitute 3–5% of all plasma cell neoplasms. Approximately 75% of SPB patients progress to plasma cell myeloma (PCM), or additional bone lesions develop with a median survival of 10 years. Conversely, EP cases have better prognosis with only 15% progressing to plasma cell myeloma.

❑ Who Should Be Suspected?
Middle-aged patients with bone pain, pathologic fractures, or neurologic symptoms related to nerve compression should be suspected for SPB. Patients with EP usually present with epistaxis, rhinorrhea, and nasal obstruction related to the tumor mass. Other manifestations depend on the location of EP.

❑ Laboratory Findings
- *Bone marrow biopsy and aspirate* are usually normal. They are necessary to rule out PCM.
- *Biopsy of SPB or EP*: Monoclonal plasma cells are seen. Some plasma cells can have plasmablastic or anaplastic morphology. EP cases might pose a diagnostic challenge, as they might be difficult to distinguish from lymphoplasmacytic lymphomas.
- *CBC* is usually normal.
- *Serum protein electrophoresis and immunofixation* may reveal a monoclonal protein (κ or λ) and identify a specific heavy chain (EP patients commonly have IgA).
- *Urine protein electrophoresis and immunofixation* may reveal M protein (BJ protein).
- *Serum free light chain ratio* is useful for predicting prognosis.
- *Renal function tests* may be abnormal in the presence of monoclonal light chain proteinuria.
- *Immunophenotype* is similar to that of PCM.
- *Cytogenetics*: Genetic abnormalities are similar to those described for PCM but are demonstrated infrequently.

Suggested Reading
Swerdlow SH, Campo E, Harris NL, et al. *WHO Classification of Tumours of Haematopoietic and Lymphoid Tissues*, 4th ed. Lyon, France: International Agency for Research on Cancer; 2008:208–209.

IMMUNOGLOBULIN LIGHT CHAIN AMYLOIDOSIS (ILCA)

❑ **Definition**

Amyloidosis is a heterogeneous group of diseases characterized by the deposition of amyloid fibrils in soft tissues. The fibrils are either intact or fragments of Ig light chains in the form of insoluble antiparallel β-pleated sheet configuration. More than 28 types of amyloid have been identified, all of which stain positively with Congo red. A previously used nomenclature consisted of three types of amyloidosis: primary, secondary, and hereditary. A new system uses an abbreviation of the native amyloid protein. For the practical purpose of this textbook, I will focus on ILCA (AL), previously referred as primary amyloidosis (PA). Genetic mutations often with an amino acid substitution can result in an amyloidogenic protein. Secondary amyloidosis (AA amyloidosis) can be seen with prolonged inflammatory conditions and infections, including transmission by prions, and in familial periodic fever. Another form of amyloidosis is seen in Alzheimer disease where the amyloid fibrils are present exclusively in the central nervous system.

- PA occurs in the setting of plasma cell dyscrasias—MGUS and PCM or lymphoplasmacytic lymphoma. Currently, it is also classified as amyloidosis-AL (associated with light chain) type, which should be differentiated from secondary amyloidosis or amyloidosis-AA type. Light chain deposition disease (LCDD) is a different entity characterized by deposition of light chains without formation of amyloid β sheets.

❑ **Who Should Be Suspected?**

Middle-aged (median age 64) male patients with clinical or laboratory findings of MGUS, PCM, or Waldenström macroglobulinemia. Common clinical manifestations include edema due to cardiac failure (restrictive cardiomyopathy) and nephrotic syndrome, malabsorption, macroglossia, hepatomegaly, purpura, bone pain, peripheral neuropathy, and carpal tunnel syndrome. Bleeding diathesis may be seen due to increased fragility of blood vessels resulting from amyloid deposition, in combination with factor X deficiency (due to binding to amyloid fibrils), decreased synthesis of clotting factors, or acquired von Willebrand disease.

❑ **Laboratory Findings**

- Confirmation and typing of amyloid are essential to initiate type-specific treatment. These are achieved by sophisticated techniques that may not be available in a routine clinical practice.
  - ▼ *Bone marrow biopsy and aspirate*: Evidence of overt myeloma or lymphoplasmacytic lymphoma along with replacement by amyloid is seen. β sheets stain pink with Congo red. New technologies (e.g., tandem mass spectrometry–based proteomic analysis) for the typing of amyloidosis in biopsy specimens are being developed.
  - ▼ *Tissue biopsy of involved organs*, for example, kidney or liver, have the highest yield in showing amyloid deposition in specific locations. The most accessible site is periumbilical fat. The diagnosis is established by demonstrating amyloid deposition by Congo red staining. LCCD is negative for Congo red staining but positive for anti-κ or anti-λ antibody staining. Secondary amyloidosis (AA) is negative for both.
  - ▼ *CBC*: Usually rouleaux formation (due to paraproteinemia) may be seen.

9

- ▼ Hypogammaglobulinemia may be present.
- ▼ *Immunofixation* reveals a monoclonal light chain (λ in 70% cases) in nearly 90% of cases. By contrast, serum protein electrophoresis demonstrates a localized band in <50% of patients with AL amyloidosis.
- ▼ *Urine protein electrophoresis and immunofixation* demonstrate M protein (Bence Jones protein), which is composed of urine light chains. Secretion of λ light chain is associated with poor prognosis.
- ▼ *Serum free light chain immunoassay*: Altered κ:λ ratio is present in PA.
- ▼ *Renal function tests* may be abnormal in cases of monoclonal light chain proteinuria. Urine albumin should be assessed regularly in patients with MGUS or plasma cell myeloma considered at risk to develop amyloidosis. Increased serum creatinine is associated with poor prognosis.
- ■ NT-proBNP, cardiac troponin-T, and echocardiography are tests of choice in the early detection and staging with respect to heart involvement in patients predisposed to amyloidosis.
  - ▼ *Immunophenotype*: Plasma cell immunophenotype is similar to that of PCM and MGUS.
  - ▼ *Cytogenetics*: There are no single chromosomal abnormalities typical for ILCA. Monosomy of chromosome 18 was recently found to be the most common cytogenetic abnormality in bone marrow biopsies. Trisomy of a variety of chromosomes was also found to be common. t(11;14), del(13q14) and gain of 1q21 have also been described.
- ■ *Mass spectrometry and gene sequencing*: Amyloid typing and genetic sequencing of amyloid fibrils are recommended because numerous different proteins can cause systemic amyloidosis. Each may require distinct therapeutic modalities.

❏ Prognosis

- ■ In PA, the median survival is approximately 2 years from diagnosis, with cardiac failure being the major cause of death.

Suggested Readings

Leung N, Nasr SH, Sethi S. How I treat amyloidosis: the importance of accurate diagnosis and amyloid typing. *Blood.* 2012;120:3206–3213.
Merlini G, Wechalekar AS, Palladini G. Systemic light chain amyloidosis: an update for treating physicians. *Blood.* 2013;121:5124–5130.

CRYOGLOBULINEMIA

❏ Definition

Cryoglobulins (CG) are proteins that precipitate in the body at low temperature or on storage of serum at refrigerated temperature. They are insoluble at 4°C and may aggregate at up to 30°C. CG are either immunoglobulins or a mixture of immunoglobulins and complement components. CG can fix complement and initiate inflammatory reactions. The term cryoglobulinemia is often used to refer to a systemic inflammatory syndrome that generally involves small- to medium-sized vessels due to CG-containing immune complexes. The majority of individuals with CG are asymptomatic, except for the symptoms attributable to the underlying disease. CG can also be detected in patients with chronic infection and/or inflammation.

❑ **Classification**

▪ *Type I:* monoclonal immunoglobulin, especially IgG or IgM κ type.
  ▼ May cause hyperviscosity syndrome in 5–25% of cases, or thrombosis.
  ▼ Most commonly associated with plasma cell myeloma and Waldenström macroglobulinemia (lymphoplasmacytic lymphoma); other lymphoproliferative neoplasms with M components; it may be idiopathic.
  ▼ The CGs are often present in great amounts (5–10 mg/dL) with cryocrits >70%. The blood may gel when drawn.
  ▼ Severe symptoms (Raynaud syndrome, gangrene without other causes).
  ▼ Skin, kidney, and bone marrow are predominantly involved.
▪ *Type II (essential mixed cryoglobulinemia):* monoclonal immunoglobulin mixed with at least one other type of polyclonal immunoglobulin, typically IgM or IgA and polyclonal IgG; always associated with rheumatoid factor (RF).
  ▼ Causes 40–60% of cases.
  ▼ Associated most often with chronic HCV or HIV infection; less often with HBV, EBV, bacterial and parasitic infections, autoimmune diseases, Sjögren syndrome, and syndrome of essential mixed cryoglobulinemia, immune complex nephritis.
  ▼ High-titer RF without definite rheumatic disease.
  ▼ C4 levels are decreased.
▪ *Type III:* mixed polyclonal immunoglobulin, most commonly IgM–IgG, occasionally IgA–IgG combinations, usually with RF. Types II and III generally produce 1–5 mg/dL CG.
  ▼ Causes 40–50% of cases.
  ▼ Most commonly associated with connective tissue disorders (SLE, Sjögren syndrome), persistent infections (HIV, HCV), and rarely with lymphoproliferative disorders.
  ▼ In types II and III, the skin, peripheral nervous system, and kidneys are predominantly involved.

❑ **Who Should Be Suspected of CG?**

Patients with cutaneous manifestations (erythematous macules, purpuric papules of the lower extremities, ulcers), the hyperviscosity syndrome, vasculitis, sensitivity to cold including Raynaud phenomenon, and the Meltzer triad: arthralgia, purpura, and weakness.

❑ **Laboratory Findings**

▪ CG are tested on serum (to distinguish from cryofibrinogen, which is tested on plasma [below]). The blood is obtained in test tubes without anticoagulant, prewarmed at 37°C, and let to clot at the same temperature. Serum is incubated at 4°C to detect turbidity or precipitate after 24–72 hours. That is compared with an aliquot of the same patient's serum kept at 37°C, which should have no precipitate.
▪ The normal value is <80 µg/dL CG in serum (40% of normal individuals may have CG in their serum). The pathologic values found in cryoglobulinemia range from 500 to 5,000 mg/dL. To determine the nature of the CG, they must be redissolved by warming, and the sample analyzed for the various components of the immune complexes. This helps to classify the various cryoglobulinemia types.

9

- *Other pertinent laboratory findings*
  - ▼ Serologic evidence of hepatitis C, rarely B, and liver disease.
  - ▼ Decreased serum early complement components.
  - ▼ Serologic evidence of HIV infection.
  - ▼ Renal disease (e.g., membranoproliferative glomerulonephritis) with proteinuria or hematuria.
  - ▼ Skin biopsy may show cutaneous vasculitis.
  - ▼ ESR and C-reactive protein are generally elevated.

❏ **Limitations**
- False-negative results may occur if the blood was cooled below 37°C during collection; if the blood clotted right away, centrifugation may remove the CG with the clot. The centrifugation too must be performed in a temperature-controlled centrifuge.
- The presence of CG may cause erroneous WBC counts on electronic counters.

Suggested Reading
Peng SL, Schur PH. Overview of cryoglobulins and cryoglobulinemia. In: Basow DS (ed). *UpToDate*, Waltham, MA: UpToDate, Inc.; 2013.

CRYOFIBRINOGENEMIA

❏ **Definition**
Cryofibrinogen (CF) is generated by a mixture of fibrinogen, fibrin, fibronectin, and other proteins that precipitate reversibly at cold temperatures in plasma, but not in serum. Cryofibrinogenemia may be classified as primary (essential, idiopathic) or secondary. The secondary form occurs in association with hepatitis C, other infections, malignancies, and inflammatory processes.

❏ **Who Should Be Suspected?**
Patients with cold-induced thrombotic events or patients with painful ulcers, purpura, livedo reticularis, and painful or pruritic erythema of the extremities. The disease is common in patients with HCV. An individual whose plasma, but not serum, forms a cryoprecipitate has cryofibrinogenemia. Some individuals may be asymptomatic, and CF may be discovered accidentally in the laboratory.

❏ **Laboratory Findings**
Refer to Cryoglobulins in chapter 16.

Suggested Reading
Peng SL. Cryofibrinogenemia. In: Basow DS (ed). *UpToDate*, Waltham, MA: UpToDate, Inc.: 2013.

 DISORDERS OF HEMOSTASIS AND THROMBOSIS

DISORDERS OF PLATELETS: THROMBOCYTOPENIAS

Thrombocytopenias represent a reduction in the number of circulating platelets below the lower limit of normal set by the laboratory (see p. 1083). They may be classified in various ways. First one must determine if the condition is congenital

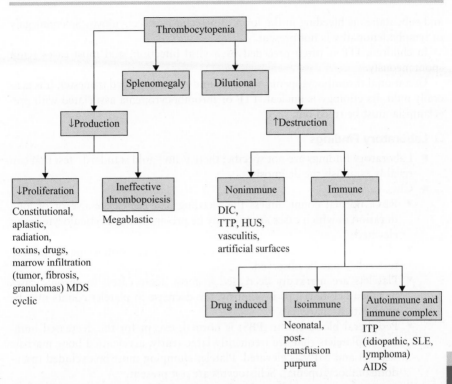

Figure 9-3 *The etiology of thrombocytopenia. DIC, disseminated intravascular coagulation; HUS, hemolytic uremic syndrome; TTP, thrombotic thrombocytopenic purpura; MDS, myelodysplastic syndromes.*

or acquired. Acquired thrombocytopenias may be acute or chronic. The causes of thrombocytopenias can be classified by etiology (Figure 9-3): increased destruction, decreased production, artifactual, and miscellaneous. TTP/HUS is discussed separately (see p. 467).

IMMUNE THROMBOCYTOPENIC PURPURA (ITP)

❑ Definition
ITP is an autoimmune disease characterized by a low platelet count (<150 × 10⁹/L) due to their accelerated destruction and impaired platelet production. Typically, thrombocytopenia is isolated without other hematopoietic lineages being affected. Depending on the severity of thrombocytopenia and other contributing factors, patients with ITP are at increased risk for bleeding. There is marked interpatient variability in the clinical presentation of ITP. Although the onset may be abrupt, it is more often insidious. ITP is a heterogeneous group of disorders. Most cases are considered primary, whereas others are secondary to drugs, other autoimmune conditions such as SLE, or HIV, HCV CMV, and VZV infections.

❑ Who Should Be Suspected?
Individuals with no previous history of bleeding and no hematologic disease who complain of mucosal (especially epistaxis, gum, or excessive menstrual bleeding)

and subcutaneous bleeding in the form of petechiae or ecchymosis. Splenomegaly or lymphadenopathy is not present.

In children, ITP is often preceded by a viral infection, and most cases remit spontaneously.

Gestational thrombocytopenia occurs in mid-second to third trimester. It is generally mild. Its etiology is unclear. TTP or thrombocytopenia associated with preeclampsia must be ruled out.

❏ **Laboratory Findings**

- Laboratory findings are not specific; there is no "gold standard" test that can reliably establish the diagnosis.
- CBC.
  - ▼ RBC: normal count, unless the bleeding had been excessive or of long duration in which cases anemia may be present and the reticulocyte count elevated.
  - ▼ WBC is normal; in cases with severe hemorrhage, a shift to the left (immature cells) may be observed.
  - ▼ Platelets are markedly decreased in most acute cases. In chronic cases or when ITP develops insidiously, the decrease in platelet counts may be moderate to marginal.
  - ▼ Peripheral blood smear (PBS) is normal, except for the decreased number of platelets that are frequently large (early, accelerated bone marrow release) and MPV is elevated. Platelet clumping must be excluded (pseudothrombocytopenia). Schistocytes are not present.
- Bone marrow is not indicated unless an underlying hematologic disease is suspected. Bone marrow examination should be performed in patients over the age of 60 to rule out a myelodysplastic syndrome. In ITP patients, there are an increased number of megakaryocytes, with a shift toward younger cells that do not seem to release platelets.
- Coagulation: All tests are normal.
- Serology to rule out SLE is mandatory in adult ITP. ANA may also be helpful.
- Platelet antibody detection and identification assays are available through reference laboratories. ELISA and flow cytometry methods are offered. However, because of the high frequency of false-positive and false-negative tests (antibodies are detected in only 60% of patients), serologic tests for platelet antibodies are not recommended.
- Microbiology: HIV and hepatitis C infections need to be ruled out in populations at risk. *Helicobacter pylori* testing may have pertinence since the elimination of certain strains may eradicate ITP.
- Blood group Rh (D) typing is necessary if anti-D Ig is being considered for therapy.

Suggested Readings

Gernsheimer T, James AH, Stasi R. How I treat thrombocytopenia in pregnancy. *Blood.* 2013;121:38–47.

Liebman HA, Pullarkat V. Diagnosis and management of immune thrombocytopenia in the era of thrombopoietin mimetics. *Hematology Am Soc Hematol Educ Program.* 2011;2011: 384–390.

DRUG-INDUCED THROMBOCYTOPENIA, IMMUNE

❏ Definition

Accelerated platelet destruction caused by drug-dependent, platelet-reactive antibodies. Decreased platelet production by megakaryocytes may be a contributory factor.

❏ Who Should Be Suspected?

A bleeding patient with *isolated* thrombocytopenia and a history of medication known to result in drug-induced thrombocytopenia. The most common offenders are: quinine,*** quinidine, heparin (discussed separately as HIT, see below), sulfa drugs, digoxin, GPIIb/IIIa antagonists, vancomycin, gold compounds, β-lactam antibiotics, valproic acid, levodopa, procainamide, and vaccines against measles–mumps–rubella. Criteria for diagnosis include a candidate drug administered shortly before the episode, especially if it was the only drug used, and exclusion of other causes for the acute thrombocytopenia.

❏ Laboratory Findings

- CBC: Severe thrombocytopenia with normal red and white cell counts.
- Laboratory tests to demonstrate the presence of specific antibodies are used in research laboratories but have not been validated for general use.
- The gold standard for diagnosis is recovery from thrombocytopenia following discontinuation of the drug, which is usually prompt.

HEPARIN-INDUCED THROMBOCYTOPENIA (HIT)

❏ Definition

HIT is a complication of heparin therapy resulting in a reduction in platelet count. HIT is an immune-mediated thrombocytopenia, with antibodies developing against the complex of heparin and platelet factor 4 (PF4). HIT develops in about 3% of patients treated with unfractionated heparin but rarely (0.2%) in those receiving low molecular weight heparin (but there is cross-reactivity of the antibodies between the two). It is extremely rare with the use of fondaparinux. It develops more frequently in surgical rather than medical patients, particularly after cardiac surgery. Its seriousness is underlined by the frequent complication of venous (approximately 60% of HIT patients) and arterial (14% of HIT patients in one study) thrombosis resulting in up to 20% mortality and limb loss rates of 2–3%. The term HITT is used for HIT associated with thrombosis. Skin necrosis at the site of heparin injection is a known complication related to HIT.

❏ Diagnosis

- The clinical diagnosis of HIT is based on the "4Ts" criteria:
  1. >50% fall in platelet count, or platelet nadir 20–100,000/μL;
  2. Onset between days 5 and 10 following initiation of heparin, or <1 day in patients with exposure to heparin within the previous 100 days;
  3. New thrombosis, skin necrosis, or acute systemic reaction post–heparin bolus;
  4. No other obvious cause for fall in platelet count.

***Quinine is present in certain soft drinks.

9

There are exceptions to these rules. One such situation is seen in patients who develop HIT after discontinuation of heparin (delayed onset HIT). In patients with typical HIT, the platelet count generally recovers within 1 week after discontinuing heparin administration.

❑ **Laboratory Findings**

- There are two types of assays: immunologic and functional. Some patients may develop specific antibodies without clinical manifestations of HIT. In these cases, the immunoassays are positive, but the functional ones are not. The immunoassays are sensitive in detecting HIT antibodies, but none is completely specific. To increase the specificity of immunoassays, manufacturers have developed IgG-specific assays. The resulting assays have a very high negative predictive value.
- Immunoassays presently available to coagulation laboratories:
  - ▼ PF4 IgG^M is an ELISA assay designed to detect IgG antibodies reactive with PF4. This assay has both excellent negative predictive value (with a cutoff <0.4 optical density [OD]) and high positive predictive value. A good relationship with the serotonin release assay (see below) has been found at OD readings of >1.4. Successful performance of the assay requires high technical skills.
  - ▼ Flow cytometry for detecting PF4 antibodies is available in research laboratories.
  - ▼ C^{14}-platelet serotonin release (PSR) is considered the gold standard for the diagnosis of HIT. It has excellent sensitivity and specificity. Because it uses radioactive serotonin as its principal reagent, this assay is performed only in a few reference laboratories. Because of the delay in obtaining results, the assay is useful only for final confirmation of the diagnosis.
  - ▼ Heparin-induced platelet aggregation is an alternative to the PSR. The assay can be performed in laboratories that offer platelet aggregometry, but it is not well standardized, and although it has excellent specificity (>90%), it lacks sensitivity.

NEONATAL THROMBOCYTOPENIA

❑ **Classification**

Thrombocytopenias in the newborn can be classified as due to increased destruction or decreased production.

Increased Destruction

- Neonatal alloimmune thrombocytopenia (NAIT) occurs when fetal platelets contain an antigen inherited from the father that the mother lacks. Fetal and neonate thrombocytopenia is the platelet equivalent of Rh disease; the most commonly involved platelet antigen is HPA-1a or Pl^{A1}. When the mother is exposed to fetal platelets during pregnancy, anti-HPA-1a antibodies are generated; they traverse the placenta, and the result is fetal thrombocytopenia. Intracranial hemorrhage is a potentially serious complication.
- Laboratory studies
  - ▼ Platelet counts in the neonate are often <50,000/μL.

▼ Platelet antigens are tested in mother and father to establish the incompatibility. HPA 1, 3, and 5 should be screened in all potential cases, as well as HPA 4 if the patient is of Asian descent. Testing must demonstrate both a platelet antigen incompatibility between the parents and a maternal antibody directed against the antigen. The assays must be performed in very experienced laboratories. It is unclear if antenatal screening should be instituted.

- Autoimmune thrombocytopenia in the newborn is the result of the mother having ITP with antibodies that cross the placenta and react with the platelets of the fetus.

- Most neonates whose mothers have ITP have mild thrombocytopenia (counts >50,000/μL), but occasionally they may be severely affected.

- Other causes of thrombocytopenia due to increased platelet destruction in the neonate:
  - ▼ Disseminated intravascular coagulation (DIC) as a complication of an acute underlying illness or as the result of consumption in large hemangiomas (Kasabach-Merritt syndrome)
  - ▼ Severe infection
  - ▼ Hypersplenism
  - ▼ Drug-related thrombocytopenia in the mother
  - ▼ Hypersplenism in neonates with an an enlarged spleen
  - ▼ Necrotizing enterocolitis

- Laboratory studies are directed to the underlying condition and monitoring the platelet counts.

Decreased Production

- Genetic disorders: thrombocytopenia-absent radius syndrome; congenital megakaryocytic thrombocytopenia; Fanconi anemia; certain chromosome abnormalities; congenital platelet disorders; lipid storage diseases

- Acquired causes: bone marrow diseases (neonatal leukemia, neuroblastoma); toxic injury to megakaryocytes due to drugs or infections; neonates whose mothers have preeclampsia; birth asphyxia; following exchange transfusion

❏ Laboratory Findings

- Serial platelet counts
- Maternal studies for thrombocytopenia
- DIC screening in infants at risk for DIC

PSEUDO (SPURIOUS) THROMBOCYTOPENIA

❏ Definition

A false decrease in reported platelet counts. It may be due to:

- Platelet clumping induced by collection of blood in EDTA (the routine anticoagulant used for CBC); it is the most common cause for spurious thrombocytopenia. In a good laboratory, the technicians observe all CBC tubes flagged for low platelets for the presence of clots and review stained peripheral blood smear (PBS) for clumps.

- Platelet satellitosis (platelets form rosettes around white cells).
- Platelet cold agglutinins.
- Giant platelets missed by automated counters.
- Very elevated RBC count.
- Artifacts due to inappropriate technique in blood collection (clotted blood, overfilling vacuum tubes).

Suggested Readings

Bussel J. Diagnosis and management of the fetus and neonate with alloimmune thrombocytopenia. *J Thromb Haemost.* 2009;7(Suppl 1):253–257.

Pouplar C, Gueret P, Fouassier M, et al. Prospective evaluation of the "4Ts" score and particle gel immunoassay specific to heparin/PF4 for the diagnosis of heparin-induced thrombocytopenia. *J Thromb Haemost.* 2007;5:1373–1379.

Warkentin TE, Sheppard JI, Moore JC, et al. Quantitative interpretation of optical density measurements using PF4-dependent enzyme-immunoassay. *J Thromb Haemost.* 2008;6: 1304–1312.

DISORDERS OF PLATELET FUNCTION: INHERITED AND ACQUIRED

Disorders of platelet function are also referred as thrombocytopathies. The platelets' major physiologic role is in hemostasis, where they arrest bleeding in small blood vessels. To perform this function optimally, the platelets' number as well as function must be normal. Thrombocytopathies can be congenital, but more commonly, they are acquired. In most acquired thrombocytopathies, the platelet counts are normal. In some of the congenital disorders, the platelet count is reduced as well. Individuals who present with recent or life-long mucocutaneous bleeding should be suspected. Because thrombocytopathies and most von Willebrand disease cases have similar presentations, workup for the two conditions should be initiated simultaneously.

INHERITED THROMBOCYTOPATHIES

Defects in platelet–platelet interaction (aggregation defects)

- *Glanzmann thrombasthenia* is the most common inherited (autosomal recessive) disorder of platelet function. Affected patients have a lifelong hemorrhagic syndrome, mostly mucocutaneous, although their platelet count and size are normal. The bleeding severity differs considerably between patients. It depends in part on the severity of the genetic defect (absence or reduction of the platelet integrin receptor GPIIb-IIIa [$\alpha_{2b}\beta_3$]). Affected genes coding for this integrin have been identified. The genotypic/phenotypic, that is, bleeding, do not correlate entirely. Moreover, the severity of bleeding declines with age. Bleeding results from the platelets' inability to bind fibrinogen. There is absence, or reduction in aggregation with all agonists, but platelets agglutinate normally with ristocetin (Table 9-4). There is normal release with strong agonists, such as thrombin. Complete absence of clot retraction was described in the severe type of disease.

TABLE 9–4. Abnormalities of Platelet Function

Disorder	Features	Collagen	ADP and Epinephrine	Arachidonic Acid	Ristocetin
Glanzmann thrombasthenia	Absent clot retraction	↓	↓↓	↓	N
Storage pool disorders	Absence of α or δ platelet granules	↓	N ↓	N	N
Aspirin ingestion and aspirin-like storage pool disorder	Decreased thromboxane 2 generation	↓	N ↓	↓↓	N
Bernard-Soulier syndrome	Thrombocytopenia and giant platelets	N	N	N	↓
von Willebrand disease, except type 2B	Plasmatic defect that affects platelet function. Normal platelet count	N	N	N	↓ or N
von Willebrand disease type 2B	Thrombocytopenia	N	N	N	↑↑
Platelet-type von Willebrand disease	Thrombocytopenia	N	N	N	↑

- Afibrinogenemia: In the absence of fibrinogen, platelet cannot adhere resulting in lack of aggregation.
- Disorders of secretion and signal transduction include storage pool deficiencies of platelet granules, or granule contents, as well as primary transduction defects. The bleeding is usually mild.
  - ▼ In the *gray platelet syndrome*, platelets are deficient in α granules. Platelet aggregation studies have produced variable results. Aggregation induced by ADP, epinephrine, arachidonic acid, and agglutination with ristocetin is normal (or only mildly impaired), but aggregation with collagen has been reported to be decreased or absent. Platelet count varies from 20,000 to 150,000/μL. On the peripheral blood smear (PBS), platelets are large and appear gray or gray-blue, are vacuolated, or look ghost-like. These patients have a tendency to develop myelofibrosis, splenomegaly, and progressive thrombocytopenia.
- Δ-storage pool diseases are characterized by the absence of dense bodies. In most cases, the second wave aggregation with ADP and epinephrine is absent. There are several subtypes:
  - ▼ Δ-storage pool disease without other associations: autosomal dominant.
    - ● Hermansky-Pudlak syndrome: autosomal recessive inheritance due to deficiency of dense bodies. It is associated with oculocutaneous albinism. Hermansky-Pudlak syndrome has a high prevalence in northwest Puerto Rico and is the most common cause of oculocutaneous albinism in Japan.
    - ● Chédiak-Higashi syndrome: autosomal recessive deficiency of dense bodies; associated with oculocutaneous albinism. Giant cytoplasmic granules are present in neutrophils, monocytes, and lymphocytes.

9

- Thrombocytopenia-absent radius syndrome: autosomal recessive. It is associated with hypomegakaryocytic thrombocytopenia.
- Wiskott-Aldrich syndrome: X-linked recessive condition due to deficiencies of dense bodies and cytoskeletal regulation. It is associated with thrombocytopenia with small platelets, eczema, and T-cell immune deficiency.
- May-Hegglin anomaly is an autosomal dominant abnormality of granulocytes and platelets, associated with thrombocytopenia, giant platelets, Döhle-like bodies in neutrophils, and chronic renal disease.

- Signal transduction defects due to abnormal platelets receptors. It is uncertain to what extent single receptor defects result in clinical bleeding.
  - ▼ Integrin α2β1 and GPVI (collagen receptor defects)
  - ▼ P2Y12 (ADP receptor) defect
  - ▼ Epinephrine receptor defect
  - ▼ Thromboxane A$_2$ receptor deficiency
- Signal transduction defects due to abnormalities in arachidonic acid pathways and thromboxane A$_2$ synthesis.
  - ▼ Patients with abnormal thromboxane A$_2$ synthesis have an aspirin-like defect.
  - ▼ Impaired release of arachidonic acid.
  - ▼ Cyclooxygenase deficiency.
  - ▼ Thromboxane synthase deficiency.
- Disorders of platelet–vessel wall interaction (platelet adhesion defects).
  - ▼ *Bernard-Soulier* syndrome is an autosomal recessive disorder, caused by absence or abnormalities in the platelet receptor complex GPIb-IX-V. It presents with moderate to severe thrombocytopenia and *giant platelets*. Platelets aggregate normally with ADP, epinephrine, collagen, and arachidonic acid but show delayed aggregation with thrombin and no response to ristocetin (see Table 9-4).
  - ▼ *Platelet-type von Willebrand disease* autosomal dominant condition associated with intermittent thrombocytopenia, normal platelet morphology, and decreased levels of high molecular weight vWF multimers. It must be distinguished from von Willebrand disease type 2B.
- Disorders of platelet function related to other defects.
  - ▼ *Quebec platelet disorder*: excessive fibrinolysis resulting from increased expression and storage of the fibrinolytic enzyme urokinase plasminogen activator in platelets. The defect results in delayed-onset bleeding after trauma or surgery.
  - ▼ *Scott syndrome*: autosomal recessive disorder due to a defect in platelets' membrane resulting in inability to assemble prothrombinase and intrinsic tenase complexes.
  - ▼ The Montreal platelet syndrome was recently documented to be a variant of type 2B von Willebrand disease.

ACQUIRED THROMBOCYTOPATHIES

❏ Drug Induced

Most clinical circumstances leading to an acquired platelet functional defect are drug induced, either for a desired therapeutic effect or for an adverse effect of medications. The following drugs are associated with reduced platelet function:

- Strong effect
  - ▼ Aspirin and nonsteroidal anti-inflammatory drugs (NSAIDs). Aspirin affects platelets by irreversible acetylation of cyclooxygenase (COX)-1. This inhibition impairs formation of thromboxane A2 required for full activation with weak agonists. NSAIDs affect the same pathways, but without permanent acetylation. The effect of aspirin on platelets lasts for approximately 7–10 days, whereas the effect of an NSAID is of short duration, 24–48 hours.
  - ▼ The P2Y12 antagonists clopidogrel and ticagrelor inhibit platelet response to ADP by blocking its receptor. The full effect of clopidogrel, the most commonly drug used for this purpose, requires 4–7 days for full effectiveness, and its ADP blocking persists for up to 7 days after it is discontinued.
  - ▼ Anti-IIb-IIIa agents are used mainly in acute coronary syndromes during cardiopulmonary bypass surgery: abciximab, eptifibatide, tirofiban.
  - ▼ Dipyridamole: mild platelet function inhibitor; unknown mechanism of action.
  - ▼ Antibiotics, especially when administered in large doses: penicillin, carbenicillin, ampicillin, ticarcillin, nafcillin, azlocillin, mezlocillin, cephalosporins, and nitrofurantoin.
  - ▼ Plasma volume expanders: dextran, hydroxyethyl starch.
- Weak or inconsistent effect
  - ▼ Chemotherapeutic drugs: bis-chloronitrosourea (BCNU), anthracyclines, mithramycin
  - ▼ Cardiovascular drugs: β-blockers, calcium-channel blockers, nitroglycerin
  - ▼ Alcohol
  - ▼ Anticonvulsants: valproic acid
  - ▼ Tricyclic antidepressants: imipramine, amitriptyline
  - ▼ Phenothiazines: chlorpromazine, trifluoperazine
  - ▼ Anesthetics: halothane
  - ▼ Epsilon aminocaproic acid administered in large doses
  - ▼ Radiographic contrast agents
  - ▼ Certain foods (onions, garlic, ginger, black tree fungus) and food supplements

❏ Disease Induced

- Myeloproliferative neoplasms: moderately severe defect.
- Myelodysplastic syndromes usually mild defect.
- Uremia: defect due to accumulation of guanidinosuccinic acid. It is partially corrected by dialysis. Platelet counts are normal.
- Liver disease: normal platelet counts, except in cases with hypersplenism. Dysfunctional platelets may contribute to bleeding risk.
- Dysproteinemias as seen in multiple myeloma and Waldenström macroglobulinemia: normal platelet counts, except in advanced cases, or as the result of chemotherapy.
- DIC affects platelet function mostly due to the effect of fibrin degradation products (FDP) on platelets.

- Cardiopulmonary bypass surgery causes marked platelet dysfunction, as well as temporary thrombocytopenia.
- CBC
  - ▼ Platelet count may be normal, decreased, or increased, depending on the etiology (see above).
  - ▼ The peripheral blood smear (PBS) may show normal platelets, or large platelets and thrombocytopenia, depending on etiology.

❏ **Assays for Thrombocytopathies**

- Platelet aggregation and release studies with various agonists (ADP, epinephrine, collagen, thrombin, and arachidonic acid) and agglutination studies with ristocetin are presently the best assays to evaluate platelet function. Mixing studies in the presence of ristocetin (the patient's platelets with normal plasma and normal platelets with the patient's plasma) are used to differentiate von Willebrand disease type 2b from platelet-type von Willebrand disease (see Table 9-4).
- PFA-100 is a device used for rapid diagnosis of platelet functional defects.
- The PFA-100 was shown to be sensitive for aspirin-induced defects, Glanzmann thrombasthenia, and von Willebrand disease. If positive, the diagnosis should be refined by studies of platelet aggregation.
- Flow cytometry is a sensitive tool to examine platelet function, but it may not be readily available.
- Electron microscopy may determine the status of platelet granules, but its utility is mostly for research purposes.

Suggested Readings

Kottke-Marchant K, Corocoran G. The laboratory diagnosis of platelet disorders. An algorithmic approach. *Arch Path Lab Med.* 2002;126:133–146.

Nurden AT, Flore M, Nurden P, et al. Glanzmann's thrombasthenia: a review of ITGA2B and ITGB3 defects with emphasis on variants, phenotypic variability, and mouse models. *Blood.* 2011;118:5996–6005.

DISORDERS DUE TO COAGULATION FACTOR DEFICIENCIES: CONGENITAL CLOTTING DEFECTS

HEMOPHILIA

❏ **Definition**

Hemophilia A (factor VIII [F VIII] deficiency) and hemophilia B (factor IX [F IX] deficiency) are congenital bleeding disorders, both inherited as X chromosome–linked recessive conditions, hence limited almost exclusively to males. Hemophilia A prevalence is 1:10,000 live male births, and hemophilia B is 1:30,000. Factor XI deficiency was classified in the past as hemophilia C; it will be presented separately. Acquired hemophilia is a severe bleeding diathesis, resulting from the development of autoantibodies against factor VIII or rarely IX, in a patient with no previous bleeding history. Hemophilia affects both males and females.

❏ **Who Should Be Suspected?**

A male with a bleeding family history in other males on the maternal side (one third of cases have a negative family history due to new mutations) and with a personal history of spontaneous major bleeding episodes (mostly in joints, skeletal muscles, gastrointestinal tract, and occasionally in the central nervous system or in other organs). Recurring joint bleeding may result in chronic disability or even fatalities if not treated promptly. In infants bleeding at circumcision, on tooth eruption, or when first standing (in knee joints) should raise the suspicion of hemophilia. The severity of bleeding is similar for the same levels of factor deficiency in hemophilia A and B. The development of alloantibodies (either against F VIII or IX) is suspected in hemophiliacs multiply infused with the respective factor, who become refractory to replacement therapy. They develop in 15–30% of hemophilia A and 3–5% of hemophilia B patients. The majority develop before age 20. Acquired hemophilia should be suspected in bleeding postpartum females, patients with lymphoproliferative neoplasms, or in the elderly without other predisposing factors except age.

❏ **Laboratory Findings**

- Screening tests: Platelet counts, PT, and PTT are recommended as the initial workup of patients presenting with a bleeding diathesis. Of those, the platelet count and PT are normal in hemophiliacs, whereas the PTT is variably prolonged.
- Definitive tests: Factor VIII and IX levels are established by quantitation of factor VIII or IX, respectively. Severe hemophiliacs have factor VIII or IX levels below 1%, moderate hemophiliac have factor levels between 1% and 5%, and the mild cases >5%. Patients in the latter group do not bleed spontaneously but may have severe bleeding on traumatic events, sometimes surprisingly, since they have no previous bleeding history. Mild hemophilia A individuals may develop inhibitors without having been ever infused with factor VIII preparations.
- Obligate female carriers are mothers to more than one hemophiliac son or daughters of a hemophiliac. Carriers usually have coagulant factor VIII levels around 50%, but there is a wide scatter in these levels, and when skewed to low levels, may result in clinical bleeding (a "female hemophiliac"). A more definitive diagnosis in suspected carriers or as prenatal diagnosis may be obtained through genetic analysis using DNA-based techniques. The most common abnormality found in carriers of severe hemophilia A is intron 22 inversion in the factor VIII gene. The genetic diagnosis is easier in factor IX carriers because of a large deletion in the factor IX gene.
- The diagnosis of inhibitors to factor VIII or IX is established by specific assays, and inhibitor titers are reported in Bethesda units.

❏ **Limitations**

- Type III and severe 2 N von Willebrand disease have the same clinical presentation as hemophilia, and both may have very low F VIII values. Detailed laboratory assays are necessary to distinguish these two conditions from hemophilia. Moreover, they are also present in females.

Suggested Readings

Verbruggen B, Meijer P, Novakova I, et al. Diagnosis of factor VIII deficiency Haemophilia. 2008;14(Suppl 3):76–82.
Whelan SFJ, Hofbauer CJ, Horling FM, et al. Distinct characteristics of antibody response against factor VIII in healthy individuals and in different cohorts of hemophilia A patients. *Blood.* 2013;121:1039–1048.

VON WILLEBRAND DISEASE (VWD)

❏ Definition

Willebrand Factor (vWF) resulting in excessive mucocutaneous bleeding. In severe cases, coagulation-type defect is present. It is the most common inherited bleeding diathesis, seen in up to 1% of the Caucasian population. vWF is synthesized in endothelial cells and megakaryocytes and released as large multimers. It is acted on by a metalloprotease, ADAMTS 13, to form variably sized multimers. It mediates platelet adhesion through a platelet receptor, GP1b. It also functions as a carrier for factor VIII. Inheritance of vWD is autosomal recessive in most cases.

❏ Who Should Be Suspected?

Patients with a personal or family history of mucosal bleeding (except for VWD type 3, where the bleeding is severe, and type 2N that mimics hemophilia) (see below). Females with severe menorrhagia presenting at menarche. Although VWD is relatively common, not all patients are diagnosed because not all have a marked bleeding history.

❏ Laboratory Findings

- Because the clinical manifestations of VWD and platelet defects are similar, the laboratory workup for platelet function and for VWD should be initiated simultaneously, except for cases with a definite family history.
- One should keep in mind that there is a continuum of vWF levels between the normal population and patients with genuine VWD. Better-defined criteria to establish separation cutoff levels, as well as genetic assays, are being developed.
- First-tier tests:
  1. vWF Ag (vWF:Ag).
  2. Factor VIII coagulant.
  3. Ristocetin cofactor (vWF:RCo) assay measures vWF activity. A ratio vWF:RCo/vWF:Ag <0.7 is indicative of a qualitative vWF defect.
  4. VWF activity: A new latex immunoassay for the quantitation of vWF has recently become commercially available (HemosIL™). It was demonstrated to have very high sensitivity and specificity for vWF activity.
  5. The collagen-binding assay is another functional assay used by some laboratories.
- Second-tier tests:
  1. VWF multimers is a useful assay to determine various subtypes of the disease. It should be ordered only when the vWD diagnosis has been established.
  2. Ristocetin-induced platelet aggregation (RIPA). In this assay, the patient's platelets and plasma are used as a source of vWF.
  3. Genetic tests are now being developed.
- *Seven clinical variants* have been described based on laboratory results and clinical history:
  1. VWD type 1 (70–80% of cases) is a quantitative defect with mild bleeding. The diagnosis can be challenging and might require repeated testing.
  2. VWD type 2A (10–15% of cases) is a qualitative defect with moderate to severe bleeding. There is absence of high molecular weight VWF multimers.

3. VWD type 2B is a rare qualitative defect with a "gain-of-function" point mutation in the GP1b binding domain of VWF. Patients have spontaneous platelet agglutination resulting in thrombocytopenia. There is absence of high molecular weight VWF multimers. DDAVP administration is contraindicated.

4. VWD type 2M is a rare, mostly autosomal dominant, qualitative defect with moderate to severe bleeding. There is a defect in the GP1b binding domain of VWF, preventing binding to platelets.

   In types 2A, 2B, and 2 M, there is a low ratio (<0.7) of VWF activity to antigen.

5. VWD type 2N is a rare qualitative defect with moderate to severe bleeding. There is a defect in the FVIII binding domain of vWF. It simulates hemophilia.

6. VWD type 3 is a rare quantitative defect with severe bleeding. These patients may develop alloantibodies to VWF after receiving multiple transfusions.

7. Platelet-type VWD is not a genuine VWD variant (see p. 450), but a qualitative defect in platelets caused by a gain of function in the GP1b receptor on platelets. That leads to increased avidity for VWF resulting in spontaneous platelet agglutination and thrombocytopenia. Platelet-type VWD can be differentiated from VWD type 2B by mixing or cryoprecipitate studies. Platelets from Bernard-Soulier syndrome (see p. 450) do not aggregate in the presence of ristocetin. The condition must be differentiated from VWD.

- Acquired VWD is seen in lymphoproliferative neoplasms, multiple myeloma, MGUS, autoimmune diseases, hypothyroidism, aortic stenosis due to sheer stress-enhanced proteolysis, ventricular septal defects, and GI telangiectasia.
- The major patterns to differentiate various types of VWD are described in Table 9-5.

❑ **Limitations**
- vWF Ag and activity levels run 20–30% lower in blood group O than in individuals with other blood groups.

TABLE 9–5. Subtypes of von Willebrand Disease

Type	vWF Ag	FVIII	Ristocetin Cofactor	Ristocetin-Induced Platelet Aggregation	Multimers
1	↓	↓	↓	N/↓	N (globally ↓)
2A	↓/N	↓/N	↓	↓	HMW absent
2B	↓/N	↓/N	↓/N	↑	HMW absent
2 M	N	N	↓	↓	N
2 N	N	↓	N	N	N
3	↓	↓	↓	↓	↓ (globally low)
Platelet type	↓/N	↓/N	↓	↑	N

N, normal; ↓, decreased; ↑, increased with low-dose ristocetin; HMW, high molecular weight multimers.

- VWF levels fluctuate. Both the VWF and factor VIII are acute-phase reactants. Levels may increase two to five times from baseline in the third trimester of pregnancy, with strenuous exercise and severe stress. Other preanalytic variables (collection of sample, storage) must be considered. Repeated testing may be required.

Suggested Readings

Branchford BR, Paola JD. Making a diagnosis of VWD. *Hematology Am Soc Hematol Educ Program.* 2012;2012:161–167.

Favaloro EJ, Mohammed S, Mcdonald J. Validation of improved performance for the automated von Willebrand factor ristocetin cofactor activity assay. *J Thromb Haemost.* 2010;8:2842–2844.

Nichols WL, Hultin MB, James AH, et al. von Willebrand disease (VWD): evidence-based diagnosis and management guidelines, the National Heart, Lung, and Blood Institute (NHLBI) expert panel report (USA). *Hemophilia.* 2008;14:171–232.

FACTOR XII (F XII) DEFICIENCY

❏ Definition

The intrinsic pathway of coagulation is initiated by F XII in a reaction involving high molecular weight kininogen and plasma kallikrein. F XII deficiency was first described preoperatively in Mr. Hageman (hence the synonym Hageman factor) who was found to have a prolonged PTT, no bleeding history, and no deficiency of any known clotting protein. He succumbed to a thrombotic event. Affected patients have no bleeding diathesis. The fact that patients with severe deficiency of F XII, prekallikrein, and low molecular weight kininogen do not bleed, even when exposed to severe trauma or surgery, suggests that these proteins play no, or a minimal, role in hemostasis, although they may have other physiologic roles.

❏ Laboratory Findings Test

- Patients have normal PT, but variably prolonged PTT, depending on the severity of deficiency. A definitive diagnosis (necessary to exclude other etiologies for a prolonged PTT) is established by determining the factor's level in plasma.
- F XII is not affected by vitamin K deficiency or oral anticoagulants.

❏ Decreased Levels

- Congenital: Autosomal recessive inheritance: Levels of F XII are 40–60% in heterozygous state and are undetectable in homozygotes.
- Acquired
  - ▼ Septic shock
  - ▼ Severe liver disease
  - ▼ Nephrotic syndrome
  - ▼ Type II hyperlipoproteinemia
  - ▼ Patients with anticardiolipins may have circulating antibodies to F XII in addition to falsely decreased F XII levels. This situation may be encountered in patients with lupus anticoagulant.

Suggested Reading

Rennee T, Schmaier AH, Nickel KF, et al. In vivo roles of factor XII. *Blood.* 2012;120:4296–4303.

FACTOR XI (F XI) DEFICIENCY

Factor XI deficiency is, in most cases, an inherited autosomal recessive disorder. More than 100 mutations have been described in the F XI gene. Although F XI deficiency is rare in the population at large, it is common in Ashkenazi Jews and in some Arab groups. Bleeding is highly variable since the deficient phenotype does not follow the laboratory level of the factor with respect to bleeding. Patients with mild F XI deficiency can experience bleeding complications, and those with severe deficiencies may not bleed excessively. In general, the homozygous patients display a severe deficiency of measurable F XI, from <1% to 20%. It is not usually associated with spontaneous hemorrhage, but these individuals may bleed excessively after injury or surgery, particularly of areas with high fibrinolytic activity, such as dental surgery. Spontaneous abortions have been seen in one patient with severe F XI deficiency by the author. F XI-deficient patients seem to be protected against ischemic stroke and deep vein thrombosis. On the other hand, individuals with high F XI levels are at increased risk of venous and arterial thrombosis. Patients with F XI deficiency have a normal PT, but a variably prolonged PTT. The definitive diagnosis is made by establishing F XI levels in each suspected patient. F XI is not affected by vitamin K deficiency or oral anticoagulants.

FACTOR XIII (F XIII) DEFICIENCY

❏ Definition

Factor XII lends to increase stability of the fibrin clot. Factor XIII deficiency is a rare condition inherited in an autosomal recessive manner. It may lead to a bleeding diathesis of varying intensity. Typically, the affected individuals bleed from the umbilical stump during the first few days of life, postoperatively, and intracranially. It is also associated with recurrent pregnancy loss and delayed wound healing disorder.

- Congenital
  - ▼ A variety of mutations lead to F XIII deficiency. Most patients deficient in F XIII lack the factor in plasma and in platelets.
- Acquired
  - ▼ Liver disease, prematurity, plasmacytoma, surgery, DIC.
  - ▼ Acute promyelocytic and some chronic leukemias.
  - ▼ Alloantibodies may develop in severely deficient patients after therapeutic exposure to the antigen. Antibody inhibitors may develop after exposure to certain drugs such as phenytoin, isoniazid, penicillin, or valproic acid. The development of antibodies against F XIII may lead to severe bleeding.

❏ Laboratory Findings

- A qualitative assay investigates the clot solubility in five molar urea. A plasma clot from a patient deficient in F XIII is easily dissolved in urea, acids, and bases, whereas in a normal control, the clot remains solid. If the test is positive, mixing studies are recommended to rule out a factor XIII inhibitor. If no inhibitor is detected, the deficiency should be confirmed by a quantitative test.
- Deficiency of F XIII does not affect PT (INR), PTT, thrombin time, or fibrinogen levels.
- F XIII is unaffected by vitamin K deficiency or oral anticoagulants.

Suggested Reading

Lorand L. Factor XIII and the clotting of fibrinogen: from basic research to medicine. *J Thromb Haemost.* 2005;3:1337–1348.

 # ACQUIRED HEMORRHAGIC DISORDERS OF MULTIFACTORIAL ETIOLOGY

DISSEMINATED INTRAVASCULAR COAGULATION (DIC)

❑ Definition

DIC is an acquired, systemic, complex syndrome, producing both hemorrhages and thrombosis. It is a secondary condition that develops as a complication to a variety of disorders (Table 9-6).

DIC consists of the systemic activation of coagulation, resulting in multiple thrombi in the microcirculation, consumption of clotting proteins and platelets, in turn leading to a hemorrhagic diathesis. Intravascular fibrin deposition is the result of tissue factor–mediated thrombin generation. The fibrinolytic mechanism becomes activated in parallel, exacerbating the hemorrhagic tendency. Most cases of DIC are fulminant. In cases of chronic and low-grade DIC, blood coagulation is continuously or intermittently activated by small amounts of tissue factor, such as may be released from disseminated malignancies.

❑ Who Should Be Suspected

In most cases of acute DIC, the condition should be suspected in an intensive care patient with end organ failure, bleeding, and thrombotic events, especially in the small vasculature and at the site of catheters. The underlying diagnosis that leads to

TABLE 9–6. Common Underlying Etiologies of Disseminated Intravascular Coagulation (DIC)

Infections	Bacterial septicemias, gram positive and negative
	High prevalence in meningococcemia
	Viremia
Shock	Septic
	Hemorrhagic
Metabolic abnormalities	Acidosis
Obstetrical accidents	Eclampsia, amniotic fluid embolism, retained dead fetus, abruptio placentae
Neoplasms	Metastatic neoplasms, especially pancreas, prostate; adenocarcinomas
Hematologic conditions	Acute leukemias, especially promyelocytic
	Intravascular hemolysis due to mismatched transfusions
	Myeloproliferative disorders
Physical injuries	Massive or blunt trauma with extensive tissue injury; extensive surgery
	Burns
Vascular malformation (chronic disseminated intravascular coagulation)	Capillary hemangiomas (Kasabach-Merritt syndrome); giant hemangiomas; large aortic aneurysm
Toxins	Snake bites, brown recluse spider bites

the suspicion of acute DIC is one of the following: sepsis, trauma, cancer, obstetrical complications, and severe immunologic reactions.

❏ Laboratory Findings

- The laboratory findings of DIC are variable. They depend on the underlying etiology and stage of the syndrome. Fibrinogen, an acute-phase reactant protein, may be elevated early on but decrease progressively due to its consumption, as the condition progresses. Pathologic fibrinolysis, invariably present initially, may diminish or disappear in very severe cases when the fibrinolytic proteins are completely consumed.

- Conversely, primary fibrinolysis may develop without DIC, as with direct infusion of thrombolytic agents and in a patient with prostate cancer.

- Because DIC is primarily a bedside diagnosis in a severely ill patient, it should be considered when, in addition to bleeding and thrombotic events, end-organ injury is documented.

- Repeated laboratory studies are more useful than a single determination. The findings described below are categorized in three groups.

  1. Procoagulant activation and consumption
     - PT, PTT, and thrombin time may be variably prolonged but are non-specific and hence of limited diagnostic value.
     - Fibrinogen is useful when obtained serially, since it can demonstrate a dynamic process of consumption coagulopathy by its progressive decline.
     - Platelet counts may be decreased, but thrombocytopenia is nonspecific. In cases of thrombocytopenia and thrombosis, HIT may have to be excluded.
     - Best markers of hypercoagulability are elevated D-dimer. To avoid false-positive results, a less sensitive assay, such as semiquantitative latex, is recommended rather than the ELISA-type supersensitive D-dimer tests used to rule out DVT and PE.
     - The following assays are reproducible and have a high positive predictive value but are not available in most hospital laboratories: increased prothrombin fragments (F1 and F2), fibrinopeptides A and B, thrombin–antithrombin complexes, and soluble fibrin.
     - Many clotting factors and the inhibitory proteins, protein C and S, are decreased because of their consumption. The most sensitive and undergoing highest decrease are factors V and VIII. Their determination is not necessary for the diagnosis of DIC.
     - Because DIC is a microangiopathic syndrome, hemolytic anemia with schistocytes on the peripheral blood smear develops in severe cases.
     - Laboratory evidence of organ failure is mandatory for the diagnosis and entails in most cases the typical chemistry profile of renal or other organ failure.

  2. Fibrinolytic activation: Increased levels of fibrin(ogen) degradation products (FDP), latex D-dimer (see above). In primary fibrinolysis, FDP are greatly elevated, whereas D-dimers are not and platelet counts are normal.

  3. Inhibitor consumption
     - Progressive decrease in antithrombin (ATIII).
     - Increased levels of thrombin–antithrombin and plasmin–antiplasmin.
     - Decrease in α2 antiplasmin (not necessary for diagnosis).

❑ Recommendations

- We have suggested a simple, selective "DIC profile" based on the three categories mentioned above: titration of latex D-dimer, FDP, and ATIII. Serial ATIII assays are useful for observing the evolution of the syndrome, since its marked decrease connotes a poor prognosis. FDP and D-dimers are elevated in chronic DIC as well. In addition to the above panel, chemistry panels to assess end-organ injury are mandatory.
- Other recommendations have been published by the International Society on Thrombosis and Haemostasis in 2003 and reviewed in 2007 and by the Japanese Ministry of Health and Welfare in 1987.

Suggested Readings

Takemitsu T, Wada H, Hatada T, et al. Prospective evaluation of three diagnostic criteria for disseminated intravascular coagulation. *J Thromb Haemost.* 2011;105:40–44.

Yu M, Nardella A, Pechet L. Screening tests of disseminated intravascular coagulation: guidelines for rapid and specific laboratory diagnosis. *Crit Care Med.* 2000;28:1777–1780.

HEREDITARY HEMORRHAGIC TELANGIECTASIA (HHT)

❑ Definition

HHT is an autosomal vascular disease manifested by epistaxis, mucocutaneous and gastrointestinal telangiectasias, and arteriovenous malformations in the pulmonary, cerebral, or hepatic circulation. It was previously described under the acronym Osler-Weber-Rendu disease. This rare disease is the result of abnormal angiogenesis due mostly to two mutations: endoglin (ENG) and ACVLR1 (ALK1) genes leading to HHT1 and HHT2, respectively. In addition, rare cases present with a mutation in the MADH4 gene encoding the transcription factor SMAD4.

❑ Who Should Be suspected?

- Patients who present with three out of the following four criteria:
  - ▼ Spontaneous, recurrent epistaxis
  - ▼ Multiple telangiectasias (lips, oral cavity, fingers, nose)
  - ▼ Family history in first-degree relative(s)
  - ▼ Visceral lesions with telangiectasias or arteriovenous fistulas

❑ Laboratory Findings

- *Molecular testing*: Genetic tests are available for the endoglin, ACVRL1, and SMAD4 genes. One of these mutations is found in 90% of patients with the clinical diagnosis of HHT. Molecular diagnosis is recommended also for screening suspected first-degree relatives.
- *CBC and serum iron studies* will detect iron deficiency anemia in most patients with recurrent bleeding manifestations.
- A definitive diagnosis is imperative since antiangiogenic treatments are being developed.

Suggested Reading

Dupuis-Girod S, Bailly S, Plauchau H. Hereditary hemorrhagic telangiectasia: from molecular biology to patient care. *J Thromb Haemost.* 2010;8:1447–1456.

HEMOSTATIC FAILURE IN CARDIOPULMONARY BYPASS SURGERY

❑ Definition and Etiology

Bleeding is a common complication in patients undergoing open heart surgery (approximately 30% of patients require red cell transfusions after CABG). The etiology of bleeding is multifactorial, as reflected in multiple laboratory abnormalities. Platelets, the fibrinolytic system, both the extrinsic and intrinsic coagulation pathways, and the complement system are activated, resulting in bleeding, and possibly thrombosis. The principal causes of bleeding in bypass surgery are excess heparin, fibrinolysis, and decrease in platelet number and function. Another cause of bleeding resulting in the need for transfusions are the antiplatelet and antithrombotic drugs used in addition to heparin: clopidogrel or prasugrel, anti-GPIIb/IIIa such as abciximab, and aspirin. Venous thromboembolism (DVT and PE) is often present but may be difficult to recognize.

❑ Laboratory Findings

- Hemostasis, platelet function, and fibrinolysis can be monitored by conventional techniques, or at the surgical room site, by a thromboelastogram.
  - ▼ Thrombocytopathy (functional platelet defect): frequent occurrence due to platelet activation during bypass; exacerbated by the use of drugs that interfere with platelet function.
  - ▼ Thrombocytopenia: platelets decline temporarily. By the end of surgery, their number is typically reduced by 40–60% due to hemodilution, activation, and consumption during bypass procedure. Occasionally, the decline may be more profound and compromise hemostasis.
  - ▼ Hyperfibrinolysis: elevated fibrin(ogen) degradation products (FDP).
  - ▼ Bleeding caused by heparin is frequently related to incomplete inactivation by protamine. "Heparin rebound" is a term that refers to delayed release of heparin from the lymphatic system after protamine has already been cleared from plasma. It may result in bleeding after completion of surgery. "Heparin resistance" may be secondary to antithrombin deficiency. Excessive infusion of protamine may itself result in bleeding.
  - ▼ DIC: The concentrations of D-dimer and of fibrinopeptides A and B are increased.

THE COAGULOPATHY OF LIVER DISEASE

❑ Definition

A syndrome of excessive *bleeding,* occasionally *thrombosis,* resulting from severe liver disease. The coagulopathy is multifactorial, due to the liver's many functions in hemostasis and thrombosis. Most coagulation factors are decreased, with the exception of fibrinogen, factor VIII, and von Willebrand factor (VWF). While fibrinogen becomes severely decreased in advanced liver disease, the latter two are often greatly increased. The VWF cleaving protease ADAMTS13 is reduced in liver cirrhosis. Naturally occurring anticoagulants (protein C, S, antithrombin) are decreased. These changes lead to rebalancing of coagulation and often to poor correlation between measured levels of clotting factors and clinical bleeding or thrombosis.

- Decreased synthesis in clotting factors → bleeding. Prekallikrein and factor VII are one of the earliest clotting proteins to be decreased in liver disease. Fibrinogen is one of the last ones.
- Decreased clearing of activated clotting factors (especially factor Xa) → tendency to DIC.
- Decreased synthesis of plasminogen and protein C, S, antithrombin → tendency to thrombosis.
- Decreased synthesis of fibrinolytic inhibitors → excessive fibrinolysis with increased bleeding, but counterbalanced by decreased plasminogen.
- Synthesis of abnormal clotting factors → bleeding; occasionally risk of thrombosis.
- Hypersplenism → thrombocytopenia that exacerbates bleeding.
- The coagulopathy of liver transplantation is extremely complex, with DIC and pathologic fibrinolysis predominating.

❑ Laboratory Findings

- PT is prolonged (INR is not recommended to evaluate liver function or the bleeding diathesis of liver disease).
- PTT is prolonged, but less consistently than PT.
- Factors V, VII, II, IX, and X are decreased.
- Antithrombin is decreased.
- Fibrinolytic inhibitors: thrombin activatable fibrinolysis inhibitor (TAFI), plasminogen activator inhibitor-1 (PAI-1), and α2-antiplasmin are decreased.
- DIC screen may be positive. The differentiation between DIC and excessive fibrinolysis may be difficult. The two conditions may coexist.

Suggested Readings

Lisman T, Porte RJ. Rebalanced hemostasis in patients with liver disease: evidence and clinical consequences. *Blood.* 2010;116:878–885.
Tripodi A, Mannucci PM. The coagulopathy of chronic liver disease. *N Engl J Med.* 2011;365:147–156.

ANTICOAGULANTS, CIRCULATING

❑ Definition

Circulating anticoagulants are antibodies that inhibit the function of specific coagulation factors, most commonly factors VIII or IX. The anticoagulants may be acquired following multiple transfusions in hemophiliacs (alloantibodies), or spontaneous (autoantibodies), most commonly against factor VIII. Lupus anticoagulant is not an anticoagulant, but prothrombotic.

❑ Who Should Be Suspected?

A circulating anticoagulant is suspected under two conditions:

- A patient with hemophilia A or B or, rarely, another congenital clotting factor deficiency, who has had multiple transfusions and whose bleeding does not stop on infusion of the missing factor.
- A middle-aged person, especially if suffering from lymphoma, or a postpartum patient who develops unprovoked hemorrhages: autoantibodies to factor VIII in most cases.

❏ Laboratory Findings and Interpretation

- In a patient with hemophilia, determinations of the missing factor show no elevations following infusions.
- In a patient with no previous bleeding history, the finding of a prolonged PTT should raise the suspicion of an acquired circulating anticoagulant. If incubation at 37°C of half normal plasma mixed with half the patient's plasma for 1–2 hours does not correct the prolonged PTT, the presence of a circulating anticoagulant is proven.
- Specific titration of the inhibitor's potency is performed either for factor VIII or IX inhibitors and the results reported in Bethesda Inhibitor units.

 # THROMBOTIC DISORDERS

THROMBOPHILIA

❏ Definition
Thrombophilia may be defined as a hereditary or acquired tendency to develop thrombotic episodes due to an abnormality in the coagulation system (i.e., a hypercoagulable state). The thrombosis may have a predilection for arteries or veins. Fifty percent of thrombotic events in patients with inherited thrombophilia occur in the setting of an acquired risk factor.

❏ Who Should Be Suspected?
1. Suspect inherited thrombophilia
   A. Venous thrombophilia
      - A family history of VTE and VTE at a young age (<45 years)
      - Recurrent VTE
      - VTE following minimal or no provocation
      - VTE at an unusual site (upper extremity, mesenteric vein, cerebral vein)
      - Pulmonary embolism (PE) without obvious etiology
      - Neonatal purpura fulminans
      - Warfarin-induced skin necrosis
   B. Arterial thrombophilia
      - Patients with unexpected/unexplained arterial thrombotic events.
2. Suspect acquired hypercoagulability
      - Patients with unprovoked venous or arterial thromboembolism in the absence of a known family history. Some patients may have both venous and arterial thrombotic events.

❏ Laboratory Findings
When should inherited thrombophilia tests be performed, in whom, and which tests?

There is no urgency in obtaining thrombophilia tests for patients who present with an acute venous thromboembolism (VTE), because this information does not alter acute therapy decisions. Consider obtaining a thrombophilia workup, if indicated, when the patient has recovered from the acute event and ideally when warfarin and/or heparin administration have been discontinued for at least 2–4 weeks.

9

I. *Suspected inherited thrombophilia.*
  - ▪ *Testing for inherited thrombophilia serves only a limited purpose and should not be performed on a routine basis: patients who have had one episode of VTE and have thrombophilia are only at a slight risk of recurrent events.*
    - ▼ *Exceptions are to identify asymptomatic immediate family members of patients with VTE who test positive for thrombophilia.*
  - A. Venous thrombophilia: The most common causes of inherited venous thrombophilia are the factor V Leiden and the prothrombin gene mutations. Protein C and S deficiencies, antithrombin deficiency, and dysfibrinogenemia are very rare. Elevated factor VIII coagulant activity is now accepted as an independent marker of increased risk for thrombosis.
    - ● *First-tier tests.*[†††]
      - • Activated protein C resistance (APCR): functional assay
      - • Prothrombin G20210A: genetic assay
      - • Protein C activity[‡‡]: functional assay
      - • Protein S activity functional assay
      - • Antithrombin (AT) activity: functional assay
    - ● *Second-tier tests.*
      - • Factor V Leiden mutation (if APCR is abnormal): genetic assay
      - • Protein C antigen (if functional test is low)
      - • Protein S antigen (total and free) (if functional test is low)
      - • AT antigen (if functional test is low), except in DIC, heparin therapy, or liver disease: Immunologic assays are rarely necessary
    - ● *Third-tier tests.*
      - • Thrombin time and fibrinogen for dysfibrinogenemia
      - • Factor VIII coagulant
    - ● Other selected clotting factors (fibrinogen, factors VII, IX, vWF) to assess marked elevations—their usefulness is not well documented. Fibrinogen may also be investigated for dysfibrinogenemia.
      - • Homocysteine (may be of value for congenital arterial thrombophilia as well)
  - B. Arterial thrombophilia[§§§]
    - ● Lipid profile
    - ● Lipoprotein a
    - ● Homocysteine

II. *Suspected acquired hypercoagulability*
  - ▪ First-tier tests:
    - ▼ Lupus anticoagulant
    - ▼ Anticardiolipin and anti-β2 glycoprotein 1 antibodies (IgG and IgM)
    - ▼ Antinuclear antibodies (ANA)
  - ▪ DIC (recommended DIC panel: FDP, Latex D-dimer, antithrombin)
  - ▪ Heparin-induced thrombocytopenia (HIT) must be ruled out

---

[†††]It may be advantageous to order together the five first-tier tests, because inherited venous thrombophilia cases are often due to a polygenic effect.

[‡‡]Warfarin therapy reduces vitamin K–dependent factors including proteins C, S, and Z and will result in spuriously low values in these patients. Testing for protein Z is not recommended at this time.

[§§§]There is no documented indication to order the tests suggested for venous thrombophilia in cases of arterial thrombophilia (except for APCR in pediatric thrombophilia with idiopathic ischemic stroke).

▼ DVT/PE: an ELISA-sensitive, quantitative assay for D-dimers to be used in relation with a probability algorithm
▼ Lipid profile
▼ Homocysteine
■ Second-tier tests:
▼ Comprehensive investigation of possible underlying neoplasm or a myelo-proliferative disorder, including JAK-2 mutation.
▼ To be considered as risk factors.
▼ Pregnancy.
▼ Paroxysmal nocturnal hemoglobinuria (PNH)–flow cytometry.
▼ Drugs: chemotherapy, thalidomide, lenalidomide, tamoxifen, contraceptive, and hormone replacement therapy.
■ If TTP is strongly suspected, start therapy and order ADAMTS 13 assay.
■ Chronic renal disease and the nephrotic syndrome
■ If promyelocytic leukemia is suspected, order diagnostic tests (FISH, karyotype, flow cytometry) on bone marrow aspirate and start therapy promptly.

Suggested Readings

Dahlback B. Advances in understanding pathogenic mechanisms of thrombophilic disorders. *Blood.* 2008;112:19–27.
Huisman MV, Klok FA. How I diagnose acute pulmonary embolism. *Blood.* 2013;121:4443–4448.
Middeldorp S. Is thrombophilia testing useful? *Hematology Am Soc Hematol Educ Program.* 2011;2011:150–155.

ANTIPHOSPHOLIPID ANTIBODY SYNDROME (APS)

9

❏ Definition

APS is an autoimmune prothrombotic disorder that can affect both the venous and arterial circulation. The other major clinical manifestations are obstetrical. The laboratory criteria are the presence of a *lupus anticoagulant (LA)* (see below), β2 *glycoprotein 1* ELISA and *anticardiolipin* antibodies of the IgG or IgM isotype (see pp. 806–807). The diagnosis of APS requires both clinical features and laboratory confirmation with the persistence of antibodies for at least 12 weeks. Lupus anticoagulants are more commonly associated with thrombotic events than are the anticardiolipin antibodies (ACA). Antiphospholipid antibodies (APLA) are directed against phospholipid-binding plasma proteins. APLA comprise a heterogeneous family of auto- and alloantibodies (IgG and IgM subclasses) directed against specific plasma proteins with *affinity* for phospholipid surfaces. The antigenic targets are β2 glycoprotein 1, factor II (prothrombin), and possibly protein C, protein S, kininogens, complement factor H, and annexin V. The most commonly detected subgroups of APLA include ACLA, antiprothrombin antibodies, and anti-β2 glycoprotein I antibodies (anti-β2 GP 1).

❏ Who Should Be Tested for APS?

Medical patients: APS occurs either as a primary condition or in the setting of an underlying disease, most commonly systemic lupus erythematosus (SLE), or other connective tissue disorders, infections, or drugs. The deep veins of the lower limbs and the cerebral arterial circulation are the most common thrombotic sites. *Catastrophic APS* develops in a small group of patients and leads to multiorgan failure with a high mortality.

Obstetrical patients: unexplained fetal death of morphologically normal fetus at or after 10 weeks of gestation; pregnancy loss at or before the 34th week of gestation due to severe preeclampsia, eclampsia, or placental insufficiency; early onset (second or early third trimester) of severe intrauterine growth retardation and premature birth.

LABORATORY EVALUATION

❏ Laboratory Findings

There is no pathognomonic single test for APS. A panel of tests should be ordered. Typically, one screens for APL with coagulation-based tests to detect the presence of a LA. Anticardiolipin antibodies (ACA) and anti-β2 GP 1 should be done in parallel.

LA are identified by coagulation-based tests in which the antibodies prolong the clotting time of a PT or PTT. The PT is commonly prolonged, but it may be only borderline prolonged, or even normal. Not all reagents for the PTT assay will demonstrate a prolongation, because many are insensitive to the LA.

Coagulation-based tests for LA:

1. PT is used mostly to rule out the effect of oral or other anticoagulants. This is followed by two screening tests.
2. PTT using a LA-sensitive PTT reagent.
3. PT using a dilute reagent confirms the suspicion of a LA if elongated. If either is prolonged, proceed with a confirmatory test.
4. Staclot LA test, this reagent inhibits the LA antibodies by hexagonal phase phospholipid. If a LA is present, the prolonged clotting time in the PT or PTT assay is corrected, and the diagnosis of LA is confirmed.
5. A second test, the dilute Russell's viper venom time (dRVVT) is recommended. This reagent activates clotting factor X. If the dRVVT is prolonged, a LA is suspected. A confirmatory test confirms the presence of LA if the clotting time shortens.
6. *Factor II* level determination is indicated in patients with greatly prolonged PT and/or bleeding manifestations. In these patients, antibodies to factor II may be present.

Immunoassays

- ELISA tests are used for the detection of IgG or IgA ACA. Their usefulness is now being debated.
- Anti-β2 GP 1 ELISA.
- ANA assay may be positive in low titers (1:40 to 1:160) in half the patients with the APS.
- Biologically false-positive serologic test for syphilis.
- CBC to assess possible anemia, leukopenia, and especially *thrombocytopenia*.
- *Serology for SLE.*
- *Renal function* investigation.

❏ Limitations

The detection of the LA is more difficult (but not impossible) in the presence of heparin or oral anticoagulant therapy. *The laboratory should be notified of antico-agulant therapy* when the assays are ordered.

Suggested Readings

Giannakopoulos B, Krilis SA. Mechanism of disease: the pathogenesis of the antiphospholipid syndrome. *N Engl J Med.* 2013;368:1033–1044.

Giannakopoulos B, Passam F, Ioannou Y, et al. How we diagnose the antiphospholipid antibody syndrome. *Blood.* 2009;113:985–994.

Rand JH, Wolgast LR. Dos and don'ts in diagnosing antiphospholipid syndrome. *Hematology Am Soc Hematol Educ Program.* 2012;2012:455–459.

THROMBOTIC THROMBOCYTOPENIC PURPURA/HEMOLYTIC UREMIC SYNDROME (TTP/HUS)

❑ Definition

TTP and HUS are severe thrombotic microangiopathies characterized by systemic platelet aggregates causing ischemia in multiple organ systems, thrombocytopenia, and fragmentation of red cells. These conditions are expressed by microangiopathic hemolytic anemia, thrombocytopenia, and occasionally neurologic, and renal involvement. TTP and HUS are disorders with many similarities. There are, however, sufficient differences between these conditions to be considered separately.

❑ Who Should Be Suspected?

TTP

- Classically, patients with TTP were described as presenting with the following pentad: fever, microangiopathic hemolytic anemia, thrombocytopenia, and impaired renal and neurologic function. In reality, most patients have some, but not all, of the components of the pentad, and the pentad criteria are no longer used.

- TTP may be congenital, or acquired, resulting from antibodies against ADAMTS 13 (Figure 9-4). The hereditary form, much less common, is known as the Upshaw-Schulman syndrome; it is the result of homozygous or compound heterozygous ADAMTS13 gene mutation.

- ADAMTS13 is a metalloprotease that cleaves very large molecular weight components of the pro-vWF, thereby reducing the propensity of the pro-vWF to agglutinate platelets in vivo. Its absence results in release into the circulation of thrombogenic very high molecular weight vWF multimers.

- TTP can be broadly divided into two categories: the acute idiopathic (classic) TTP, seen in about one third of cases, and secondary TTP (in two thirds of cases), those in which a causative condition or agent can be identified: bacterial or viral (including AIDS) infections, pregnancy (especially during the third trimester and postpartum period), certain drugs: ADP inhibitors of platelet function (ticlopidine [rarely used now] and infrequently clopidogrel), quinine, mitomycin C, cisplatinum, bleomycin, α-interferon, cyclosporine, tacrolimus, other immunosuppressive or chemotherapeutic agents, disseminated malignancy, and allogeneic stem cell transplantation. Classic TTP occurs primarily in adults and has a higher incidence in women.

HUS

- HUS is predominantly a pediatric disease. It presents commonly in a child who recently had abdominal pain and bloody diarrhea and develops acute microangiopathic hemolytic anemia, thrombocytopenia, and acute renal failure.

9

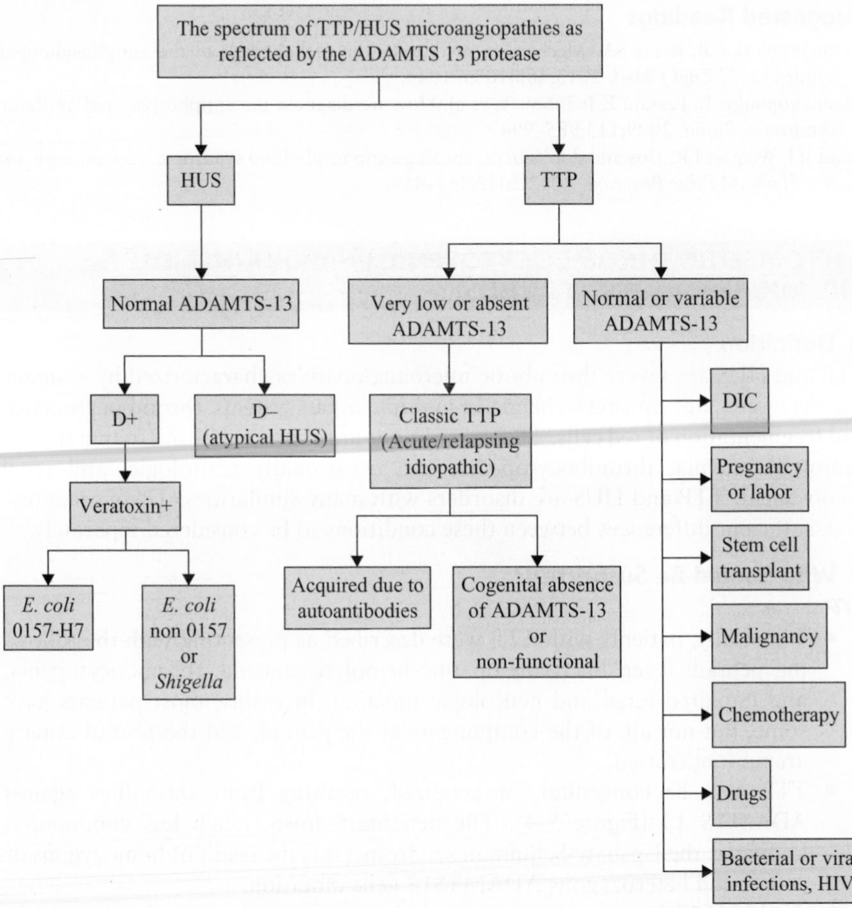

Figure 9–4 *The spectrum of thrombotic thrombocytopenic purpura (TTP)/hemolytic uremic syndrome (HUS) microangiopathies as reflected by the ADAMTS 13 protease. E. coli, Escherichia coli.*

It is a complication of an infection caused by a verotoxin-producing strain of *E. coli* 0157:H7 (most common cause in the United States) or *Shigella* (see Figure 9-4). In different countries, other bacteria have been found to be the etiologic agent in HUS. HUS is a self-limited disease.

■ Atypical HUS, which comprises approximately 10% of cases, is a term now reserved for HUS caused by complement regulatory abnormalities. In these patients, a low serum C3 level may be detected.

❏ **Laboratory Findings**
TTP
■ CBC.
▼ Microangiopathic hemolytic anemia with Hb <8 g/L.
▼ WBC may be increased (with neutrophilia) or normal counts.

- ▼ Platelets: severe thrombocytopenia (usually <20,000/μL) rapidly responsive to effective therapy.
- ▼ Peripheral blood smear (PBS): Fragmented red cells (schistocytes) (see p. 1121) represent >1% of RBC (or two or more per HPF); they decrease with response to therapy (schistocytes are absent in rare cases). Characteristics: nucleated red cells; basophilic stippling; polychromasia resulting from reticulocytosis.
- LDH is very elevated (>1,000 U/L at presentation is not unusual); LDH levels decrease with therapy and are useful in assessing response.
- Haptoglobin is decreased.
- Indirect bilirubin is elevated.
- Direct Coombs test is negative.
- Coagulation studies are normal and help in ruling out DIC (see p. 458).
- Increased creatinine may occur, but marked increase favors HUS.
- Serology for HIV is necessary to rule out HIV as a causative agent.
- ADAMTS13 (see Figure 9-4).
  - ▼ ADAMTS 13 measurements are most helpful retroactively to confirm the diagnosis of TTP and for follow-up because the assay provides useful prognostic information. Newer, "second-generation" assays are easier to perform, available in some commercial laboratories, and have a short turnaround time.
  - ▼ *Under no circumstances should the clinician wait for results of ADAMTS13 levels or its antibodies before starting therapy when other criteria for TTP are present.* Extremely low plasma levels of ADAMTS13 (<5–10%) are characteristic for TTP but not entirely specific since they are found occasionally in non-TTP microangiopathic anemia cases. The absence of ADAMTS13 at the time of diagnosis is predictive of relapsing episodes in nearly half of cases.
  - ▼ In thrombotic microangiopathies associated with allogeneic stem cell transplantation, chemotherapy and other drugs, as well as in HUS (see below), the levels of the protease are in most cases normal. Because 94% to 97% of idiopathic TTP cases are acquired and due to anti-ADAMTS13 antibodies, the antibodies assay should be performed at the same time with the measurement of the enzyme.

HUS

- CBC, LDH, haptoglobin, indirect bilirubin, direct Coombs and coagulation results are similar to those of TTP.
- Creatinine is very elevated at presentation in most cases.
- Urinalysis may show proteinuria and red cell casts.
- ADAMTS13 is normal in most cases of HUS.

Suggested Readings

George JN. How I treat patients with thrombotic thrombocytopenic purpura: 2010. *Blood.* 2010;116:4060–4069.

Kremer Hovinga JA, Lammle B. Role of ADAMTS13 in the pathogenesis, diagnosis, and treatment of thrombotic thrombocytopenic purpura. *Hematology Am Soc Hematol Educ Program.* 2012;2012:610–616.

MISCELLANEOUS DISORDERS

IRON OVERLOAD DISORDERS (IOD) AND HEREDITARY HEMOCHROMATOSIS (HH)

❑ Definition
The term IOD refers to patients with increased iron stores resulting from iron supply that exceeds the body's ability to eliminate it. Due to iron toxicity, its excess results in tissue damage (liver cirrhosis often followed by hepatocellular carcinoma, diabetes, and cardiomyopathy). IOD may be primary, commonly hereditary, or secondary (acquired). The most common form of primary IOD in North America and Western Europe is HH.

Hereditary (primary) hemochromatosis

- HH is an HLA-linked autosomal recessive defect, caused by increased duodenal absorption of iron from dietary sources, leading to excess iron deposition in various organs. HH is the result of an abnormal gene present in 10% of the Caucasian population (see below under Genetic studies). The manifest disease, in contrast with the genotypical or biochemical phenotype, is quite rare. Excess iron is toxic to cells due to excess production of free radicals and the Fenton reaction.
- Other genetic forms of hemochromatosis are juvenile hereditary hemochromatosis, neonatal hemochromatosis aceruloplasminemia, mutations in transferrin receptor-22 or ferroportin-1, and African iron overload (combined hereditary increased absorption and excess intake, seen particularly in Bantu

Secondary hemochromatosis

- Increased, long-term intake of iron medication
- Anemias with ineffective erythropoiesis and/or extravascular hemolysis (especially if associated with multiple transfusions): sickle cell anemia, β-thalassemia major, aplastic anemia, myelodysplastic syndromes
- Chronic hemodialysis
- Porphyria cutanea tarda (minor)
- Alcoholic liver disease (iron deposited in Kupffer cells) and other chronic liver disorders
- Following portosystemic shunts

❑ Who Should Be Suspected?
IOD should be suspected in individuals with a family history of HH, or in its absence, in those with chronic liver disease, skin hyperpigmentation, or diabetes without predisposing factors and in patients with unexplained arthritis, cardiomyopathy, or hypogonadism. Weakness and lethargy can also be presenting manifestations of HH. Individuals with the secondary form of IOD have usually a history of a disease predisposing to increased iron stores or of multiple RBC transfusions.

❑ Laboratory Findings
- The presence of IOD is established by the demonstration of increased body iron using serum iron studies, radiologic techniques (MRI using special techniques), *liver biopsy*, and assessment of response to phlebotomy if clinically indicated. When one of the hereditary forms is suspected, genetic studies are helpful.

- Transferrin saturation is the best method for screening populations of North European ancestry suspected for IOD. A persistent value of >45% starting early in life remains the best predictive phenotypic test for the homozygous C282Y mutation (see below). Percent transferrin saturation is frequently >70% and may reach 100%.
- Total iron binding capacity is an assay similar to transferrin saturation, and parallels it, increasing with increase in iron store.
- Increased serum ferritin is found in approximately two thirds of patients with IOD. Levels >300 µg/L in men and >200 µg/L in women with no evidence of inflammatory or autoimmune disease are the recommended thresholds for further screening for IOD. The serum ferritin is usually >1,000 µg/L at the time of diagnosis, and it indicates biochemical accumulation of tissue iron. The critical threshold associated with the development of liver cirrhosis is unknown.
- Serum iron is usually increased (>200 µg/dL in women and >250 µg/dL in men), but it is a less reliable test, especially if performed alone.
- Other laboratory tests explore damage to various organs:
  - ▼ Studies for diabetes
  - ▼ Chondrocalcinosis (pseudogout)
  - ▼ Pituitary dysfunction
  - ▼ Liver function tests
- Genetic tests for HH. Note: phenotypic analysis should be the first step in screening for HH, with screening strategies including measurement of transferrin saturation and serum ferritin, before resorting to genetic testing.
  - ▼ HFE genetic hemochromatosis.
  - ▼ In most patients of European ancestry, HH is the result of mutations in two specific genes known as HFE, found within the major histocompatibility locus on chromosome 6. The HFE gene has two common missense mutations: the C282Y (rare in non-Caucasian populations) and the H63D found in both Caucasians and non-Caucasians) but with a less well-defined role in HH.
  - ▼ Patients with a C282Y/C282Y genotype are homozygous for HH and are at risk for the phenotypic HH disease. The disease seems to have a low penetrance. The reason for the occurrence of the fully expressed penetrance of these genes remains unknown. The homozygous are generally found to have a higher prevalence of abnormal liver function tests independent of other manifestations of HH. Modifier factors may be genetic, gender, and high iron or alcohol intake. *Genetic population screening for these mutations in individuals with no clinical or biochemical signs of hemochromatosis is not recommended. Screening of families with one proband documented for HH may be helpful for discovering other members affected with the same mutations.*
  - ▼ Patients with a C282Y/wild-type genotype are heterozygous for HH and have less risk of iron overload.
  - ▼ Patients with a C282Y/H63D genotype (one allele with each mutation) have a 60% chance of intermediate-degree IOD, and 35% have normal iron stores.

9

- Non-HFE genetic hemochromatosis
  - ▼ Juvenile hemochromatosis (JH) is the result of a mutation in the gene HJV at chromosome 1q21. This is a rare autosomal recessive disorder similar to HH, but with onset in the second decade of life; a severe form of JH is caused by mutations in HAMP, the gene for hepcidin (in its wild form hepcidin becomes elevated in order to block iron absorption when iron stores become increased).
  - ▼ Mutations in the gene for ferroportin cause autosomal dominant HH.
  - ▼ Mutations in the genes for transferring and ceruloplasmin produce autosomal recessive disorders of iron overload.

❏ Limitations

- Serum ferritin may be increased in severe inflammatory conditions and in hepatic necrosis, in the absence of IOD. In HH patients, it becomes elevated later in life than transferrin saturation.
- Serum iron levels fluctuate diurnally, with lowest values in the evening and highest between 7 AM and noon.

Suggested Readings

Adams PC, Barton JC. How I treat hemochromatosis. *Blood.* 2010;116:317–325.

Camaschella C. Treating iron overload. *N Engl J Med.* 2013;368:2325–2327.

Fleming RE, Ponka P. Iron overload in human disease. *N Engl J Med.* 2012; 366:348–359.

Hoffbrand AV, Taher A, Cappelini MD. How I treat transfusional hemochromatosis. *Blood.* 2012;120:3657–3669.

Genetic disorders are conditions caused by absent or defective genes or by chromosomal aberrations. Genetic disorders can be tested at the level of DNA, RNA, or protein. A genetic test is the analysis of human DNA, RNA, mitochondrial DNA, chromosomes, proteins, or certain metabolites in order to detect alterations that may be inherited or acquired. This can be accomplished by directly examining the DNA or RNA that makes up a gene (direct testing), looking at markers coinherited with a disease-causing gene (linkage testing), enzyme activity or metabolites (biochemical testing), or examining the chromosomes (cytogenetic testing) (www.genetests.org). The results of a genetic test can confirm or rule out a suspected genetic condition, determine an individual's risk of developing disorders, identify carriers, or assess gene variants influencing an individual's rate of drug metabolism. Hundreds genetic tests are currently in use and more are being developed. Genetic testing may be undertaken as part of the process of treating or advising patients.

 # OVERVIEW

MOLECULAR DIAGNOSIS: TYPES OF GENETIC TESTING

- *Diagnostic genetic testing*: Confirmatory test for symptomatic individuals.
- *Presymptomatic genetic testing*: Carried out in people without symptoms for estimating the risk of developing (e.g., Huntington disease).
- *Carrier testing*: Performed to determine whether an individual carries one copy of an altered gene for a particular recessive disease. Autosomal recessive diseases occur only if an individual receives two copies of a gene that have a disease-associated mutation; therefore, each child born to two carriers of a mutation in the same gene has a 25% risk of being affected with the disorder.
- *Risk factor testing (susceptibility tests)*: Gene variants have been discovered that are associated with common diseases such as Alzheimer disease, Parkinson's disease and diabetes.
- *Pharmacogenetic testing*: Determining differences an individual's response to drugs.
- *Preimplantation testing*: Preimplantation diagnosis is used following in vitro fertilization to diagnose a genetic disease or condition in a preimplantation embryo.
- *Prenatal testing*: Used to diagnose a genetic disease or condition in a developing fetus.
- *Newborn screening*: Performed in newborns by in place of in state public health programs to detect certain genetic diseases for which early diagnosis and interventions are available.

GENETIC COUNSELING

Genetic testing is often accompanied by genetic counseling. Genetic counseling is the process by which patients or relatives, at risk of an inherited disorder, are advised of the consequences and nature of the disorder, the probability of developing or transmitting it, and the options open to them in management and family planning in order to prevent, avoid, or ameliorate it. A instead of any person may seek genetic counseling for a condition he or she have inherited from his or her biologic parents. A woman may be referred for genetic counseling if pregnant and undergoing prenatal testing or screening. Genetic counselors educate the patient about their testing options and inform them of their results.

If a prenatal screening or test is abnormal, the genetic counselor evaluates the risk of an affected pregnancy, educates the patient about these risks, and informs the patient of their options. A person may also undergo genetic counseling after the birth of a child with a genetic condition. In these instances, the genetic counselor explains the condition to the patient along with recurrence risks in future children. In cases of a positive family history for a condition, the genetic counselor can evaluate risks and recurrence and explain details about the condition.

INFORMED CONSENT

Informed consent is the process by which a health care provider discloses appropriate information to a competent patient so that the patient may make a voluntary choice to accept or refuse treatment, and thus be an informed participant in health care decisions. In this way, an individual receives information about their health condition and treatment options, and he/she is able to decide what health care treatment they want to receive and give consent to actually receive it.

"*Request for Release of Medical Information*" is a written consent document for the requested release of a person's genetic information or the release of medical records containing such information. Such a written consent form shall state the purpose for which the information is being requested and shall be distinguished from written consent for the release of any other medical information.

"*Genetic information*" is any written or recorded individually identifiable result of a genetic test. In many instances, a laboratory receiving a request to conduct a genetic test from a facility, a physician, or a health care provider may conduct the requested test only when the request is accompanied by a signed statement of the medical practitioner ordering the test warranting that the appropriate prior written consent has been obtained from the patient.

FACTORS TO CONSIDER WHEN ORDERING GENETIC TESTS

1. *Family history*—is an important source of information about risks of genetic disease. Factors to consider are the mode of inheritance of the diseases, ethnicity, possibility of a new mutation, the presence of inherited susceptibility, consanguinity of the parents, adoption, the use of artificial insemination by donor sperm, and multiple sexual partners.
2. *Risk factors*—the age and past or present exposure to an environment that is more likely to result in disease in those with genetic predispositions.
3. *Availability of treatment or preventive therapy.*
4. *Possibility of modification of patient behavior*—preventive behavior
5. *The test needs to be beneficial for the patient,* - if the test result could inflict "psychological harm," pre- and posttesting, genetic counseling must be available, (such as in the case of Huntington disease). At-risk individuals may want to make informed reproductive and career decisions at a time when a disease is not yet clinically detectable.

GENETIC NONDISCRIMINATION LEGISLATURE

Most European countries have since 1990 enacted genetic nondiscrimination legislation for life or health insurance to address concerns about potential misuse of genetic information. There is no specific genetic legislation at EU level except data protection and discrimination provisions related to handling and using genetic data: "genetic data pertaining health are 'sensitive data' under EU data protection directive and is thus to be treated confidentially."

The U.S. 2008 Genetic Nondiscrimination Act: Title I: Genetic nondiscrimination in health insurance (Sec. 101): amends the Employee Retirement Income Security Act of 1974 (ERISA), the Public Health Service Act (PHSA), and the Internal Revenue Code to prohibit a group health plan from adjusting premium or contribution amounts for a group on the basis of genetic information.

U.S. Genetic Nondiscrimination Act Title II:

- Prohibits employment discrimination on the basis of genetic information (Sec. 202). Prohibits, as an unlawful employment practice, an employer, employment agency, labor organization, or joint labor–management committee from limiting, segregating, or classifying employees, individuals, or members because of genetic information in any way that would deprive or tend to deprive such individuals of employment opportunities or otherwise adversely affect their status as employees.
- Prohibits, as an unlawful employment practice, an employer, employment agency, labor organization, or joint labor-management committee from requesting, requiring, or purchasing an employee's genetic information, except for certain purposes, which include where (1) such information is requested or required to comply with certification requirements of family and medical leave laws; (2) the information involved is to be used for genetic monitoring of the biologic effects of toxic substances in the workplace; and (3) the employer conducts DNA analysis for law enforcement purposes as a forensic laboratory or for purposes of identification of human remains.

MOLECULAR TESTS USED FOR DETECTION AND MONITORING INFECTIOUS DISEASES

The sample should be collected before starting treatment.

- Qualitative: Detection of the presence of viral particles or confirmation of positive viral antibody test; reported as "positive" or "negative"; highly sensitive low limit of detection.
- Quantitative: Measurement of the amount of virus to monitor the effectiveness of a treatment (copies/mL, IU/mL, log).
- Genotyping: Determination of the viral type or subtype when considering antiviral therapy. Genotype testing is available and is useful in treatment planning and for determining length and possible response to treatment. Genotype testing should be done as part of the patient's initial evaluation once infection has been confirmed. It may aid in identifying the source of infection.
- High sensitivity of molecular assays allows early detection of infection when other markers are negative and detection of infection in immunocompromised patients (antibodies negative). In additional to monitoring the patient's response to therapy, the molecular test will be negative before antibodies are negative.
- Molecular tests allow for high specificity of the tests by using conserved regions of genomic sequence of organisms' species and subspecies.

GENETIC DISEASES

 DISORDERS OF THE IMMUNE SYSTEM

FAMILIAL MEDITERRANEAN FEVER (FMF)

❏ Definition
Familial Mediterranean fever (FMF) is an inherited inflammatory disease caused by mutations in the MEFV gene, encoding a protein that has been named pyrin or marenostrin.

❏ Who Should Be Suspected?
Classic familial Mediterranean fever (FMF) is an autosomal recessive disorder, MIM #249100, associated with homozygous or compound heterozygous mutations in the MEFV gene and characterized by recurrent attacks of fever and inflammation in the peritoneum, synovium, or pleura and accompanied by pain. As a complication, patients may develop amyloidosis. Familial Mediterranean fever (FMF), autosomal dominant form of FMF, MIM #134610, is associated with heterozygous mutation in the MEFV gene and characterized by recurrent bouts of fever and abdominal pain, and amyloidosis in some patients. MEFV mutations lead to reduced amounts of pyrin or a malformed form of pyrin protein, and as a result, there is not enough normal protein to control inflammation, leading to an inappropriate or prolonged inflammatory response.

❏ Relevant Tests and Diagnostic Value
Mutation analysis of the MEFV gene; however, there are some patients with FMF for whom mutations have not been identified.

❏ Other Considerations
Some evidence suggests that another gene, called SAA1, can modify the risk of developing amyloidosis among people with the M694V mutation.

 METABOLIC DISORDERS

FAMILIAL HYPERINSULINISM (FHI)

❏ Definition
Familial hyperinsulinism (FHI) is a disorder that causes abnormally high levels of insulin. Familial hyperinsulinemic hypoglycemia-1 (HHF1; **MIM #256450**) or persistent hyperinsulinemic hypoglycemia of infancy (PHHI) is caused by mutations in the ABCC8 gene, encoding the SUR1 subunit of the pancreatic beta cell inwardly rectifying potassium channel.

HHF2 (**MIM #601820**) is caused by mutations in the KCNJ11 gene encoding the Kir6.2 subunit of the pancreatic beta cell potassium channel.

HHF3 (**MIM #602485**) is caused by mutations in the glucokinase gene (GCK).

HHF4 (**MIM #609975**) is caused by mutations in the HADH gene.

HHF5 (**MIM #609968**) is caused by mutations in the insulin receptor gene (INSR).

HHF6 (**MIM #606762**) is caused by mutations in the GLUD1 gene.

HHF7 (**MIM #610021**) is caused by mutations in the SLC16A1.

Other genes that may be involved in hyperinsulinism: HNF4A and UCP2.

❑ Who Should Be Suspected?

People with this condition have frequent episodes of low blood sugar (hypoglycemia). Although it affects mainly infants and children, numerous cases have been reported in adults but at a much lower incidence.

❑ Relevant Tests and Diagnostic Value

- Blood and urine testing obtained during an episode of spontaneous hypoglycemia
- Histologic: abnormal pancreatic beta cell types: "diffuse," "focal," and "atypical" or "mosaic"
- Fluorodopa positron emission tomography (F-DOPA-PET) scanning
- Diagnostic molecular testing:
  - ▼ Targeted mutation analysis ethnic specific: Ashkenazi individuals may be tested initially for the two, ABCC8 mutations: Phe1387del and c.3989-9G>A; Finnish individuals for the founder mutations in ABCC8: p.Val187Asp and p.Glu1506Lys.
  - ▼ Sequence analysis: Comprehensive molecular genetic testing may focus on selected genes or on a multigene panel. Individuals with elevated serum ammonia should first be tested for mutations in GLUD1. Individuals with neonatal onset of severe disease should be tested for ABCC8 and KCNJ11 first.
- Carrier testing: Requires prior identification of the disease-causing mutations in the family
- Prenatal diagnosis and preimplantation genetic diagnosis (PGD): Requires prior identification of the disease-causing mutations in the family

❑ Other Considerations

In approximately 50% of cases, the genetic cause of hyperinsulinism is unknown.

Suggested Reading

Glaser B. Familial hyperinsulinism. In: Pagon RA, Adam MP, Bird TD, et al., eds. *GeneReviews™ [Internet]*. Seattle, WA: University of Washington, Seattle; 2003:1993–2013 [Updated 2013 Jan 24]. Available from: http://www.ncbi.nlm.nih.gov/books/nbk1375/

MAPLE SYRUP URINE DISEASE (MSUD)

MIM #248600

❑ Definition

- Maple syrup urine disease (MSUD) is an inherited disorder in which the body is unable to process three amino acids: leucine, isoleucine, and valine. MSUD can be caused by homozygous or compound heterozygous mutation in at least three genes: BCKDHA (MSUD type 1A), BCKDHB (MSUD type 1B), and DBT (MSUD type 2). These genes encode two of the catalytic components of the branched-chain alpha-ketoacid dehydrogenase (BCKD), which catalyzes the metabolism of the branched-chain amino acids, leucine, isoleucine, and valine. People with MSUD have a defective BCKD protein complex resulting in buildup of toxic levels of these amino acids in the body.

❑ Who Should Be Suspected?

MSUD causes loss of appetite, fussiness, and sweet-smelling urine. The elevated levels of amino acids in the urine generate the smell, which is suggestive of maple syrup.

❑ Relevant Tests and Diagnostic Value

Biochemical testing:

- ■ Quantitative plasma amino acid analysis.
- ■ Tandem mass spectrometry (MS/MS)–based amino acid profiling. Newborn screening (NBS) programs that employ tandem mass spectrometry detect MSUD.
- ■ BCKAD enzyme activity.

Molecular diagnostic testing:

- ■ Gene sequencing and mutation analysis of the three genes: BCKDHA, BCKDHB, and DBT
- ■ Deletion/duplication analysis of the three genes BCKDHA, BCKDHB, and DBT

Molecular carrier testing: Targeted mutation analysis if the mutation is known.

Molecular prenatal testing: Targeted mutation analysis after familial mutation has been identified.

Suggested Reading

Strauss KA, Puffenberger EG, Morton DH. Maple syrup urine disease. In: Pagon RA, Adam MP, Bird TD, et al., eds. *GeneReviews™ [Internet]*. Seattle, WA: University of Washington, Seattle; 2006:1993–2013 [Updated 2013 May 9]. Available from: http://www.ncbi.nlm.nih.gov/books/NBK1319/

PHENYLKETONURIA (FOLLING DISEASE; PKU)

MIM #261600

❑ Definition

- ■ Phenylketonuria (PKU) is an autosomal recessive inborn error of metabolism resulting from a deficiency of phenylalanine hydroxylase (PAH), an enzyme that catalyzes the hydroxylation of phenylalanine to tyrosine, the rate-limiting step in phenylalanine catabolism. If untreated causes mental retardation, but with early diagnosis, it is treatable with dietary therapy.

❑ Relevant Tests and Diagnostic Value

PAH deficiency can be diagnosed by newborn screening based on detection of the presence of hyperphenylalaninemia using a blood spot obtained from a heel prick. Normal blood phenylalanine levels are 58 ± 15 μmol/L in adults, 60 ± 13 μmol/L in teenagers, and 62 ± 18 μmol/L (mean $\pm$ SD) in childhood. In the newborn, the upper limit of normal is 120 μmol/L (2 mg/dL). In untreated classical PKU, blood levels as high as 2.4 mM/L can be found.

Molecular genetic testing of PAH is used primarily for genetic counseling purposes to determine carrier status of at-risk relatives and for prenatal testing.

Suggested Readings

Blau N, van Spronsen FJ, Levy HL. Phenylketonuria. *Lancet.* 2010;376:1417–1427.
Scriver CR. The PAH gene, phenylketonuria, and a paradigm shift. *Hum Mutat.* 2007;28: 831–845.

 # LYSOSOMAL STORAGE DISORDERS

CANAVAN DISEASE

MIM #271900

❏ Definition
Canavan disease is an autosomal recessive disorder caused by mutations in the gene encoding aspartoacylase (ASPA) that results in progressive damage of nerve cells in the brain. This disease belongs to a group of genetic disorders called leuko-dystrophies, which are characterized by degeneration of myelin.

❏ Relevant Tests and Diagnostic Value
The diagnosis of neonatal/infantile Canavan disease is possible by demonstration of very high concentration of N-acetyl aspartic acid (NAA) in the urine. In mild/ juvenile Canavan disease, NAA may only be slightly elevated. The aspartoacylase enzyme activity is not a reliable test. *Molecular genetic testing*—the diagnosis relies on molecular genetic testing of ASPA gene.

- Targeted mutation analysis—testing for three mutations in the ASPA gene: Glu285Ala, p.Tyr231X, and p.Ala305Glu detect 98% of disease alleles in the Ashkenazi population and 30–60% of disease alleles in the non-Ashkenazi European population.
- Sequence analysis of the ASPA coding region is recommended for individuals in whom mutations were not identified by targeted mutation analysis.
- Deletion/duplication analysis—is recommended when mutations were not found by sequence analysis. There are known cases of complete deletion and of partial deletions in ASPA gene.

Suggested Reading

Matalon R, Michals-Matalon K. Canavan disease. In: Pagon RA, Adam MP, Bird TD, et al., eds. *GeneReviews™ [Internet].* Seattle, WA: University of Washington, Seattle; 1999:1993–2013 [Updated 2011 Aug 11]. Available from: http://www.ncbi.nlm.nih.gov/books/NBK1234/

CYSTINOSIS (CYSTINOSIS, NEPHROPATHIC; CTNS)

MIM #219800

❏ Definition
Cystinosis is an autosomal recessive inherited disease caused by impaired transport of cystine from lysosomes to cytoplasm that results in intralysosomal accumulation of cystine. There are three clinical forms of cystinosis: infantile (nephropathic) cystinosis; late-onset cystinosis; and benign cystinosis.

❏ Who Should Be Suspected?

Infantile cystinosis is the most severe and the most common type of cystinosis. Children with nephropathic cystinosis appear normal at birth, but by 9–10 months of age, have symptoms that include excessive thirst and urination and failure to thrive. The abnormally high loss of phosphorus in the urine leads to rickets. The longer-term manifestations of cystinosis, primarily in older patients and as a result of renal transplantation, include pancreatic endocrine and exocrine insufficiency, and recurrent corneal erosions, CNS involvement, and severe myopathy.

❏ Relevant Tests and Diagnostic Values

- Cystine measurement in blood cells, amniotic fluid cells, and chorionic villi.
- Sequence analysis of the *CTNS* gene (chr17p13.2) is clinically available; >50 mutations have been identified. However, in approximately 20% of patients, no mutation is identified.
- FISH analysis detects a relatively common 57 kb deletion in the *CTNS* gene.

❏ Other Considerations

- Kidney biopsy can demonstrate cystine crystals and destructive changes to the kidney cells and structures.

Suggested Reading

Bendavid C, Kleta R, Long R, et al. FISH diagnosis of the common 57 kb deletion in CTNS causing cystinosis. *Hum Genet*. 2004;115:510–514.

FABRY DISEASE (ANGIOKERATOMA CORPORIS DIFFUSUM, ANDERSON-FABRY DISEASE)

MIM #301500

❏ Definition

Fabry disease is a rare X-linked recessive lysosomal storage disease caused by a deficiency of α-galactosidase A (α-gal A) that results in progressive accumulation of globotriaosylceramide (Gb3) and related glycosphingolipids in plasma and vascular endothelium. This glycosphingolipid accumulation leads to ischemia and infarction in various organs (e.g., kidney, heart, brain, eye, nerves). Characteristic findings include angiokeratomas of skin and a whorl-like corneal pattern of cream-colored lines. Heterozygous females are not just carriers, and they may have mild or severe disease.

❏ Relevant Tests and Diagnostic Value

- α-Galactosidase measurement in blood cells in male patients.
- Sequence analysis of the *GLA* gene (Xq22.1) is clinically available. Females should have DNA testing, as enzyme assay testing is not generally useful for diagnosing Fabry disease in females.
- Measurement of globotriaosylceramide (Gb3) increased concentrations of globotriaosylceramide (Gb3).

❏ Other Considerations

Enzyme replacement therapy is available.

Suggested Reading

Aerts JM, Groener JE, Kuiper S, et al. Elevated globotriaosylsphingosine is a hallmark of Fabry disease. *Proc Nat Acad Sci U S A*. 2008;105:2812–2817.

FARBER DISEASE (FARBER LIPOGRANULOMATOSIS; ACID CERAMIDASE DEFICIENCY)

MIM #22800

❑ **Definition**

This disease is a rare autosomal recessive lysosomal storage disease caused by deficiency of acid ceramidase (also called N-acylsphingosine amidohydrolase). Mutations in the acid ceramidase gene, located at 8p22, result in a defect in glycolipid degradation (ceramide), causing accumulation of ceramide, leading to abnormalities in the joints, liver, throat, tissues, and CNS.

❑ **Classification**

Type 1 (classic): The diagnosis can be made by noting the triad of subcutaneous nodules, arthritis, and laryngeal involvement.

Types 2 and 3: Patients survive longer. The liver and lung appear not to be involved. Normal intelligence in many of these patients and the postmortem findings suggest that brain involvement is limited or not present. Several patients with type 3 disease may survive in relatively stable condition well into the second decade.

Type 4: Patients present with hepatosplenomegaly and severe disability in the neonatal period and die before 6 months of age. Massive histiocytic infiltration of the liver, spleen, lungs, thymus, and lymphocytes is found at autopsy.

Type 5: Characterized particularly by psychomotor deterioration beginning at age 1–2.5 years.

❑ **Relevant Tests and Diagnostic Value**

Biochemical testing:

- Enzyme assay: Acid ceramidase assay of skin fibroblasts.
- Analyte: based on giving cultured cells ^{14}C-stearic acid sulfatide and determining the amount of radiolabeled ceramide accumulating in cultured cells after 3 days.
- Histologic appearance is granulomatous. In the nervous system, both neurons and glial cells are swollen with stored material characteristic of nonsulfonated acid mucopolysaccharide.

Molecular testing:

- Sequence analysis: Analysis of the entire coding region of the *ASAH* gene

Suggested Readings

Li CM, Park JH, He X, et al. The human acid ceramidase gene (ASAH): structure, chromosomal location, mutation analysis and expression. *Genomics.* 2000;62:223–231.

MIM, Online Mendelian Inheritance in Man, John Hopkins University: Farber Lipogranulomatosis, http://www.ncbi.nlm.nih.gov/mim

10

GAUCHER DISEASE (ACID BETA-GLUCOSIDASE DEFICIENCY; GBA DEFICIENCY)

MIM #230800

❑ **Definition**

Gaucher disease, the most common lysosomal storage disorder, is caused by the autosomal recessively inherited deficiency of acid β-glucosidase (glucocerebrosidase;

GBA). Mutations in the GBA gene, located at 1q21, result in accumulation of the glycosphingolipid glucosylceramide within lysosomes, predominantly in macrophages.

❏ Who Should Be Suspected?

Among individuals of Ashkenazi Jewish descent, the incidence of type 1 Gaucher disease is approximately 1 in 500–1,000, with a carrier frequency of approximately 1 in 15 individuals. In contrast, Gaucher disease is seen in only 1 in 50,000–100,000 individuals in the general population.

❏ Classification

Type 1 (nonneuronopathic) is the most common form of the disease and does not involve the CNS. The clinical manifestations of type 1 Gaucher disease are heterogeneous, can come to attention from infancy to adulthood, and can range from very mildly affected individuals to those having rapidly progressive systemic abnormalities.

Type 2 is very rare, rapidly progressive, and affects the brain as well as the organs affected in type 1 Gaucher disease. It is usually fatal by 2 years of age.

Type 3. The signs and symptoms appear in early childhood, with onset much later than type 2. Some patients have ophthalmoplegia as the only neurologic abnormality, but more severe presentations are variable and include supranuclear horizontal ophthalmoplegia, progressive myoclonic epilepsy, cerebellar ataxia, spasticity and dementia, as well as the signs and symptoms seen in type 1.

❏ Relevant Tests and Diagnostic Value

Biochemical testing—enzyme assay: Acid β-glucosylceramidase activity in WBCs (lymphocytes) or skin cells (fibroblasts). The overlap in the range of GBA enzyme activity values between noncarriers and Gaucher disease carriers makes enzyme testing only about 90% accurate for identification of carriers.

Molecular testing:

■ Targeted mutation analysis: Available for four common mutations (N370S, L444P, 84GG, and IVS2 + 1G>A), which account for approximately 90% of the disease-causing alleles in the Ashkenazi Jewish population and 50–60% in non-Jewish populations. Some laboratories offer testing for additional seven "rare" mutations (V394L, D409H, D409V, R463C, R463H, R496H, and a 55-base-pair deletion in exon 9). DNA testing needs to distinguish mutations in the functional GBA gene from sequences present in the highly homologous GBA pseudogene.

■ Sequence analysis: Analysis of the entire coding region or exons. More than 150 GBA gene mutations have been described. Non-Jewish individuals with Gaucher disease tend to be compound heterozygotes that include one common mutation.

Suggested Readings

Beutler E, Nguyen NJ, Henneberger MW, et al. Gaucher disease: gene frequencies in the Ashkenazi Jewish population. *Am J Hum Genet.* 1993;52(1):85–88.

Horowitz M, Pasmanik-Chor M, Borochowitz Z, et al. Prevalence of glucocerebrosidase mutations in the Israeli Ashkenazi Jewish population. *Hum Mutat.* 1998;12(4):240–244. [Erratum in: *Hum Mutat.* 1999;13(3):255.]

Tsuji S, Choudary PV, Martin BM, et al. A mutation in the human glucocerebrosidase gene in neuronopathic Gaucher disease. *N Engl J Med.* 1987;361:570–575.

GLYCOGEN STORAGE DISEASE, TYPE I (GLUCOSE-6-PHOSPHATASE DEFICIENCY, VON GIERKE DISEASE)

MIM #232200

❑ **Definition**

Glycogen storage disease (GSD) type I is the most common of the glycogen storage disorders. This genetic disease results from deficiency of either the enzyme glucose-6-phosphatase (type Ia) or a glucose-6-phosphate translocase transporter (type Ib). The lack of either glucose-6-phosphatase catalytic activity or glucose-6-phosphate translocase activity in the liver leads to inadequate conversion of glucose-6-phosphate into glucose through normal glycogenolysis and gluconeogenesis, resulting in hypoglycemia, lactic acidosis, hyperuricemia, hyperlipidemia, hepatomegaly, and renomegaly.

❑ **Relevant Tests and Diagnostic Value**

Chemistry:

- Fasting blood glucose concentration <60 mg/dL (reference range: 70–120 mg/dL)
- Blood lactate >2.5 mmol/L (reference range: 0.5–2.2 mmol/L)
- Blood uric acid >5.0 mg/dL (reference range: 2.0–5.0 mg/dL)
- Triglycerides >250 mg/dL (reference range: 150–200 mg/dL)
- Cholesterol >200 mg/dL (reference range: 100–200 mg/dL)

Biochemical testing:

- Glucose-6-phosphatase enzyme activity in the liver: In most individuals with type Ia disease, the activity of the glucose-6-phosphatase is <10% (normal is 3.50 ± 0.8 μmol/minute/g tissue). In rare individuals with higher residual enzyme activity and milder clinical manifestations, the enzyme activity could be higher (>1.0 μmol/minute/g tissue).
- Glucose-6-phosphate translocase (transporter) activity: Most clinical diagnostic laboratories refrain from offering this enzyme activity assay because fresh (unfrozen) liver is often needed to assay enzyme activity accurately.

Molecular testing:

The two genes known to be associated with type I disease are *G6PC* (type Ia) and *SLC37A4* (type Ib). Mutations in *G6PC* (type Ia) are responsible for 80% of GSD type I, while mutations in the *SLC37A4* (type Ib) transporter gene are responsible for 20% of GSD type I.

- Targeted mutation analysis
  - ▼ *G6PC* gene: Arg83Cys and Gln347X or larger panels of mutations
  - ▼ *SLC37A4* gene: Trp118Arg, 1042_1043delCT, and Gly339Cys
- Gene sequence analysis
  - ▼ *G6PC:* Detects mutations in up to 100% of affected individuals in some homogeneous populations, but in mixed populations (e.g., in the United States), the detection rate is approximately 94%.
  - ▼ *SLC37A4:* Detects mutations in up to 100% of affected individuals in some homogeneous populations, but in mixed populations (e.g., in the United States), the detection frequency could be lower because both mutations may not be detected in some individuals.

10

Suggested Readings

Bali DS, Chen YT. Glycogen storage disease type I. In: Pagon RA, Bird TC, Dolan CR, et al., eds. *GeneReviews [Internet]*. Seattle, WA: University of Washington, Seattle; 1993–2006 Apr 19 [updated 2008 Sep 02].

Ekstein J, Rubin BY, Anderson SL, et al. Mutation frequencies for glycogen storage disease Ia in the Ashkenazi Jewish population. *Am J Med Genet.* 2004;129A:162–164.

GLYCOGEN STORAGE DISEASE, TYPE II (POMPE DISEASE; ACID ALPHA-GLUCOSIDASE DEFICIENCY; ACID MALTASE DEFICIENCY)

MIM #606800

❑ Definition

GSD, type II, is an autosomal recessive disorder caused by mutations in the acid alpha-glucosidase gene (17q25.3) that result in the deficiency or dysfunction of the lysosomal hydrolase acid alpha-glucosidase (GAA). This enzymatic defect results in lysosomal glycogen accumulation in multiple tissues, with cardiac and skeletal muscle tissues most severely affected.

❑ Classification

- Classic infantile onset: May be apparent in utero but more often presents in the 1st month of life with hypotonia, motor delay/muscle weakness, cardiomegaly and hypertrophic cardiomyopathy, feeding difficulties, failure to thrive, respiratory distress, and hearing loss.
- Nonclassic infantile onset: Usually presents within the 1st year of life with motor delays and/or slowly progressive muscle weakness.
- Late onset (i.e., childhood, juvenile, and adult onset) is characterized by proximal muscle weakness and respiratory insufficiency without cardiac involvement; these patients may have residual GAA activity <40% of normal when measured in skin fibroblasts.

❑ Relevant Tests and Diagnostic Value

Chemical tests

- Serum CK: Elevated as high as 2,000 IU/L (normal: 60–305 IU/L) in classic infantile onset and in the childhood and juvenile variants but may be normal in adult-onset disease. However, because serum CK concentration is elevated in many other conditions, this test is nonspecific.
- Urinary oligosaccharides: Elevation of a certain urinary glucose tetrasaccharide is highly sensitive in Pompe disease but is also seen in other glycogen storage diseases. In addition, it may be normal in late-onset disease.

Biochemical testing

- Acid α-GAA enzyme activity in cultured skin fibroblasts, whole blood, or dried bloodspot (confirmation by a second method is preferred). Activity <1% of normal controls (complete deficiency) is associated with classic infantile-onset Pompe disease. Activity 2–40% of normal controls (partial deficiency) is associated with the nonclassic infantile-onset and the late-onset forms.

Muscle biopsy: Glycogen storage may be observed in the lysosomes of muscle cells as vacuoles of varying severity that stain positively with periodic acid–Schiff.

However, 20–30% of individuals with late-onset type II GSD with documented partial enzyme deficiency may not show these muscle-specific changes.

Molecular testing: GAA is the only gene known to be associated with GSD II.

- Targeted mutation analysis: Depending on ethnicity and phenotype, an individual could be tested first for one of the three common mutations—Asp645Glu, Arg854X, and IVS1—13T>G—before proceeding to full-sequence analysis.
- Gene sequence analysis: In 83–93% of individuals with confirmed reduced or absent GAA enzyme activity, two mutations can be detected by sequencing genomic DNA.
- Deletion/duplication analysis: Deletion of exon 18 was seen in approximately 5–7% of alleles; single-exon deletions as well as multiexonic deletions have been seen rarely.

❑ Other Considerations

Histochemical evidence of glycogen storage in muscle is supportive of a glycogen storage disorder but not specific for Pompe disease. CK, AST, ALT, and LDH if elevated, may be useful in the initial evaluation of a patient but must be considered nonspecific.

Suggested Readings

ACMG Work Group on Management of Pompe Disease. Pompe disease diagnosis and management guideline. *Genet Med.* 2006;8(5):382.

Tinkle BT, Leslie N. Glycogen storage disease type II (Pompe Disease). In: Pagon RA, Bird TC, Dolan CR, et al., eds. *GeneReviews [Internet].* Seattle, WA: University of Washington, Seattle; 1993–2007 Aug 31 [updated 2010 Aug 12].

GM₁ GANGLIOSIDOSIS (LANDING DISEASE, SYSTEMIC LATE INFANTILE LIPIDOSIS, BETA-GALACTOSIDASE-1 DEFICIENCY)

MIM #230500

❑ Definition

GM_1 gangliosidosis is an autosomal recessive lysosomal storage disease characterized by accumulation of ganglioside substrates in lysosomes due to a deficiency of beta-galactosidase-1 (GLB1).

❑ Classification

The three main clinical presentations have variable residual beta-galactosidase activity and show different degrees of neurodegeneration and skeletal abnormalities.

- Type I, or infantile form, shows rapid psychomotor deterioration within 6 months of birth, generalized CNS involvement, hepatosplenomegaly, facial dysmorphism, macular cherry-red spots, skeletal dysplasia, and early death.
- Type II, or late-infantile/juvenile form, has onset between 7 months and 3 years, shows generalized CNS involvement with psychomotor deterioration, seizures, localized skeletal involvement, and survival into childhood. Hepatosplenomegaly and cherry-red spots are usually not present.
- Type III, or adult/chronic form, onsets from 3 to 30 years and is characterized by skeletal involvement and localized CNS abnormalities, such as dystonia or gait or speech disturbance. There is an inverse correlation between disease severity and residual enzyme activity.

❏ **Relevant Tests and Diagnostic Value**

▪ Assay of lysosomal acid beta-galactosidase enzyme in leukocytes, cultured fibroblasts, or brain tissue
▪ Prenatal diagnosis by enzyme assay in cultured amniotic fluid cells or by HPLC analysis of galactosyl oligosaccharides in amniotic fluid
▪ Sequence analysis of gene mutations

❏ **Other Considerations**

▪ Tissue biopsy or culture of marrow or skin fibroblasts shows accumulation of GM$_1$ ganglioside.

Suggested Reading

Suzuki Y, Oshima A, Nanba E. Beta-galactosidase deficiency (beta-galactosidosis): GM1 gangliosidosis and Morquio B disease. In: Scriver CR, Beaudet AL, Sly WS, et al., eds. *The Metabolic and Molecular Bases of Inherited Disease. Vol. II.* 8th ed. New York: McGraw-Hill; 2001:3775–3809.

HUNTER SYNDROME (MUCOPOLYSACCHARIDOSIS II; IDURONATE-2-SULFATASE DEFICIENCY)

MIM #309900

❏ **Definition**

Mucopolysaccharidosis II arises from iduronate-2-sulfatase (I2S) deficiency, which results in tissue deposits of mucopolysaccharides and urinary excretion of large amounts of chondroitin sulfate B and heparitin sulfate. This sex-linked type of mucopolysaccharidosis differs from mucopolysaccharidosis I in being on the average less severe and in not showing corneal clouding. Features are dysostosis with dwarfism, grotesque facies, hepatosplenomegaly from mucopolysaccharide deposits, cardiovascular disorders from mucopolysaccharide deposits in the intima, deafness, and excretion of large amounts of chondroitin sulfate B and heparitin sulfate in the urine.

❏ **Relevant Tests and Diagnostic Value**

▪ Quantitation of total glucosaminoglycans in urine and accumulation of keratan sulfate in tissues
▪ Definitive diagnosis is established by iduronate-2-sulfatase enzyme assay in cultured fibroblasts, leukocytes, amniocytes, or chorionic villi
▪ Sequence analysis of the iduronate-2-sulfatase gene

❏ **Other Considerations**

Hunter syndrome is clinically similar to Hurler syndrome but milder, with no corneal opacity. Maternal serum shows increased activity of iduronate sulfate sulfatase with a normal or heterozygous fetus but no increase if fetus has Hunter syndrome.

Suggested Reading

Jonsson JJ, Aronovich EL, Braun SE, et al. Molecular diagnosis of mucopolysaccharidosis type II (Hunter syndrome) by automated sequencing and computer-assisted interpretation: toward mutation mapping of the iduronate-2-sulfatase gene. *Am J Hum Genet*. 1995;56:597–607.

HURLER SYNDROME (MUCOPOLYSACCHARIDOSIS 1H, MPS1-H)

MIM #607014

❑ **Definition**

Hurler syndrome is an autosomal inherited disorder caused by mutations in the gene encoding alpha-L-iduronidase (IDUA) at 4p16.3 that hydrolyzes the terminal alpha-L-iduronic acid residues of the glycosaminoglycans dermatan sulfate and heparan sulfate. The accumulation of partially degraded glycosaminoglycans interferes with cell, tissue, and organ function.

❑ **Who Should Be Suspected?**

Deficiency of alpha-L-iduronidase can result in a wide range of phenotypic involvement with three major recognized clinical entities: Hurler (mucopolysaccharidosis IH), Scheie (mucopolysaccharidosis IS), and Hurler-Scheie (mucopolysaccharidosis IH/S) syndromes. Hurler and Scheie syndromes represent phenotypes at the severe and mild ends of the mucopolysaccharidosis I clinical spectrum, respectively, and the Hurler-Scheie syndrome is intermediate in phenotypic expression.

❑ **Relevant Tests and Diagnostic Value**

- Urinary excretion of glycosaminoglycans.
- Definitive diagnosis is established by alpha-L-iduronidase enzyme assay using artificial substrates (fluorogenic or chromogenic) in cultured fibroblasts, leukocytes, amniocytes, or chorionic villi.
- Sequence analysis of the IDUA gene.

Suggested Reading

Hall CW, Liebaers I, Di Natale P, et al. Enzymic diagnosis of the genetic mucopolysaccharide storage disorders. *Methods Enzymol.* 1978;50:439–456.

10

I-CELL DISEASE (MUCOLIPIDOSIS II)

MIM #252500

❑ **Definition**

I-cell disease is an autosomal recessive disorder resulting from mutations in GNPTAB gene (12q23.2) causing deficient activity of N-acetylglucosamine-1-phosphotransferase. This results in abnormal lysosomal enzyme localization and phosphorylation and buildup of lysosomal substrates.

❑ **Who Should Be Suspected?**

Clinical features resemble Hurler syndrome, but without corneal changes or increased mucopolysaccharides in urine. Congenital dislocation of the hip, thoracic deformities, hernia, and hyperplastic gums are evident soon after birth.

❑ **Relevant Test and Diagnostic Value**

Sequence analysis of the N-acetylglucosamine-1-phosphotransferase gene.

Suggested Readings

Canfield WM, Bao M, Pan J, et al. Mucolipidosis II and mucolipidosis IIIA are caused by mutations in the GlcNAc-phosphotransferase alpha/beta gene on chromosome 12p. (Abstract.) *Am J Hum Genet.* 1998;63:A15.

Tiede S, Storch S, Lubke T, et al. Mucolipidosis II is caused by mutations in GNPTA encoding the alpha/beta GlcNAc-1-phosphotransferase. *Nature Med.* 2005;11:1109–1112.

KRABBE DISEASE (GLOBOID CELL LEUKODYSTROPHY; GALACTOCEREBROSIDASE DEFICIENCY)

MIM #234200

❏ Definition

Krabbe disease is an autosomal recessive disorder caused by mutations in the galactosylceramidase (*GALC*) gene (14q31) with pathology involving the white matter of the CNS as well as abnormalities of the peripheral nervous system. Although most patients present within the first 6 months of life ("infantile" or "classic" disease); others present later in life, including in adulthood.

❏ Relevant Tests and Diagnostic Value

Biochemical testing—enzyme assay: GALC activity is deficient (0–5% of normal) in leukocytes isolated from whole heparinized blood or in cultured skin fibroblasts. However, measuring GALC enzyme activity for carrier testing is unreliable because of the wide range of enzymatic activities observed in carriers and noncarriers.

Molecular testing

- Targeted mutation analysis: The 809G>A mutation is often found in individuals with the late-onset form of Krabbe disease.
- Sequence analysis of the entire coding region, intron–exon boundaries, and 5′-untranslated region: Detects 100% of the disease-causing mutations and polymorphisms.
- Deletion/duplication analysis: Deletions involving single exons and multiple exons have been detected. A 30-kb deletion accounts for approximately 45% of the mutant alleles in individuals of European ancestry and 35% of the mutant alleles in individuals of Mexican heritage with infantile Krabbe disease.

❏ Other Considerations

Conjunctival biopsy shows characteristic ballooned Schwann cells. Brain biopsy (massive infiltration of unique multinucleated inclusion-containing globoid cells in white matter due to accumulation of galactosylceramide; also diffuse loss of myelin, severe astrocytic gliosis).

CSF protein electrophoresis shows increased albumin and α-globulin and decreased β- and γ-globulin (same as in metachromatic leukodystrophy).

Suggested Readings

Svennerholm L, Vanier, MT, Hakansson G, et al. Use of leukocytes in diagnosis of Krabbe disease and detection of carriers. *Clin Chim Acta.* 1981;112:333–342.

Wenger DA, Rafi MA, Luzi P, et al. Krabbe disease: genetic aspects and progress toward therapy. *Molec Gen Metab.* 2000;70:1–9.

Wenger DA, Sattler M, Hiatt W. Globoid cell leukodystrophy: deficiency of lactosyl ceramide beta-galactosidase. *Proc Nat Acad Sci U S A.* 1974;71:854–857.

MAROTEAUX-LAMY SYNDROME (ARYLSULFATASE B DEFICIENCY; MUCOPOLYSACCHARIDOSIS VI)

MIM #253200

❑ **Definition**

Mucopolysaccharidosis type VI is an autosomal recessive lysosomal storage disorder resulting from a deficiency of N-acetylgalactosamine-4-sulfatase (arylsulfatase B; ARSB)

❑ **Who Should Be Suspected?**

Clinical features and severity are variable but usually include short stature, hepatosplenomegaly, dysostosis multiplex, stiff joints, corneal clouding, cardiac abnormalities, and facial dysmorphism. Intelligence is usually normal.

❑ **Relevant Tests and Diagnostic Value**

- Measurement of residual N-acetylgalactosamine-4-sulfatase in fibroblasts
- Sequence analysis of the *ARSB* gene (5q14.1)

Suggested Reading

Litjens T, Brooks DA, Peters C, et al. Identification, expression, and biochemical characterization of N-acetylgalactosamine-4-sulfatase mutations and relationship with clinical phenotype in MPS-VI patients. *Am J Hum Genet.* 1996;58:1127–1134.

METACHROMATIC LEUKODYSTROPHY (ARYLSULFATASE A DEFICIENCY)

MIM #250100

10

❑ **Definition**

Metachromatic leukodystrophy is a rare autosomal recessive lipidosis caused by a deficiency of arylsulfatase A (ARSA). There are infantile and adult forms caused by the inability to degrade sphingolipid, sulfatide, or galactosylceramide that results in accumulation of sulfatide. The metachromatic leukodystrophies comprise several allelic disorders, including late infantile, juvenile, and adult forms; partial cerebroside sulfate deficiency; and pseudoarylsulfatase A deficiency; and two nonallelic forms: metachromatic leukodystrophy due to saposin B deficiency and multiple sulfatase deficiency or juvenile sulfatidosis, a disorder that combines features of a mucopolysaccharidosis with those of metachromatic leukodystrophy.

❑ **Relevant Tests**

Biochemical testing

- *ARSA activity*: Measured in leukocytes or cultured fibroblasts or amniocytes; <10% enzyme activity compared to normal controls is suggestive of metachromatic leukodystrophy. However, this test is not diagnostic due to possible ARSA pseudodeficiency that is 5–20% of normal controls. Pseudodeficiency is difficult to distinguish from true ARSA deficiency by biochemical testing. Therefore, one of the other tests needs to be used for diagnosis confirmation.

- *Urinary excretion of sulfatides*: Measured by thin-layer chromatography, HPLC, and/or mass spectrometric techniques. Amount of sulfatides in metachromatic leukodystrophy is 10- to 100-fold higher than in controls. Urinary sulfatide excretion is referenced on the basis of urinary excretion in 24 hours or to another urinary component such as creatinine (which is a function of muscle mass) or sphingomyelin (newer approach).
- *Metachromatic lipid deposits in a nerve or brain biopsy*: Highly invasive approach used only in exceptional circumstances (such as confirmation of a prenatal diagnosis of *metachromatic leukodystrophy following pregnancy termination*).

Molecular methods

- *Targeted mutation analysis*: Four most commonly tested mutations in the ARSA gene (22q13.33) are c.459 + 1G>A, c.1204 + 1G>A, Pro426Leu, and Ile179Ser. These four mutations account for 25–50% of the ARSA mutations in European and North American populations. Pseudodeficiency variants (ARSA-PD) are common polymorphisms that result in lower than average but sufficient enzyme activity to avoid sulfatide accumulation and thus do not cause MLD. The two most commonly tested ARSA-PD mutations are missense mutations: c.1049A>G mutation and the polyadenylation-site mutation c.1524 + 96A>G.
- *Gene sequence mutation analysis*: >150 mutations in the *ARSA* gene associated with arylsulfatase A deficiency have been reported. Sequencing is expected to detect 97% of ARSA mutations including small deletions, insertions, and inversions within exons.
- *Deletion/duplication analysis*: Gene deletion is rare; no cases of full gene duplication are known. A case of dispermic chimerism has been reported where two ARSA genes were obtained from the father, one with a metachromatic leukodystrophy–causing mutation and the other normal.

❏ **Diagnostic Value**

- Absence of ARSA activity in the urine is useful for early diagnosis.
- Keratan sulfate is increased in urine (often two to three times normal).
- Urine sediment may contain metachromatic lipids (from breakdown of myelin products).

❏ **Other Considerations**

Biopsy of dental or sural nerve stained with cresyl violet showing accumulation of metachromatic sulfatide is diagnostic; also increased in the brain, kidney, and liver. Pseudoarylsulfatase A deficiency refers to a condition of apparent ARSA enzyme deficiency and cerebroside sulfatase activity in leukocytes in persons without neurologic abnormalities in a metachromatic leukodystrophy family. Conjunctival biopsy shows metachromatic inclusions within Schwann cells.

Suggested Reading

Polten A, Fluharty AL, Fluharty CB, et al. Molecular basis of different forms of metachromatic leukodystrophy. *N Eng J Med*. 1991;324:18–22.

MORQUIO SYNDROME (MUCOPOLYSACCHARIDOSIS IVA; GALNS DEFICIENCY)

MIM #253000

❑ **Definition**

Morquio syndrome, mucopolysaccharidosis type IVA, is an autosomal recessive lysosomal storage disease characterized by intracellular accumulation of keratan sulfate and chondroitin-6-sulfate.

❑ **Who Should Be Suspected?**

Key clinical features include short stature, skeletal dysplasia, dental anomalies, and corneal clouding. Intelligence is normal, and there is no direct CNS involvement, although the skeletal changes may result in neurologic complications.

❑ **Relevant Tests and Diagnostic Value**

- Enzyme assay in fibroblasts, leukocytes, or amniocytes
- Sequence analysis of the *GALNS* gene (16q24.3)

Suggested Reading

Sukegawa K, Nakamura H, Kato Z, et al. Biochemical and structural analysis of missense mutations in N-acetylgalactosamine-6-sulfate sulfatase causing mucopolysaccharidosis IVA phenotypes. *Hum Mol Genet.* 2000;9:1283–1290.

MUCOLIPIDOSIS III (*N*-ACETYLGLUCOSAMINE-1-PHOSPHATE TRANSFERASE DEFICIENCY; PSEUDO-HURLER DYSTROPHY)

MIM #252600

❑ **Definition**

Mucolipidosis III alpha/beta (classic pseudo-Hurler polydystrophy) is caused by mutation in the gene encoding the alpha/beta-subunits precursor gene of *N*-acetylglucosamine-1-phosphotransferase (GNPTAB; GlcNAc-phosphotransferase; 12q23). The clinical features of autosomal recessive type III mucolipidosis resemble those of Hurler syndrome but without increased mucopolysaccharides in urine due to a defect in recognition or catalysis and uptake of certain lysosomal enzymes due to deficient activity of N-acetylglucosamine-1-phosphotransferase.

❑ **Relevant Tests and Diagnostic Value**

- Enzyme assay in fibroblasts or leukocytes
- Sequence analysis of the *GNPTAB* gene

❑ **Other Considerations**

- Mucolipidosis II alpha/beta, or I-cell disease, is also caused by mutations in the GNPTAB gene.
- Mucolipidosis II has been renamed mucolipidosis II alpha/beta, mucolipidosis IIIA has been renamed mucolipidosis III alpha/beta, and mucolipidosis IIIC has been renamed mucolipidosis III gamma.

Suggested Reading

Bargal R, Zeigler M, Abu-Libdeh B, et al. When mucolipidosis III meets mucolipidosis II: GNPTA gene mutations in 24 patients. *Mol Genet Metab.* 2006;88:359–363.

NIEMANN-PICK DISEASE, TYPES A AND B (SPHINGOMYELINASE DEFICIENCY)

MIM #257200

❏ Definition and Classification

- Niemann-Pick disease (NPD) types A and B are allelic autosomal recessive disorders that result from a deficiency of acid sphingomyelinase (ASM; also called sphingomyelin phosphodiesterase, SMPD1) and the subsequent accumulation of sphingomyelin in lysosomes of the macrophage and monocytes.
  - ▼ Type A (NPD-A) is neuronopathic with death in early childhood.
  - ▼ Type B (NPD-B) is nonneuronopathic.

❏ Relevant Tests and Diagnostic Value

- *Biochemical testing*: ASM enzyme activity measured in peripheral blood lymphocytes or cultured skin fibroblasts; <10% enzyme activity compared to normal controls diagnoses ASM deficiency. However, it was reported that individuals with the *SMPD1* gene mutation Q292K may have apparently normal enzymatic activity when artificial substrate is used.
- *Bone marrow examination*: Reveals lipid-laden macrophages. However, this procedure is not necessary for diagnosis and should not be performed unless specific clinical indications are present.
- *Molecular testing*
  - ▼ Sequence analysis of *SMPD1* detects mutations in 99% of individuals with enzymatically confirmed ASM deficiency. Over 100 mutations causing ASM deficiency have been published.
  - ▼ Targeted mutation analysis
    - ● NPD-A mutations are more prevalent in the Ashkenazi Jewish population where the combined carrier frequency for the three common *SMPD1* gene mutations is between 1:80 and 1:100. Three mutations (R496L, L302P, and fsP330) account for approximately 90% of NPD-A disease–causing alleles in individuals of Ashkenazi Jewish background.
    - ● NPD-B mutations are panethnic. Testing for one mutation p.R608del (also known as deltaR608) may account for almost 90% of NPD-B mutant alleles in individuals from North Africa (Tunisia, Algeria, and Morocco), 100% of NPD-B mutant alleles in Gran Canaria Island, and about 20–30% of the NPD type B mutant alleles in persons of North African descent in the United States.

Suggested Readings

Brady RO, Kanfer JN, Mock MB, et al. The metabolism of sphingomyelin. II. Evidence of an enzymatic deficiency in Niemann-Pick disease. *Proc Natl Acad Sci U S A.* 1966;55(2): 366–369.

McGovern MM, Schuchman EH. Acid sphingomyelinase deficiency. In: Pagon RA, Bird TC, Dolan CR, et al., eds. *GeneReviews [Internet]*. Seattle, WA: University of Washington, Seattle; 1993–2006 Dec 07 [updated 2009 Jun 25].

NIEMANN-PICK DISEASE, TYPE C (NIEMANN-PICK DISEASE WITH CHOLESTEROL ESTERIFICATION BLOCK)

MIM #257220

❏ Definition and Classification

Niemann-Pick disease type C (NPD-C) is an autosomal recessive lipid storage disorder caused by mutations in the *NPC1* or *NPC2* genes involved in lipid trafficking, particularly cholesterol, from late endosomes or lysosomes and characterized by progressive neurodegeneration.

- NPD type C1, which is responsible for 95% of cases of NPD-C, is caused by mutations in the *NPC1* gene (18q11.2).
- NPD type C2, which is responsible for 5% of cases of NPD-C, is caused by mutations in the *NPC2* gene (18q11.2).

In addition, the term NPD type D used in a previous edition of this book describes a genetic isolate from Nova Scotia that is biochemically and clinically indistinguishable from NPD-C and that also results from mutation of the *NPC1* gene. Therefore, the previous NPD type D currently is NPD type C1.

❏ Relevant Tests and Diagnostic Value

Biochemical testing

- The diagnosis of NPD-C can be confirmed by demonstrating impaired exogenously supplied cholesterol esterification in cultured fibroblasts or by cytologic technique—filipin staining—to demonstrate the intracellular accumulation of cholesterol in cultured fibroblasts.
- Note: These methods are unreliable for carrier testing due to significant overlap of results between patients and controls.

Histology: Tissue biopsies and tissue lipid analysis are now rarely needed. These tests include examination of the bone marrow, spleen, and liver, which contain foamy cells (lipid-laden macrophages); sea-blue histiocytes may be seen in the marrow in advanced cases.

Electron microscopy: The skin, rectal neurons, liver, or brain may show polymorphous cytoplasmic bodies.

Imaging: MRI of the brain is usually normal until the late stages of the illness. At that time, marked atrophy of the superior/anterior cerebellar vermis, thinning of the corpus callosum, and mild cerebral atrophy may be seen. Increased signal in the periatrial white matter, reflecting secondary demyelination, may also occur. Magnetic resonance spectroscopy may be more sensitive in NPD-C than standard MRI.

Molecular methods:

- Sequence analysis: Detects 80–90% of mutations in *NPC1* gene and close to all mutations in *NPC2* gene. Approximately 200 mutations have been described in NPD-C1. Most affected individuals with NPD-C1 have mutations unique to their family.

10

- Deletion/duplication analysis: Few partial and whole gene deletions have been reported for NPD-C1. No large insertions or deletions have been reported in NPD-C2.

❏ **Other Considerations**

Cholestatic jaundice occurs in some patients. Foamy Niemann-Pick cells and "sea-blue" histiocytes with distinctive histochemical and ultrastructural appearances are found in the bone marrow. In the childhood-onset form, death usually occurs at age 5–15. Adult-onset forms, with insidious onset and slower progression, have also been reported (NPD-E and -F).

Suggested Readings

Argoff CE, Kaneski CR, Blanchette-Mackie EJ, et al. Type C Niemann-Pick disease: documentation of abnormal LDL processing in lymphocytes. *Biochem Biophys Res Commun.* 1990;171:38–45.
Patterson M. Niemann-Pick disease type C. In: Pagon RA, Bird TC, Dolan CR, et al., eds. *GeneReviews [Internet].* Seattle, WA: University of Washington, Seattle; 1993–2000 Jan 26 [updated 2008 Jul 22].

SANFILIPPO TYPE A SYNDROME (HEPARAN SULFATASE DEFICIENCY; MUCOPOLYSACCHARIDOSIS IIIA)

MIM #252900

❏ **Definition**

The Sanfilippo syndrome is an autosomal recessive lysosomal storage disease due to impaired degradation of heparin sulfate caused by mutations in the gene encoding N-sulfoglucosamine sulfohydrolase (SGSH; 17q25,3).

❏ **Who Should Be Suspected?**

The clinical features are severe mental defect with relatively mild somatic features (moderately severe claw hand and visceromegaly, little or no corneal clouding or skeletal [e.g., vertebral] change). The presenting problem may be marked overactivity, destructive tendencies, and other behavioral aberrations in a child of 4–6 years of age. Onset of clinical features usually occurs between 2 and 6 years; severe neurologic degeneration occurs in most patients between 6 and 10 years of age, and death occurs typically during the second or third decade of life. Type A usually presents as the most severe, with earlier onset and rapid progression of symptoms and shorter survival.

❏ **Relevant Tests and Diagnostic Value**

Measurement of heparin sulfate in the urine is diagnostic.

❏ **Other Considerations**

- Mucopolysaccharidosis III includes four types, each due to the deficiency of a different enzyme: heparan N-sulfatase (type A); alpha-N-acetylglucosaminidase (type B); acetyl CoA:alpha-glucosaminide acetyltransferase (type C); and N-acetylglucosamine-6-sulfatase (type D).
- A Dachshund canine model of Sanfilippo syndrome type A is available.

Suggested Readings

Esposito S, Balzano N, Daniele A, et al. Heparan N-sulfatase gene: two novel mutations and transient expression of 15 defects. *Biochim Biophys Acta.* 2000;1501:1–11.

Schmidt R, von Figura K, Paschke E, et al. Sanfilippo's disease type A: sulfamidase activity in peripheral leukocytes of normal, heterozygous and homozygous individuals. *Clin Chim Acta.* 1977;80:7–16.

TAY-SACHS DISEASE (GM$_2$ GANGLIOSIDOSIS, TYPE I; HEXOSAMINIDASE A DEFICIENCY)

MIM #272800

❑ **Definition**

Tay-Sachs disease is an autosomal recessive lysosomal storage disease caused by mutations in the alpha subunit of the hexosaminidase A (*HEXA*) gene (15q23). It occurs predominantly in Ashkenazi Jews, French Canadians, and Cajuns.

❑ **Who Should Be Suspected?**

This disease is a progressive neurologic disorder which, in the classic infantile form, is characterized by psychomotor deterioration, blindness, macula cherry-red spot, and an exaggerated extension response to sound, with death usually by age 2 years. There is also a juvenile form (with death by age 15) and a chronic form in adults.

❑ **Relevant Tests and Diagnostic Value**

- Enzyme assay for HEXA in serum, plasma, leukocytes, and cultured amniotic cells and skin fibroblasts
- Sequencing for mutation analysis
- Accumulation of ganglioside GM$_2$ in the brain

❑ **Other Considerations**

Macula cherry-red spots appear only in the infantile form. Pseudodeficiency alleles 739C-T and 745C-T cause reduced HEXA activity but do not cause illness, and serum acid phosphatase is normal.

Suggested Reading

De Braekeleer M, Hechtman P, Andermann E, et al. The French Canadian Tay-Sachs disease deletion mutation: identification of probable founders. *Hum Genet.* 1992;89:83–87.

WOLMAN DISEASE (CHOLESTERYL ESTER STORAGE DISEASE, LAL DEFICIENCY, CHOLESTERYL ESTER HYDROLASE DEFICIENCY)

MIM #278000

❑ **Definition**

Wolman disease is an autosomal recessive disorder resulting from the deficiency of lysosomal acid lipase (LIPA; LAL) activity, causing accumulation of total cholesterol and triglycerides throughout body tissues. Two major disorders, the severe infantile-onset Wolman disease and the milder late-onset cholesteryl ester storage disease (CESD), are caused by mutations in different parts of the LIPA gene (10q23.21).

❑ **Relevant Tests and Diagnostic Value**

- Sequence analysis of the LIPA gene for mutations

- Assay of acid lipase activity in leukocytes, cultured fibroblasts, or cultured amniocytes

❏ **Other Considerations**

- Peripheral blood smear shows prominent vacuolation (in the nucleus and cytoplasm) of leukocytes. Abnormal liver function tests are caused by lipid accumulation.
- There is decreased adrenal cortical function with diffuse calcification on CT scan.

Suggested Readings

Anderson RA, Byrum RS, Coates PM, et al. Mutations at the lysosomal acid cholesteryl ester hydrolase gene locus in Wolman disease. *Proc Natl Acad Sci U S A.* 1994;91:2718–2722.

Assmann G, Fredrickson DS. Acid lipase deficiency (Wolman's disease and cholesteryl ester storage disease). In: Stanbury JB, Wyngaarden JB, Fredrickson DS, et al., eds. *Metabolic Basis of Inherited Disease.* 5th ed. New York: McGraw-Hill; 1983:803–819.

 # PEROXISOMAL DISORDERS

ADRENOLEUKODYSTROPHY (ALD)

MIM #300100

❏ **Definition**

Adrenoleukodystrophy is an X-linked disorder caused by mutation in the ABCD1 gene resulting in the defect of peroxisomal beta-oxidation and the accumulation of the saturated very long-chain fatty acids (VLCFA) in all tissues of the body. The manifestations of the disorder occur primarily in the adrenal cortex, the myelin of the central nervous system, and the Leydig cells of the testes. Even though men are largely affected with ALD, approximately 40% of X-ALD heterozygous females develop mild neurologic symptoms in their late 30s–40s.

❏ **Relevant Tests and Diagnostic Value**

Imaging studies: MRI is always abnormal in males with neurologic symptoms caused by ALD
  Very long-chain fatty acids (VLCFA) testing:

- Plasma concentration of VLCFA is abnormal in 99% of males; measurement of VLCFA is sufficient to establish the diagnosis in majority of man with ALD.
- Concentration of VLCFA is increased in plasma and/or cultured skin fibroblasts in approximately 85% of affected females.

Molecular genetic testing—recommended when the measurement of VLCFA is inconclusive, for identification of familial mutation, and for prenatal testing when the familial mutation was established.

- Sequence analysis of the entire coding region
- Deletion/duplication analysis

Suggested Readings

Steinberg SJ, Moser AB, Raymond GV. X-linked adrenoleukodystrophy. In: Pagon RA, Adam MP, Bird TD, et al., eds. *GeneReviews™ [Internet]*. Seattle, WA: University of Washington,

Seattle; 1999:1993–2013 [Updated 2012 Apr 19]. Available from: http://www.ncbi.nlm.nih.gov/books/NBK1315

BATTEN DISEASE (CLN3, BATTEN-SPIELMEYER-VOGT DISEASE, NEURONAL CEROID LIPOFUSCINOSIS)

MIM #204200

❏ **Definition**

The neuronal ceroid lipofuscinoses (NCLs or CLNs) are a clinically and genetically heterogeneous group of neurodegenerative disorders characterized by the intracellular accumulation of autofluorescent lipopigment storage material in different patterns ultrastructurally.

❏ **Who Should Be Suspected?**

The clinical course includes progressive dementia, seizures, and progressive visual failure. CLN3 is especially prevalent in Finland with an incidence of 1:21,000 live births and a carrier frequency of 1 in 70.

❏ **Relevant Tests and Diagnostic Value**

- Enzyme testing for CLN1 or CLN2 is useful before ordering DNA mutation screening for affected individuals. Enzyme testing is not a reliable carrier test.
- Sequence analysis for mutations.
- Detection of a 1.02-kb deletion in the CLN3 gene at 16p11.2 present in the majority of Batten disease cases.
- The hallmark of CLN3 is the ultrastructural pattern of lipopigment with a "fingerprint" profile, which can have three different appearances: pure within a lysosomal residual body; in conjunction with curvilinear or rectilinear profiles; and as a small component within large membrane-bound lysosomal vacuoles. The combination of fingerprint profiles within lysosomal vacuoles is a regular feature of blood lymphocytes from patients with CLN3.

❏ **Other Considerations**

Presentations of CLN are caused by mutations in eight genes. The CLNs were originally classified broadly by age at onset: CLN1 as the infantile-onset form or the infantile-onset Finnish form, having first been described in that population; CLN2 as the late infantile-onset form; CLN3 as the juvenile-onset and most common form; and CLN4 as the adult-onset form. With the identification of molecular defects, the CLNs are now classified numerically according to the underlying gene defect. For example, CLN1 refers to CLN caused by mutations in the *PPT1* gene, regardless of the age at onset.

Suggested Readings

International Batten Disease Consortium. Isolation of a novel gene underlying Batten disease, CLN3. *Cell.* 1995;82:949–957.

Mole SE, Williams RE, Goebel HH. Correlations between genotype, ultrastructural morphology and clinical phenotype in the neuronal ceroid lipofuscinoses. *Neurogenetics.* 2005;6: 107–126.

NEUROLOGIC DISORDERS

ALZHEIMER DISEASE (PRESENILE AND SENILE DEMENTIA)

MIM #104300

❑ **Definition**

Alzheimer disease (AD) is a progressive adult-onset dementia that typically begins with subtle memory failure that becomes more severe and incapacitating. Pathologic findings include cerebral cortical atrophy, beta-amyloid plaque formation, and intraneuronal neurofibrillary tangles. A genetic mutation in amyloid precursor protein (APP) that significantly decreases the amount of beta-amyloid by about 40% confers protection from developing Alzheimer's.

❑ **Who Should Be Suspected?**

- Early-onset familial Alzheimer disease (EOFAD) is associated with multiple affected family members having onset before 65 years (often before 55 years) and/or a mutation in the APP (AD1; 21q21.3), PSEN1(AD3), or PSEN2(AD4) genes that is are known to be associated with EOFAD.
- EOFAD is inherited in an autosomal dominant manner. Children of an affected parent have a 50% chance of inheriting a mutation causing EOFAD and genetic counseling can be helpful to at-risk individuals.
- Additional disease causing mutations remain to be identified.

❑ **Relevant Tests and Diagnostic Value**

- Sequence analysis for the A673T mutation in the APP gene that protects against Alzheimer disease and cognitive decline in the elderly without Alzheimer disease.
- Sequence analysis of the PSEN1 gene entire coding and associated intronic regions to detect missense and splice site mutations. Deletion/duplication analysis screening of the entire gene to detect deletions, including the 4,555 bp Finnish population mutation.
- Sequence analysis of the PSEN2 gene entire coding region to detect mutations causing EOFAD.
- Sequence analysis of APP gene exons 16 and 17 identifies most pathologic missense, nonsense, or indel mutations. FISH and other deletion/duplication analysis is useful to detect the <1% pathogenic duplication mutations in APP.

Suggested Readings

American College of Medical Genetics/American Society of Human Genetics Working Group on ApoE and Alzheimer's disease. Statement on use of apolipoprotein E testing for Alzheimer's disease. *JAMA.* 1995;274(20):1627–1629.

Bird TD. Early-onset familial Alzheimer disease. In: Pagon RA, Adam MP, Bird TD, et al., eds. *GeneReviews™ [Internet].* Seattle, WA: University of Washington, Seattle; 1999:1993–2013 [Updated 2012 Oct 18]. Available from: http://www.ncbi.nlm.nih.gov/books/NBK1236

Cao G, Bales KR, DeMattos RB, et al. Liver X receptor-mediated gene regulation and cholesterol homeostasis in brain: relevance to Alzheimer's disease therapeutics. *Curr Alzheimer Res.* 2007;4(2):179–184.

Jonsson T, et al. A mutation in *APP* protects against Alzheimer's disease and age-related cognitive decline. *Nature.* 2012;488:96–99.

ANGELMAN SYNDROME (AS)

MIM #105830

❑ **Definition**

Angelman syndrome is a neurodevelopmental disorder characterized by developmental delay, lack of speech, seizures, excessive laughter, jerky movements, and walking and balance disorders. Most cases are caused by absence of a maternal contribution to the imprinted region on chromosome 15q11-q13. Approximately 70% of AS cases result from de novo maternal deletions involving chromosome 15q11.2-q13; approximately 2–3% result from paternal uniparental disomy of 15q11.2-q13; 3–5% result from imprinting defects; 5–10% of cases are caused by mutations or deletions in the gene encoding the ubiquitin-protein ligase E3A gene (UBE3A); 1–2% by other chromosomal rearrangements; and 10–15% by unknown causes.

❑ **Relevant Tests and Diagnostic Value**

Laboratory diagnostic testing for AS can be complex. The evaluation of an individual suspected of AS may be initiated with DNA methylation analysis of the AS/PWS imprinting center region.

If the methylation test is positive, additional studies are needed to define which of these genetic mechanisms is present and causes the disease:

- The large common deletion can be tested by FISH (fluorescent in situ hybridization) or array-based comparative genomic hybridization [CGH]).
- Uniparental disomy—additional molecular testing involving parental bloods.
- Defects in the imprinting center (IC).

If the methylation test is negative, mutation analysis of the UBE3A gene may detect an abnormality.

Suggested Reading

Williams CA, Peters SU, Calculator SN. *Facts About Angelman Syndrome.* 7th ed. Aurora, IL: Angelman Syndrome Foundation Inc., 2009. Available from: http://www.angelman.org/understanding-as/facts-about-angelman-syndrome

10

FAMILIAL DYSAUTONOMIA

MIM #223900

❑ **Definition**

Familial dysautonomia (hereditary sensory and autonomic neuropathy type III, sometimes called Riley-Day syndrome) is an autosomal recessive disorder almost completely limited to persons of Ashkenazi Jewish heritage. It affects the development and survival of sensory, sympathetic, and parasympathetic neurons, resulting in variable symptoms including insensitivity to pain, inability to produce tears, poor growth, and labile blood pressure and leads to decreased life expectancy in affected individuals.

❑ **Relevant Tests and Diagnostic Value**

- Currently, the diagnosis of familial dysautonomia is established by molecular genetic testing of the *IKBKAP* (inhibitor of kappa light polypeptide gene enhancer in B cells, kinase complex–associated protein) gene.

- Targeted mutation analysis—available for two mutations, c.2204 + 6T>C (VS20 + 6T>C) and pR696P (Arg696Pro), which account for >99% of mutant alleles in individuals of Ashkenazi Jewish descent affected with familial dysautonomia.
- Sequence analysis: Analysis of the entire coding region of the *IKBKAP* gene.

Suggested Reading

Blumenfeld A, Slaugenhaupt SA, Liebert CB, et al. Precise genetic mapping and haplotype analysis of the familial dysautonomia gene on human chromosome 9q31. *Am J Hum Genet.* 1999;64:1110–1118.

FRAGILE X SYNDROME OF MENTAL RETARDATION/FMR1-RELATED DISORDERS

(MIM #300624)

❑ Definition

Fragile X syndrome is the most common form of inherited mental retardation. It is caused by loss of function of the *FMR1* gene on the X chromosome (Xq27.3). Most affected individuals carry an expansion of a triplet CGG repeat in the *FMR1* gene; rarely, other causes of loss-of-function gene mutations (point mutations, deletions, abnormal gene methylation) are causal.

❑ Who Should Be Suspected?

Typically, male full-expansion carriers are affected with mental retardation in the moderate range; there is some variation in the extent of methylation on the expanded allele leading to some variation in phenotype. Female full-expansion carriers frequently manifest disease symptoms but typically in a milder form. Premutation (allele expansion is greater than normal but less than the full expansion associated with fragile X syndrome) is associated with increased risk of premature ovarian failure and may cause fragile X–associated tremor/ataxia syndrome (FXTAS), a late-onset neurodegenerative disorder, mostly affecting male carriers.

❑ Relevant Tests and Diagnostic Value

Molecular Testing: Direct diagnosis by DNA analysis using Southern blotting, PCR, and methylation analysis. This can be performed for pre- and postnatal diagnosis and to detect asymptomatic carriers. Diagnostic value: identifies affected males and heterozygous/affected females.

Stretches of CGG repeats without an AGG "anchor" are more likely to expand than those with interspersed AGG interruptions. Normal size of the CGG sequence is between 5 and 44 repeats. Between 45 and 54 CGG repeats is considered a grey or intermediate zone. Individuals with 55 to 200 CGG repeats are considered premutation carriers. Most individuals with Frag X syndrome have an expansion of more than 200 CGG repeats that causes loss of function of *FMR1*.

Other: Full-sequence analysis is required to detect rare loss-of-function mutations such as point mutations/small deletions. Methylation results from a chorionic villus sample may or may not reflect the accurate future status in the child.

HUNTINGTON DISEASE

MIM #143100

❑ **Definition**

Huntington disease (HD), autosomal dominant progressive neurodegenerative disorder, is caused by an expanded trinucleotide repeat (CAG)n, encoding glutamine, in the gene encoding huntingtin (HTT) on chromosome 4p16.3. HTT alleles are classified based on the size of the expansion:

- Normal alleles: 26 or fewer CAG repeats.
- Intermediate alleles: 27–35 CAG repeats. An individual with an allele in this range is not at risk of developing symptoms of HD, but because of instability in the CAG tract, may be at risk of having a child with an allele in the HD-causing range.
- HD-causing (full mutation) alleles: 36 or more CAG repeats. Individuals who have an allele with full mutation are considered at risk of developing HD in their lifetime.

❑ **Relevant Tests and Diagnostic Value**

- HTT (HD) is the only gene known to cause Huntington disease. A CAG repeat expansion is the only mutation observed.
- Clinical testing:
  - ▼ PCR method to detect number of CAG trinucleotide repeats.
  - ▼ Southern blot is used for confirmation of homozygous genotype and identification of large expansions.
- Predictive testing for at-risk asymptomatic adult family members requires prior confirmation of the diagnosis in the family using molecular genetic testing.
- Prenatal diagnosis and preimplantation genetic diagnosis (PGD) for at-risk pregnancies require prior confirmation of the diagnosis in the family using molecular genetic testing.

Suggested Reading

Warby SC, Graham RK, Hayden MR. Huntington disease. In: Pagon RA, Adam MP, Bird TD, et al., eds. *GeneReviews™ [Internet]*. Seattle, WA: University of Washington, Seattle; 1998:1993–2013 Oct 23 [Updated 2010 Apr 22]. Available from: http://www.ncbi.nlm.nih.gov/books/NBK1305/

LESCH-NYHAN SYNDROME

MIM #300322

❑ **Definition**

Lesch-Nyhan syndrome is an X-linked recessive disorder with almost complete absence of hypoxanthine–guanine phosphoribosyltransferase (HGPRT), which catalyzes hypoxanthine and guanine to their nucleotides. Mutations in *HPRT1* (Xq26-q27.2) cause an accumulation of purines.

❑ **Who Should Be Suspected?**

Affected males manifest with neurologic dysfunction, cognitive and behavioral disturbances (choreoathetosis, mental retardation, and tendency to self-mutilation), and uric acid overproduction. Clinical manifestations are due to secondary gout (tophi after 10 years, crystalluria, hematuria, urinary calculi, UTI, gouty arthritis, response to colchicine). Patients die of renal failure by age 10 years unless treated. Orange crystals or sand is seen in infants' diapers.

❏ Relevant Tests and Diagnostic Value

- A urinary urate-to-creatinine ratio >2.0 is characteristic for affected male patients who are younger than 10 years of age but is not considered diagnostic. Neither hyperuricuria nor hyperuricemia (serum uric acid >8 mg/dL; 600–1,000 mg/24 hour in patients weighing ≥15 kg) is specific for diagnosis.
- Hypoxanthine–guanine phosphoribosyltransferase (HPRT) enzyme activity in male patients <1.5% of normal in blood cells, cultured fibroblasts, amniocytes, or lymphoblasts is diagnostic. The assay is possible on erythrocytes in anticoagulant or on dried blood spots on filter paper. Enzyme assay is not helpful in female patients.
- Sequence analysis of the *HPRT1* gene is available. More than 200 mutations (primarily missense and nonsense mutations and small deletions/insertions) have been identified.

❏ Other Considerations

- Variants with partial deficiency of HGPRT show 0–50% of normal activity in RBC hemolysates and >1.2% in fibroblasts; accumulate purines but no orange sand in diapers or abnormality of CNS or behavior.
- Probenecid and other uricosuric drugs designed to reduce the serum concentration of uric acid are contraindicated because they augment the delivery of uric acid into the urinary system and raise the risk of acute anuria from deposition of uric acid crystals in the renal collecting system.

Suggested Readings

Jinnah HA, Harris JC, Nyhan WL, et al. The spectrum of mutations causing HPRT deficiency: an update. *Nucleosides Nucleotides Nucleic Acids.* 2004;23:1153–1160.

Lesch M, Nyhan WL. A familial disorder of uric acid metabolism and central nervous system function. *Am J Med.* 1964;36:561–570.

MENKES SYNDROME (KINKY HAIR)

MIM #309400

❏ Definition

Menkes syndrome is an X-linked recessive disorder of copper metabolism caused by gene mutations in the gene encoding Cu^{2+}-transporting ATPase, alpha polypeptide (ATP7A) that result in a block of copper transport from intestinal mucosa cells to blood, causing generalized copper deficiency.

❏ Who Should Be Suspected?

It is a syndrome of neonatal hypothermia, feeding difficulties, and sometimes prolonged jaundice; at 2–3 months, seizures and progressive hair depigmentation and twisting take place. The syndrome also includes a striking facial appearance, increasing mental deterioration, infections, failure to thrive, death in early infancy, and changes in the elastica interna of arteries.

❑ **Relevant Tests and Diagnostic Value**

- Decreased copper in serum and liver; normal in RBCs; increased copper in amniotic fluid, cultured fibroblasts, and amniotic cells
- Decreased serum ceruloplasmin

❑ **Other Considerations**

Carrier status for the Menkes disease gene can usually be determined by examination of multiple hairs from scattered scalp sites for pili torti. Changes in the metaphyses of the long bones resemble scurvy. Ascorbic acid oxidase is copper dependent.

Suggested Reading

Moller LB, Bukrinsky JT, Molgaard A, et al. Identification and analysis of 21 novel disease-causing amino acid substitutions in the conserved part of ATP7A. *Hum Mutat.* 2005;26:84–93.

PARKINSON'S DISEASE (PD)

MIM #168600

❑ **Definition**

Alpha-synuclein is a highly conserved and abundant protein in neurons, and aggregated alpha-synuclein proteins form brain lesions that are hallmarks of PD regardless of the patient's genotype. Accumulation of alpha-synuclein, a major component of Lewy bodies, results in loss of dopaminergic neurons in the substantia nigra.

❑ **Who Should Be Suspected?**

Clinical manifestations of Parkinson's include resting tremor, muscular rigidity, bradykinesia, and postural instability. Multiple combinations of genetic and/or environment causes can result in sporadic or late-onset Parkinson's.

❑ **Relevant Tests and Diagnostic Value**

10

- There is a wide genetic heterogeneity in Parkinson disease (PD). Mutations in the LRRK2 gene (12q12) are the most common genetic component, while mutations in the SNCA gene (4q22.1) encoding alpha-synuclein are found in several families with a high prevalence of PD. Mutations in the Parkin gene (6q26) have been identified in cases of autosomal recessive juvenile PD (MIM #600116), and multiple additional genes have been implicated in cases of autosomal dominant or autosomal recessive PD.
- Sequence analysis of entire coding regions; targeted mutation analysis; deletion/insertion analysis.
- Gene dosage analysis of SNCA. FISH analysis.
- Many other diseases have parkinsonian motor features ("parkinsonism"), and accurate diagnosis may depend on the presence of Lewy bodies on pathologic examination.
- Individuals that carry a Gaucher disease mutation (GBA gene mutation) have an approximately fivefold increased risk of developing Parkinson's disease.

Suggested Readings

Feany MB. New genetic insights into Parkinson's disease. *New Eng J Med.* 2004;351:1937–1940

Gandhi PN, Wang X, Zhu X, et al. The Roc domain of leucine-rich repeat kinase 2 is sufficient for interaction with microtubules. *J Neurosci Res.* 2008;86:1711–1720.

Michael J. Fox Foundation for Parkinson's Research. Available from: https://www.michaeljfox.org/

Polymeropoulos MH, Lavedan C, Leroy E, et al. Mutation in the alpha-synuclein gene identified in families with Parkinson's disease. *Science.* 1997;276:2045–2047.

Shimura H, Schlossmacher MG, Hattori N, et al. Ubiquitination of a new form of alpha-synuclein by parkin from human brain: implications for Parkinson's disease. *Science.* 2001;293:263–269.

Sidransky E, Nalls MA, Aasly JO, et al. Multicenter analysis of glucocerebrosidase mutations in Parkinson's disease. *New Eng J Med.* 2009;361:1651–1661.

PRADER-WILLI SYNDROME (PWS)

MIM #176270

❑ **Definition**

Prader-Willi syndrome (PWS) results from deletion of the paternal copies of the imprinted SNRPN gene, the necdin gene, and possibly other genes within the chromosome region 15q11-q13.

❑ **Who Should Be Suspected?**

Prader-Willi syndrome is characterized by diminished fetal activity, obesity, muscular hypotonia, mental retardation, short stature, hypogonadotropic hypogonadism, and small hands and feet. There are three genetic reasons of PWS: (1) paternal deletion—about 70% of all cases of PWS, (2) maternal uniparental disomy (UPD)—about 25% of cases, and (3) imprinting defect—<5% of cases

❑ **Relevant Tests and Diagnostic Value**

- Molecular testing:
  - ▼ FISH—typical deletions, large and small, can be detected—if the FISH test is positive (a deletion is found), the diagnosis of PWS is confirmed.
  - ▼ DNA methylation test—confirms or rules out PWS as a diagnosis with over 99% accuracy. Normal results show both paternal and maternal DNA imprinting pattern. In PWS, there is only a maternal pattern, but the positive result does not tell whether the cause of PWS is deletion, uniparental disomy (UPD), or an imprinting defect.
  - ▼ DNA polymorphism study is done to confirm UPD. It requires blood samples from both parents and child. If both chromosomes are from the mother, the PWS is confirmed.

Suggested Readings

Driscoll DJ, Miller JL, Schwartz S, et al. Prader-Willi syndrome. In: Pagon RA, Adam MP, Bird TD, et al., eds. *GeneReviews™ [Internet].* Seattle, WA: University of Washington, Seattle; 1998: 1993–2013 Oct 6 [Updated 2012 Oct 11]. Available from: http://www.ncbi.nlm.nih.gov/books/NBK1330

http://www.pwsausa.org/syndrome/Genetics_of_PWS.htm

www.faseb.org/genetics/acmg/pol-22htm

RETT SYNDROME

MIM #312750

❑ **Definition**

The majority of females presenting with clinical consensus criteria for Rett Syndrome have mutations in the transcription repressor MECP2 gene (Xq28). However, not all patients with MECP2 mutations have all the necessary clinical criteria for Rett syndrome diagnosis, and MECP2 mutations have not been found in some Rett patients.

❑ Who Should Be Suspected?

Classic Rett syndrome is characterized by abnormal psychomotor development usually beginning in the first 6 months of life, followed by loss of purposeful hand skills and spoken language, gait abnormalities, and appearance of stereotypic hand movements.

❑ Relevant Tests and Diagnostic Value

Sequence analysis of entire coding region, especially C-terminal; deletion/insertion analysis.

Suggested Reading

Neul JL, Kaufmann WE, Glaze DG, et al. Rett syndrome: revised diagnostic criteria and nomenclature. *Ann Neurol.* 2010;68:944–950.

SPINAL CEREBELLAR ATAXIAS

SPINOCEREBELLAR ATAXIA TYPE 1 (SCA1; OLIVOPONTOCEREBELLAR ATROPHY 1; OPCA1)

MIM #164400

❑ Definition

The clinical manifestations of autosomal dominant inherited spinocerebellar ataxias are caused by the variable pathologic involvement of the brain stem and spinal cord, that results in cerebellar degeneration. Spinocerebellar ataxia-1 (SCA1) is caused by expansion of a CAG trinucleotide repeat in the ataxin-1 gene (ATXN1; 6p22.3).

❑ Relevant Tests and Diagnostic Value

Polymerase chain reaction (PCR) and fragment analysis by capillary electrophoresis of CAG triplet repeat expansion in the *AATXN1* gene; normal: ≤ 35 CAG trinucleotide repeats.

Suggested Readings

Margolis RL. Dominant spinocerebellar ataxias: a molecular approach to classification, diagnosis, pathogenesis and the future. *Expert Rev Mol Diagn.* 2003;3:715–732.

Orr HT, et al. Expansion of an unstable trinucleotide CAG repeat in spinocerebellar ataxia type 1. *Nat Genet.* 1993;4:221–226.

van de Warrenburg BP, et al. Age at onset variance analysis in spinocerebellar ataxias: a study in a Dutch-French cohort. *Ann Neurol.* 2005;57:505–512.

WILSON DISEASE (HEPATOLENTICULAR DEGENERATION)

MIM #277900

❑ Definition

Wilson disease is an autosomal recessive disorder caused by mutations in the ATPase, Cu^{2+}-transporting, beta polypeptide gene (ATP7B) at 13q14 that encodes a polypeptide functioning as a plasma membrane copper transport protein. This disorder is characterized by buildup of intracellular hepatic copper that results in cirrhosis and neurologic abnormalities. There is a wide range in the age of onset of Wilson disease, including early childhood. Diagnosis of Wilson disease is dependent on both clinical and laboratory evidence of abnormal copper metabolism. A deep copper-colored Kayser-Fleischer ring may be present at the periphery of the cornea.

❏ Relevant Tests and Diagnostic Value

- Low serum ceruloplasmin and/or high urinary copper.
- Mutation detection: Sequence analysis of the entire coding regions; deletion/duplication analysis; targeted mutation analysis.
- MRI may show increased signal intensities in the basal ganglia.

Suggested Readings

De Bie P, Muller P, Wijmenga C, et al. Molecular pathogenesis of Wilson and Menkes disease: correlation of mutations with molecular defects and disease phenotypes. *J Med Genet.* 2007;44:673–688.

Gow PJ, Smallwood RA, Angus PW, et al. Diagnosis of Wilson's disease: an experience over three decades. *Gut.* 2000;46:415–419.

 # NEUROMUSCULAR DISORDERS

AMYOTROPHIC LATERAL SCLEROSIS (ALS; LOU GEHRIG DISEASE)

MIM #105400

❏ Definition

Diagnosis of ALS is dependent on a thorough medical and neurologic examination, as well as clinical and laboratory diagnostic testing, to rule out treatable diseases that have symptoms similar to ALS. Clinical testing can include electrodiagnostic tests: electromyography (EMG) and nerve conduction velocity (NCV), x-rays, magnetic resonance imaging (MRI), spinal tap, myelogram of the cervical spine, and muscle and/or nerve biopsy. Determination of family history and genetic counseling are important. Ninety percent of ALS patients have no family history (sporadic ALS; SALS), and inheritance patterns can be autosomal dominant, autosomal recessive, or X-linked. The most common inheritance pattern in approximately 10% of patients having familial ALS (FALS) is autosomal dominant. Mutations in the SOD1 (21q22.11), TARDBP (1p36; encodingTDP-43), FUS (16p11.2), C9ORF72 (9p21.2), and UBQLN2 (Xp11.21) genes have been identified in approximately 50% of FALS patients.

❏ Who Should Be Suspected?

The initial hallmark sign in ALS is muscle weakness, occurring in approximately 60% of patients. The onset and nature of symptoms in ALS is very variable, but since it is a disease of upper and lower motor neurons, the senses of touch, hearing, taste, smell, and sight are not affected. Although therapy can in some cases slow the progression of disease, as the disease progress, weakness and paralysis spread to the muscles of the trunk, speech, swallowing, chewing, and breathing, and ultimately patients require permanent breathing support to survive.

❏ Relevant Tests and Diagnostic Value

- Mutation detection by analysis of the entire coding regions by single-strand conformation polymorphism (SSCP) or sequence analysis of genes associated with FALS, including SOD1, TARDBP (TDP-43), FUS, C9ORF72, and UBQLN2
- Blood, urine, and CSF studies including high-resolution serum protein electrophoresis, thyroid, and parathyroid hormone levels and 24-hour urine collection for heavy metals

Suggested Readings

ALS Association. Available from: http://www.alsa.org/about-als/genetic-testing-for-als.html

McKinnon WC, Baty BJ, Bennett RL, et al. Predisposition testing for late-onset disorders in adults: a position paper of the National Society of Genetic Counselors. *JAMA*. 1997;278:1217–1220.

Turner MR, et al. Controversies and priorities in amyotrophic lateral sclerosis. *Lancet Neurol*. 2013;12(3):310–322.

CHARCOT MARIE TOOTH HEREDITARY NEUROPATHY (CMT)

MIM #118220

❑ Definition

At least 27 types of CMT can be identified by DNA testing, but a negative result does not rule out the diagnosis as some mutations remain to be identified. More than 40 different genes/loci are associated with CMT, and inheritance can be autosomal recessive, autosomal dominant, or X-linked dominant. Clinical diagnosis is based on family history, neurologic examination, EMG/NCV testing, and in some cases sural nerve biopsy.

❑ Who Should Be Suspected?

Charcot-Marie-Tooth disease (CMT) typically presents during adolescence and early adulthood with distal muscle weakness and atrophy often accompanied by sensory loss, depressed tendon reflexes, and high-arched feet.

❑ Relevant Tests and Diagnostic Value

- Duplication/deletion testing in the PMP22 gene as the most common cause of CMT, and, if negative for PMP22 gene mutations, followed by sequencing other genes associated with a patient's clinical presentation.

Suggested Readings

England JD, et al. Practice parameter: evaluation of distal symmetric polyneuropathy: role of laboratory and genetic testing (an evidence-based review): report of the American Academy of Neurology, American Association of Neuromuscular and Electrodiagnostic Medicine, and American Academy of Physical Medicine and Rehabilitation. *Neurology*. 2009;72:185–192.

Saifi GM, Szigeti K, Snipes GJ, et al. Molecular mechanisms, diagnosis, and rational approaches to management and therapy for Charcot-Marie-Tooth disease and related peripheral neuropathies. *J Investig Med*. 2003;51:261–283.

Saporta AS, Sottile SL, Miller LJ, et al. Charcot-Marie-Tooth disease subtypes and genetic testing strategies. *Ann Neurol*. 2011;69:22–33.

10

MUSCULAR DYSTROPHY, DUCHENNE TYPE; DMD

MIM #310200

MUSCULAR DYSTROPHY, BECKER TYPE; BMD

MIM #300376

❑ Definition

Duchenne muscular dystrophy (DMD) is an X-linked disorder resulting from mutations in the dystrophin gene (Xq21.2-Xq21.1). Onset of gait difficulty usually occurs by age 3 years, with patients developing cardiomyopathy, wheelchair limited by age 12, and dying by age 20 years. Female heterozygotes of a mutation can develop progressive cardiac abnormalities.

Becker muscular dystrophy (BMD) presents with a similar but milder and more slowly progressive course compared to DMD. Age of onset can be as early as age 12 years or much later, with loss of ambulation occurring in adolescence onward, and survival into the fourth or fifth decade.

❏ **Relevant Tests and Diagnostic Value**

- Markedly elevated serum creatine kinase levels
- Western blot testing for dystrophin: Absent in DMD; abnormal size; normal amount in BMD
- Sequence analysis of the entire coding region and deletion/duplication analysis of the dystrophin gene

Suggested Readings

Beggs AH, Kunkel LM. Improved diagnosis of Duchenne/Becker muscular dystrophy. *J Clin Invest.* 1990;85:613–619.

Emery AEH. The muscular dystrophies. *Lancet.* 2002;359:687–695.

Tuffery-Giraud S, et al. Genotype-phenotype analysis in 2,405 patients with a dystrophinopathy using the UMD-DMD database: a model of nationwide knowledgebase. *Hum Mutat.* 2009;30:934–945.

MYOTONIC DYSTROPHY TYPE 1

MIM #160900

❏ **Definition**

Myotonic dystrophy (DM1) clinically presents with myotonia, muscular dystrophy, cataracts, hypogonadism, frontal balding, and an abnormal EKG. In contrast to DMD, DM1 initially affects head and neck muscles, extraocular muscles, and the distal muscles of the extremities, and only later involves proximal musculature. DM1 results from the autosomal dominant inherited expansion of a CTG trinucleotide repeat sequence in the 3′- untranslated region of the dystrophia myotonica protein kinase gene (DMPK; 19q13.3).

❏ **Relevant Tests and Diagnostic Value**

Determination of CTG repeat size by polymerase chain reaction (PCR) amplification of the repeat region or by Southern blot analysis. Repeat size of <37 repeats is normal; 36–49 repeats are premutations; and 50 or more repeats are consistent with myotonic dystrophy type 1. A negative result does not rule out this diagnosis, and a diagnosis of myotonic dystrophy type 2 (DM2) associated with an expansion of a CCTG repeat in intron 1 of the zinc finger protein 9 (ZNF9) gene should also be considered.

Suggested Readings

Groh WJ, et al. Electrocardiographic abnormalities and sudden death in myotonic dystrophy type 1. *New Eng J Med.* 2008;358:2688–2697.

Modoni A, Silvestri G, Pomponi MG, et al. Characterization of the pattern of cognitive impairment in myotonic dystrophy type 1. *Arch Neurol.* 2004;61:1943–1947.

Musova Z, et al. Highly unstable sequence interruptions of the CTG repeat in the myotonic dystrophy gene. *Am J Med Genet.* 2009;149A:1365–1374.

FRIEDREICH ATAXIA (FRDA)

MIM #229300

❏ **Definition**

FRDA1 results from mutations in the frataxin gene (FXN; 9q21.11). The most common mutation is a GAA trinucleotide repeat expansion in intron 1 of the FXN gene, and it is found in over 95% of FRDA1 patients. In normal individuals, there are 5–30 GAA repeat expansions, while FRDA1 patients have 70 or more GAA repeats.

❏ **Who Should Be Suspected?**

Friedreich ataxia (FRDA1) is an autosomal disorder with onset in the first or second decade characterized by progressive gait and limb ataxia, and limb muscle weakness. Clinical manifestations include lower limb areflexia, extensor plantar responses, dysarthria, and decreased vibratory sense and proprioception.

❏ **Relevant Tests and Diagnostic Value**

- Polymerase chain reaction (PCR), fragment analysis, and Southern blot for GAA repeat detection
- Sequence analysis of the entire coding region; targeted mutation analysis; deletion/duplication analysis

Suggested Readings

Lodi R, et al. Deficit of in vivo mitochondrial ATP production in patients with Friedreich ataxia. *Proc Natl Acad Sci U S A.* 1999;96:11492–11495.

Pandolfo M. Friedreich ataxia *Arch Neurol.* 2008;65:1296–1303.

SPINAL MUSCULAR ATROPHY (SMA)

❏ **Definition and Classification**

Spinal muscular atrophy (SMA) refers to a group of neuromuscular autosomal recessive diseases of the motor nerves that cause muscle weakness and atrophy (wasting). The four types of SMA types I–IV, classified according to the age of onset, muscular activity achieved, and survivorship, are caused by mutations in the SMN1 (survival motor neuron 1) gene:

- SMA type I **MIM #253300**, severe infantile acute SMA, or Werdnig-Hoffman disease
- SMA type II **MIM #253550** or infantile chronic
- SMA type III **MIM #253400**, juvenile SMA, or Wohlfart-Kugelberg-Welander disease
- SMA type IV **MIM #271150** or adult-onset SMA

The copy number of the SMN2 (survival motor neuron 2) gene (homologous to SMN1 but impaired functionally) is known to modify the phenotype of SMA through low level expression of each copy of the SMN2 gene. SMA is the second most common lethal, autosomal recessive disease in Caucasians. Mutations in the SMN1 gene can occur by deletion of SMN1 exon 7, other large deletions, or point mutations.

❑ Diagnostic Criteria

- Clinical diagnosis: The child's physical appearance, history of motor difficulties, weakness at birth, a delay in the developmental milestones, such as holding the head up, rolling over, sitting independently, standing, or walking later than, would be expected.
- Molecular genetic diagnosis: The two genes associated with SMA are SMN1 and SMN2. About 95–98% of individuals with SMA are homozygous for a deletion or truncation of SMN1 and about 2–5% are compound heterozygotes for an SMN1 deletion or truncation and an SMN1 intragenic mutation.

❑ Relevant Tests

- Methods used in molecular diagnostic testing:
  - ▼ Targeted mutation analysis—to detect deletion of exon 7 of SMN1.
  - ▼ Sequence analysis of all SMN1 exons and intron/exon borders to identify the intragenic SMN1 mutations.
  - ▼ Gene dosage analysis—a PCR-based dosage assay, which can determine the number of SMN1 and SMN2 copies.
- SMA carrier testing—gene dosage analysis of SMN1 copy number is performed by measuring the number of exon 7–containing SMN1 copies. However, intragenic mutations will not be detected by this test. In addition, molecular tests will not indicate if the two copies of the normal SMN1 gene are located on one chromosome, making the individual a carrier with no SMN1 gene on another chromosome (approximately 4% of the population). Furthermore, 2% of individuals with SMA have one de novo mutation, meaning that only one parent is a carrier.
- Because of these difficulties in SMA carrier test interpretation, SMA carrier testing should be provided in the context of formal genetic counseling.

❑ Other Considerations

To help to distinguish SMA from other disorders of nerve or muscle that may look similar to SMA, the following tests may be performed:

- Electromyography (EMG), a test that measures the electrical activity of muscle
- Muscle biopsy, looks for the presence of the specific ultrastructural changes
- Creatine kinase (CK), an elevated level indicates muscle disease

Other rare forms of SMA with different genetic causes:

- Spinal muscular atrophy respiratory distress (SMARD) inherited in an autosomal recessive pattern is caused by mutations in the IGHMBP2 gene.
- Spinal muscular atrophy type V/distal hereditary motor neuropathy, autosomal dominant disorder caused by mutations in the BSCL2 and GARS genes.
- Kennedy disease, X-linked autosomal recessive disease known as X-linked recessive bulbospinal neuropathy or X-linked spinal and bulbar atrophy, is associated with an increase in the number of CAG repeats encoding a polyglutamine stretch within the androgen receptor.

Suggested Readings

http://www.fsma.org/FSMACommunity/UnderstandingSMA/

Prior TW, Russman BS. Spinal muscular atrophy. In: Pagon RA, Adam MP, Bird TD, et al., eds. GeneReviews™ [Internet]. Seattle, WA: University of Washington, Seattle; 2000:1993–2013 [Updated 2011 Jan 27]. Available from: http://www.ncbi.nlm.nih.gov/books/NBK1352/

PULMONARY SYSTEM

ALPHA-1 ANTITRYPSIN DEFICIENCY (A1ATD)

MIM #613490

❑ **Definition**

Alpha-1 antitrypsin deficiency, an autosomal recessive disorder caused by mutations in the protease inhibitor 1 gene, SERPINA1. Mutations in the SERPINA1 gene can lead to a shortage (deficiency) of alpha-1 antitrypsin or an abnormal form of the protein that cannot control neutrophil elastase. Without enough functional alpha-1 antitrypsin, neutrophil elastase destroys alveoli and causes lung disease. Abnormal alpha-1 antitrypsin can accumulate in the liver and cause damage. One of the clinical manifestations of A1ATD is liver disease in childhood and cirrhosis and/or hepatocellular carcinoma (HCC) in adulthood. Alpha-1 antitrypsin deficiency is commonly overlooked cause of lung disease.

Suggested Reading

http://alpha-1foundation.org/what-is-alpha-1

CYSTIC FIBROSIS AND RELATED DISORDERS

MIM #219700

❑ **Definition**

Cystic fibrosis (CF) is an autosomal recessive disorder with abnormal ion transport caused by mutations in the cystic fibrosis conductance regulator gene (CFTR) located on chromosome 7 that commonly affect the lungs and digestive system of patients. CF is the most common genetic disease in the Caucasian population in the United States. The disease occurs in 1 in 2,500–3,500 Caucasian newborns. CF is less common in other ethnic groups, affecting about 1 in 17,000 African Americans and 1 in 31,000 Asian Americans. Cystic fibrosis affects the epithelia of the respiratory tract, exocrine pancreas, intestine, male genital tract, hepatobiliary system, and exocrine sweat glands, resulting in complex multisystem disease. Respiratory symptoms include fatigue, cough, wheezing, recurrent pneumonia or sinus infections, excess sputum, and shortness of breath. Mutations in the CFTR gene can also cause congenital absence of the vas deferens (CAVD).

❑ **Diagnostic Criteria for CF**

- Presence of two disease-causing mutations in CFTR.
- Sweat chloride values (>60 mEq/L) accurately diagnosis approximately 90% of cases.
- Transepithelial nasal potential difference (NPD) measurements characteristic of CF.
- In newborn screening, immunoreactive trypsinogen (IRT) assays are performed on blood spots; abnormal IRT results are further evaluated through sweat testing and/or molecular genetic testing of the CFTR gene.

❑ **Diagnostic Criteria for CAVD**

- Azoospermia
- Low volume of ejaculated semen
- Absence of the vas deferens on clinical or ultrasound examination
- And at least one disease-causing mutation in the CFTR gene

❏ **Relevant Tests**

- Quantitative pilocarpine iontophoresis for sweat chloride concentrations remains the primary test for the diagnosis of CF.
- Molecular testing—the CFTR gene is the only gene known to be associated with the CFTR-related disorders, CF, and CAVD.
  - ▼ Diagnostic testing for symptomatic individuals should be performed if needed for family studies, for confirmation of diagnosis when results from the other tests are unavailable or uninformative, and for epidemiologic purposes. Some CF patients may have unidentified mutations when tested by a target mutation panel and may need sequencing of the whole gene and/or testing for deletion/duplication.
  - ▼ Carrier testing in at-risk relatives and their reproductive partners is recommended. Also carrier testing for pregnant or planning pregnancy women is offered.
  - ▼ Prenatal testing is recommended for pregnancies at risk for CF when the parental mutations are known and for pregnancies in which fetal echogenic bowel has been identified.
  - ▼ Preimplantation genetic diagnosis for pregnancies at increased risk for CF is possible when the parental mutations are known.
- Transepithelial nasal potential difference (NPD) measurements are recommended to confirm the diagnosis of CF in symptomatic individuals with borderline or nondiagnostic sweat tests in whom only one or no CFTR disease–causing mutation has been detected.

❏ **Other Considerations**

Individuals who test negative in carrier testing for a panel of CFTR mutations have their carrier risk reduced (though not eliminated). Carrier risk before testing and residual risk after carrier testing are calculated by the laboratories based on the patient's family history and mutation detection rate of the testing panel and carrier frequency, which depends on the patient's ethnicity. An increased prevalence of CFTR mutations has been noted in individuals with idiopathic pancreatitis, bronchiectasis, allergic bronchopulmonary aspergillosis, and chronic rhinosinusitis. At present, DNA testing is of unknown and unclear utility for these conditions.

Suggested Reading

Moskowitz SM, Chmiel JF, Sternen DL, et al. CFTR-related disorders. In: Pagon RA, Adam MP, Bird TD, et al., eds. *GeneReviews™ [Internet]*. Seattle, WA: University of Washington, Seattle; 2001:1993–2013 [Updated 2008 Feb 19]. Available from: http://www.ncbi.nlm.nih.gov/books/NBK1250/

 DISORDERS OF HEARING AND VISION

DEAFNESS, AUTOSOMAL RECESSIVE 1 (DFNB1)

OMIM #220290

❏ **Definition**

Nonsyndromic hearing loss and deafness (DFNB1; NSHL) is characterized by autosomal inheritance of congenital, nonprogressive, mild to severe sensorineural hearing impairment and is unaccompanied by other medical abnormalities. Autosomal recessive deafness-1A (DFNB1A) is caused by mutations in the GJB2 gene (13q11-q12) encoding the gap junction beta-2 protein connexin-26 (CX26) or compound heterozygote mutations in both the GJB2 and the allelic gap junction beta-6 protein GJB6 gene encoding connexin-30. NSHL from homozygous mutations in only the GJB6 gene is rare.

❏ Relevant Tests and Diagnostic Value

- Sequencing of the entire coding regions of *GJB2* and *GJB6* detects more than 99% of autosomal recessive deafness-causing mutations in these genes. Testing should include detection of the splice site mutation in exon 1 of *GJB2* and large deletions in *GJB6* by assays such as PCR or MLPA.
- Sequencing of mtDNA.

Suggested Readings

Petersen MB, Willems PJ. Non-syndromic, autosomal-recessive deafness. *Clin Genet.* 2006;69:371–392.

Schimmenti LA, et al. Infant hearing loss and connexin testing in a diverse population. *Genet Med.* 2008;10:517–524.

LEBER OPTIC ATROPHY (LEBER HEREDITARY OPTIC NEUROPATHY; LHON)

MIM #535000

❏ Definition

Leber optic atrophy (LHON) is caused by mutations in multiple genes in complex I, III, and IV polypeptides encoded by the mitochondrial genome (mtDNA), suggesting that LHON results from a defect in the respiratory chain. The vulnerability of retinal ganglion cells to mitochondrial dysfunction leads to midlife, acute or subacute, painless, central vision loss (scotoma). Depending on the mutation, final visual acuity can range from 20/50 to no light perception. The maternal transmission is due to mtDNA mutations, but the incomplete penetrance and male bias remain puzzling. Three primary mutations at base pairs 11,778, 3,460, and 14,484 are present in at least 90% of families. However, a significant percentage of individuals with an LHON mutation do not develop the disorder. More than 50% of males and more than 85% of females with a mutation never experience vision loss due to LHON.

❏ Relevant Tests and Diagnostic Value

Complete and targeted sequence of the mitochondrial genome.

Suggested Readings

Kirkman MA, et al. Gene-environment interactions in Leber hereditary optic neuropathy. *Brain.* 2009;132:2317–2326.

Yu-Wai-Man P, et al. Inherited mitochondrial optic neuropathies. *J Med Genet.* 2009;46:145–158. Note: Erratum: *J Med Genet.* 2011;48:284 only.

NONSYNDROMIC SENSORINEURAL DEAFNESS, MITOCHONDRIAL

MIM #500008

❏ Definition

Mitochondrial nonsyndromic sensorineural deafness has a wide range of penetrance manifested by broad variability in severity, age-at-onset, and audiometric abnormalities of hearing impairment. Mitochondrially inherited NSHL can result from mutations in any of several mitochondrial genes (mtDNA), frequently involving the 12S rRNA and tRNA genes. The mtDNA mutations account for only about 2% of NSHL and show dominant maternal inheritance.

❑ **Relevant Tests and Diagnostic Value**
Sequence analysis of the complete mitochondrial genome.

Suggested Reading
Chaig MR, et al. A mutation in mitochondrial 12S rRNA, A827G, in Argentinean family with hearing loss after aminoglycoside treatment. *Biochem Biophys Res Commun.* 2008;368:631–636.

USHER SYNDROME TYPE 1A (USH1)

MIM #276900
❑ **Definition**
Usher syndrome is the most common type of autosomal recessive syndromic hearing loss and the most common genetic cause of combined deafness and blindness. The variably progressive deafness is accompanied by a variable age of onset and progression of night blindness and loss of peripheral vision through progressive degeneration of the retina (retinitis pigmentosa, RP).

❑ **Who Should Be Suspected?**
Usher syndrome type I, the most severe form, is characterized by congenital, severe sensorineural hearing loss, vestibular dysfunction, and the onset of RP by the age 10 years. Type I is further subdivided into five types, where the pathogenic variants in the *MYO7A* (the most common), *USH1C, CDH23, PCDH15, and USH1G (SANS)* genes cause type 1B, type 1C, type 1D, type 1F, and type 1G, respectively. Additional Usher presentations result from mutations in the *USH2A, GPR98, DFNB31,* and *CLRN1* genes.

❑ **Relevant Tests and Diagnostic Value**
- Next-generation sequencing of the coding regions and splice sites for detection of mutations in genes associated with Usher syndrome
- Microarray targeted mutation analysis of genes associated with Usher syndrome
- Individual targeted gene sequencing, deletion/duplication testing, ethnicity-based testing

Suggested Reading
Reiners J, et al. Molecular basis of human Usher syndrome: deciphering the meshes of the Usher protein network provides insights into the pathomechanisms of the Usher disease. *Exp Eye Res.* 2006;83(1):97–119.

 # SKELETAL DYSPLASIA

ACHONDROPLASIA (ACH)

MIM #100800
❑ **Definition**
Achondroplasia (ACH) is the most frequent form of short-limb dwarfism, with clinical manifestations including short stature, shortening of the limbs, frontal bossing, lumbar lordosis, genu varum, and trident hand. ACH is an autosomal

dominant disorder, caused by mutations in the fibroblast growth factor receptor-3 gene (FGFR3; 4p16.3), with the majority of cases resulting from de novo mutations.

❑ Relevant Tests and Diagnostic Value

Targeted sequencing mutation analysis of *FGFR3* exons 10, 13, and 15 detects the majority of ACH mutations, as well as many mutations associated with hypochondroplasia; sequence analysis of the entire coding region.

Suggested Reading

Shiang R, et al. Mutations in the transmembrane domain of FGFR3 cause the most common genetic form of dwarfism, achondroplasia. *Cell.* 1994;78:335–342.

ELLIS-VAN CREVELD (EVC MIM #225500) AND WEYERS ACROFACIAL DYSOSTOSIS (MIM #193530)

MIM #193530 AND #193530

❑ Definition

Ellis-van Creveld syndrome is an autosomal recessive skeletal dysplasia characterized by short limbs, short ribs, postaxial polydactyly, and dysplastic nails and teeth. Congenital cardiac defects, most commonly a defect of primary atrial septation producing a common atrium, occur in 60% of affected individuals. Weyers acrofacial dysostosis (Curry-Hall syndrome) is an autosomal dominant inheritance syndrome of postaxial polydactyly with anomalies of the lower jaw, dentition, and oral vestibule. Both EVC and Weyers are caused by mutations in the EVC1 and/or EVC2 genes.

❑ Relevant Tests and Diagnostic Value

Sequencing of the EVC1 and EVC2 genes identifies mutations in individuals with EVC and Weyers acrofacial dysostosis in about 70% of cases.

Suggested Reading

Galdzicka M, England JA., Ginns EI. EVC and EVC2 and Ellis-van Creveld Syndrome, Second Edition of CJ Epstein, RP Erickson, A Wynshaw-Boris (eds.) Inborn Errors of Development: the molecular basis of clinical disorders of morphogenesis, Oxford University Press, New York (2008).

OSTEOGENESIS IMPERFECTA (OI; BRITTLE BONE DISEASE)

MIM #166200

❑ Definition

Osteogenesis imperfecta type I (OI) is a generalized connective tissue disorder characterized by bone fragility and blue sclerae. Mutations in the collagen, type I, alpha-1 (COL1A1; 17q21.33) or the collagen, type I, alpha-2 (COL1A2; 7q21.3) gene result in OI, but lack of finding a mutation does not rule out OI.

❑ Relevant Tests and Diagnostic Value

Protein analysis demonstrating reduced amounts of normal collagen I.

Suggested Reading

Kuivaniemi H, et al. Mutations in fibrillar collagens (types I, II, III, and XI), fibril-associated collagen (type IX), and network-forming collagen (type X) cause a spectrum of diseases of bone, cartilage, and blood vessels. *Hum Mutat.* 1997;9:300–315.

CONNECTIVE TISSUE DISORDERS

MARFAN SYNDROME (MFS)

MIM #154700
❑ **Definition**
Marfan syndrome is a disorder of fibrous connective tissue having autosomal dominant inheritance. There is marked clinical variation manifestations observed in the skeletal, ocular, and cardiovascular tissues that include increased height, disproportionately long limbs and digits, anterior chest deformity, joint laxity, scoliosis and thoracic lordosis, a narrow, arched palate, ectopia lentis, and aortic root/aneurysm pathology.

MFS results from heterozygous mutations in the fibrillin-1 gene (FBN1) located at 15q21.1.

❑ **Relevant Tests and Diagnostic Value**
Sequence analysis of the entire coding region; deletion/duplication analysis.

Suggested Readings
Attias D, et al. Comparison of clinical presentations and outcomes between patients with TGFBR2 and FBN1 mutations in Marfan syndrome and related disorders. *Circulation.* 2009;120:2541–2549.
Pyeritz RE, McKusick VA. Basic defects in the Marfan syndrome. (Editorial). *New Eng J Med.* 1981;305:1011–1012.
Tiecke F, et al. Classic, atypically severe and neonatal Marfan syndrome: twelve mutations and genotype-phenotype correlations in FBN1 exons 24–40. *Eur J Hum Genet.* 2001;9:13–21.

 ONCOLOGIC HEREDITARY DISORDERS

BRCA1 AND BRCA2 HEREDITARY BREAST AND OVARIAN CANCER

MIM #604370 (BRCA1) AND #612555 (BRCA2)
❑ **Definition**
Familial breast and/or ovarian cancer are autosomal dominant multifactorial disorders and are caused by mutations in the BRCA1 and BRCA2 genes. BRCA1 and BRCA2 are tumor suppressor genes. The proteins produced from these two genes are involved in repairing damaged DNA, preventing cells from growing and dividing too rapidly in an uncontrolled way. Lifetime risk of breast cancer in BRCA1 mutation carriers is 80–90% and ovarian cancer 40–50%. Lifetime risk of breast cancer in BRCA2 mutation carriers is 60–85% and ovarian cancer 10–20%. Lifetime risk of breast cancer in male with BRCA mutation is 6%. Mutations in these genes are rare in the general population and are estimated to account for no more than 5–10% of breast and ovarian cancer cases overall.

❑ **Relevant Tests and Diagnostic Value**
- Genetic testing for mutations in BRCA1 and BRCA2, two genes predisposing to breast and ovarian cancers, is available to women with a relevant family history. Testing of the family member with breast or ovarian cancer is recommended first. If a BRCA1 or BRCA2 mutation is found, other family

members can be tested for the specific BRCA mutation. If no mutation is found, the cancer is probably not due to an inherited BRCA1 and BRCA2 gene mutation, and other family members should not be tested for mutations in these genes.

- No currently available technique can guarantee the identification of all cancer-predisposing mutations in BRCA1 or BRCA2.
- Mutations of uncertain clinical significance may be identified.
- Mutations in the genes p53 and PTEN/MMAC1 increase breast cancer risk.
- Clinical testing
  - ▼ Targeted mutation analysis—may be used when familial mutation is known and in ethnic-specific studies, which include mutations known to be found at greater frequencies in individuals of certain ethnic backgrounds. In persons of Ashkenazi Jewish heritage, three founder germ line mutations are observed: c.68_69delAG (BRCA1), c.5266dupC (BRCA1), and c.5946delT (BRCA2). One in 40 Ashkenazi individuals have one of these three founder mutations.
  - ▼ Sequence analysis—can detect both common and family-specific BRCA1 and BRCA2 mutations.
  - ▼ Deletion/duplication or rearrangements analysis—recommended in patients in which sequencing did not identified any mutation.
  - ▼ Both sequence analysis and deletion analysis may be required to detect complex BRCA1 or BRCA2 alleles.
  - ▼ Next-generation sequencing (NGS) testing for hereditary breast and ovarian cancer syndrome is being developed for routine diagnostics to improve genetic testing for BRCA1 and BRCA2 diagnosis due to its huge sequencing capacity and cost-effectiveness.

❏ **Other Considerations**

Options for lowering the risk of breast cancer for women at high risk:

- Taking a risk-lowering drug (tamoxifen or raloxifene)
- Having a prophylactic mastectomy
- Having a prophylactic oophorectomy

Suggested Readings

National Cancer Institute Fact Sheet. Available from: http://www.cancer.gov/cancertopics/factsheet/Risk/BRCA

Susan G. 2013. Komen® at http://ww5.komen.org/understandingbreastcancerguide.html

 # DUPLICATION/DELETION SYNDROMES

KLINEFELTER SYNDROME

Males with the 47,XXY karyotype have a fairly well-defined phenotype known as Klinefelter syndrome. They are tall and thin with long legs. Physical appearance is fairly normal until puberty, during which a characteristic eunuchoid habitus develops. Secondary sexual characteristics are underdeveloped, and testes remain small, with azoospermia and subsequent infertility. Gynecomastia can be a feature of this syndrome. IQ is reduced in this population of patients, and two thirds of patients have educational problems, particularly dyslexia.

TRISOMY 13 (PATAU SYNDROME)

❏ Definition

Trisomy 13 is the third most common viable autosomal trisomy. It has a clinically severe phenotype with severe mental retardation and CNS malformations, often including holoprosencephaly and arhinencephaly. Most trisomy 13 conceptions abort spontaneously; about half of trisomy 13 liveborns die in the 1st month of life. Trisomy 13 is usually caused by meiotic nondisjunction resulting in a karyotype of 47,XX (or XY), +13 with minimal recurrence risk. Risk, as for other autosomal trisomies, increases with advancing maternal age. Other causes may include the presence of a robertsonian translocation in combination with two free copies of chromosome 13; in such cases, one of the parents often is a balanced carrier of the robertsonian translocation. Recurrence risk is low, but significant, and depends on the specific robertsonian translocation and sex of the carrier parent. Prenatal diagnosis (chromosome analysis) should be offered to all Robertsonian translocation carriers.

❏ Relevant Tests and Diagnostic Value

- Prenatal screening: Maternal serum screening is not applicable for detection of trisomy 13. Fetal abnormalities are significant, however, and are almost always detected with a second-/third-trimester ultrasound scan.
- Chromosome analysis: Chromosome analysis is diagnostic for trisomy 13 and can be performed on chorionic villus, amniotic fluid, and peripheral blood.
- FISH: Interphase FISH may be performed for rapid enumeration on chorionic villus, amniotic fluid, and peripheral blood.
- Non-invasive prenatal testing (NIPT) is available.

TRISOMY 18 (EDWARDS SYNDROME)

❏ Definition

Trisomy 18 is the second most common viable autosomal trisomy. Occurrence is usually sporadic and caused by meiotic nondisjunction; it carries minimal recurrence risk. Risk of trisomy 18 increases with advancing maternal age. This trisomy has a severe phenotype with mental retardation and failure to thrive. Classic clenching of fists may be detected on fetal ultrasound examination. Most trisomy 18 conceptuses abort spontaneously, and about 90% of liveborns die in the 1st year.

❏ Relevant Tests and Diagnostic Value

- Maternal serum screen: Risk of trisomy 18 may be calculated with either first- or second-trimester maternal serum screening. Because trisomy 18 is rare, detection rates are not as precise as for Down syndrome, but with a 0.4% false-positive rate, detection rates reportedly range from 60 to 80%.
- Chromosome analysis: Chromosome analysis is diagnostic for trisomy 18 and can be performed on chorionic villus, amniotic fluid, and peripheral blood.

- FISH: Interphase FISH may be performed for rapid enumeration on chorionic villus, amniotic fluid, and peripheral blood.
- Non-invasive prenatal testing (NIPT) is available.

TRISOMY 21 (DOWN SYNDROME)

❑ **Definition**

Trisomy 21 is the most common viable autosomal trisomy. Individuals with Down syndrome have moderate mental retardation, characteristic dysmorphic features, increased risk of leukemia, and early Alzheimer disease. Cardiac anomalies are common. Risk of trisomy 21 increases with advancing maternal age.

❑ **Etiology**

- Usual causes involve meiotic nondisjunction, resulting in a karyotype of 47,XX(or XY),+21. For these cases, recurrence risk is small, approximately 1% greater than age-related risk for women younger than 35 and no significant risk increase over age-related risk for women older than age 35.
- Other causes include presence of a robertsonian translocation in combination with two free copies of chromosome 21. Often in such cases, one parent is a balanced carrier of the robertsonian translocation. Recurrence risk of trisomy 21 depends on the specific robertsonian translocation and the sex of the carrier parent. Prenatal diagnosis (chromosome analysis) should be offered to all robertsonian translocation carriers.

❑ **Relative Tests and Diagnostic Value**

- Prenatal maternal screening: Risk of trisomy 21 may be calculated with first-trimester, second-trimester, or both semester (integrated/sequential) screening modalities that include measurement of maternal serum analytes and fetal ultrasound. Detection rates vary depending on the screening modality and on the false-positive rate. The second-semester maternal quad screen can detect 80% of affected pregnancies with a 5% false-positive rate; integrated testing can detect 90% with a 5% false-positive rate.
- Chromosome analysis: Diagnostic for trisomy 21 and can be performed on chorionic villus, amniotic fluid, and peripheral blood.
- FISH: Interphase FISH may be performed for rapid enumeration on chorionic villus, amniotic fluid, and peripheral blood.
- Non-invasive prenatal testing (NIPT) is available.

TURNER SYNDROME (45,X KARYOTYPE AND VARIANTS)

❑ **Definition**

Turner syndrome is widely known as 45,X, although approximately 50% of individuals with Turner syndrome have a variation of this karyotype. About 15% of patients carry one normal X chromosome and one structurally aberrant X chromosome. Approximately 25–30% of patients are mosaic with one 45,X cell line and a second cell line that might contain, among others, two normal X chromosomes (i.e., 45,X/46,XX), one normal and one abnormal X chromosome (i.e., 45,X/46,X,i(Xq)), or one X and one Y chromosome (i.e., 45,X/46,XY).

❑ Who Should Be Suspected?

A number of phenotypic abnormalities are pathognomonic for Turner syndrome. The most characteristic findings are short stature (under 5 ft or 150 cm) and gonadal dysgenesis (usually streak gonads). Fetal cystic hygroma is common, resulting from lymphedema and leading to postnatal neck webbing. Other associated anomalies include low posterior hairline, shield chest with widely spaced nipples, cubitus valgus, cardiac anomalies (frequently coarctation of the aorta), and renal anomalies.

❑ Relevant Tests and Diagnostic Value

- Obtaining the karyotype of patients with Turner syndrome is clinically important. Although many of the individual symptoms of Turner syndrome seem to be randomly distributed with respect to different deletions throughout the X chromosome, some correlations with phenotype can be made. Most individuals with breakpoints distal to Xq25 have few abnormalities except occasional secondary amenorrhea or premature menopause. Short stature is almost always associated with deletions of the distal portion of the short arm; it is seen less often with long arm deletions.
- Determination of the presence of Y chromosomal material is of critical medical importance because its presence leads to an increased risk for gonadoblastoma in sex-reversed individuals. As such, molecular studies for detection of Y chromosomal DNA should be performed. In addition, rare patients with features of Turner syndrome are determined to have a 46,XY karyotype missing a portion of the Y chromosome. These individuals also have an increased risk of gonadoblastoma.

Suggested Readings

Levilliers J, et al. Exchange of terminal portions of X- and Y-short arms in human XY females. *Proc Natl Acad Sci U S A.* 1989;86:2296–3000.

Therman E, Susman B. The similarity of phenotypic effects caused by Xp and Xq deletions in the human female: a hypothesis. *Hum Genet.* 1990;85:175–183.

GLOSSARY FOR MOLECULAR METHODS TERMINOLOGY

Array comparative genomic hybridization (aCGH): A microarray-based technique to detect abnormalities in DNA copy number (i.e., missing or extra pieces of chromosomes) that can detect smaller abnormalities than a standard chromosomal analysis but will not detect balanced chromosomal rearrangements, such as translocations. It is used as an adjunct or replacement to chromosome analysis; does not detect single-gene mutations.

Allele-specific oligonucleotide (ASO) testing: Detection of a specific mutation using a synthetic segment of DNA approximately 20 base pairs in length (an oligonucleotide) that binds to and hence identifies the complementary sequence in a DNA sample.

bDNA testing: Branched DNA testing is a test in which a phosphorescent chemical that is known to bind to RNA is added to the suspect DNA. The more brightly the test sample glows, the greater amount of RNA that is present in the sample; this test is used to directly measure the amount of RNA in a sample (e.g., viral load).

Bead array: Array consisting of addressable beads either impregnated with different concentrations of fluorescent dye or labeled with some type of bar code. The addressable beads enable the identification of specific oligonucleotide binding to the bead's surface. The combination of specific oligonucleotide bound to a specific bead is decoded to determine the presence or absence of a particular target DNA sequence.

Chromosome analysis: Provides an overview of the genome through microscopic visual inspection of banded mitotic chromosomes. It requires cells to be in metaphase; therefore, cells must be *cultured* and chemically arrested in metaphase to obtain chromosomes that can be visualized. Aberrations must be at least 5–10 Mb to be appreciated.

Denaturing gradient gel electrophoresis (DGGE): Detects changes in DNA sequence based on differences in energy required for separation during electrophoresis of double-stranded DNA fragments of the same size into single-stranded DNA on a polyacrylamide gel with gradient of denaturant (chemical denaturants as formamide and urea) at elevated temperatures. DNA fragments are progressing through the gel according to their melting (denaturing) temperature, which is dependent on the ratio of GC to AT base pairs that make up a particular segment of DNA. A confirmatory test is required for mutation analysis.

Denaturing high-performance liquid chromatography (DHPLC)—a large-scale chromatographic method used for identification of sequence variation allows rapid detection of mutations by heteroduplex formation between wild-type and mutant DNA. Exon sequencing is required to characterize the mutation.

Diagnostic test: Test performed to confirm the presence of a specific medical condition. Molecular tests are used currently as an aid in evaluation of patients suspected of/with infectious diseases, genetic disorders, and other disorders where there are established known genetic risk factors. Also in the last few years, pharmacogenetic testing has evolved, creating personalized approached to drug choices and dosing based on the individual's variants.

Fluorescence in situ hybridization (FISH): Molecular hybridization of a fluorescently labeled, cloned sequence to a mitotic chromosome or to an interphase nucleus. FISH is used to interrogate a specific region of the genome, designed to detect chromosome rearrangements or aberrations that are least 100 kb in size.

Fluorescence-based fragment size analysis: A method for detection of mutations/variants that cause change in the size of a DNA fragment, such as expansion or contraction of tandem repeats. The size of fluorescently labeled fragments, amplified by PCR, is detected using the capillary electrophoresis and then interpreted using the analysis software. Multiple-colored fluorescent dyes can be detected in one sample. One of the dye colors is used for a labeled size standard that is added to each lane. The analysis software uses the size standard to create a standard curve for each lane and then determines the length of each dye-labeled fragment by comparing it with the standard curve for that specific lane.

Fluorescence resonance energy transfer (FRET): Mechanism describing energy transfer between two chromophores.

Genome: Complete DNA sequence, containing the entire genetic information, of a gamete, an individual, a population, or a species.

Genomics: Field of genetics concerned with structural and functional studies of the genome.

Genotyping: Process of determining the genetic makeup of an individual, usually with methods such as PCR, DNA sequencing, ASO probes, and hybridization to DNA microarrays or beads.

Haplotype analysis: Determination of the extent of association to a trait of a set of closely linked loci such as a group of genes that occupy a specific position on one chromosome that tend to be inherited together.

Hybridization: Used to determine the degree of sequence identity, as well as specific sequences between nucleic acids by interacting single-stranded DNA or RNA in solution or with one component immobilized so that complexes called hybrids are formed by molecules with similar, complementary sequences.

Invader chemistry: Composed of two simultaneous isothermal reactions, a primary reaction that detects mutation and secondary reaction that amplifies the signal. The fluorescent signal is generated by the cleavage of a synthetic oligonucleotide probe labeled with FRET.

Karyotype: Ordered pairing of chromosomes that aids in detecting abnormalities.

Ligase chain reaction (LCR): DNA amplification technology based on the ligation of two pairs of synthetic oligonucleotides, which hybridize at adjacent positions to complementary strands of a target DNA.

Linkage analysis: Testing DNA sequence polymorphisms (normal variants) that are near or within a gene of interest to track inheritance of a disease-causing mutation.

Microarray: Consists of the hybridization of a nucleic acid sample (target) to a very large set of oligonucleotide probes, which are attached to a solid support or in solution, to determine sequence, or to detect variations in a gene sequence or expression or for gene mapping.

Multiplex ligation–dependent probe amplification (MLPA): Detects deletions and duplications, determines the copy number of all or selected exons within a gene with high sensitivity.

Mutation scanning: A search for novel sequence variants within a specific DNA fragment.

Next-generation sequencing (Next Gen, NGS): The bases of DNA fragments are sequentially identified from signals emitted as each fragment is resynthesized from a DNA template across millions of reactions in a massively parallel fashion; multiple, fragmented sequence reads are assembled together on the basis of their overlapping location. This advance enables rapid sequencing of large stretches of DNA base pairs spanning entire genomes.

- *The automated Sanger methodology* is referred to as a "first-generation technology," and NGS technologies are essentially grouped into second-generation (2G) and third-generation (3G) approaches. Several 2G approaches are commercially available (e.g., Roche-454, Illumina-Solexa, Applied Biosystems-SOLiD). The third-generation (3G) platforms are represented by the Helicos HeliScope, the Pacific Bioscience, and Oxford Nanopore Technologies.

- *Second-generation (2G) platforms* use either "emulsion PCR" (Roche-454, Applied Biosystems-SOLiD) or "bridge PCR" (Illumina) for target amplification, followed by cyclic-array sequencing, the sequencing of DNA on a dense array, for example, streptavidin beads (Roche-454), flow cells (Illumina), or glass surfaces (Applied Biosystems-SOLiD) by alternating cycles of enzyme-driven biochemistry and imaging-based data collection. All 2G technologies are engineered to obtain massively parallel output.

- *3G technologies* use a single molecule template approach, do not use PCR amplification step, and avoid the cyclic-array approach and thereby enable further massive parallelization. These methods (Read-out) include differential conductance across nanopores (Oxford Nanopore Technology) and single molecule real-time sequencing using Fluorescence Resonance Energy Transfer (Applied Biosystems) or zero-mode waveguide detectors (Pacific Biosciences). Current applications of NGS include de novo sequencing, resequencing, epigenetics, and metagenomics.

Non-Invasive Prenatal Testing (NIPT): Cell-free fetal DNA circulating in maternal blood, is analyzed for trisomy 21 and other fetal chromosomal aneuploidies.

Northern blot: Used to study gene expression by detection of RNA with a hybridization probe complementary to part of or an entire size-separated RNA sample.

Oligonucleotide ligation assay (OLA): Rapid, sensitive, and specific method for the detection of known SNPs that is based on the joining of two adjacent oligonucleotide probes (capture and reporter oligos) using a DNA ligase while they are annealed to a complementary DNA target. The detection of an SNP occurs by the ability of DNA ligase to join probes that are perfectly matched to a complementary target sequence, whereas a 3′ mismatch in the capture probe prevents ligation.

Polymerase chain reaction (PCR): Molecular technique by which a short DNA (or RNA following reverse transcription) sequence is amplified by two flanking oligonucleotide primers used in repeated cycles of primer extension and DNA synthesis with DNA polymerase.

Proteome: All the proteins expressed by the genome in a given cell or tissue at a given time under specific conditions.

Proteomics: Field of biochemistry/genetics encompassing the comprehensive analysis and cataloging of the structure and function of the proteome.

Pyrosequencing: Method for sequencing single-stranded DNA by synthesizing the complementary strand along it, one base pair at a time, and detecting which base was actually added at each step by detecting the activity of DNA polymerase (a DNA-synthesizing enzyme) with another chemiluminescent enzyme.

Real-time PCR (quantitative PCR): Used to quantify DNA or messenger RNA (mRNA) in a sample by using sequence specific, fluorescently labeled primers to determine the relative (between tissue or relative to a specific housekeeping gene) or absolute number of copies of a particular DNA or RNA sequence in a sample. The quantification arises by measuring the amount of amplified product at each stage during the PCR cycle.

Restriction enzymes (RE): Part of the system that bacteria use to protect themselves against viruses by cutting up DNA at specific sequences. Many RE are used to digest DNA into specific fragments that can be used for genotyping.

Reverse hybridization (line probe assay; LIPA): Biotinylated amplified PCR product is hybridized to oligonucleotides that are immobilized as parallel lines on membrane (e.g., nitrocellulose) strips. Unhybridized PCR product is washed off the strip, and a reporter such as alkaline phosphatase–labeled streptavidin conjugate is bound to the biotinylated hybrid, followed by chromogen substrate (such as BCIP/NBT) visualization of the banding pattern. The top band of the membrane strip usually contains a positive control.

Reverse transcription: Synthesis of a complementary DNA sequence from an RNA template; uses an enzyme, reverse transcriptase, which is an RNA-dependent DNA polymerase.

Restriction fragment length polymorphism (RFLP) analysis: Procedure in which the DNA sample is digested into smaller fragments by restriction enzymes, and the resulting fragments are separated according to their lengths. RFLP is used for determination of mutations and paternity testing.

Sequence analysis: Determination of the nucleotide sequence in a DNA sample. Sequencing is a gold standard for mutation analysis detection of single base changes and microdeletions and/or microinsertions.

Single nucleotide polymorphism (SNP): Change in which a single nucleotide in the genomic DNA differs from the usual nucleotide at that position. Some SNPs are responsible for disease, whereas other SNPs are variations without functional significance.

Southern blot: Used to identify and identify electrophoresed size-separated, membrane-immobilized DNA sequences that are complementary to a DNA fragment used as a hybridization probe.

Single-stranded conformation polymorphism (SSCP): Detects changes in DNA sequence based on differences in electrophoretic mobility under nondenaturing conditions and constant temperature. The method can be used for mutation screening but requires mutation confirmation by another method such as sequencing.

Targeted mutation analysis: Testing for either one or more specific mutations.

Temperature gradient gel electrophoresis (TGGE): Detects changes in DNA sequence based on differences in energy required for separation of double-stranded DNA fragments of the same size into single-stranded DNA strands (unzipping) during electrophoresis on a polyacrylamide gel using only a temperature gradient (DGGE also uses denaturants). A confirmatory test is required for mutation analysis.

Transcription-mediated amplification (TMA): Isothermal target nucleic acid amplification method that uses RNA transcription (using RNA polymerase) and DNA synthesis (using reverse transcriptase) to produce an RNA amplicon from a target nucleic acid. TMA can be used to amplify both an RNA and DNA, and produces 100–1,000 copies per cycle; in contrast to PCR and LCR that produce only two copies per cycle.

CHAPTER 11

Infectious Diseases

Michael J. Mitchell

This chapter reviews some of the major infectious diseases caused by bacterial, fungal, viral, and parasitic pathogens. Pathogenic agents are arranged in alphabetical order in each section. Information regarding infections of specific organ systems may be found in the appropriate organ-specific chapters. For example, information regarding TB can be found in Chapter 13, Respiratory, Metabolic, and Acid–Base Disorders.

The diagnosis of specific infectious diseases is typically based on a combination of clinical signs and symptoms, exposure history, specific risk factors, and laboratory testing. Molecular diagnostic testing is playing an increasingly important role in the diagnosis of infectious diseases. See Chapter 17, Infectious Disease Assays, for detailed information regarding specific diagnostic testing for infectious diseases. Refer to http://www.fda.gov/MedicalDevices/ProductsandMedicalProcedures/InVitroDiagnostics/ucm330711.htm for an updated listing of FDA-approved nucleic acid based diagnostic tests.

INFECTIOUS DISEASES CAUSED BY BACTERIAL PATHOGENS

Bacterial pathogens may be classified by criteria such as Gram stain characteristics (gram-positive or gram-negative), shape (cocci, bacilli, coccobacilli, curved bacilli, spiral bacteria), growth atmosphere (aerobic, anaerobic, microaerophilic, CO_2 supplemented), optimal growth temperature (25, 35, 42°C), growth rate, inhibition on selective agar (e.g., MacConkey), required enrichment (e.g., heme, cysteine), and other factors. Definitive identification and characterization may depend on biochemical, serologic, molecular, or other testing.

Mycobacteria and other acid-fast organisms are discussed in a separate section.

- *Gram-negative bacilli, nonfastidious*: The pathogens in this group grow within 24–48 hours on routine laboratory media, like sheep blood agar (SBA). Inoculation of selective and differential media, like MacConkey (MAC) agar, may facilitate isolation from contaminated specimens. Aerobic gram-negative bacteria (GNBs) may be grouped on the basis of their ability to ferment glucose. Glucose-fermenting pathogenic GNBs include the "enterics," like *Escherichia coli* and *Salmonella*, as well as the *Vibrio* spp. Glucose nonfermenters (nGNBs) include *Pseudomonas aeruginosa* and *Acinetobacter* spp. Gram staining demonstrates avidly staining organisms. These GNBs demonstrate a variety of resistance mechanisms. Standardized susceptibility testing is required to guide treatment for most infections caused by this group of pathogens.

- *Gram-negative bacilli, fastidious*: Organisms in this group are usually capable of growth in vitro but require enriched media or special techniques for isolation.

- *Gram-negative cocci*: Organisms in this group usually grow well and rapidly on routine laboratory media but may require chocolate or other enriched media for isolation. Selective media may be used to improve isolation from specimens likely to be contaminated with endogenous flora. Empirical therapy is usually successful, but susceptibility testing is recommended for patients who fail to respond or in regions with decreased rates of susceptibility to standard treatments. Serologic testing does not play a role in routine diagnosis or management.

- *Gram-positive bacilli*: The gram-positive bacilli (GPB) usually grow within 24–48 hours on routine laboratory media, like SBA. Inoculation of selective and differential media, like Columbia colistin–nalidixic acid (CNA) or phenylethyl alcohol agar (PEA), may facilitate isolation from contaminated specimens.

- *Gram-positive cocci*: Gram-positive cocci (GPCs) cause a wide variety of infections in immunocompromised and immunocompetent hosts. Organisms grow well and rapidly on media routinely inoculated for bacterial infections. Selective media improve detection of carriage from specimens with mixed flora, as for methicillin-resistant *Staphylococcus aureus* or vancomycin-resistant enterococci (VRE). Standardized susceptibility testing may be required for management of some infections because of unpredictable susceptibility patterns. Molecular methods are playing an increasing role in diagnosis of some infections. Serologic testing does not play a role in diagnosis of acute infection.

- *Intracellular bacterial pathogens*: These organisms are unable to proliferate independently outside of host eukaryotic cells, limiting the use of routine culture for diagnosis; some agents may grow in eukaryotic cell culture, such as used for virus isolation. Infection may be confirmed by direct detection, serologic response, or molecular diagnostic methods.

- *Spiral bacteria*: The spiral bacteria form a large, metabolically diverse group of microorganisms. The organisms in this group do not grow or are difficult to grow, in vitro. In addition, special staining techniques, like silver staining, dark-field, or immunofluorescent microscopy, are needed for direct detection in specimens. Therefore, serologic techniques play a major role in specific diagnosis of these infections. Molecular diagnostic techniques are also emerging as important diagnostic tools.

- *Cell wall–deficient bacteria*: These pathogens lack the rigid outer cell wall that is typical of bacteria. They do not stain by Gram staining but may be visualized by special stains, like acridine orange. Agents are not isolated by routine culture techniques; serologic testing and molecular diagnostic testing are important methods when specific diagnosis is required.

ACINETOBACTER INFECTION

❑ Definition
Acinetobacter baumannii is a nonfastidious, glucose nonfermenting GNB. This species is the second most frequently isolated nGNB in the clinical laboratory, playing an important role in the etiology of nosocomial infections.

❑ Who Should Be Suspected?
Acinetobacter species are able to survive in very diverse environments. Although *Acinetobacter* species may be isolated as culture contaminants, they are now well established as important primary and nosocomial pathogens. Infections in virtually all organ systems have been described. Major infections include the following:

- *Wounds*: *Acinetobacter baumannii* emerged as a significant cause of infection in battlefield injuries during the Vietnam conflict and recently in casualties from Afghanistan and Iraq. It is now established as an important cause of wound and burn infections in nonmilitary patients.
- *Hospital-acquired pneumonia*: *Acinetobacter baumannii* causes a significant minority (approximately 10%) of nosocomial pneumonias, both as isolated infections or epidemic outbreaks.
- *Meningitis*: *Acinetobacter baumannii*, along with other gram-negative rods (GNRs), is playing an increasing role as a complication of neurosurgery and external CSF drain placement.
- *Nosocomial bloodstream infection*: *Acinetobacter baumannii* is responsible for up to 2% of nosocomial bloodstream infection, usually in ICU patients. The reported mortality rate is approximately 40%, exceeded only by *Pseudomonas aeruginosa* and *Candida*.
- *UTI*: *Acinetobacter baumannii* is an established, but uncommon, cause of nosocomial UTI, usually in patients with indwelling catheters.

Treatment of *A. baumannii* infections poses a significant challenge to clinicians because of intrinsic and acquired resistance. Carbapenem antibiotics are usually effective. Isolates often develop resistance to drugs used to treat these infections. Resistance may quickly emerge to the preferred agents used for nosocomial infections. Definitive treatment should be determined by susceptibility testing of the initial isolate; retesting, to detect emerging resistance, is recommended for subsequent isolates recovered during therapy.

ANAPLASMOSIS AND EHRLICHIOSIS

❏ Definition
The agents of ehrlichiosis and anaplasmosis are small, obligate intracellular bacterial pathogens. Infection is transmitted primarily by the bite of ticks. Specific diseases show restricted geographic distribution based on arthropod vector ranges.

Human granulocytotropic anaplasmosis (HGA) is caused by *Anaplasma phago-cytophilum*, transmitted by *Ixodes scapularis* or *Ixodes pacificus* (black legged tick). Disease occurs in New England and the North Central and Pacific United States. Like *Borrelia burgdorferi*, HGA may cause coinfection with other agents transmitted by *Ixodes* ticks. Deer and the white-footed mouse are the primary reservoir for HGA in the United States.

Human monocytotropic ehrlichiosis (HME) is caused by *Ehrlichia chaffeensis* and is transmitted by the lone star tick, *Amblyomma americanum*. Disease is seen in the South and mid-Atlantic, the Central United States, and some areas of New England. The white tail deer is the primary reservoir for HME.

HME and HGA are national notifiable diseases, reportable to the CDC and local departments of public health.

❏ Who Should Be Suspected?
Disease develops 1–2 weeks after the tick bite. Fever is present in most infected patients, but asymptomatic or mild disease is common. Nonspecific symptoms are common, including headache, malaise, myalgias, arthralgias, and nausea and vomiting. Rash occurs in a significant minority of patients with HME but is unusual in HGA. Rash caused by coinfection, like rickettsiosis or Lyme disease, should be considered. Mental status changes or meningeal signs may occur in a minority of patients. Renal and respiratory failures have been described infrequently.

❏ Laboratory Findings
Culture: not available for routine diagnostic testing.

Direct examination of peripheral blood or buffy coat smear stained by routine hematologic methods: Examination may demonstrate organism-filled vacuoles (morulae) in the cytoplasm of infected cells. Inclusions in granulocytes may be seen in 20–80% of patients with confirmed HGA but in a minority (1–20%) of monocytes in patients with HME. The diagnosis of HGA or HME is not ruled out by a negative smear examination. Disease should be confirmed by specific serology or other definitive test. When HME or HGA is suspected, manual differential examination should be specifically ordered. Automated methods are unlikely to detect abnormalities or trigger manual examinations.

Immunochemical staining: Immunohistochemical staining may be useful in severe or fatal cases, or for patients with early antimicrobial therapy, which may delay the immune response. Specific staining may be used on affected tissues, like bone marrow, or postmortem tissues, including the spleen, liver, lung, kidney, heart, or brain.

NAAT: Molecular diagnostic tests have been developed for diagnosis of HME, HGA, and related organisms. PCR may be positive in serum or CSF in acute stage, but moderate sensitivity (60–85%) may limit the utility of these tests; infection is not ruled out by a negative result.

11

Serology: Specific antibody response may provide an accurate diagnosis; IFA is the serologic method of choice. Patients are usually negative for specific IgG and IgM in the first week of disease. Therefore, testing paired acute serum sample and another collected 2–3 weeks later is recommended.

A probable case designation may be achieved in patients with a compatible illness in whom a single serum specimen, collected in early acute infection, shows an IFA titer that exceeds a cutoff established by the laboratory that is performing the test. Diagnosis is established by demonstration of a fourfold increase (or decrease) in IFA titer of specific IgG (*A. phagocytophilum*, *E. chaffeensis*, or other *Ehrlichia* species) in paired serum specimens. IgM testing has not been shown to be superior to paired IgG studies.

Core laboratory: Leukopenia (with left shift of PMNs), thrombocytopenia, and elevation of serum aminotransferases are commonly seen but are nonspecific findings in patients with HME and HGA.

CSF findings: Pleocytosis and protein elevation are commonly seen in patients with neurologic complications of HME; CSF is usually normal in HGA patients with neurologic complications.

ANTHRAX (*BACILLUS ANTHRACIS*)

❏ Definition
Anthrax is caused by infection with *Bacillus anthracis*, a large, spore-forming grampositive rod (GPR). Naturally occurring anthrax is a zoonotic disease associated with grazing animals in regions without effective vaccination programs; humans may be infected as secondary hosts, usually through contact with spores. In the United States, sporadic infection has been associated with contact with animal products imported from regions with endemic infection.

Anthrax has been recognized as a potential agent of bioterrorism or biologic warfare because of the ability to "weaponize" the organism and the severity of disease caused by airborne spores.

Anthrax is a national notifiable infectious disease. Reporting to public health departments is mandated for all suspected or confirmed cases of *B. anthracis* infection.

❏ Who Should Be Suspected?
There are three major anthrax syndromes, cutaneous, alimentary tract, and inhalational, depending on the route of transmission. Other organ systems may be infected by spread from a primary site of infection. The diagnosis of anthrax requires a high index of suspicion. Early recognition and antibiotic treatment are critical for successful management of patients with GI, pulmonary, or other invasive infections.

❏ Laboratory Findings
Cultures: Specimens may include vesicular fluid, swab, or tissue from below the leading edge of cutaneous lesions, lower respiratory secretions/sputum, feces, or CSF, or specimens from other infected sites. Blood cultures should be submitted for all patients with suspected anthrax.

Gram stain: Shows large GPBs; may form short chains. Capsules may be apparent. Spores may be seen in subcultures.

BARTONELLOSIS

❏ Definition
Bartonellosis refers to a range of syndromes caused by infection with *Bartonella* species, fastidious GNBs. The bacteria may be isolated from a wide range of animals, which serve as the likely reservoir for human infection.

❏ Who Should Be Suspected?
Bartonella henselae infection most commonly manifests as cat scratch disease (CSD). CSD is most commonly manifested by self-limited lymphadenopathy, but a number of organ systems may be involved. *Bartonella henselae* should be strongly suspected on the basis of typical clinical presentation after exposure to cats, especially if flea infested.

Almost all patients with CSD present with a cutaneous lesion at the site of inoculation and regional lymphadenopathy. Skin lesions appear within 3–10 days after inoculation and may show vesicular, erythematous, and papular phases. Lesions are minimally symptomatic and resolve after several weeks, healing without scarring. Primary lesions may occur on the mucous membranes or conjunctiva. Tender solitary lymphadenopathy, typically with overlying erythema, develops in the 2nd or 3rd week after infection but may be delayed up to several months. In uncomplicated cases, lymphadenopathy usually resolves within 1–4 months.

Bartonella quintana was associated with trench fever during World War I. Trench fever is transmitted by the body louse; patients present with fever, malaise, sweats and chills, conjunctivitis, retro-orbital pain, back and neck pain, and anterior tibial pain. In recent years, *B. quintana* has emerged as a cause of "urban trench fever" in indigent populations with bacteremia and endocarditis, peliosis, and bacillary angiomatosis, primarily in patients with AIDS. Suspect infection in patients with culture-negative endocarditis, vascular proliferative lesions (bacillary angiomatosis [BA]), and cystic lesions of the liver or other internal organs (peliosis).

❏ Laboratory Findings
Direct examination and histopathology: Histopathologic examination may provide strong support for diagnosis of bartonellosis. Demonstration of typical granulomas and typical organisms (Warthin-Starry stain) strongly supports the diagnosis of CSD. Histologic appearance of excised lymph node, skin lesions, and so on may be characteristic but are nonspecific. In BA, there is H&E staining of vascular proliferation. Lesions show eosinophilic debris; Warthin-Starry staining reveals masses of small bacteria.

Molecular diagnosis: Sensitive and specific molecular diagnostic assays have been described. PCR and related methods are playing an increasing role in the diagnosis of infections caused by *Bartonella* species, when available. There are no FDA-approved methods, however.

Culture: Isolation of *Bartonella* in culture provides a definitive diagnosis, but special culture techniques and prolonged incubation are required. Cultures are often negative in infected patients. In addition, most clinical laboratories cannot perform the testing required for specific identification, so isolates must be sent to a reference laboratory for further characterization. The lysis centrifugation method is recommended for blood cultures to detect *Bartonella* bloodstream infections.

11

Serology: The sensitivity and specificity of serologic assays are not high, limiting their utility for the diagnosis of bartonellosis. There may be cross-reactions with other *Bartonella* species and other, unrelated organisms. The prevalence of seropositivity in general populations may be significant, suggesting that asymptomatic *Bartonella* infection is common. In CSD, *B. henselae* IFA IgG titer of ≥1:256 is consistent with recent infection, supporting a diagnosis of CSD. Titers ≥1:64 to 128 are suggestive but should be repeated after 2 weeks to confirm diagnosis; titers <1:64 indicate that recent infection is unlikely. A positive reaction for *B. henselae* IgM strongly supports recent infection, but IgM production is typically brief.

General laboratory: ESR and CRP are usually increased in bartonellosis. WBC count is usually normal but may be slightly elevated ≤13,000/μL; eosinophils may be increased. Other laboratory findings are related to specific organ involvement.

BORDETELLA PERTUSSIS

See Chapter 13, Respiratory, Metabolic, and Acid–Base Disorders.

BOTULISM (*CLOSTRIDIUM BOTULINUM*)

❑ **Definition**
Botulism describes a toxin-mediated paralytic disease caused by heat-labile toxins of *Clostridium botulinum*. Botulism toxins bind to the synaptic vesicles of cholinergic nerves, preventing release of acetylcholine into the neurosynaptic cleft. Botulism intoxication results in acute, symmetrical, flaccid paralysis. Patients usually present with impairment of cranial nerves and muscles of the head and neck. Symptoms progress to symmetrical paralysis of the musculature of the trunk, progressing to the extremities. Respiratory paralysis is usually the most life-threatening manifestation of botulism.

Several distinct botulism syndromes have been described. Foodborne botulism usually presents in adults after ingestion of preformed toxin in *C. botulinum*–contaminated food. Infant botulism, the most commonly encountered form of botulism, results from the ingestion of *C. botulinum* organisms or spores that proliferate and produce toxin within the infant's gut. Wound botulism is a rare form of botulism in which toxin is formed in vivo by *C. botulinum* organisms causing wound infection.

Clinicians must be alert to patients presenting with signs and symptoms compatible with botulism because they may represent an index case of a bioterror incident. Reporting to public health authorities is mandated for suspected or documented botulism.

❑ **Laboratory Findings**
Culture: In the proper clinical setting, diagnosis may be established by isolation of *C. botulinum* or botulinum toxin from patient specimens or food. Isolation of *C. botulinum* by anaerobic culture may be attempted for infected patient specimens or feces. Isolation from food should only be attempted by specialized reference laboratories.

Toxin detection: Typical specimens include any food suspected in an outbreak, serum (15–20 mL in adults; 2–3 mL in infants), gastric contents or vomitus, and feces (as much as possible, up to approximately 50 g). Toxin detection is performed by specialized reference or public health laboratories.

Core laboratory: Routine laboratory tests are usually normal.

BRUCELLA

❑ Definition
Brucella species are fastidious, slowly growing GNRs. Isolates are highly infectious and pose a serious risk of laboratory-acquired infections; clinicians should alert the laboratory when brucellosis is suspected. The CDC has classified *Brucella* species as potential bioterror agents, and reporting is mandated when *Brucella* infection is suspected or confirmed.

❑ Who Should Be Suspected?
Brucellosis causes a wide spectrum of clinical disease with acute and chronic forms. In affected patients, fever, chills, night sweats, malaise, headache, and other non-specific symptoms are common and may mimic other acute or chronic illness or fever of unknown origin (FUO). Bacteremia often occurs and may result in second-ary localized infections; suppurative lesions may affect any organ system, including bone and joints, liver, and spleen.

❑ Laboratory Findings
Cultures: *Brucella* species primarily infect the RE system with secondary spread to other organ systems. Therefore, blood and bone marrow cultures are specimens of choice for diagnosis. Other infected patient samples may also be submitted for culture.

Serology: Acute serum samples should be collected, followed by conva-lescent samples several weeks later. IgM titers are increased within the first 1–2 weeks of acute infection; there is a transition to IgG production after the 2nd week. Titers fall in response to effective therapy.

BURKHOLDERIA INFECTIONS

❑ Definition
Burkholderia species are nonfastidious, glucose nonfermenting GNBs. *Burkholderia pseudomallei* and *Burkholderia cepacia* are the species most commonly associ-ated with human disease. *Burkholderia pseudomallei* has a fairly restricted, geo-graphically limited incidence; primary infection in the United States is uncommon. *Burkholderia cepacia* has been isolated from numerous environmental sources.

Burkholderia mallei (a primary pathogen of horses) and *B. pseudomallei* have been classified by the CDC as potential bioterror agents. Reporting is mandated as soon as *B. mallei* or *B. pseudomallei* infection is suspected or confirmed.

❑ Who Should Be Suspected?
Burkholderia pseudomallei causes melioidosis, an infection with a restricted geo-graphic distribution; disease is largely confined to Southeast Asia and northern Australia. Direct contact with or inhalation of contaminated soil or water is the most common mode of transmission. Most infections are asymptomatic or mini-mally symptomatic with a flu-like syndrome but may present with acute or chronic

11

illness, including pneumonia, skin and soft tissue infections, chronic suppurative infections, and bacteremia.

Burkholderia cepacia has emerged as a significant pathogen, primarily causing disease in patients with CF and chronic granulomatous disease. In patients with CF, respiratory tract colonization may be associated with a rapid decline in pulmonary function and an increased mortality in the year following acquisition.

❑ Laboratory Findings

Culture: *Burkholderia pseudomallei* or *mallei* may be isolated by routine bacterial culture but may require additional incubation time. Selective media should be used for isolation of *B. cepacia* from lower respiratory specimens collected from CF patients.

Susceptibility: *Burkholderia cepacia* is intrinsically resistant to aminoglycosides but typically susceptible to TMP/SMX.

CAMPYLOBACTER GASTROENTERITIS

❑ Definition

Campylobacter species are microaerophilic, curved GNBs. *Campylobacter* species cause diarrheal infections globally and are the most common bacterial cause of significant diarrheal illness in most countries. *Campylobacter jejuni* is the most important human pathogen. In developed countries, asymptomatic infection is uncommon.

❑ Who Should Be Suspected?

Infection is usually acquired by contact with animals, mainly poultry, in which *Campylobacter* species are common components of endogenous gut flora. Person-to-person transmission is uncommon. Most infections resolve within 7 days. *Campylobacter* GI infection typically results in diarrhea with fever, cramping, and vomiting. Blood may be present in the stools. A nonspecific colitis, with marked fecal leukocytes, is common. Guillain-Barré syndrome has been associated with campylobacteriosis. Disease outside the GI tract is uncommon. Septic arthritis, bacteremia, proctocolitis, meningitis, and other infections have been reported.

❑ Laboratory Findings

Culture: The special culture procedures required for isolation of *Campylobacter* species are included in routine stool culture protocols in clinical microbiology laboratories.

CHLAMYDIA AND CHLAMYDOPHILA INFECTIONS

❑ Definition

Chlamydia and *Chlamydophila* species are obligate intracellular bacterial pathogens.

❑ Who Should Be Suspected?

The Chlamydiaceae are responsible for a number of distinctive disease syndromes, including

- *Chlamydia genital tract infection*. *Chlamydia trachomatis* is the most common cause of sexually transmitted bacterial infections in industrialized nations; serovars D through K are responsible for these genital infections.

Serovars L1, L2 (including a and b variants), and L3 are responsible for lymphogranuloma venereum (LGV), a systemic STD most commonly encountered in developing countries.

Most sexually transmitted *C. trachomatis* infections are asymptomatic, contributing to their spread. Common clinical manifestations include urethritis, mucopurulent cervicitis, ascending infections, female genital tract conditions (PID, endometritis, salpingitis, perihepatitis syndrome), male genital tract problems (epididymitis), conjunctivitis (nonscarring), and proctitis. Complications of *C. trachomatis* genital infection may include scarring of the fallopian tubes, infertility, and ectopic pregnancy. Maternal *C. trachomatis* infection at the time of delivery may result in neonatal infection, which typically manifests as conjunctivitis or pneumonia. Acute, nonscarring inclusion conjunctivitis occurs in 18–50% of infants of mothers with untreated genital infection.

- *Trachoma*: Trachoma refers to chronic *C. trachomatis* conjunctivitis, usually caused by serovars A, B1, B2, and C. Infection leads to corneal scarring and, in late stages, blindness.
- *Chlamydophila pulmonary infections* (*Chlamydophila pneumoniae* and *Chlamydophila psittaci*): *C. pneumoniae* is most commonly associated with lower and upper respiratory tract infections (e.g., pneumonia, bronchitis, sinusitis). This pathogen has been implicated in a significant minority (approximately 15%) of community-acquired cases of pneumonia.

Chlamydophila psittaci infection causes psittacosis. Birds are the natural reservoir for this organism; infectious forms may remain viable in the environment for extended periods. Human infection is easily transmitted by inhalation of infectious organisms directly shed from birds or from organisms in their environment. Patients usually present with nonspecific symptoms in acute infection, including flu-like illness: fever, severe headache, hepatomegaly, splenomegaly, and GI symptoms. Chronic pneumonitis may develop.

❏ Laboratory Findings

Molecular diagnostic testing: NAATs are considered the gold standard for the diagnosis of genital *C. trachomatis* infections. FDA-approved kits are available for endocervical, urine, urethral specimens, and liquid-based Pap test specimens. The sensitivities reported for NAATs range from approximately 90 to 97%; the specificities are >99%. NAATs have been described for detection of *C. pneumoniae* and *C. psittaci*, but FDA-approved kits are not available, and their performance has not been clearly defined.

Culture: Isolation of *C. trachomatis* in culture remains an important technique for diagnosis of nongenital infections and is considered the standard for evidence in medicolegal cases, such as rape and child abuse. For optimal isolation, it is critical to collect samples that contain the host cells infected by chlamydia and to transport in conditions that will maintain the viability of the organisms. For detection of genital infections, the sensitivity of tissue culture is approximately 65–85%, with specificity near 100%.

Direct detection: DFA staining kits are available for direct detection of *C. trachomatis* from genital specimens. Slides require examination by an experienced laboratorian, and slides must be carefully evaluated to ensure adequate specimen collection (i.e., the presence of columnar epithelial cells). Under optimal conditions, the sensitivity of DFA is approximately 60–80% with specificity >98%. Typical intracytoplasmic inclusions in epithelial cells of Giemsa-stained smears from conjunctival scrapings are found in 50% of patients with *C. trachomatis* conjunctivitis.

EIA detection: A number of EIA kits for the diagnosis of *C. trachomatis* genital infection are commercially available. Sensitivities of approximately 60% are reported for cervical infections. Reported specificity is high, but false-positive reactions are possible for tests based on detection of *C. trachomatis* lipopolysaccharide.

Serology: Serologic testing is not helpful for the diagnosis of acute genital infection caused by *C. trachomatis*. Serology may be useful to document diagnosis of psittacosis, LGV, and respiratory tract infections.

- *Complement fixation (CF) assays* target response to LPS common to all members of the Chlamydiaceae, so positive results must be interpreted in the context of disease. CF testing is most useful for LGV, where titers ≥256 are considered diagnostic.
- *Microimmunofluorescence (MIF) assays* are useful for the diagnosis of neonatal pulmonary infection because they allow specific detection of IgM and IgG. An IgM titer of ≥32 supports the diagnosis. In LGV, an IgG titer of ≥128 provides strong support for diagnosis. *Chlamydophila pneumoniae* infection may be documented by a fourfold increase in titer between acute and convalescent specimens, an IgM titer ≥16 or an IgG titer ≥512.
- *EIA assays*, based on synthetic peptides, have been developed to simplify the technically demanding MIF procedure. In general, results have compared favorably to results of MIF testing.

CLOSTRIDIAL INFECTIONS: GENERAL

Clostridium species are anaerobic, spore-forming gram-positive bacilli. The formation of spores results in efficient survival of clostridia in the environment; the spores serve as the source of infections of exogenous origin (e.g., *Clostridium difficile* colitis, *Clostridium perfringens* food poisoning). Clostridia may also cause infections of endogenous origin (e.g., myonecrosis). *Clostridium* species produce some of the most potent toxins, which are responsible for some clostridial diseases (e.g., tetanus). Botulinum toxin is considered to have significant potential for use as a bioterror agent.

Clostridia grow well and rapidly on media for anaerobic culture, but selective media may be needed for contaminated specimens. The interpretation of cultures positive for *Clostridium* species is usually straightforward, but because of the ubiquitous distribution of clostridia in the environment, positive cultures must be interpreted in the context of the clinical presentation. Standardized susceptibility testing is available using specialized techniques, but many laboratories do not offer the testing in-house.

CLOSTRIDIAL GAS GANGRENE, CELLULITIS, AND PUERPERAL SEPSIS

❏ Definition

These syndromes may be caused by a number of clostridial species of endogenous or exogenous origin. Most cases of clostridial gangrene are caused by *C. perfringens*, *Clostridium novyi*, and *Clostridium septicum*.

❏ Who Should Be Suspected?

Patients present with rapidly progressive tissue necrosis, tissue liquefaction, and gas formation. Gas formation in tissue is not specific for clostridial infections and may be formed by other bacterial pathogens. Clostridial myonecrosis should be considered a medical emergency, and rapid and effective communication with clinical personnel, especially surgeons, is critical.

❏ Laboratory Findings

Direct detection: Gram stain typically shows massive tissue necrosis, a lack of PMNs, and the presence of typical organisms (usually large "box-car" GPBs; the absence of spores on Gram stain is common and does not rule out clostridial infection; other bacterial morphotypes may be seen in mixed infections).

Culture: Blood cultures may be positive.

Core laboratory: WBC count is increased (15,000–40,000/μL). Platelets are decreased in 50% of patients. Protein and casts are often present in urine. Renal insufficiency may progress to uremia. Laboratory findings typical for underlying diseases (e.g., DM) or complications of clostridial infection are seen. In postabortion sepsis, sudden severe hemolytic anemia is common with conditions such as hypoglobulinemia, hemoglobinuria, increased serum bilirubin, spherocytosis, and increased osmotic and mechanical fragility.

CLOSTRIDIUM DIFFICILE INFECTION (CDI) AND ASSOCIATED (PSEUDOMEMBRANOUS) COLITIS

❏ Definition

Clostridium difficile is a major cause of antibiotic-associated diarrhea and colitis. It is the most important cause of pseudomembranous colitis. CDI is usually acquired nosocomially.

❏ Who Should Be Suspected?

Several factors are associated with increased risk for *C. difficile* disease, including recent or current antimicrobial (or antineoplastic) therapy, age (>65 years), suppression of gastric acid production, and debilitating underlying medical conditions.

❏ Laboratory Findings

Culture: Specific laboratory diagnosis is based on the growth of *C. difficile* from stool culture or by detection of *C. difficile*–specific antigen, toxins, or DNA. Testing should be performed only on liquid stool specimens; asymptomatic carriage may be seen. Formed stool should be rejected if submitted for testing. Isolation of toxigenic *C. difficile*, using selective anaerobic culture, is considered the "gold standard" for diagnosis. Toxin production by isolates must be documented and may be confirmed by PCR, antigen, or cytotoxicity assays. The complexity and turnaround time required for toxigenic culture assays have limited their use for routine testing.

Cytotoxicity assays: These assays are based on detection of the cytotoxic effect of *C. difficile* toxin B on cultured eukaryotic cells. Testing may be performed on stool filtrate or *C. difficile* culture supernatant.

Toxin EIA: A number of enzyme immunoassays are commercially available for rapid detection of *C. difficile* toxin B or both toxins A and B. Because of their simplicity and rapid turnaround time (<1 hour), EIA tests have been widely used for diagnosis of CDI. EIA assays have shown high specificity (>95%), but the sensitivity of different assays is variable, ranging from approximately 60 to 95%, which has limited their use in critically ill patients or infection control investigations.

Antigen detection: Detection of *C. difficile*–specific glutamate dehydrogenase (GDH) antigen may be used to screen stools for *C. difficile*. The sensitivity of the GDH assay depends on the reference standard; sensitivities ranging from approximately 70 to >95% have been reported. Toxin must be documented in GDH antigen–positive specimens because nontoxigenic *C. difficile* strains are detected by this assay.

Molecular diagnostic testing: PCR assays that target the toxin B gene have emerged as clinically important assays for the diagnosis of *C. difficile* GI infection. Several FDA-approved methods are commercially available. Reported performance of molecular diagnostic assays has shown S/S both in the range approximately 95–99%. The use of real-time PCR assays provides for results within 24 hours.

Combination tests: Some laboratories have combined EIA, GDH antigen, and/or PCR testing in simultaneous or sequential test algorithms to improve the S/S and cost-effectiveness of these test methods.

CLOSTRIDIUM TETANI INFECTION

❑ Definition
Tetanus describes disease caused by a heat-labile toxin (tetanospasmin) elaborated by *Clostridium tetani*. Infection typically results from "dirty" traumatic injuries (e.g., deep puncture wounds, crush injuries) contaminated by spores of *C. tetani*. Toxin diffuses from the site of infection into the circulation, where it gains access to peripheral motor neurons. Toxin is transported through the neurons to the CNS, where it blocks inhibitory signals from the CNS to motor neurons. Tetanospasmin also binds to receptors at the myoneural junctions (different from the receptors for botulinum toxin), inhibiting the release of acetylcholine. Tetanus has been essentially eliminated in populations with an effective vaccination program, but sporadic cases occur in unvaccinated populations.

❑ Who Should Be Suspected?
Patients present with spasm of flexor and extensor muscles. Patients develop pathologic hyperresponsiveness to minor stimuli. Common features include "lock jaw," risus sardonicus, and back spasms resulting in relentless arching.

❑ Laboratory Findings
Diagnosis is usually made on the basis of typical clinical findings. Culture from an infected site usually has poor sensitivity and is usually noncontributory. Core laboratory findings are usually normal.

DIPHTHERIA

See Chapter 13, Respiratory, Metabolic, and Acid–Base Disorders.

ENTEROCOCCAL INFECTIONS

❑ **Definition**

Enterococcus species are aerobic GPCs that form pairs and short chains. *Enterococcus* species are universal components of the endogenous lower GI tract flora in healthy humans; colonization of the urogenital mucosa is common. Enterococci are moderately virulent, but the mechanisms are not clearly understood.

Enterococci may demonstrate intrinsic and acquired resistance to antibiotics, including vancomycin. This characteristic is at least partially responsible for the emergence of enterococci as significant nosocomial pathogens. *Enterococcus faecalis* and *E. faecium* are the species most commonly associated with human infection.

❑ **Who Should Be Suspected?**

Enterococci may cause infection in virtually any organ system; common infections include UTIs, bacteremia, endocarditis, intra-abdominal infections, and wound infections. Hospitalized patients who are rectal carriers of VRE may transmit these pathogens to other patients that may be at high risk for invasive VRE infection.

❑ **Laboratory Findings**

Culture: Isolates grow in 24–48 hours on media for GPC isolation under standard incubation conditions. Susceptibility testing must be performed for significant clinical isolates.

ESCHERICHIA COLI INFECTION

❑ **Definition**

Escherichia coli is a nonfastidious, glucose-fermenting GNB. *E. coli* is the most common clinical isolate in most microbiology laboratories. It is a ubiquitous component of the GI bacterial flora and is the most common cause of community-acquired UTI in normal hosts. *Escherichia coli* is a major cause of nosocomial infections and infections in immunocompromised patients. *Escherichia coli* isolates may cause enteritis or gastroenteritis by a number of mechanisms, including toxin production and adherence to mucosal epithelial cells of the colon.

❑ **Who Should Be Suspected?**

Escherichia coli should be considered in any patient with UTI. *Escherichia coli* may also be suspected in patients with "traveler's diarrhea" (abrupt onset, with profuse, watery diarrhea after travel to an endemic area). Enterohemorrhagic *E. coli* infection may be suspected in patients with diarrhea, especially in patients who develop HUS after diarrheal illness. See the discussion of foodborne causes of diarrhea in Chapter 5, Digestive Diseases.

Escherichia coli is responsible for a wide spectrum of opportunistic and nosocomial infections. It is a major cause of nosocomial pneumonia, bloodstream infection, surgical site infection, and UTI. It is also responsible for a significant proportion of severe neonatal infections, including sepsis and meningitis.

❑ **Laboratory Findings**

Culture: Recognition of *E. coli* strains that cause enterohemorrhagic gastroenteritis may be improved by the use of the differential sorbitol–MAC agar. These strains produce Shiga toxin 1 and/or toxin 2, which may be directly detected in stool specimens by antigen testing or NAAT.

Serotyping: In the United States, most isolates are serotype O157:H7. Although there are tests that can be used to identify other types of diarrheagenic *E. coli*, testing is not widely available. Specific diagnosis is rarely needed for patient management.

FRANCISELLA TULARENSIS INFECTION

❑ Definition
Tularemia is caused by *F. tularensis*, a fastidious, tiny gram-negative coccobacillus. Naturally acquired tularemia is a zoonotic, tick-transmitted infection. The normal host species include rabbits, rodents, squirrels and other small mammals, and deer. Domestic livestock, especially sheep, are also susceptible to infection. Human infection is transmitted by direct contact with an infected animal or through the bite of an intermediate arthropod vector.

Francisella tularensis is highly infectious and poses a serious risk for laboratory-acquired infections; clinicians should alert the laboratory when tularemia is suspected so that appropriate precautions and culture techniques are used. The CDC has classified *F. tularensis* as a potential bioterror agent. Possible or confirmed *F. tularensis* infections must be reported to state departments of health.

❑ Who Should Be Suspected?
Disease usually occurs 2–10 days after exposure, with ulceration at the site of tick bite and painful regional adenopathy. Nonspecific symptoms are common, including fever, chills, headache, sweats, severe conjunctivitis, and regional adenopathy. Approximately 20% of patients present with acute onset of fever and abdominal symptoms, including nonbloody diarrhea, vomiting, pain, and tenderness.

❑ Laboratory Findings
Gram stain: Tiny faintly staining coccobacilli.

Culture: Samples of blood, bone marrow, primary ulcers, lymph node aspirates, or other infected tissue. Cysteine is required for growth.

HAEMOPHILUS INFECTIONS

❑ Definition
Haemophilus species are fastidious gram-negative coccobacilli and are responsible for a variety of infectious syndromes. They are common components of the endogenous flora of the mouth and upper respiratory tract. Most of the respiratory species have limited virulence and are able to cause disease only when normal host defenses are compromised. Strains of *Haemophilus influenzae* may be encapsulated (serotypes a, b, c, d, e, and f). The serotype b capsular material is a virulence factor and is responsible for the ability of *H. influenzae* type b (Hib) to cause severe, invasive infections. *Haemophilus ducreyi* causes the STD chancroid.

❑ Who Should Be Suspected?
Most *Haemophilus* infections present as localized infections of the pararespiratory structures, like sinusitis or otitis media. Acute sinusitis is usually manifested by nasal congestion with purulent discharge, which may be unilateral. See the discussion of sinusitis in Chapter 13. Respiratory, Metabolic, and Acid–Base Disorder.

Haemophilus influenzae may cause an acute lobar pneumonia, but lower respiratory disease is most commonly manifested as bronchitis in patients with underlying lung disease. These patients typically present with nonproductive cough, wheezing, and increasing shortness of breath. In these patients, *Haemophilus* infection may cause significant deterioration of pulmonary function tests, hypoxemia, and dyspnea. Low-grade fever may be seen.

Epiglottitis, cellulitis of the supraglottic structures, is a life-threatening manifestation of Hib infection. The tissue may be directly seeded by posterior pharyngeal organisms or as a result of bacteremia. There is typically an abrupt onset of fever, malaise, severe sore throat, and dysphagia. Dyspnea, inspiratory stridor, and drooling develop with progression to severe disease, caused by obstruction of the airway by the swelling of the supraglottic tissue. Attempts to collect swab specimens for culture may stimulate acute obstruction, so they are contraindicated prior to securing a protected airway. Lateral x-ray studies of the hypopharyngeal region demonstrate swelling of the epiglottis. Culture of blood commonly yields *H. influenzae*.

Encapsulated strains, especially type b, may cause meningitis or invasive disease. Culture and analysis of blood and CSF should be submitted to establish the diagnosis. Other localized infections associated with bacteremic disease include septic arthritis, osteomyelitis, and cellulitis. Buccal and periorbital cellulitis have been commonly, but not exclusively, associated with Hib. Buccal cellulitis presents with swelling of the cheek with deep red discoloration. Periorbital cellulitis presents with signs and symptoms of pus accumulation in the orbital tissues and a characteristic purple discoloration of the lids and skin surrounding the affected eye. *Haemophilus influenzae* may also cause acute conjunctivitis and endophthalmitis. *Haemophilus influenzae* biogroup *aegyptius* has been implicated in conjunctivitis and Brazilian purpuric fever, a bacteremia syndrome with fever and hypotension, purpuric rash, vomiting, and abdominal pain.

Haemophilus ducreyi causes chancroid, an ulcerative STI that occurs primarily in tropical regions. Disease is manifested by multiple genital and perineal ulcers. Unlike the chancres of syphilis, the ulcers of chancroid are painful and have ragged borders with minimal induration. Inguinal adenopathy is common and may progress to draining buboes. Like other genital ulcerative diseases, chancroid increases the risk of transmission of HIV infection.

❏ Laboratory Findings

Gram stain: Diagnosis of *Haemophilus* infection depends primarily of Gram stain and culture of infected specimens. Gram staining shows small, pleomorphic, faintly staining gram-negative rods; some end-to-end pairing or small filamentous forms may be present.

Culture: *Haemophilus* species are fastidious but are efficiently isolated on chocolate agar and in routine blood culture media. Positive cultures from the upper respiratory tract must be interpreted with caution because *Haemophilus* species, including encapsulated strains, are common components of the endogenous flora. Specimens for the diagnosis of chancroid are collected from the margin and undermined base of fresh ulcers. *Haemophilus ducreyi* is difficult to isolate by culture, requiring specialized enriched media that should be inoculated at bedside.

Antigen detection (for detection of Hib from CSF, serum, or urine): Use of antigen detection is not recommended, having been shown to rarely contribute to the clinical management of patients.

HELICOBACTER PYLORI INFECTION

❏ **Definition**

Helicobacter pylori is a fastidious, curved GNB. *Helicobacter pylori* infection shows a global distribution.

Most infections are transmitted by the fecal–oral route.

❏ **Who Should Be Suspected?**

Helicobacter pylori is the cause of most gastric and duodenal ulcers through disruption of the protective mucous layer. This organism is epidemiologically linked to gastric adenocarcinoma and lymphoma.

❏ **Laboratory Findings**

Helicobacter pylori may be diagnosed by several invasive or noninvasive means:

- *Histologic examination of gastric mucosa*: Organisms stain poorly with H&E but may be demonstrated with Giemsa or silver staining.
- *Culture of gastric mucosa*: Special culture techniques are required for isolation. The organism is microaerophilic and capnophilic and yields growth within 5 days on enriched media.
- *Urease activity* (direct tissue or breath test): Strongly positive.
- *Specific antigen*: A commercially available assay for detection of *H. pylori* antigen in feces shows a sensitivity of approximately 90% and specificity of approximately 95% for detection of active infection. *Helicobacter pylori* antigen may be useful for monitoring response to therapy.
- *Serology*: *Helicobacter pylori* antibody IgG is typically measured. Positive response is predictive of active infection in patient populations where the prevalence of active infection is not high. Antibody levels may remain persistently positive for a period after successful therapy, so serology may have a limited role in early test of cure.

KLEBSIELLA PNEUMONIAE INFECTION

❏ **Definition**

Klebsiella pneumoniae is a nonfastidious, glucose-fermenting GNB. *Klebsiella pneumoniae* is widely distributed in nature as well as the normal fecal flora of humans. It is a common isolate in the clinical laboratory, often associated with nosocomial infection or infection of immunocompromised hosts.

❏ **Who Should Be Suspected?**

Klebsiella pneumoniae is associated with severe pneumonia, especially in alcoholics. The pneumonia results in necrosis and hemorrhage; mucoid, "currant jelly" sputum is classic. Bacteremia is seen in a significant number of cases. *Klebsiella pneumoniae* is also associated with primary or hospital-acquired UTI, nosocomial bloodstream, ventilator-associated, or other extraintestinal infection. *Klebsiella pneumoniae* isolates are of particular importance in hospital-acquired infections because of their intrinsic and acquired resistance to antimicrobial agents.

❏ **Laboratory Findings**

Cultures: *Klebsiella pneumoniae* isolates often produce mucoid colonies due to production of capsular material.

Susceptibility: All *Klebsiella* species are intrinsically resistant to ampicillin and ticarcillin. Many hospital isolates have additional resistance through acquisition of plasmids that carry resistance genes. Extended-spectrum beta-lactamases confer resistance to third-generation cephalosporins and most other beta-lactam antibiotics. *Klebsiella pneumoniae* carbapenemases confer resistance to imipenem, ertapenem, and meropenem in addition to most beta-lactam antibiotics.

LISTERIA INFECTION

❑ Definition
Listeriosis is caused by infection with *Listeria monocytogenes*, an aerobic, pleomorphic gram-positive bacillus. This organism is widely distributed in nature, and up to 5% of asymptomatic, healthy adults carry *L. monocytogenes* as a component of their endogenous fecal flora. CNS and placental tissue are predisposed to *Listeria* infection. Most infections are thought to occur as a result of oral ingestion, followed by invasion across the gut mucosa and systemic spread. Disease may occur in a sporadic or epidemic pattern.

❑ Who Should Be Suspected?
- *Listeria* is responsible for a small proportion of foodborne infections, and most cases are sporadic, but the case–fatality rate is relatively high. Outbreaks have been caused by a variety of types of food, including delicatessen meats, unpasteurized cheeses, smoked seafood, and processed meat spreads. Ingestion of contaminated food may cause self-limited gastroenteritis in normal hosts, with onset typically several days after exposure. Symptoms include fever, nausea, vomiting, and diarrhea. Flu-like symptoms are common.
- Risk factors associated with increased infection risk and severity include immunocompromise, age ≥70 years, alcoholism, glucocorticoid therapy, kidney disease, nonhematologic malignancy, neonatal infection, and pregnancy.
- In normal hosts, complete recovery is typical after several days of illness. During pregnancy, listeriosis usually presents with flu-like symptoms and may resolve spontaneously. Severe listeriosis may occur in the third trimester where placental infection and transmission to the fetus or neonate may occur. The signs and symptoms of *Listeria* sepsis are not distinctive, and diagnostic cultures are critical for specific diagnosis. Patients present with fever and malaise that may progress to shock and sepsis. Symptoms of meningoencephalitis are nonspecific and may include meningeal signs, mental status changes, or focal neurologic defects (e.g., ataxia, cranial nerve abnormalities, and deafness). Direct hematogenous seeding of the brain parenchyma may result in cerebritis or brain abscess, most typically manifested by stroke-like symptoms or focal neurologic defects.

❑ Laboratory Findings
Culture (blood): Most reliable diagnostic test; culture of CSF and other infected tissue is indicated on the basis of clinical presentation. Isolation of *Listeria* from suspected food samples requires special techniques performed at reference laboratories.

Gram stain: CSF Gram stain is only positive in about one third of patients with meningoencephalitis and lower in localized CNS infections. *Listeria* may be misidentified as *Streptococcus pneumoniae*, diphtheroids, or even *H. influenzae*.

CSF findings: Pleocytosis is typical (100 to 10,000 WBCs/µL). Significant CSF lymphocytosis (>25%) may be seen on CSF WBC differential prior to antibiotic therapy. CSF protein concentration is typically moderately elevated; CSF glucose is reduced in only approximately 40% of patients with CNS infection. CSF findings may lead to misdiagnosis as viral infection, syphilis, Lyme disease, or TB.

Serology: Not usually useful for diagnosis of acute listeriosis.

LYME DISEASE

❑ Definition

Lyme disease is a systemic, chronic borreliosis caused by *Borrelia burgdorferi*, a fastidious spiral bacterium. Infection is transmitted by the bite of *Ixodes* ticks. A variety of clinical manifestations are seen. Recurrent clinical disease may be caused by reinfection. Lyme disease is reportable in the Nationally Notifiable Infectious Diseases Surveillance System. Criteria for case definition may be seen on the CDC Web site: ⟨http://www.cdc.gov/ncphi/disss/nndss/casedef/lyme_disease_2008.htm⟩.

❑ Who Should Be Suspected?

- Acute disease occurs about 1–4 weeks after tick bite, manifested by non-specific febrile symptoms that may be confused with a "viral syndrome." Erythema migrans (EM) is characteristic for Lyme disease and occurs in 60–80% of infected patients. EM typically begins as a red papule with surrounding erythema that expands over days to weeks. The central region commonly clears, resulting in a bull's-eye appearance. Secondary EM lesions may appear. Other common acute symptoms include fever, headache, and fatigue. Myalgias, arthralgias, and mild meningeal signs may occur. EM is diagnostic for Lyme disease in patients at epidemiologic risk, but its absence does not exclude this diagnosis. Laboratory confirmation is recommended for patients with EM with no known exposure or for patients with nonspecific signs and symptoms of Lyme disease.
- Late symptoms are typically manifested by musculoskeletal, cardiovascular, or nervous system signs and symptoms. Chronic, intermittent arthritis affecting one or a few large joints is a common manifestation of late, chronic infection and may occur weeks to years after acute infection. The knee is commonly involved. Progressive arthritis or symmetric polyarthritis is not typical and should prompt consideration or another diagnosis. Nonspecific findings include arthralgias or myalgias.
  - ▼ Carditis is usually manifested by acute second- or third-degree atrioventricular conduction defects that typically resolve in days to weeks. Myocarditis may accompany the conduction abnormalities. Nonspecific findings may be seen, including bradycardia or palpitations.
  - ▼ A variety of nervous system abnormalities may be seen, including acute meningitis, cranial neuritis (facial nerve palsy), radiculopathy, or encephalomyelitis. The triad of aseptic fluctuating meningoencephalitis, Bell palsy, and peripheral neuropathy is very suggestive of Lyme disease. Nonspecific findings may be seen, including fatigue, headache, or paresthesias.

❏ Laboratory Findings

Culture: Not widely available and usually positive only early during the acute infection.

Serology: Not helpful or necessary at the early, acute stage; tests are only 40–60% sensitive, and diagnosis is not ruled out by a negative test. Testing should be ordered only to support clinical diagnosis, not for screening persons with nonspecific symptoms because of their intrinsic poor sensitivity and specificity. Vaccination produces seropositivity. See Chapter 17, Infectious Disease Assays for details of serologic testing for *B. burgdorferi* infection.

- A negative EIA or IFA result usually excludes Lyme disease, but testing paired acute- and convalescent-phase serum samples may be needed for patients with a high index of suspicion and negative results of initial testing. Patients with disseminated or chronic Lyme disease are usually strongly positive for specific anti-*B. burgdorferi* IgG.
- Specific IgM antibodies usually appear 2–4 weeks after EM and peak after 3–6 weeks of illness. IgM usually declines to undetectable levels after 4–6 months. In some patients, IgM remains elevated for many months or reappears late in illness, indicating continued infection. A negative test within 2 weeks of onset of symptoms does not rule out infection.
- Specific IgG titers rise more slowly, usually appearing 4–8 weeks after rash. IgG titers peak after 4–6 months and may remain high for months or years, even with successful antibiotic therapy. A single increased IgG titer may be due to previous infection or vaccination and must be interpreted in the context of clinical symptoms. An IgG titer ≥1:800 usually indicates active infection; a titer of 1:200 to 1:400 is indeterminate. Titers <1:100 are considered negative.
- Paired acute and convalescent sera at 4- to 6-week intervals may demonstrate a significant rise in titer, indicating active infection. Testing of paired serum samples may be needed to confirm infection in patients with compatible symptoms, but without a known tick bite or rash, who have been in endemic area.
- RF may cause false-positive result for IgM. False-positive IgG in high titers may be caused by antibodies from spirochetal diseases (syphilis, relapsing fever, yaws, pinta); low titers may be found in infectious mononucleosis, hepatitis B, autoimmune diseases (e.g., SLE, RA), periodontal disease, ehrlichiosis, rickettsiosis, other bacteria (e.g., *H. pylori*). Five percent to fifteen percent of persons in endemic areas may be seropositive without any signs or symptoms of active infection.

Western blot assays: Used to confirm initial serologic testing with EIA or IFA. IgG WB assays may not become positive until after many months of illness; negative WB should be repeated in 2–4 weeks if Lyme disease is strongly suspected.

Molecular tests: PCR plays a limited role in the diagnosis of Lyme disease and is not recommended in seronegative patients. PCR may be positive for CSF in acute lymphocytic meningitis (not encephalomyelitis or other neurologic syndrome) or for synovial fluid of joints with active disease. PCR is not reliable for other types of specimens.

Synovial fluid of affected joints: Shows mild to moderate increased WBCs, typically with granulocyte predominance.

CSF findings: Patients with Lyme encephalomyelitis show lymphocytic pleocytosis, slightly increased protein and globulin, and normal glucose. Oligoclonal bands may be demonstrated. Intrathecal antibody production may be demonstrated by higher titer in CSF than in serum. Almost all of these patients will have positive serum serologic tests.

Core laboratory: Findings related to dysfunction of infected organs may be seen. Nonspecific laboratory findings include increase of ESR, lymphopenia, cryoglobulinemia, and increase of hepatic enzymes. Treponemal tests for syphilis may be positive, but nontreponemal tests should be nonreactive.

MYCOPLASMA PNEUMONIAE AND UREAPLASMA UREALYTICUM INFECTIONS

❑ Definition

Mycoplasma and *Ureaplasma* species are cell wall–deficient organisms. Cells are surrounded by a trilayer cell membrane. They are the smallest free-living human pathogens.

❑ Who Should Be Suspected?

- *Mycoplasma pneumoniae* is a significant cause of community-acquired pneumonia, typically presenting with upper respiratory tract symptoms and tracheobronchitis. Extrapulmonary symptoms are presumably caused by an autoimmune response to primary pulmonary infection. Extrapulmonary manifestations include arthritis, hemolytic anemia, and neurologic diseases (meningoencephalitis, cranial nerve palsy, ascending paralysis, transverse myelitis).

- *Ureaplasma urealyticum* may be detected in the microflora of genital mucosa in healthy adults, but there is evidence to link *U. urealyticum* to genital tract and neonatal infections. Infections include epididymitis, neonatal infections (pneumonia, bacteremia), nongonococcal urethritis, and orchitis.

❑ Laboratory Findings

Direct detection: Because of the lack of a rigid cell wall, *M. pneumoniae* and *U. urealyticum* do not stain with Gram stain. A DNA stain, like acridine orange, may demonstrate organisms in infected tissue.

Culture: Culture of the organism from sputum, nasopharynx, or other infected specimen shows good sensitivity but requires special culture techniques that are not widely available.

Molecular diagnostic testing: An FDA-approved assay is available for *M. pneumoniae*.

Serology: Serologic assays have been described for both *M. pneumoniae* and *U. urealyticum*. EIA methods are most widely used and provide good sensitivity and specificity. Accurate detection may require testing of both acute and convalescent specimens, especially in adults. EIA methods have been adapted for the detection of specific IgM.

IgM increases in the first week, peaks in the 3rd to 5th week, begins to decrease in 4–6 months but may persist ≤1 year; the interpretation of acute infection based on a positive IgM reaction, therefore, must be made with caution. The presence of IgM (>1:64) or a fourfold rise in IgG titer indicates recent infection. IgG peaks approximately 5 weeks after acute infection. IgG is unusual in the first week of infection, so repeat testing of convalescent serum is recommended. IgG titers increase for several years after acute infection.

Core laboratory: Patients may show nonspecific signs of inflammation (mildly elevated WBCs, increased ESR) on routine laboratory testing. Cold agglutinins (agglutination of type O, Rh-negative RBCs at 4°C) may be seen in approximately 50% of patients with *M. pneumoniae* infection. Cold agglutinins, however, are not specific, and this test is not recommended for diagnosis of *M. pneumoniae* infection.

NEISSERIA GONORRHOEAE INFECTION

❑ Definition
Neisseria gonorrhoeae isolates are moderately fastidious gram-negative cocci that typically form pairs with characteristic "coffee bean" morphology. Diseases caused by *N. gonorrhoeae* are almost exclusively transmitted by sexual contact or exposure to infected genital secretions. *Neisseria gonorrhoeae* is never considered normal flora; isolates are always considered to represent infection.

❑ Who Should Be Suspected?
- Gonorrhea is an STD of adults. Infection in neonates may be acquired by exposure to contaminated secretions during childbirth. Infections in other prepubertal children must be investigated as a possible indication of child abuse.
- Males with gonorrhea most commonly present with urethritis, manifested by dysuria and urethral discharge. In the absence of specific antimicrobial therapy, spontaneous resolution is common. Complications include "ascending" infection (epididymitis and seminal vesiculitis, regional adenitis, abscess formation, and urethral stricture) and distant infection by contaminated secretions (e.g., conjunctivitis).
- Anorectal and pharyngeal gonorrhea may occur in men who have sex with men. Anorectal infections may be asymptomatic but often present with proctitis or rectal pain with purulent discharge and painful defecation. Pharyngeal infection may be asymptomatic but usually occurs as an acute, suppurative pharyngitis with regional adenopathy.
- Most women with *N. gonorrhoeae* infection present with cervical and urethral infection. Symptoms include vaginal and urethral discharge, pelvic pain, and abnormal vaginal bleeding. Adjacent structures, like Bartholin glands, may become infected by local spread. Ascending infection, resulting in pelvic inflammatory disease (PID) (e.g., salpingitis, endometritis, tuboovarian abscess, perihepatitis), occurs in 10–20% of patients. Anorectal infection in women is most commonly acquired by autoinfection by infected vaginal secretions. PID increases the risk of sterility and tubal pregnancy. *N. gonorrhoeae* infection during pregnancy may result in premature delivery or spontaneous abortion, chorioamnionitis, and transmission of infection (conjunctival or pharyngeal) to the neonate.

11

❑ **Laboratory Findings**

Direct detection: Gonorrhea may be diagnosed accurately by Gram stain of urethral secretions from symptomatic males. The detection of typical gram-negative diplococci within PMNs is diagnostic (S/S of approximately 95%). Gram stain examination of endocervical secretions may support a diagnosis of gonorrheal cervical or anorectal infection if many intracellular gram-negative diplococci are seen (sensitivity approximately 50%), but smears must be interpreted with caution because of the presence of nonpathogenic gram-negative organisms in the endogenous flora of these sites.

Culture: The gold standard for diagnosis of nongenital *N. gonorrhoeae* infections. Swabs of secretions of anal crypts should be submitted for diagnosis of anorectal gonorrhea; rectal swabs (heavily contaminated with feces) should not be submitted. Cultures are required for other types of specimens and for medicolegal specimens (e.g., child abuse, rape).

Molecular diagnosis: Considered the gold standard for diagnosis of *N. gonorrhoeae* genital infection. Several advantages of nucleic acid testing include the ability to detect nonviable organisms and increased sensitivity, allowing diagnostic testing on urine specimens. Tests with S/S >98% are available, depending on the assay and specimen type.

NEISSERIA MENINGITIDIS INFECTION

❑ **Definition**

Neisseria meningitidis is a moderately fastidious gram-negative diplococcus with characteristic "coffee bean" morphology. *Neisseria meningitidis* may be isolated as components of the endogenous respiratory flora of healthy individuals. In meningococcal disease, infection is usually transmitted by the respiratory route. In susceptible patients, bacteremia may occur by passage of organisms across the epithelial barrier. Infection in multiple organ systems is common in meningococcal disease.

❑ **Who Should Be Suspected?**

Common infectious syndromes include the following:

- Meningococcemia: Meningococcemia may result in sustained bacteremia and seeding of various organ systems. Sustained bacteremia is typically associated with fever, malaise, and leukocytosis. Fulminant disease is usually associated by seeding of the CNS and other organs, DIC, adrenal insufficiency, and multiorgan failure. Meningitis should be actively ruled out by clinical and laboratory evaluation in patients in whom meningococcemia is documented.
- CNS infection (meningitis and meningoencephalitis):
  - ▼ More than 90% of adults with clinically significant meningococcal infections have meningitis. Patients with CNS disease usually present with typical signs and symptoms of meningitis.
  - ▼ The clinical presentation may be dominated by symptoms of fulminant disease and multiorgan failure. Overwhelming disease may be associated with shock, petechial rash, purpura fulminans, gangrenous necrosis of the distal extremities, or the Waterhouse-Friderichsen syndrome (3–4% of patients).

❑ Laboratory Findings

Direct detection: CSF Gram stain is diagnostic in 50–70% of patients with meningitis; pyogenic meningitis in which bacteria cannot be found in smear is more likely to be caused by meningococcus than to other bacteria.

Core laboratory: Increased WBC count (12,000–40,000/µL). Urine may show albumin, RBCs; occasional glycosuria. Laboratory findings of predisposing conditions such as asplenia (e.g., sickle cell anemia) or immunodeficiency (e.g., complement, immunoglobulin). Laboratory findings due to complications (e.g., DIC) and sequelae (e.g., subdural effusion) may be seen.

CSF findings: Markedly increased WBC count (2,500–10,000/µL), almost all PMNs; increased protein (50–1,500 mg/dL); decreased glucose (0–45 mg/dL).

PASTEURELLA MULTOCIDA INFECTION

❑ Definition

Pasteurella multocida, a fastidious aerobic GNR, is a common part of the endogenous oral flora of domesticated cats and dogs, as well as other domesticated and wild animals.

❑ Who Should Be Suspected?

Infection is usually manifested as cellulitis or wound infections associated with cat bites or scratches. Close contact with animals and underlying medical conditions, especially hepatic disease and malignancy, predispose to infection. Infections at the site of inoculation are painful with marked erythema and swelling. Because of the nature of cat bites (deep penetrating wounds), deep soft tissue infection, septic arthritis, and osteomyelitis are common complications. Localized infection may progress to bacteremia with hematogenous spread to other organ systems, including endocarditis and CNS infections. Colonization of the upper respiratory tract predisposes to pneumonia and pararespiratory abscesses, like sinusitis or empyema.

❑ Laboratory Findings

Gram staining: Possibly small, faintly staining gram-negative coccobacilli.

Cultures: Isolates grow well on SBA or chocolate agar incubated in increased CO_2.

PSEUDOMONAS AERUGINOSA INFECTION

❑ Definition

Pseudomonas aeruginosa is a nonfastidious, glucose nonfermenting GNB that is intrinsically virulent for humans; it is capable of producing a wide range of localized and systemic infections. This organism can metabolize a variety of substrates and can be isolated from many environmental reservoirs, including water sources (e.g., sink traps), aqueous solutions, disinfectant solutions, and condensates in respirators, contributing to its role in nosocomial infections. *Pseudomonas aeruginosa* exhibits intrinsic and acquired resistance to commonly used antibiotics.

❑ Who Should Be Suspected?

Pseudomonas aeruginosa may cause such infections as bacteremia/endocarditis and systemic infection in neutropenic and ICU patients, burn wound infection with sepsis, chronic pneumonia in patients with CF, keratoconjunctivitis due to contaminated contact lens solutions and other eye infections, nosocomial pneumonia, osteomyelitis due to nail puncture injuries or hematogenous spread (especially in IV drug abusers), otitis externa (swimmer's ear and malignant otitis externa), and/or UTI.

❑ **Laboratory Findings**
Culture: *Pseudomonas aeruginosa* grows well on routine laboratory media after overnight incubation. Special selective media are recommended to improve isolation of *P. aeruginosa* from lower respiratory specimens submitted from patients with CF.

Susceptibility: Susceptibility testing should be performed on all significant isolates. Isolates may develop resistance during prolonged therapy with any antibiotic; testing of repeat isolates may be indicated. Reported susceptibility to beta-lactam and beta-lactam/beta-lactamase combinations implies the need for high-dose therapy for serious infections; combination therapy is often recommended.

Q FEVER (*COXIELLA BURNETII*)

❑ **Definition**
Q fever describes zoonotic infections caused by *Coxiella burnetii*, a small, obligately intracellular gram-negative bacterium. Cattle, sheep, and goats are the primary reservoir for organisms, which are very stable in the environment. Human infection is usually acquired by inhalation of organisms from environments contaminated with urine, feces, products of gestation, or other materials from infected animals. Infection may also be acquired by ingestion of unpasteurized dairy products.

❑ **Who Should Be Suspected?**
Coxiella infection may cause acute or chronic infection, but many infections remain asymptomatic. Acute infection is usually manifested by flu-like illness, hepatitis, and/or pneumonitis. Endocarditis may develop, usually in patients with preexisting valve disease. Chronic disease is defined as infection lasting >6 months and is usually manifested by endocarditis, aneurism, or infection of prosthetic material.

❑ **Laboratory Findings**
Histology: "Doughnut" granulomas in liver biopsy or bone marrow are highly suggestive but not pathognomonic.

Culture: *C. burnetii* may be isolated by special eukaryotic cell culture, but this testing is not widely available.

Serology: The basis of definitive diagnosis. IFA testing is more sensitive (approximately 91%) than CF testing (78%). Serum (1:50 dilution) is screened for anti-phase II anti-immunoglobulin. Positive specimens are tested for anti-phase I and anti-phase II IgG, IgM, and IgA, with titer. Single phase IgG titer ≥1:800 by immunofluorescence is diagnostic and strongly suggests *C. burnetii* endocarditis; any positive IgM titer is diagnostically significant. High specific IgM titer suggests hepatitis. High specific IgA titer is common in chronic Q fever and suggests culture-negative endocarditis. ELISA testing is sensitive (approximately 94%) in early convalescence.

Molecular diagnostics: PCR techniques have been described, but there is no FDA-approved kit for NAA.

ROCKY MOUNTAIN SPOTTED FEVER

❏ **Definition**

This disorder is an infectious vasculitis due to *Rickettsia rickettsii*, an intracellular bacterium. RMSF is transmitted by infected ticks, primarily of the *Dermacentor* genus in the United States.

❏ **Who Should Be Suspected?**

Most patients present approximately 7 days after exposure with nonspecific symptoms, including fever, headache, malaise, and muscle and joint pains. Nausea and abdominal pain may be significant. Rash appears in approximately 90% of patients, usually 3–7 days after onset of illness. Rash typically starts on the wrists and ankles and then spreads widely, including the palms and soles. The rash becomes petechial; itching is not characteristic. Disease may progress to involve multiple organ systems, including gangrene, CNS manifestations, and other organ dysfunction.

❏ **Laboratory Findings**

Culture: Requires special conditions and is rarely performed.

   Histology: DFA of skin biopsy for antigen has S/S of approximately 70%/100% and is the only specific test in early stages of disease. Sensitivity declines after the initiation of antimicrobial therapy.

   Molecular tests: PCR has been used to detect *R. rickettsii* DNA in blood and tissues.

   Serology: Sera should be collected during acute infection and then 2–4 weeks later for both IgG and IgM. A ≥4 times increase in IgG or total antibody, or specific IgM, is evidence of recent infection. IgM appears by days 3–8, peaks at 1 month, and lasts 3–4 months. IgG appears within 3 weeks, peaks at 1–3 months, and lasts for >12 months.

   Core laboratory: WBC is mildly elevated; thrombocytopenia may be severe.

SALMONELLA AND *SHIGELLA* INFECTIONS

See Chapter 5, Digestive Diseases.

STAPHYLOCOCCUS AUREUS INFECTION

❏ **Definition**

Staphylococci are nonfastidious, aerobic GPCs that form clusters. The genus *Staphylococcus* is composed of several species that are implicated in human infection. *Staphylococcus aureus* is a frequent cause of pyogenic infection. Staphylococcal disease may also be caused by the elaboration of several potent toxins.

❏ **Who Should Be Suspected?**

Staphylococcus aureus is able to cause disease in virtually all organ systems. The many clinical presentations of *S. aureus* infection include the following:

- *Pneumonia*: Pulmonary infections may be caused by aspiration of organisms from the upper respiratory tract or by hematogenous seeding from another primary site of infection. *Staphylococcus aureus* pneumonia may represent a severe complication of viral infection (e.g., measles, influenza), CF, or debilitating underlying disease.

■ *Acute osteomyelitis, septic arthritis*: Osteomyelitis in adults is usually a result of a direct extension of local infection, often at the site of a surgical or traumatic wound. The vertebral column is a common site of infection of hematogenous origin. Septic arthritis in adults is usually of hematogenous origin.

■ *Pyomyositis*: *Staphylococcus aureus* infection of skeletal muscle is usually caused by trauma or direct extension from an adjacent site.

■ *Bacteremia and endocarditis*: Bacteremia may occur as a complication of localized pyogenic infection. Metastatic foci of infection are common. Patients generally present with acute sepsis syndromes, often with signs and symptoms due to localized infections. Endocarditis may be caused by seeding of valves during a primary bacteremia or by organisms directly introduced into the blood stream (e.g., intravascular catheter, injection drug use). Patients with endocarditis may present with subacute or acute symptoms. Normal cardiac valves are commonly affected. *Staphylococcus aureus* endocarditis causes rapid, severe damage to valves, producing acute mechanical heart failure (e.g., rupture of chordae tendineae, perforation of valve, valvular insufficiency) in addition to the physiologic effects of severe infection. Typical stigmata of endocarditis (e.g., Janeway lesions, splinter hemorrhages, Roth spots) are common.

■ *Food poisoning*: Staphylococcal food poisoning is caused by ingestion of food tainted by enterotoxin-producing strains of *S. aureus*. Symptoms, including crampy abdominal pain, nausea and vomiting, and diarrhea, occur early (2–6 hours after ingestion). Patients are symptomatic for 8–10 hours after onset of illness. Aggressive fluid management forms the mainstay of therapy. Suspected clusters of foodborne gastroenteritis must be reported to state boards of public health.

■ *Impetigo*: A superficial skin infection commonly affecting the face: seen most commonly in infants. The rash of impetigo presents with red macules that mature into vesicles, which may shed honey-colored serous fluid prior to drying. Most cases of impetigo are caused by *S. aureus*.

■ *Meningitis*: CNS infection with *S. aureus* may occur in traumatic or surgical wounds, by hematogenous spread from other primary site of infection, or contamination of an intraventricular pressure monitoring device or other foreign body. Signs and symptoms are similar to those caused by other pathogens.

■ *Toxic shock syndrome (TSS)*: This syndrome is caused by the action of TSS toxin-1 (or related toxin), a pyrogenic superantigen elaborated by a colonizing strain of *S. aureus*. Note that several other species, like group A *Streptococcus*, may elaborate similar toxins that produce an identical clinical presentation. Patients present acutely with vascular congestion, increased permeability of capillaries, and decreased vascular resistance. Hypotension and tissue hypoxia develop as a consequence of the loss of the intravascular blood volume. ARDS and DIC are common complications in patients with severe disease. Staphylococcal TSS is defined by fever >38.9°C, diffuse macular rash, desquamation, and hypotension (systolic blood pressure ≤90 mm Hg for adults).

Diagnosis is possible when signs and symptoms of disease are seen in three organ systems (muscular, GI, liver, bone marrow, CNS, kidney, skin/mucous membranes). TSS is probable when five organ systems are involved and confirmed if all six organ systems are affected.

❏ **Laboratory Findings**

Direct detection: In pyogenic infections, Gram stain usually demonstrates many GPCs in clusters, with a brisk PMN response.

Culture: *Staphylococcus aureus* grows on standard media after overnight incubation. In patients with bacteremia, the persistence of positive blood cultures at 72–96 hours after the initiation of appropriate antimicrobial therapy is a predictor of a complicated recovery course and predicts the need for prolonged treatment.

Susceptibility testing: Should be performed on significant *S. aureus* isolates because resistance to primary therapeutic agents is common; resistance or intermediate susceptibility to vancomycin is uncommon but has been well documented.

STENOTROPHOMONAS MALTOPHILIA INFECTION

❏ **Definition**

Stenotrophomonas maltophilia is a commonly isolated glucose nonfermenting GNB in clinical laboratories. Organisms may colonize a variety of hospital and environmental sources, which serve as the reservoir for human colonization and infection.

❏ **Who Should Be Suspected?**

Stenotrophomonas maltophilia infections have been reported for all organ systems; however, most infections occur in patients with some type of innate or acquired immune defect. Isolates from patient specimens must be carefully evaluated for clinical significance because *S. maltophilia* may be isolated at a component of endogenous or contaminating flora. True *S. maltophilia* infection is associated with increased mortality. Typical syndromes include the following:

11

- *Lower respiratory tract infection*: *Stenotrophomonas maltophilia* is most commonly isolated from respiratory specimens and may cause approximately 5% of nosocomial pneumonias, especially in intubated patients with significant prior exposure to broad-spectrum antibiotics.
- *Bacteremia*: *Stenotrophomonas maltophilia* bacteremia is most commonly nosocomial, caused by indwelling catheter or other site of primary infection.
- *Wound infections*: *Stenotrophomonas maltophilia* is a relatively common cause of traumatic wound and soft tissue infections. Metastatic cellulitis has been described in oncology patients with neutropenia.

❏ **Laboratory Findings**

Culture: *S. maltophilia* grows well on routine laboratory media after overnight incubation.

Susceptibility: With few exceptions, penicillins (including beta-lactam/beta-lactamase combinations), cephalosporins, quinolones, and aminoglycosides are ineffective for *S. maltophilia* infections. TMP/SMX is the treatment of choice; alternative agents include ceftazidime, chloramphenicol, levofloxacin, minocycline, or ticarcillin–clavulanate.

STREPTOCOCCUS AGALACTIAE (GROUP B) INFECTION

❏ Definition

Streptococcus agalactiae (GBS) isolates are nonfastidious GPCs that grow on routine media under aerobic or anaerobic conditions. Staining shows GPCs that form moderate length chains. GBS is a component of the GI and vaginal flora of healthy adults, which serve as the primary reservoir for infection. Intermittent rectovaginal carriage is seen in approximately 25% of pregnant women. Infant prophylaxis, based on results of screening for maternal carriage at 35–37 weeks of gestation, has resulted in a significant decline in the rate of neonatal GBS infections. Adult disease is playing an increasing role in the spectrum of GBS disease.

❏ Who Should Be Suspected?

- Adult disease: UTI and bacteremia are the most common manifestation of GBS infection in adults, but any organ system may be affected. Pregnancy, advanced age, and significant underlying medical conditions (e.g., cirrhosis, DM, malignancy) are risk factors for acquisition of GBS disease in adults.
- Neonatal and perinatal disease: Vaginal colonization at the end of gestation may lead to neonatal infection, either by ascending intrauterine infection after rupture of membranes or by exposure during passage through the birth canal. Risk factors include prolonged rupture of membranes, amnionitis, and maternal bacteremia.

❏ Laboratory Findings

Culture: GBS isolates grow well on routine media incubated in aerobic conditions; selective cultures improve detection from specimens likely to be contaminated with endogenous flora. Most strains demonstrate β-hemolysis on SBA. Gram stain shows gram-positive cocci that form chains of moderate length.

The CDC and American College of Obstetrics and Gynecology now recommend that decisions regarding prophylactic antimicrobial treatment for the prevention of neonatal GBS infection be based on cultures to detect maternal GBS carriage. See Group B Streptococcus Vaginal–Rectal Culture Screen in Chapter 17, Infectious Disease Assays for recommendations for GBS carrier detection in pregnant women.

Susceptibility testing: GBS isolates are predictably susceptible to penicillin and related antibiotics, the drugs of choice for these infections. Susceptibility testing of GBS must be performed for other antibiotics, as for use in penicillin-allergic patients.

Antigen detection: Commercially available agglutination tests for GBS are available for direct detection of GBS and other CNS pathogens using CSF, serum, and urine specimens. Reported sensitivity of assays has ranged from poor to good, and false-positive reactions are well documented. One clinical study showed that the clinical management of patients was not affected by the results of these antigen tests. Bacterial antigen testing for preliminary detection of CNS pathogens is not recommended.

Molecular diagnostics: FDA-approved PCR testing is available for detection of GBS in rectovaginal specimens or enrichment culture.

STREPTOCOCCUS PNEUMONIAE INFECTION

❑ Definition

Streptococcus pneumoniae isolates are nonfastidious GPCs that grow on routine media under aerobic or anaerobic conditions. Staining shows GPCs in pairs and short chains. *Streptococcus pneumoniae* is a common component of the endogenous upper respiratory flora of healthy humans (approximately 10%) that serves as the source for most infections. Carriage may be transient. The disease may be of endogenous or exogenous origin.

❑ Who Should Be Suspected?

- Most serious infections occur in children and the elderly. Underlying conditions, like DM, AIDS, alcoholism, and chronic lung disease, increase the risk of infection. Current or recent respiratory viral infection also predisposes to *S. pneumoniae* infection.
- The upper respiratory tract is the most common source of infecting organisms. *Streptococcus pneumoniae* may cause infection in any organ system, usually as a result of bacteremic spread from a primary site of infection. Common infections include the following:
- *Respiratory tract infections*, including pneumonia (community acquired), otitis media, and sinusitis: Abrupt onset of fever and shaking chills with cough with purulent sputum production. Severe disease may lead to respiratory failure, sepsis, and death.
- *Bacteremia*: *Streptococcus pneumoniae* is a significant pathogen in the etiology of bacteremia and sepsis. Bacteremia may occur secondary to a primary site of infection (e.g., otitis media in children, pneumonia in adults) or may be the primary infection.
- *Meningitis*: *Streptococcus pneumoniae* is one of the most common causes of bacterial meningitis in all age groups. Hematogenous dissemination is the most common route of infection, but direct invasion from infected sinuses is also well described; basilar skull fracture may cause recurrent *S. pneumoniae* meningitis.

❑ Laboratory Findings

Gram stain: The typical Gram stain of sputum from patients with pneumococcal pneumonia shows many PMNs and many lancet-shaped GPCs in pairs (diplococci).

Culture: *Streptococcus pneumoniae* grows on routine media after overnight incubation but may lose viability after or during transport or storage. Culture of sputum for isolation of *S. pneumoniae* has a sensitivity of approximately 45% of patients with community-acquired pneumonia. Collection of blood cultures may improve detection in critically ill patients with pneumonia; blood cultures are positive in approximately 25% of untreated patients. Pleural effusions yield organisms in approximately 15% of patients. *Streptococcus pneumoniae* is a well-documented cause of spontaneous bacterial peritonitis in patients with alcoholic cirrhosis; bedside inoculation of peritoneal fluid directly into blood culture media improves isolation compared to culture onto solid media in the laboratory.

Susceptibility testing: Testing of *S. pneumoniae* isolates must be performed for significant clinical isolates.

Urine antigen detection: Antigen testing for direct detection of *S. pneumoniae* is available as an adjunct for diagnosis of *S. pneumoniae* respiratory infections. See *Streptococcus pneumoniae* Urine Antigen Test in Chapter 17, Infectious Disease Assays for information.

STREPTOCOCCUS PYOGENES (GROUP A) INFECTION

❏ Definition

Streptococcus pyogenes (GAS) isolates are nonfastidious GPCs that grow on routine media under aerobic or anaerobic conditions. Staining shows GPCs that form moderate-length chains. GAS colonizes the upper respiratory tract and skin, and infections at these sites are the most common manifestations of GAS disease. Invasive pyogenic infections are commonly caused by GAS; infections in all organ systems have been described. In addition to primary GAS infections, GAS may cause clinically significant superinfections (e.g., GAS pneumonia complicating influenza, GAS cellulitis complicating chicken pox). GAS infections may result in suppurative complications, immune-mediated nonsuppurative sequelae, and toxin-mediated disease.

Diseases caused by GAS include the following:

- *Pharyngitis*: see Chapter 13, Respiratory, Metabolic, and Acid–Base Disorders
- *Cellulitis and soft tissue infections*: Impetigo describes a superficial vesicular rash, usually presenting in children. The vesicles evolve into pustules, which break down and scab over the following week. Erysipelas is a soft tissue infection that most often affects adults, who present with fever and erythematous, edematous areas of inflammation with well-demarcated edges, usually on the face. GAS may also cause cellulitis in tissue surrounding infected wounds or trauma.
- *Acute rheumatic fever*: This disorder is a nonsuppurative complication following prior GAS pharyngitis (2–5 weeks). Common manifestations include carditis, chorea, erythema marginatum, polyarthritis, and subcutaneous nodules.
- *Acute poststreptococcal GN (PSGN)*: Acute GN is a nonsuppurative complication following GAS pharyngitis (>10 days) or GAS skin infections (3–6 weeks). Clinical symptoms include headache, malaise, fatigue, edema, hypertension, and encephalopathy.
- *Group A streptococcal toxic shock–like syndrome*: This disorder may develop in patients infected with GAS strains capable of elaborating streptococcal pyrogenic exotoxins. The syndrome is often preceded by nonspecific symptoms (fever, chills, malaise). There may be prominent symptoms at the site of primary infections. Disease progresses to shock and multiorgan failure.

❏ Laboratory Findings

Culture: GAS isolates grow well on routine media incubated in aerobic or anaerobic conditions; selective cultures improve detection from specimens likely to be contaminated with endogenous flora. Most strains demonstrate β-hemolysis on SBA. Gram stain shows gram-positive cocci that form chains of moderate length.

Susceptibility testing: Group A *Streptococcus* isolates are predictably susceptible to penicillins and related antibiotics, the drugs of choice for these infections.

For penicillin-allergic patients, susceptibility testing of GAS must be performed for other antibiotics.

Serology: Not recommended for diagnosis of acute GAS infection but may be used for diagnosis of infection in the recent past in patients with symptoms of GN or RF. Several specific assays are most useful for detection of GAS antibodies. See: Streptozyme, Antistreptococcal Antibodies, Antistreptolysin O [ASO], Anti-DNase-B [ADB] in Chapter 17, Infectious Disease Assays.

- *Antistreptolysin O (ASO)*: ASO antibody testing is the most commonly used and standardized test to diagnose prior GAS infection. Antibody response is brisk after upper respiratory tract infection: detectable antibodies appear approximately 1 week after acute infection and reach maximum titers 3–6 weeks after acute infection. Skin infections (impetigo, pyoderma), however, do not stimulate a good ASO response, so this assay is not recommended for patient evaluation following skin infections. There are several causes for false-positive test results, including multiple myeloma, hypergammaglobu-linemia, rheumatoid factor, or infection with group C or G *Streptococcus*.
- *Anti-DNase B*: The anti-DNase B assay is most useful for the evaluation of patients with acute rheumatic fever or glomerulonephritis after impetigo, pyoderma, or other skin infection. Antibody titers are usually detectable approximately 2 weeks after acute infection and reach peak titers 6–8 weeks after infection. Factors causing false-positive ASO titers do not affect anti-DNase B testing, but false-positive anti-DNase B results may be seen in acute hemorrhagic pancreatitis.
- *Streptozyme*: This assay is based on agglutination of RBCs coated with a number of GAS antigens. The reagents have not been well standardized, so lot-to-lot variation has been documented, in terms of both sensitivity and specificity, limiting the value of this testing.

Rapid GAS detection: Throat swab for rapid direct antigen testing for GAS has a sensitivity of 70–90% compared to culture on SBA; specificity is approximately 95%. Antigen testing may provide results within minutes, but cultures are recommended in children when antigen testing is negative. A positive antigen test result means the patient has GAS pharyngitis or is a GAS carrier.

Molecular diagnostics: The sensitivity of the Gen-Probe Group A Strep Direct Test is 89–95%, with >97% specificity. Sensitivity of the LightCycler Strep-A real-time PCR assay is approximately 93%, with specificity approximately 98%. The high sensitivity of these molecular assays for detection of GAS pharyngitis obviates culture in direct assay–negative specimens.

Core laboratory: In patients with PSGN, abnormal urinalysis (RBCs, WBCs, and casts), anemia, decreased total complement, and C3 and/or increased ESR are typical.

TREPONEMAL DISEASE: SYPHILIS

❑ Definition
Syphilis is a chronic disease caused by infection with the spirochete *Treponema pallidum*, an unculturable spiral bacterium. Syphilis has a global distribution. *Treponema pallidum* is an obligate pathogen of humans; there are no known

animal or reservoirs that serve as a source of infection. The disease is transmitted by exposure of a susceptible individual to active lesions of an infected patient or by transplacental transmission. Congenital or neonatal syphilis may be transmitted directly by contact with infectious lesions or by transplacental transmission, which may occur at any time during pregnancy.

❑ **Who Should Be Suspected?**

- In venereal syphilis, a local infection, usually manifested as painless ulcer (chancre), forms at the site of inoculation. There is a high concentration of spirochetes in the ulcer exudate. Wide dissemination of organisms occurs during the phase of primary syphilis. Chancres generally heal spontaneously within several weeks.
- Signs and symptoms of secondary syphilis occur several weeks to months after resolution of primary syphilis. The rash of secondary syphilis is most characteristic, typically involving the palms and soles. A wide variety of non-specific symptoms may also be seen, including fever, malaise, headache, lymphadenopathy, and eye involvement (e.g., uveitis). The symptoms of secondary syphilis usually resolve spontaneously.
- Latent phase: The patient is typically asymptomatic.
- In late (tertiary) syphilis, symptoms related to chronically infected organ systems manifest, most commonly cardiovascular disease (e.g., aortitis), CNS disease (e.g., tabes dorsalis, paresis), and gummatous disease (nodular lesions of the skin, bone, or other tissues).
- Patients with AIDS are at increased risk for severe *T. pallidum* infection.
- There is a high rate of fetal loss or stillbirth. Fetal hydrops may be apparent.
- Most neonates are asymptomatic at birth but may show stigmata of infection, including skin lesions (including the palms, soles, and mucous membranes), hepatosplenomegaly, jaundice, and anemia. Radiographic abnormalities may be seen (e.g., periostitis).
- Untreated, damage cause by congenital syphilis may manifest by the Hutchinson triad (abnormal upper incisors, interstitial keratitis, 8th nerve deafness), as well as such conditions as frontal bossing, saddle nose, and high arched palate.

❑ **Laboratory Findings**

Direct microscopic detection: Direct detection techniques may be used on exudates of active cutaneous or genital specimens during the primary or secondary phases of disease.

- *Dark-field microscopy*: Dark-field microscopy may be used to detect typical organisms; specimens must be examined immediately by an experienced microscopist. Documentation of the characteristic morphology and motility of organisms is critical. Dark-field microscopy should not be performed on oral lesions because of the presence of nonpathogenic, endogenous spirochetal flora.
- *DFA for T. pallidum (DFA-TP)*:
  - ▾ This test is performed on exudate from chancres. Antibody reagent is used to detect *T. pallidum* in the material. Advantages of DFA-TP are that viable organisms are not required; immediate examination is not necessary.

DFA-TP may be positive on chancre exudate in the first week, before a serologic reaction has occurred.

▼ The use of polyclonal antibody reagents may limit the utility of DFA testing if they are not preabsorbed (e.g., Reiter treponemes) to eliminate binding to antigens common to nonpathogenic treponemes.

■ *Histopathology*: Tissue sections stained using a silver stain, or other technique for spirochetes, may demonstrate organisms and may provide support for diagnosis in immunocompromised patients who do not mount an antibody response to infection.

■ *Serology*: Detectable antibodies develop during primary infection and increase in titer during the secondary phase of syphilis. Titers decline during the latent phase. The interpretation of serologic testing of neonates may be complicated by the presence of transplacental maternal antibodies. See Syphilis Serology Tests in Chapter 17, Infectious Disease Assays for information about these tests.

■ Non-Treponemal tests

▼ The VDRL-CSF assay is the only nontreponemal assay for detection of antibodies in CSF. VDRL on CSF is highly specific but lacks sensitivity (40–60%); therefore, it should be used to rule in, but not rule out, neurosyphilis. The VDRL-CSF cannot be used to follow response to therapy.

▼ The RPR card test is positive in 75–100% of patients with primary syphilis, 100% with secondary syphilis; 95–100% with latent syphilis, and approximately 75% with late, tertiary syphilis. Specificity is approximately 98%.

▼ Acute (<6 months' duration) false-positive tests may occur in acute viral illnesses (e.g., infectious mononucleosis, hepatitis, measles), chlamydia infection, malaria, *Mycoplasma pneumoniae* infection, pregnancy, and recent immunization.

▼ Chronic (>6 months) false-positive tests may be caused by increased age (>70 years), infection caused by non–*T. pallidum* spirochetal infections, IV drug abuse, medications, and rheumatologic disease and/or underlying disease (e.g., collagen vascular diseases, leprosy, malignancy).

■ Treponemal tests

▼ These tests use *T. pallidum*, or specific *T. pallidum* antigens, to detect antibodies. Particle agglutination and EIA formats are most commonly used. Treponemal tests have been used traditionally to confirm the specificity of positive reactions of nontreponemal assays. However, development of assays adapted for efficient testing of large numbers of patient samples, like EIA assays, has led to increasing use of these assays as primary screening tests.

▼ Treponemal assays are also used for diagnosis of late latent or tertiary syphilis in untreated patients, when nontreponemal assays may have become nonreactive.

▼ Treponemal tests usually remain reactive for many years after successful therapy, so these assays are not reliable for measuring response to therapy or to assess the possibility of reinfection.

▼ *Treponema pallidum*–specific IgG EIA is positive in 90–95% of patients with primary syphilis and 99–100% positive in patients with secondary, latent, or late syphilis.

VIBRIO INFECTION

❑ Definition

Vibrio species are nonfastidious, glucose-fermenting GNBs. *Vibrio cholerae* is the cause of cholera, a severe diarrheal disease. Risk of infection is significant in populations with poor sanitation related to water sources. Transmission is primarily caused by ingestion of contaminated water or poorly cooked seafood. Continued transmission may result by fecal contamination of potable water sources or food. Disruption of potable water sources by natural disaster or civil disruption increases the risk of epidemic disease. Asymptomatic carriage is rare.

❑ Who Should Be Suspected?

- Young children are most commonly infected and most susceptible to severe infection. After ingestion, symptoms usually begin within 2–4 days. Initial symptoms of nausea, vomiting, and abdominal discomfort are followed by severe diarrhea. Without aggressive rehydration, life-threatening dehydration may ensue, with neuromuscular symptoms, hypoglycemia, acute renal failure, or other complications.

- Noncholera *Vibrio* species may also cause human infection, most commonly diarrheal syndromes, albeit typically less severe than classic cholera. Extraintestinal infection is uncommon but well described. *Vibrio vulnificus* may cause significant infection after ingestion of contaminated seafood or traumatic inoculation. Preexisting liver disease, as seen with alcoholic cirrhosis, hepatitis, and hemochromatosis, predisposes patients to invasive infection. Cellulitis with formation of bullae is characteristic. Secondary *V. vulnificus* bacteremia is associated with high mortality.

❑ Laboratory Findings

Culture: Isolates grow on routine laboratory media after overnight incubation; isolation is improved by the use of specific selective and differential media (e.g., TSCB) for specimens likely to be contaminated, like stool.

Core Laboratory: In cholera, careful monitoring of core laboratory values to assess the patient's state of hydration and metabolic status is critical.

YERSINIA INFECTION

❑ Definition

Yersinia species are nonfastidious, glucose-fermenting GNBs, but growth in culture may be slow. Yersiniosis is usually caused by infection with *Yersinia enterocolitica* presenting with acute gastroenteritis. *Yersinia enterocolitica* is widely distributed in nature and transmitted by the oral route. Swine have been implicated as a reservoir for human infections.

Yersinia pestis is a significant pathogen. In naturally occurring infection, humans are incidental hosts, acquiring infection by exposure to the epizootic cycle between fleas and rodents (e.g., flea bite, contact with infected animal carcasses) or through care of patients with pneumonic plague. *Yersinia pestis* infection is now rare due to control of the normal rodent reservoir, but *Y. pestis* is considered a potential risk for development as a bioterror agent; public health officials must be contacted immediately if *Y. pestis* infection is suspected.

❑ Who Should Be Suspected?

Symptoms of *Y. enterocolitica* infection include acute enteritis (diarrhea and abdominal pain), mesenteric adenitis, and pseudoappendicitis.

There are three major clinical manifestations of human *Y. pestis* infection:

- *Bubonic* (approximately 90% of reported cases): Sudden onset of fever, chills, malaise. Patients develop pain and swelling of a regional lymph node, usually with edema and erythema. The inguinal nodes are most commonly affected, although the upper extremity or cervical nodes may be more commonly involved in infection transmitted by cats.
- *Septicemic* (approximately 10% of cases): Patients present with fever and sepsis without specific or localized symptoms. DIC and multiorgan failure develop as late complications.
- *Pneumonic*: Pneumonic plague may develop as a complication of bubonic plague through hematogenous spread or by direct inhalation of infectious aerosols. Patients present with a sudden onset of dyspnea, cough, and fever.

❑ Laboratory Findings

Culture: Laboratories should have procedures in place for recognition and limitation of handling of *Y. pestis* isolates. The appropriate public health department should be alerted as soon as *Y. pestis* infection is suspected on the basis of clinical or laboratory findings. Further diagnostic testing should be performed under the direction of public health officials.

Yersinia gastroenteritis is diagnosed by culture of infected material. Isolates may grow slowly on MAC and show an optimum incubation temperature of 25–32°C. Isolation may be improved by the use of special selective media and incubation, like cold enrichment, but in acute yersiniosis, the bacterial load is high in stool and is usually detected by routine enteric cultures if the laboratory has been alerted to rule out *Yersinia*. Because of their growth characteristics, automated identification and susceptibility testing may be unreliable.

Stool may contain increased WBCs and RBCs, but grossly bloody stool is uncommon. Bacteremia is uncommon but may occur in patients with disorders leading to iron overload, like beta-thalassemia.

Suggested Readings

Ben-Ami R, Ephros M, Avidor B, et al. Cat-scratch disease in elderly patients. *Clin Infect Dis.* 2005;41:969–974.

Brouwer MC, van de Beek D, Heckenberg SGB, et al. Community-acquired *Listeria monocytogenes* meningitis in adults. *Clin Infect Dis.* 2006;43:1233–1238.

Cetinkaya Y, Falk P, Mayhall CG. Vancomycin-resistant enterococci. *Clin Microbiol Rev.* 2000;13:686–707.

Coenye T, Vandamme P, Govan JRW, et al. Taxonomy and identification of the *Burkholderia cepacia* complex. *J Clin Microbiol.* 2001;39:3427–3436.

Denton M, Kerr KG. Microbiological and clinical aspects of infection associated with *Stenotrophomonas maltophilia. Clin Microbiol Rev.* 1998;11:57–80.

Gaynes R, Edwards JR; the National Nosocomial Infections Surveillance System. Overview of nosocomial infections caused by gram-negative bacilli. *Clin Infect Dis.* 2005;41:848–854.

Gottlieb SL, Martin DH, Xu F, et al. Summary: the natural history of *Chlamydia trachomatis* genital infection and implications for chlamydia control. *J Infect Dis.* 2010;201:S190–S204.

Klein JO. Danger ahead: politics intrude in Infectious Diseases Society of America Guideline for Lyme disease. *Clin Infect Dis.* 2008;47:1197–1199.

11

Kuehnert MJ, Doyle TJ, Hill HA, et al. Clinical features that discriminate inhalational anthrax from other acute respiratory illnesses. *Clin Infect Dis.* 2003;36:328–336.

Maragakis LL, Perl TM. *Acinetobacter baumannii*: epidemiology, antimicrobial resistance, and treatment options. *Clin Infect Dis.* 2008;46:1254–1263.

Mundy LM, Sahm DF, Gilmore M. Relationships between enterococcal virulence and antimicrobial resistance. *Clin Microbiol Rev.* 2000;13:513–522.

Munoz-Price LS, Weinstein RA. *Acinetobacter* infection. *N Engl J Med.* 2008;358:1271–1281.

Newman LM, Moran JS, Workowski KA. Update on the management of gonorrhea in adults in the United States. *Clin Infect Dis.* 2007;44:S84–S101.

Parola P, Paddock CD, Raoult D. Tick-borne rickettsioses around the world: emerging diseases challenging old concepts. *Clin Microbiol Rev.* 2005;18:719–756.

Parola P, Raoult D. Ticks and tickborne bacterial diseases in humans: an emerging infectious threat. *Clin Infect Dis.* 2001;32:897–928.

Peterson LR, Robicsek A. Does my patient have *Clostridium difficile* infection? *Ann Intern Med.* 2009;151:176–179.

Reimer LG. Q Fever. *Clin Microbiol Rev.* 1993;6:193–198.

Rosenstein NE, Perkins BA, Stephens DS, et al. Meningococcal disease. *N Engl J Med.* 2001;344:1378–1388.

Swartz MN. Recognition and management of anthrax—an update. *N Engl J Med.* 2001;345:1621–1626.

Swindells J, Brenwald N, Reading N, et al. Evaluation of diagnostic tests for *Clostridium difficile* infection. *J Clin Microbiol.* 2010;48:606–608.

Waites KB, Katz B, Schelonka RL. Mycoplasmas and ureaplasmas as neonatal pathogens. *Clin Microbiol Rev.* 2005;18:757–789.

Waites KB, Talkington DF. *Mycoplasma pneumoniae* and its role as a human pathogen. *Clin Microbiol Rev.* 2004;17:697–728.

Walker DH. Rickettsiae and rickettsial infections: the current state of knowledge. *Clin Infect Dis.* 2007;45:S39–S44.

Weinstein A. Laboratory testing for Lyme disease: time for a change? *Clin Infect Dis.* 2008;47:196–197.

Winn WC Jr, Allen SD, Janda WM, et al. Gram positive cocci, part I: staphylococci and related gram-positive cocci. In: *Koneman's Color Atlas and Textbook of Diagnostic Microbiology*, 6th ed. Baltimore, MD and Philadelphia, PA: Lippincott Williams & Wilkins; 2006.

Wormser GP. Discovery of new infectious diseases—*Bartonella* species. *N Engl J Med.* 2007;356:2346–2347.

INFECTIOUS DISEASES CAUSED BY ACID-FAST BACTERIAL PATHOGENS (AFB)

The organisms in this group contain mycolic acids in their cell walls, which renders the cells relatively resistant to both staining and destaining. Therefore, special techniques are used for direct visual detection of these organisms in specimens. *Mycobacterium* species, in general, are resistant to strong decolorization procedures with acid–alcohol. *Nocardia* and *Rhodococcus* species have a lower cell wall mycolic acid content and are acid-fast only when weaker decolorizing procedures are used.

Diseases caused by organisms in this group are usually diagnosed by isolation in culture. Specialized culture procedures are required, with prolonged incubation. Because of the slow growth rate of many isolates, molecular methods are increasingly used for direct detection and speciation of isolates. Tests that measure a patient's cellular immune response (e.g., TSTs and IGRA tests) may be used to screen for TB; serologic testing is not otherwise useful for diagnosis.

See Chapter 17, Infectious Disease Assays for information about AFB culture and staining, and IGRA screening tests.

MYCOBACTERIUM TUBERCULOSIS

See Chapter 13, Respiratory, Metabolic, and Acid–Base Disorders.

NOCARDIA INFECTION

❑ **Definition**

Nocardiosis describes infections caused by species of the genus *Nocardia*. These bacteria are aerobic gram-positive organisms that form delicate filaments that show branching and fragmentation. *Nocardia* species are widely distributed in nature worldwide and are involved in the decay of organic material. Human infections are usually seen in patients with immunocompromising or debilitating underlying medical conditions. Pulmonary infections acquired by inhalation, or cutaneous infections acquired by direct or traumatic inoculation, represent most primary infections. Local spread and systemic dissemination are common. *Nocardia* have tropism for the CNS. Recurrent or progressive infection may occur despite appropriate antimicrobial therapy. *Nocardia asteroides* is the most common species associated with invasive human infections. *Nocardia brasiliensis* is predominantly associated with cutaneous infections.

❑ **Who Should Be Suspected?**

These organisms have a low intrinsic virulence; infection most commonly occurs in immunocompromised patients, but no underlying condition is found in 10–20% of patients. Factors that increase the risk of nocardiosis include AIDS, alcoholism, chronic lung disease, DM, glucocorticoid therapy, malignancy, and solid organ or hematopoietic stem cell transplantation.

❑ **Laboratory Findings**

Direct stain: Gram positive or gram variable; modified acid-fast positive.

   Culture: Most nonselective media for bacterial, fungal, and mycobacterial isolation will support the growth of *Nocardia* but may require up to 6-week incubation for isolation. Noninvasively obtained specimens may be inadequate for sensitive detection of nocardiae. Sputum is positive in only 30% of cases of pulmonary infection. Blood culture is rarely positive. All patients with nocardiosis should be evaluated for possible disseminated, including CNS, infection.

   Susceptibility: Sulfonamides, including TMP/SMX, are considered the drug of choice of nocardiosis because of the low rate of resistance and extensive clinical experience. Susceptibility testing is recommended, however, for life-threatening infections and for patients allergic to sulfa drugs.

RAPIDLY GROWING MYCOBACTERIA

❑ **Definition**

Rapidly growing mycobacteria (RGM) are widely distributed in environmental water sources, dust, and soil. Although exposure to these organisms is common, disease is uncommon because of their low intrinsic pathogenicity in normal

11

hosts. RGM produce mature colonies within 7 days after subculture. The clinical significance of culture isolates must be interpreted carefully to rule out contamination. Factors to be considered include site, quantity of growth, number of positive cultures, and signs of inflammation and host immune status.

❑ **Significant Species**
Three species are most commonly associated with clinical disease: *Mycobacterium abscessus, Mycobacterium fortuitum*, and *Mycobacterium chelonae.*

- *Mycobacterium abscessus* usually causes pulmonary disease. Patients with underlying pulmonary disease are most commonly infected, but disease may also occur in patients with no pulmonary disease.
- *Mycobacterium fortuitum* usually causes skin and soft tissue infection after direct inoculation. Infections include surgical site, catheter-related, and other infections. Pulmonary isolates may represent transient infection or colonization.
- *Mycobacterium chelonae* may cause a variety of infections in immunocompromised patients.

❑ **Laboratory Findings**
AFB staining and culture: Diagnosis is usually established by culture of infected material: RGM may be positive only with modified acid-fast staining. American Thoracic Society criteria (ATS) should be used to assess the significance of isolates.

SLOW-GROWING, NONTUBERCULOUS MYCOBACTERIA

❑ **Definition**
There are a large number of nontuberculous mycobacteria (NTM). These organisms are ubiquitous in the environment. A number of these species are able to cause human disease but usually in patients with immune defects.

❑ **Who Should Be Suspected?**
Most infections are acquired from environmental sources; human-to-human transmission occurs rarely, if ever. NTM are increasingly implicated in nosocomial infections and pseudo-outbreaks in health care settings. Although this patient population may be at increased risk for NTM infection, culture isolates must be interpreted cautiously because of the frequency of isolation as culture contaminants. *Mycobacterium gordonae*, for example, is a fairly common isolate in AFB cultures, like BAL specimens, and virtually always represents a culture contaminant.

❑ **Significant Species**
- *Mycobacterium avium* complex (MAC): This complex includes two genetically related species: *Mycobacterium avium* and *Mycobacterium intracellulare*. Organisms are widely distributed in nature, being prevalent in soil and water with low pH and oxygen content, and they are relatively chlorine resistant. MAC has been isolated from municipal water supplies and hospital hot water systems and shower heads.
  - ▾ In patients with AIDS or other immune defects, mycobacteremia, manifested with fever, fatigue, night sweats, anemia, diarrhea, failure to thrive,

or other nonspecific symptoms, is the most common type of infection. Other sites may be secondarily infected, but pulmonary infection is relatively uncommon. Risk of MAC increases with decreasing CD4$^+$ cell count.

▼ The isolation of NTM from respiratory specimens is well described for patients with CF. *Mycobacterium avium* complex isolates are most common, followed by *M. abscessus* in a significant minority of patients, although there may be significant variability of the etiology globally. The virulence of NTM in CF patients also shows variability. CF patients, from whom NTM are isolated tend to be older, have better lung function and have a lower frequency of chronic *P. aeruginosa* infection (but higher rate of *S. aureus*) compared to patients without NTM infection.

▼ In immunocompetent patients, pneumonia is the most common disease caused by MAC. A syndrome similar to TB has been described in elderly men with underlying pulmonary disease. Patients present with chronically progressive cough and weight loss. Upper lobe cavitation is well described, and parenchymal damage may be significant. A second common syndrome is described in women, usually older than 50, without underlying lung disease. Patients present with insidious onset of cough and sputum production; systemic symptoms are not prominent.

■ *Mycobacterium kansasii*: *M. kansasii* infection presents as pulmonary disease that may be difficult to distinguish from TB. Most patients present with chest pain and fever. Hemoptysis, fever, and night sweats are also common. Cavitation is commonly seen on chest x-ray. *Mycobacterium kansasii*, in contrast to other NTM, is not found in soil or natural water sources but is associated with tap water in cities where the organism is endemic.

■ *Mycobacterium marinum*: *M. marinum* is well described as a cause of chronic cutaneous infection after exposure to water sources, the so-called fish tank granuloma.

▼ Organisms enter through traumatic or preexisting breaks in the skin surface. Several weeks after exposure, a nodular or ulcerating lesion develops at the site of infection, with subsequent spread along lymphatic channels. Infections usually occur on the extremities, most often the hands. The infection may be locally invasive but usually only in immunocompromised patients.

▼ Diagnosis may be established by AFB smear and culture. Note that *M. marinum* (and other NTM that are mainly associated with cutaneous infection) grows optimally in cultures incubated at 30°C, so special AFB cultures should be requested. Histopathologic examination shows granuloma formation.

❑ **Laboratory Findings**

AFB smear and culture of lower respiratory samples. ATS/Infectious Disease Society of America (IDSA) criteria to confirm NTM pulmonary infection:

■ Positive culture from two or more expectorated sputum samples
■ Positive culture from one or more BAL or bronchial wash samples
■ Lung biopsy consistent with mycobacterial infection (granulomatous inflammation or AFB), confirmed by positive culture of tissue or respiratory specimen
■ Positive culture from a normally sterile, nonpulmonary site of infection

AFB smear and culture of infected material from nonpulmonary sites: When NMT infection is suspected, AFB smear and culture of specimens taken from infected, nonpulmonary sites, especially normally sterile sites, are recommended. Ensure that an adequate quantity of sample is submitted for AFB culture; repeat testing of sequential specimens is likely to improve isolation.

Blood culture: The diagnosis of disseminated NTM infection is usually efficiently established in immunocompromised patients by submission of AFB blood cultures. AFB culture of bone marrow may also be diagnostic, especially in immunocompromised patients with hematologic abnormalities.

Susceptibility testing:

- MAC: clarithromycin only
- *Mycobacterium kansasii*: rifampin only
- RGM: amikacin, imipenem (*M. fortuitum*), doxycycline, fluoroquinolones, sulfonamide or TMP/SMX, cefoxitin, clarithromycin, linezolid, tobramycin (*M. chelonae*)

Core laboratory: Laboratory tests related to specific organ systems infected by NTM. HIV serology or other diagnostic testing should be considered in any patient who is diagnosed with significant or severe infection with these mycobacteria.

Suggested Readings

Brown-Elliott BA, Brown JM, Conville PS, et al. Clinical and laboratory features of the *Nocardia* spp. based on current molecular taxonomy. *Clin Microbiol Rev.* 2006;19:259–282.

Lederman ER, Crum NF. A case series and focused review of nocardiosis, Clinical and microbiologic aspects. *Medicine (Baltimore).* 2004;83:300–313.

 DISEASES CAUSED BY FUNGAL PATHOGENS

Fungi are eukaryotic organisms widely distributed in the environment; specific pathogens, like *Coccidioides*, may show a restricted geographic distribution. The fungal pathogens in this section may be initially characterized as yeasts (e.g., reproduce by binary fission with minimal cellular differentiation) or molds (e.g., formation of multicellular mycelia with differentiation of cells within the mycelial structure: vegetative hyphae, aerial hyphae, reproductive structures).

Direct examination of patient specimens (e.g., histopathology, KOH wet mount, staining) may provide initial presumptive evidence of infection. Detection of specific (e.g., cryptococcal antigen) or nonspecific (e.g., galactomannan) fungal antigens also supports a diagnosis of fungal disease. Definitive diagnosis of fungal infections, however, is primarily based on isolation of a pathogen in culture. Serologic testing may be useful for epidemiologic studies but are rarely used for the diagnosis of acute infection. See Chapter 17, Infectious Disease Assays for additional information related to diagnostic testing for fungal infection.

- *Molds*: A huge variety of mold species are ubiquitous in nature, with a global distribution; humans are exposed on a daily basis. In immunocompetent individuals, infection is rare. A number of common mold species have emerged as significant opportunistic pathogens in immunocompromised patients. In these patients, infection is usually acquired by inhalation or direct inoculation. Disseminated or locally invasive disease may ensue.

A definitive diagnosis of infection is most reliably established by some combination of histopathology, imaging studies, and isolation of the pathogen by culture. Although septate hyphae may be distinguished from aseptate hyphae histologically, identification of different pathogens within these groups cannot be reliably established by standard histologic staining techniques alone. Definitive species identification is usually based on examination of culture isolates. Opportunistic mold species usually grow well and rapidly on nonselective fungal media. Some species may be inhibited by cycloheximide. Serology does not play a significant role in the diagnosis of opportunistic invasive fungal infections.

- Laboratory findings are consistent with dysfunction of organ systems affected by fungal infection as well as predisposing diseases (e.g., diabetes, neoplasms, IV drug use, and malnutrition).
- *Yeasts*: Yeasts behave more like bacteria than mold in the clinical laboratory; they are often isolated on bacterial culture media. Infection is usually based on microscopic morphology and biochemical testing. Antigen detection may support the diagnosis. Standardized susceptibility testing methods are available for common pathogens.
- *Dimorphic fungi*: This group of fungi includes species with intrinsic pathogenicity. Most exhibit different forms depending on their growth conditions. In the environment, the spore-forming mold form predominates. In the patient, organisms differentiate into a tissue (usually yeast) form. These organisms may be widely distributed in the environment, but the geographic distribution varies by species. Most infection is transmitted by inhalation of spores, but direct inoculation is well described.

ASPERGILLOSIS

❑ Definition
Species of the genus *Aspergillus* cause a variety of diseases referred to as aspergillosis. These fungi are nonpigmented, septate mold species. Humans are frequently exposed to hyphal fragments or spores, usually by inhalation. Such exposure may result in disease by invasive proliferation (infection), colonization of aerated spaces (fungus ball, otomycosis), or by immunologic response to *Aspergillus* antigens.

❑ Who Should Be Suspected?
- Risk factors for invasive aspergillosis include advanced AIDS, allogeneic hematopoietic stem cell and solid organ transplantation, chronic granulomatous disease, glucocorticoid therapy, graft versus host disease, hematologic malignancy, and/or prolonged profound neutropenia. Infection has been associated with exposure to construction sites, presumably due to increased dispersal of spores.
- The respiratory tract is the common portal of entry and disease most commonly involves the lungs or pararespiratory tissues. Secondary infection may be seen in any organ system, although the CNS, kidney, liver, and spleen are most commonly affected.
- Patients with invasive sinusitis due to *Aspergillus* usually present with fever, epistaxis, nasal congestion, facial edema, and pain over the affected sinuses.

Infection may extend to the cavernous sinus, orbit (blurred vision, proptosis, chemosis), or CNS (mental status changes and a variety of specific symptoms related to the affected area). Endocarditis, endophthalmitis, skin infection, and GI infection are well-described infections associated with invasive aspergillosis, presumably due to hematologic dissemination from a primary site of infection.

- *Aspergillus* species may cause noninvasive diseases in immunocompetent patients. Allergic bronchopulmonary aspergillosis (APBA) occurs in 1–2% of patients with chronic asthma. Patients present with exacerbation of asthma symptoms, including increased and recurrent bronchial obstruction. Fever and malaise are common. Brownish mucous plugs or blood may be seen in expectorated sputum. APBA may respond to glucocorticoid therapy. Diagnosis is usually based on a number of major criteria, including history of asthma, immediate skin test reactivity to *Aspergillus* antigens, precipitin antibodies to *Aspergillus* species, total serum IgE >1,000 ng/mL, peripheral blood eosinophilia >500/mm^3, radiographic abnormalities, and elevation of serum anti-*Aspergillus* IgE and IgG.
- Fungus balls may form by colonization and proliferation of *Aspergillus* species in lung cavities formed by unrelated disease. Disease may result from erosion into critical structures.

❏ **Laboratory Findings**

Culture: Blood cultures are rarely positive, even in patients with evidence of hematogenous spread.

Histopathology: The morphology of *Aspergillus* is fairly characteristic, usually demonstrating nonpigmented, narrow, septate hyphae with acute angle branching. Angioinvasion is commonly demonstrated. The morphology, however, is not specific; other molds, like *Scedosporium* or *Fusarium*, may show a similar histopathology.

Core laboratory: Laboratory studies related to the function of affected organs should be submitted. Eosinophilia (>1,000/µL; often >3,000/µL) is common in ABPA.

BLASTOMYCOSIS

❏ **Definition**

Blastomycosis is caused by the thermally dimorphic fungus *Blastomyces dermatitidis*. Most cases are reported from the North America; endemic areas include southeastern, south central and midwestern states (especially around the Mississippi and Ohio River basins), north central states and Canadian provinces bordering the Great Lakes, and St. Lawrence River basin. Blastomycosis is also endemic in regions of Africa and may occur sporadically in patients in other areas.

❏ **Who Should Be Suspected?**

- The scope of pulmonary infection ranges from asymptomatic or mild infection to acute or chronic pulmonary infection to disseminated extrapulmonary disease. Immunocompromised patients are more susceptible to severe, extrapulmonary, and recurrent disease. Infection may spread to secondary sites.

- Conditions associated with increased risk include AIDS, cytotoxic and immunosuppressive therapy, hematologic malignancy, pregnancy, and solid organ transplantation.

❏ **Laboratory Findings**

- Direct detection: Wet mount or calcofluor white preparation has moderate sensitivity for early diagnosis of blastomycosis. Sensitivity is improved by the use concentrated specimens.
- Histopathology: Frequently demonstrates pyogranulomas in infected tissues. Visualization of characteristic yeast forms is improved by the use of fungal stains, like periodic acid–Schiff or methenamine silver stains.
- Culture: Isolation of *B. dermatitidis* in culture provides definitive diagnosis of blastomycosis. Cultures of sputum, BAL aspirate, or infected tissue should be positive in most patients with active infection.
- Serology: Specific antibody detection has played a minor role in diagnosis of blastomycosis because of poor S/S. Sensitivity is reported approximately 90% and specificity approximately 80%.
- Routine laboratory: WBC and ESR are increased. Mild normochromic anemia is present; serum globulin may be slightly increased and/or serum ALP may be increased with bone lesions.

CANDIDIASIS

❏ **Definition**

- Candidiasis describes disease caused by any of several species within the fungal genus *Candida*. *Candida* species are globally distributed yeast, and those that cause infection form a part of the human endogenous flora, as well as the normal flora of other warm-blooded animals. *Candida* spp. are common inhabitants of the GI tract but may also be found on other mucosal surfaces, including the oral and genital tracts, and skin surfaces, including under the fingernails and toenails and intertriginous areas. Disease may occur when an individual's local host defense mechanisms or systemic immunity is compromised. The incidence of invasive candidiasis has increased in the recent decades as a result of increasing use of broad-spectrum antibacterial agents and the emergence of AIDS and other immunocompromising conditions.
- *Candida albicans* is the most common cause of candidiasis. This species causes most infections of the genital, oral, and cutaneous sites. Candidiasis can also be caused by a number of other *Candida* species, most frequently: *Candida glabrata*, *Candida krusei*, *Candida lusitaniae*, *Candida parapsilosis*, and *Candida tropicalis*. *Candida dubliniensis* is a recently identified species that may mimic *C. albicans* in commonly used identification algorithms.
- Although several organism factors contribute to the ability of *Candida* species to cause infection, the most important factor is the status of the host's immunity. Most infections are endogenous, usually caused by organisms from the individual's GI flora. Most infections of deep tissues result from hematogenous spread from a primary site of infection. Disease processes that

result in the breakdown of the integrity of the gut mucosa or skin surface are predisposing factors for hematogenous spread.

❑ Who Should Be Suspected?

- Mucosal and cutaneous candidiasis may occur in normal hosts with minor predisposing conditions, like recent antibiotic therapy. However, more serious conditions should be considered (e.g., HIV infection, DM).
- Genital (see discussion of vaginitis and vaginosis in Chapter 8, Gynecologic and Obstetric Disorders).
- Oropharyngeal: "Thrush" is a common infection in healthy infants after antibiotic exposure but also occurs in patients with defects in cell-mediated immunity, like AIDS. In addition to recent antibiotic treatment, risk is increased by chemotherapy or head and neck radiation. Patients with dentures are also at increased risk. Oropharyngeal candidiasis usually presents with characteristic white plaques on the tongue, buccal mucosa, palate, or posterior oropharynx. Patients may be asymptomatic. Some patients complain of odynophagia or painful stomatitis, frequently seen in patients with dentures.
- Esophageal: Esophageal candidiasis is an AIDS-defining illness in patients with HIV infection. Patients may have oropharyngeal candidiasis. Odynophagia and retrosternal pain are common complaints. White plaques are seen by endoscopic examination, the scrapings of which show budding yeast with pseudohyphae.
- Skin and nails: Superficial infection may occur, typically in intertriginous or other warm, moist areas. Infection presents with erythema, pruritus, and characteristic rash. *Candida albicans* and *C. parapsilosis* are the most common causes of onychomycosis of the fingers and may be associated with paronychia. Congenital candidiasis may present in neonates as a generalized erythematous desquamating rash. Chronic mucocutaneous candidiasis is uncommon but may occur in patients with congenital autoimmune syndromes or other defects in cell-mediated immunity. Conditions commonly misdiagnosed as cutaneous candidiasis include psoriasis, chronic nail trauma, squamous carcinoma of the nail bed, "yellow-nail syndrome," or other conditions that should be considered and ruled out as appropriate. In skin and nail involvement in children, congenital hypoparathyroidism and Addison disease should be ruled out.
- Candidemia: Invasive candidiasis is most commonly caused by hematogenous spread of endogenous *Candida* in immunocompromised patients, often associated with a break in the integrity of the mucosal barrier of the bowel or indwelling central venous catheter. Symptoms may be variable, ranging from low fever and malaise to a full-blown sepsis syndrome. The incidence of candidemia is increasing as a result of HIV infection and other acquired immunodeficiency diseases, increasing use and potency of immunosuppressive therapies, intensive care interventions, increased survival of premature infants, increased use of chronic IV nutrition, and other factors. *Candida albicans* is the most common isolate, but other *Candida* species are playing an increasing role in candidemia, resulting in an increased rate of resistance to antifungal agents in candidemic patients. *Candida* species play a significant role in the etiology of nosocomial bloodstream infections, causing up to 10% of these infections. Candidemia has a high attributable mortality.

Cofactors contributing to poor outcome include older age, disseminated candidiasis, and severe and persistent neutropenia.

- Pneumonia: Though *Candida* species are commonly isolated from cultures of lower respiratory samples, they are usually contaminants; primary *Candida* pneumonia is extremely rare, even in intubated patients. Secondary *Candida* pneumonia occurs rarely in candidemic patients, but diagnosis may require invasive techniques and histopathologic confirmation.
- Cardiovascular: Endocarditis, myocarditis, or pericarditis may occur. *Candida* is responsible for <5% of cases of endocarditis, but *C. albicans* is responsible for >50% of the cases of fungal endocarditis. Risk factors include presence of prosthetic valves, IV drug abuse, major surgery, preexisting valve disease, and chronic placement of deep IV catheters or pacemakers. The presentation of *Candida* endocarditis cannot be distinguished from bacterial endocarditis on the basis of clinical presentation alone. Patients with *Candida* endocarditis are at high risk for embolization; the brain, eye, kidney, liver, skin, and spleen are common sites.
- CNS: Infections are uncommon but may arise as secondary infections in candidemic patients or as complication of neurosurgery or chronic ventricular shunting. The clinical presentation is not distinctive.
- Ocular: Chorioretinitis or endophthalmitis is usually caused by hematogenous spread and may be the first sign of invasive candidiasis. Keratitis and some cases of chorioretinitis or endophthalmitis are caused by trauma or surgery. Patients present with pain and loss of visual acuity. Ophthalmologic examination is recommended for all patients with candidemia. Characteristic findings are confirmed by culture.
- Bone and joint: Infections may be due to direct trauma, joint injection or surgery, or secondary to hematogenous seeding. These infections may present many months after the infectious incident; onset is often gradual and subtle. The vertebrae are most commonly affected in the elderly, whereas infection of the long bones is most common in children. Diagnosis is established by isolation of *Candida* from specimens collected from the bone or joint.
- Abdominal: *Candida* species, as common components of the endogenous GI microflora, may be isolated in almost any infectious process of the abdomen. Specific *Candida* peritonitis may be seen in patients undergoing chronic peritoneal dialysis. *Candida* infection is a fairly common complication in patients recovering from acute pancreatitis from other causes. Hepatosplenic candidiasis may complicate resolution of neutropenia in patients on chemotherapeutic regimens for hematologic malignancies. The liver and spleen may have been seeded during a recognized or unrecognized episode of candidemia, although there is the possibility that *Candida* was introduced by the portal vasculature. Patients present with fever, nausea, vomiting, anorexia, and right upper quadrant pain. Discrete microabscesses form in the liver and spleen, which may be detected by a variety of imaging techniques.

11

❑ Laboratory Findings
Culture: Positive cultures from normally sterile sites support the diagnosis, but cultures must be interpreted with caution to rule out contamination with endogenous flora. The detection of candiduria in patients with bladder catheters in place most likely represents colonization. In patients without foreign bodies in the urinary tract, however,

significant candiduria may be a marker of obstruction, DM, or other serious condition. There is not a clear relationship between the quantity of *Candida* in urine (CFU/mL) and clinical significance, as is seen with bacteria. Isolation of *Candida albicans* from sputum and other respiratory specimens is common but rarely associated with pulmonary infection. In CNS infection, isolation of *Candida* from CSF is diagnostic, but the concentration of organisms may be very low, so repeat testing and submission of a large volume of CSF per sample may be needed to establish the diagnosis.

Direct detection of organisms in tissue or clinical specimens: When associated with signs of inflammation or tissue damage, this may provide reliable detection of infection. Diagnosis of oropharyngeal, esophageal, or vulvovaginal candidiasis may be made on the basis of clinical appearance and risk factors. Confirmation may be established by wet mount or Gram stain examination of scrapings from the affected sites. Negative direct examination does not rule out mucosal candidiasis.

Histopathology: Shows yeast cells and mycelial forms, epithelial disruption with organisms invading through mucosal cells, and submucosal inflammation in mucosal candidiasis. Deep tissue candidiasis shows organisms invading and disrupting infected tissue.

Serology: Antibody detection has played a limited role in diagnosis of candidiasis.

Core laboratory: ALP levels are increased in patients with hepatosplenic candidiasis.

COCCIDIOIDOMYCOSIS

❑ Definition
Coccidioidomycosis is caused by dimorphic fungi in the genus *Coccidioides* (*Coccidioides immitis* and *Coccidioides posadasii*). *Coccidioides* species are endemic in the desert regions of the Western hemisphere, including the Southwestern United States and California. Infection is acquired by inhalation of arthroconidia produced by the mycelial form in the environment.

❑ Who Should Be Suspected?
- There is a wide spectrum of disease. Asymptomatic or mild disease is common as judged by seroepidemiologic studies. The risk of clinical infection is increased with increasing exposure to dust (i.e., in the dry periods following periods of rain) in endemic regions and in immunocompromised patients. Disease usually develops 1 to 4 weeks after exposure.
- Disease resolves spontaneously in most patients, resulting in lifelong immunity. However, it is likely that recovery is not associated with a complete microbiologic cure: recrudescent infection is well documented in patients as a result of acquired immunocompromise, as seen in malignancies, HIV infection, and immunosuppressive therapy.
- "Valley fever" is the most common presentation of disease. This syndrome is usually associated with low-grade fever and pneumonia, with cough, and pleuritic chest pain. Systemic symptoms, including fatigue and arthralgias, are common. Cutaneous findings may be seen, including erythema nodosum or erythema multiforme. Hoarseness is uncommon. Severe and chronic disease may be seen in a minority of normal hosts but is more common in immunocompromised patients and in those with specific conditions (e.g., chemotherapy, glucocorticoid therapy, hematologic malignancy, HIV infection,

immunosuppressive therapy for autoimmune disease, preexisting chronic lung disease, and/or solid organ transplant).

- Signs and symptoms of severe and chronic disease are related to the organ system affected and degree of tissue damage. Common manifestations of progressive disease include cutaneous dissemination, extensive pulmonary disease, meningitis, osteomyelitis, and/or septic arthritis.

❏ Laboratory Findings

Culture: *Coccidioides* species grow on most routine microbiologic media, including those used for bacterial culture, often within several days. It is important to alert the laboratory when a specimen is submitted from a patient in whom coccidioidomycosis is suspected; *Coccidioides* is a significant risk factor for laboratory-acquired infection. Blood cultures are rarely positive for *Coccidioides*, even with evidence of hematogenous spread.

- *Direct detection*: Detection of spherules, the tissue form of *Coccidioides*, is a strong, specific predictor of infection.
- *Serology*: Most, but not all, patients develop specific anticoccidioidal antibodies in response to infection. The appearance of antibodies may be delayed for months after the onset of acute infection. Failure or delay in seroconversion is increased in immunocompromised patients; the diagnosis of coccidioidomycosis is not ruled out by negative results. Titers may fall to undetectable levels during the course of illness in patients who resolve their acute infections. Repeat testing is recommended in patients with negative results if a high index of suspicion remains. Several serologic methods are available:
  - ▼ *CF antibodies*: CF assays primarily reflect the presence of IgG antibody. These antibodies typically develop later but are more persistent than precipitin antibodies. High CF titers are more commonly seen in patients with extensive infection. Changes in CF titer may be used to predict progression or regression of disease.
  - ▼ *EIA*: EIA techniques have been developed and are sensitive and specific for detection of IgG and IgM antibodies in serum and CSF. EIA methods represent the most efficient serologic method, but results may not correlate exactly with other methods.
  - ▼ *LA*: These methods are convenient in resource-limited settings, but the increased occurrence of false-positive reactions limits their use.
  - ▼ *Precipitin antibodies*: Carbohydrate cell wall antigen reagents are used to detect specific antibody by precipitin formation. Precipitin antibodies are primarily of the IgM class. Approximately 90% of patients develop precipitin antibodies in the first weeks of symptomatic infection, but levels fall with resolution of infection. Cross-reactions with *Histoplasma capsulatum* and *B. dermatitis* are reported.
  - ▼ *Skin test reactivity*: Patients with coccidioidomycosis develop a hypersensitivity to specific antigens, manifested by erythema and induration at the site of intradermal injection. Skin testing may be useful for seroepidemiologic studies. The utility of testing is limited for acute disease because skin test reactivity cannot differentiate between acute and past infection; many patients with coccidioidomycosis may be anergic on the basis of their underlying disease or therapy.

11

Routine laboratory: Most routine laboratory tests are unremarkable. Decreased peripheral blood lymphocyte count, increased ESR, or slight elevation of WBC is often seen; eosinophilia may be seen.

Radiology: Abnormal radiologic studies are common in pulmonary and extrapulmonary disease and help delineate the extent of disease. Bone scans can be used to screen for osteomyelitis.

- *Septic arthritis*: Arthroscopy with synovial biopsy may be used to establish infection.
- *Meningitis*: Culture is usually negative. Mononuclear pleocytosis (100–200 WBCs/μL), decreased glucose, increased protein. Detection of IgG-specific antibody is diagnostic of meningitis in undiluted CSF and is detected in approximately 75% of patients with *Coccidioides* meningitis. Serology may be used to document response to antifungal therapy. Detection of specific IgG may be used to document relapse for 1–2 years after end of therapy. Serum titers are often negative or only borderline positive.

CRYPTOCOCCOSIS (*CRYPTOCOCCUS NEOFORMANS*)

❑ Definition

Several species of the genus *Cryptococcus*, including *Cryptococcus neoformans* and *Cryptococcus gattii*, are capable of causing disease in humans. The typical geographic distribution of *C. gattii* is restricted to tropical and subtropical regions with eucalyptus trees. *Cryptococcus neoformans*, on the other hand, has a worldwide distribution and is responsible for most cases of cryptococcosis worldwide. Organisms are able to survive in the gut of pigeons and in dried pigeon droppings; this is likely responsible for wide distribution through the environment. Infection is acquired by inhalation of organisms present in the environment, and person-to-person transmission does not occur.

❑ Who Should Be Suspected?

In immunocompetent individuals, exposure usually results in self-limited asymptomatic or mild disease; progressive and chronic disease is uncommon. Immunocompromised patients, however, are at risk for more severe disease with progression to extrapulmonary tissues. Conditions associated with increased risk of disseminated cryptococcosis include AIDS, glucocorticoid therapy, organ transplantation, malignancy, and/or sarcoidosis. Types of infection include the following:

- *Pulmonary*: Symptoms of pulmonary cryptococcosis include chest pain, cough, dyspnea, fever, sputum production, and weight loss. Hematogenous dissemination may occur.
- *CNS*: A significant proportion of AIDS patients with clinically significant pulmonary cryptococcosis progress to cryptococcal meningoencephalitis or infection in other organs. Frequent symptoms include altered mental status, fever, headache, seizures, and visual disturbances.
- *Bone and joint*: Osteomyelitis usually occurs in vertebrae or bony prominences due to hematogenous spread from a primary pulmonary infection. Cryptococcal arthritis may occur by spread from a contiguous osteomyelitis.
- *Lymphadenopathy*: usually cervical or supraclavicular.

- *Prostate*: Asymptomatic, persistent infection of the prostate may occur, most commonly in AIDS patients, and serves as a reservoir for recurrent infection.
- *Skin*: May represent primary infection but usually represents hematogenous dissemination from a primary pulmonary infection. A wide variety of cutaneous lesions have been described.

❑ Laboratory Findings

Radiology: In immunocompetent patients, solitary or few noncalcified nodules are most commonly seen. Cavitation is uncommon. In AIDS patients, bilateral interstitial infiltrates, which may mimic *Pneumocystis jirovecii* or other opportunistic infection, are common.

Gram stain: Gram stain may demonstrate yeast consistent with *C. neoformans*.

Culture: *Cryptococcus neoformans* may be isolated from 90 to 100% of infected specimens submitted from patients with cryptococcosis. Coinfection with other opportunistic pathogens has been reported in pulmonary cryptococcosis in AIDS patients.

Histopathology: *Cryptococcus neoformans* cells may be seen in biopsy material using a variety of stains, including H&E, silver, Fontana-Masson, and mucicarmine.

Serology: Serology is not useful for diagnosis of acute cryptococcal infection.

Cryptococcal antigen (CA): Detection of specific polysaccharide antigen is sensitive and specific for diagnosis of cryptococcosis. LA assays are most commonly used and provide rapid results. CA can be detected in CSF >90% of patients with cryptococcal meningitis. Serum CA may also be used as a less sensitive screen for meningitis or cryptococcal infection at other sites but should be confirmed by culture of the infected site.

CSF CA titers are useful for predicting outcome and monitoring therapy in AIDS patients with cryptococcal meningoencephalitis. Patients with an initial titer of ≤1:2,048 predict a favorable outcome. Relapse is likely in patients with persistently elevated CA titers in spite of effective antifungal therapy. False-positive CA tests may be caused by RF, cross-reaction with *Trichosporon beigelii*, or *Capnocytophaga canimorsus* or syneresis fluid from culture media. The EIA does not show a prozone effect and is not affected by RF. The turnaround time for EIA results is longer than for LA testing.

Laboratory findings (cryptococcal meningitis): Meningitis should be considered, regardless of symptoms, in immunocompromised patients with pulmonary cryptococcosis, and relevant diagnostic testing performed. Relapse is less frequent when increase in protein and cells is marked rather than moderate. Poor prognosis is suggested if initial CSF examination shows positive India ink preparation, low glucose (<20 mg/dL), and low WBC count (<20/µL). CBC and ESR usually remain normal.

CSF findings: Positive culture is related to CSF volume submitted and is improved when ≥10 mL is available. Protein is increased in 90% of patients (<500 mg/dL). Glucose is moderately decreased in approximately 55% of patients. CSF cell count is almost always increased, but ≤800 cells (more lymphocytes than leukocytes).

FUSARIOSIS

❑ Definition

Fusariosis is caused by infection with species of the genus *Fusarium*. These fungi form septate, nonpigmented hyphae. These fungi are saprophytic with a wide distribution in the environment. Disease is transmitted primarily by inhalation or direct inoculation, usually at a site of trauma. Proliferation at the site of inoculation may result in localized infection or disseminated disease.

❑ Who Should Be Suspected?

Major risk factors for invasive infection include hematologic malignancy, especially in patients with hematopoietic stem cell transplantation, glucocorticoid treatment, prolonged neutropenia, and disruption of skin integrity (e.g., burns, long-term central venous catheter placement, trauma). Significant disease is uncommon in immunocompetent patients. As with other opportunistic molds, broad range of disease may be caused by *Fusarium*, from superficial and allergic, to locally invasive, to disseminated, multiorgan disease. Affected patients and clinical manifestations include the following:

- *Immunocompetent patients*: Localized infection is most commonly seen; onychomycosis and keratitis are the most common types of infection. Infections at other sites, including sinusitis, pulmonary infection, and foreign body–associated infection, are described but occur infrequently. Keratitis occurs almost exclusively in contact lens users and may be associated with use of specific lens solutions.

- *Immunocompromised patients*: Invasive and disseminated infection is most common in immunocompromised patients; patients with severe and prolonged neutropenia are at greatest risk. Immunocompromised patients with fusariosis usually present with sepsis, associated with positive blood cultures and skin lesions. Skin lesions may occur as a primary site of infection but are the most common site of disseminated infection, occurring in a significant majority of patients with systemic disease. Patients typically present with multiple, painful lesions. Papular or nodular lesions are most common on the extremities. They commonly develop central necrosis with surrounding erythema.

❑ Laboratory Findings

Histopathology: Hyaline, segmented hyphae with acute and right-angle branching are seen in tissues. Hyphae cannot be confidently differentiated from other opportunistic fungi, like *Aspergillus* and *Scedosporium*, but the presence of adventitious sporulation in vivo is not seen in *Aspergillus* and suggests *Fusarium* or *Scedosporium* infection. Angioinvasion may be evident, with distal necrosis due to vascular compromise.

Culture: *Fusarium* species grow well on nonselective media for fungal isolation. Accurate speciation relies on specialized testing, like nucleic acid sequencing or specific PCR, and is not widely available. Standardized antifungal susceptibility testing is available.

Other: The $(1,3)$-β-D-glucan assay is usually positive in invasive disease but is not specific for fusariosis. The galactomannan test is negative.

HISTOPLASMOSIS

❑ **Definition**
Histoplasmosis is caused by the thermally dimorphic fungus *Histoplasma capsulatum*. There are two variants, *H. capsulatum* var *capsulatum* and *H. capsulatum* var *duboisii*. *Histoplasma capsulatum* var *capsulatum* is endemic in the eastern United States (Mississippi, Ohio, and St. Lawrence River basins) and Latin America. *Histoplasma capsulatum* var *duboisii* occurs in Africa (Gabon, Uganda, and Kenya) and is associated with a lower frequency of pulmonary infection but more frequent skin and bone infection. The natural habitat of *H. capsulatum* is soil with high nitrogen content, such as found near roosting areas of birds or in caves, where the organism proliferates in its mold phase. Infection is transmitted by inhalation of conidia or mycelial fragments.

❑ **Who Should Be Suspected?**
Most infections are asymptomatic. Patients with defects in T-cell–mediated immune mechanisms are at increased risk for dissemination, reactivation of latent infection, or reinfection. Heavy exposure may result in acute pulmonary histoplasmosis and increased risk of disseminated disease. Conditions associated with disseminated disease include AIDS, chemotherapy for malignancy, glucocorticoid therapy, primary immunodeficiency disease, solid organ transplantation, and treatment with tumor necrosis factor blockers. Pulmonary histoplasmosis may mimic TB, other endemic mycoses, or other subacute or chronic pulmonary diseases. Histoplasmosis should be considered in patients with pneumonia at epidemiologic risk.

❑ **Laboratory Findings**
Direct detection: Direct detection is most useful for acute histoplasmosis by detection of yeast-like cells in infected patient specimens. Small budding yeast (2–5 μm), often within mononuclear cells, may be seen by wet mount preparations or histology.

Culture: Culture of the lung, skin, and mucosal lesions, sputum, BAL, gastric washings, blood, or bone marrow may provide a specific diagnosis. Fungal culture of blood is recommended for all patients with histoplasmosis. Two or three specimens may be needed for sensitive detection. Fungal culture of bone marrow is positive in a majority of patients with cytopenias or other signs of marrow failure. Blood and bone marrow cultures are positive in 50–70% of patients. Respiratory culture is positive in <40% of acute pulmonary cases but in up to 85% of patients with chronic pulmonary disease. Culture of tissue from infected sites is positive in 25–30% of patients. Culture is positive in approximately 50% of patients with meningitis, but a large volume of CSF is needed to detect CNS histoplasmosis by culture. Repeat culture on several occasions is recommended. Cultures may take up to 8 weeks to yield positive results, so initial therapeutic decisions are often based on clinical and other laboratory results.

Histology: Granulomas, lymphohistiocytic aggregates, and mononuclear cell infiltrates are most commonly seen histopathologically using routine staining methods; staining to enhance fungi, like methenamine silver or periodic acid–Schiff, improves detection of yeast cells in tissue. Biopsy (specially stained) of skin and mucosal lesions, bone marrow, and RE system provides initial diagnosis in approximately 45% of cases. Demonstration of *H. capsulatum* in smears of peripheral blood, buffy coat, bone marrow (25–60% positive), or respiratory secretions is often the most rapid method of diagnosis; fungal culture is recommended to improve sensitivity of detection.

Antigen detection:

- *Histoplasma capsulatum*–specific antigen may provide accurate diagnosis in early acute histoplasmosis, especially in patients with severe and progressive disease. The sensitivity of antigen detection is increased by submission of urine, blood, BAL fluid, and specimens from other potentially infected sites. Antigen may be detected in ≥75% of patients with diffuse acute pulmonary histoplasmosis.
- Antigen detection is especially useful in disseminated disease in which patients may not show significant antibody response. Urine antigen is positive in approximately 90% of patients with disseminated disease, approximately 20% of patients with acute self-limited disease, and <10% of patients with chronic pulmonary cavitary disease.
- Serum antigen testing is less sensitive than urine and is positive in approximately 70% of patients with disseminated disease. Antigen is detected in CSF in <50% of patients with meningitis; positive antigen must be interpreted with caution, as cross-reactions are seen in coccidioidal meningitis. (CSF antibodies may also cross-react.) Antigen is positive in BAL fluid in approximately 70% of patients with pulmonary histoplasmosis.
- Increasing antigen titer, or reconversion to antigen positivity, may be a sign of relapse. Antigen becomes undetectable after antifungal therapy. Cross-reactions may rarely be seen in patients with blastomycosis, coccidioidomycosis, paracoccidioidomycosis, or other invasive fungal disease.

Serology

- CF and immunodiffusion (ID) tests are most useful for diagnosis of histoplasmosis. EIA screening methods are less sensitive and less specific. Positive CF and ID reactions are markers of active histoplasmosis; background seropositivity in endemic areas is low. Positive reactions, however, may be due to asymptomatic, self-limited disease. Results of serologic tests must be interpreted with consideration of clinical and other laboratory information.
- Detection in specific *H. capsulatum* antibody is seen in approximately 90% of patients with acute pulmonary infection, but because seroconversion may not occur for several months after onset of infection, negative tests should be repeated after 4–6 weeks. Virtually, all patients with chronic pulmonary or disseminated disease are seropositive.
- CF titers are slightly more sensitive but less specific than the immunodiffusion test for diagnosis of histoplasmosis. A single serum CF titer ≥1:32 or a fourfold increase in CF titer is highly suggestive of active histoplasmosis; a CF titer <1:8 is considered negative. Rising CF titers occur in >95% of patients with symptomatic primary infections. A CSF CF titer ≥1:8 is evidence for meningeal histoplasmosis. CSF antibodies, however, may not be detected until the 3rd to 6th week of infection. Positive CF titers persist for months or years. Prognosis is not indicated by level or changes in titers. IgG and IgM detection is not clinically useful because of high false-positive and false-negative results.

Core laboratory: Increased serum aminotransferases and bilirubin suggest hepatic involvement. Anemia, leukopenia, and thrombocytopenia are more common (60–80% of cases) in acute than in subacute or chronic disseminated types. Increased serum LDH may be clue to disseminated form in AIDS patients.

CSF findings: Lymphocytic pleocytosis, increased protein, and decreased glucose

MUCORMYCOSIS

❑ Definition
Mucormycosis describes diseases caused by opportunistic aseptate molds of the *Mucorales* order. Species of the genus *Rhizopus* are responsible for most clinical infection, followed by *Mucor*. Most species grow very rapidly in culture. Clinical infection is often associated with high mortality, loss of function, and disfigurement. Most infections are acquired through the respiratory tract, causing local infection and subsequent dissemination. Organisms from the upper respiratory tract may be swallowed, resulting in GI infection. Organisms are able to proliferate in the presence of high concentrations of glucose, and they have the ability to invade blood vessels, resulting in tissue infarction. Nosocomial transmission, infection due to ingestion of contaminated food, and traumatic inoculation are less common but well-described modes of transmission. Person-to-person transmission does not occur.

❑ Who Should Be Suspected?
Although any organ may be involved in mucormycosis, the respiratory tract is the most common site of primary infection. Disseminated infection may follow primary infections. A high index of suspicion is required for efficient diagnosis of mucormycosis; early diagnosis is critical for appropriate intervention and antifungal therapy. Factors predisposing to infection include AIDS, deferoxamine therapy, DM, glucocorticoid therapy, hematologic malignancies, immunosuppressive therapy, neutropenia, renal failure, and solid organ transplantation. Common sites of infection include the following:

- *Rhinocerebral*: Rhinocerebral disease is the most common manifestation of mucormycosis, occurring in about 50% of patients. Primary infection is initiated in the nasal mucosa and then may spread through the palate, sinuses, orbit, other facial structures, or brain. Patients usually present with symptoms similar to bacterial sinusitis with fever, purulent discharge, and headache. Infection is commonly unilateral. Eschar forms on affected mucosa, and nasal discharge may be bloody. Ipsilateral extension may result in ulceration and necrosis of sinuses or palate. Ocular involvement manifests with orbital pain, proptosis, ophthalmoplegia, visual abnormalities, conjunctivitis, and inflammation and edema of the eyelid. The brain may be involved by spread of infection across the dura, causing cavernous sinus thrombosis and cerebral disease. Cerebral mucormycosis is manifested by cranial nerve palsies, change in level of consciousness, or severe disruption of cerebral function. Blood vessel involvement may result in symptoms of stroke.
- *Pulmonary*: Pulmonary disease represents about 10% of mucormycosis cases, occurring primarily in immunocompromised patients. Patients may present with FUO and respiratory symptoms unresponsive to antibiotic

therapy. Rapidly progressive pulmonary disease may present with a variety of patterns and may mimic pulmonary aspergillosis. Pulmonary necrosis may result in massive hemoptysis. Infection may progress into contiguous spaces and tissues, including the diaphragm, mediastinum, and heart.

- *GI*: GI disease occurs in <10% of patients. Symptoms and signs depend on the GI tissue involved and the type of pathology. Symptoms are nonspecific, including abdominal pain and diarrhea. Ulcerative lesions are common and may lead to perforation or massive bleeding with hematemesis or lower GI bleed.
- *Cutaneous*: Cutaneous infection is caused by direct inoculation of infectious mold into tissue or dissemination from the sites of primary infection. About 15% of cases of mucormycosis are cutaneous. Nodular lesions may show bruising with surrounding pallor. Lesions may be chronic or rapidly progressive. The extremities are most commonly involved, but 35–40% of cases occur on the head, neck, or thorax. The mortality is higher in central lesions.
- *Disseminated*: Disseminated infection occurs in about 5% of patients; the signs and symptoms depend on the extent of dysfunction of affected tissues. Specific organ disease may be apparent but nonspecific. Therefore, a high index of suspicion, based on patients underlying disease and clinical findings, is critical.

❏ Laboratory Findings

Histopathology: Infected tissue is necrotic, hemorrhagic, thrombotic, or pale depending on the degree and type of vascular compromise. Inflammation is not prominent in acute infection. Angioinvasion may be seen.

Culture: Specimens should be submitted for fungal culture, but cultures may be negative, depending on the location and type of infection and processing of specimens. Vigorous processing may damage hyphae, resulting in false-negative cultures. Therefore, when mucormycosis is suspected, the laboratory should be alerted to use gentle processing protocols, like gentle mincing of tissue rather than tissue homogenization. Cultures may be positive from acutely infected nasal sinus or turbinate tissue or nasal discharge. Cultures from CSF are rarely contributory. Mucormycosis cannot be excluded by negative cultures. In addition, positive cultures must be interpreted with caution to rule out possible contamination.

PARACOCCIDIOIDOMYCOSIS (*PARACOCCIDIOIDES BRASILIENSIS*)

❏ Definition

Paracoccidioidomycosis is caused by the thermally dimorphic fungus *Paracoccidioides brasiliensis*. This organism is endemic in wet, heavily vegetated, high-humidity areas of South America and Central America. The incidence of paracoccidioidomycosis is highest in Brazil.

❏ Who Should Be Suspected?

Most infections remain asymptomatic or mild, but clinical recovery may not be associated with microbiologic cure. Dormant infection may lead to recurrent, symptomatic infection at the time of acquired immunodeficiency. Disease is uncommon in children. Most symptomatic infections occur in men with occupations or other activities that put them in close contact with the environment. Symptoms are nonspecific and mimic TB, histoplasmosis, or other conditions. Symptoms include fever, chronic cough, sputum production, dyspnea, chest pain, weight loss, and malaise. The risk of infection is increased in patients who smoke, those who are alcoholic, or those who have AIDS. Person-to-person transmission does not occur.

❏ Laboratory Findings

Direct detection: Deep respiratory specimens, CSF, or tissue from granulomas, ulcers, lymph nodes, or other infected sites show the characteristic large yeast cells with multiple narrow-based buds (mariner's wheel). A mixed granulocytic, monocytic response is typical.

Culture: Routine fungal culture yields growth in the mold phase, which shows characteristic, but not specific, mycelial and conidial morphology.

Serology: The diagnosis is supported by demonstration of specific antibodies using CF, ID, and other antibody detection techniques. Successful therapy is associated in significant decrease in antibody titers when acute and convalescent serum samples are tested. The quantitative ID assay is sensitive (>95%) and specific (near 100%) for diagnosis and is recommended.

Routine laboratory: Morning cortisol levels and ACTH stimulation testing are recommended because of the frequency of adrenal gland involvement. Routine laboratory testing to evaluate the function of infected organs is recommended. Common findings include anemia, eosinophilia, hypoalbuminemia, hyperbilirubinemia, hypergammaglobulinemia, and mildly elevated transaminases.

PNEUMOCYSTIS JIROVECII (FORMERLY P. CARINII)

See Chapter 13, Respiratory, Metabolic, and Acid–Base Disorders.

SPOROTRICHOSIS

11

❏ Definition

Sporotrichosis is a subacute to chronic infection caused by the thermally dimorphic fungus *Sporothrix schenckii*. Sporotrichosis occurs mainly in North and South America and Japan, but scattered cases are seen worldwide. In the environment, this organism exists in its mold phase and is associated with soil and thorned plants, like roses. Infection is transmitted most commonly by traumatic inoculation or inoculation of nonintact skin surfaces. Most infections, therefore, are related to outdoor recreational or occupational activities. Infection may disseminate from the site of primary infection.

❏ Who Should Be Suspected?

Extracutaneous infection is most commonly seen in patients with underlying illnesses that may compromise immune function, including alcoholism, DM, COPD, and AIDS (uncommon).

- *Lymphocutaneous sporotrichosis*: A papular lesion, with overlying erythema, initially forms at the site of inoculation. The lesion commonly ulcerates. Similar lesions develop along the lymphatic drainage path from the primary site of infection. The lesions of lymphocutaneous sporotrichosis are usually only minimally painful. Systemic symptoms are usually absent.

- *Pulmonary sporotrichosis*: Pulmonary sporotrichosis usually occurs in alcoholic men. Signs and symptoms may mimic TB. Chest radiography commonly shows upper lobe disease with cavitation, fibrosis, or nodular densities. Respiratory symptoms include cough, dyspnea, and sputum production (may be bloody).
- *Osteoarticular sporotrichosis*: Osteoarticular sporotrichosis is usually caused by hematogenous spread from a primary cutaneous infection in alcoholic men. Joint infection is usually seen in the extremities: the knee, elbow, ankle, and wrist are most commonly affected. Osteomyelitis may occur as a result of local invasion. Patients present with pain, swelling, and decreased range of motion.
- *CNS sporotrichosis*: CNS infection is rare and occurs mainly in patients with AIDS or other T-cell defects. CNS infection has a subacute presentation with fever and headache.

❑ Laboratory Findings

Direct detection: Histopathologic examination of infected tissue shows a mixed pyogenic and granulomatous response. Typical "cigar-shaped" budding yeast may be seen. Detection is improved by use of fungal stains, like periodic acid–Schiff or methenamine silver stains. H&E staining may demonstrate "asteroid bodies"—basophilic yeast surrounded by eosinophilic material that probably represents antigen–antibody complex.

Culture: Isolation of *S. schenckii* in culture provides definitive diagnosis of sporotrichosis. The organism is readily isolated from biopsy or aspirated material from infected sites. Growth usually appears during the first week of incubation, but cultures are usually incubated for 4 weeks before being signed out as negative.

Serology: Does not play a significant role in the diagnosis of active infection.

CSF findings: Patients with meningitis have a lymphocytic pleocytosis, low glucose, and increased protein.

Suggested Readings

Chapman SW, Dismukes WE, Proia LA, et al. Clinical Practice Guidelines for the Management of Blastomycosis: 2008 Update by the Infectious Diseases Society of America. *Clin Infect Dis.* 2008;46:1801–1812.

Cuellar-Rodriguez J, Avery RK, Lard M, et al. Histoplasmosis in solid organ transplant recipients: 10 years of experience at a large transplant center in an endemic area. *Clin Infect Dis.* 2009;49:710–716.

Dromer F, McGinnis MR. Chapter 12: Zygomycosis. In: Anaissie EJ, McGinnis MR, Pfaller MA, (eds). *Clinical Mycology*. Philadelphia, PA: Churchill Livingstone; 2003.

Galgiani JN, Ampel NM, Blair JE, et al. Coccidioidomycosis. *Clin Infect Dis.* 2005;41:1217–1223.

Hage CA, Bowyer S, Tarvin SE, et al. Recognition, diagnosis, and treatment of histoplasmosis complicating tumor necrosis factor blocker therapy. *Clin Infect Dis.* 2010;50:85–92.

Kauffman CA. Sporotrichosis. *Clin Infect Dis.* 1999;29:231–237.

Kauffman CA, Bustamante B, Chapman SW, et al. Clinical Practice Guidelines for the Management of Sporotrichosis: 2007 Update by the Infectious Diseases Society of America. *Clin Infect Dis.* 2007;45:1255–1265.

Koo S, Bryar JM, Page JH, et al. Diagnostic performance of the $(1 \rightarrow 3)$-β-D-glucan assay for invasive fungal disease. *Clin Infect Dis.* 2009;49:1650–1659.

Nucci M, Anaissie E. *Fusarium* infections in immunocompromised patients. *Clin Microbiol Rev.* 2007;20:695–704.

Pera S, Patterson TF. Chapter 15 endemic mycoses. In: Anaissie EF, McGinnis MR, Pfaller MA, (eds). *Clinical Mycology*. Philadelphia, PA: Churchill Livingstone; 2003.

Perfect JR, Dismukes WE, Dromer F, et al. Clinical Practice Guidelines for the Management of Cryptococcal Disease: 2010 Update by the Infectious Diseases Society of America. *Clin Infect Dis*. 2010;50:291–322.

Ribes JA, Vanover-Sams CL, Baker DJ. Zygomycetes in human disease. *Clin Microbiol Rev*. 2000;13: 236–301.

Rex JH. Galactomannan and the diagnosis of invasive aspergillosis. *Clin Infect Dis*. 2006;42:1428–1430.

Segal BH. Aspergillosis. *N Engl J Med*. 2009;360:1870–1884.

Sun H-Y, Wagener MM, Singh N. Cryptococcosis in solid-organ, hematopoietic stem cell, and tissue transplant recipients: evidence-based evolving trends. *Clin Infect Dis*. 2009;48:1566–1576.

Yozwiak ML, Lundergan LL, Kerrick SS, et al. Symptoms and routine laboratory abnormalities associated with coccidioidomycosis. *West J Med*. 1988;149:419–421.

INFECTIOUS DISEASES CAUSED BY VIRAL PATHOGENS

This section reviews viral pathogens that are responsible for a very wide and diverse range of diseases. Viral pathogens are incapable of multiplication outside of host eukaryotic cells, but many do not require human cells for proliferation. Other mammals, arthropods, or other species may serve as intermediate or definitive hosts for pathogenic viruses. Most viral infections are mild, self-limited diseases and are presumptively diagnosed on the basis of clinical signs and symptoms. Serologic testing is most commonly used when definitive diagnosis is required and may be used for diagnosis of acute or past infection or to determine the immune status of a host. Viral infection may also be established presumptively by typical histopathologic findings; specific identification may be made by specific immunostaining. Isolation of virus in eukaryotic cell culture provides definitive diagnosis, but the sensitivity of culture for isolation usually falls significantly after acute symptoms resolve, and some viral pathogens cannot be isolated in culture. Molecular diagnostic procedures are playing an increasing role in the diagnosis of viral infections. Molecular methods may be used for diagnosis, predicting response to antiviral agents, monitoring disease activity or response to treatment, or other purposes.

CYTOMEGALOVIRUS INFECTION

❏ Definition

Human cytomegalovirus (CMV) is member of the *Herpesviridae*, subfamily *Betaherpesvirinae*. CMV is ubiquitous with a worldwide distribution. Although CMV infection can be demonstrated in a significant majority of individuals in developing and developed countries, clinical disease is uncommon in immunocompetent hosts. Acute infection with CMV, as characteristic of herpesviruses, results in long-term latent infection with periodic reactivation to a replicative phase of infection.

❏ Who Should Be Suspected?

- Immunocompetent patients who develop acute disease most often present with a mononucleosis syndrome with pharyngitis, lymphadenopathy, and splenomegaly. Laboratory studies may show elevated atypical lymphocytes and transaminases.

- Fetal and neonatal disease is the result of vertical transmission during acute or recurrent maternal infection. Neonatal infection may also be transmitted by breast milk. Most infected neonates are asymptomatic at birth but are at risk (10–15%) for development of hearing loss, learning disability, and/ or other organ dysfunction. Congenital CMV disease may manifest at birth with a variety of clinical features, alone or in combination, including intrauterine growth retardation, microcephaly, intracranial calcifications, hepatosplenomegaly, jaundice, retinitis, thrombocytopenia, and purpura.

- Disease in immunocompromised patients may be caused by acute, newly acquired infection or by reactivation of latent infection. CMV disease may cause life-threatening systemic or organ-specific disease. Primary infection poses the greatest risk for severe disease in immunocompromised patients, but there is also significant risk associated with CMV reactivation, especially in bone marrow transplant patients. Fever is a constant feature of disease. Other disease manifestations include CNS disease (encephalitis, polyradiculopathy), GI infection (colitis, esophagitis), hepatitis, myelosuppression/thrombocytopenia, pneumonitis, and retinitis.

- Transmission of CMV by blood transfusion and organ transplantation is well described.

❏ **Laboratory Findings**

Culture: Routine viral culture provides strong evidence for viral replication in vivo and can be performed on a variety of specimen types. Cell cultures, however, may take up to 3-week incubation to provide final results. The shell vial technique, with early staining for proteins produced early in the CMV replicative phase using tagged monoclonal antibodies, markedly decreases turnaround time (48–72 hours) while maintaining good sensitivity. Within the first 2 weeks, viral culture of urine is the most sensitive and specific means for diagnosis of congenital CMV infection. Viral cultures of CSF are usually negative in CNS infections.

Antigenemia: Tagged monoclonal antibodies may be used to detect CMV antigens associated with active replication. The CMV pp65 antigenemia assay can be used to detect active CMV replication associated with emerging or active disease in transplant patients with good sensitivity and specificity.

Molecular diagnostics: Viral load testing has provided the most important indicator for the presence (or emergence) of active infection in immunocompromised patients. The viral load is directly proportional to the potential severity of disease. Low viral loads must be interpreted with caution because they may represent transient dysregulation of latent infection rather than progressive, active replication.

Histopathology: Histopathologic examination demonstrates characteristic changes, including intranuclear and intracytoplasmic inclusions. Specimens may be stained using H&E, other nonspecific stain, or with specific immunologic or nucleic acid reagents.

Serology: May be used to diagnose acute infection or to document immune status.

Core laboratory: Laboratory findings due to predisposing or underlying conditions are seen. Characteristic laboratory changes are seen with infection of the liver, kidney, or adrenal gland.

ENCEPHALITIS VIRUSES

See Chapter 4, Central Nervous System Disorders, for a discussion of encephalitis and causal viral pathogens.

ENTEROVIRUS, COXSACKIEVIRUS, AND ECHOVIRUS

❏ Definition

Coxsackieviruses and echoviruses are species in the genus *Enterovirus*, family *Picornaviridae*. Enteroviruses show broad serologic diversity. Enteroviruses are very stable in the environment, allowing them to survive for long periods in water and sewage. Humans are the only natural host for enteroviral infections. As the name implies, enteroviruses initiate infection in the intestines. Infection is usually acquired by fecal–oral transmission. Infections occur worldwide.

❏ Who Should Be Suspected?

Children are most frequently infected, although enterovirus infections occur in all ages. The humoral immune response seems to be most important for control of enteroviral infections; agammaglobulinemic patients are at risk for more severe or chronic disease. Common clinically significant disease syndromes include myocarditis disease, myalgia, pleurodynia, neonatal infection, aseptic meningitis, conjunctivitis, hand-foot-mouth disease, herpangina, and upper and lower respiratory tract infections.

❏ Laboratory Findings

Most enteroviral infections are mild and self-limited and may be diagnosed without specific laboratory testing. For severe disease, possible diagnostic tests include the following:

Viral culture: Isolation of virus in culture has been the traditional method for specific diagnosis of enteroviral infection. Growth of specific enteroviruses is variable in different cell lines, and the pattern of growth in culture may provide preliminary presumptive identification for a specific group. Some group A coxsackieviruses do not grow in cell culture. Isolation of an *Enterovirus* species from CSF establishes a diagnosis of enteroviral meningitis. Although isolation of enteroviruses from stool or the nasopharynx is commonly seen in patients with severe enteroviral disease, like meningitis, positive cultures from these sites must be interpreted with caution: transient "colonization" may be seen unrelated to the clinical syndrome for which the specimen was collected.

Molecular diagnostic tests: A number of commercially available diagnostic tests have been shown to provide very sensitive and specific detection of enteroviral infections. NAATs have proven to be especially useful to diagnose aseptic meningitis and help rule out bacterial meningitis in children presenting with fever and meningeal signs in summertime.

Serology: Not useful for diagnosis.

Typical core laboratory: CBC and WBC counts are typically normal or show only mild, nonspecific abnormalities.

CSF findings: Enteroviral meningitis shows moderate pleocytosis (<1,000 mononuclear cells; may see PMN predominance early), normal or slightly reduced glucose, normal or slightly increased protein.

EPSTEIN-BARR VIRUS INFECTIONS

❏ Definition

Epstein-Barr virus (EBV) is a lymphocryptovirus in the *Herpesviridae* family. EBV infections are widespread and occur worldwide. In developing regions, primary EBV infections usually occur in younger children. In developed countries, primary infections usually occur in adolescents and young adults. The rate of seropositivity is high (>90%) by middle age. Infections are primarily transmitted by oropharyngeal secretions. After exposure, oropharyngeal epithelial cells and tonsillar B lymphocytes are thought to be the first cells infected. Infection is spread to lymphoid cells throughout the body by memory B cells.

❏ Who Should Be Suspected?

Most primary EBV infections are asymptomatic, but EBV infection may cause a variety of mild to severe diseases:

- *Acute infectious mononucleosis (AIM)*: AIM is the most common manifestation of primary EBV infection, usually occurring in adolescents. Patients commonly present with fever, pharyngitis, posterior lymphadenopathy, and lethargy. Headache and malaise are also common, and rash, anorexia, nausea, and other nonspecific "viral" symptoms occur less frequently. A palpable spleen may be present in a significant proportion of patients, and splenic rupture, although uncommon, is a serious potential complication of AIM. The development of a morbilliform rash following amoxicillin or ampicillin treatment is highly suggestive of EBV AIM in patients with febrile pharyngitis syndromes.

  Acute symptoms usually resolve within 2 weeks, but fatigue may persist for months. Note that mononucleosis syndromes are not agent specific for EBV. Heterophile-negative mononucleosis syndrome may be found in other infectious diseases, especially CMV, toxoplasmosis, and HSV. Atypical lymphocytes may be seen in other acute illnesses (e.g., rubella, roseola, mumps, acute viral hepatitis, acute HIV, drug reactions).

- *Nasopharyngeal carcinoma*: EBV DNA is consistently detected in nasopharyngeal carcinoma cells.
- *Lymphoproliferative diseases*: EBV infection is associated with a number of lymphoproliferative diseases, including:
  - ▼ *Burkitt lymphoma*: EBV has been implicated as a cause of endemic Burkitt lymphoma in equatorial Africa. EBV is seen less frequently in sporadic cases outside of endemic areas.
  - ▼ *Hodgkin disease*: EBV DNA may be detected in malignant cells of Hodgkin disease. The frequency of detection varies in different geographic regions but is almost universal in Hodgkin disease associated with AIDS.
  - ▼ *Lymphomas associated with HIV infection*: The incidence of non-Hodgkin lymphoma is markedly increased compared to nonimmunocompromised patients, and EBV is associated with a majority of these malignancies. Most EBV-related non-Hodgkin lymphomas in HIV-infected patients present in the CNS.
  - ▼ *Posttransplant lymphoproliferative disease (PTLD)*: The severity of PTLD after allograft transplantation may range from benign B-cell proliferation

to aggressive B-cell lymphoma. The severity of disease is related to the degree of immunosuppression. Fever, pharyngitis, and nonspecific symptoms may occur during the development of PTLD.

▼ *X-linked lymphoproliferative syndrome (XLP)*: XLP, manifested by a severe or fatal mononucleosis or immunodeficiency syndrome, is essentially a selective defect in immunity to EBV infection. Mutation in the gene implicated in XLP, *SH2D1A*, results in defective activation–induced cell death in CD8 T lymphocytes, with subsequent uncontrolled proliferation.

❑ Laboratory Findings

Histopathology: The use of EBV-specific immunohistochemical staining to detect EBV proteins may provide improved sensitivity and specificity for establishing EBV as the specific cause of disease when the etiology of the syndrome is broad.

Serology:

- AIM is diagnosed by detection of heterophile antibodies (Paul-Bunnell test), which provide moderate to good sensitivity and high specificity for detection of AIM during the acute, symptomatic phase of disease. This "spot" test has an overall sensitivity ≤92% and specificity >96%, except in children <4 years old, where the slide test is less sensitive. Heterophile agglutination is positive in 60% of young adults by 2 weeks and 90% by 4 weeks after onset of clinical infectious mononucleosis (therefore, they may be negative when hematologic and clinical findings are present). Low titers may persist for a year. False-positive slide tests may occur in leukemia, malignant lymphoma, malaria, rubella, hepatitis, and pancreatic carcinoma, and they may be present for years in some persons with no known explanation. In adults, false positive results in approximately 2% of patients and false negative results in approximately 5%.

- Specific EBV antibody tests: Specific tests are rarely required; most patients are heterophile antibody positive, and clinical illness is usually self-limited and relatively mild. Specific tests may be useful, however, in atypical mononucleosis syndromes or for very severe cases, especially in young children or immunocompromised patients. See Epstein-Barr Virus (EBV) Serology Screen Antibody Profile in Chapter 17, Infectious Disease Assays.

- Anti-EA-R is high and correlated with tumor burden in Burkitt lymphoma. Anti-EA-D is high and correlated with tumor burden in nasopharyngeal carcinoma.

Nucleic acid–based testing: Qualitative or quantitative PCR may be valuable for diagnosis or disease management in EBV-associated diseases.

Core laboratory:

- In AIM, hematologic findings of absolute (>4,500/μL) and relative lymphocytosis (≥50%) in 70% of cases, with ≥10% (often ≤70%) characteristic atypical lymphocytes. Leukopenia and granulocytopenia are evident during the first week. Later, WBC is increased (usually 10,000–20,000/μL) because of increased lymphocytes; peak changes occur in 7–10 days; may persist for 1–2 months. Increased number of bands and >5% eosinophilia are frequent. Mild thrombocytopenia is seen in about 50% of early cases, and platelet dysfunction is frequent. Hemolytic anemia is rare.

- Evidence of mild hepatitis (e.g., increased serum transaminases, increased urine urobilinogen) is very frequent but may be transient. Increased serum bilirubin in ≤30% of adults and <9% of children. Bilirubin/enzyme dissociation (serum bilirubin normal or <2 mg/dL with moderate increase of ALP, GGT, AST, ALT) occurs in 75% of cases. If no liver function abnormalities can be found, another diagnosis should be sought.
- T-cell response: AIM is associated with an oligoclonal expansion of CD8+ T lymphocytes.

HEPATITIS VIRUSES

See Chapter 5, Digestive Diseases.

HERPES SIMPLEX VIRUS INFECTIONS

❏ Definition
Herpes simplex viruses (HSV) are members of the family *Herpesviridae*, subfamily *Alphaherpesvirinae*. Humans serve as the normal reservoir for HSV infections, and HSV disease has a global distribution. The viruses are transmitted by close personal contact. There is no evidence for epidemics of HSV, although clusters of infections may occur. There is no clear seasonal pattern in the incidence of HSV disease. Genital infections are most commonly caused by HSV-2; genital infections caused by HSV-1 tend to be milder and associated with a lower rate of recurrence.

❏ Who Should Be Suspected?
HSV infection is associated with a number of syndromes, including:

- *Primary oropharyngeal*: HSV disease is usually asymptomatic or associated with mild symptoms. Severe symptoms may occur, including vesicular gingivostomatitis and pharyngitis with lymphadenopathy. Nonspecific symptoms are common, including fever and malaise. Adolescents and adults may present with a mononucleosis syndrome. Specific antibodies are usually detectable within the first week following onset of infection, but virus may continue to shed for several weeks. Outbreaks of recurrent lesions, usually at the vermilion border of the lip, are usually preceded by pain, itching, or other symptoms. Lesions usually crust over within 4–5 days.
- *Primary genital*: Disease is manifested as a papulovesicular eruption of the genital mucosa and surrounding skin. Primary infections are usually associated with painful lesions and systemic symptoms, including fever, headache, and malaise. Patients may complain of dysuria, and inguinal lymphadenopathy may be evident. Neurologic symptoms, including aseptic meningitis, sacral radiculopathy, and neuralgias, are not uncommon. Vesicles may persist for 3 weeks in primary infection but usually resolve within 1 week in recurrent outbreaks. Primary infections are associated with more lesions and a higher virus burden compared to recurrent disease. Genital or oropharyngeal HSV infection in pregnant women is of particular importance; it may result in disseminated disease in the mother, leading to complications including necrotizing hepatitis, meningoencephalitis, and coagulopathy. Genital HSV

infection in pregnant women is also a primary risk factor for neonatal HSV infection in the offspring.

- *Neonatal*: Disease may occur at any time between birth and 4 weeks of age. Most neonatal HSV infections are acquired from infected maternal genital secretions during labor and delivery. A number of factors increase the risk of transmission and severity of neonatal disease: Primary maternal infection at or near the time of labor and delivery, maternal seronegativity for the infecting type of HSV, prolonged (>6 hours) rupture of fetal membranes prior to delivery, and/or the use of fetal scalp monitor. There are three common presentations of neonatal disease: (a) disseminated disease of multiple organ systems; (b) localized CNS disease; and (c) localized infection of the skin, eyes, and mouth. Early intrauterine infection may rarely be seen, presenting with vesicles or scarring of skin, various ocular abnormalities, and CNS abnormalities, including microcephaly and hydranencephaly.
- *HSV keratoconjunctivitis*: Manifested by photophobia, tearing, chemosis, lid edema, and preauricular lymphadenopathy. Visual acuity may be decreased. Slit-lamp examination typically shows characteristic branching dendritic lesions.
- *Skin*: Infections occur most commonly in patients with eczema. Outbreaks may be localized or disseminated (Kaposi varicella-like eruption). Infection localized to the digits (herpetic whitlow) is associated with direct inoculation of virus, often acquired by health care manipulation.
- *CNS*: HSV is the most common cause of severe sporadic encephalitis. Patients typically present with focal encephalitis and neurologic abnormalities related to the region of brain affected. Patients also typically present with other symptoms, including fever, behavior changes, and decreased level of consciousness.

❏ Laboratory Findings

Cell culture: HSV may be isolated by viral culture of vesicles, ulcers, or infected tissues. Culture of specimens from lesions of recurrent disease is much less sensitive. Positive viral cultures for HSV must be interpreted in the context of clinical presentation because HSV may rarely be shed in chronic infection in the absence of overt clinical disease.

Histology: Direct cytologic examination of scrapings of lesions (Wright-Giemsa stain) shows multinucleated giant cells with intranuclear inclusions (Tzanck smear). Skin vesicles produce a positive smear in 66% and positive viral culture in 100% of cases; pustules produce a positive smear in 50% and a positive viral culture in 70% of cases; crusted ulcers produce a positive smear in 15% and a positive viral culture in 34% of cases. Multinucleated cells may also be identified in routine Pap smear of cervix. A negative direct test does not rule out this diagnosis.

Molecular diagnosis: NAAT techniques may be used for detection of HSV DNA in tissue, CSF, and other specimen types. PCR is the diagnostic test of choice if CNS infection is suspected, with sensitivity and specificity >95%.

Serology: Serologic testing is of limited value for the management of acute infection but may be useful in assessing past infection or a patient's risk for infection. Immunoblot IgG has sensitivity >80% and specificity of 95%. See Herpes Simplex Virus (HSV) Serology Tests, Type 1– and Type 2–Specific Antibodies, IgG and IgM in Chapter 17, Infectious Disease Assays.

Core laboratory: In patients with HSV encephalitis, CSF shows increased WBC count with mononuclear cell predominance; RBC count is usually increased. CSF protein is increased.

HIV-1 INFECTION AND ACQUIRED IMMUNODEFICIENCY SYNDROME

❏ Definition

- Human immunodeficiency virus (HIV) infection is the cause of acquired immunodeficiency syndrome (AIDS), as well as symptomatic disease prior to the development of AIDS. HIV infection now has a global distribution, and most disease is caused by HIV-1. HIV-2 infection is more geographically restricted, primarily occurring in western Africa.

- HIV-1 viruses fall into three genetic groups: M, O, and N. Group M viruses, which can be further subdivided into clades (A–D, F–H, J, and K), are the predominant viruses responsible for the global epidemic. In the United States, Europe, and Australia, the B clade predominates. Other clades may be predominant in other geographic locations. HIV-2 is genetically distinct. This discussion will focus on disease caused by HIV-1.

- HIV transmission is due to direct contact with infected body fluids, primarily blood, semen, vaginal and cervical secretions, breast milk, and amniotic fluid. This contact is usually mediated by sexual contact, IV drug abuse, blood exposure (transfusion, transplantation, needlestick injury), and vertical transmission (pregnancy, childbirth, and nursing). The relative contribution of these modes shows regional variability. The risk of transmission depends on a number of factors, including viral load in infected fluid, presence of other STDs, sexual history, having an infected partner who is uncircumcised, and genetic factors.

- HIV is able to infect cells that express CD4 on their surfaces, primarily CD4$^+$ T lymphocytes and macrophages.

❏ Who Should Be Suspected?

HIV-1 infection may be divided into three clinical phases:

- *Acute phase*: During the acute phase, which usually occurs between 1 and 4 weeks after exposure, there is viremia with infection of cells throughout the body. The HIV-1 plasma viral load is markedly elevated, typically >10^6 copies/mL. The level of CD4$^+$ T lymphocytes is reduced, due to destruction and sequestration.
  - ▼ Thirty to seventy percent of patients develop nonspecific symptoms. A mononucleosis-type syndrome is common. Symptoms include headache, fever, malaise, pharyngitis, myalgias, and arthralgias. A nonpruritic macular rash commonly develops on the face and trunk. Generalized lymphadenopathy is common. Other symptoms include ulcerations of skin and mucous membranes, nausea, vomiting, and diarrhea. Neurologic symptoms, including aseptic meningoencephalitis and neuropathy, may develop.
  - ▼ Symptoms typically resolve within 4 weeks.

- *Asymptomatic or minimally symptomatic phase*: The acute phase is followed by a phase, typically prolonged, where the patient is not severely immuno-compromised and symptoms may be absent or mild. During this time, there is continued viral replication and CD4+ T-lymphocyte depletion. The rate of loss of CD4 cells is related to the HIV-1 viral load.
  - ▼ During this phase, fatigue and lymphadenopathy may be seen. Other manifestations may include bacillary angiomatosis, cervical dysplasia or carcinoma in situ, chronic diarrhea, oral leukoplakia, progressive fatigue, progressive weight loss, night sweats, recurrent shingles or zoster in multiple dermatomes, and/or vaginal or oral candidiasis.
  - ▼ This second phase of infection usually lasts for 8–10 years before progression to AIDS.
- *AIDS/symptomatic phase*: The relentless depletion of CD4 cells eventually results in profound immunosuppression and the clinical manifestations of AIDS. A specific diagnosis of AIDS is based on laboratory findings and the presence of AIDS-defining infections or malignancies, including candidiasis, cervical cancer, recurrent infections, coccidiomycosis, cryptococcosis, cryptosporidiosis, encephalopathy, histoplasmosis, Kaposi sarcoma, lymphoma, *Mycobacterium tuberculosis* infection, progressive multifocal leukoencephalopathy, *Pneumocystis* pneumonia, CNS toxoplasmosis, and wasting syndrome (unintentional loss of >10% of body weight).

❏ Diagnosis and Staging

The CDC and WHO have established diagnostic criteria for HIV infection status and AIDS diagnosis to be used for surveillance criteria. See: http://www.cdc.gov/hiv/pdf/research_mmp_MRA_MHF_2012_v710.pdf. Testing for diagnosis of HIV infection: See Human Immunodeficiency Virus 1,2 Antibody Screen and Human Immunodeficiency Virus (HIV-1) Confirmatory Western Blot Assay in Chapter 17, Infectious Disease Assays. CDC criteria for staging of HIV-1 infected patients. See: http://www.cdc.gov/mmwr/preview/mmwrhtml/rr5710a1.htm

- Stage 1: No AIDS-defining illness and either CD4+ T lymphocytes ≥500 cells/μL or CD4+ T-lymphocyte percentage of total lymphocytes >29.
- Stage 2: No AIDS-defining illness and either CD4+ T lymphocytes 200–499 cells/μL or CD4+ T-lymphocyte percentage of total lymphocytes 14–28.
- Stage 3 (AIDS): CD4+ T lymphocytes <200 cells/μL or CD4+ T-lymphocyte percentage of total lymphocytes <14 or documentation of an AIDS-defining condition (http://www.cdc.gov/mmwr/preview/mmwrhtml/rr5710a2.htm) regardless of CD4+ T-lymphocyte level or percentage of total lymphocytes.
- In 2012, a revision of the CDC case definition, including a stage 0 for patients with recent diagnosis, was recommended but not implemented. See http://www.cdc.gov/hiv/pdf/statistics_HIV_Case_Def_Consult_Summary.pdf

❏ Laboratory Findings

Serology: Most HIV-1–infected patients are diagnosed by HIV serology. Virtually all infected patients develop antibodies to HIV-1 antigens, and final diagnosis of HIV-1 should be based on detection of antibodies. Fourth-generation assays are able to detect both HIV antigen (p24) and antibody (HIV-1 group M, HIV-1 group O, and HIV-2) formation 14 days after infection, significantly earlier than second- and third-generation assays. Most patients become positive for HIV-1 antibody testing within 1–2 months after infectious exposure; >95% of patients are seropositive within 6 months. Note that seropositivity for HIV-1 does not imply immunity.

- The specificity of HIV-1 EIA assays is very high, but when they are used to screen low-prevalence populations, the PPV may be <80%. Therefore, positive EIA assays should be confirmed with a second highly specific assay, such as a WB assay using standardized interpretive criteria. Using a combination of diagnostic tests, false-positive test results can be almost completely eliminated.

- Patients with repeatedly reactive HIV EIA tests, but negative or equivocal WB, should have repeat WB testing after 4–6 weeks. Testing for HIV-1 RNA, proviral DNA, or p24 antigen may be informative. If unresolved, infection with HIV-2 or uncommon HIV-1 subtypes (O or N) might be considered.

Testing to monitor disease and therapy:

- See Human Immunodeficiency Virus Type 1 (HIV-1) RNA, Quantitative Viral Load (Molecular Assay) in Chapter 17, Infectious Disease Assays.

- Patients diagnosed with HIV-1 infection should be initially tested and subsequently monitored with HIV-1 viral load and CD4$^+$ T-lymphocyte cell count or fraction of total lymphocytes. Viral load testing is recommended just before and then at 8–12 weeks following initiation of antiretroviral treatment. A two-$\log_{10}$ decrease in viral load is expected within 8 weeks. The viral load should fall below the detection level of the viral load assay within 6 months. Successful therapy is also associated with an increase in the number, or fraction, of CD4$^+$ T lymphocytes. The rate of fall of viral load and recovery of CD4 T lymphocytes is slower in patients after changes in treatment due to therapeutic failure.

- Successful antiretroviral therapy should result in a new viral load baseline, ideally at an undetectable level. Changes in viral load from the baseline should be interpreted with caution. Small changes, up to 0.3–0.4 $\log_{10}$ copies/mL, may be seen as a result of variability of immunologic control of viral replication or to false-positive results at viral loads near the lower level of detection. These results should be repeated and interpreted with CD4 cell levels and clinical findings. Viral load changes >0.5–0.7 $\log_{10}$ copies/mL are more predictive of treatment failure and worsening disease.

Antiviral drug resistance testing:

- See Human Immunodeficiency Virus Type 1 (HIV-1) Genotype (Molecular Assay) in Chapter 17, Infectious Disease Assays.

- Numerous studies have demonstrated improved patient outcome when therapy is guided by results of antiviral resistance testing, especially for initial treatment in areas with a high circulation of resistant viruses and for patients who fail a therapeutic regimen. HIV-1 reverse transcriptase, protease inhibitors, and substrate analogs are the most common types of antiviral agents used for treatment of HIV-1 infection and are most commonly reported in antiviral drug resistance testing. Development of drugs targeting other essential steps in HIV-1 infection, like fusion and integrase functions, as well as relevant resistance testing, is ongoing.

- Resistance to antiviral agents can be determined by phenotypic or genotypic methods. Both methods require the amplification of informative sequences from HIV-1 RNA isolated from the patient plasma.
  - ▼ In genotypic assays, mutations in genes whose products are the targets of specific antiviral agents are detected. Most commonly, these mutations are detected by sequencing amplicons. Resistance interpretations for specific drugs or drug classes are maintained in frequently updated databases.
  - ▼ For phenotypic assays, the target sequences of a "reagent" HIV-1 virus are replaced by the genes amplified from HIV-1 RNA from the patient's plasma. The recombinant virus is used to infect cell cultures in the presence of different antiviral agents, with results interpreted on the basis of the drug's ability, or not, to prevent infection of the cell line. An advantage of phenotypic assays is that they do not depend on knowledge of specific mutations for interpretation of drug efficacy and they are efficient in detecting how multiple mutations in the patient's HIV-1 RNA interact in terms of inhibiting or enhancing the activity of an antiviral agent.
  - ▼ Both methods are limited in their ability to yield results when the patient's viral load is low (<1,000 copies/mL), primarily due to technical limitations of the laboratory processing. Resistant "quasispecies" may emerge due to selective pressure during antiviral therapy. Neither genotypic nor phenotypic assays are efficient in detecting relevant resistance in these quasispecies until they contribute more than approximately 30% of the HIV-1 RNA in the patient's plasma.

❑ Diagnostic Challenges

HIV viral load tests have a low rate of false-positive results, virtually all with levels <10,000 copies/mL. If viral load testing is performed in patients who are negative by HIV antibody testing (e.g., to evaluate possible infection during the "window phase" or for patients with positive HIV antigen in a fourth-generation screening test, but negative WB), positive results must be confirmed by subsequent antibody testing before an unequivocal diagnosis is established.

Placental transfer of HIV-1 IgG from an infected mother to her fetus complicates the diagnosis of HIV infection in the infant after delivery. In infants at risk for HIV-1 infection, viral culture or molecular diagnostic tests are recommended for diagnosis. Sequential testing at 48 hours after birth, at age 1–2 months, and at 3–6 months has been recommended. Testing for plasma HIV-1 RNA is reported to provide the greatest sensitivity for HIV-1 infection in the neonate. Positive results must be confirmed with subsequent testing. Detection of p24 antigen may be an alternative to HIV culture or molecular diagnostic testing, especially in areas where this testing is not immediately available, although this test is less sensitive and less specific compared to the other virologic assays. An ultrasensitive method for p24 antigen detection using dried blood spots has been described (see Knuchel et al. in Suggested Readings). Infants with negative virologic studies should be assessed serologically. Two negative HIV-1 serology tests, performed at least 1 month apart after 6 months of age, essentially excludes a diagnosis of HIV-1 infection in the infant. Specific testing may be needed for diagnosis of HIV-2 and non–M HIV-1 infections.

❑ **Other Considerations**

■ Greater severity and persistence of symptoms during primary infection and severe depression of CD4+ T lymphocytes beyond 2–3 months are associated more rapid progression to severe immunosuppression and AIDS.

■ The HIV-1 viral load at baseline is the best predictor of severity and progression early in disease; the CD4+ T-lymphocyte count is the best predictor of progression in late disease.

■ The risk of progression to AIDS is related to the baseline HIV-1 viral load after seroconversion. Plasma viral load >100,000 copies/mL at 6 months after seroconversion are associated with a 10-fold greater risk of progression to AIDS within 5 years, compared to patients with lower baseline levels.

■ Although the results of HIV-1 viral load assays are correlated, there may be proportional differences in the results from laboratories performing testing using different platforms. It is recommended that viral load testing to monitor patients be performed in the same laboratory using the same platform. If the testing platform is changed, unexpected changes in viral load must be interpreted with caution. It may be important to "rebaseline" the patient with sequential testing on the new platform.

■ Patients with HIV infection are at high risk for coexisting infections. Patients should be carefully evaluated to rule out the following infections: hepatitis B, hepatitis C, CMV, *Toxoplasma gondii*, syphilis, and TB.

HUMAN PAPILLOMAVIRUS (HPV) INFECTION

❑ **Definition**

Papillomaviruses are nonenveloped DNA viruses that cause a spectrum of diseases of epithelial tissues, ranging in severity from benign plantar warts to genital tract cancers. The papillomaviruses are widespread in vertebrate hosts, but individual viruses are narrowly species specific. HPVs have a supercoiled, nonsegmented circular double-stranded DNA genome. They are classified by genotype, with different genotypes associated with different clinical diseases (Table 11-1).

TABLE 11–1. Disease Associations of Specific Human Papillomavirus (HPV) Genotypes

Lesion	Common HPV Type
Common warts	1, 2, 4
Plantar warts	1, 2
Flat warts	3, 10
Butcher warts	2, 7
Epidermodysplasia	5, 8, 9, 12, 14,15, 17
Respiratory, recurrent papillomas	6, 11
Genital warts, low risk	6, 11, 26, 42, 43, 44, 53, 54, 55, 62, 66
Genital warts, moderate risk	33, 35, 39, 51, 52, 56, 58, 59, 68
Genital warts, high risk	16, 18, 31, 45

❏ Who Should Be Suspected?

Three types of warts are most common: common warts, plantar warts, and flat warts.

- Common warts often occur in groups and are round, hyperkeratotic papules that usually occur on the dorsum of the hand or on the fingers. Common warts are painless.
- Plantar warts are usually solitary and occur on the weight-bearing locations of the foot. Plantar warts are circular and commonly show a keratotic ring surrounding a roughened, dark-speckled center. They are deep-set and usually painful.
- Flat warts usually occur as multiple, painless smooth papules on the face or hands. Immunocompromised patients are at increased risk for the occurrence and severity of cutaneous warts. In immunocompetent patients, cutaneous warts typically resolve spontaneously.

Papillomavirus infections of squamous epithelial tissues of the anogenital tract are responsible for genital warts and carcinomas. These infections are primarily sexually transmitted, and the risk of infection is most strongly related to the patient's life-time number of sexual partners and history of other STIs. Most infections are acquired in the teens and early 20s.

- Condylomata acuminata are multiple hyperkeratotic papules that commonly develop irregular surfaces. Groups of venereal warts may coalesce to form cobblestone patches. Warts may occur at any genital site, including the distal urethra. In males, lesions usually appear on the shaft of the penis. In women, most warts occur at the posterior introitus. Warts may also occur in anal and perianal surfaces. Genital warts are usually asymptomatic, but patients may complain of itch or burning pain.
- Anogenital papillomavirus infections are associated with malignant transformation. Globally, HPV-16 and HPV-18 are the genotypes most strongly associated with invasive cervical carcinoma, but there is variability in the genotypes less frequently associated with cervical cancer in different geographic regions.

❏ Laboratory Findings

Most cutaneous warts are diagnosed clinically, and specific laboratory confirmation is not required. The diagnosis of papillomavirus infections at anogenital and other sites can often be made clinically, but specific diagnostic testing may be warranted.

Culture: Isolation of HPV by viral culture is not available.

Serology: Not useful for diagnosis of HPV infection.

Cytologic or histologic examination: These techniques can be considered "gold standard" for confirmation of HPV disease; however, they do not provide HPV type determination.

NAAT assays: Most sensitive detection of HPV infection and may provide information about the genotype (or risk category) of the infecting virus if type-specific primers are used. See Human Papillomavirus (HPV) Molecular Testing in Chapter 17, Infectious Disease Assays.

MUMPS

❏ Definition

Mumps is usually a mild, self-limited viral infection caused by mumps virus. The virus is highly contagious and transmitted by respiratory droplets. Humans are the only natural reservoir, and children, especially in the pre–vaccination era, were the primary targets of infection. The incidence of mumps dropped >99% since the introduction of live vaccine in 1967, but recent outbreaks have occurred in the United States.

❏ Who Should Be Suspected?

- After exposure, there is a 1- to 2-week incubation period followed by onset of prodromal symptoms. Prodromal symptoms are nonspecific, including fever, malaise, myalgias, anorexia, and headache. Ninety-five percent of patients develop the characteristic swelling and tenderness of the parotid glands. Parotid swelling may last for 7–10 days. Subtle disease may develop in a minority of patients, usually adults, consisting of predominantly respiratory symptoms. Virus shedding and secondary transmission begin during the prodromal period and peak in the days before the onset of parotitis.
- Mumps is associated with several common complications.
  - ▼ Up to 10% of patients develop symptomatic aseptic meningitis with typical symptoms of headache, mild nuchal rigidity, and low-grade fever.
    - CSF profile typically shows pleocytosis with lymphocyte predominance, normal or slightly elevated protein, and normal or slightly decreased glucose. Full recovery without sequelae is the rule. Less than 0.1% of patients develop mumps encephalitis, with fever and altered levels of consciousness, seizure, paralysis, ataxia, or other CNS abnormalities. Parotitis may be absent in 20–60% of patients. The peripheral WBC count is usually normal. A mild CSF mononuclear pleocytosis is typical (average 250 cells/mL); protein is usually normal or slightly elevated ($\leq$100 mg/dL); glucose concentration is usually normal but is decreased in $\leq$29% of cases.
    - Simultaneous serum and CSF specimens show increased mumps IgG antibody index (in 83% of patients) and mumps IgM antibody index (in approximately 67% of patients with IgM in CSF). Oligoclonal Ig in CSF is detected in 90% of cases. Virus can be isolated from CSF by culture. PCR has been reported to provide more rapid and sensitive diagnosis compared to culture. Recovery is usually complete.
  - ▼ Sensorineural deafness, with occasional vestibular symptoms, is a well-documented complication of mumps.
  - ▼ Orchitis, manifested by high fever and severe testicular pain with testicular and scrotal swelling, occurs in 30–40% of postpubertal males with mumps infection. Symptoms typically occur approximately 10 days after onset of parotitis. There may be unilateral or bilateral involvement. WBC count and ESR are typically elevated. Full sterility is rare following mumps orchitis, but impaired fertility may be seen in a minority of patients. Oophoritis occurs in 5–10% of postpubertal females.
  - ▼ Other uncommon complications of mumps include arthritis, pancreatitis, and myocarditis. Mumps infection in pregnant women is not associated with congenital anomalies.

❏ Laboratory Findings

Viral culture: Mumps virus may be isolated from saliva, urine, or CSF early in acute disease. Viral culture is usually used for complicated infection or when a virus isolate is needed, as for epidemiologic investigation.

Serology: Mumps is confirmed by a positive mumps-specific IgM result or a significant change in mumps-specific IgG titer in acute and convalescent (2–4 weeks after acute onset) serum samples. IgM usually peaks at approximately day 7 of acute disease and persists for 6 weeks or longer. IgM response may be blunted in previously immunized patients and a negative result does not exclude mumps infection in this population. Detectable IgG levels usually peak at 2–4 weeks and persist for years. See Mumps Serology Screen (Mumps IgG and IgM) in Chapter 17, Infectious Disease Assays.

Molecular diagnosis: Real-time PCR for specific mumps sequences has been shown to improve detection of mumps encephalitis.

Core laboratory: WBC and ESR are normal in acute infection. There may be a slight relative lymphocytosis. Serum and urine amylase are increased during the first week of parotitis; therefore, increase does not always indicate pancreatitis. Serum lipase is normal.

NOROVIRUS GASTROENTERITIS (NORWALK AGENT)

❑ Definition

Novovirus has been identified as the major cause of epidemic and endemic gastro-enteritis. The Norwalk agent was discovered by immune EM of stool in patients with diarrhea. These viruses have subsequently been classified by molecular techniques as a member of the family *Caliciviridae*. The virus is nonenveloped with a single positive-strand RNA genome. Genetic and immunologic diversity in clinical isolates is significant. Humans are thought to be the only host for *Norovirus*. Infections occur globally and affect individuals of all ages.

❑ Who Should Be Suspected?

Disease outbreaks have been associated with a wide variety of exposures, including day care centers, long-term care facilities, cruise ships, and restaurants. Persons living in high-density conditions are at high risk. Clinical disease usually presents with abrupt onset of vomiting and/or diarrhea 10 hours to 2 days after exposure. Abdominal cramping is common. Patients often have nonspecific symptoms, including low-grade fever, headache, myalgias, and fatigue. Disease is self-limited in most patients, spontaneously resolving after several days. Prolonged symptomatic and more severe disease may be seen in young children, the elderly, and immunocompromised patients.

❑ Laboratory Findings

Because most patients have relatively mild, self-limited disease, they do not require specific diagnostic testing. Diagnostic testing may be necessary for patients with severe diseases or to establish the cause of an outbreak.

Molecular testing: Real-time PCR has emerged as the most widely used assays for diagnosis of *Norovirus* infection. Virus-specific RNA may be detected for several weeks after onset of illness.

Antigen detection assays: Use of antiserum reagents elicited against recombinant viral antigens has been described, but the sensitivity of available assays is relatively poor.

PARVOVIRUS B19 (ERYTHEMA INFECTIOSUM, FIFTH DISEASE, TRANSIENT APLASTIC ANEMIA)

❑ Definition

Parvovirus B19 is a single-strand, nonenveloped DNA virus. It is the cause of the erythematous childhood rash erythema infectiosum (fifth disease). Parvovirus B19 infections occur worldwide, causing endemic and epidemic disease. Humans are the only natural host for the virus, with the bone marrow being the primary target of infection. Serologic surveys demonstrate that infection is common. Infection is usually transmitted by respiratory droplets.

❑ Who Should Be Suspected?

Parvovirus B19 infections occur most commonly in children. The classic presentation involves a confluent, erythematous rash, especially on the cheeks with circumoral pallor (slapped face appearance) with viral syndrome symptoms, like fever, malaise, myalgias, headache, cough, and pharyngitis. Arthralgias develop in some patients. The facial rash fades in several days, followed by formation of a lacy rash affecting the extremities and trunk. Complications of parvovirus B19 infection are uncommon and include hepatitis, myocarditis, and meningoencephalitis. Adults diagnosed with parvovirus B19 infection present more frequently with viral syndrome and arthropathy, and rash is less common. Complications of parvovirus infection during pregnancy include fetal hydrops and congenital anemia; specific IgM is detected in cord blood. Chronic infection may cause severe anemia in immunocompromised persons. Pure erythrocyte aplasia and persistent infection may develop in patients with immunodeficiency or underlying hemolytic anemias, like sickle cell disease, hereditary spherocytosis, pyruvate kinase deficiency, and beta-thalassemia.

❑ Laboratory Findings

Serology: Usual diagnostic method. Specific IgM is formed very early in infection, closely followed by IgG. IgM levels begin to wane after 1–2 months but may be detectable for 6 months after acute infection. IgG antibody typically remains detectable for years.

POLIOMYELITIS

❑ Definition

Poliomyelitis is caused by poliovirus species (types 1–3), in the genus *Enterovirus*. The transmission of polio has been greatly reduced in areas with effective vaccination programs; however, wild-type virus continues to occur sporadically in developing countries. The attenuated virus used in the oral polio vaccine has caused paralytic disease in immunocompromised patients. It is mandated to report paralytic poliomyelitis in all states in the United States. Public health officials should be contacted as soon as paralytic poliomyelitis is suspected. Public health officials may provide guidance regarding confirmatory testing.

❑ Who Should Be Suspected?

- During poliovirus outbreaks, most infected patients remain asymptomatic or have mild, self-limited disease. A minority of patients (<2%), however, develop paralytic poliomyelitis or occasionally meningitis or encephalitis without paralysis. Illness may be preceded by fever, myalgias, and nonspecific "viral" symptoms.

- Poliomyelitis is caused by infection of the anterior horn cells of the spinal cord, resulting in acute flaccid paralysis of associated muscle groups. Spinal poliomyelitis may vary in severity from isolated paresis to paralysis of the limbs, quadriplegia, and paralysis of the diaphragm or other muscle groups. Cranial nerve nuclei may be involved resulting in bulbar poliomyelitis, with paralysis of muscles involved in swallowing or destruction of cells regulating central respiration. Infected patients may develop disease related to both spinal and bulbar poliomyelitis. Cerebral function is typically unaffected.

- Five to ten percent of patients die, usually as a result of respiratory failure. Most children recover; however, a majority are left with residual sequelae ranging in severity from mild motor weakness to complete paralysis.

❏ **Laboratory Findings**
Poliomyelitis may be suspected on the basis of clinical signs and symptoms in appropriate clinical settings.

Culture: The diagnosis is usually confirmed by isolation of virus in culture. Several samples of stool and throat for viral culture, obtained at least 24 hours apart, should be collected early in the course of disease.

Serology of acute and convalescent sera: May be submitted to support a diagnosis of poliomyelitis, but test interpretation may be difficult.

CSF findings: Nonspecific. Cell count is usually 25–500/µL; rarely is normal or markedly elevated. At first, most are PMNs; after several days, most are lymphocytes. Protein may be normal at first, increased by 2nd week (usually 50–200 mg/dL), and normal by 6th week. Glucose is usually normal.

Core laboratory: Blood shows early moderate increase in WBC (≤15,000/µL) and PMNs. WBC returns to normal within 1 week. Increased AST in 50% of patients is caused by the associated hepatitis.

11

RESPIRATORY VIRUSES

See Chapter 13, Respiratory, Metabolic, and Acid–Base Disorders, for a detailed discussion of viral respiratory tract pathogens, including adenovirus, influenza viruses, parainfluenza viruses, and RSV.

RUBELLA (GERMAN MEASLES)

❏ **Definition**
Rubella virus causes German measles, one of the classic viral exanthems of childhood (the "third disease"). The virus primarily infects the respiratory epithelial cells. Infection is transmitted by respiratory droplets. The virus has a global distribution, although endemic virus circulation has been greatly reduced or eliminated in countries with widespread vaccination programs. Humans are the only natural host.

❏ Who Should Be Suspected?

▪ Rubella infection is usually mild and self-limited. Viremia typically occurs after 5–7 days, and clinical infection may ensue around 14 days after exposure with a nonspecific "viral" syndrome, including fever, malaise, mild respiratory symptoms, and lymphadenopathy. The characteristic, nonconfluent rash starts on the face and then progresses to the trunk and extremities. The rash resolves in 3–5 days. Up to 50% of infected children may remain asymptomatic.

▪ The congenital rubella syndrome is caused by transplacental infection of a fetus during the viremic phase of illness. Maternal infection early in gestation is associated with more severe disease (approximately 80% incidence with maternal rubella in the first trimester). Virtually, all fetal organ systems are susceptible to infection, and infection may lead to stillbirth or premature delivery. The most common anomalies include cardiac defects, cataracts and other ocular defects, deafness, bone defects, hepatitis, microcephaly and mental retardation, splenomegaly, and thrombocytopenia. Subacute arthritis is a common (70%) complication of rubella infection in adult women. Fingers, wrists, and knees are the most commonly affected joints, and symptoms may last up to 1 month.

▪ Rubella is preventable by vaccination, with a primary goal of reducing the incidence of the congenital syndrome. Vaccine-induced protection may wane over time; improved vaccines have improved the durability of the immune response. Since 1993, 70% of patients with rubella fall into the 15- to 39-year age group, reflecting this declining immunity. Therefore, significant public health resources have been dedicated to ensuring that adolescents, especially girls, have been immunized.

❏ Laboratory Findings

Culture: Detection of rubella virus in cell culture is slow and technically challenging. There is little CPE in cell lines. Rubella infection can be inferred by interference assays, such as inhibition of enterovirus superinfection of cell lines infected by rubella virus from a specimen. Rubella-specific neutralization or immunostaining techniques are used for confirmation.

Serology: Serologic diagnosis is most commonly used to document rubella infection. See Rubella Serology Screen (Rubella IgG and IgM) in Chapter 17, Infectious Disease Assays.

▪ Infection is confirmed by demonstration of a positive reaction for rubella IgM (acute primary infection) or by change in rubella IgG titers in acute (7–10 days) and convalescent (14–21 days) serum specimens. IgM antibodies are detected and peak within several days after appearance of rash and then rapidly fall below detectable levels after approximately 8 weeks. IgG usually appears around 2 weeks after onset of rash and usually remain detectable, at lower levels, for life.

▪ In congenital infection, IgM can be detected at birth and persists for ≤6 months in >90% of infants. During the first 6 months of life, IgM is the best test for congenital or recent infection. After age 7 months, assess persistence of IgG. IgG appears 15–25 days after infection and >25 to 50 days after vaccination; <33% of persons may show no detectable IgG after 10 years. Absence of IgG in infant excludes congenital infection.

RUBEOLA (MEASLES)

❑ **Definition**

Measles is caused by the measles virus in the family *Paramyxoviridae*, genus *Morbillivirus*. It is a single-stranded RNA virus. The virus is transmitted by respiratory droplets and infects epithelial cells of the respiratory tract of exposed individuals. Measles is highly contagious, and outbreaks are well documented. The disease is preventable by vaccination. Imported infections are transmitted to nonimmune individuals in regions with a low endemic rate.

❑ **Who Should Be Suspected?**

- Clinical disease develops after an incubation period of 10–14 days. In typical measles, the characteristic morbilliform rash appears after 4–5 days of prodromal symptoms, which include cough, coryza, and conjunctivitis, with fever and malaise. Local lymphadenopathy may develop. Koplik spots, the characteristic enanthem, appear on the buccal mucosa 1 day or 2 before the appearance of the rash. The blanching rash first appears behind the ears and forehead and spreads over the trunk and limbs over the ensuing several days. Otitis media, diarrhea, and pneumonitis occur relatively frequently in uncomplicated measles.
- Pregnant women are at risk for more severe measles-associated pneumonia. Although not associated with congenital anomalies, measles may be transmitted to the fetus, and neonates may develop mild to severe clinical infection. Patients with defects of cell-mediated immunity are susceptible to severe measles virus pneumonia and progressive encephalitis demonstrating typical inclusion bodies in neurons and glial cells.
- Neurologic complications are uncommon in patients with normal immunity, but acute postinfectious measles encephalomyelitis and subacute sclerosing panencephalitis (SSPE) are rare complications of measles infections.
  - ▼ Acute postinfectious encephalomyelitis, an autoimmune reaction, usually occurs in the week following onset of rash. Patients present with headache, irritability, and change in mental status progressing to seizures, obtundation, and coma. CSF lymphocytic pleocytosis and protein elevation are seen. Mortality is as high as 20%, and many survivors have neurologic sequelae.
  - ▼ SSPE is a progressive neurologic complication with a high mortality rate. It usually occurs 5–10 years after primary measles. SSPE is more common when primary infection occurred before 2 years of age. The onset is subtle with personality changes, declining intellectual function and loss of coordination, which usually progress relentlessly. Death usually occurs within several years of onset. There are characteristic EEG changes (Rodermacker complexes). CSF analysis shows oligoclonal bands and intrathecal production of antimeasles antibodies.

❑ **Laboratory Findings**

Viral culture: Measles virus can be isolated in cell culture from respiratory, nasopharyngeal, conjunctival, blood, or urine specimens.

Pathology/cytology: Epithelial cells from the respiratory tract, conjunctiva, or urine (early disease), or infected tissues (acute or chronic disease), may be stained to demonstrate multinucleated giant cells with intranuclear and cytoplasmic inclusion bodies.

Serology: Most infections are diagnosed serologically in the setting of typical clinical findings. See Measles Serology Screen (Measles [Rubeola] IgG and IgM) in Chapter 17, Infectious Disease Assay.

- Detection of measles virus–specific IgM or a fourfold or greater rise in measles virus–specific IgG in paired acute and convalescent serum specimens are diagnostic.
- IgG antibody levels develop in the week after onset of rash and usually peak in the first month after appearance of the rash. IgM antibodies can usually be detected in the first week of infection and become undetectable after 2 months.

NAAT assays: May be useful in diagnosis of CNS infection in immunocompromised patients.

SMALLPOX (VARIOLA VIRUS)

❑ Definition

Smallpox is caused by the variola virus. Historically, smallpox is a highly infectious viral infection associated with significant morbidity and mortality. Humans are the primary natural host for variola virus. An aggressive global vaccination effort eliminated naturally occurring smallpox by 1980. Because the complication rate of smallpox vaccination using the vaccinia virus is relatively high, widespread vaccination is no longer practiced, resulting in a presumed return of widespread susceptibility to this disease. Ominously, laboratory-proliferated variola virus could be weaponized, and this virus is one of the most feared potential bioterror agents. Any patient suspected of having smallpox must be immediately isolated and reported to the relevant Department of Health officials. Case evaluation, management, and diagnostic testing will be directed by state and federal agencies.

❑ Who Should Be Suspected?

- Smallpox was usually acquired by inhalation of infectious droplets. Spiking fever, headache, and malaise precede the appearance of rash. The typical rash appears about 10 days after exposure and resolves in 4–5 weeks in survivors. The rash progresses from macules to papules to umbilicated pustules. At 2–3 weeks, the host immune response results in scabbing over of pustules and healing of lesions. Scarring, especially on the face, is common in survivors.
- Smallpox is differentiated from chickenpox by the increased toxicity of patients and the pattern of rash. In smallpox, skin lesions appear simultaneously and are more prominent on the face and distal extremities. A rare hemorrhagic form of smallpox was described, most commonly in pregnant women, with a petechial rash, hemorrhage, severe toxicity, and high mortality. Previously vaccinated patients with waning immunity have developed mild disease with few skin lesions that resolved rapidly.

VARICELLA-ZOSTER VIRUS INFECTIONS

❑ Definition

Varicella-zoster virus (VZV) is the agent responsible for varicella (chickenpox) and zoster (shingles). Chickenpox is the common manifestation of VZV infection, whereas zoster represents a reactivation of latent VZV. VZV may also cause disseminated infection in immunocompromised patients as well as neonatal infections. VZV is a member of the family *Herpesviridae*. There is only one serotype of VZV; all clinical isolates are antigenically related. VZV infections occur worldwide, and most adults in temperate climates have serologic evidence of prior infection even those with no history of chickenpox. Historically, the incidence of chickenpox has been highest in children. Widespread use of varicella vaccine, however, has had an impact on the normal epidemiology with an increasing number of primary infections occurring in young adults.

❏ Who Should Be Suspected?

- Varicella and zoster are usually relatively mild and self-limited diseases. Morbidity and mortality are low, but more severe disease is often seen in adults, pregnant women, and immunocompromised.

- Clinical disease typically occurs about 14 days after exposure. Most patients with primary varicella show an abrupt onset with the appearance of asynchronous "crops" of vesicular lesions appearing over several days, mainly on the head and trunk. Lesions at various stages, papular, vesicular, ulcerative, and crusted, are all seen at any time during active infection. Fever and nonspecific symptoms may occur. Lesions typically heal without scar formation.

- The most common complication of primary varicella is bacterial superinfection, especially with *Streptococcus pyogenes*. Although involvement of the respiratory tract may occur in a significant minority of patients, clinically significant pneumonia is an uncommon, but potentially serious, complication in a small number of patients, especially adults. Meningoencephalitis, cerebellar ataxia, and other CNS complications occur rarely. Hemorrhagic varicella is an uncommon complication in immunocompetent patients.

- Zoster occurs, mainly in the elderly, decades after primary VZV infection. It usually presents with a localized, unilateral eruption of vesicles restricted to one or several adjacent dermatomes, reflecting the role of dorsal root or cranial nerve ganglia as the source of viruses. Aseptic meningitis with minimal CSF abnormalities may be seen in patients with zoster. Most patients recover spontaneously within 2 weeks. Localized cutaneous HSV infection may mimic zoster.

- Postherpetic neuralgia is a common complication of zoster and may develop in a significant minority of elderly patient after resolution of the rash. Motor deficits occur at the affected dermatome in about 1% of patients. This may manifest as bladder dysfunction or intestinal ileus. Zoster related to cranial nerves may result in retinitis or other ocular abnormalities, Ramsay Hunt syndrome, facial palsies, or other abnormalities of cranial nerve function.

- Congenital varicella syndrome may occur in maternal infections during the first or early trimester of pregnancy. The embryopathy is manifested primarily by skin scars, limb atrophy, ocular abnormalities, mental retardation, or fetal loss. Maternal varicella after 20 weeks of gestation is usually not associated with congenital varicella syndrome, although "silent" infection occurs in the fetus. When maternal infection occurs between 2 and 5 days prior to delivery, however, severe neonatal varicella may develop.

❏ Laboratory Findings

The diagnosis of varicella and zoster can accurately be made clinically. Laboratory testing is usually required only for immunocompromised patients or patients with atypical disease. See the various diagnostic tests for Varicella-Zoster in Chapter 17, Infectious Disease Assays.

Culture: VZV may be reliably isolated by cell culture of vesicle fluid or scrapings from the base of wet ulcerative lesions. Culture results are usually positive after 3–5 days. The sensitivity of viral culture of CSF and other specimen types is lower.

NAAT: Standard and real-time PCR methods may be used for diagnosis of acute VZV infections. Molecular diagnostic methods provide sensitive and specific results for a variety of types of specimens.

Serology: Humoral and cell-mediated responses are brisk after primary infection, occurring within several days of clinical disease. Levels peak within 3 months and then decline but are detectable for years. A bump in specific antibody subsets may be seen in patients after an outbreak of zoster.

- A positive IgM result or fourfold or greater increase in VZV IgG or total antibody titer in acute and convalescent samples is diagnostic of VZV infection. Silent fetal infection may be inferred by persistence of positive VZV antibody titers beyond 8 months of life.
- The fluorescent antibody to membrane antigen assay (FAMA) is the most sensitive assay, if available, to document immunity after natural infection or vaccination. Detection of VZV antibodies in CSF is diagnostic of aseptic meningitis, even without skin lesions.

Histology: Demonstration of specific VZV antigen by immunofluorescent staining of cells from vesicular lesions is diagnostic of acute VZV infection and is more sensitive than viral culture. DFA testing allows prompt diagnosis.

Core laboratory: Core laboratory tests are generally not required unless severe disease is present. Clinical or subclinical hepatitis may occur in primary or systemic VZV infections. Elevation of transaminases, without hyperbilirubinemia, is typical. WBC count is usually decreased with absolute and relative lymphocytosis early in primary infection. Thrombocytopenia may be seen, especially in severe disease.

CSF findings: In patients with CNS complications of VZV infection, the CSF parameters are usually normal or only mildly abnormal. Forty percent of zoster patients show increased cells (<300 mononuclear/µL) in CSF.

Suggested Readings

Arvin AM. Varicella-Zoster virus. *Clin Microbiol Rev.* 1996;9:361–381.
Bonnez W. Chapter 28, Papillomavirus. In: Richman DD, Whitley RJ, Hayden FG. *Papillomavirus in Clinical Virology*, 3rd ed. Washington, DC: ASM Press; 2009.
Cohen JI. Epstein-Barr virus Infection. *N Engl J Med.* 2000;343:481–492.
Corey L, Wald A. Maternal and neonatal herpes simplex virus infections. *N Engl J Med.* 2009;361:1376–1385.
Crough T, Khanna R. Immunobiology of human cytomegalovirus: from bench to bedside. *Clin Microbiol Rev.* 2009;22:76–98.
Glass RI, Parashar UD, Estes MK. Norovirus gastroenteritis. *N Engl J Med.* 2009;361:1776–1785.
Gnann JW, Whitley RJ. Herpes zoster. *N Engl J Med.* 2002;347:340–346.
Guatelli JC, Siliciano RF, Kuritzkes DR, et al. Human immunodeficiency virus. In: Richman DD, Whitley RJ, Hayden FG. *Clinical Virolog*, 3rd ed. Washington, DC: ASM Press; 2009.

Howley PM, Lowy DR. Chapter 62, Papillomaviruses. In: Knipe DM, Howley PM, eds. *Fields Virology.* 5th ed. Philadelphia, PA: Lippincott Williams & Wilkins; 2007.

Kimberlin DW. Chapter 55, Rubella virus. In: Richman DD, Whitley RJ, Hayden FG. *Clinical Virology.* 3rd ed. Washington DC: ASM Press; 2009.

Kimberlin DW, Rouse DJ. Genital herpes. *N Engl J Med.* 2004;350:1970–1977.

Knuchel MC, Jullu B, Shah C, et al. Adaptation of the ultrasensitive HIV-1 p24 antigen assay to dried blood spot testing. *J Acquir Immune Defic Syndr.* 2007;44:247–253.

Lambert JS, Harris DR, Stiehm ER, et al. Performance characteristics of HIV-1 culture and HIV-1 DNA and RNA amplification assays for early diagnosis of perinatal HIV-1 infection. *J Acquir Immune Defic Syndr.* 2003;34:512–519.

Lane JM, Ruben FL, Neff JM, Millar JD. Complications of smallpox vaccination 1968; national survey in the United States. *N Engl J Med.* 1969;281:1201–1208.

Markowitz LE, Preblud SR, Orenstein WA, et al. Patterns of transmission in measles outbreaks in the United States, 1985–1986. *N Engl J Med.* 1989;320:75–81.

Poggio GP, Rodriguez C, Cisterna C, et al. Nested PCR for rapid detection of mumps virus in cerebrospinal fluid from patients with neurological diseases. *J Clin Microbiol.* 2000;38: 274–278.

Young NS, Brown KE. Parvovirus B19. *N Engl J Med.* 2004;350:586–597.

INFECTIOUS DISEASES CAUSED BY PARASITIC PATHOGENS

Parasites are eukaryotic pathogens; they may be single celled or multicelled. Parasites are responsible for an enormous disease burden worldwide. Infection and disease are especially common in developing nations, in which large segments of the population may be infected, and infection with multiple pathogens may be frequent. Improved sanitation and control of vector populations have reduced, but not eliminated, the burden of parasitic diseases in industrialized nations.

Parasites may have complicated life cycles, and there are varied modes of transmission to humans. Oral transmission is a common route for spread of infection; enteric parasites are responsible for the greatest burden of parasitic infection. Arthropod-transmitted parasites, such as *Plasmodium* spp., are also responsible for an enormous disease burden. Some parasites may be transmitted by direct invasion, as through skin, or other means of infection. Immunocompromised patients, like patients with AIDS, are at increased risk for severe disease.

Most parasitic disease is diagnosed by direct detection of organisms in infected specimens. Detection of specific antigens provides sensitive and specific diagnosis for several common parasitic pathogens, like *Giardia* and *Cryptosporidium.* Serologic assays may contribute to diagnosis and may be useful for epidemiologic studies. Isolation of parasites in culture is restricted to a few pathogens and is not widely available for routine diagnosis. Molecular diagnostic strategies are playing an increasingly important role in diagnosis and definitive speciation.

Common human parasites may be divided into different, genetically related groups:

- *Protozoa:* Protozoan species are single-celled parasites. There are four groups: amoeboid protozoa, ciliated protozoa, flagellated protozoa, and sporozoans.
- *Helminths:* Helminth species are parasitic worms. There are three major groups: cestodes (segmented tapeworms), nematodes (roundworms) and trematodes (flukes).

See: Macroscopic Examination, Parasites; Ova and Parasite Examination, Stool; Blood Parasite Examination in Chapter 17, Infectious Disease Assays.

AMEBIASIS

❏ Definition

Invasive amebiasis is caused by the protozoan parasite *Entamoeba histolytica*. *Entamoeba histolytica* is primarily seen in Central and South America, Africa, and the Indian subcontinent. *Entamoeba histolytica* is transmitted by ingestion of fecally contaminated water or food. The trophozoites are able to invade into the intestinal mucosa, leading to the formation of flask-shaped ulcers. Trophozoites may gain access to the central circulation, providing access to distant organs, most commonly the liver, but also brain, lung, and others. During multiplication, some amebae revert to the cyst form, which is excreted in stool, leading to continuing transmission of infection.

❏ Who Should Be Suspected?

- Amebiasis is a symptomatic, but self-limited, disease in approximately 90% of infected patients; asymptomatic disease occurs in about 10% of patients. Most symptomatic patients present with GI disease manifested by low fever, abdominal pain, and diarrhea, which may be bloody. Organisms are able to penetrate into, and through, the intestinal mucosa, causing dysentery or extraintestinal disease. The liver abscess is the most common site of extraintestinal infection.
- Risk for symptomatic infection depends in part on immunity; travelers from nonendemic areas are at greatest risk when visiting endemic regions. In asymptomatic patients, it may be important to differentiate *E. histolytica* from *Entamoeba dispar*. The latter does not require eradication, but *E. histolytica* "carriage" poses a significant risk of progression to invasive disease, even after months of asymptomatic infection.

❏ Laboratory Findings

Culture: Culture is the gold standard for diagnosis of amebiasis, but it is not widely available.

Direct detection: Detection of trophozoites or cysts in stool is the most common diagnostic procedure. The sensitivity of a single stool specimen is <50%. At least three samples, collected on consecutive days, should be examined before ruling out amebiasis. The observation of phagocytized RBCs is specific for *E. histolytica* and provides differentiation from *E. dispar*. Motile trophozoites may be detected in saline wet mounts if stool can be examined immediately. The finding of many RBCs, but minimal WBCs, on microscopic examination of stool helps to differentiate amebiasis from bacillary dysentery.

Serology and antigen testing: The indirect hemagglutination assay for *E. histolytica* antibody is 99% sensitive in patients with liver abscess and 88% sensitive for intestinal disease. Tests remain positive for years and cannot distinguish acute from past infection. Detection of stool antigen is sensitive (95%) and specific (93%) for *E. histolytica*.

Histology: Endoscopic biopsy or smear of exudate of sigmoid ulcers may show *E. histolytica* in 50% of cases. Collect from six or more lesions for permanent staining. Tissue diagnosis for amebic liver abscess is rarely performed; imaging studies and serologic and antigen studies can usually confirm this diagnosis. When sampled, amoebae are usually located in the abscess wall, not in the necrotic contents of the abscess. Parasites are identified in abscess material in <20% of cases.

Core laboratory: Liver abscess should be suspected in patients with risk factors who present with fever (90%), leukocytosis, increased ALP, and right upper quadrant pain and tenderness (85%). The right hemidiaphragm may be elevated. Many patients (60%) with liver abscess have no history of intestinal disease; stool for O&P is positive in <20–40% of patients with hepatic abscess. Eosinophilia is uncommon.

ASCARIASIS (ASCARIS LUMBRICOIDES)

❑ Definition
Ascaris lumbricoides is a large intestinal roundworm with a global distribution. After ingestion, embryonated eggs hatch, releasing second-stage larvae in the intestinal lumen. These penetrate into the capillaries and lymphatics of the intestinal mucosa. From the circulation, they are deposited in the lungs where they develop into fourth-stage larvae. Fourth-stage larvae migrate up the trachea and are swallowed, returning to the small intestine, where they develop into mature adults.

❑ Who Should Be Suspected?
Most infections are asymptomatic, but mild, nonspecific pulmonary or abdominal symptoms may occur. Symptoms may be caused by immune response, effects of larval migration, large worm burden, and nutritional impact. Pneumonitis may occur (e.g., Loeffler syndrome) during migration. With high worm burden, malnutrition or intestinal, biliary, or pancreatic obstruction may occur. Nausea, vomiting, diarrhea, and other conditions may develop.

❑ Laboratory Findings
Direct detection: Identification of eggs by routine O&P examination is the usual method of identification. Larvae are occasionally seen in sputum or gastric aspirates. In pneumonitis associated with a primary infection, stool examination for eggs may be negative.

Radiology: Abnormalities associated with pneumonitis may be transient.

Core laboratory: Eosinophilic reaction is common during symptomatic disease.

BABESIOSIS

❑ Definition
Babesia microti, a protozoan blood parasite, is transmitted by the tick Ixodes scapularis, which is also the vector for Lyme borreliosis and human granulocytic ehrlichiosis. Sexual reproduction occurs in the tick. After the infective forms enter the host during a blood meal, they enter erythrocytes, where asexual reproduction occurs. Most cases of babesiosis occur in the Northeastern and Great Lakes states in the United States and are caused by Babesia microti. Other Babesia species cause infections in other regions of the United States as well as in Europe, and these infections may differ in their clinical presentation. Transmission of babesiosis by transfusion is well described.

❏ Who Should Be Suspected?

■ Most *Babesia* infections are likely to be asymptomatic or subclinical. In symptomatic infections, influenza-like symptoms with fever, accompanied by sweats and chills, malaise, fatigue, weakness, and joint pain are seen with onset in the first month after tick bite or 1–2 months after transmission by transfusion. Fever and severe symptoms generally resolve within several weeks, but milder malaise and fatigue may linger for months.

■ Severe disease can occur in patients with asplenia or other immunocompromising condition. These patients may develop very high parasitemia levels, leading to hemolysis and jaundice, anemia, renal failure, DIC, ARDS, hypotension, and other complications.

■ Infections caused by *Babesia divergens* almost always occur in splenectomized patients. Disease is rapidly progressive and severe and is associated with high mortality. After an incubation period of 1–4 months, high fevers, malaise, myalgias, headache, hypotension, jaundice, intravascular hemolysis, and renal failure may occur. Diarrhea, nausea, and vomiting are prominent symptoms. Coma and death occur within 1 week after onset of symptoms in almost 50% of patients.

❏ Laboratory Findings

Direct detection: Most diagnoses are made by examination of thin and thick blood smears. Multiple smears should be examined to rule out infection. Parasites may be seen inside or outside of erythrocytes.

Serology: Antibody detection is limited by poor overall sensitivity and specificity; serologic tests are not widely available but are rarely needed or used for diagnosis.

Core laboratory: Hemolytic anemia may last days to months; most patients have thrombocytopenia. Concurrent infection with *B. burgdorferi* (Lyme disease) and *A. phagocytophilum* (HGA) should be considered. Patients should be monitored closely for complications of primary babesiosis, with coagulation, renal, liver, and pulmonary function tests.

BEEF TAPEWORM (*TAENIA SAGINATA*)

❏ Definition

Beef tapeworm disease is caused by ingestion of viable metacestodes (cysticerci) of *Taenia saginata*.

❏ Who Should Be Suspected?

Most beef tapeworm infections are asymptomatic, but intestinal, biliary, or pancreatic obstruction may occur in heavy infection.

❏ Laboratory Findings

Direct detection: Detection is usually achieved by identification of ova, proglottids, strobila, or scolices from feces. Tapeworm ova are detected in the stool in 50–75% of patients but cannot be distinguished from those of *Taenia solium* (see below for specific discussion). Definitive identification is usually achieved by examination of the uterine morphology of gravid proglottids. Because *T. saginata* proglottids actively migrate though the anus to deposit eggs on the perianal skin, proglottid segments may be available for examination, significantly improving species identification.

Core laboratory: Eosinophils may be slightly increased.

CRYPTOSPORIDIOSIS AND OTHER COCCIDIA INFECTIONS

❏ Definition
Coccidia infections are caused by protozoon parasites, including *Cryptosporidium parvum*, *Isospora belli*, and *Cyclospora cayetanensis*. These parasites are capable of causing severe diarrheal illness in patients with AIDS. These organisms infect microvillus epithelial cells of the GI tract.

- Cryptosporidiosis is very infectious, and diarrheal disease occurs in most infected patients. Outbreaks linked to day care centers and recreational water activities are well described. Springtime is the season of peak incidence.
- Humans serve as the only known reservoir for infection with *Isospora belli*. There is global distribution, but the highest prevalence is in tropical and subtropical areas. The oocytes of *Isospora* mature to infectious forms in the environment several days after excretion, so person-to-person transmission is less efficient.
- *Cyclospora* infection is probably acquired by ingestion of contaminated water. Because the oocysts of *Cyclospora* must mature to infectious forms in the environment for several days after excretion, direct person-to-person transmission is uncommon. *Cyclospora* may cause endemic disease during the rainy season in developing countries. Epidemic disease is well described in developed countries; consumption of fecally contaminated foods is usually implicated.

❏ Who Should Be Suspected?
Coccidial infections manifest with watery diarrhea, crampy abdominal pain, and anorexia. Nonspecific systemic symptoms are common. RBCs and WBCs are typically absent from stool. Chronic and intermittent diarrheal illness may occur in immunocompromised patients.

❏ Laboratory Findings
Direct detection: Routine O&P examination is insensitive for detection of coccidian protozoan pathogens. All are acid-fast and are detected in stool using an acid-fast stain modified for staining stool smears for parasites. Multiple stool samples should be examined to rule out infection. Sensitivity of staining may be increased by concentration techniques. Staining of *Cyclospora* may be variable, but *Cyclospora* may be detected by its characteristic autofluorescence.

Histology: Biopsy of the duodenal or proximal jejunal mucosa may demonstrate *Isospora* when stool acid-fast stains are negative.

Serology and immunology: DFA staining techniques have been described and may improve detection compared to acid-fast staining. Commercially available EIA methods also provide sensitive and specific diagnosis. Kits combining reagents for multiple intestinal parasites, like *Cryptosporidium*, *Giardia*, and *E. histolytica*, are available.

Core laboratory: Eosinophilia may be seen in patients with *Isospora* infection.

CYSTICERCOSIS (PORK TAPEWORM, *TAENIA SOLIUM*)

❏ **Definition**

Pork tapeworm disease is caused by ingestion of viable metacestodes (cysticerci) or the eggs of *Taenia solium*. Ingestion results in small bowel infection by adult tapeworms.

❏ **Who Should Be Suspected?**

Most infections caused by adult pork tapeworms are asymptomatic, but intestinal, biliary, or pancreatic obstruction may occur in heavy infection. Neurocysticercosis is caused by hematologic spread of larvae to the brain. Cysticercosis is a significant cause of intracranial masses, with related symptoms, in endemic areas.

❏ **Laboratory Findings**

The diagnosis of cysticercosis relies on a combination of epidemiologic, imaging, histopathologic, and laboratory studies.

Direct detection: Detection is usually achieved by identification of ova, proglottids, strobila, or scolices from feces. Tapeworm ova may be identified by O&P examination but cannot be distinguished from ova of *T. saginata*. Examination of portions of adult worms, like the uterine morphology of gravid proglottids, is required for speciation.

Serology: The presence of detectable antibodies depends on the number and condition of cysticerci. Antibody detection using serum may be more sensitive than CSF for diagnosis of neurocysticercosis, especially in cases with degenerating cysts. ELISA detects antibody in serum or CSF in 75–80% with few or calcified cysts and 93% with severe CNS disease. Enzyme-linked immunoelectrotransfer blot (EITB) on serum or CSF has S/S of >94% with multiple CNS lesions and approximately 72% with single lesions. Change in titers is not reliable for judging cure. Solitary CNS lesions may not consistently induce antibody production.

Core laboratory: Eosinophils may be slightly increased. Marked increase in ESR is unusual and suggests another diagnosis.

CSF findings: May show increased eosinophils (in 10–77% of cases), increased mononuclear cells (≤300/μL), slightly increased protein, normal or mildly decreased glucose; parasites are not found.

GIARDIASIS

❏ **Definition**

Giardiasis is caused by infection with the flagellate protozoan *Giardia lamblia*. This pathogen has a worldwide distribution but is more prevalent in warmer climates. Infection is most commonly acquired by ingestion of cysts, with an incubation period of 2–3 weeks. After excystation and maturation, the trophozoites typically attach to the crypts of the duodenal mucosa by means of ventral disks. They do not penetrate the intestinal mucosa and typically cause minimal pathologic changes; villous atrophy may be seen in severe, chronic disease. Organisms are released and may encyst or pass in the feces as trophozoites.

❏ **Who Should Be Suspected?**

Children are most commonly infected. Although immunocompromised patients are at risk for severe disease, most infections occur in immunocompetent individuals.

Acute infection may manifest with nausea, anorexia, and explosive, watery diarrhea. Systemic signs and symptoms are common with fever, malaise, and chills. The acute phase may be accompanied by a subacute or chronic phase, manifested by recurrent diarrhea. Chronic giardiasis may be complicated by weight loss, malabsorption, and electrolyte imbalance.

❑ Laboratory Findings

Direct detection: Stool O&P testing should be performed on up to six specimens. Organisms may be excreted intermittently in chronic infection. Stool should be concentrated by centrifugation and permanent stains prepared. Examination of duodenal mucus, collected by duodenal aspirate or an enteric string capsule, may be used as an adjunct to stool O&P testing.

Serology: Not useful for diagnosis because positive results cannot distinguish between acute and past infections.

Antigen detection: Stool antigen detection or fluorescent staining provides rapid, sensitive, and specific detection of *Giardia*; sensitivity is greater than that of routine O&P examination. Antigen testing should not replace O&P testing. Multiple specimens should be examined by antigen testing to rule out giardiasis.

LARVA MIGRANS (CUTANEOUS AND VISCERAL)

❑ Definition

- Cutaneous larva migrans (CLM) is a skin eruption caused by migration of animal hookworms (usually *Ancylostoma caninum* or *Ancylostoma braziliense*) through the upper dermis. Filariform larvae of animal hookworms in the soil penetrate skin, usually of the feet or lower extremities, and then begin a sinuous migration through the upper dermis, causing inflammation with intense itching. These larvae cannot mature to adult stage hookworms, so they die out within several weeks.

- Visceral larva migrans (VLM) infections are caused by animal nematode larvae that are unable to mature into adult stage worms. Disease is caused by the migration of larvae through human organs. VLM occurs worldwide. Toxocariasis and classic VLM syndromes are caused by *Toxocara canis* and less commonly by *Toxocara cati*. Both of these ascarid nematodes have complex life cycles in dogs and cats, respectively, involving vertical transmission to pups and kittens, which excrete large numbers of embryonated eggs in their feces. When ingested by humans, the eggs hatch and the resulting larva is able to penetrate through tissues and migrate through different organs.

❑ Who Should Be Suspected?

Children are at highest risk for disease. Symptoms depend on the organ primarily affected; the liver is involved most commonly (approximately 85%). Severe VLM may be characterized by fever, wheezing and bronchopneumonia, hepatosplenomegaly, anemia, or other symptoms. Arthritis and vasculitis have been described. CNS invasion may occur with severe consequences, including eosinophilic meningitis, encephalitis, and other abnormalities. Ocular larva migrans is based on clinical findings and examination.

❏ **Laboratory Findings**
Direct detection: Eggs are not detected by O&P examination.
   Histology: Larvae may rarely be found in biopsy of granulomatous lesions.
   Serology: Not useful for diagnosis of CLM. For VLM, *Toxocara*-specific ELISA has a sensitivity approximately 75% with specificity >90%. Specificity may be improved by immunoblot testing and may be less sensitive in ocular than in visceral disease.
   Core laboratory: Significant eosinophilia (>30%) is seen in VLM but not CLM. Leukocytosis, increased IgE, and hypergammaglobulinemia are common.

LEISHMANIASIS

❏ **Definition**
Leishmaniasis is used to describe a wide variety of diseases caused by protozoan species (more than 20) of the genus *Leishmania*. The disease is transmitted by the bite of female sandflies (genus *Lutzomyia* in the Americas and *Phlebotomus* elsewhere). It has a wide geographic distribution. In humans, disease is caused by the intracellular proliferation of the amastigote stage of the pathogen.

❏ **Who Should Be Suspected?**
There are three common syndromes: cutaneous (oriental sore), mucosal, and visceral. The epidemiology and clinical characteristics depend on the species and vectors endemic to specific regions.

- In cutaneous leishmaniasis, the vectors are *Phlebotomus* flies. A nodule develops at the bite site, eventually ulcerating. Wet lesions have a raised border with a granulating, exudate-covered base. Dry lesions are typically smaller and crusted over. Resolution of cutaneous lesions occurs in weeks or months, leaving an atrophic scar. Some patients develop fever and systemic symptoms and may develop regional adenopathy. Diffuse cutaneous leishmaniasis, caused by *Leishmania aethiopica* in Africa and *Leishmania amazonensis* in South America, results from wide dissemination of amastigotes, forming plaques and nodules.
- Mucosal leishmaniasis (espundia) occurs only in the Americas. In a small subset of patients, mucosal leishmaniasis develops months or years after resolution of primary cutaneous leishmaniasis. Ulceration of the nasal mucosa develops and may be followed by involvement of the lips, soft palate, and pharynx or other adjacent tissues.
- Visceral leishmaniasis is caused by *Leishmania chagasi* in Latin America and *Leishmania donovani* and *Leishmania infantum* in Mediterranean regions, Africa, and Asia. Most infections are asymptomatic or show only mild symptoms. A minority of patients progress to fulminant disease (kala-azar), presenting with fever, malaise, weight loss, and hepatosplenomegaly. Patients have decreased granulocyte levels and increased globulins. The course may be complicated by malnutrition and failure to thrive, edema, and bleeding diatheses. Immunocompromised patients are at greatest risk for visceral leishmaniasis.

❏ **Laboratory Findings**
Histology: Definitive diagnosis is made by the identification of *Leishmania* in tissues. The raised border of cutaneous lesions should be biopsied. For visceral leishmaniasis, aspirate of the liver, spleen, or bone marrow, buffy coat, or biopsy of affected organ is used for diagnosis.

Culture: Leishmania may be isolated in culture, but the special techniques required are not widely available.

Serology: Serology or the leishmanin skin tests (cutaneous, mucosal, or resolved visceral disease) are useful for diagnosis of leishmaniasis. IFA and EIA methods are most commonly used. Tests based on the rK39 antigen of *L. chagasi* are sensitive for active visceral leishmaniasis, but cross-reactions may limit their utility.

Core laboratory: In visceral leishmaniasis, serum globulin (IgG) levels are markedly increased with decreased albumin and reversed A/G ratio. ESR is increased, caused by increased serum globulin. Anemia, leukopenia, and thrombocytopenia may be seen due to hypersplenism and decreased marrow production. Proteinuria and hematuria may be seen. Laboratory findings due to amyloidosis may be seen in chronic cases.

MALARIA

❏ Definition

Malaria is caused by infection by protozoan pathogens of the genus *Plasmodium*. Four species account for most human infections: *Plasmodium vivax*, *Plasmodium falciparum*, *Plasmodium malariae*, and *Plasmodium ovale*. *Plasmodium knowlesi* is emerging as an increasingly reported cause of malaria. Malaria is endemic in tropical regions of sub-Saharan Africa, Central and South America, and Asia. *Plasmodium falciparum* and *P. malariae* show a worldwide distribution. *Plasmodium vivax* is less common in equatorial Africa, whereas *P. ovale* is uncommon outside of Africa. *Plasmodium knowlesi* is the cause of a significant proportion of cases of malaria acquired in Southeast Asia. Regions with chloroquine-resistant *P. falciparum* are fairly well defined geographically, emphasizing the importance of determining where infection was acquired for therapeutic decisions. The Duffy blood group antigen serves as the erythrocyte binding ligand for *P. vivax*.

❏ Who Should Be Suspected?

- Fever, sweats, anemia, and splenomegaly are the usual signs and symptoms of acute malaria. The classical presentation of malaria is the malarial paroxysm, which occurs cyclically with erythrocyte lysis, but these fever cycles are often not seen. Fevers recur every 48 hours in *P. vivax* and *P. ovale* infection and every 72 hours with *P. malariae* infection. *Plasmodium falciparum* infections also have a 48-hour cycle, but erythrocyte lysis is usually not synchronized. The erythrocyte cycle for *P. knowlesi* is only 24 hours. Nonimmune individuals and pregnant women are at greatest risk for severe and complicated infection.

- *Plasmodium falciparum* infection is associated with the greatest risk of severe and complicated disease. Anemia is common and may be severe with high levels of parasitemia. Hypoglycemia and acidosis are seen as a complication of severe malaria. Hyperthermia (T >41°C) may be seen, especially related to severe anemia, hypoglycemia, and cerebral malaria. Cerebral malaria, usually manifested by coma and/or seizures, is caused by multiple factors, including microvascular obstruction by parasites and metabolic disorders. Cerebral malaria is associated with high morbidity. Oliguric renal failure (blackwater fever) may complicate severe malaria and is associated with high mortality. Pulmonary edema, caused by capillary leak syndrome, may be seen, usually in combination with other symptoms of complicated malaria. Microvascular sequestration of parasitized erythrocytes may cause intestinal dysfunction, resulting in diarrhea. The complications of falciparum malaria are not well correlated to the level of parasitemia.

❑ Laboratory Findings

Direct detection:

- Diagnosis is usually achieved by examination of thin and thick blood smears stained with Giemsa, Wright, or Wright-Giemsa stain. Giemsa is recommended because most morphologic descriptions are based on Giemsa staining. Thick smears of peripheral blood or bone marrow provide the most sensitive method for detection, and the thin smears are used for speciation.
- Multiple specimens should be examined to rule out malaria. Smears should be made every 6–12 hours for 3 consecutive days. Requests for malaria diagnosis should be considered as representing a potential medical emergency, so specimens should be transported and tested in a "stat" manner. Capillary blood is recommended if thin and thick smears can be prepared at the bedside. EDTA-anticoagulated blood may be used, but stippling may be lost if the smears are not prepared quickly.

Serology: Limited value in acute infection.

Molecular tests: PCR methods have been developed that are very sensitive and species specific, but FDA-approved tests are not yet available.

Core laboratory: Hemolytic anemia (average 2.5 million erythrocytes per microliter in chronic cases); usually hypochromic; may be macrocytic in severe chronic disease. Reticulocyte count is increased. Thrombocytopenia is commonly seen. Leukocytes may be decreased. ESR is increased. There is increased serum indirect bilirubin and other evidence of hemolysis. Serum globulin is increased (especially euglobulin fraction); albumin is decreased. Biologic false-positive test for syphilis is frequent. Proteinuria and hematuria may be seen. Renal complications of malaria may result in acute tubular necrosis with casts on microscopic examination, azotemia, and oliguria progressing to anuria. Liver function tests may be moderately elevated.

MICROSPORIDIOSIS

❑ Definition

The microsporidia are obligate intracellular protozoan species capable of infecting a wide variety of vertebrate and invertebrate species. *Enterocytozoon bieneusi* is the most common human pathogen. Infection is usually acquired by oral ingestion of the microsporidia, rarely by inhalation.

❑ Who Should Be Suspected?

- *Enterocytozoon bieneusi* has emerged as a significant pathogen for patients with AIDS. Clinical disease is similar to that of *Cryptosporidium* and *Isospora*, with frequent, watery diarrhea with nausea and anorexia. Stools are not bloody. Complications of diarrhea may occur in severe cases, with dehydration, hypovolemia, electrolyte imbalance, and malabsorption. A significant number of patients with proven intestinal microsporidiosis may be coinfected with *Cryptosporidium*. Microsporidia have been identified in lower respiratory secretions of AIDS patients.

- Self-limited intestinal disease has been described in patients with intact immune systems. Microsporidia other than *E. bieneusi* are more likely to be responsible for extraintestinal microsporidiosis (e.g., keratoconjunctivitis, hepatitis, sclerosing cholangitis, peritonitis, respiratory tract infection, sinusitis, myositis, kidney disease).

❑ Laboratory Findings

- See Microsporidia Examination in Chapter 17, Infectious Disease Assays.
- *Direct detection*: EM is the gold standard for confirming infection and speciation, if needed. Several modified trichrome stains have been described for detection of microsporidia in stool. Stool smears should be very thin to help avoid artifacts. Optical brightening agents, like calcofluor, stain microsporidia in stool but are nonspecific.
- *Histology*: Microsporidia may be identified by a number of histologic stains, like H&E, periodic acid–Schiff, and silver stains. Staining may be inconsistent. Detection may be improved by examination of stained touch preparations.

PINWORM INFECTION (*ENTEROBIUS VERMICULARIS*)

❑ Definition
Enterobius vermicularis is a small roundworm with global distribution. Enterobiasis may be more common in temperate climates. Female worms migrate through the anus at night to deposit embryonated eggs on perianal skin. The worms develop into infective stage 3 larvae within the egg. The worms and eggs cause intense pruritus ani. The host fingers are contaminated during scratching, facilitating fecal–oral transmission. Once ingested, the eggs hatch and then mature to adult worms in the large intestine. Female worms can produce over 10,000 eggs per day.

❑ Who Should Be Suspected?
Poor hygiene and crowding are predisposing factors. Most infections are asymptomatic. Perianal itching is the most common symptom.

❑ Laboratory Findings
Pinworm Examination: See Chapter 17, Infectious Disease Assays.

Direct detection: Detection of adult female worms or eggs is the usual method of diagnosis. Because release into stool is relatively uncommon, collection of specimens from perianal skin using cellophane tape or "pinworm paddles" is recommended. Collection of multiple night or first-morning specimens is recommended. Three tests detect 90% of cases, and five tests detect 95% of cases.

Core laboratory: Pinworm infection is not associated with eosinophilia.

SCHISTOSOMIASIS

❑ Definition
Schistosomiasis is caused by infection by species in the *Schistosoma* genus. The major pathogens are *Schistosoma mansoni*, *Schistosoma japonicum*, and *Schistosoma haematobium*. There is a very wide geographic distribution of schistosomiasis in tropical and subtropical areas.

11

Humans acquire infection when cercaria penetrates through skin while wading or swimming in an infected water source. Most disease manifestations are due to the host immune reaction to the worms and their eggs.

❑ Who Should Be Suspected?

▪ Cercarial dermatitis, a pruritic, papular rash of skin exposed to contaminated water, is a frequent manifestation of acute infection. Dermatitis is usually associated with *S. mansoni* and *S. haematobium*. Symptoms of acute infection develop 2–4 weeks after exposure and are most commonly seen with *S. japonicum* and *S. mansoni* infections. Symptoms include fever (Katayama fever), with chills and sweats, abdominal pain, diarrhea, headache, and cough. Hepatosplenomegaly and lymphadenopathy may be seen. Eosinophilia is typical. Biopsy or serologic testing is used for diagnosis of acute infection.

▪ *Schistosoma japonicum* infection, also known as Oriental blood fluke, is seen in Japan, China, Indonesia, and the Philippines. Clinical symptoms are similar to those of *S. mansoni* infection but may be more severe because of the higher egg production by female–male pairs. Hepatocellular and colorectal carcinomas have been associated with *S. japonicum* infection. Severe disease in the large intestine is typical. This may be associated with lower abdominal pain and cycles of diarrhea and constipation. Hepatosplenic disease, similar to *S. mansoni* but more severe, is common. CNS disease, manifested by a wide variety of symptoms, occurs in <5% of patients.

▪ *Schistosoma haematobium* infection is seen in the Nile River valley. After infection, larvae migrate most commonly through the hemorrhoidal and pudendal veins to reside in the vesicle and pelvic plexuses. Eggs are most commonly embedded in the bladder and distal ureters, resulting in fibrosis and ulceration. Calcification, significant hematuria, obstructive uropathy, renal failure, chronic bacterial UTIs, and bladder carcinoma are complications of severe urologic disease. Genital involvement is common, manifesting with heavy egg deposition in the cervix, vagina, and vulva. Friable "sandy patches" are described in the lower genital tract. Bacteremic infections with *Salmonella* species are seen. Schistosomal appendicitis is well described with *S. haematobium*. Hepatosplenomegaly, due to portal fibrosis and pulmonary, CNS, and cardiac diseases, is described but uncommon.

❑ Laboratory Findings

Direct detection: Eggs are seen but may be absent in the first several months after acute infection. Eggs are most commonly found in stool in *S. mansoni* and *S. japonicum* infections. For *S. haematobium* diagnosis, urine specimens, ideally collected between noon and 3 pm when egg excretion is highest, are used. The examination of multiple samples is recommended.

▪ Egg morphology is used as the basis for speciation, which is an important guide to therapy.

▪ Note: *Schistosoma haematobium* ova are sometimes found in stool, and *S. mansoni* eggs are sometimes found in urine, especially in heavy infection. Treated patients should have O&P examinations for at least 1 year to ensure sustained cure.

Histology: Rectal or bladder biopsy is useful for diagnosis in light or inactive infections. Unstained rectal or bladder mucosa, examined microscopically, may show viable or dead ova when stools or urine O&P examinations are negative; granulomatous lesions may be present. Biopsy may identify eggs in affected organs.

Serology: Serologic testing may be useful for diagnosis of infection in patients from nonendemic areas or to support a diagnosis in infection with low egg counts. A specific ELISA, confirmed by immunoblot, is recommended. Positive serology is not useful for distinguishing between acute and chronic infection.

Antigen detection: May be more promising, but utility is hampered by low specificity and cross-reactions with other helminth parasites. Sensitive and specific methods have been described for *S. mansoni*, *S. japonicum*, and *S. haematobium*. An immunoblot assay to detect schistosome antigen is reported to have high sensitivity (approximately 95%) and specificity (approximately 100%).

Core laboratory: Eosinophilia occurs in 20–60% of acute cases. ESR is increased. Hematuria is an important early sign of *S. haematobium* infection. Immunoglobulin levels, especially IgE, are elevated. Liver function tests are usually normal, even in chronic infection. Signs and symptoms related to inflammatory damage of other organs, like the lung (cough, hemoptysis, pulmonary hypertension), brain (seizures), and the spinal cord (myelopathy), may be present. Anemia, eosinophilia, increased serum globulin and decreased albumin, hematuria, proteinuria, hydronephrosis, azotemia, and squamous cell carcinoma of the bladder may occur.

STRONGYLOIDIASIS (*STRONGYLOIDES STERCORALIS*)

❏ Definition
The parasitic roundworm *Strongyloides stercoralis* has a global distribution in tropical and subtropical regions.

❏ Who Should Be Suspected?
- Strongyloidiasis should be considered in any patient who has traveled to an endemic area at any time in the past regardless of local disease prevalence. As in patients who host other successful intestinal parasites, most infected patients are asymptomatic or have minimal, nonspecific symptoms. Patients may complain of epigastric pain, bloating, dyspepsia, diarrhea (sometimes with blood), or constipation. Patients with chronic infection may develop urticarial rashes or the syndrome of larva currens, caused by migration of larvae in the dermal layer.
- The hyperinfection syndrome occurs in immunodeficient patients, including those with HIV and HTLV-1 infections. In the hyperinfection syndrome, severe, bloody diarrhea may result, with malnutrition and intestinal dysfunction. Septic complications may result from the damage to intestinal mucosa. Pulmonary complications, including pneumonia and pulmonary hemorrhage, are common in the hyperinfection syndrome. CNS involvement may result in gram-negative or mixed bacterial meningitis.
- Note that the morphology of larvae of *S. stercoralis* is similar to that of the larvae of hookworms, and care must be taken if endemic infection for both is possible.

❏ **Laboratory Findings**

Direct detection: The identification of stage 1 rhabditiform larvae in stool has formed a primary method for diagnosis, but sensitivity is limited in patients with asymptomatic, uncomplicated infection. A single stool O&P examination shows a sensitivity of 30–60%. Sensitivity is improved by multiple O&P examinations. Sensitivity may also be improved by examination of duodenal fluid collected by endoscopy or other method (sensitivity: 60–80%). In the hyperinfection syndrome, adult and larval forms may be detected in a variety of affected organs.

Serology: May be useful, but the performance of different assays, based on different antigen preparations, has not been standardized.

Core laboratory: Eosinophilia is seen in approximately 70% of infected patients.

TOXOPLASMOSIS

❏ **Definition**

Toxoplasmosis is used to describe diseases caused by the intracellular protozoan parasite *Toxoplasma gondii*. Infection is most commonly transmitted by ingestion of oocytes (sporozoites) in cat feces or by ingestion of cysts (bradyzoites) in raw or undercooked meat of infected animals (e.g., lamb, pork, goat). Acute infection most commonly occurs in the muscle, liver, spleen, lymph nodes, and CNS. Infected monocytes die, resulting in an inflammatory reaction in the affected organ. Bradyzoite-filled cysts are formed, but organ function usually returns to normal in immunocompetent hosts. Indications for serologic screening of asymptomatic patients include pregnancy, new diagnosis of HIV-1 infection, transplant donors and recipients, and patients who will be treated with immunosuppressive drugs.

WHO SHOULD BE SUSPECTED?

- Most infections are asymptomatic.
- Acute infection may be manifested by adenopathy and fever. Occasionally patients develop malaise, headache, myalgias, and hepatosplenomegaly. Atypical lymphocytosis may be seen on blood differential, suggesting mononucleosis syndrome, which may last for weeks or months. Toxoplasmosis may cause up to 15% of cases of unexplained lymphadenopathy.
- Congenital infection may occur when the mother acquires acute infection during pregnancy (which is usually clinically unapparent). The risk of transmission is 15–25% for maternal infections in the first trimester, 30–45% in the second, about 65% in third trimester, and near 100% at term. Severe congenital disease is more likely with fetal infection in the first trimester, with high mortality; 90% have CNS sequelae. Most infected infants (85%) eventually develop sequelae, even if asymptomatic at birth, some years later. Neurologic sequelae include seizures, psychomotor retardation, hydrocephalus, microcephalus, ocular abnormalities (e.g., retinal necrosis and granulomatous inflammation of the choroid, optic atrophy), deafness, and other abnormalities. Intracerebral calcifications are common. Infants may show fever, jaundice, vomiting and diarrhea, hepatosplenomegaly, pneumonitis, and other symptoms.

❏ **Laboratory Findings**

Histology: Organisms may be identified by histologic examination of infected tissues. Detection is improved by the use of specific immunohistologic staining.

Direct detection is low yield for specimens other than tissue. Organisms may be seen in Giemsa-stained BAL or CSF specimens.

Serology

- See: Toxoplasma Serology Screen (*Toxoplasma gondii* IgG and IgM) in Chapter 17, Infectious Disease Assays.
- Serology is the diagnostic method of choice for most patients. Results of serologic tests must be interpreted based on patient age, clinical status, and other factors, including performance characteristics of the test method.
- Diagnosis of acute or congenital infection is more difficult.
  - ▼ Acute infection may be documented by detection of specific IgM or a fourfold rise in antibody titer between acute and convalescent titers. IgM reactivity usually appears within 2 weeks of primary infection. IgG usually develops within 4 weeks. Peak titers usually occur between 4 and 8 weeks after primary infection. A fourfold increase in the IgG titer supports a diagnosis of acute infection. IgG levels usually reach a titer of 1:1,000 or greater. Specific IgM appears in the first week of infection and peaks within 1 month. Reactivity usually disappears in 3–5 months (as early as 1 month) but may persist for up to 2 years in IgM capture assays.
  - ▼ In congenital infection, IgM is usually present, but a negative result does not rule out toxoplasmosis. IgG in the absence of infection, due to transplacental transfer, should disappear within 6–12 months. In retinochoroiditis, IgG is positive and IgM is negative. In reactivation of latent disease in immunocompromised patients, IgG is positive but IgM typically negative. In acute toxoplasmosis in immunocompromised patients, positive IgG and IgM reactions, or an increased IgG titer, usually develop. A negative reaction for IgG in serum occurs in 3% of AIDS patients with toxoplasma encephalitis.
- ANAs and RF may cause false-positive IgM-IFA tests. IgM antibodies may be detectable for more than a year after acute infection. IgG reactivity remains detectable for life.
- A number of tests may be needed to determine the timing of infection. If IgG is positive and IgM is negative, it is likely that infection was acquired >6 months previously. If IgG and IgM are both positive, primary infection may have been only as recent as the previous 2 years. An IgG avidity test may be helpful. Low avidity suggests acute infection within the prior 3 months.

Molecular tests: PCR techniques have proven to be sensitive for the diagnosis of toxoplasmosis, especially for prenatal diagnosis. PCR of amniotic fluid has a sensitivity >97% and NPV >99% for intrauterine toxoplasmosis.

Core laboratory: Atypical lymphocytosis, increased or decreased WBC, anemia, and decreased platelets. Increased globulin concentration and signs of specific organ dysfunction occur in severe disease.

CSF findings: Pleocytosis and increased protein.

TRICHINOSIS (TRICHINELLOSIS; *TRICHINELLA SPIRALIS*)

❑ Definition

Trichinosis is caused by *Trichinella spiralis* and related species. A foodborne zoonotic infection with a global distribution, trichinosis most commonly occurs in Europe and North America. All mammals are susceptible to disease. Swine and rats form the major host reservoir for *T. spiralis*. When infected meat is ingested, the capsule is digested, allowing the larvae to emerge and invade into the epithelium of the small intestine.

❏ Who Should Be Suspected?

Clinical infection shows two phases.

- The first phase, correlated with the entry and activity of adult worms in the small intestine, is often mild.
- The second phase, caused by the circulation of larvae, is associated with fever, myalgias, weakness, malaise, diarrhea, and periorbital and facial edema (approximately 50% of cases) and other symptoms.

Headache is very common. Neurologic symptoms occur in 10–20% of patients and suggest a more severe course. Myalgias, fatigability, headache, and ocular symptoms may persist for decades in chronic infection.

❏ Laboratory Findings

Diagnosis is usually made on the basis of clinical symptoms, dietary history, and serologic testing.

Direct detection: Definitive diagnosis, if needed, is achieved by demonstration of larvae in striated muscle. The deltoid muscle is often biopsied. Muscle biopsy may show the encysted larvae beginning 10 days after ingestion. Direct microscopic examination of compressed specimen is superior to routine histologic preparation. Stool O&P examination is rarely contributory, but adult worms may be seen in acute illness with diarrhea.

Serology: Useful, but seroconversion may not occur for several weeks after acute infection. Serologic tests become positive 1 week after onset of symptoms in only 20–30% of patients and reach a peak in 80–90% of patients by 4th to 5th week. Rise in titer in acute and convalescent phase sera is diagnostic. Titers may remain negative in overwhelming infection. False-positive results may occur in polyarteritis nodosa, serum sickness, penicillin sensitivity, infectious mononucleosis, malignant lymphomas, and leukemia. EIA is method of choice; it peaks in 3 months and may still be detected at 1 year. Specificity is >95%. IHA is also used. Previously used tests include CF, bentonite flocculation, precipitin, and latex fixation.

Core laboratory:

- Eosinophilia develops in >50% of patients and may be one of the earliest laboratory abnormalities supporting a clinical diagnosis. Eosinophilia appears with values of ≤85% on differential count and 15,000/μL on absolute count. It occurs about 1 week after the eating of infected meat and reaches maximum after 3rd week. It usually subsides in 4–6 weeks but may last up to 6 months and occasionally for years.
- Laboratory signs indicating muscle damage (e.g., increased concentrations of creatine phosphokinase, LDH, aldolase, aminotransferases) are frequently seen.
- Decrease in serum total protein and albumin occurs in severe cases between 2 and 4 weeks and may last for years. Increased (relative and absolute) gamma globulins parallel titer of serologic tests. The increase occurs between 5 and 8 weeks and may last 6 months or more. ESR is normal or only slightly increased. Urine may show albuminuria with hyaline and granular casts in severe cases. With meningoencephalitis, CSF may be normal or ≤300 lymphocytes/μL with increased protein with higher antibody level in CSF than in serum.

TRICHOMONIASIS

See discussion of vaginitis and vaginosis in Chapter 8, Gynecologic and Obstetric Disorders.

Suggested Readings: Parasitic Pathogens

Ash LR, Orihel TC. *Ash and Orihel's Atlas of Human Parasitology*, 5th ed. Chicago, IL: ASCP Press; 2007.

Barratt JL, Harkness J, Marriott D, et al. Importance of nonenteric protozoan infections in immunocompromised people. *Clin Microbiol Rev.* 2010;23:795–836.

Garcia LS. *Diagnostic Medical Parasitology*. Washington, DC: ASM Press; 2007.

Gottstein B, Pozio E, Nöckler K. Epidemiology, diagnosis, treatment and control of trichinellosis. *Clin Microbiol Rev.* 2009;22:127–145.

Hunter PR, Nichols G. Epidemiology and clinical features of *Cryptosporidium* infection in immunocompromised patients. *Clin Microbiol Rev.* 2002;15:145–154.

Okhuysen PC. Traveler's diarrhea due to intestinal protozoa. *Clin Infect Dis.* 2001;33:110–114.

Ross AGP, Bartley PB, Sleigh AC, et al. Schistosomiasis. *N Engl J Med.* 2002;16:1212–1220.

Stark D, Barratt JLN, van Hal S, et al. Clinical significance of enteric protozoa in the immunosuppressed human population. *Clin Microbiol Rev.* 2009;22:634–650.

Tanyuksel M, Petri WA. Laboratory diagnosis of amebiasis. *Clin Microbiol Rev.* 2003;16:713–729.

APPENDIX: TABLES FOR REFERENCE

Nosocomial Infections

- *Acinetobacter baumannii*
- *Candida* species
- *Clostridium difficile*
- *Escherichia coli*
- *Klebsiella pneumonia*
- *Mucor* species
- *Mycobacterium avium*
- *Mycobacterium intracellulare*
- *Pseudomonas aeruginosa*
- *Stenotrophomonas maltophilia*
- *Rhizopus* species

Insect Bites

- *Anaplasma phagocytophilum*
- *Babesia microti*
- *Babesia divergens*
- *Borrelia burgdorferi*
- *Ehrlichia chaffeensis*
- *Francisella tularensis*
- *Leishmania* species
- Malaria species

11

Foodborne Illness

- *Ascaris lumbricoides*
- *Bacillus cereus*
- *Campylobacter* species
- *Clostridium botulinum*
- *Clostridium perfringens*
- *Cryptosporidium* and *Coccidia* infections
- *Cyclospora cayetanensis*
- *Entamoeba histolytica*
- *Escherichia coli*
- *Giardia lamblia*
- *Listeria monocytogenes*
- *Microsporidiosis*
- *Rhizopus* species
- *Staphylococcus aureus*
- *Taenia* species
- *Trichinella spiralis*
- *Vibrio cholera*
- *Vibrio vulnificus*
- *Yersinia enterocolitica*

Bioterrorism Agents

Category A

These high-priority agents can be easily transmitted and disseminated and result in high mortality.

- *Bacillus anthracis* (anthrax)
- *Clostridium botulinum* (botulinum toxin)
- *Francisella tularensis* (tularemia)
- Variola virus (smallpox)
- Viral hemorrhagic fever agents
- *Yersinia pestis* (bubonic plague)

Category B

Category B agents are moderately easy to disseminate and have low mortality rates.

- *Brucella* species (brucellosis)
- *Burkholderia mallei* (glanders)
- *Burkholderia pseudomallei* (melioidosis)
- *Clostridium perfringens* (epsilon toxin)
- *Coxiella burnetii* (Q fever)

Category C

Emerging pathogens that might be engineered for mass dissemination because of their availability, ease of production and dissemination, high mortality rate, or ability to cause a major health impact.

- Nipah virus
- Hantavirus
- SARS
- H1N1
- HIV/AIDS

A complete list of agents can be found on the CDC Web site: http://www.bt.cdc.gov/agent/agentlist.asp.

Table Describing Groups of Microorganisms by Morphology

Aerobic (Facultative) Gram-Negative Bacilli

- *Acinetobacter*
- *Burkholderia*
- *Citrobacter*
- *Enterobacter* and *Pantoea*
- *Escherichia coli*
- *Klebsiella*
- *Morganella*
- *Proteus*
- *Pseudomonas*
- *Salmonella* and *Shigella*
- *Serratia*
- *Stenotrophomonas*
- *Yersinia*

Aerobic (Facultative) Gram-Negative Curved and Spiral Bacilli

- *Borrelia*
- *Campylobacter*
- *Helicobacter pylori*
- *Leptospira*
- *Treponema*
- *Vibrio*

Aerobic Gram-Negative Coccobacilli

- Bartonella
- Bordetella pertussis
- *Brucella*
- *Francisella tularensis*
- HACEK organisms
- *Haemophilus influenzae*
- *Legionella*
- *Pasteurella*

Aerobic Gram-Negative Cocci

- *Branhamella*
- *Neisseria gonorrhoeae*
- *Neisseria meningitidis*

Aerobic Gram-Positive Bacilli

- *Arcanobacterium*
- *Bacillus anthracis*
- *Corynebacterium diphtheriae*
- *Erysipelothrix*
- *Gardnerella vaginalis*
- *Lactobacillus*
- *Listeria*

(Continued)

11

Table Describing Groups of Microorganisms by Morphology (*Continued*)

Aerobic Gram-Positive Cocci

Staphylococci
- Nonaureus staphylococci
- *Staphylococcus aureus*

Streptococci
- Group A *Streptococcus*
- Group B *Streptococcus*
- Other β-hemolytic streptococci
- *Streptococcus pneumoniae*
- Other viridans streptococci

Enterococci

Obligate Anaerobes

Anaerobic Gram-Negative Bacilli

- *Bacteroides*
- *Fusobacterium*
- *Porphyromonas*
- *Prevotella*

Anaerobic Gram-Positive Bacilli

- *Actinomyces*
- *Clostridium*
- *Propionibacterium acnes*

CHAPTER 12

Renal Disorders

M. Rabie Al-Turkmani

This chapter provides the latest information on diagnosis of common renal disorders. It also reviews congenital disorders and tumors of the kidney as well as renal involvement in selected diseases. Each entry is organized with a brief definition of the disorder, information regarding clinical presentation, and laboratory findings.

Infectious renal and urinary tract diseases are discussed elsewhere in this book (see Chapter 7, Genitourinary System Disorders and Chapter 11, Infectious Diseases).

ACUTE KIDNEY INJURY (ACUTE RENAL FAILURE)

❑ **Definition**

- Acute kidney injury (AKI), previously known as acute renal failure (ARF), is characterized by a rapid decline in kidney function that limits its ability to maintain homeostasis and eliminate nitrogenous waste. AKI is found in 7% of all hospitalized patients and up to 30% of critically ill patients.
- AKI is defined as any of the following:
  - ▼ Increase in serum creatinine by ≥0.3 mg/dL within 48 hours.
  - ▼ Increase in serum creatinine to ≥1.5 times baseline, which is known or presumed to have occurred within the prior 7 days.
  - ▼ Urine volume of <0.5 mL/kg/hour for 6 hours.
- AKI is staged for severity based on serum creatinine level and urine output (see Table 12-1).
- Causes of AKI can be divided into three categories:
  - ▼ Prerenal: hypovolemia (e.g., hemorrhage, dehydration, burns), anaphylactic or septic shock, heart failure, or decreased renal perfusion due to drugs or toxins
  - ▼ Renal (intrinsic): acute tubular necrosis due to renal ischemia, nephrotoxic drugs or toxins, or acute renal diseases (e.g., acute glomerulonephritis, pyelonephritis)
  - ▼ Postrenal: due to obstruction of the urinary flow

❑ **Who Should Be Suspected?**

Patients with AKI present in a variety of ways:

- Patients with symptoms suggestive of uremia. The term uremia describes the clinical syndrome associated with retention of the end products of nitrogen

TABLE 12–1. Staging of Acute Kidney Injury

Stage	Serum Creatinine	Urine Output
1	1.5–1.9 times baseline OR ≥0.3 mg/dL(≥26.5 µmol/L) increase	<0.5 mL/kg/h for 6–12 h
2	2.0–2.9 times baseline	<0.5 mL/kg/h for ≥ 12 h
3	3.0 times baseline OR Increase in serum creatinine to ≥4.0 mg/dL (≥353.6 µmol/L) OR Initiation of renal replacement therapy OR, In patients <18 y, decrease in eGFR to <35 mL/min/1.73 m²	<0.3 mL/kg/h for ≥24 h OR Anuria for ≥12 h

eGFR, estimated glomerular filtration rate.
Source: Kidney Disease: Improving Global Outcomes (KDIGO) Acute Kidney Injury Work Group.
KDIGO clinical practice guideline for acute kidney injury. *Kidney Int.* 2012;2(Suppl):1–138.

metabolism due to severe reduction in renal function. It can be a consequence of either acute or chronic renal disease.

■ Patients with oliguria (urine output of <500 mL/day) or anuria (urine output <100 mL/day).

■ Patients with an elevated serum creatinine level.

■ Hospitalized patients with severe losses of extracellular fluid or patients exposed to nephrotoxic drugs, sepsis, or radiographic contrast agents who demonstrate the symptoms or findings described above.

❑ **Laboratory Findings**

■ Urinalysis is the most important noninvasive test in the diagnosis of AKI and its etiology (see Figure 12-1). Microscopic examination is normal in most cases of prerenal disease. The presence of RBC casts or dysmorphic RBCs

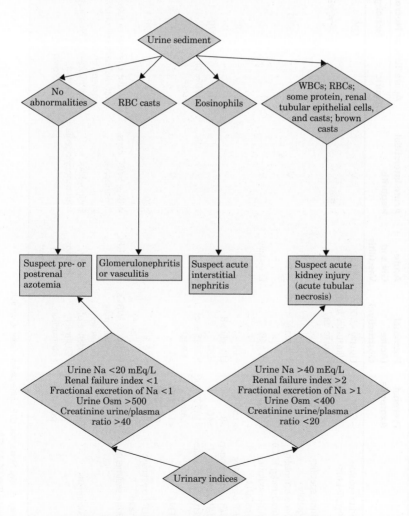

Figure 12–1 *Algorithm for the diagnosis of acute kidney injury.*

TABLE 12–2. Urinary Diagnostic Indices in Acute Kidney Injury

	Prerenal Azotemia	Postrenal (Acute Obstructive)	Acute GN and Vasculitis	Acute Interstitial Nephritis	Acute Tubular Necrosis		Renal Vascular Occlusion	
					Oliguric	Nonoliguric	Arterial	Venous
Urine volume (mL/24 hrs)	~500*	Usually <500; fluctuates from day to day	<500	V	<350	1,000–2,000	V; Anuria if bilateral/complete	V
Urine specific gravity	H; >1.015				L; <1.010			
Urine osmolality (mOsm/kg H$_2$O)	>500	V; usually <500	<500	V	<350	<350	V	V
Urine sodium (mEq/L)	L; <20	H; >40	L; usually <20	V	>40	V	V	V
U/P osmolality	>1.5	<1.2			<1.2	<1.2		
U/P urea nitrogen	>8	Usually >8	>8		<3	<8		
U/P creatinine	>40	<20	>40		<20	<20		
Renal failure index	<1 (90% of cases)	>2 (95% of cases)	<1		>2 (90% of cases)	>3		
FENa	<1 (≤94% of cases)	>1	<1	V	>1	>1	V	V
BUN:creatinine ratio	>20:1	>20:1	>20:1	<20:1	<20:1	<20:1	<20:1	<20:1
Urine sediment	Hyaline casts	N; RBCs, WBCs, crystals may be present	RBCs, RBC casts	WBCs, WBC casts, eosinophils	Granular casts, renal tubular epithelial cells, cell debris, pigment, crystals		V	V
Comments	Decreased renal perfusion	Evidence of GU tract obstruction	Biopsy findings classify disease	Eosinophilia; thrombocytopenia	Renal hypoperfusion; nephrotoxin	Nephrotoxin	Aortic injury; atheromatous emboli	Renal vein occlusion with nephrotic syndrome

H, high; L, low; N, normal; U/P, urine/plasma ratio; V, variable.

*Polyuria may be present.

Sources: Andreoli TE, et al., eds. *Cecil Essentials of Medicine*, 2nd ed. Philadelphia, PA: WB Saunders; 1990;212; Okum DE. On the differential diagnosis of acute renal failure. *Am J Med.* 1981;71:916; Schrier RW. Acute renal failure: pathogenesis, diagnosis, and management. *Hosp Pract.* 1981;16:93–98; Miller TR, et al. Urinary diagnostic indices in acute renal failure: a prospective study. *Ann Intern Med.* 1978;89:47.

indicates glomerular disease, whereas finding cellular debris or granular casts suggests ischemic or nephrotoxic AKI. Urine specific gravity is of limited value in establishing the etiology of AKI.

- Glomerular filtration rate (GFR) gives an approximate estimation of the number of functioning nephrons and may be markedly reduced in patients with AKI. Estimation of GFR has a prognostic rather than diagnostic utility in AKI.
- Serum creatinine level is elevated at diagnosis and continues to rise. The rate of rise may be helpful in determining the etiology of AKI.
- Blood urea nitrogen (BUN)/serum creatinine ratio is normal in intrinsic renal disease (10–15:1) and elevated (>20:1) in prerenal azotemia.
- Urine-to-serum creatinine ratio is high in patients with prerenal disease and low with renal causes of AKI.
- Patients with postrenal disease are diagnosed based on clinical presentation and imaging studies.
- Several protein biomarkers have been found to signal AKI prior to the rise in serum creatinine. These candidate biomarkers include, but not limited to, kidney injury molecule-I (KIM-1), N-acetyl-β-glucosaminidase (NAG), neutrophil gelatinase–associated lipocalin (NGAL), retinol-binding protein and interleukin (IL)-18.
- See Table 12-2.

Suggested Readings

Kidney Disease: Improving Global Outcomes (KDIGO) Acute Kidney Injury Work Group. KDIGO clinical practice guideline for acute kidney injury. *Kidney Int.* 2012;(Suppl 2):1–138. http://www.kdigo.org/clinical_practice_guidelines/pdf/KDIGO%20AKI%20Guideline.pdf

Vaidya VS, Ferguson MA, Bonventre JV. Biomarkers of acute kidney injury. *Annu Rev Pharmacol Toxicol.* 2008;48:463–493.

ACUTE TUBULAR NECROSIS

❏ Definition

- Acute tubular necrosis (ATN) is an acute disorder of kidney function associated with injury to the renal tubular epithelial cells.
- ATN develops in the context of renal ischemia (ischemic ATN) or exposure to nephrotoxins (nephrotoxic ATN). It is associated with high mortality rate.
- Prerenal disease and ATN are the most common causes of hospital-acquired AKI.

12

❏ Who Should Be Suspected?

Candidates for investigation include patients (in most cases hospitalized) with exposure to a nephrotoxin (e.g., therapy with aminoglycoside or amphotericin B, radiologic contrast materials, heavy metals, cisplatin, ethylene glycol, or heme pigments such as free hemoglobin or myoglobin), severe trauma, hemorrhage, hypotension, surgery or sepsis, and recent-onset oliguria or anuria.

❏ Laboratory Findings

- Urinalysis: sloughed renal tubular epithelial cells muddy brown epithelial and granular casts; hyaline casts may be seen. Urine volume is typically, but not invariably, low.

- Urine osmolality is typically below 400 mOsm/kg.
- Fractional excretion of sodium (FENa) is an accurate test to differentiate between prerenal disease (<1%) and ATN (>1%). There are few limitations, however, to the use of FENa in determining the cause of AKI since it may be <1% in some ATN cases (e.g., when ATN is associated with a chronic prerenal disease such as heart failure), or >1% in some prerenal disease cases (e.g., patients treated with diuretics).
- Sudden elevation in serum creatinine with normal BUN/creatinine ratio (10–15:1).

CHRONIC KIDNEY DISEASE

❏ Definition

- Chronic kidney disease (CKD) occurs when there is a progressive, irreversible alteration in kidney structure and function, as reflected by a gradual decrease in GFR and increase in BUN and creatinine, and/or albuminuria. This condition becomes more prevalent with increasing age.
- CKD is defined by the Kidney Disease Outcomes Quality Initiative (KDOQI) as
  - ▼ Kidney damage for ≥3 months as defined by structural or functional abnormalities of the kidney, with or without decreased GFR, manifested by either pathologic abnormalities or markers of kidney damage
  - ▼ GFR <60 mL/minute/1.73 m² for ≥3 months, with or without kidney damage
- CKD is divided into five stages based on GFR (see Table 12-3). Stage 5 or kidney failure is the most advanced stage. The term end-stage renal

TABLE 12–3. Classification and Clinical Action Plan for Chronic Kidney Disease

Stage	Description	GFR (mL/min/1.73 m²)	Action*
	At increased risk	≥60 (with CKD risk factors)	Screening, CKD risk reduction
1	Kidney damage with normal or ↑ GFR	≥90	Diagnosis and treatment, Treatment of comorbid conditions, Slowing progression, CVD risk reduction
2	Kidney damage with mild ↓ GFR	60–89	Estimating progression
3	Moderate ↓ GFR	30–59	Evaluating and treating complications
4	Severe ↓ GFR	15–29	Preparation for kidney replacement therapy
5	Kidney failure	<15 (or dialysis)	Replacement (if uremia present)

Shaded area identifies patients who have chronic kidney disease; unshaded area designates individuals who are at increased risk for developing chronic kidney disease.
*Includes actions from preceding stages.
GFR, glomerular filtration rate; CKD, chronic kidney disease; CVD, cardiovascular disease.
Source: National Kidney Foundation. K/DOQI clinical practice guidelines for chronic kidney disease: evaluation, classification and stratification. *Am J Kidney Dis.* 2002;39(Suppl 1):S1–S266.

disease (ESRS) refers to chronic kidney failure treated with either dialysis or transplantation.

- CKD is usually asymptomatic in its early stages (1–3). Symptoms and metabolic complications (e.g., anemia, hyperparathyroidism, water and electrolyte imbalance) usually appear at later stages when GFR drops below 30 mL/minute/1.73 m^2.
- Another staging system uses urine albumin-to-creatinine ratio (mg/g): stage 1: <30 mg/g; stage 2: 30–299 mg/g; stage 3 ≥ 300 mg/g.
- The distinction between acute, subacute, and chronic kidney disease is not always well defined but may be important, since AKI may be reversible, whereas CKD is not. A reduced size of the kidney (demonstrated by ultrasound) indicates a chronic phase.
- The majority of CKD cases are due to glomerular disease, tubular or interstitial disease, or long-standing obstructive uropathy.

❏ Who Should Be Suspected?

- Patients who have had acute renal injury or glomerulonephritis.
- Patients with diseases that can initiate or propagate kidney disease, such as diabetes or hypertension.
- Those in whom symptoms develop insidiously suggesting uremia (easy fatigability, anorexia, vomiting, mental status changes, seizures) or generalized edema.
- Those in whom renal function or urinalysis abnormalities are discovered incidentally.
- Those with a family history of CKD or have a congenital renal abnormality.

❏ Laboratory Findings

Laboratory studies are indicated once renal disease is suspected. Until renal insufficiency is severe, adaptation of tubular function allows excretion of relatively normal amounts of water and sodium.

- Serum creatinine and BUN increase in parallel.
- Creatinine clearance, established via well-accepted formulas, is used to estimate the GFR (estimated GFR or eGFR). This parameter is generally considered the best index of overall kidney function and repeated determinations, in conjunction with creatinine measurement, establish whether the patient has stable or progressive disease. GFR has no etiologic diagnostic value.
- Albuminuria is a marker of kidney damage that is commonly determined by measuring albumin/creatinine ratio (ACR) in untimed "spot" urine. An ACR cutoff of 30 mg/g indicates abnormality (see Figure 12-2).
- Urinalysis
  - ▼ Microscopic examination is an important tool in determining the etiology of CKD. WBCs, RBCs, and casts are usually found.
  - ▼ Dipstick examination for albumin, glucose, pH, nitrate, and blood contribute to determining the etiology of CKD.
- Blood pH measurement can be helpful since acidosis is a frequent complication of advanced CKD.

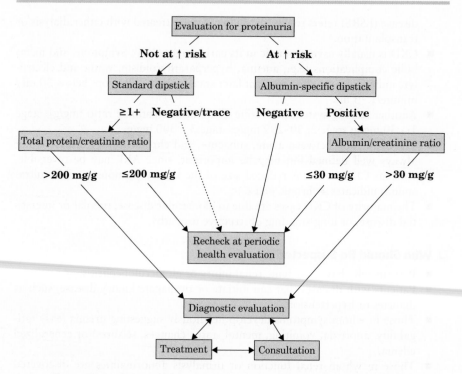

Figure 12-2 *Evaluation of proteinuria in patients not known to have kidney disease.*

■ Serum abnormalities include hyperphosphatemia, hyperkalemia, hyponatremia, hypocalcemia, and hypermagnesemia. Uric acid and amylase may also be increased.

■ Hypoalbuminemia and hyperlipidemia (increased triglycerides, cholesterol, and VLDL lipoprotein levels) may occur, and they are common in the nephrotic syndrome. Hypergammaglobulinemia with monoclonal gammopathy suggests myeloma kidney as the etiology of CKD.

■ Anemia is caused by reduction in the synthesis of erythropoietin and usually develops with reduction of renal function to 30–50% of normal.

■ Coagulation studies may be affected by uremic by-products such as guanidinosuccinic acid and exuberant production of nitrous oxide by uremic vessels, resulting in abnormal platelet function.

Suggested Readings

National Kidney Foundation. K/DOQI clinical practice guidelines for chronic kidney disease: evaluation, classification and stratification. *Am J Kidney Dis.* 2002;39(Suppl 1):S1–S266. http://www.kidney.org/professionals/kdoqi/pdf/ckd_evaluation_classification_stratification. pdf

Stevens PE, Levin A, et al. Evaluation and management of chronic kidney disease: synopsis of the kidney disease: improving global outcomes 2012 clinical practice guideline. *Ann Intern Med.* 2013;158(11):825–830.

FOCAL SEGMENTAL GLOMERULOSCLEROSIS

❑ **Definition**

- Focal segmental glomerulosclerosis (FSGS) is a histologic lesion that is commonly found to underlie the nephrotic syndrome. It accounts for 20% of nephrotic syndrome cases in children and 40% of such cases in adults. In addition, it is the most common pathology identified in patients with ESRD.
- Classified as
  - ▼ Primary (idiopathic): commonly presents with nephrotic syndrome and accounts for approximately 80% of FSGS cases
  - ▼ Secondary: due to diseases (e.g., vasculitis, SLE), infections (e.g., HIV, hepatitis B), drugs, toxins, malignancies, or genetic abnormalities (familial). Patients present with slowly progressing renal insufficiency over time.

❑ **Laboratory Findings**

- Marked proteinuria; nephrotic range (>3.5 g/day) in primary FSGS and non-nephrotic in secondary FSGS.
- Hypoalbuminemia (more common in primary FSGS).
- Hypercholesterolemia and peripheral edema can occur.
- Hematuria, microscopic and macroscopic.
- Serum level of soluble urokinase receptor is elevated.
- Histologic findings are used to confirm the diagnosis.

Suggested Reading

D'Agati VD, Kaskel FJ, Falk RJ. Focal segmental glomerulosclerosis. *N Engl J Med*. 2011;365(25): 2398–2411.

GLOMERULONEPHRITIS

❑ **Definition and Classification**

- Glomerulonephritis (GN) is a renal disease characterized by inflammation of the glomeruli and hematuria. It can be acute or chronic and is often associated with decreased GFR, proteinuria, edema, hypertension, and sometimes oliguria.
  - ▼ Acute GN is defined as the sudden onset of hematuria, proteinuria, and RBC casts.
    - • Chronic GN can develop over years and, in a subset of patients, can ultimately lead to renal failure.
- GN disorders can be grouped into nonproliferative and proliferative types.
- Non-proliferative GN disorders include
  - ▼ Focal segmented glomerulosclerosis
  - ▼ Membranous glomerulopathy
  - ▼ Minimal change disease
- Proliferative GN disorders include
  - ▼ IgA nephropathy
  - ▼ Postinfectious GN
  - ▼ Membranoproliferative GN
  - ▼ Rapidly progressive GN

12

- GN can be a primary disorder due to causes intrinsic to the kidney or secondary to autoimmune disorders, infections, diabetes, or drug treatment.
- Conditions associated with GN can be also classified as antibody-mediated or cell-mediated, infectious or noninfectious, or hypocomplementemic or normocomplementemic.

Antibody Mediated

- For example, anti–glomerular basement membrane (GBM) disease (Goodpasture syndrome), following renal transplantation
- Immune complex–mediated diseases (typically show hypocomplementemia): for example, IgA nephropathy, systemic lupus erythematosus (SLE), acute postinfectious GN, membranoproliferative GN

Cell Mediated

- Examples include Wegener granulomatosis, polyarteritis.

Infectious

- Acute poststreptococcal (group A beta-hemolytic GN)
- Non-poststreptococcal: bacterial (e.g., infective endocarditis, bacteremia), viral (e.g., HBV, HCV, CMV infections), parasitic (e.g., trichinosis, toxoplasmosis, malaria), or fungal

Noninfectious

- Multisystem (e.g., SLE, Henoch-Schönlein purpura, Goodpasture syndrome, Alport syndrome)
- Primary glomerular disease (e.g., IgA nephropathy, membranoproliferative GN)

Hypocomplementemic

- Intrinsic renal diseases (especially poststreptococcal, membranoproliferative GN)
- Systemic (e.g., SLE, cryoglobulinemia)

Normocomplementemic

- Intrinsic renal diseases (e.g., IgA nephropathy, idiopathic rapidly progressive GN)
- Systemic (e.g., polyarteritis nodosa, Wegener granulomatosis)
- See Table 12-4.

❏ Various Clinical Courses of GN

The clinical spectrum of GN comprises:

- Asymptomatic subnephrotic proteinuria without hematuria.
- Asymptomatic proteinuria with hematuria: the coexistence of asymptomatic proteinuria and hematuria substantially increases the risk of significant glomerular damage, hypertension, and progressive renal dysfunction in comparison to the situation of isolated asymptomatic proteinuria.
- Nephrotic syndrome: proteinuria in excess of 3.5 g in 24 hours, accompanied by edema, hypoalbuminemia, hyperlipidemia, and lipiduria.
- Nephritic syndrome: nonnephrotic proteinuria, hematuria, and appearing tendency to GFR lowering.
- Course of rapidly progressive glomerulonephritis, including non-nephrotic proteinuria, hematuria with rapid GFR decline, and acute renal failure.

TABLE 12–4. Serum Complement in Acute Nephritis

Disorder	Approximate Percentage of Cases
Depressed Serum C3 or Hemolytic Complement Levels	
Systemic disease	
SLE (focal)	75
SLE (diffuse)	90
Subacute bacterial endocarditis	90
"Shunt" nephritis	90
Cryoglobulinemia	85
Renal disease	
Acute poststreptococcal GN	90
Membranoproliferative GN	
Type I	50–80
Type II	80–90
Normal Serum Complement Level	
Systemic disease	
Polyarteritis nodosa	
Wegener granulomatosis	
Hypersensitivity vasculitis	
Henoch-Schönlein purpura	
Goodpasture syndrome	
Visceral abscess	
Renal disease	
IgG–IgA nephropathy	
Idiopathic rapidly progressive GN	
Anti–glomerular basement membrane disease	
Immune complex disease	
Negative immunofluorescence findings	

- Macroscopic hematuria associated with glomerular diseases, appearing mainly in children and young adults as a symptom of IgA nephropathy and postinfectious GN. The characteristic feature of IgA nephropathy is episodic frank hematuria occurring simultaneously with an upper respiratory tract infection, whereas in postinfectious GN, there is a 2- to 3-week period of latency between infection and hematuria.
- See Figure 12-3.

12

Suggested Reading

Klinger M, Mazanowska O. Primary idiopathic glomerulonephritis: modern algorithm for diagnosis and treatment. *Pol Arch Med Wewn.* 2008;118(10):567–571.

GLOMERULONEPHRITIS, MEMBRANOPROLIFERATIVE

❑ **Definition**

- Membranoproliferative GN (MPGN) accounts for approximately 10% of all cases of biopsy-confirmed glomerulonephritis and ranks as the third leading cause of end-stage renal disease among the primary glomerulonephritides.

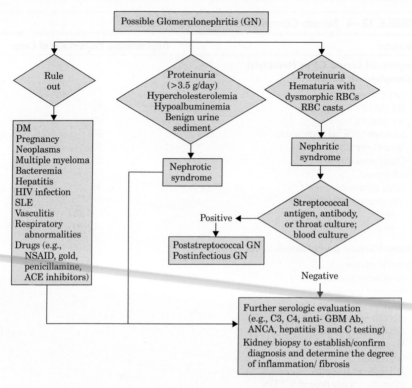

Figure 12–3 *Algorithm for evaluation of glomerulonephritis.*

- MPGN can be primary or secondary to systemic diseases (e.g., SLE), neoplasms, monoclonal gammopathy, or infections (especially HCV with cryoglobulinemia).
- MPGN most commonly presents in childhood but can occur at any age. Patients can present with a variety of findings ranging from microscopic hematuria to severe glomerulonephritis associated with hypertension and nephrotic syndrome. The clinical course may be clinically active, or there may be periods of remission. Approximately 50% of untreated patients have chronic renal insufficiency in 10 years.
- On the basis of the electron microscopical findings, MPGN is traditionally classified as type I (idiopathic, most common), type II, or type III (rare). In another classification that is more useful and based on the pathogenetic process, MPGN can be classified as immune complex mediated, complement mediated, or MPGN without immunoglobulin or complement deposition.

❑ **Laboratory Findings**

- Variable degree of proteinuria, which can be marked or reach the nephrotic range.
- Hematuria is present in patients with active disease.
- Decreased serum levels of complement C3. C4 may be normal or decreased. Clinical course is not related to serum complement levels.
- GFR <80 mL/minute/1.73/m² in two thirds of patients.

- Relevant tests for the detection of secondary causes may be helpful (e.g., serologic testing and culture to detect infections, anti-GBM antibodies, cryoglobulins, serum protein electrophoresis and immunofixation, and antinuclear antibody testing).

Suggested Reading

Sethi S, Fervenza FC. Membranoproliferative glomerulonephritis—a new look at an old entity. *N Engl J Med.* 2012;366(12):1119–1131.

GLOMERULONEPHRITIS, MEMBRANOUS

❏ Definition

- Membranous GN is an antibody-mediated disorder in which immune complexes localize between the outer aspect of glomerular basement membrane and epithelial cells. These complexes are formed by binding of antibodies to antigens that are part of the basement membrane, or deposited from elsewhere by the systemic circulation.
- It usually occurs in adults and is the second most common cause of nephrotic syndrome.
- It may be primary (≥75% of cases) or secondary. Secondary membranous GN may be due to autoimmune diseases (e.g., SLE), infections (e.g., HBV, syphilis, malaria, schistosomiasis, leprosy), drugs (e.g., NSAIDs, penicillamine), or neoplasms (e.g., non-Hodgkin lymphoma, leukemia, carcinomas, melanoma).
- Approximately 20% of patients will progress to ESRD in 20–30 years.

❏ Laboratory Findings

- Marked proteinuria; nephrotic syndrome is found in many patients.
- Microscopic hematuria may be present.
- Autoantibodies against phospholipase-A2 receptor (PLA2R-Ab), mostly of the IgG4 class, can be found in 70% of patients with primary membranous GN and levels correlate with the clinical course and proteinuria.
- Definitive diagnosis is by renal biopsy showing diagnostic findings by light, immunofluorescence, and electron microscopy.

Suggested Reading

Floege J. Primary glomerulonephritis: a review of important recent discoveries. *Kidney Res Clin Pract.* 2013;32(3):103–110.

12

GLOMERULONEPHRITIS, POSTINFECTIOUS

❏ Definition

- Postinfectious GN (PIGN) occurs after infection, usually with a nephritogenic strain of group A β-hemolytic *Streptococcus* (poststreptococcal GN [PSGN]).
- It is the most common glomerular disorder in children between 5 and 15 years.
- Pathogenesis is thought to be related to deposits of immune complexes in the glomerular basement membrane causing glomerular damage. Only 1–2% of cases progress to chronic GN.

❑ **Laboratory Findings**

- Evidence of infection with group A β-hemolytic *Streptococcus* by throat culture.
- **Serologic findings:** Anti-streptolysin O (ASO) is the most common laboratory test to confirm recent streptococcal infection. ASO titers remain elevated for several months in 50–80% of patients. Anti- DNase B is anther serologic test to confirm a previous group A streptococcal infection.
- **Urinalysis:**
  - ▼ Hematuria: gross or microscopic. Microscopic hematuria may occur during the initial febrile upper respiratory infection and then reappear with nephritis in 1–2 weeks and lasts for 2–12 months.
  - ▼ RBC casts and dysmorphic RBCs show glomerular origin of hematuria.
  - ▼ WBC casts and WBCs show inflammatory nature of the lesion.
  - ▼ Granular and epithelial cell casts are present.
  - ▼ Fatty casts and lipid droplets occur several weeks later and are not related to hyperlipidemia.
  - ▼ Oliguria is frequent.
- Random urinary protein/creatinine ratio is usually between 0.2 and 2 but may occasionally be in the nephrotic range.
- Phenolsulfonphthalein (PSP) excretion is normal in cases of mild to moderate severity and increases with progression of disease. Azotemia with high urine specific gravity and normal PSP excretion usually indicates acute GN.
- **Blood Findings:**
  - ▼ Azotemia is found in approximately 50% of patients.
  - ▼ Leukocytosis and increased ESR.
  - ▼ There is mild anemia, especially when edema is present (may be caused by hemodilution, bone marrow depression, or increased destruction of RBCs).
  - ▼ Serum proteins are normal, or there is nonspecific decrease in albumin and increase in alpha-2 and sometimes beta and gamma regions.
  - ▼ Serum C3 and total hemolytic complement activity (CH50) fall during the active disease and return to normal within 6–8 weeks in 80% of cases. If C3 is low for more than 8 weeks, lupus nephritis or MPGN should be considered.
  - ▼ Serum cholesterol may be increased.
- Renal biopsy shows characteristic findings with EM and immunofluorescence microscopy.
- Chronic renal insufficiency is reported in ≤20% of patients.

GLOMERULONEPHRITIS, RAPIDLY PROGRESSIVE (CRESCENTIC)

❑ **Definition**

- Rapidly progressive GN (RPGN) is characterized by progressive loss of renal function and severe oliguria and renal failure that develop over a period of few weeks.
- The histopathologic term "crescentic" refers to crescent formation, a nonspecific response to severe injury to the glomerular capillary wall. Patients

may have rapidly progressive GN in association with anti–glomerular membrane (anti-GBM) antibody disease (Goodpasture syndrome), a condition in which circulating antibodies are directed against an antigen in the glomerular basement membrane, resulting in progressive glomerulonephritis and, in approximately 60% of patients, pulmonary hemorrhage. RPGN can also be associated with Wegener granulomatosis, small vessel vasculitis, SLE, or cryoglobulinemia. Depending on the specific disorder, antineutrophil cytoplasmic antibodies (ANCA) can be present in the serum of RPGN patients.

❑ **Who Should Be Suspected?**

- Candidates include patients with rapidly developing oliguria or anuria and acute onset of hematuria and edema, especially in the presence of an underlying immunologically mediated systemic illness, or following an infection or administration of certain drugs (e.g., allopurinol, hydralazine, rifampin, D-penicillamine).
- Three types of RPGN can be distinguished according to the underlying mechanism of the glomerular injury:
  - ▼ Type I: mediated by anti-GBM antibodies (<5% of RPGN cases; ≤40 of patients are ANCA positive).
  - ▼ Type II: mediated by immune complexes (45% of cases; <5% of patients are ANCA positive).
  - ▼ Type III (pauci-immune RPGN): glomerulonephritis is associated with few or no immune deposits by immunofluorescence or electron microscopy (50% of cases; up to 90% of patients are ANCA positive).

❑ **Laboratory Findings**
Laboratory workup is urgent to initiate therapy since untreated patients progress rapidly to ESRD. Renal biopsy findings establish the diagnosis and prognosis.

- **Urinalysis**
  - ▼ Oliguria, with urine volume often <400 mL/day.
  - ▼ Gross hematuria: RBCs, WBCs, RBC casts.
  - ▼ Proteinuria starts approximately 3 days after injury and may not be marked because of the severe reduction in GFR.
- **Rapid, progressive rise in creatinine and BUN.**
- Laboratory tests to determine underlying etiology (e.g., ANCA, anti-GBM antibodies, antinuclear antibodies) can be helpful. Other tests include serology testing for HIV and hepatitis B and C.

12

HEPATORENAL SYNDROME

❑ **Definition**

- Progressive renal failure that develops in patients with decompensated liver cirrhosis or fulminant hepatic failure.
- Classified as
  - ▼ Type I: serum creatinine increases to >2.5 mg/dL within 2 weeks
  - ▼ Type II: less severe and associated with gradual increase in serum creatinine (1.5–2.5 mg/dL) over few weeks or months

❑ Who Should Be Suspected?

- Patients with liver cirrhosis and ascites, especially following fluid loss (e.g., GI hemorrhage, diarrhea or forced diuresis) or an intercurrent infection.
- Patients with other liver conditions that are associated with portal hypertension such as severe alcoholic hepatitis.

❑ Laboratory Findings

- Progressive increase in serum creatinine (>1.5 mg/dL) and decrease in GFR.
- No improvement in serum creatinine after volume expansion with intravenous albumin.
- Urinalysis
  - ▼ Oliguria: concentrated urine with high specific gravity
  - ▼ Protein excretion <500 mg/day
  - ▼ Less than 50 RBCs per high-power field
  - ▼ Decreased urine sodium (<10 mEq/L)
- Hyponatremia.
- Markedly abnormal liver function tests.

Suggested Reading

Salerno F, Gerbes A, Gines P, et al. Diagnosis, prevention and treatment of hepatorenal syndrome in cirrhosis. *Gut.* 2007;56:1310–1318.

HYPERCALCEMIC NEPHROPATHY

❑ Definition

This renal condition is caused by increased levels of calcium in the blood due to conditions such as hyperparathyroidism, sarcoidosis, vitamin D intoxication, milk-alkali syndrome, or multiple myeloma or other malignancies.

❑ Laboratory Findings

- Increased serum calcium level (12–15 mg/dL).
- Decreased urine osmolality due to reduced renal concentrating ability manifested by polyuria and polydipsia.
- Proteinuria is usually slight or absent.
- Later findings include decreased GFR, decreased renal blood flow, and azotemia.
- Renal insufficiency is slowly progressive and may sometimes be reversed by correcting hypercalcemia.

HYPERCALCIURIA

- See calculi in Chapter 7, Genitourinary System Disorders.
- Hypercalciuria is the most common disorder found in patients with nephrolithiasis (40–50% of cases). It is defined as urinary calcium excretion of >300 mg/day in men and >250 mg/day in women assuming a regular, unrestricted diet. It can also be defined as urinary calcium excretion of >4 mg/kg of body

weight per day (for either sex or children) or a urinary concentration of more than 200 mg of calcium per liter.

- Types of hypercalciuria:
  - ▼ Renal: due to abnormal renal tubular reabsorption. It is one tenth as common as the absorptive type.
  - ▼ Absorptive: due to primary increase in intestinal calcium absorption.
  - ▼ Resorptive: due to primary hyperparathyroidism.
  - ▼ Idiopathic: the most common cause of hypercalciuria and defined as an excess urinary calcium excretion without an apparent underlying etiology. As a result, diagnosis requires exclusion of all other causes of hypercalciuria. This condition is familial in nature and present in 2–6% of asymptomatic children.
- Patients with absorptive hypercalciuria will have lowered urine calcium with dietary restriction and therefore can be differentiated from patients with renal or resorptive hypercalciuria.

❑ **Laboratory Findings**

- Increased urinary calcium excretion (see definition above) and urinary calcium/creatinine ratio.
- Blood calcium level is typically normal. Other laboratory tests such as serum creatinine, phosphorus, parathyroid hormone (PTH), and vitamin D levels help identify the cause of hypercalciuria.

HYPERTENSIVE NEPHROSCLEROSIS

❑ **Definition**

- This condition is characterized by thickening and luminal narrowing of the large and small arteries and arterioles of the kidney and sclerosis of the glomeruli secondary to hypertension.
- It is classified as benign or malignant (rare) depending the severity of hypertension and rapidity of the arteriolar change. With the malignant form, severe high blood pressure can lead to acute kidney injury and hematuria.

❑ **Who Should Be Suspected?**

- Patients with long history of hypertension presenting with slowly progressive elevations in serum BUN and creatinine levels and mild proteinuria.
- Blacks, patients with marked elevations of blood pressure, and patients with diabetic nephropathy are at higher risk.

❑ **Laboratory Findings**

- Benign nephrosclerosis: elevated BUN and creatinine, mild proteinuria (usually <1 g/day), and normal or near-normal urine sediment.
- Malignant nephrosclerosis: hematuria, azotemia, and proteinuria (minimal or marked).
- Renal biopsy is rarely indicated; diagnosis is mainly based on the clinical features.

12

IgA NEPHROPATHY

❏ **Definition**

- This immune-mediated condition, also referred to as Berger disease, is the most common cause of glomerulonephritis and the primary chronic glomerular disease worldwide. It is characterized by prominent deposition of IgA in the glomerular mesangium.
- Progressive decline in renal function occurs in approximately 40% of cases; half of these reach ESRD in 5–25 years. Up to 30% of cases have a benign course with persistent microscopic hematuria.

❏ **Who Should Be Suspected?**

- Presenting conditions may include persistent or intermittent hematuria (visible or microscopic) that can be associated with proteinuria. Episodes of visible hematuria occur in 75% of children and young adult cases and often start few days following upper respiratory infection.
- Few cases (<10%) can have a more severe presentation that is similar to nephrotic syndrome or rapidly progressive GN (edema, renal insufficiency, and hematuria).
- IgA deposits are frequently associated with Henoch-Schönlein purpura (IgA vasculitis) and may also be found with diseases of the GI tract (e.g., celiac disease), skin (e.g., dermatitis herpetiformis), liver (e.g., cirrhosis), carcinomas (e.g., lung, pancreas), autoimmune diseases (e.g., SLE, RA), and infections (e.g., HIV, leprosy).

❏ **Laboratory Findings**

- Diagnosis is based on renal biopsy finding by immunofluorescence microscopy showing predominant mesangial IgA deposits alone or with IgG, IgM, or both. Complement C3 and properdin are almost always present, and C1q is usually absent.
- Urinalysis shows RBCs and RBC urinary casts.
- Proteinuria is usually <2 g/day.
- Serum IgA level is increased in ≤50% of patients.
- Serum complement is normal.
- Serum galactose-deficient IgA1 concentration is frequently elevated.
- Serum levels of glycan-specific IgG antibodies have been found to correlate with urinary protein excretion and risk of progression to ESRD or death.

Suggested Reading

Wyatt RJ, Julian BA. IgA nephropathy. *N Engl J Med*. 2013;368(25):2402–2414.

INTERSTITIAL NEPHRITIS

❏ **Definition**

- This immune-mediated condition is characterized by the presence of inflammatory infiltrate in the kidney interstitium. The onset can be acute or chronic.
- Drug therapy is responsible for more than 75% of acute interstitial nephritis (AIN) cases. The major causative drugs include antibiotics (e.g., beta lactams, cephalosporins, rifampin), sulfonamide diuretics, and NSAIDs.

- Other causes include
    - Infections (5–10% of cases): group A β-hemolytic streptococcal infections, diphtheria, brucellosis, leptospirosis, infectious mononucleosis, toxoplasmosis
    - Systemic diseases (10–15% of cases): SLE, Sjögren syndrome, sarcoidosis
    - Tubulointerstitial nephritis and uveitis (TINU syndrome)
    - Toxic substances

❏ **Who Should Be Suspected?**

- Patients with nonspecific signs of renal dysfunction, especially when associated with symptoms of allergic-type reaction after initiation of a new drug therapy. Disease onset ranges from few days to several months following drug exposure.
- The clinical triad of rash, fever, and eosinophilia is found in approximately 10% of patients with acute interstitial nephritis.
- Patients with chronic interstitial nephritis can present with nausea, vomiting, fatigue, and weight loss.

❏ **Laboratory Findings**

- **Blood:**
    - Serum creatinine is increased. Serum IgG is usually increased, and serum complement is normal. Patients with IgG4-related disease may have elevated IgG4 levels.
    - CBC may show increased WBCs, neutrophils, and bands. Eosinophilia and increased blood IgE levels are seen in approximately one third of patients. Anemia may be present with no evidence of hemolysis or iron deficiency. Anemia resolves when renal functionn becomes normal.
    - Indirect Coombs test is negative, and bone marrow is typically normal.

- **Urine:**
    - May be oliguric or nonoliguric. Urinary indices similar to those seen in ATN.
    - Microscopic hematuria, sterile pyuria, and WBC casts. RBC casts are rare.
    - Eosinophiluria (eosinophils >1% of urinary WBCs). Sensitivity of eosinophiluria for the detection of AIN is 40% and the positive predictive value is 38%.
    - Proteinuria is usually mild to moderate (<1.0 g/24 hours). Nephrotic-range proteinuria may occur (rare).
- FENa >1% indicates tubular damage.
- Hyperchloremic metabolic acidosis suggests tubulointerstitial injury.
- Kidney biopsy confirms the diagnosis.

MINIMAL CHANGE DISEASE

❏ **Definition**

This condition is the most common cause of nephrotic syndrome in the pediatric population, accounting for 70–90% of cases in children <10 years and 50% of cases in older children. It is also an important cause of nephrotic syndrome in adults (10–15% of cases).

❏ Who Should Be Suspected?

Candidates are patients with sudden onset of nephrotic syndrome, which may be a primary occurrence or secondary to drugs, infections, autoimmune disorders, or malignancies, particularly hematologic malignancies (Hodgkin disease, non-Hodgkin lymphoma, or leukemia).

❏ Laboratory Findings

- Marked proteinuria (>3.5 g/day), mostly albuminuria.
- Hypoalbuminemia (<2 g/dL) and, in most cases, hyperlipidemia.
- Normal findings by light microscopy and absence of immunoglobulin or complement deposits by immunofluorescence microscopy.
- Diffuse effacement of the podocyte foot processes is visible on EM. Microscopic hematuria occurs in less than one third of patients.

NEPHRITIC SYNDROME

❏ Definition

- Acute nephritic syndrome is an immune disorder characterized by glomerulonephritis and acute onset of hematuria, proteinuria, and declining renal function.
- Two patterns can be distinguished:
  - ▼ Focal nephritic: generally associated with inflammatory regions in less than one half of glomeruli. Patients often present with asymptomatic hematuria and proteinuria.
  - ▼ Diffuse nephritic: heavy proteinuria, edema, and hypertension may be observed.

❏ Causes

- Renal: can be postinfectious (due to certain nephritogenic strains after streptococcal, staphylococcal, or pneumococcal infections, mumps, measles, chickenpox, hepatitis B and C) or due to MPGN or anti–glomerular membrane disease.
- Systemic: due to SLE, vasculitides, IgA nephropathy, or Henoch-Schönlein purpura.

❏ Laboratory Findings

- Urinalysis: oliguria (<400 mL/day), proteinuria (usually <3.5 g/day), and hematuria, with RBC casts.
- Uremia and azotemia.
- Complement C3 level is usually decreased. Immunologic tests (e.g., anti-GBM antibodies, ASO) can help in the differential diagnosis.
- Renal biopsy establishes the diagnosis.

NEPHROTIC SYNDROME

This syndrome presents as heavy proteinuria, hypoalbuminemia, hyperlipidemia, lipiduria, and edema.

❏ Causes

- Primary glomerular diseases are responsible for >50% of all nephrotic syndrome cases. Systemic diseases such as diabetic glomerulosclerosis, SLE (14% of all cases), and amyloidosis (6% of cases) can also be associated

TABLE 12–5. Major causes of Nephrotic Syndrome

Primary renal diseases
   Membrane nephropathy (MN) (33%)
   Focal glomerulosclerosis (FSGS) (33%)
   IgA nephropathy (IgA) (10%)
   Minimal change disease (MCD) (15%)
   Membranoproliferative glomerulonephritis (MPGN) (2–5%)
   Other (e.g., proliferative glomerulonephritis) (5–7%)
Systemic diseases*
   Diabetes
   Amyloidosis
   Systemic lupus erythematosus
   Dysproteinemias
      Multiple myeloma
      Immunotactoid/fibrillary glomerulonephritis
      Light chain deposition disease
      Heavy chain deposition disease
Infections
   Human immunodeficiency virus disease (FSGS)
   Hepatitis B (MN)
   Hepatitis C (MPGN)
   Syphilis (MN)
   Malaria (MN)
   Schistosomiasis (MN)
   Tuberculosis (Amyloid)
   Leprosy (MN)
Malignant neoplasms
   Solid adenocarcinomas, for example, lung, breast, colon (MN)
   Hodgkin lymphoma (MCD)
   Other malignant neoplasms
Drugs or toxins
   Nonsteroidal anti-inflammatory drugs (MCD)
   Gold (MN)
   Penicillamine (MN)
   Probenecid (MN)
   Mercury (MN)
   Captopril (MN)
   Heroin (intravenous, FSGS)
   Heroin ("skin poppers," amyloid)
Others
   Preeclampsia
   Chronic allograft rejection
   Vesicoureteral reflux (FSGS)
   Bee sting

*Lesions that resemble primary glomerular diseases are indicated in parentheses.
Source: Madaio MP, Harrington JT. The diagnosis of glomerular diseases: acute glomerulonephritis and the nephrotic syndrome. *Arch Intern Med.* 2001;161(1):25–34.

with nephrotic syndrome. Other causes include infections, neoplasms (10% of adult cases), and drugs or toxins (see Table 12-5).

❑ Laboratory Findings

- Urinalysis: Marked proteinuria: >3.5 g/24 hour in adults (normal protein excretion is <150 mg/24 hour) and >50 mg/kg/day in children. Albumin is the main urinary protein. Total protein-to-creatinine ratio (mg/mg) in a random urine specimen correlates closely with daily protein excretion in g/1.73 m² of body surface area. Minimal hematuria and azotemia may present but not part of the syndrome. Granular and epithelial cell casts are present in the urine.

■ Decreased serum albumin (usually <2.5 g/dL) and total protein. Serum α_2 and β-globulins are markedly increased, γ-globulin is decreased, and α_1-globulin is normal or decreased. If γ-globulin is increased, systemic diseases (e.g., SLE) should be ruled out.

■ Changes secondary to proteinuria and hypoalbuminemia such as decreased serum calcium, decreased serum ceruloplasmin, and increased fibrinogen may be present.

■ Hyperlipidemia: increased serum cholesterol, usually >350 mg/dL. Low or normal serum cholesterol levels may occur with poor nutrition and suggest poor prognosis. Serum triglycerides and total lipids are increased.

■ Helpful serologic studies can be evaluated based on the clinical settings and may include ANA testing, complement (C3, C4), serum free light chains, and urine protein electrophoresis/immunofixation, syphilis and hepatitis B and C serology.

■ Antithrombin III levels can be decreased in the blood due to its loss in the urine resulting in hypercoagulability. In addition, platelet hyperreactivity is found in 70% of patients and other abnormalities in coagulation factors, clotting inhibitors, and fibrinolytic system have been also described. Associated renal vein thrombosis has been reported in approximately 25% of cases.

■ Renal biopsy establishes the diagnosis.

Suggested Reading

Loscalzo J. Venous thrombosis in the nephrotic syndrome. *N Engl J Med*. 2013;368(10):956–958.

RADIATION NEPHROPATHY

❑ **Definition**

■ This type of nephritis involves exposure of one or both kidneys to ionizing radiation (>2,000 rad). The injury is related to total dose and duration of radiation, and it affects approximately 20% of patients receiving radiation to kidneys.

■ Latent period is 6–12 months for acute radiation nephropathy. Most affected individuals progress after >10 years to chronic nephritis with diminishing renal function and severe hypertension.

❑ **Laboratory Findings**

■ Acute: abrupt onset of hematuria, proteinuria (non-nephrotic range), severe hypertension, and severe normochromic, normocytic anemia.

■ Chronic: stable isolated proteinuria, mild to moderate hypertension and slow progression to renal failure.

RENAL ABSCESS

See Urinary Tract Infections in Chapter 7, Genitourinary System Disorders

RENAL ARTERY STENOSIS

❑ **Definition**

- Narrowing of one or both renal arteries or their branches.
- Caused by atherosclerosis and, less frequently, by fibromuscular dysplasia.
- Often leads to hypertension and chronic renal insufficiency. Ischemic nephropathy with irreversible parenchymal damage and renal failure may also occur.

❑ **Who Should Be Suspected?**

- Candidates include patients with new-onset hypertension, rapid blood pressure swings, or increase in severity of known hypertension, especially if it becomes refractory to antihypertensive therapy.
- Old age, other atherosclerotic lesions, and the presence of chronic kidney disease are risk factors.

❑ **Laboratory Findings**

- Laboratory findings are nonspecific. Diagnosis is established by imaging studies.
- Mild proteinuria is common.
- BUN and creatinine may show recent increase.
- Plasma rennin activity (PRA) in peripheral veins is often increased.

RENAL INFARCTION

❑ **Definition**

- Renal infarction commonly results from either thromboemboli, usually originating from clots in the heart or aorta, or an in situ renal artery thrombosis (less common).
- Renal artery injury and atrial fibrillation are two common causes of renal infarction. Other causes include dissecting aneurysm of the aorta or renal artery, renal artery vasculitis (e.g., polyarteritis nodosa), or having hypercoagulable state (e.g., antiphospholipid syndrome).

❑ **Who Should Be Suspected**

Candidates are patients with acute onset of flank or abdominal pain, frequently accompanied with nausea, vomiting, and fever.

❑ **Laboratory Findings**

- Urinalysis: microscopic or gross (less common) hematuria. Proteinuria may occur.
- Plasma renin activity (PRA) may rise on the 2nd day and remain elevated for more than a month.
- Increased serum creatinine concentration, particularity in patients with a large embolus.
- Serum LDH is markedly increased (>400 U/L).
- WBCs, CRP, and ESR are usually increased.
- CT scan helps establish the diagnosis and asses the infarction.

12

RENAL TUBULAR ACIDOSIS

- Renal tubular acidosis (RTA) refers to a group of disorders in which metabolic acidosis develops due to defects in the kidney's ability to appropriately acidify the urine.
- All forms of RTA (1–4) are characterized by normal anion gap and hyperchloremic metabolic acidosis.

❏ Distal RTA (Type 1)

- Characterized by impaired secretion of H^+ and therefore ammonium by the collecting ducts.
- It should be suspected in any patient with metabolic acidosis with normal anion gap (AG) and inappropriately high urine pH.
- Major causes in adults include autoimmune disease (e.g., Sjögren syndrome, SLE, rheumatoid arthritis) and hypercalciuria (e.g., vitamin D intoxication, hyperparathyroidism). In addition, drugs (e.g., ifosfamide, amphotericin B) or other diseases (pyelonephritis, Hodgkin disease, cryoglobulinemia, amyloidosis, sarcoidosis, medullary sponge kidney) can also cause distal RTA. In children, hereditary distal RTA is the most common cause.

❏ Laboratory Findings

- High urine pH (>5.3; usually in the 6.5–7 range) regardless of serum bicarbonate concentration. Urinary pH below 5.3 generally excludes distal (but not proximal) RTA. Urine sodium concentration is typically >25 mEq/L. Urine ammonium excretion is reduced and can be estimated indirectly by measurement of the urine anion gap or osmolal gap. This parameter can distinguish patients with distal RTA from those who have normal anion gap metabolic acidosis and hypokalemia due to other causes.
- Blood potassium level is usually low.
- Hyperchloremic acidosis and low serum bicarbonate concentration (may be <10 mEq/L).
- Ammonium loading test shows inability to acidify urine below pH 5.3.

❏ Proximal RTA (Type 2)

- This condition results from defective bicarbonate reabsorption in the proximal tubule, causing bicarbonate wasting in the urine. This wasting continues until serum bicarbonate concentration reaches a level that is low enough to allow all of the filtered bicarbonate to be reabsorbed.
- It can be present as an isolated disorder or in association with a generalized proximal tubular dysfunction called Fanconi syndrome, in which reabsorption of other solutes such as phosphate, glucose, uric acid, and amino acids is impaired resulting in bone demineralization (osteomalacia or rickets) due to phosphate wasting.
- Most commonly due to increased excretion of light chains in multiple myeloma and other monoclonal gammopathies. Other causes of proximal RTA include drugs (e.g., carbonic anhydrase inhibitors, ifosfamide, aminoglycosides), heavy metals (e.g., lead, mercury), and vitamin D deficiency. Primary causes of proximal RTA can be idiopathic or familial

(e.g., bicarbonate transfer mutations, tyrosinemia, galactosemia, Wilson disease, cystinosis, and carbonic anhydrase type 2 deficiency).

❏ Laboratory Findings

- Variable urine pH, depending on whether the patient is treated with alkali therapy or not (generally elevated with alkali therapy and appropriately 5.3 or less in untreated patients in whom filtered bicarbonate level is below the bicarbonate reabsorptive threshold).
- Low serum bicarbonate concentration (12–20 mEq/L) with hyperchloremic acidosis. Intravenous (IV) infusion of sodium bicarbonate (0.5–1.0 mEq/kg/hour) causes an increase in serum bicarbonate concentration toward normal (18–20 mEq/L) and a rapid increase in urine pH (>7.5) and fractional excretion of bicarbonate (>15–20%).

❏ Combined or Mixed RTA (Type 3)

Mixed RTA is most often applied to a rare autosomal recessive syndrome that results from carbonic anhydrase II deficiency and has features of both proximal and distal RTA.

❏ Hyperkalemic RTA (Type 4)

- This type results from either aldosterone deficiency (e.g., primary adrenal insufficiency, ACE inhibitors, severe illness, inherited disorders) or tubular resistance to aldosterone action (e.g., pseudohypoaldosteronism).
- Characterized by mild hyperchloremic metabolic acidosis and hyperkalemia.
- Major laboratory findings: serum bicarbonate concentration typically >17 mEq/L, urine pH <5.3, and increased plasma potassium.
- See Table 12-6.

Suggested Reading

Kelepouris E, Agus ZS. Overview of renal tubular acidosis. In: Basow DS (ed). *UpToDate*. Waltham, MA: UpToDate; 2013.

TABLE 12–6. Characteristics of Different Types of Renal Tubular Acidosis

	Distal RTA (Type 1)	Proximal RTA (Type 2)	Hyperkalemic RTA (Type 4)
Primary defect	Impaired distal acidification	Defective proximal bicarbonate reabsorption	Decreased aldosterone secretion or resistance to aldosterone action
Hyperchloremic acidosis	Yes	Yes	Yes (mild)
Urine pH	>5.3	Variable (depending on serum bicarbonate level)	<5.3
Serum bicarbonate	Usually reduced (may be <10 mEq/L)	12–20 mEq/L	>17 mEq/L
Serum potassium	Reduced (corrects with alkali therapy)	Reduced (decreases further with alkali therapy)	Increased

RENAL VEIN THROMBOSIS

❑ Definition
- This condition is characterized by the formation of a thrombus that obstructs one or both renal veins.
- Most commonly associated with nephrotic syndrome and severe dehydration. Other causes include trauma, DIC, tumors, oral contraceptives, and hypovolemia (especially in infants).

❑ Who Should Be Suspected?
- Infants with acute loss of renal function.
- Patients with subacute or chronic deterioration of renal function in the appropriate setting, including those with thrombophilia or an underlying renal disease.
- Frequently associated with deep vein thrombosis or pulmonary embolism.
- Acute onset is associated with pain in the lower back and sides of the abdomen, fever, decreased urine output, and bloody urine.

❑ Laboratory Findings
- Diagnosis is made by imaging studies.
- Urinalysis shows mild proteinuria and RBCs.
- Fibrin degradation products and D-dimer can be elevated.
- Various findings according to the underlying disease.

Suggested Reading
Wysokinski WE, Gosk-Bierska I, Green EL, et al. Clinical characteristics and long-term follow-up of patients with renal vein thrombosis. *Am J Kidney Dis.* 2008;51:224–232.

URIC ACID NEPHROPATHY

❑ Definition
Hyperuricemia causes several renal conditions due to kidney deposition of uric acid. These conditions can be divided into three types:
- Chronic urate nephropathy: a rare form of renal insufficiency caused by deposition of urate crystals in the kidney's medullary interstitium, resulting in chronic inflammatory response.
- Acute uric acid nephropathy: a reversible cause of renal insufficiency that results from deposition of large amounts of uric acid crystals in the renal tubules and characterized by severe oliguria or anuria.
- Uric acid nephrolithiasis: may develop as a consequence of persistently low urine pH and sometimes hyperuricemia. Kidney stones caused by uric acid crystals occur in approximately 15% of patients with gout (compared to 8% in people without gout) and may cause kidney damage. Large stones can block one of the ureters, thus preventing the kidney from removing wastes and causing genitourinary tract infections.

❑ Who Should Be Suspected?
- Chronic urate nephropathy can be considered in patients with chronic renal insufficiency and severe hyperuricemia that is out of proportion to the degree of renal insufficiency.

- Acute uric acid nephropathy is suspected in patients with acute onset of oliguria or anuria, especially following chemotherapy or radiation therapy for a hematologic malignancy or, less commonly, a nonhematologic tumor (tumor lysis syndrome). It can be also suspected in patients with Lesch-Nyhan disease, which results in overproduction of uric acid, and in those with decreased uric acid reabsorption in the proximal tubules (Fanconi-like syndrome).
- Uric acid nephrolithiasis is mainly suspected in patients with gout and those on uricosuric drugs, in subjects exposed to dehydration or chronic diarrhea, and in those with diabetes, metabolic syndrome, or myeloproliferative neoplasms.

❏ Laboratory Findings

- Urinalysis: twenty-four–hour urine collection may reveal hyperuricemia. Uric acid crystals may be visualized in the urine sediment. Calcium oxalate and amorphous urate crystals can also be seen.
- Serum uric acid may be increased and is greatly elevated in the tumor lysis syndrome.
- Early renal damage is indicated by decreased renal concentrating ability, mild proteinuria, and decreased phenolsulfonphthalein (PSP) excretion. Later renal damage is indicated by slowly progressive azotemia with slight albuminuria.
- In uric acid nephrolithiasis, urinary pH is low (5.5 or lower).
- In acute uric acid nephropathy, uric acid-to-creatinine ratio (mg/mg) is >1.0 in a random urine sample, whereas in most forms of AKI with decreased urinary output the ratio is <1.0. Hyperkalemia, hyperphosphatemia, and hypocalcemia may also accompany acute uric acid nephropathy, especially when it is the result of severe tissue destruction (e.g., tumor lysis syndrome).

Suggested Reading

Wiederkehr MR, Moe OW. Uric acid nephrolithiasis: a systemic metabolic disorder. *Clinic Rev Bone Miner Metab.* 2011;9:207–217.

CONGENITAL KIDNEY DISORDERS

ECTOPIC KIDNEY

- Ectopic kidney or renal ectopy is a birth defect in which a kidney is located below, above, or on the opposite side of its usual position. The incidence is 1:1,000.
- The ectopic kidney generally has decreased function compared to the normal kidney, but the majority of patients are asymptomatic. In symptomatic patients, findings are mainly related to associated complications such as urinary tract infections, kidney stones, obstruction, or kidney damage.
- Diagnosed by imaging studies.

HEREDITARY NEPHRITIS (ALPORT SYNDROME)

- A genetic disorder caused by mutations in the genes encoding the alpha chains of type IV collagen. Approximately 85% of cases are due to mutations in the *COL4A5* gene located on the X chromosome (X-linked inheritance), which encodes the α_5 chain of type IV collagen. The remaining cases result from mutations at the *COL4A3/COL4A4* locus on chromosome 2, encoding the α_3 and

α_4 chains of type IV collagen. Inheritance of Alport syndrome caused by these mutations is autosomal recessive or, much less commonly, autosomal dominant.

- The initial renal manifestation during childhood is persistent microscopic hematuria, which may become gross hematuria after upper respiratory infection. Later in life, patients demonstrate progressive renal insufficiency and proteinuria. ESRD may develop during adulthood.
- In addition to renal abnormalities, patients often exhibit systemic manifestations, the most common of which are hearing impairment and ocular abnormalities.
- Diagnosis is based on family history and the specific manifestations such as renal failure and hearing loss. Renal biopsy findings by electron microscopy are essential for the diagnosis.

Suggested Reading

Haas M. Alport syndrome and thin glomerular basement membrane nephropathy: a practical approach to diagnosis. *Arch Pathol Lab Med.* 2009;133(2):224–232.

HORSESHOE KIDNEY

- This congenital disorder involves fusion of two kidneys across midline, usually at the lower poles.
- Incidence is 1 in 500 or less; higher in females with Turner syndrome (15%).
- Usually asymptomatic, though patients with this condition have increased risk of renal abnormalities such as renal obstruction, infections, stones, and tumors. Laboratory abnormalities are usually due to these renal complications.

MEDULLARY CYSTIC KIDNEY DISEASE

- Medullary cystic kidney disease (MCKD), also known as autosomal dominant interstitial kidney disease (ADIKD), is inherited in an autosomal dominant pattern and characterized by progressive kidney disease and adult-onset renal failure. It is similar to juvenile nephronophthisis but occurs in older patients and is limited to the kidneys with no extrarenal organ involvement. Fluid-filled medullary cysts can be present in some cases.
- Three types of MCKD have been described based on the genetic mutations:
  ▼ Mutations in the *UMOD* gene, which encodes uromodulin (Tamm-Horsfall mucoprotein): this condition is also called MCKD type 2 or uromodulin-associated kidney disease (UAKD) and presents in the majority of MCKD cases. It is characterized by hyperuricemia that results from reduced urate excretion.
  ▼ Mutation in the *REN* gene, which encodes renin.
  ▼ Mutations in the *MUC1* gene, which encodes mucin 1 (also referred to as MCKD type 1).
  ▼ Mutations in *REN* and *MUC1* genes have been described in only some families. Additional mutations of other unidentified genes may account for some other cases.
- UAKD patients typically present during their teenage years with gout, hyperuricemia, and mild elevation in serum creatinine. ESRD typically develops between the ages of 20 and 70 years. Urinalysis is typically bland with minimal or no proteinuria.

- Similar to UAKD, patients with *REN* mutations also develop early-onset gout, but their CDK progresses more slowly and ESRD occurs after age 40. Additionally, these patients demonstrate anemia and may have hyperkalemia.
- Patients with *MUC1* mutations present with slowly progressive CKD with no early onset of gout.
- Diagnosis of all types is based on family history and clinical presentation. Definitive diagnosis is achieved by genetic testing.

Suggested Reading

Bleyer A. Autosomal dominant interstitial kidney disease (medullary cystic kidney disease). In: Basow DS (ed). *UpToDate*. Waltham, MA: UpToDate; 2013.

MEDULLARY SPONGE KIDNEY

❏ Definition

This congenital condition is characterized by cystic dilation and malformation of the collecting tubules as well as cyst formation in the medulla. The evidence for genetic transmission is little, and a positive family history is usually absent.

❏ Who Should Be Suspected?

Most patients are asymptomatic, and the condition may be discovered incidentally after a radiologic testing. Symptomatic patients often present with hematuria, kidney stones, and UTI.

Diagnosis is confirmed by imaging studies.

NEPHRONOPHTHISIS

❏ Definition

Nephronophthisis (NPHP) is inherited in an autosomal recessive fashion and characterized by decreased urine concentration ability, chronic nephritis, and progression to ESRD at an early age (typically <20 years). It is the most common genetic cause of ESRD in the first two decades of life.

❏ Who Should Be Suspected?

Patients typically present with polyuria, polydipsia, anemia, and mild proteinuria. Urine sediment is typically bland. Depending on the specific gene defect, patients may also have extrarenal symptoms such as retinal defects, liver problems, and skeletal defects.

❏ Laboratory Findings

Depending on the median age of onset of ESRD, three clinical variants have been described: infantile (median age 4 years), juvenile (the most common variant; median age 13 years), and adolescent (median age 19 years).

- Eleven different mutations in the genes encoding components of the primary cilia or renal epithelial cells have been identified (*NPHP1–NPHP11*). Mutations of the *NPHP1* gene are most common (20% of cases) and characterized by ESRD at a mean age of 13 years (juvenile NPHP). Mutations in the other genes contribute to only <3% of cases each. The main causative gene is still unknown in approximately 70% of individuals with NPHP. Mutations in the *NPHP2* gene are associated with the infantile form and those in the

NPHP3 gene are rare and associated with the adolescent form. The juvenile form is associated with mutations in all the *NPHP* genes except *NPHP2*.

▪ Pathologic studies demonstrate sever tubular damage and a thickened basement membrane. NPHP histology findings are similar to those found in MCKD.

Suggested Reading
Wolf MT, Hildebrandt F. Nephronophthisis. *Pediatr Nephrol.* 2011;26(2):181–194.

POLYCYSTIC KIDNEY DISEASE

Polycystic kidney disease (PKD) is a genetic disorder characterized by the growth of numerous cysts in the kidney and has two major forms—autosomal dominant and autosomal recessive.

❑ Autosomal Dominant Polycystic Kidney Disease (ADPKD)

▪ It is the most common hereditary kidney disease affecting 1–2:1,000 live births.
▪ Approximately 85–90% of ADPKD mutations occur in the *PKD1* gene located on chromosome 16, whereas the remaining mutations (10–15%) occur in the *PKD2* gene located on chromosome 4. Patients with *PKD2* gene mutations generally have a less severe phenotype.
▪ Symptoms usually develop during the fourth decade of life, but can start earlier. ADPKD leads to progressive renal failure due to continued enlargement of the cysts and replacement of normal kidney tissue. In addition, patients suffer from other complications such as hypertension, hematuria, renal infarction, kidney stones, and renal infections.
▪ Diagnosis is based on a family history of ADPKD and imaging studies demonstrating the presence of kidney cysts. Cysts can also be found in other organs such as the liver and pancreas. Genetic testing can distinguish between *PKD1* and *PKD2* mutations.

❑ Autosomal Recessive Polycystic Kidney Disease (ARPKD)

▪ Less common than ADPKD with an incidence of 1: 20,000 live births. It is caused by mutations of the *PKHD1* (polycystic kidney and hepatic disease 1) gene and typically identified during the first few weeks after birth.
▪ Children born with ARPKD often develop kidney failure before reaching adulthood. In addition, they demonstrate liver scarring and can have nephrolithiasis, hypertension, and urinary tract infections.
▪ Kidney and liver imaging studies of the fetus or newborn establish the diagnosis.

Suggested Reading
Harris PC, Torres VE. Polycystic kidney disease. *Annu Rev Med.* 2009;60:321–337.

RENAL PARENCHYMAL MALFORMATION

❑ Definition
This condition causes failure of normal nephron development and results from genetic and environmental factors. Genetic factors include mutations in the genes expressed during kidney development (e.g., *EYA1, SIX1, TCF2, SALL1, FRAS1, PAX2*); environmental factors include exposure to teratogens and nutritional deficiencies.

❏ Laboratory Findings

- Renal parenchymal malformation disorders can be distinguished based on histologic examinations and they include:
  - ▼ Renal hypoplasia: the number of structurally normal nephrons is decreased. Renal size is typically reduced by 2 standard deviations from the mean size for the age.
  - ▼ Renal dysplasia: characterized by the presence of malformed kidney tissue elements. Dysplastic kidneys are variable in size but usually smaller than normal.
  - ▼ Renal agenesis: defined as congenital absence of renal parenchymal tissue. The majority of patients with unilateral renal agenesis are asymptomatic.
  - ▼ Multicystic dysplasia: characterized by a nonfunctioning dysplastic kidney with multiple cysts.
  - ▼ Renal tubular dysgenesis: very rare disorder characterized by the absence or poor development of proximal tubules.
- Imaging and genetic studies establish the diagnosis.

THIN BASEMENT MEMBRANE NEPHROPATHY (BENIGN FAMILIAL HEMATURIA)

❏ Definition

- This relatively common familial disorder affects approximately 1% of the general population and is considered, along with IgA nephropathy and Alport syndrome, a common cause of hematuria in children and adults.
- In addition to hematuria, patients with thin basement membrane nephropathy (TBMN) have uniformly thinned glomerular basement membrane as determined be electron microscopy.
- The genetic defect is similar to that of hereditary nephritis (Alport syndrome). Approximately 40% of patients with TBMN have heterozygous mutations at the *COL4A3/COL4A4* locus and thus can be considered carriers of autosomal recessive Alport syndrome.
- Prognosis is benign and hematuria clears spontaneously with time.

❏ Who Should Be Suspected?

Possible candidates are patients with a family history of hematuria (noted in 30–50% of patients). Macroscopic hematuria can happen and may be associated with flank pain but without evidence of renal disease.

❏ Laboratory Findings

- Laboratory diagnosis is directed to exclude other glomerular disorders that may cause isolated hematuria, such as IgA nephropathy and Alport syndrome.
- Urinalysis: microscopic hematuria can be persistent or intermittent and is usually asymptomatic. Urinary dysmorphic RBCs and RBC casts may present.
- Renal function and urinary protein excretion are frequently normal.
- Diagnosis requires the demonstration of diffusely thin GBMs by electron microscopy. If these are found, it is necessary to rule out Alport syndrome by immunohistologic and genetic studies.

Suggested Reading

Haas M. Alport syndrome and thin glomerular basement membrane nephropathy: a practical approach to diagnosis. *Arch Pathol Lab Med.* 2009;133(2):224–232.

VON HIPPEL-LINDAU DISEASE

❑ Definition
Von Hippel-Lindau disease (VHLD) is a rare genetic disorder inherited in an autosomal dominant manner and caused by mutations of the von Hippel-Lindau tumor suppressor gene on the short arm of chromosome 3. Approximately 20% of VHLD patients have a de novo mutation and do not have a family history of the disease.

❑ Who Should Be Suspected?
- Clinical hallmarks are the development of retinal and central CNS hemangioblastomas, pheochromocytomas, multiple visceral cysts in the pancreas and kidneys, and an increased risk for malignant transformation of renal cysts into renal cell carcinoma, which is the leading cause of death in VHLD patients.
- Classified in two types, depending on the likelihood of developing pheochromocytoma:
  - ▼ Type 1: results from deletion or nonsense mutations. Patients mainly have hemangioblastomas; renal cell carcinoma and pheochromocytoma are rare.
  - ▼ Type 2: results from missense mutations and subdivided into 2A, 2B, and 2C. Patients with this type are at high risk of developing pheochromocytoma. Type 2A patients are at risk of hemangioblastomas and pheochromocytomas, but not renal cell carcinomas; type 2B patients are at risk of all three tumors with a high risk of renal cell carcinoma; type 2C patients are at risk for only pheochromocytoma.

❑ Laboratory Findings
- Complete blood count (CBC) to look for evidence of polycythemia vera due to increased erythropoietin production.
- Urinalysis: to detect hematuria. Analysis of catecholamine metabolites in the urine (metanephrine, normetanephrine, dopamine, and vanillylmandelic acid) may aid to detect pheochromocytoma. Urine cytology may detect renal cell carcinoma.
- Diagnosis is also based on family history, imaging studies, and genetic testing.

Suggested Reading

Maher ER, Neumann HP, Richard S. von Hippel-Lindau disease: a clinical and scientific review. *Eur J Hum Genet.* 2011;19(6):617–623.

 # KIDNEY TUMORS

JUXTAGLOMERULAR CELL TUMOR

❑ Definition
This very rare rennin-secreting tumor is a benign tumor that mainly affects adolescents and young adults, with peak prevalence in the second and third decades of life.

❑ **Who Should Be Suspected?**

The main characteristics of this tumor are hypertension and hyperaldosteronism secondary to excessive rennin secretion by tumor cells. Patients typically present with headache, retinopathy, double vision, dizziness, nausea, polyuria, and proteinuria.

❑ **Laboratory Findings**

- Plasma rennin activity (PRA) is increased, with levels significantly higher in the renal vein from the affected side.
- Hyperaldosteronism and hypokalemia.

RENAL CELL CARCINOMA

❑ **Definition**

Renal cell carcinoma (RCC) originates from the lining of the proximal tubule. It is the most common type of kidney cancer, responsible for 80–85% of primary renal neoplasms and 2–3% of all malignant diseases in adults.

❑ **Who Should Be Suspected?**

- RCC is more common in males than females (2:1 ratio), with a typical presentation in the sixth and seventh decades of life. Many patients are asymptomatic until later stages of the disease. The classic triad of RCC (hematuria, flank pain, and palpable renal mass) occurs in only 9% of patients and usually suggests advanced disease.
- At least four hereditary syndromes associated with renal cell carcinoma have been recognized, including von Hippel-Lindau syndrome, hereditary papillary renal carcinoma, familial renal oncocytoma, and hereditary renal carcinoma.

❑ **Laboratory Findings**

- Urinalysis: microscopic or gross hematuria, which can be associated with the presence of clots.
- Complete blood count (CBC) shows anemia, either normal or microcytic; anemia usually precedes the diagnosis of RCC by several months. Erythrocytosis is found in up to 5% of patients due to increased production of erythropoietin.
- Serum testing may show hypercalcemia and increased serum ferritin.

Suggested Reading

Rini BI, Campbell SC, Escudier B. Renal cell carcinoma. *Lancet.* 2009;373(9669):1119–1132.

WILMS TUMOR

❑ **Definition**

- It is the most common renal malignancy in childhood (95% of cases are diagnosed before 10 years of age).
- This tumor has been associated with loss-of-function mutations of a number of tumor suppressor genes including the *WT1, FTW1, FTW2,* and *p53* genes.
- Diagnosis is by histologic examination of a renal biopsy or the tumor removed surgically.

❏ **Who Should Be Suspected?**

Candidates are children between the ages of 3 and 10 years, with an abdominal mass, hematuria, abdominal pain, or hypertension.

❏ **Laboratory Findings**

- Urinalysis may show proteinuria in some cases.
- Serum creatinine may be elevated. Liver function tests, if abnormal, may indicate the presence of hepatic metastasis. Hypercalcemia may accompany other associated syndromes.
- Studies for Von Willebrand disease (vWD) are indicated since up to 8% of affected children have acquired vWD disease and may bleed at surgery.
- Genetic studies of tumor suppressor genes can be helpful.

 RENAL DISORDERS IN SELECTED DISEASES

AMYLOIDOSIS-ASSOCIATED KIDNEY DISEASE

❏ **Overview**

- See primary amyloidosis.
- This condition, which involves amyloid deposition in the kidneys, is one of the most frequent complications of AA, AL, and several hereditary forms of amyloidosis.

❏ **Who Should Be Suspected?**

Candidates include patients with known systemic amyloidosis who develop proteinuria or, in the absence of this diagnosis, individuals with new-onset proteinuria, renal insufficiency, or nephrotic syndrome of unknown etiology.

❏ **Laboratory Findings**

- Urinalysis: persistent proteinuria, associated with glomerular deposits of amyloid. Proteinuria varies from mild, with or without hematuria, to massive with urinary protein excretion rate in the nephrotic range (>3.5 g/day) and may exceed 20 g/day. Urinary protein is mostly albumin. Urine sediment is typically benign.
- GFR is reduced, and serum creatinine concentration is moderately elevated.
- Hypoalbuminemia and other findings secondary to the nephrotic syndrome are seen in advanced cases. ESRD develops in 20% of renal amyloidosis patients with nephrotic syndrome.
- Nephrogenic diabetes insipidus (DI) and renal tubular acidosis may result from tubular deposition of amyloid.

Suggested Reading

Dember LM. Amyloidosis-associated kidney disease. *J Am Soc Nephrol*. 2006;17:3458–3471.

DIABETIC NEPHROPATHY

❏ **Overview**

- See diabetes mellitus (DM).
- Diabetic nephropathy (DN), also referred to as diabetic kidney disease or Kimmelstiel-Wilson disease, is characterized by persistent proteinuria and

TABLE 12–7. Evolution of Renal Disease in Insulin-Dependent Diabetes Mellitus (IDDM)

Stage	Time of Onset	Laboratory Finding*	Morphologic Findings	% of Cases Progress
Early	At time of diagnosis	↑ GFR	Kidney size ↑	100
Renal lesion; no clinical signs	2–3 y after diagnosis	↑ GFR; albuminuria cannot be detected	↑ thickness of glomerular and tubular capillary basement membrane; glomerulosclerosis	35–40
Incipient nephropathy	7–15 y after diagnosis	Albuminuria 0.03–0.3 g/d. N or sl ↑ GFR; beginning to decline	Glomerulosclerosis progressing	80–100
Clinical diabetic nephropathy	10–30 y after diagnosis	Albuminuria >0.3 g/d N or sl D GFR; steady fall	Glomerulosclerosis widespread	>75
End stage renal disease	20–40 y after diagnosis	GFR <10 mL/min; serum creatinine ≥10 mg/dL		

D, decreased; GFR, glomerular filtration rate; I, increased; N, normal; sl, slightly.
*when albuminuria is 0.075–0.1 g/d in IDDM, significant renal disease is present and albuminuria will progress to clinical nephropathy. GFR declines—10 mL/min/y after nephropathy is established.
Source: Selby JV, Fitz-Simmons SC, Newman M, et al. The natural history and epidemiology of diabetic nephropathy. *JAMA.* 1990;263:1954–1960.

progressive renal insufficiency in diabetic patients in the absence of other renal diseases. Approximately one third of patients with diabetes develop DN years after diagnosis. DN is the most common cause of ESRD in the United States and Europe, with ESRD incidence of 30% in type 1 DM and up to 20% in type 2 DM (see Table 12-7).

- Microalbuminuria is an early sign of the development of DN and has very high specificity and positive predictive value for subsequent DN. It is also associated with a longer duration of diabetes, poorer glycemic control, higher blood pressure, development of more advanced retinopathy and neuropathy, subsequent renal failure, increased vascular damage, and risk for cardiovascular disease.

❏ **Who Should Be Suspected?**

- Diabetes and DN are more prevalent in blacks, Mexican Americans, Polynesians, and Maoris. Additional risk factors include poorly controlled diabetes, positive family history, and uncontrolled hypertension.
- Generally, any patient presenting with progressive renal failure or proteinuria should be investigated for the presence of DM. On the other hand, all patients with DM should have urinalysis and renal function studies performed periodically.

❏ **Laboratory Findings**

- Microalbuminuria (urinary albumin excretion between 30 and 300 mg/day, or 30–300 mg/g creatinine using a random urine sample) usually appears 5–10 years after the onset of diabetes. Macroalbuminuria, also referred to as clinical albuminuria (>300 mg/g creatinine), can occur at later stages and may in some cases develop to frank nephrotic syndrome. An elevated albumin/creatinine ratio should be confirmed with an additional first-void urine specimen collected in the next 3–6 months (see Figure 12-4).

- Urine sediment is usually bland, but hematuria may rarely occur.
- Serum protein may be decreased, especially in the advanced disease.
- BUN and creatinine rise gradually; azotemia usually develops several years after the onset of proteinuria.
- Measurement of hemoglobin A1c (HbA1c) in DM patients and maintaining it at a target value of approximately 7.0% helps prevent or delay progression of DN.

Suggested Readings

DOQI clinical practice guidelines and clinical practice recommendations for diabetes and chronic kidney disease. *Am J Kidney Dis.* 2007;49(2 Suppl 2):S12–S154. http://www.kidney.org/professionals/kdoqi/pdf/Diabetes_AJKD_FebSuppl_07.pdf

KDOQI clinical practice guideline for diabetes and CKD: 2012 update. *Am J Kidney Dis.*2012;60(5):850–886.http://www.kidney.org/professionals/KDOQI/guidelines_diabetesUp/diabetes-ckd-update-2012.pdf

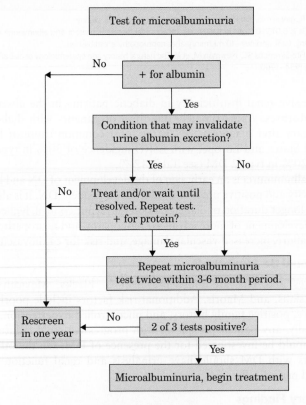

Figure 12–4 *Screening for microalbuminuria.*
Source: American Diabetes Association. Nephropathy in diabetes.
Diabetes Care. 2004 Jan;27 Suppl 1:S79–83.

HENOCH-SCHÖNLEIN PURPURA NEPHRITIS

❏ **Overview**

- See Henoch-Schönlein purpura (HSP).
- HSP, also termed IgA vasculitis, involves hypersensitivity systemic vasculitis of small vessels with deposition of IgA-containing immune complexes. It mainly affects the skin as well as other organs such as the kidneys, digestive tract, and joints. This condition can occur at any time in life, but most common in children.
- Kidney damage is the most common long-term complication of HSP. It is more frequent and tends to be more severe in adults than children. Renal involvement is typically noted shortly after the onset of systemic symptoms. Up to 30% of adults will experience CKD or kidney failure within 15 years after diagnosis.
- Diagnosis is mainly clinical.

❏ **Laboratory Findings**

- Hematuria and proteinuria are present in approximately one third of patients and usually associated with decreased GFR. Nephrotic-range proteinuria is more likely to be seen in adults than children.
- Elevated serum levels of IgA and IgA-containing immune complexes.
- Renal biopsy supports the diagnosis and assesses severity of the disease. Biopsy results are identical to those found in IgA nephropathy.

LUPUS NEPHRITIS

❏ **Overview**

- See systemic lupus erythematosus (SLE).
- Up to 60% of patients with SLE are diagnosed with lupus nephritis (LN). The prevalence is significantly higher in blacks and Hispanics than in whites, and higher in men than women. The International Society of Nephrology/Renal Pathology Society classification divides LN into six classes (I–VI) based on kidney biopsy histopathology.

❏ **Laboratory Findings**
Depend on the class of LN:

- Minimal mesangial LN (class I): patients have normal urinalysis and serum creatinine concentration.
- Mesangial proliferative LN (class II): microscopic hematuria and mild proteinuria may be present.
- Focal LN (class III): involves <50% of glomeruli and can be subdivided into subclasses depending on the activity/chronicity of the lesions. It is characterized by hematuria and proteinuria. In some patients, proteinuria may be in the nephrotic range and serum creatinine may be elevated.
- Diffuse LN (class IV): divided into subclasses similar to class III. Hematuria and proteinuria are present. Some patients may display nephrotic-range proteinuria and hypertension.
- Membranous LN (class V): most patients have nephrotic syndrome.
- Advanced sclerosing LN (class VI): characterized by sclerosis involving more than 90% of glomeruli.

12

- Titers of anti-DNA antibodies are elevated, and levels of C3 and C4 are low.
- Kidney biopsy is performed to establish the diagnosis and classify LN.

Suggested Reading

Hahn BH, McMahon MA, Wilkinson A, et al. American College of Rheumatology guidelines for screening, treatment, and management of lupus nephritis. *Arthritis Care Res.* 2012;64(6):797–808. http://www.rheumatology.org/practice/clinical/guidelines/Lupus_Nephritis_Guidelines_Manuscript.pdf

MYELOMA KIDNEY

❑ Overview

- See plasma cell myeloma.
- Myeloma kidney, or myeloma cast nephropathy, is a common complication of plasma cell myeloma in which monoclonal light chain (Bence Jones [BJ] proteins) excretion in the urine contributes to acute or chronic renal failure. Less frequently, high levels of free light chains can lead to immunoglobulin light chain amyloidosis or light chain deposition disease. These conditions are usually associated with insidious progression of renal failure rather than acute kidney injury.

❑ Laboratory Findings

- Increased urinary excretion of light chains (>100 mg/day but can be much higher; normal <30 mg/day). Bence Jones proteinuria is not detectable by urine dipstick and occurs in <50% of myeloma patients but in almost all patients with renal failure due to myeloma kidney. Kidney damage can also lead to albuminuria and azotemia.
- Protein electrophoresis and immunofixation of serum and a 24-hour urine collection help establish the diagnosis and determine the type and amount of monoclonal protein and light chains.
- Severe anemia out of proportion to azotemia occurs.
- Altered renal tubular function may result in hypophosphatemia, oliguria, and nephrogenic diabetes insipidus. Urine sediment is typically bland.
- Kidney biopsy can be helpful if a definitive diagnosis is needed.

Suggested Reading

Dimopoulos MA, Terpos E, Chanan-Khan A, et al. Renal impairment in patients with multiple myeloma: a consensus statement on behalf of the International Myeloma Working Group. *J Clin Oncol.* 2010;28(33):4976–4984. http://myeloma.org/pdfs/IMWG-Renal-Impairment.pdf

POLYARTERITIS NODOSA, RENAL DISEASE

❑ Overview

- See polyarteritis nodosa.
- Renal involvement occurs in 75% of polyarteritis nodosa patients and is associated with renal insufficiency and hypertension. Renal infarction can also be seen in severe cases.

❑ Laboratory Findings

- Mild azotemia that is slowly progressive.
- Albuminuria and hematuria are common. Fat bodies are frequently present in urine sediment.

RENAL TUBERCULOSIS

See chapter 7, Genitourinary System Disorders.

SCLERODERMA, RENAL DISEASE

❑ **Overview**

- See scleroderma.
- Renal involvement occurs in more than 50% of scleroderma patients and is associated with increased mortality.
- Scleroderma renal crisis (SRC) is the most severe renal condition associated with scleroderma. SRC is seen in approximately 10–20% of diffuse cutaneous scleroderma patients and in only 1% of patients with limited cutaneous scleroderma. It is characterized by acute onset of hypertension, thrombotic microangiopathy, progressive renal failure, and a 5-year survival rate of 65%.

❑ **Laboratory Findings**

- Progressive renal insufficiency with mild proteinuria (often <2 g/day). Urine sediment is typically normal.
- SRC is associated with acute kidney injury that is characterized by oliguria and sudden onset of proteinuria or hematuria. Microangiopathic hemolytic anemia and thrombocytopenia are also seen in some patients.
- Plasma renin activity is markedly elevated in SRC patients.
- Anti-RNA polymerase III autoantibodies are detected in one third of patients with SRC.

Suggested Reading

Bussone G, Bérezné A, Pestre V, et al. The scleroderma kidney: progress in risk factors, therapy, and prevention. *Curr Rheumatol Rep.* 2011;13(1):37–43.

SICKLE CELL NEPHROPATHY

❑ **Overview**

- See sickle cell disease.
- Renal function abnormalities are common in sickle cell disease patients, and they include glomerular and tubular disorders. These abnormalities are mainly caused by sickling of RBCs in the microvasculature and usually associated with increased mortality.
- Generally, renal manifestations are more severe in patients with sickle cell disease (SCD) than those with sickle cell trait or combined hemoglobinopathies.

❑ **Laboratory Findings**

- Urinalysis: proteinuria is present in 15–40% of SCD patients and can be in the nephrotic range. Asymptomatic hematuria (microscopic, macroscopic, or gross) is common in SCD. Early decrease in the kidney concentrating ability is evident in patients with SCD leading to polyuria. This finding is less pronounced in patients with sickle cell trait.

- Low serum creatinine level due to hypersecretion in the proximal tubule and glomerular hyperfiltration is a common finding in young patients with SCD. Later in life, progressive decrease in GFR due to glomerular injury occurs with increased serum levels of BUN and creatinine.
- Urinary acidification capacity can be altered, resulting in renal tubular acidosis.
- Renal failure occurs in approximately 5–18% of SCD patients.
- Papillary necrosis, renal infarction, and renal medullary carcinoma can develop in affected patients.

Suggested Reading

Da Silva GB Jr, Libório AB, Daher Ede F. New insights on pathophysiology, clinical manifestations, diagnosis, and treatment of sickle cell nephropathy. *Ann Hematol.* 2011;90(12):1371–1379.

 # KIDNEY TRANSPLANTATION

❑ Overview

- Kidney transplantation is the most effective form of renal replacement therapy and treatment of choice for end-stage renal disease.
- It has been recommended that transplantation should not proceed unless the measured or calculated GFR is <20 mL/minute, and there is evidence of progressive and irreversible deterioration in renal function over the previous 6–12 months.
- Initial evaluation of potential kidney recipients and living donors includes medical and surgical history, physical examination, chest x-ray and imaging studies, electrocardiogram, and laboratory testing.

❑ Laboratory Evaluation of Recipients and Donors

- ABO blood type and HLA typing.
- Urinalysis and urine culture, GFR, and protein excretion.
- Serologic testing for HIV, HBV, HCV, HAV, cytomegalovirus, Epstein Barr virus, herpes simplex virus, varicella virus, and syphilis testing.
- Other laboratory tests include CBC, electrolytes, BUN, creatinine, uric acid, albumin, calcium, phosphorus, lipid panel, and liver function tests.
- For deceased donors, history of active viral infection, malignancy, renal disease, and hypertension is obtained.

❑ Exclusion Criteria for Donors

- Kidney problems: impaired renal function, proteinuria, hematuria, kidney disease, or vascular abnormalities of the kidney or urinary tract
- Diabetes mellitus
- Active viral infection (HIV, HBV, HCV or CMV)
- Active or history of malignancy
- Presence of chronic disease (pulmonary, cardiac, neurologic, hepatic, autoimmune)
- Sever hypertension
- Pregnancy

❑ HLA Testing in Kidney Transplantation[1]

HLA testing has been an indispensable component in transplantation since the recognition that antibodies, directed against lymphocytes, were associated with allograft failure. This crucial finding led to the discovery of the MHC and the appreciation of the importance of HLA testing in transplantation. Early approaches focused on the importance of HLA matching and were an important aspect of deceased donor organ allocation. As a direct result of improvements in immunosuppression in recent years, we are now challenged with selecting donor–recipient pairs based on acceptable mismatches, especially for patients with HLA alloantibodies. Therefore, routine HLA testing for kidney transplantation is more comprehensive, including both HLA typing/matching and antibody identification. Posttransplant monitoring also becomes a common practice to provide early antibody-mediated rejection warning. The testing plan listed below is recommendation only. Developing a testing agreement with the transplant team is a requirement by the United Network for Organ Sharing (UNOS) and can be unique to each transplant center.

A. New patient testing

▼ All new transplant candidates and potential donors are prospectively typed for HLA-A, HLA-B (include Bw4/6), HLA-C, HLA-DRB1, HLA-DQA1, HLA-DQB1, and HLA-DRB345. HLA-DPB1 typing is performed for all patients and their potential donors if the patient has DPB1 antibodies or is enrolled in a paired exchange program.

▼ All new transplant candidates are screened for the presence of anti-HLA IgG antibodies. All confirmed positive screens should have multiple samples and assays to assign antibody specificity, monitor antibody strength, and identify possible interference, such as IgM, endogenous complement masking, or prozone effect.

▼ Auto and allo prospective T- and B-cell cross-matches by complement-dependent cytotoxicity (CDC), Anti-human globulin (AHG)-enhanced CDC methods are performed for all new transplant candidates. Serum collected within 2 months is used in the preliminary cross-match. If a sensitization event is documented, a serum collected within 2–3 weeks after should be used for cross-match.

▼ Flow T- and B-cell allo cross-matches are performed on all sensitized and/or retransplant patients. Additionally, auto prospective T and B Flow cross-matches will be done for patients in whom autoimmune disease as the cause of ESRD is communicated at the time of new patient evaluation.

▼ Alternative cross-match: For patients with >80% cPRA, the donor's HLA typing via buccal swab can be requested instead of cross-matching. Donors can be ruled out if unacceptable donor-specific antigens are present.

▼ The extent of sensitization of each patient at the time of his/her initial evaluation and the following of potentially sensitizing events are monitored by the transplant coordinator and communicated to the histocompatibility laboratory. The pretransplant coordinator should obtain serum samples 2–3 weeks after known sensitizing events and have them sent to the HLA laboratory for storage or testing. Such information is recorded in the HLA management database.

12

[1]The HLA Testing in Kidney Transplantation section was contributed by Neng Yu, MD.

▼ Results of this comprehensive evaluation are submitted to the transplant program within 1 week of the initial visit, and the patient will be listed with UNOS if qualified. The kidney donor options are live donor (both related and unrelated), deceased donor (UNOS waitlist), and paired exchange program.

B. Monthly antibody screening program

▼ All renal transplant candidates are required to submit monthly serum to be screened or used for cross-match. Rotated regularly sera under the program is screened by single antigen bead assay or PRA antibody screen.

▼ Changes in specificity or strength are reviewed and updated in the UNET. All negative-to-positive conversion has to be confirmed by the single antigen bead assay.

C. Interim antibody screen and cross-match

In the case of a sensitizing event after the completion of preliminary patient donor workup, an interim antibody screening by single antigen bead assay is advised to reassess the patient's antibody specificities and identify possible donor-specific antibody (DSA). The pretransplant coordinator will obtain the serum sample 2–3 weeks after known sensitizing events and have them sent to the HLA laboratory. If antibody profile changes, the Laboratory Director and the transplant team may require interim cross-match by CDC and/or flow.

D. Final cross-match

Prior to transplant

▼ Complete DNA typing for both the patient and donor.

▼ Two HLA antibody samples from two separate appointments and one preliminary CDC/AHG-CDC cross-match with the donor.

Final XM (performed within 2 weeks of scheduled transplant):

▼ Allo T- and B-cell CDC, AHG-CDC, and Flow cross-match, antibody screen on Patient.

▼ Auto T- and B-cell CDC, AHG-CDC (optional).

Serum selection:

Selection of sera for final cross-matching of patients should address the impact of historic and current sensitizing events. Selection recommendations:

▼ Current serum (collected within 2 weeks).

▼ Historic serum if the patient is sensitized with preference to serum that contains DSA that were defined by single antigen bead assay (collected within 6 months, preferably).

▼ The serum sample collected 2–3 weeks after a known sensitizing event should be included in cross-match if available. Most often, the current sample would meet this requirement.

Results of the final cross-matches are reported to the transplant program before renal transplantation or combined organ and tissue transplants in which a kidney is to be transplanted, except for emergencies. If emergency transplants are performed before the cross-match test results are available, information provided by the transplant candidate's physician to the laboratory as to the reason for the emergency transplant is documented.

DSA: Donor-specific antibody is determined based on the patient's HLA antibody profile and the potential donor's HLA type. The DSA specificity can change when patients change their potential donors. Since patients and donors are fully typed during initial evaluation, HLA antibody analysis can identify DSA for each patient–donor pair.

E. Deceased donor transplant HLA testing

Deceased kidneys must be allocated according to the UNOS policies. The final decision to accept a particular organ will remain the choice of the transplant surgeon and/or physician responsible for the care of the candidate. This allows physicians and surgeons to exercise their medical judgment regarding the suitability of the organ being offered for a specific candidate, to be faithful to their personal and programmatic philosophy about such controversial matters as the importance of cold ischemia time and anatomic anomalies, and to give their best assessment of the prospective recipient's medical condition at the moment. If an organ is declined for a candidate, a notation of the reason for that decision must be made on the appropriate form and submitted to the UNOS promptly.

The minimum typing requirements for both recipient and donor are antigens. When reporting DR antigens, DRBI and DRB3/4/5 must be reported. The lab is encouraged to report splits for all loci.

Calculated PRA (cPRA) is the percentage of donors expected to have one or more of the unacceptable antigens indicated on the waiting list for the candidate. Sensitized waiting list candidates with defined unacceptable HLA antigens that yield a cPRA of 80% or greater will be assigned points on the waitlist based on the current allocation policy. Each transplant center may define the criteria for unacceptable antigens that are considered as contraindications for transplantation. Unacceptable antigens that are defined by laboratory detection of HLA-specific antibodies must be determined using at least one solid-phase immunoassay using purified HLA molecules. It is the prerogative of the transplant center to establish criteria for additional unacceptable antigens, such as repeat transplant mismatches. The cPRA will be calculated automatically when the unacceptable antigens are listed or updated on the waiting list. The cPRA will be derived from the HLA antigen/allele group and haplotype frequencies for the different racial/ethnic groups in proportion to their representation in the national deceased donor population.

A prospective cross-match is mandatory for all candidates, except where clinical circumstances support its omission. The transplant program and its histocompatibility laboratory must have a joint written policy that states when the prospective cross-match may be omitted. Guidelines for policy development, including assigning risk and timing of cross-match testing, are set out in UNOS Appendix D to Policy 3.

F. UNET waitlist maintenance and transplant support

The UNOS has developed an online database system, called UNET, to collect, store, analyze, and publish all Organ Procurement and Transplantation Network (OPTN) data that pertain to the patient waiting list, organ matching, and transplants. Launched on October 25, 1999, this system contains data regarding every organ donation and transplant event occurring in the United States since 1986. UNET is a fail-safe, 24/7, secure internet-based transplant information database. It enables the nation's organ transplant institutions to register patients for transplants, match donated organs to waiting patients, and manage the time-sensitive, life-critical data of all patients before and after their transplants.

When a new patient is listed in the UNET by the Transplant Program, the data will be verified by HLA staff using most current typing and antibody results. Double review is required for any UNET edits, and the documentation will be signed and stored in the patient file indefinitely.

As required by the UNOS, the UNET Waitlist histocompatibility data for each patient for whom the laboratory performed testing are reviewed and verified monthly or as needed by the HLA lab staff. Documentation of such reviews is kept for at least 3 years or the interval required by local, state, and Federal regulations, whichever is longer. They are available for audit by the UNOS. The unacceptable antigen list is uploaded to the UNET each month to establish cPRA value.

G. Posttransplant monitoring
Risk Stratification:

▼ High risk: DSA+, both to live or deceased current donor
▼ Intermediate risk: DSA- and cPRA >80%, HLA-mismatched transplant only
▼ Low risk: DSA- and cPRA <80% or 0 mismatched transplant
▼ Clinical risk: prior transplant; low-risk patient with clinical indications

Monitoring schedule:

Group	Frequency
High Risk	Week 1, 2, 4, 8, then Every 6 months to 5 years
Intermediate Risk	Every 6 months to 5 years
Clinical Risk	As needed
Low Risk	Annual

❑ Acute Renal Allograft Rejection

▪ Although 0 HLA-mismatched grafts generally have superior transplant outcomes compared to ≥1 HLA-mismatched grafts, some 0 HLA mismatches may be complicated by acute rejection, possibly due to incompatibilities at other minor HLA loci or the imperfect tissue typing methods used routinely. On the other hand, some ≥1 HLA-mismatched grafts have excellent graft outcomes, suggesting that certain HLA mismatches may be permissible under certain circumstances.

▪ HLA-DR mismatches are associated with the highest risk of acute rejection after kidney transplantation compared to mismatches at the HLA-A and HLA-B loci. Additionally, HLA mismatches exert their effects at different times posttransplant (e.g., the maximum effect of HLA-DR mismatching occurs within the first 6 months, whereas that of HLA-B mismatching arises 2 years posttransplant).

▪ The most common form of acute allograft rejection involves activation of recipient T cells directed against donor MHC antigens. Additionally, B cells may play an important role in the immune response to an allograft through the production of antibodies that either mediate acute or chronic rejection of the allograft (antibody-mediated rejection) or, in the case of acute cellular rejection, support recipient T cells.

- Acute renal allograft rejection is associated with acute deterioration in allograft function and specific pathologic changes in the graft. Most episodes of acute rejection occur during the first 6 months after transplantation, with many episodes occurring early after surgery.
- Although most patients who have acute rejection episodes are asymptomatic, some patients occasionally present with fever, malaise, oliguria, hypertension, and graft pain or tenderness. Differential diagnoses in symptomatic patients include viral infection (BK, CMV, and adenovirus), bacterial pyelonephritis, and urinary leak or obstruction.
- An acute rise in serum creatinine level over the patient's baseline is the main laboratory finding in patients with acute allograft rejection. This finding, however, occurs relatively late in the course of rejection and usually indicates the presence of significant histologic damage. Other laboratory findings reported with acute rejection include decreased urinary output, proteinuria, appearance of urinary cellular or granular casts, decreased urine osmolality, and hyperchloremic renal tubular acidosis.
- Kidney biopsy is the gold standard for diagnosing acute rejection among transplant patients with deteriorating kidney function. The biopsy may show either cellular- or antibody-mediated rejection or both.
- Other noninvasive candidate methods for the diagnosis of acute kidney rejection include
  - ▼ Sequential measurement of subsets of activated T cells by flow cytometry.
  - ▼ Measurement of urinary concentration of mRNAs for the cytotoxic proteins perforin, granzyme B, and cyclophilin B by PCR (increased in acute rejection).
  - ▼ Other biomarker candidates for determining acute rejection have been identified by urinary proteomic analysis by mass spectrometry, and they demonstrate good diagnostic performance.

Suggested Readings

Clark B, Unsworth DJ. HLA and kidney transplantation. *J Clin Pathol.* 2010;63(1):21–25.

Murphey CL, Forsthuber TG. Trends in HLA antibody screening and identification and their role in transplantation. *Expert Rev Clin Immunol.* 2008;4(3):391–399.

Tait BD, Süsal C, Gebel HM, et al. Consensus guidelines on the testing and clinical management issues associated with HLA and non-HLA antibodies in transplantation. *Transplantation.* 2013;95(1):19–47.

UNOS Policy. http://optn.transplant.hrsa.gov/PoliciesandBylaws2/policies/pdfs/policy_7.pdf

UNOS, OPTN, Appendix D to Policy 3. http://optn.transplant.hrsa.gov/PoliciesandBylaws2/policies/pdfs/policy_109.pdf

12

Respiratory, Metabolic, and Acid–Base Disorders

Lokinendi V. Rao and Michael J. Mitchell

RESPIRATORY DISORDERS

Respiratory diseases include diseases of the lung, pleural cavity, bronchial tubes, trachea, and upper respiratory tract and diseases of the nerves and muscles of breathing. These conditions range from mild and self-limiting such as the common cold to life threatening such as bacterial pneumonia or pulmonary embolism. The symptoms of respiratory disease differ depending on the disease. Common symptoms are cough with or without the production of sputum, hemoptysis, and dyspnea, which usually occurs with exercise, chest pain, noisy breathing (either wheeze or stridor), somnolence, loss of appetite, weight loss, cachexia, and cyanosis. In some cases, respiratory disease is diagnosed in the absence of symptoms during the investigation of another disease or through a routine check.

Respiratory diseases can be classified in many different ways: by the organ involved, by the pattern of symptoms, or by the cause of the disease.

- *Obstructive lung diseases* are diseases of the lung in which the bronchial tubes become narrowed, making it difficult to move air in and especially out of the lung.
- *Restrictive lung diseases* (also known as interstitial lung diseases) are a category of respiratory diseases characterized by a loss of lung compliance, causing incomplete lung expansion and increased lung stiffness.

Respiratory tract infections can affect any part of the respiratory system. They are traditionally divided into upper respiratory tract infections (URTIs) and lower respiratory tract infections (LRTIs). The most common URTI is the common cold. However, infections of specific organs of the upper respiratory tract such as sinusitis, tonsillitis, otitis media, pharyngitis, and laryngitis are also considered URTIs. *Streptococcus pneumoniae* is the most common cause of severe, community-acquired bacterial pneumonia. Worldwide, TB is an important cause of pneumonia, usually presenting as a chronic infection. Other pathogens such as viruses and fungi can cause pneumonia, for example, severe influenza and *Pneumocystis* pneumonia. Tumors of the respiratory tract are either malignant or benign. Benign tumors are relatively rare causes of respiratory disease. Malignant tumors, or cancers of the respiratory system, particularly lung cancers, are a major health problem responsible for 15% of all cancer diagnoses and 29% of all cancer deaths. The majority of respiratory system cancers are attributable to smoking tobacco.

There are a wide range of symptoms due to the intrathoracic effects of various respiratory diseases, the most common of which are dyspnea, cough, and infections.

13

COUGH

Cough is a forced expulsive maneuver, usually against a closed glottis and which is associated with a characteristic sound. It is a natural respiratory defense mechanism to protect the respiratory tract and one of the most common symptoms of pulmonary disease. Most cases of troublesome cough reflect the presence of an aggravating factor (asthma, drugs, environmental, gastroesophageal reflex, upper airway pathology) in a susceptible individual. A cough can be classified by its duration, character, quality, and timing and is somewhat arbitrary. A cough lasting <3 weeks is termed "acute," between 3 and 8 weeks is "subacute," and one lasting >8 weeks is defined as "chronic."

❑ Acute Cough

Acute cough is defined as a cough lasting <3 weeks. Most frequently, it presents in primary care settings and is commonly associated with URTIs. In most cases, it is benign and self-limiting and most commonly related to virus induced, postnasal drip, throat clearing secondary to laryngitis or pharyngitis. It is frequently associated with acute exacerbations and hospitalizations with asthma and COPD. Symptoms associated with acute cough that require further investigation include hemoptysis, breathlessness, fever, chest pain, and weight loss. Common serious conditions presenting with isolated cough include neoplasms, infections (e.g., TB), foreign body inhalation, acute allergy–anaphylaxis, and interstitial lung disease.

❑ Subacute Cough

Subacute cough is defined as a cough lasting 3–8 weeks. The gray area between 3 and 8 weeks of cough is difficult to define etiologically, since all chronic cough will have started as acute cough, but the diagnostic group of chronic cough is diluted by the patients with postviral cough (a URTI cough lingering for >3 weeks). Cough after infection is the most common cause of subacute cough (48%), postnasal drip is the second most common (33%), and cough variant asthma is the third most common (16%). In a significant percentage of patients, subacute cough (34%) is self-limited and will resolve without treatment. Most patients with subacute cough that spontaneously resolves had a postinfection cough.

❑ Chronic Cough

Chronic cough is defined as a cough lasting >8 weeks. It is reported by 10–20% of adults and is common in women and obese people. Most patients present with a dry or minimally productive cough. The presence of significant sputum production usually indicates primary lung pathology.

Chest radiograph and spirometry are recommended. Bronchial provocation testing should be performed in patients without a clinically obvious etiology. Bronchoscopy should be undertaken in all patients with chronic cough in whom inhalation of foreign body is suspected. A cough can be dry or productive, depending on whether sputum is coughed up. Dry cough, that is, there is no "phlegm" and is caused by a virus infection, cold, or dry air or air pollutants such as cigarette smoke, smog, and dust. Productive coughs are coughs that produce phlegm and can be associated with tuberculosis, bacterial pneumonia, and bronchitis.

 PULMONARY DISEASES ASSOCIATED WITH COUGH

INFECTIOUS RESPIRATORY DISEASES

ACUTE BRONCHITIS

❑ Definitions

Acute bronchitis is a disease caused by infection and inflammation of the bronchial mucosa. Acute bronchitis is caused by respiratory viruses (e.g., influenza virus, parainfluenza virus, rhinovirus, RSV, adenovirus, corona viruses). There is little evidence to implicate bacteria as a significant cause of acute bronchitis, though atypical respiratory bacterial pathogens (*Bordetella pertussis, Mycoplasma pneumoniae, Chlamydophila pneumoniae*) cause a small proportion of cases.

❑ **Who Should Be Suspected?**

▪ Patients initially present with cold symptoms but progress to cough that persists for more than 5 days. Purulent sputum may be described; purulent sputum alone is not a reliable indication of bacterial infection and should not be used as the sole indication for antibiotic treatment. Cough resolves within 2–3 weeks in most patients.

▪ Wheezing and bronchospasm develop in some patients.

▪ Fever and systemic symptoms are unusual in uncomplicated acute bronchitis; these symptoms may suggest pneumonia or influenza.

❑ **Diagnosis**

Pertussis should be ruled out for patients with suggestive clinical signs and symptoms. Acute bronchitis is a self-limited viral infection in the vast majority of patients and does not require testing for effective management. Influenza testing might be considered during "flu season" for patients at risk for complicated influenza.

▪ Radiographic and laboratory testing may be considered in patients if clinical presentation suggests pneumonia (cough, fever, sputum production, and systemic symptoms) or chronic bronchitis (cough and sputum production on most days for at least 3 months during 2 consecutive years).

▪ There is little evidence that outcome is improved by antibiotic therapy of *M. pneumoniae* or *C. pneumoniae* infection; specific diagnostic testing for these agents is not recommended.

Suggested Reading

Wenzel RP, Fowler AA III. Acute bronchitis. *N Engl J Med*. 2006;355:2125–2130.

CROUP (LARYNGOTRACHEITIS)

❑ **Definition**

Croup refers to inflammation of the upper airway below the glottis and has been used to describe a variety of upper respiratory conditions in children, including laryngitis, laryngotracheitis, laryngotracheobronchitis, bacterial tracheitis, or spasmodic croup. Croup is usually caused by viral infection, especially parainfluenza virus, but it is occasionally caused by bacteria or an allergic reaction. It typically occurs in children 6 months to 3 years of age, usually during winter and early spring. Epiglottitis may result in acute airway obstruction and should be considered a medical emergency. A stable airway should be assured prior to collection of diagnostic specimens. Bacterial causes of epiglottitis include type b *Haemophilus influenzae*, *S. pneumoniae*, and beta-hemolytic streptococci. The clinical picture in infectious mononucleosis or diphtheria may resemble epiglottitis. TB may cause chronic laryngitis.

❑ **Who Should Be Suspected?**

▪ The hallmark of croup in infants and young children is the barking cough. In older children and adults, hoarseness predominates. Croup is usually a mild and self-limited illness, although significant upper airway obstruction, respiratory distress, and, rarely, death can occur. Symptoms usually begin with nasal irritation, congestion, and coryza. Symptoms generally progress over 12–48 hours to include fever, hoarseness, barking cough, and stridor. Respiratory distress increases as upper airway obstruction becomes more severe. Rapid progression or signs of lower airway involvement suggest a more serious illness.

- Symptoms typically persist for 3–7 days, with a gradual return to normal.
- Usually caused by viruses (80%). Parainfluenza virus (type 1–3) is the most common etiology.

❑ **Diagnostic and Laboratory Findings**

Laboratory studies are of limited diagnostic utility but may help guide management in more severe cases.

- CBC: WBC counts can be low, normal, or elevated; WBC counts >10,000 cells/μL are common. CBC differential shows neutrophil or lymphocyte predominance. The presence of a large number of band-form neutrophils is suggestive of primary or secondary bacterial infection.
- Chemistries: Not associated with any specific alterations in serum tests.
- Microbiology: Confirmation of etiologic diagnosis is not necessary, as croup requires only symptomatic therapy. Identification of a specific viral etiology may be necessary to make decisions regarding isolation for patients requiring hospitalization, for initiation of antiviral therapy, or for epidemiologic monitoring purposes.
- Culture: Diagnosis of a specific viral etiology may be made by viral culture of secretions from the nasopharynx or throat.

Suggested Readings

Cherry JD. Croup (Laryngitis, laryngotracheitis, spasmodic croup, laryngotracheobronchitis, bacterial tracheitis, and laryngotracheobronchopneumonitis). In: Feigin RD, Cherry JD, Demmler-Harrison GJ, et al. (eds). *Textbook of Pediatric Infectious Diseases*, 6th ed. Philadelphia, PA: Saunders; 2009.

Rihkanen H, Rönkkö EB, Nieminen T, et al. Respiratory viruses in laryngeal croup of young children. *J Pediatr.* 2008;152:661–665.

PERTUSSIS (WHOOPING COUGH)

❑ **Definition**

Pertussis, a syndrome characterized by prolonged and severe cough, is usually caused by the bacterium *B. pertussis*; however, *B. parapertussis*, *B. holmesii*, and *B. bronchiseptica* may also cause a pertussis syndrome. Infection is highly communicable, with potential for epidemic spread. Infection is transmitted by the direct respiratory route through exposure to droplets generated by an infected individual. Historically, the association of pertussis as a significant cause of morbidity and mortality in infants and children is well described. Implementation of routine immunization resulted in a significant reduction in the incidence of pertussis. However, since a nadir in the 1970s (0.5 cases/100,000), the incidence of pertussis has been increasing (13.4 cases/100,000 in 2012); outbreaks continue to occur in the United States. This increased incidence is likely due to multiple factors, including waning immunity among vaccines, improved diagnostics, and improved reporting. The incidence of pertussis continues to be highest among infants, followed by older children and adolescents. Spread of infection is limited by vaccination, timely diagnosis and reporting to Public Health officials, antimicrobial therapy and prophylaxis, and measures to prevent further transmission by infected patients.

❏ Who Should Be Suspected/Who Should Be Tested

- The most important issue in pertussis diagnosis is clinical recognition. Typical cases of pertussis demonstrate three phases:
- Catarrhal (7–10 days): Runny nose; mild cough; low-grade fever. The burden of *B. pertussis* is highest in the catarrhal phase.
- Paroxysmal (1–6 weeks): Severe, paroxysmal coughing spells; inspiratory whoop; cyanosis; posttussive vomiting.
- Recovery (2–4 weeks): Decreasing severity of symptoms.

Infants and patients who are unvaccinated, are immunocompromised, or have underlying medical conditions are more likely to have more severe symptoms.

- Clinical case definition: Recognition of the pertussis syndrome is critical for diagnosis. A clinical case is defined as a cough illness lasting at least 2 weeks (without other cause), with at least one of the following features: paroxysms of coughing, inspiratory "whoop" (most common in infants), posttussive vomiting.
- In the context of a pertussis epidemic, any patient with a prolonged cough illness, regardless of other symptoms, may be suspected.

❏ Diagnostic and Laboratory Findings

A number of test methods are available for detection of *B. pertussis* infection.

Tests recognized by the CDC for confirmation of pertussis:

Culture: Culture should be obtained from all suspected cases of pertussis. Isolation of *B. pertussis* confirms the diagnosis (specificity: approximately 100%), but cultures are frequently negative (sensitivity: 15–35%). Nasopharyngeal aspirate or swab (not cotton) specimens should be collected in the first 2 weeks of illness. Specimens should be directly plated onto supportive media, like Regan-Lowe or Bordet-Gengou, or inoculated into supportive media, like half-strength Regan-Lowe charcoal–blood media, for immediate transport to the laboratory. Negative cultures may be due to a number of factors including collection of specimen >2 weeks after the onset of illness, improper collection (e.g., site, swab type), delayed or improper transport conditions, prior antibiotic therapy, and recent vaccination.

PCR: Though there is no FDA-approved test for *B. pertussis*, PCR is playing an increasingly important role in diagnosis. Testing performed by a Public Health Laboratory is recommended. PCR methods have high sensitivity (93–95%) and specificity (97–99%) when performed on appropriate patients. PCR testing should only be performed on patients with a clinical diagnosis of pertussis. PCR should not be performed on asymptomatic contacts or other asymptomatic patients. Nasopharyngeal aspirate or swab (Dacron, rayon, or nylon) should be collected within the first 3 weeks after the onset of illness. Antibiotic therapy may result in false-negative PCR results.

Tests not recognized by the CDC for confirmation of pertussis:

DFA: Though very specific (>95%), the sensitivity of DFA, compared to PCR, is low (10–50%). For initial clinical management, if timely PCR testing is not available, DFA may be considered.

Serology: Serologic testing has limited utility for the diagnosis or management of patients with suspected pertussis. Serologic responses in patients usually occurs

13

2 or more weeks after the onset of cough (after the time when antibiotic therapy may be useful). Performance characteristics of commercially available tests have not been well defined for diagnosis of pertussis, and Public Health officials do not accept them for confirmation of pertussis. However, a single-point test has been validated by the Massachusetts Public Health Laboratory and is accepted by the CDC for confirmation of pertussis. This assay cannot be used for vaccinated children <11 years old or in adults vaccinated within 2 years.

❏ **Interpretation of Test Results**

Confirmed:

- Clinical: Any cough illness; lab: isolation of *B. pertussis* by culture
- Clinical: Meets CDC Clinical Case Definition; lab: positive PCR for *B. pertussis*
- Clinical: Meets CDC Clinical Case Definition and epidemiologic link to a case confirmed by culture or PCR

Probable:

- Clinical: Meets CDC Clinical Case Definition, but not confirmed by culture or PCR, and is not epidemiologically linked to a laboratory-confirmed case. Positive *B. pertussis* DFA or serology supports but does not confirm diagnosis.

Suggested Readings

Best Practices for Health Care Professionals on the Use of Polymerase Chain Reaction (PCR) for Diagnosing Pertussis. Atlanta, GA: Centers for Disease Control and Prevention; 2012. See: http://www.cdc.gov/pertussis/clinical/diagnostic-testing/diagnosis-pcr-bestpractices.html. Accessed July, 2013.

Faulkner A, Skoff T, Martin S, et al. *Chapter 10: Pertussis. Centers for Disease Control and Prevention. Manual for the Surveillance of Vaccine-Preventable Diseases*, 5th ed. Atlanta, GA: Centers for Disease Control and Prevention; 2012. See: http://www.cdc.gov/vaccines/pubs/surv-manual/index.html. Accessed July, 2013.

Loeffelholz MJ, Thompson CJ, Long KS, et al. Comparison of PCR, culture, and direct fluorescent-antibody testing for detection of *Bordetella pertussis*. *J Clin Microbiol*. 1999;37:2872–2876.

Tilley PAG, Kanchana MV, Knight I, et al. Detection of *Bordetella pertussis* in a clinical laboratory by culture, polymerase chain reaction, and direct fluorescent antibody staining; accuracy, and cost. *Diagn Microbiol Infect Dis*. 2000;37:17–23.

She RC, Billetdeaux E, Phansalkar AR, et al. Limited applicability of direct fluorescent-antibody testing for *Bordetella* sp. and *Legionella* sp. specimens for the clinical microbiology laboratory. *J Clin Microbiol*. 2007;45:2212–2214.

 NONINFECTIOUS RESPIRATORY DISEASES

SARCOIDOSIS

❏ **Definition**

- Sarcoidosis is a multiorgan disorder of unknown etiology, characterized by granuloma formation, predominantly in the lungs and intrathoracic lymph nodes. It can affect all individuals with any race, sex, and age, but commonly affects middle-aged adults.

- In the United States, the incidence of sarcoidosis ranges from 5 to 40 cases for 10,0000 populations. The age-adjusted incidence for whites is 11 cases per 10,0000 population. Incidence is higher in African American (34/10,0000) and seems to experience more severe and chronic disease. Also, in African Americans, siblings and parents of sarcoidosis cases have about 2.5-fold increased risk for developing the disease.

- Internationally, the incidence is 20 cases per 10,0000 in Sweden, 1.3 cases per 10,0000 in Japan, and low in China, Africa, India, and other developing countries and could be hidden and misdiagnosed as tuberculosis.

- Incidence peaks in persons aged 25–35 years, and a second peak occurs for women aged 45–65 years. Male-to-female ratio is approximately 2:1. Morbidity, mortality, and extrapulmonary involvement are higher in affected females.

- Several studies have reported on association between environmental factors and occurrence of sarcoidosis. These include wood-burning stoves, tree pollen, soil exposures, inorganic particles, insecticides, and moldy environment. Also, several occupational associations are also observed, that include ship's servicemen, navy, metal work, building supplies, fire workers, hardware, and gardening materials.

❏ Who Should Be Suspected?

- Clinical presentation of sarcoidosis is variable and depends on ethnicity, duration of illness, site and extent of organ involvement, and activity of the granulomatous process.

- Sarcoidosis typically presents with bilateral hilar lymphadenopathy, pulmonary infiltration, and skin and ocular lesions.

- Sarcoidosis can be clinically classified as
  - ▼ *Asymptomatic sarcoidosis*: Incidentally detected on chest imaging. Thirty to 50% of patients found to be asymptomatic at the time of diagnosis.
  - ▼ *Sarcoidosis with nonspecific constitutional symptoms*: Observed more frequently in African Americans and Asian Indians. The nonspecific symptoms include fever (39–40°C), weight loss (2–6 kg), fatigue, and malaise.
  - ▼ *Sarcoidosis with symptoms related to specific organ involvement*: Acute sarcoidosis has sudden onset, more frequently seen in Caucasians and may part as Lofgren syndrome (bilateral hilar adenopathy, erythema nodosum, and ankle arthritis) and constitutional nonspecific symptoms. Organ-related symptoms, often related to pulmonary infiltration (cough and dyspnea).
    - ● *Pulmonary sarcoidosis*: Asymptomatic (30–60%), but chest radiograph abnormalities are high (85–95%). Clinical course is very heterogenous, with 2/3 patients show spontaneous remissions and can be chronic and progressive about 10–30% of patients causing destruction of lung and permanent loss of lung function. Seventy-five percent of patients have bilateral lymphadenopathy.
    - ● *Extrapulmonary*: Common but is almost always associated with lung involvement. May involve entire length of respiratory tract airways causing obstructive airway disease and broad spectrum of airway dysfunction. Common in African Americans than in Caucasians, and

13

in addition, the eyes, bone marrow, extrapulmonary lymph nodes, and skin are more frequently involved.

● *Cutaneous disease:* Skin lesions can be divided into specific and non-specific on the basis of the presence or absence of granulomatous inflammation on histopathology. Erythema nodosum, lupus pernio, and violaceous rash on the cheek or more are common.

● *Ocular disease:* Most common ocular manifestation is anterior uveitis, which can manifest with blurred vision, red, painful eyes, and photophobia. Conjunctiva can be affected in 6–40% of cases. Optic neuropathy is rare but can cause rapid, permanent loss of vision or color vision.

● *Hepatic disease:* Hepatic sarcoidosis is usually asymptomatic, but the common features are abdominal pain, pruritus, fever, weight loss, and jaundice. Biopsy-based studies showed presence of granulomas is 50–65% of patients and serology-based studies showed abdominal liver function tests in 35% of patients.

● *Cardiac disease*: Known to give rise to heart failure, arrhythmias, sudden cardiac death, and granulomatoses, inflammation in the heart is present in 25% of patients.

● *Renal disease*: Common, although clinically important involvement is occasional. Glomerular involvement is rare. Most patients remain asymptomatic, but nephrolithiasis (1–14%), nephrocalcinosis (observed in half of patients with renal insufficiency), and polyuria are potential complications. Hypercalciuria and hypercalcemia due to hyperabsorption of dietary calcium are most often responsible for renal involvement, but granulomatous interstitial nephritis, glomerular disease, obstructive uropathy, and rarely end-stage renal disease may occur.

❏ **Diagnostic and Laboratory Findings**

▪ Diagnosis requires biopsy in most cases. Endobronchial biopsy via bronchoscopy is often done.

▪ Routine laboratory evaluation is often unrevealing, but possible abnormalities include hypercalcemia, hypercalciuria, and elevated alkaline phosphatase and angiotensin-converting enzyme (ACE) levels.

▪ *Kveim-Siltzbach test:* This is a skin test specially designed for the diagnosis of sarcoidosis. It involves intradermal injection of sarcoid tissue preparation resulting in a specific localized granulomatous response (firm red papules) in patients with sarcoidosis. This test is poorly standardized and rarely used.

▪ Pulmonary function test: Spirometry and diffusing capacity of the lung for the carbon monoxide (DLCO) are commonly used.

▪ Serologic tests: A variety of laboratory and biologic markers are available such as ACE, lysozyme, neopterin, soluble IL-2 receptor, soluble intercellular adhesion molecules (ICAM-1, IFN-8), or in bronchoalveolar lavage (BAL) fluid, such as high lymphocytes, activation of marker expression on T cells, CD4/CD8 ratio, macrophages, TNF-alpha release, collagen III peptide, vitronectin, fibronectin, and hyaluronan. None of the mentioned markers are clinically recommended as routine assessment, except for serum ACE.

▪ Serum ACE is elevated in 40% of patients who have clinically active disease. It has limited value in the diagnosis, but useful in monitoring the course of disease and treatment.

Suggested Reading
Dastoori M. et al. Sarcoidosis—a clinically oriented review. *J Oral Pathol Med.* 2013;42:281–289.

UPPER AIRWAY COUGH SYNDROME

❑ Definition
Upper airway cough syndrome (UACS) is the newly recommended term to replace postnasal drip syndrome, referring to cough associated with upper airway conditions, because it is unclear whether the mechanism of cough is postnasal drip, direct irritation, or inflammation of the cough receptors in the upper airway. Postnasal drip is the drainage of secretions from the nose or paranasal sinuses into the pharynx. UACS, which is secondary to a variety of rhinosinus conditions, is the most common cause of chronic cough. It includes a variety of diseases: allergic rhinitis, perennial nonallergic rhinitis, nonallergic rhinitis with eosinophilia (NARES), bacterial sinusitis, and allergic fungal sinusitis, rhinitis due to anatomic abnormalities, rhinitis due to physical or chemical irritants, and occupational rhinitis.

❑ Who Should Be Suspected?
Clinically, the diagnosis depends on the reporting of the patient of a sensation of having something drip down into the throat, nasal discharge, or frequent throat clearing. The presence of mucoid, mucopurulent secretions, or cobblestoning of the mucosa during nasopharyngeal or oropharyngeal examination is also suggestive of UACS. It is the most common cause of the chronic condition.

❑ Diagnostic Findings
- In patients with chronic cough, the diagnosis of UACS-induced cough should be determined by considering a combination of criteria, including symptoms, physical examination findings, radiographic findings, specific allergen testing (to check whether acquired hypogammaglobulinemia is present) and, ultimately, the response to specific therapy. Because UACS is a syndrome, no pathognomonic findings exist.
- Specific therapy is instituted when the cause of chronic cough is apparent; empiric therapy should be considered in cough of unknown etiology.

Suggested Reading
Pratter MR. Chronic upper airway cough syndrome secondary to rhinosinus diseases (previously referred to as postnasal drip syndrome): ACCP evidence-based clinical practice guidelines. *Chest.* 2006;129(1 Suppl): 63S–71S.

13

 DYSPNEA

❑ Definition
"Dyspnea" is a term used to characterize a subjective experience of breathing discomfort that comprises qualitatively distinct sensations that vary in intensity (American Thoracic Society guidelines, 2012). The experience derives from interactions among multiple physiologic, psychological, social, and environmental factors and may induce secondary physiologic and behavioral responses. It is a common symptom that afflicts millions of patients with pulmonary disease.

- The majority of patients with chronic dyspnea of unclear etiology have one of four diagnoses: asthma, COPD, interstitial lung disease, or myocardial dysfunction. Mild dyspnea is common. Dyspnea is a common chief complaint among patients who come to the emergency department. The majority of life-threatening causes of dyspnea are classified below.
- Life-threatening upper airway causes: tracheal foreign objects, angioedema, anaphylaxis, infections of the pharynx, and neck and airway trauma
- Life-threatening pulmonary causes: pulmonary embolism, COPD, asthma, pneumothorax, pulmonary infections, ARDS, direct pulmonary injury, and pulmonary hemorrhage
- Life-threatening cardiac causes: ACS, flash pulmonary edema, high-output heart failure, cardiomyopathy, cardiac arrhythmia, valvular dysfunction, and cardiac tamponade.
- Life-threatening neurologic causes: stroke, neuromuscular disease
- Life-threatening toxic and metabolic causes: poisoning, salicylate poisoning, carbon monoxide poisoning, DKA, sepsis, anemia, and acute chest syndrome
- Other miscellaneous causes include lung cancer, pleural effusion, ascites, pregnancy, hyperventilation, anxiety, and massive obesity.
- The combination of all historical elements and physical examination findings is helpful in diagnosing the cause of both acute and chronic dyspnea.
- Advanced cardiopulmonary exercise testing is the most accurate way to diagnose dyspnea. Many standard diagnostic tests for shortness of breath, including noninvasive cardiopulmonary testing, EKG, CT, and pulmonary function testing, provide inconclusive results or misdiagnosis.
- There are relatively few blood tests that are necessary in the initial evaluation of a patient with dyspnea. Hemoglobin and hematocrit to exclude anemia, and ABG measurements may be a value in managing severe underlying cardiopulmonary disease. D-Dimer is a component of the evaluation of patients with suspected PE. For patients with acute dyspnea, especially those who come to ER, BNP or NT-pro BNP may be useful for the evaluation of heart failure as the cause of dyspnea.

PULMONARY DISEASES ASSOCIATED WITH DYSPNEA

INFECTIOUS RESPIRATORY SYNDROMES ASSOCIATED WITH DYSPNEA

LOWER RESPIRATORY TRACT SYNDROMES

BRONCHIOLITIS

❏ **Definition**

Bronchiolitis is an inflammatory disease of the small airways and may be caused by a variety of infectious or noninfectious conditions. Infectious bronchiolitis is usually caused by viral pathogens and is primarily a disease of infants and young children. *Respiratory syncytial virus* (RSV) is the primary cause of bronchiolitis (approximately 75%), especially severe bronchiolitis that requires medical attention or hospitalization. Rhinovirus and other respiratory viral pathogens may causes bronchiolitis, including parainfluenza virus (type 3), human metapneumovirus, influenza virus, and adenovirus. Monoclonal antibody therapy or antiviral therapies may be considered for infants with severe RSV infection.

❏ **Who Should Be Suspected?**
■ Bronchiolitis usually occurs in the fall and winter, during the peak times of circulation of seasonal respiratory viruses. The peak incidence is in children 2–6 months of age. Children with cardiac or pulmonary disease, immunodeficiency, and history of premature birth are at increased risk for serious disease.
■ There may be nonspecific findings of viral respiratory infection, like rhinitis. The major clinical manifestation is air trapping due to expiratory obstruction. Wheezing is common.
■ Infants present with an increased respiratory rate and obvious difficulty breathing marked by nasal flaring. Severely affected infants may be cyanotic. Fever is not a prominent feature.

❏ **Diagnostic and Laboratory Findings**
Diagnostic studies are not required for the management of most infants with clinical signs and symptoms of bronchiolitis; testing should be reserved for patients for whom results are likely to affect management decisions, like decisions regarding the need for antibiotic therapy.

Chest radiograph: May be indicated to rule out pneumonia.

Core labs: ABGs may be monitored in infants with severe disease. Core laboratory tests are usually normal, although fluid status must be monitored carefully because of the risk of dehydration due to tachypnea.

Molecular tests: Commercially available assays, which include testing for a panel of respiratory viruses, are recommended for establishing a specific diagnosis. These assays show improved sensitivity and specificity compared to viral culture or antigen testing; they also enable detection of a broader range viruses.

Antigen detection: Detection of specific antigen in nasopharyngeal secretions is available for several relevant viruses, like influenza viruses A and B, RSV, and human metapneumovirus. Assays based on DFA staining are useful for evaluation of specimen quality and have shown improved sensitivity compared to IFA assays. Because of the rapid turnaround time and reasonable specificity, antigen detection assays may be helpful in establishing a diagnosis. Infection cannot be ruled out by antigen assays because of their limited sensitivity and the limited scope of viruses tested.

Culture: Most of the relevant viruses may be isolated by viral culture, but turnaround time is slow. Therefore, viral culture is usually not helpful for acute clinical management.

LEGIONELLA INFECTION (LEGIONNAIRES DISEASE)

❏ **Definition**
Legionella species have been documented as a relatively common cause of community-acquired and nosocomial pneumonia. Infection is usually caused by *Legionella pneumophila*, a fastidious aerobic gram-negative bacillus, but several other species may also cause disease. Respiratory infections are the primary manifestation of legionellosis.

❑ Who Should Be Suspected?

The pulmonary signs and symptoms of *Legionella* pneumonia are fairly nonspecific and are characterized by progressive respiratory distress (dyspnea, cough, and minimal sputum production). Symptoms outside the respiratory tract may increase the likelihood of legionellosis. GI symptoms, including diarrhea, nausea and vomiting, hepatic dysfunction, and abdominal pain, occur frequently and may be prominent. Patients often develop confusion or other neurologic findings. Hyponatremia occurs more frequently in legionellosis and in other types of pneumonia.

❑ Laboratory Findings

Specific diagnosis is most reliably based on culture isolation and antigen detection.

Culture: Isolation requires the use of special media, usually a combination of selective and nonselective buffered charcoal yeast extract (BCYE) agars. Using pleural fluid, lung biopsy, or transtracheal or bronchial aspirate, organisms may require 3–7 days' incubation for isolation.

Direct antigen detection and serology: Urine antigen testing is an important method for diagnosis of Legionnaires diseases caused by *L. pneumophila* serogroup 1 (approximately 90% of community-acquired and approximately 60% of nosocomial respiratory *Legionella* respiratory infections). The specificity of the urine antigen test is approximately 99%. Antigen may be detected in urine for several days after the initiation of antimicrobial therapy. The sensitivity of urine antigen testing depends on the probability of infection with *L. pneumophila* serogroup 1 and the severity of infection. About 90% of patients with severe legionellosis that requires hospitalization should show a positive urine antigen test, whereas only about 50% of outpatients with milder legionellosis will yield a positive urine antigen test. The specificity of the urine antigen test is approximately 99%.

Serologic testing may be a useful adjunct to diagnostic testing, but serologic testing plays a limited role in acute patient management because of the time required to provide definitive results. Serum IFA testing is recommended and allows detection of immunoglobulin subclasses. Testing for total antibody as well as specific IgM and IgG is recommended. Seroresponse may not be detectable for weeks to months after acute infection. Only half of infected patients will seroconvert at 2 weeks. Therefore, testing paired acute and multiple convalescent (2, 4, 6, 8, and 12 weeks) serum samples is recommended. A diagnosis is supported by detection of specific IgM or by a fourfold or greater change in titer between acute and convalescent specimens. Specificity depends on the antigen preparation used in the assay. Tests that use *L. pneumophila* serogroup 1 demonstrate the best specificity (approximately 99%), while assays that use polyvalent antigen preparations demonstrate somewhat lower (90–95%) specificity.

Direct detection: Gram stain of sputum is of little use for detection because the faintly staining organisms are frequently masked by the proteinaceous background. Patient specimens show few to moderate number of PMNs. Stains with enhanced staining of *Legionella*, like silver or Gimenez staining, also show poor overall sensitivity for detection of legionellosis. DFA staining is very specific but shows variable sensitivity (25–75%). Therefore, a negative DFA test result cannot rule out legionellosis and does not substitute for culture.

Molecular testing: PCR-based assays have been described, but FDA-approved tests are not available. Molecular assays have not been shown to be superior to culture for the diagnosis of *Legionella* infection.

Published assays show moderate to high sensitivity, depending on the type of specimen tested, and high specificity. An advantage of most molecular diagnostic tests, compared to the urine antigen assay, is their ability to detect all *Legionella* species, rather than being limited to *L. pneumophila* serogroup 1.

Core laboratory findings: WBC count is increased (10,000–20,000/µL) in 75% of cases (leukopenia is a bad prognostic sign); thrombocytopenia is common. Hypophosphatemia; hyponatremia; hypoalbuminemia (<2.5 g/dL); proteinuria (approximately 50% of patients); microscopic hematuria; and abnormal LFTs (mild to moderate increase of serum AST, ALP, LD, or bilirubin is found in approximately 50% of patients).

Suggested Readings

Fields BS, Benson RF, Besser RE. Legionella and Legionnaires' disease: 25 years of investigation. *Clin Microbiol Rev.* 2002;15:506–526.

Newton HJ, Ang DKY, van Driel IR, et al. Molecular pathogenesis of infections caused by *Legionella pneumophila. Clin Microbiol Rev.* 2010;23:274–298.

BACTERIAL PNEUMONIA

❏ Definition
Pneumonia describes infection of the pulmonary parenchyma. Bacteria most commonly gain access to lower respiratory tract directly, by inhalation or aspiration, or by hematogenous seeding from a distal site of infection. *Streptococcus pneumoniae* is the most common cause of serious community-acquired bacterial pneumonia. Viruses are implicated in about 30% of cases of community-acquired pneumonia. Other pathogens, like *H. influenzae, Moraxella catarrhalis, M. pneumoniae, Legionella,* and *C. pneumoniae,* are also significant pathogens. *Staphylococcus aureus* and gram-negative bacilli are often implicated in nosocomial pneumonias.

❏ Who Should Be Suspected?
- A broad range of conditions predispose to bacterial pneumonia, including underlying medical conditions (e.g., alcoholism, decreased level of consciousness, malnutrition, immune compromise, uremia), toxic exposure (e.g., inhalants, tobacco smoke, environmental pollutants), structural or functional defects of normal pulmonary defense mechanisms (e.g., COPD, cystic fibrosis, bronchiectasis, ciliary dysfunction), and age >65 years.
- Common symptoms include dyspnea, shortness of breath, pleuritic chest pain, cough, and sputum production, typically purulent. Systemic signs include fever and malaise; a significant minority of patients report rigors.
- Physical examination may demonstrate diffuse or localized abnormalities, including rales, ronchi, and diminished breath sounds.

❏ Diagnostic and Laboratory Findings
- Pneumonia is generally diagnosed on the basis of clinical signs and symptoms and CXR.
- Diagnostic testing depends on the severity of disease and specific risk factors. Healthy outpatients may be managed without additional laboratory testing.

13

For patients with significant infection or risk for complications of respiratory tract infection, CBC, blood culture, sputum Gram stain, and culture are recommended. High-resolution CT scanning may be requested in patients with negative CXR.

- The diagnosis of tuberculosis should be considered and ruled out as appropriate. Special culture techniques (e.g., *Legionella* culture) or urine antigen testing (e.g., *Legionella*, *S. pneumoniae*) might be considered. Additional respiratory pathogens may be considered on the basis of epidemiologic risk and clinical presentation.

- Sputum specimens should be collected prior to initiation of antibiotic treatment. Patients should be instructed on how to produce a "deep" specimen and avoid mixing saliva with the specimen. Abstaining from eating for several hours and rinsing the mouth prior to collection may improve the quality of expectorated sputum specimens.

- The value of lower respiratory culture is limited by the quality of the specimen submitted, and results must be carefully interpreted. Criteria for accepting sputum, based on the presence of PMN and bacteria, and the absence of SECs should be established for routine bacterial cultures in order to avoid inoculation of contaminated specimens. Quantitative culture of BAL specimens may improve diagnosis for patients who are unable to provide a good-quality expectorated sputum sample or when unusual pathogens are suspected.

- Informative cultures should show moderate to heavy growth of a bacterial pathogen as the predominant growth in culture. Cultures that yield growth of three or more species in comparable quantities are more likely to be contaminated and are of limited value for managing patients. A specific pathogen can only be identified by culture in about half of patients with community-acquired pneumonia that requires hospitalization. Blood culture is positive in approximately 20% of these patients; pneumococcal urinary antigen is positive in approximately 50%.

- PCR may demonstrate improved sensitivity, but the impact on patient management has not been demonstrated.

- *Core laboratories*: Leukocytosis (>15,000 with left shift) is typical for acute bacterial pneumonia. Leukopenia is associated with poor prognosis. Serial measurement of ABGs, electrolytes, and other analytes should be collected to monitor the respiratory and metabolic status of patients with severe infection. Abnormalities typical for underlying medical conditions or severity of disease should be evaluated.

Suggested Readings

Mandell LA, Wunderink RG, Anzueto A, et al. Infectious Diseases Society of America/American Thoracic Society consensus guidelines on management of community-acquired pneumonia in adults. *Clin Infect Dis.* 2007;44:S27–S72.

Reimer LG, Carroll KC. Role of the microbiology laboratory in the diagnosis of lower respiratory tract infections. *Clin Infect Dis.* 1998;26:742–748.

van der Eerden MM, Vlaspolder F, de Graaff CS, et al. Value of intensive diagnostic microbiological investigation in low- and high-risk patients with community-acquired pneumonia. *Eur J Clin Microbiol Infect Dis.* 2005;24:241–249.

PNEUMOCYSTIS PNEUMONIA (PCP)

❏ Definition
Pneumocystis jirovecii (formerly *Pneumocystis carinii*) infection is almost exclusively restricted to pulmonary disease in immunocompromised patients. Its role as an opportunistic pathogen was described after World War II in malnourished children affected by atypical pneumonia and subsequently as a rare cause of pneumonia in patients with hematologic malignancies. The incidence of PCP increased dramatically in the 1980s in association with HIV infection. Though the incidence of *P. jirovecii* pneumonitis has decreased in recent years, due to the use of highly active antiretroviral therapy and prophylaxis in susceptible patients, PCP remains an important cause of pulmonary disease in immunocompromised patients. PCP is an opportunistic infection in patients with HIV infection and is an AIDS-defining illness in these patients. The incidence of PCP has fallen dramatically in patients compliant with highly active antiretroviral treatment.

❏ Who Should Be Suspected?
Radiology: Most patients with *Pneumocystis* pneumonitis show bilateral, diffuse interstitial infiltrates on CXR. Some patients with PCP have no abnormality on CXR. In such patients, high-resolution CT scans have high sensitivity for detecting the characteristic ground-glass abnormalities of PCP.

HIV-infected patients: The onset of PCP is usually slowly progressive with fever, shortness of breath, tachypnea, and nonproductive cough. Fatigue, weight loss, and other symptoms are common. Chest x-rays most commonly demonstrate diffuse, bilateral abnormality usually consisting of interstitial infiltrates; other patterns may be seen. Gallium scanning shows intense diffuse uptake. The risk of PCP is inversely related to CD4 counts; patients with HIV infection are at highest risk when the CD4 count falls below 200 cells/mm^3.

Non–HIV-infected patients: These patients typically present with acute onset of respiratory failure, fever, and nonproductive cough. Glucocorticoid use and defects in cell-mediated immunity are the most common predisposing factors for infection. Conditions associated with increased risk for PCP in patients without HIV infection include

- Immunosuppressive drug therapy
- Malignancy (usually hematologic)
- Organ transplantation (hematopoietic or solid organ)
- Primary immunodeficiency
- Rheumatologic or inflammatory diseases

The risk of PCP is reduced in patients taking effective prophylactic therapy.

❏ Diagnostic Testing
Definitive diagnosis of *P. jirovecii* depends on the demonstration of organisms in respiratory specimens taken from patients at risk for PCP with typical signs, symptoms, and radiographic findings.

Specimens: It is critical to sample alveolar contents or lung tissue for sensitive diagnosis of PCP. Induced sputum (IS) samples are relatively noninvasive and sensitive (50–90%). The sensitivity of bronchoalveolar lavage (BAL) for PCP diagnosis approaches 100%. The sensitivity of lung biopsy is very high, but biopsy is rarely

13

needed for diagnosis. Lung biopsy may be collected for diagnosis of other infections (e.g., fungi) or diseases (e.g., lymphoma) that may be in the differential diagnosis. Organisms are rarely detected in routine expectorated sputum or bronchial wash specimens. The sensitivity of detection may be reduced in non-HIV patients or patients on antifungal prophylaxis.

Direct detection: Definitive diagnosis is achieved by microscopic demonstration of organism in respiratory secretions or lung tissue. A variety of stains may be used to demonstrate characteristic cyst forms (like calcofluor white, Gomori silver, toluidine blue) or troph forms (like Wright-Giemsa or Papanicolaou) of *Pneumocystis*. A commercially available fluorescein-conjugated monoclonal antibody is available that provides sensitive detections of both cyst and troph forms.

Nucleic acid amplification: Methods have been developed for PCP diagnosis, but none are FDA approved. The increased sensitivity of PCR testing may allow for sensitive detection using noninvasively collected specimens, like saliva. However, the increased cost and turnaround time for PCR, and small (if any) incremental sensitivity compared to visual detection, are likely to limit wide implementation of PCR for PCP diagnosis. In addition, false-positive results have been reported for PCR.

Culture: Effective in vitro culture techniques are not available.

Serum beta-D-glucan assay: May be used as a sensitive test to screen for PCP in HIV-infected patients. The performance of the assay depends on the definition used for a positive result as well as the population studied, but sensitivity >90% for detection of PCP has been demonstrated. The specificity is limited by reactivity in infections caused by other fungi.

Serology: Testing does not play a role in PCP diagnosis.

Core laboratory: Elevated LDH is typical; the degree of LDH elevation and increasing LDH despite therapy are poor prognostic signs.

Suggested Readings

Azoulay E, Bergeron A, Chevret S, et al. Polymerase chain reaction for diagnosing pneumocystis pneumonia in non-HIV immunocompromised patients with pulmonary infiltrates. *Chest.* 2009;135:655–661.

Fischer S, Gill VJ, Kovacs J, et al. The use of oral washes to diagnose *Pneumocystis carinii* pneumonia: a blinded prospective study using a polymerase chain reaction-based detection system. *J Infect Dis.* 2001;184:1485–1488.

Sax PE, Komarow L, Finkelman MA, et al. Blood (1->3)-beta-D-glucan as a diagnostic test for HIV-related *Pneumocystis jiroveci* pneumonia. *Clin Infect Dis.* 2011;53:197–202.

Stringer JR. *Pneumocystis carinii*: what is it, exactly? *Clin Microbiol Rev.* 1996;9:489–498.

Thomas CF, Limper AH. Pneumocystis pneumonia. *N Engl J Med.* 2004;350:2487–2498.

VIRAL PNEUMONIA

❑ Definition

Viral pneumonia is characterized by the development of abnormal alveolar gas exchange and inflammation of the lung tissue. May be caused by a number of viral respiratory pathogens. Pneumonia is often preceded by nonspecific symptoms of URI. The etiology depends somewhat on the age and the patient's state of immunocompetence. In children, viral pneumonia is most important in patients younger than 5 years. Clinically significant, purely viral pneumonia is uncommon in immunocompetent older children and adults. The parainfluenza viruses, RSV, and human metapneumoviruses are relatively more common causes of viral pneumonia in children and infants compared to older children and adults. In older children and adults, influenza viruses, especially type A, are responsible for most cases of pneumonia. CMV is the most common, clinically significant cause of viral pneumonia in immunocompromised patients.

❑ Etiology and Diagnosis

- Specific identification may be required for optimal management of severely ill patients. Because the clinical and laboratory presentation of viral pneumonia is not specific, other etiologies, like bacteria, mycoplasmas, *P. jirovecii*, must be considered and ruled out by relevant laboratory and other evaluations.
- Common causes include influenza (adults), parainfluenza (children), RSV (immunocompromised patients), human metapneumovirus (children), adenovirus, corona viruses, CMV (primarily in immunocompromised patients and children), HSV, measles virus, and VZV.

❑ Who Should Be Suspected?

- The clinical presentation is variable and depends on the patient's age, immunocompetence, underlying medical conditions, and specific viral pathogen. Most patients have mild, self-limited disease, but viral pneumonia may present clinically with life-threatening disease, especially in high-risk patients. In immunocompetent hosts, disease is usually self-limited and mild, with resolution of symptoms within 7–10 days.
- The activity of viruses circulating in the community should be considered in the patient's initial assessment.
- The presenting findings in viral pneumonia include acute illness with fever, showing signs of hypoxemia. Cough is usually nonproductive with scant mucoid sputum. Examination typically demonstrates tachypnea, rales, and wheezing. There may be signs of viral infection in other respiratory tract tissues, like conjunctivitis and acute rhinosinusitis. Underlying medical conditions may be exacerbated by viral pneumonia; the severity of viral pneumonia is often greater in patients with underlying illness.
- Imaging studies typically demonstrate diffuse, bilateral interstitial infiltrates, although the spectrum of abnormalities is broad and nonspecific.
- Bacterial superinfection is well described and represents a significant complication of viral pneumonia. Bacterial superinfection may be suspected in patients whose initial pneumonia resolves but develop fever, cough, and dyspnea 1–2 weeks later. Bacterial pathogens associated with superinfection of viral pneumonia include *S. pneumoniae*, *H. influenzae*, and *S. aureus*.

❑ Diagnostic and Laboratory Findings

Most patients with viral pneumonia have a relatively benign, self-limited illness. Specific diagnosis is usually not required unless severe disease or complication of infection is present.

Culture: Most of the relevant viruses may be isolated by viral culture, but turnaround time is slow. Therefore, viral culture is usually not helpful for acute clinical management.

Direct antigen detection: Antigen detection kits are commercially available for a number of the relevant viruses, such as influenza viruses A and B, RSV, and human metapneumovirus. Although the specificity of these assays is usually high, sensitivity may be <80%; they may be used to confirm but cannot exclude any specific viral infection. The use of specific DFA staining is useful for evaluation of specimen quality and has shown improved sensitivity.

Molecular testing: FDA-approved assays are available for respiratory viral pathogens. These assays provide high sensitivity and specificity, a broad range of detectable viruses, and short turnaround time, but higher cost, compared to culture and antigen testing.

Serology: Serologic testing is not useful for the acute management of patients.

Core laboratory findings: ABGs, CBC, and other tests should be monitored in patients with severe or complicated viral pneumonia. Core laboratory tests are usually normal. In patients with severe respiratory distress, careful monitoring of ABGs is critical for patient management. Fluid status must be monitored carefully because of the risk of dehydration due to fever and tachypnea.

Suggested Reading

Treanor JJ. Chapter 2 Respiratory infections. In: Richman DD, Whitley RJ, Hayden FG (eds). *Clinical Virology*, 3rd ed. Washington, DC: ASM Press; 2009.

TUBERCULOSIS

Diagnosis of tuberculosis is suspected on clinical presentation, screening tests (e.g., IGRAs), and imaging studies and is confirmed by acid-fast smear and culture and other laboratory findings. See Chapter 11, Infectious Diseases for a further discussion of mycobacteria and mycobacterial diseases.

❑ Definition

Tuberculosis refers to disease caused by infection with *Mycobacterium tuberculosis* (Mtb), or, rarely, related mycobacterial species. Tuberculosis is usually transmitted by inhalation of respiratory droplets. Transmission is not efficient, typically requiring prolonged exposure on multiple occasions. Other organs may be infected by lymphohematogenous spread.

❑ Who Should Be Suspected?

Typical signs and symptoms of tuberculosis depend on the age and state of immunocompetence of the patient.

- More aggressive disease is common in young children (<5 years), with risk for extrapulmonary infection. CXR demonstrates prominent hilar and mediastinal lymphadenopathy; middle and lower lung field pneumonitis may be minimal.
- In the elderly, tuberculosis is also more aggressive and may represent new infection, with mid-field pneumonitis and hilar adenopathy, or due to reactivation of latent infection, with typical apical cavitary disease.
- In adolescents and adults, primary infection may not be clinically obvious. Apical abnormality may be seen coincidentally during latent infection or at the time of reactivation of disease.

- Patients whose primary infection is controlled by their immunologic response enter a latent, asymptomatic phase of infection. Organisms, however, continue to multiply slowly in infected tissues, leading to ongoing risk of reactivation disease.
- Common symptoms of active disease include nonspecific constitutional symptoms, like fever, anorexia, weight loss, and night sweats, and specific symptoms related to the respiratory tract or other infected organ systems, like cough with sputum production, hemoptysis, or pleuritic chest pain.

Factors associated with increased risk of acquisition and transmission of tuberculosis include living in, or emigration from, a region with a high prevalence of tuberculosis, poverty and homelessness, crowded living conditions, AIDS, and intravenous drug abuse. Patients usually become noninfectious within 2 weeks after initiation of effective therapy. Negative AFB smears for three specimens, taken at least 8 hours apart, are recommended to take patients out of respiratory isolation.

❑ Laboratory Findings

Screening tests for tuberculosis: Screening for tuberculosis is recommended for patients at high risk of tuberculosis on the basis of clinical signs and symptoms or epidemiologic factors.

Tuberculin skin test (TST): TST is performed by intradermal injection of a standardized solution of a purified protein precipitate from Mtb. Induration (not erythema) at the injection site is assessed after 48–72 hours. A 5-mm cutoff is used for immunocompromised persons and other individuals with recent exposure to patients with active tuberculosis. A 10-mm cutoff is used for individuals in other risk groups. BCG vaccination is an unlikely cause of false-positive TST, unless the vaccination was administered in the prior several years. False-positive TST may also be seen in patients with infections caused by mycobacterial species other than *Mycobacterium tuberculosis* (NTM). False-negative TST reactions may occur in HIV-infected patients with advanced immunosuppression; retesting may be performed after immune recovery associated with effective antiretroviral therapy.

Interferon-γ release assays (IGRA): These assays measure the quantity of interferon-γ released from patient's peripheral blood lymphocytes incubated with purified Mtb antigens. These assays have comparable sensitivity and specificity compared to TST assays. An advantage of IGRAs is that patients do not have to return for test interpretation; BCG vaccination does not cause false-positive IGRA reaction. The utility of IGRAs has not been established for young children (<5 years) or immunocompromised patients.

Specimens for AFB smear and culture:

- *Sputum samples*: Sputum is most commonly submitted to the laboratory for analysis. First-morning specimens are recommended as most likely to yield positive results. Submission of two or three specimens, submitted at least 8 hours apart and including at least one first-morning specimen, has been recommended for evaluation of patients. Sputum specimens of at least 5-mL volume should be submitted for AFB studies; detection is decreased in lower volume specimens. Pooled sputum is not acceptable because of the high rate of culture contamination. Sputum induced by inhalation of hypertonic saline or specimens collected by bronchoalveolar lavage (BAL) are recommended for patients who are unable to provide a good quality expectorated sputum sample and for those with a continued high suspicion for tuberculosis even

13

after negative AFB studies of expectorated sputum. First-morning gastric lavage specimens may be submitted on infants or other patients from whom sputum collection is not feasible.

- *Specimens from other potentially infected sources*, like blood, pleural fluid, urine, or CSF, should be submitted in addition to respiratory specimens.
- *Respiratory specimens, and specimens from other sources* typically contaminated with endogenous flora, are decontaminated and concentrated (centrifugation at $3,000 \times g$ for 15 minutes) for smear preparation and culture inoculation.

Culture: Isolation of *Mtb* by culture is the gold standard for diagnosis; cultures should be submitted for every patient.

- Three types of media are commonly used for AFB culture: egg-based solid (e.g., Lowenstein-Jensen), agar-based solid (e.g., Middlebrook 7H11), and liquid media (e.g., Middlebrook 7H12). Cultures are incubated in 5–10% CO_2 for up to 8 weeks.
- Cultures should include liquid media and at least one type of solid media. Growth is more rapid in liquid media. Solid media may be more sensitive for isolation of mycobacteria and can also provide information about the quantity of growth, colony morphology, and purity of culture.
- Broth systems have been used to develop automated systems for incubation and detection of growth. Automated systems have decreased turnaround time for positive cultures and are less labor intensive than traditional culture methods.

Direct detection (AFB smear):

- The acid-fast smear is used for direct detection of mycobacteria in clinical specimens; Gram stains are not reliable for detection. AFB should be quantified (e.g., 1+ to 4+) for positive smears.
- The sensitivity of AFB smears for detection of tuberculosis is variable (20–80%), depending on factors like type of disease, specimen quality, laboratory procedures, and experience; overall, at least one AFB smear is positive in 60–80% of patients with active tuberculosis and positive cultures for *Mtb*.
- Sensitivity of the AFB smear is directly related to the organism burden in the sample; detection is improved by evaluation of multiple specimens, examination of sputum samples of >5-mL volume, decontamination and concentration, use of fluorochrome staining, and following standardized methods for smear examination.
- The predictive value of a positive AFB smear for tuberculosis is >90%.

Molecular testing

- Several FDA-approved nucleic acid amplification assays are available for the direct detection of *Mtb* in clinical specimens. Good performance depends on strict adherence to the manufacturer's instructions.
- The sensitivity for detection is intermediate between AFB smear and culture; assays are useful to provide presumptive diagnosis of *Mtb* infection in patients with positive AFB smears (sensitivity: 40–77% in smear-negative patients and >95% in smear-positive patients).

Testing should only be performed on patients with a high clinical suspicion for tuberculosis. Though the specificity is high (>95%), the clinical utility may be unacceptably low in low-prevalence populations because of false-positive test results.

- Nonamplified rRNA probes are available for preliminary identification of some mycobacterial species from positive cultures, including M. *tuberculosis* complex, M. *avium* and *intracellulare*, M. *gordonae*, and M. *kansasii*. Note: The M. *tuberculosis* complex includes Mtb, M. *bovis*, M. *africanum*, M. *microti*, and several other related species.

Susceptibility testing: Should be performed on all initial Mtb isolates and repeated if cultures remain positive after 3 months of appropriate treatment. Susceptibility testing for second-line agents should be performed on rifampin-resistant isolates, on isolates resistant to any two other primary drugs, or for patients in whom a second-line agent will be used for treatment.

- *Method*: The agar proportion method, using organisms isolated in culture, is commonly used for susceptibility testing. Standardized inocula of the clinical isolate are inoculated onto Middlebrook plates containing a specific critical concentration of the drug tested, as well as drug-free control media. Antibiotics for which there is <99% reduction in organisms, compared to growth on the control media, are unlikely to be clinically effective. Susceptibility test methods adapted to use of liquid media have been developed using automated or manual methods. Testing methods have also been described for direct preparation of inocula from smear-positive specimens.
- *Primary panel*: Isoniazid (INH), rifampin (RMP), ethambutol (EMB), and pyrazinamide (PZA).
- *Second-line panel*: INH—high concentration, IMB—high concentration, amikacin, capreomycin, ethionamide, kanamycin, levofloxacin, ofloxacin, para-aminosalicylic acid, rifabutin, streptomycin.

Strains that are resistant to at least rifampin and INH are considered MDR (multiple drug resistant); strains resistant to at least rifampin, INH, a fluoroquinolone, and an aminoglycoside are considered XDR (extensively drug resistant).

- *Nonculture methods*: Specific mutations have been identified that confer resistance to drugs used to treat tuberculosis. For example, >95% of rifampin resistance is caused by mutation of the *rpoB* gene. Various methods may be used to detect relevant mutations, and several are commercially available (e.g., LIPA, molecular beacons).

Common core laboratory findings in active tuberculosis:
  CBC: normocytic, normochromic anemia; WBC and differential usually normal.
  Chemistry: Hypoalbuminemia; hypogammaglobulinemia. Hyponatremia may occur due to SIADH or adrenal gland infection.

Suggested Readings

Barnes PF. Rapid diagnostic tests for tuberculosis: progress but no gold standard. *Am J Respir Crit Care Med.* 1997;155:1497–1498.

Forbes BA, Banaiee N, Beavis KG, et al. *Laboratory Detection and Identification of Mycobacteria; Approved Guideline. CLSI Document M48-A.* Wayne, PA: Clinical and Laboratory Standards Institute; 2008.

Mase SR, Ramsay A, Ng V, et al. Yield of serial sputum specimen examinations in the diagnosis of pulmonary tuberculosis: a systemic review. *Int J Tuberc Lung Dis.* 2007;11:485–495.

Pfyffer GE, Palicova F. Chapter 28: mycobacterium: general characteristics, laboratory detection, and staining procedures. In: Versalovic J (ed). *Manual of Clinical Microbiology*, 10th ed. Washington, DC: ASM Press; 2011.

Steingart KR, Henry M, Ng V, et al. Fluorescence versus conventional sputum smear microscopy for tuberculosis: a systemic review. *Lancet Infect Dis.* 2006;6:570–581.

Woods GL, Lin SG, Desmond EP. Chapter 73: susceptibility test methods: mycobacteria, nocardia, and other actinomycetes. In: Versalovic J. *Manual of Clinical Microbiology*, 10th ed. Washington, DC: ASM Press; 2011.

NONINFECTIOUS PULMONARY DISEASES ASSOCIATED WITH DYSPNEA

ASPIRATION PNEUMONIA

❑ Definition

Aspiration pneumonia refers to pulmonary disease caused by abnormal entry of fluids into the lower respiratory tract. The fluid may be endogenous secretions (e.g., gastric contents, upper respiratory secretions) or exogenous. Development of disease usually requires defective protective mechanisms (e.g., cough reflex, glottis function, ciliary transport) and aspiration of "toxic" material (e.g., particulate matter, acidic fluid, heavy bacterial contamination). Conditions that predispose to aspiration include alcoholism, seizure, CVA, head trauma, general anesthesia, dysphagia, periodontal disease, neurologic disorder, protracted vomiting, and mechanical disruption of the usual defense barriers (nasogastric tube, endotracheal intubation, upper GI endoscopy, and bronchoscopy).

❑ Who Should Be Suspected?

- The endogenous flora of the upper respiratory and gastrointestinal tract most commonly cause bacterial aspiration pneumonia. Polymicrobial infection, including anaerobes and less virulent streptococcal species found in gingival crevices, is typical.

- Most patients present with subacute progression of symptoms over several weeks. Common symptoms include dyspnea, cough, and purulent (often putrid) sputum production, with associated fever and weight loss. Rigors are uncommon. Symptoms of complicated infection, like abscess or empyema, may be present.

❑ Diagnostic and Laboratory Findings

- Microbiology: Expectorated sputum is not reliable for diagnosis, except for possibly establishing an alternative diagnosis. Culture of specimens (e.g., transtracheal or transthoracic aspirates) collected using techniques for anaerobic isolation may be informative.

- *Fusobacterium nucleatum, Bacteroides, Peptostreptococcus,* and *Prevotella* species are most commonly implicated anaerobes. Aerobic organisms, including *S. aureus* and gram-negative bacilli, are common, especially in nosocomial aspiration pneumonias.

- Core laboratory: Anemia is typical. Laboratory abnormalities associated with underlying medical conditions should be investigated that includes ABGs.

Suggested Reading

Marik PE. Aspiration pneumonitis and aspiration pneumonia. *N Engl J Med.* 2001;344(9):665–671.

ASTHMA

❏ **Definition**

- Asthma is a highly prevalent and chronic inflammatory disorder in which the airway smooth muscle undergoes exaggerated contractions and is abnormally responsive to external stimuli. The best defined and most commonly identified cause of this inflammation is inhalation of allergens.
- Classification of bronchial asthma can be based on age, etiology-associated characteristics, or severity. The pattern of disease presenting at different ages is distinct. In the first 2 years of life, wheezing and bronchiolitis are not distinguishable, and the most common cause of these episodes is infection with the RSV. In older children and young adults, by far the most commonly identified cause of asthma is sensitization to one of the most common inhalant allergens, particularly those encountered indoors.
- Asthma that presents after 20 years of age provides a complex problem, and there is a wider differential diagnosis. Major causes include simple allergic asthma in adults, intrinsic asthma associated with chronic hyperplastic sinusitis, allergic bronchopulmonary aspergillosis, and wheezing associated with chronic obstructive lung disease.
- Among adults aged >40 years who develop severe asthma for the first time, almost 50% may have intrinsic asthma (negative skin tests to common allergens, no family history, persistent eosinophilia). Late-onset asthma, which is frequently not associated with atopy, may be linked to workplace (occupational exposure to sensitizing chemicals).

❏ **Who Should Be Suspected?**

- Classic symptoms of asthma are intermittent dyspnea, cough, and wheezing. These symptoms are nonspecific and sometimes difficult to distinguish from other respiratory diseases. Patients may present to clinics or the emergency department with acute symptoms of breathlessness, wheezing, and coughing. Alternatively, they may present between episodes with normal or near-normal lungs. Asthma may develop at any age, although new-onset asthma is less frequent in elderly compared to other age groups. Seventy-five percent of the cases are diagnosed before the age 7.
- Asthmatic symptoms characteristically come and go, with a time course of hours to days, resolving spontaneously with removal of triggering stimulus or in response to antiasthmatic medications. Characteristic triggers of asthma include cold air, exercise, and exposure to allergens. Allergens that typically trigger asthmatic symptoms include dust, molds, furred animals, cockroaches, and pollens. Viral infections are also common triggers.

❏ **Diagnostic Findings**

The diagnostic tools should include history, physical examination, pulmonary function tests (PFTs), and other laboratory evaluations.

- PFTs: Measurement of peak expiratory flow rate (PEFR) and spirometry are the two PFTs most often used in the diagnosis of asthma. Spirometry is used to measure the amount of air a person can breathe out and the amount of time taken to do so. Forced vital capacity (FVC): maximum volume of air

13

that can be exhaled during a forced maneuver. Forced expired volume in 1 second (FEV_1): volume expired in the first second of maximal expiration after a maximal inspiration. This is a measure of how quickly the lungs can be emptied. FEV_1/FVC: FEV_1 expressed as a percentage of the FVC gives a clinically useful index of airflow limitation. The ratio FEV_1/FVC is between 70% and 80% in normal adults; it is influenced by the age, sex, height, and ethnicity and is best considered as a percentage of the predicted normal value. Variability of >20% in PEFR, a reversible reduction in FEV_1 and FEV_1/FVC, and heightened sensitivity to bronchoprovocation are findings consistent with asthma.

- Chest radiography: Almost always normal in patients with asthma. It is recommended in the evaluation of severe or difficult-to-control asthma and for the detection of comorbid conditions (e.g., allergic bronchopulmonary aspergillosis, eosinophilic pneumonia, or atelectasis due to mucous plugging).
- Hematology: CBC with differential WBC analysis to screen for eosinophilia or significant anemia may be helpful in certain cases. Markedly elevated eosinophil percentages (>15%) may be due to allergic asthma but should prompt consideration of alternative diagnoses, including parasitic infections, drug reactions, and syndromes of pulmonary infiltrates with eosinophilia. An alpha-1 antitrypsin level is recommended in nonsmokers with persistent and irreversible airflow obstruction to exclude emphysema due to alpha-1 antitrypsin deficiency.
- Allergy tests: Allergic sensitivity to specific allergens can be assessed by either skin tests or blood tests for allergen-specific IgE. Aeroallergens (house dust mite, cat or dog dander, cockroach, pollen, and mold spore antigens) are most commonly implicated in asthma. Food allergens rarely cause isolated asthmatic symptoms. Total IgE levels are sometimes helpful. A very high level (>1,000 IU/mL) suggests the associated conditions of eczema or allergic bronchopulmonary aspergillosis.

Suggested Reading

National Asthma Education and Prevention Program: Expert Panel Report III: Guidelines for the Diagnosis and Management of Asthma. Bethesda, MD: National Heart, Lung, and Blood Institute, 2007. (NIH publication no. 08–4051): Full text available online: www.nhlbi.nih.gov/guidelines/asthma/asthgdln.htm.

CARDIAC HEART FAILURE

See Chapter 3, Cardiovascular Disorders.

CHRONIC OBSTRUCTIVE PULMONARY DISEASE

❑ Definition

- Chronic bronchitis with emphysema, also known as chronic obstructive pulmonary disease (COPD), is in most cases a sequel of many years of active smoking. It refers to a group of diseases that cause airflow blockage and breathing-related problems. COPD results from complex interactions between clinical and genetic risk factors. Definite or possible risk factors for COPD include inhalational exposure (e.g., smoking), increased airway responsiveness, atopy, and antioxidant deficiency. Genetic risk factors for COPD include a variety of gene polymorphisms, antioxidant-related enzyme dysfunction, metalloproteinase dysregulation, and abnormalities that cause excess elastase.

- The Global Initiative for Chronic Obstructive Lung Disease (GOLD)—a report produced by the National Heart, Lung, and Blood Institute (NHLBI) and the World Health Organization (WHO)—defines COPD as "a preventable and treatable disease with some significant extrapulmonary effects that may contribute to the severity in individual patients. Its pulmonary component is characterized by airflow limitation that is not fully reversible. The airflow limitation is usually progressive and associated with an abnormal inflammatory response of the lungs to noxious particles or gases."

- Classification of severity of COPD. *An FEV_1/FVC <70% indicates airflow limitation and the possibility of COPD.*
  - ▼ *Stage 0*—at risk: normal spirometry; chronic symptoms (cough, sputum production); FEV_1/FVC <70%.
  - ▼ *Stage I*—mild: with or without chronic symptoms (cough, sputum production); mild airflow limitation (FEV_1/FVC_1 >80% predicted).
  - ▼ *Stage II*—moderate: Worsening airflow limitation (FEV_1/FVC <70%; 50% < FEV_1 <80% predicted), with shortness of breath typically developing during exertion.
  - ▼ *Stage III*—severe: with or without chronic symptoms (cough, sputum production); further worsening of airflow limitation (FEV_1/FVC <70%; 30% < FEV_1 < 50% predicted).
  - ▼ *Stage IV*—very severe: with or without chronic symptoms (cough, sputum production); severe airflow limitation (FEV_1/FVC <70%; FEV_1 <30% predicted); or FEV_1 <50% predicted plus chronic respiratory failure. Patients may have very severe (stage IV) COPD even if the FEV_1 is >30% predicted, whenever this complication is present.

❏ Who Should Be Suspected?

The dominant symptoms of COPD are coughing and shortness of breath on activity, but some patients present with acute breathlessness and wheezing, which is difficult to distinguish from asthma. There are three typical ways that patients with COPD present. Some patients have few complaints but an extremely sedentary life style. Other patients describe chronic respiratory symptoms (e.g., dyspnea on exertion, cough). Finally, some patients present with an acute exacerbation (e.g., wheezing, cough, and dyspnea). The physical examination of chest varies with severity of COPD.

- COPD should be considered and PFTs performed in all patients who report any combination of the following: chronic cough, chronic sputum production, dyspnea or inhalational exposure to tobacco smoke, occupational dust, or occupational chemicals. COPD is confirmed when a patient who has symptoms that are compatible with COPD is found to have airflow obstruction (FEV_1/FVC <0.70), and there is no alternative explanation for the symptoms and airflow obstruction.

13

❑ **Diagnostic Findings**

- Spirometry: This is an essential test to confirm the diagnosis and establish the staging of COPD. If values are abnormal, a post–bronchodilator test may be indicated. Reversibility following bronchodilator would suggest asthma, and, if function reversed to normal, would exclude COPD. The FVC or FEV is needed to establish the presence of obstruction (see above for significance of specific values). The inspiratory capacity may decrease acutely with tachypnea due to dynamic hyperinflation. It is the best physiologic correlate of dyspnea, but it is not usually required to diagnose COPD.
- Carbon monoxide (CO) diffusing capacity: Measurement of CO diffusing capacity can help establish the presence of emphysema, but it is not necessary for the routine diagnosis of COPD.
- Chest radiography: Only diagnostic of severe emphysema but always essential to exclude other lung diseases.
- Blood gas: ABGs are not needed in mild (FEV_1 >80%) and moderate (FEV_1 65–79%) airflow obstruction. ABGs are optional except oximetry, which should be measured in moderately severe (FEV_1 50–64%) airflow obstruction. (ABGs should be measured if oxygen saturation is >88%.) ABGs should be monitored in all severe (FEV_1 30–49%) and very severe (FEV_1 <30%) airflow obstruction.
- Alpha-1-antitrypsin deficiency can cause COPD (inherited emphysema).

Suggested Reading

Documents and Resources. Global Initiative for Chronic Obstructive Lung Disease (http://www. goldcopd.org).

CYSTIC FIBROSIS*

❑ **Definition**

An autosomal recessive disorder with abnormal ion transport due to (>1,000) chromosome 7 mutation in the transmembrane conductance regulator (CFTR gene) that controls salt, especially chloride, entry/exit into cells. Incidence of 1:2,500 in non-Hispanic whites in North America with a carrier frequency of 1:20; 1:17,000 in African Americans; marked heterogeneity among patients. For more information, refer to Chapter 10, Hereditary and Genetic Diseases.

❑ **Who Should Be Suspected?**

- Respiratory symptoms include fatigue, cough, wheezing, recurrent pneumonia or sinus infections, excess sputum and/or shortness of breath.

❑ **Diagnostic Criteria**

- At least one characteristic clinical feature (respiratory, sweat, GI, GU) *or* sibling with CF *or* positive neonatal screening

  AND

- Sweat chloride ≥60 mEq/L *or* presence of two *CFTR* genes *or* positive nasal transmembrane potential difference.

---

*Written by Michael Snyder, MD and Mary Williamson, PhD.

❑ Laboratory Findings

Culture: Special culture techniques should be used in these patients. Before 1 year of age, *S. aureus* is found in 25% and *Pseudomonas aeruginosa* in 20% of respiratory tract cultures; in adults, *P. aeruginosa* grows in 80% and *S. aureus* in 20%. *Haemophilus influenzae* is found in 3.4% of cultures. *Pseudomonas aeruginosa* is found increasingly often after treatment of *Staphylococcus*, and special identification and susceptibility tests should be performed on *P. aeruginosa*. *Burkholderia cepacia* is becoming more important in older children. Increasing serum antibodies against *P. aeruginosa* can document probable infection when cultures are negative.

Molecular tests: DNA genotyping (using blood; can use buccal scrapings) to confirm diagnosis based on two mutations is highly specific but not very sensitive and supports diagnosis of cystic fibrosis (CF), but failure to detect gene mutations does not exclude CF because of large number of alleles. A substantial number of patients with CF have unidentified gene mutations. This test should be done when the sweat test is borderline or negative. It can also be used for carrier screening. Identical genotypes can be associated with different degrees of disease severity. The genotype should not be used as sole diagnostic criterion for CF. Prevalence of the 25 most common genes in the panel depends on population group (Table 13-1). Villus sampling in first trimester or amniocentesis in second or third trimester: >1,000 mutations of *CFTR* gene but the 25 most common account for approximately 90% of carriers. Fifty-two percent are homozygous for ΔF508, and 36% are heterozygous for ΔF508/other CF mutation.

Core laboratory: Serum albumin is often decreased (because of hemodilution due to cor pulmonale; may be found before cardiac involvement is clinically apparent). Serum protein electrophoresis shows increasing IgG and IgA levels with progressive pulmonary disease; IgM and IgD levels are not appreciably increased. Serum chloride, sodium, potassium, calcium, and phosphorus levels are normal unless complications occur (e.g., chronic pulmonary disease with accumulation of CO_2; massive salt loss due to sweating may cause hyponatremia). Urine electrolytes are normal. Submaxillary saliva has slightly increased chloride and sodium but not potassium; considerable overlap with normal results prevents diagnostic use.

Saliva findings: Submaxillary saliva is more turbid, with increased calcium, total protein, and amylase. These changes are not generally found in parotid saliva.

Other: Nasal electrical potential difference measurements may be more reliable than sweat tests but are much more complex; mean = −46 mV in affected persons but −19 mV in unaffected persons.

13

TABLE 13–1. Demographic Groups and Their Risk for Cystic Fibrosis

	Detection Rate of Panel (%)	Frequency of Carriers
Ashkenazi Jew	97	1/25
North European	90	1/25
South European	68–70	1/29
Black	69	1/60
Hispanic	55–57	1/45
Asian	30	1/90

❑ Considerations

Laboratory changes secondary to complications should also suggest diagnosis of CF:

- Chronic lung disease (especially upper lobes) with laboratory changes of decreased pO_2, accumulation of CO_2, metabolic alkalosis, severe recurrent infection, secondary cor pulmonale, nasal polyps, and pansinusitis; normal sinus x-rays are strong evidence against CF.
- Overt liver disease, including cirrhosis, fatty liver, bile duct strictures, and cholelithiasis, in ≤5% of cases. Neonatal cholestasis in ≤20% of affected infants may persist for months.
- Meconium ileus during early infancy; causes 20–30% of cases of neonatal intestinal obstruction; present at birth in 8% of these children. Almost all of them will develop the clinical picture of CF.

PULMONARY EMBOLISM

❑ Definition

Pulmonary embolism (PE) refers to the occlusion of the pulmonary artery or one of its branches by a blood clot, tumor, air, or fat that developed elsewhere in the body. The classic symptoms of PE are hemoptysis, dyspnea, and chest pain. PE can be classified as acute or chronic. In acute PE, patients develop symptoms and signs immediately after obstruction of pulmonary vessels. In chronic PE, patients slowly develop progressive dyspnea over a period of years due to pulmonary hypertension. The incidence of PE appears to be significantly higher in blacks than whites. Mortality rates for PE for blacks have been 50% higher than whites followed by people of other races (Asians) and Native Americans. The risk is increased in pregnancy and during the postpartum period. Other risk factors include venous stasis, various hypercoagulable states, immobilization, surgery, trauma, oral contraceptives, estrogen replacement, CHF, advanced age, and malignancy.

❑ Who Should Be Suspected?

PE should be suspected in a patient with sudden onset of dyspnea, deterioration of existing dyspnea, or the onset of pleuritic chest pain without another apparent cause. Other signs to look for include chest wall tenderness, back pain, shoulder pain, upper abdominal pain, hemoptysis, painful respiration, and new onset of wheezing. PE is a frequent consideration in emergency departments. Rule-out criteria where the prevalence is low including patient age <50 years, heart rate <100 bpm, oxyhemoglobin saturation >95%. There is no hemoptysis, estrogen use, prior deep venous thrombosis or PE, unilateral leg swelling, surgery, or trauma requiring hospitalization within last 4 weeks.

❑ Diagnostic Findings

- Pulmonary angiography: The "gold standard" in the diagnosis of PE. CT pulmonary angiography (CT-PA) is being used increasingly as a diagnostic modality in patients suspected of PE, and its accuracy appears to vary widely from institution to institution. This may be due to differences in the experience of the person interpreting images and image quality. Clinicians should consider their institution's experience and the pretest probability of PE when deciding whether to use CT-PA or to pursue additional testing.

- Chest x-rays: May be normal; suggestive findings include elevated diaphragm, pleural effusion, dilation of the pulmonary artery, abrupt vessel cut off, and atelectasis. Seventy percent of the patients with acute PE will have ECG abnormalities, most commonly nonspecific ST-segment and T-wave changes.
- Majority of the routine laboratory tests are nonspecific for the diagnosis of PE, although they may suggest another diagnosis. A hypercoagulation workup should be performed if no obvious cause of embolic disease is apparent, that includes antithrombin III deficiency, protein C and protein S deficiency, lupus anticoagulant, cardiolipin antibodies, and homocysteine
  - ▼ ABG and pulse oximetry: Have a limited role in the diagnosis. ABGs usually reveal hypoxemia, hypocapnia, and respiratory alkalosis. Room air pulse oximetry readings of <95% at the time of diagnosis are at increased risk of in-hospital complications.
- Core laboratory: BNP or NT-proBNP levels of higher in patients with PE and appear to correlate with increased risk of complications and prolonged hospitalizations in these patients. Thirty percent to 50% of patients have also have elevated troponin I or T, and they are not useful for diagnosis. Leukocytosis, increased ESR, and elevated LDH or AST with normal serum bilirubin are commonly observed.
- D-Dimer assays: Diagnosis of PE has been studied extensively. These assays have good sensitivity (95%) and negative predictive value but poor specificity (40–68%) and positive predictive value. D-Dimer levels of <500 ng/mL are sufficient to exclude PE in patients with a low or moderate pretest probability of PE.

Suggested Readings

Kruip MJ, Leclercq MG, van der Heul C, et al. Diagnostic strategies for excluding pulmonary embolism in clinical outcome studies. A systematic review. *Ann Intern Med.* 2003;138:941.

Roy PM, Colombet I, Durieux P, et al. Systematic review and meta-analysis of strategies for the diagnosis of suspected pulmonary embolism. *BMJ.* 2005;331:259.

Wolf SJ, McCubbin TR, Nordenholz KE, et al. Assessment of the pulmonary embolism rule-out criteria rule for evaluation of suspected pulmonary embolism in the emergency department. *Am J Emerg Med.* 2008;26:181.

DRUG-INDUCED PULMONARY DISEASES

❏ Definition

- Drug-induced pulmonary disease (DIPD) represents a heterogeneous group of disorders, a common clinical problem in which a patient without previous pulmonary disease develops respiratory symptoms, chest x-ray changes, deterioration of pulmonary function, histologic changes, or several of these findings in association with drug therapy. More than 150 drugs or categories of drugs have been reported to cause pulmonary disease; the mechanism is rarely known.
- Depending on the drug, drug-induced syndromes can produce asthma, bronchiolitis, hypersensitivity infiltrate, interstitial fibrosis, organizing pneumonia, asthma, noncardiogenic pulmonary edema, pleural effusions, pulmonary eosinophilia, pulmonary hemorrhage, or venoocclusive disease. DIPDs can present a variety of clinical presentations and radiographic patterns. A good

resource for details on different DIPDs and their clinical and radiographic presentation is available at www.pneumotox.com

■ Causal drugs

▼ In cardiovascular drugs, amiodarone is a classic example that caused pulmonary toxicity. In 3–20% of patients, ACE inhibitors induce a dry, persistent, and often nocturnal cough that may require discontinuation of the drug.

▼ Among anti-inflammatory agents, aspirin triad characterized by asthma, nasal polyposis, and drug sensitivity.

▼ Many chemotherapeutic and immunosuppressive drugs including bleomycin, mitomycin-C, busulfan, cyclophosphamide, and nitrosourea drugs are implicated.

❑ **Who Should Be Suspected?**

■ Many types of lung injury can result from medications, and it is often impossible to predict who will develop lung disease resulting from a medication or drug. Symptoms may vary from patient to patient. The most common symptoms include cough, wheezing, shortness of breath, chest pain, bloody sputum, and fever. Many drugs can induce alveolar inflammation, interstitial inflammation, and/or interstitial fibrosis, resulting in lung dysfunction.

❑ **Diagnostic Findings**

There is no clear-cut laboratory or radiographic testing of the clinical syndromes associated with DIPD. The diagnosis is usually one of exclusion. Plain chest x-rays may miss or underestimate the presence of lung disease at the time of initial presentation. Diagnosis is based on observation of responses to withdrawal from and, if practical, reintroduction to the suspected drug. Echocardiography may rule out cardiac disease, sputum studies may rule out infectious diseases, and ANA or RF testing may be helpful in suspected cases of collagen vascular disease.

■ Pulmonary function: Testing is useful in assessing the toxicity.

■ Hematology: CBC with differential can detect eosinophilia, which may suggest drug rash with eosinophilia and systemic symptoms (DRESS) syndrome.

Suggested Readings

Bhadra K, Suratt BT. Drug induced lung diseases: a state of the art review. *J Respir Dis.* 2009;30:1.
Ozkan M, Dweik RA, Ahmad M. Drug induced lung disease. *Cleve Clin J Med.* 2001;68:782–795.
www.pneumotox.com.

CHEMICAL PNEUMONITIS*

❑ **Definition**

Chemical pneumonitis is inflammation of the lungs or difficulty breathing following acute or chronic inhalation exposure to a foreign substance or chemical fumes. Aspiration pneumonitis (Mendelson syndrome) is a chemical injury caused by the inhalation of sterile gastric contents during general anesthesia due to abolition of the laryngeal reflexes.

---

*Written by Mary Williamson, PhD.

❏ Who Should Be Suspected?

A number of clinical features should raise the possibility of chemical pneumonitis: Abrupt onset of symptoms with prominent dyspnea; cough, low-grade fever, cyanosis, and diffuse crackles on lung auscultation; severe hypoxemia; and infiltrates on chest x-ray involving dependent pulmonary segments.

❏ Laboratory Findings

- Pulmonary function tests (PFTs): Show decreased compliance, abnormal ventilation–perfusion, and reduced diffusing capacity. Chest x-ray: Changes are noted within 2 hours. Bronchoscopy shows erythema of bronchi indicating acid injury.
- Blood gas: Studies often show that the partial pressure of oxygen is reduced to 35–50 mm Hg accompanied by a normal or low partial pressure of CO_2 with respiratory alkalosis. Lactate can be an early marker of septic shock.
- Other: Elevated WBC count and increased neutrophils may be present.

CARCINOMA OF THE LUNG

❏ Definition

The term *lung cancer*, or bronchogenic carcinoma, refers to malignancies that originate in the airways or pulmonary parenchyma. Lung cancer is the second most diagnosed cancer in men and women, but it is the number one cause of death from cancer. Eighty-seven percent of all lung cancers are smoking related. Exposure to second-hand smoke also increases the risk of developing lung cancer. Other substances including asbestos, radon, radiation exposure, TB, industrial substances, and pollutants also increase the risk. Family history/genetics also play a role in the development of cancer.

Approximately 95% of all lung cancers are classified as either small cell lung cancer (SCLC) or non–small cell lung cancer (NSCLC). This distinction is essential for staging, treatment, and prognosis. Other cell types comprise about 5% of malignancies arising in the lung. NSCLC accounts for 80% and SCLC accounts for 20% of all total lung cancers identified. There are different types of NSCLC, including:

- *Squamous cell carcinoma*: Most common type in men. Forms within the lining of bronchial tubes.
- *Adenocarcinoma*: Most common in women and nonsmokers. Found in the glands of the lungs that produce mucus.
- *Bronchoalveolar carcinoma*: Rare subset of adenocarcinoma forms near lungs air sacs.
- *Large cell undifferentiated carcinoma*: Rapidly growing cancer forms near the surface or outer edges of the lungs.

❏ Who Should Be Suspected?

- Heavy cigarette smokers who have new onset of cough, a change in the characteristics of a preexisting cough, and the presence of hemoptysis should be considered; cancer may be the cause of cough.
- Typical symptoms of lung cancer in the chest include persistent cough; pain in the chest, shoulder, or back unrelated to pain from coughing; a change in

13

color or volume of sputum; shortness of breath, changes in the voice; harsh sounds with each breath; and recurrent lung problems such as bronchitis, pneumonia, and hemoptysis.

❏ **Diagnostic Findings**

- The diagnosis of lung cancer is primarily based on evaluation of individuals with symptoms. Screening for lung cancer is not widely used, since no screening test (chest radiography, sputum cytology, or CT) has been shown to reduce mortality from lung cancer.
- Diagnostic tests should include physical and chest examination, chest x-ray, CT, positron emission tomography (PET) and spiral CT scan, MRI, sputum cytology, bronchoscopy, and biopsy. Cytologic examination of spontaneously expected or induced sputum may provide a definitive diagnosis of lung cancer. Bronchoscopy is usually indicated when there is a suspicion of airway involvement by a malignancy.
  - ▼ Molecular diagnostic tests for non–small cell lung cancer (NSCLC) included EGFR, and KRAS mutations are important for proper therapy selections.
  - ▼ Anaplastic lymphoma kinase (ALK) gene rearrangements to identify a subset of patients with NSCLC and specific treatment with ALK inhibitors.

Suggested Readings

Bach PB, Silvestri GA, Hanger M, et al. Screening for lung cancer. ACCP Evidence-Based Clinical Practice Guidelines. *Chest.* 2007;132:69S–77S.
Kvale P. Chronic cough due to lung tumors. *Chest.* 2006;129:147S–153S.
Rivera M, Detterbeck F, Mehta AC. Diagnosis of lung cancer, the guidelines. *Chest.* 2003;123:129S–136S.

EVALUATION OF PLEURAL EFFUSIONS

❏ **Definition**

Pleural effusion is defined as increased amount of fluid in the pleural cavity. The underlying cause of an effusion is usually determined by first classifying the fluid as an exudate (e.g., infections, malignant, drug reactions) or a transudate (e.g., CHF, cirrhosis, atelectasis, nephritic syndrome).

- Exudates are fluids, cells, or other cellular substances that are slowly discharged from blood vessels, usually from inflamed tissues.
- Transudates are fluids that pass through a membrane or squeeze through tissue or into the extracellular space of tissues. Transudates are thin and watery and contain few cells or proteins.

It is clinically important to classify pleural and ascitic fluids into exudates and transudates because this is indicative of the underlying pathophysiologic process involved (Figure 13-1). A transudate does not usually require additional testing, but exudates always do.

Transudate
- Causes
  - ▼ CHF (causes 15% of cases); acute diuresis can result in pseudoexudate
  - ▼ Cirrhosis with ascites (pleural effusion in approximately 5% of cases)—rare without ascites

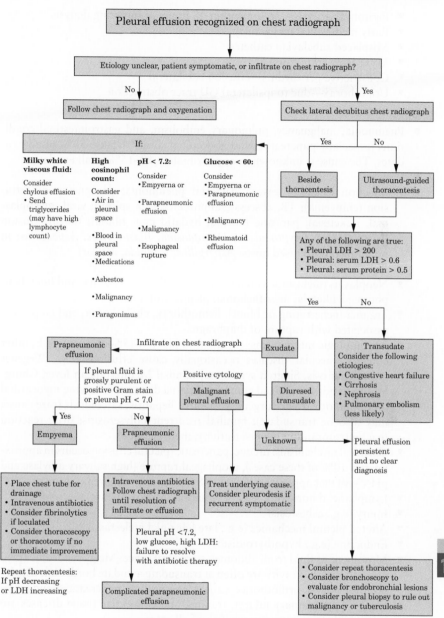

Figure 13–1 *Algorithm for the workup of patients with pleural effusion. LDH = lactate dehydrogenase.*

▼ Nephrotic syndrome
▼ Early (acute) atelectasis
▼ PE
▼ Superior vena cava obstruction
▼ Hypoalbuminemia

▼ Peritoneal dialysis—occurs within 48 hours of initiating dialysis
▼ Early mediastinal malignancy
▼ Misplaced subclavian catheter
▼ Myxedema (rare cause)
▼ Constrictive pericarditis—effusion is bilateral
▼ Urinothorax—due to ipsilateral GU tract obstruction

Exudate

■ Pneumonia, malignancy, pulmonary embolism, and gastrointestinal conditions (especially pancreatitis and abdominal surgery) cause 90% of all exudates. The cause is unknown in approximately 10–15% of all exudates.
■ Causes
  ▼ Infection (25% of cases): bacterial pneumonia; parapneumonic effusion (empyema); TB; abscess (subphrenic, liver, spleen); viral, mycoplasmal, rickettsial; parasitic (ameba, hydatid cyst, filaria); fungal effusion (*Coccidioides, Cryptococcus, Histoplasma, Blastomyces, Aspergillus*; in immunocompromised hosts: *Aspergillus, Candida, Mucor*)
  ▼ PE/infarction
  ▼ Neoplasms (metastatic carcinoma, especially breast, ovary, and lung; lymphoma; leukemia; mesothelioma; pleural endometriosis) (42% of cases)
  ▼ Trauma (penetrating or blunt): hemothorax, chylothorax, and empyema, associated with rupture of diaphragm
  ▼ Immunologic mechanisms: rheumatoid pleurisy (5% of cases), SLE; other collagen vascular diseases occasionally cause effusions (e.g., Wegener granulomatosis, Sjögren syndrome, familial Mediterranean fever, Churg-Strauss syndrome, mixed connective tissue disease); following myocardial infarction or cardiac surgery; vasculitis; hepatitis; sarcoidosis (rare cause; may also be transudate); familial recurrent polyserositis; drug reaction (e.g., nitrofurantoin hypersensitivity, methysergide)
  ▼ Chemical mechanisms: uremic, pancreatic (pleural effusion occurs in approximately 10% of these cases), esophageal rupture (high salivary amylase and pH <7.30 that approaches 6.00 in 48–72 hours), subphrenic abscess
  ▼ Lymphatic abnormality (e.g., irradiation, Milroy disease)
  ▼ Injury (e.g., asbestosis)
  ▼ Altered pleural mechanics (e.g., late [chronic] atelectasis)
  ▼ Endocrine (e.g., hypothyroidism)
  ▼ Movement of fluid from abdomen to pleural space: Meigs syndrome (protein and specific gravity are often at transudate–exudate border but usually not transudate), urinothorax, cancer, pancreatitis, pancreatic pseudocyst
  ▼ Cirrhosis, pulmonary infarct, trauma, and connective tissue diseases are responsible for approximately 9% of all cases.

Exudates That Can Present as Transudates

■ Causes
  ▼ PE (>20% of cases)—caused by atelectasis
  ▼ Hypothyroidism—caused by myxedema heart disease
  ▼ Malignancy—because of complications (e.g., atelectasis, lymphatic obstruction)
  ▼ Sarcoidosis—stages II and III

- Location
  - ▼ Typically left sided: Ruptured esophagus, acute pancreatitis, rheumatoid arthritis. Pericardial disease is left sided or bilateral; it is rarely exclusively right sided.
  - ▼ Typically right sided or bilateral: CHF (if only on left, consider that the right pleural space may be obliterated or the patient has another process [e.g., pulmonary infarction]).
  - ▼ Typically right sided: rupture of amebic liver abscess.
- Gross appearance
  - ▼ Clear, straw-colored fluid is typical of transudate.
  - ▼ Turbidity (cloudy, opaque appearance) may be caused by lipids or increased WBCs; after centrifugation, a clear supernatant indicates WBCs or debris as the cause; clear or white supernatant is caused by chylomicrons.
  - ▼ Red indicates blood; brown indicates blood has been present for a longer time. RBC count of 5,000–10,000/μL causes a blood-tinged color. If grossly bloody, Hct >50% of peripheral Hct indicates a hemothorax.
  - ▼ Bloody fluid suggests malignancy, pulmonary infarct, trauma, postcardiotomy syndrome; also uremia, asbestos, pleural endometriosis. Bloody fluid from traumatic thoracentesis should clot within several minutes, but blood present more than several hours will have become defibrinated and does not form a good clot. Nonuniform color during aspiration and absence of hemosiderin-laden macrophages also suggest traumatic aspiration. Absent of platelets suggests that the condition is not caused by traumatic thoracentesis.
  - ▼ White fluid suggests chylothorax, cholesterol effusion, or empyema.
  - ▼ Chylous (milky) is usually due to trauma (e.g., auto accident, postoperative) but may be obstruction of duct (e.g., especially lymphoma; metastatic carcinoma, granulomas) or parenteral nutrition via a central line with perforation of superior vena cava.
  - ▼ After centrifugation, supernatant is clear in empyema but cloudy or turbid in chylous effusion caused by chylomicrons, which also stain with Sudan III.
  - ▼ Pleural fluid triglycerides >110 mg/dL or triglyceride pleural fluid-to-serum ratio >2 occurs only in chylous effusion (seen especially within a few hours after eating). Triglycerides <50 mg/dL excludes chylothorax. Equivocal triglyceride levels (50–10 mg/dL) may require a lipoprotein electrophoresis of fluid to demonstrate chylomicrons, which are diagnostic of chylothorax.
  - ▼ Pseudochylous (may have lustrous sheen) appearance in chronic inflammatory conditions (e.g., rheumatoid pleurisy, TB, chronic pneumothorax therapy) is caused by either cholesterol crystals (rhomboid-shaped) in sediment or lipid-containing inclusions in leukocytes. Distinguish from chylous effusions by microscopy. Chylomicrons ≤50 mg/dL with cholesterol >250 mg/dL occurs in pseudochylous effusions.
  - ▼ Black fluid suggests *Aspergillus niger* infection.
  - ▼ Greenish fluid suggests biliopleural fistula.
  - ▼ Purulent fluid indicates infection.
  - ▼ Anchovy (dark red-brown) color is seen in amoebiasis, old blood. Anchovy paste in ruptured amebic liver abscess; amebas found in <10%.

13

- ▼ Turbid and greenish-yellow fluid is classic for rheumatoid effusion.
- ▼ Very viscous (clear or bloody) is characteristic of mesothelioma; also in pyothorax.
- ▼ Debris in fluid suggests rheumatoid pleurisy; food particles indicate esophageal rupture.
- ▼ Color of enteral tube food or central venous line infusion due to tube or catheter entering pleural space.

Odor
- Putrid due to anaerobic empyema.
- Ammonia due to urinothorax.

Protein, Albumin, Lactate Dehydrogenase
- When exudate criteria are met by LD but not by protein, consider malignancy and parapneumonic effusions.
- Very high pleural fluid LD (>1,000 IU/L) occurs in empyema, rheumatoid pleurisy, paragonimiasis; sometimes with malignancy; rarely with TB. Level indicates degree of pleural inflammation; increasing values suggest need for more aggressive therapy. Measurement of LD isoenzymes is said to have limited value.

Glucose
- Transudate has same concentration as serum.
- Usually normal but 30–55 mg/dL or pleural fluid-to-serum ratio <0.5 and pH <7.30 may be found in TB, malignancy, SLE; also esophageal rupture; lowest levels may occur in empyema and RA. Therefore, only helpful if very low level (e.g., <30). A level of 0–10 mg/dL is highly suspicious for RA. Poor prognostic sign in pneumonia. In neoplasm, lower glucose indicates greater tumor burden. Rarely found in SLE, Churg-Strauss, urinothorax, hemothorax, or paragonimiasis.

pH
- Normal pleural fluid pH is alkaline (7.60–7.66). Transudative effusions have a pH range of about 7.45–7.55, and most exudates have a pH of 7.30–7.45.
- Low pH (<7.30) always means exudate, especially empyema, malignancy, rheumatoid pleurisy, SLE, TB, esophageal rupture; may also be caused by systemic acidosis, hemothorax, urinothorax, paragonimiasis.
- pH <6.0 is consistent with but not diagnostic of esophageal rupture.
- Collagen vascular disease is the only other cause of pH <7.0.
- In a parapneumonic effusion, a pH <7.20 indicates need for tube drainage; pH >7.30 suggests that resolution with only medical therapy is possible. A pH <7.0 indicates the presence of complicated parapneumonic effusion.
- pH may fall before glucose becomes decreased.
- *Proteus* infection may increase pH because of urea splitting.
- In a malignant effusion, pH <7.30 is associated with short survival time, poorer prognosis, and increased positive yield with cytology and pleural biopsy; tends to correlate with pleural fluid glucose <60 mg/dL.

Generally, low pH is associated with low glucose and high LD; if low pH with normal glucose and low LD, the pH is probably a lab error.

Amylase

- Increased pleural fluid-to-serum ratio >1.0 and may be >5 or pleural fluid ULN for serum; should be determined only for left pleural effusions.
- Acute pancreatitis—may be normal early with increase over time.
- Pancreatic pseudocyst—always increased, may be >1,000 IU/L.
- Also perforated esophageal rupture, peptic ulcer, necrosis of small intestine (e.g., mesenteric vascular occlusion); 10% of cases of metastatic cancer.
- Isoenzyme studies
  - ▼ Pancreatic type of amylase in acute pancreatitis and pancreatic pseudocyst.
  - ▼ Salivary type of amylase is found in esophageal rupture and occasionally in carcinoma of the ovary or lung or in salivary gland tumor.
- Other chemical determinations
  - ▼ C-reactive protein ranged from 10–20 mg/dL in transudates compared to 30–40 mg/dL in exudates in one small study. Parapneumonic effusions were highest (89 ± 16 mg/dL). The pleural fluid-to-serum ratio was 0.8 ± 0.5 mg/dL in transudates and 2.8 ± 0.7 mg/dL in exudates.
  - ▼ Cholesterol and triglycerides.
  - ▼ Routine tumor markers (e.g., CEA, cancer antigen-125, acid phosphatase in prostate cancer, hyaluronic acid in mesothelioma) are not generally recommended. CEA >10 ng/mL is suggestive but not diagnostic of malignant pleural fluid; usually <10 ng/mL in lymphomas, sarcomas, mesotheliomas.
- Immune complexes (measured by Raji cell, C1q component, radioimmunoassay, etc.) are often found in exudates due to collagen vascular diseases (SLE, RA). LA tests show frequent false-positive results and should not be ordered. Occasionally, LA for bacterial antigens is useful.

 # RHINITIS/PHARYNGITIS

DISORDERS OF THE NOSE AND THROAT ASSOCIATED WITH RHINITIS/PHARYNGITIS

THE COMMON COLD

❏ **Definition**

- This infection of ciliated epithelial cells in nasal mucosa results in nasal discharge due to the inflammatory process.
- It is most commonly the result of rhinovirus infection. Other viruses may cause rhinitis, including *Coronavirus*, parainfluenza, adenovirus, *Enterovirus*, influenza, and respiratory syncytial virus.

❏ **Who Should Be Suspected?**

- Symptoms are typically mild, including nasal congestion, rhinitis, and sneezing. Fever, headache, cough, sore throat, and malaise, if present, are usually mild.
- Symptoms usually resolve within 7–10 days.
- The incidence of colds peaks in colder months, typically between September and March.

13

- Purulent nasal discharge, otitis, high fever, or other severe systemic symptoms suggest complication of infection or a different cause of infection, like influenza.

❑ **Laboratory Findings**

- Specific diagnostic testing is rarely needed but may be attempted for severe or complicated infection. Nasopharyngeal swabs or washings are recommended for diagnostic testing, if indicated.
- Direct antigen testing: Available for several viral pathogens, including influenza viruses and RSV.
- Viral culture: High sensitivity for correctly collected and transported specimens.
- Molecular tests: Available for detection of a very broad range of viral respiratory tract pathogens.
- Serology: Not useful.

PHARYNGITIS

❑ **Definitions**

Acute pharyngitis, inflammation of the posterior pharyngeal and tonsillar tissues, is a common clinical complaint, especially in children. Most episodes of acute pharyngitis are relatively mild, self-limited infectious diseases, caused by common upper respiratory tract pathogens. The etiology varies somewhat by the age of the patient and season. In general, however, viral infection is the most common cause of acute pharyngitis, both in children and adults. Detection of group A beta-hemolytic streptococcus (*Streptococcus pyogenes*) is the focus of most diagnostic testing, however, because of the risk of poststreptococcal acute RF and GN. Specific diagnosis may also guide the appropriate use, or nonuse, of antibiotics. Acute pharyngitis must be distinguished from other serious infections of the head and neck, like epiglottitis, peritonsillar abscess, and submandibular abscess. Severe symptoms and sepsis, difficulty swallowing and drooling, neck swelling and other signs suggest other sites of primary infection or local, suppurative complications of bacterial pharyngitis.

- Etiology

Viral Disease

- Acute respiratory infection is the cause of significant morbidity and mortality throughout the world. Viruses are the cause of most of these infections, and children are primarily affected. There is a clear seasonal pattern for most of the viral pathogens, especially in temperate climates where incidence peaks during the winter months. There may be differences in clinical presentations depending on the agent, age of the patient, underlying health, and other factors.
- Most nasopharyngeal viral infections present as the "common cold," manifested by mild symptoms like rhinitis, nasal congestion, sneezing, and runny nose. Mild pharyngitis and "ticklish" cough may be reported. Fever, headache, and malaise, if present, are usually mild. Most upper respiratory tract viral infections resolve completely after 7–10 days. Complications are uncommon, including otitis media, sinusitis, and exacerbations of chronic pulmonary disease.

- Specific diagnosis of viral pharyngitis or upper respiratory tract infection is rarely needed; most patients can be managed symptomatically on the basis of clinical presentation. When indicated, specific diagnosis may be pursued by virus culture, or more commonly, by molecular diagnostic testing using a respiratory virus panel. Serologic diagnostic testing is not useful.
- The common viral causes of primary pharyngitis include adenovirus, Enterovirus, rhinoviruses, HSV, EBV, CMV, influenza,, and parainfluenza viruses.

Bacterial Disease

- Group A beta-hemolytic streptococcus (GAS): GAS causes infection in a significant minority (10–30%) of patients seeking medical attention for acute pharyngitis. Most infections have an acute onset of sore throat with erythema of the tonsillar and posterior pharyngeal mucosa and exudate. Fever, headache, and abdominal pain are commonly reported. Physical examination often shows enlarged, tender anterior cervical lymph nodes, petechiae of the palate, and uvular inflammation. Conjunctivitis, rhinorrhea, cough, and sneezing are uncommon symptoms and suggest another pathogen.
- Scarlet fever may complicate "strep throat" and is characterized by formation of a typical "scarlatiniforme" rash in the first or second day of fever. The rash is characterized as fine, rough-textured (sandpaper), blanching and worse in the armpits and skinfolds. The rash resolves after several days, followed by desquamation. A bright red, "strawberry" tongue may be obvious.

❏ Who Should Be Suspected?

- Various criteria have been recommended for predicting the probability of GAS infection and need for antibiotic treatment. They have generally shown better negative than positive predictive value. For children, the following criteria have been recommended. With six criteria, the probability of a culture positive for GAS = 75%; the probability falls to 59% if only five criteria are met:
  - ▼ Age: 5–15 years
  - ▼ Season: late fall, winter, or early spring
  - ▼ Pharyngeal erythema, edema, and/or exudates
  - ▼ Anterior lymph nodes: tender, enlarged
  - ▼ Temperature: 101–103°F
  - ▼ No typical viral upper respiratory signs and symptoms
- For adults, the Centor criteria for adults are listed below. The probability of GAS infection increases with the number of criteria present: the presence of three or four is reported to have a positive predictive value up to 60%; the presence of 0 or 1 is reported to have a negative predictive value of 80%.
  - ▼ Tonsillar exudates
  - ▼ Tender anterior cervical adenopathy
  - ▼ Fever or fever history
  - ▼ Absence of cough

❏ Diagnosis

- Culture: Throat culture is the "gold standard" for the diagnosis of pharyngitis due to GAS, with sensitivity in the 90–95% range. The specificity is very high in patients with acute pharyngitis, but "false-positive" cultures, in terms of active disease, may be seen in chronic GAS carriers or after recent, successful therapy. Cultures for "test of cure" are not recommended, except for patients at very high risk for acute rheumatic fever.

▪ Direct antigen detection: Direct antigen tests are also available for rapid detection of GAS; however, these assays are not as sensitive as throat cultures. The sensitivity of antigen tests varies by technique and specific kit used, ranging from 60–95%; the specificity of most tests exceed 95%. Therefore, throat culture should be performed to confirm negative antigen tests but are not needed to confirm positive tests.

▪ *Molecular tests*: An FDA-approved molecular diagnostic assay is available for the detection of *S. pyogenes* in pharyngeal specimens. Sensitivity of the assay is 88–95% with specificity of 98–99.7%. The high sensitivity and specificity for this test allow test results to stand without the need for confirmation of positive or negative tests.

ACUTE RHINOSINUSITIS

❏ **Definitions**

Acute rhinosinusitis (ARS) is an inflammatory condition of the nasal and sinus mucosal tissues that resolves in fewer than 4 weeks, usually within 10 days. ARS is most commonly caused by respiratory viruses (like rhinovirus, parainfluenza virus, and influenza virus); bacterial superinfection (like *S. pneumonia*, *H. influenzae*, and *M. catarrhalis*) may occur in 1–2% of adults with community-acquired ARS. Bacterial superinfection occurs more frequently in children (5–10%).

❏ **Who Should Be Suspected?**

▪ Nasal congestion, purulent discharge, middle ear pain or fullness, tenderness over the maxillary sinus, and cough are common signs of uncomplicated ARS.

▪ Uncomplicated bacterial superinfection typically resolves without antibiotic treatment within 4 weeks.

▪ Serious complications are suspected in patients with high fever (>39°C), severe headache, visual changes, periorbital edema, change in mental status, or other evidence of extension of infection. These infections require urgent referral for imaging, collection of diagnostic specimens, and consideration of invasive intervention.

▪ Increased risk for severe or invasive ARS include immunodeficiency, impaired sinus drainage (e.g., foreign body, abnormal ciliary function), and mucosal irritation (e.g., allergy, intranasal drug abuse).

❏ **Diagnosis**

▪ During early ARS infection, clinical finding cannot be used to accurately differentiate patients with viral infection from those with bacterial superinfection.

▪ Because most viral and bacterial ARS infections resolve spontaneously within 10 days, specific diagnostic testing is not recommended. Testing for influenza virus may be considered if circulating in the community and if antiviral therapy would be indicated for the patient.

▪ Empiric antimicrobial therapy may be considered in patients with symptoms persisting >10 days, patients with severe symptoms (e.g., high fever for at least 3–4 days), patients with evidence of intracranial spread, and patients with worsening symptoms after a period of improvement.

- Identification of the infecting pathogen should be attempted in patients with severe disease. Nasopharyngeal and throat cultures are of no value in diagnosis. In children, sinus aspiration is the preferred method for specimen collection; in adults, endoscopic collection from an infected sinus may be used as a less invasive method for specimen collection. In addition to aerobic cultures, anaerobic cultures should be performed if a dental infection is considered as a potential source of infection.

Suggested Reading

Chow AW, Benninger MS, Brooks I, et al. IDSA clinical practice guideline for acute bacterial rhinosinusitis in children and adults. *Clin Infect Dis.* 2012;54:e72–112.

DIPHTHERIA

❏ Definition

Diphtheria is caused by infection with *Corynebacterium diphtheriae* a pleomorphic gram-positive rod that produces an exotoxin. Most patients present respiratory or cutaneous disease.

Diphtheria has a global distribution, primarily affecting unvaccinated individuals in underdeveloped, economically disadvantaged areas. Humans are the only known reservoir for *C. diphtheriae*, and transmission is mediated by contact with respiratory droplets or secretions from patients with actively infectious mucous membrane or cutaneous lesions. Disease usually occurs within 1 week after infectious contact. The lesions in untreated patients may be infectious for up to 6 weeks; treated patients become noninfectious within days. Diphtheria is a national notifiable disease, reportable to the CDC and local departments of public health.

❏ Who Should Be Suspected?

- Diphtheria usually presents as respiratory disease. The common presentation of respiratory disease is pseudomembranous pharyngitis, with formation of a gray membrane of necrotic material in the tonsillar area, which may extend to adjacent posterior pharyngeal surfaces. Patients often complain of sore throat and difficulty swallowing. There is a risk of dislodgement, with respiratory obstruction, in patients with extensive pseudomembrane formation. The underlying mucosa is friable and edematous. Local adenopathy and tissue edema (bull neck) may occur. Low-grade fever, malaise, or other nonspecific symptoms are common.
- Serious complications may develop due to the effect of exotoxin on other organ systems, usually myocarditis or neuropathy.
- Myocarditis, usually presenting in the 2nd week of infection, may be asymptomatic, but conduction defects and arrhythmias may be serious.
- Neuropathy may present as an early or late complication of infection. Cranial nerve palsy and local neuropathy are common early complications, whereas ocular palsy and limb or diaphragmatic paralysis are late complications.

13

❑ **Laboratory Findings**

■ Culture: Provides the definitive diagnosis of acute diphtheria. For respiratory diphtheria, collect swabs from the nasopharynx and throat, including the edges of the pseudomembrane. Alert the laboratory prior to submitting specimens to ensure that appropriate media are available. Specimens are planted on selective–differential media, like modified Tinsdale and Löeffler media, in addition to routine culture medium. *Corynebacterium diphtheriae* isolates must be tested for exotoxin production using the modified Elek immunodiffusion method. Culture from involved area is positive within 12 hours on Löeffler medium (more slowly on blood agar) (toxin-producing strain). Nasopharyngeal cultures should always be obtained when diphtheria is suspected. *If there has been prior antibiotic therapy, culture may be negative or take several days to grow.* Note: *Corynebacterium ulcerans* may cause diphtheria.

■ Nucleic acid amplification: Tests have been developed both for detection/identification of *C. diphtheriae* as well as the gene responsible for exotoxin production.

■ Core laboratory: Troponin and other cardiac markers may be used to identify asymptomatic cardiac disease or assess prognosis in patients with overt myocarditis. Decreased serum glucose may be seen. Albumin and casts are frequently present in urine; blood is rarely found.

■ Hematology: WBC may be moderately increased (≤15,000/μL). Moderate anemia is common.

■ Serology (EIA): Not useful for diagnosis of acute infection but may be used for epidemiologic studies. Diphtheria antibody testing may also be used to assess immune function by comparing pre- and postvaccination sera.

Suggested Readings

http://wwwnc.cdc.gov/travel/yellowbook/2010/chapter-2/diphtheria.aspx.
Bisno AL. Acute pharyngitis. *N Engl J Med.* 2001;344:205–211.
Coyle MB, Lipsky BA. Coryneform bacteria in infectious diseases: clinical and laboratory aspects. *Clin Microbiol Rev.* 1990;3:227–246.
Kneen R, Dung NM, Hoa NTT, et al. Clinical features and predictors of diphtheritic cardiomyopathy in Vietnamese children. *Clin Infect Dis.* 2004;39:1591–1598.

NONINFECTIOUS RESPIRATORY DISORDERS

ALLERGIC RHINITIS

❑ **Definition**

Rhinitis can be defined as symptoms of nasal irritation, sneezing, rhinorrhea, and nasal blockage lasting for at least 1 hour a day on most days. It occurs mostly in patients aged 15–25 years.

Allergic rhinitis (AR), one of the rhinitis syndromes, is a chronic inflammatory disease of the upper airways and can be seasonal or perennial. In allergic rhinitis, there is usually a clear relationship with exposure to known allergens—most frequently to pollens in seasonal rhinitis and house dust mites or household pets in perennial rhinitis. In general, allergic rhinitis can result in either inflammatory or noninflammatory causes. Many patients with allergic rhinitis have a nonallergic contribution (mixed rhinitis). Underlying causes of nonallergic rhinitis include vasomotor rhinitis, rhinitis medicamentosa, nonallergic rhinitis with nasal eosinophilia syndrome, and miscellaneous other disorders.

❏ Who Should Be Suspected?

- Typical patient presentation includes nasal irritation, sneezing, rhinorrhea, and nasal blockage, symptoms that may be seasonal or perennial. The dominant symptoms may differ from one patient to another. There is also a wide individual variation in terms of tolerability of nasal symptoms. Conjunctival symptoms of itching and increase in tear fluid are also very common in association with allergic rhinitis.
- A new classification system of AR was designed based on frequency and severity of symptoms. Frequency (intermittent (<4 days/week or <4 consecutive weeks) versus persistent (4 days/week and >4 consecutive weeks). Severity of AR can be classified as mild, moderate to severe based on whether AR symptoms result in impairment of daily activities and degree of symptoms.

❏ Diagnostic Findings

The diagnosis of rhinitis in a patient complaining of upper airway problems consists of obtaining a detailed history and performing physical examination supplemented by critical tests.

- Hematology: High numbers indicate that atopy is present. The usefulness of eosinophilia and determination of total IgE are limited in the diagnosis of allergic rhinitis, because to some degree, they are dependent on the size of the organ.
- Allergen-specific testing: The use of diagnostic testing to identify culprit allergens has been associated with improved patient outcomes.
- Skin testing: When carefully performed by well-trained individual, immediate hypersensitive skin testing (skin prick tests [SPTs]) is a safe way to identify the presence of allergen-specific IgE. Skin testing is useful among patients with
  - ▼ Unclear diagnosis based on the history and physical examination
  - ▼ Poorly controlled symptoms, such as persistent nasal symptoms and/or an inadequate clinical response to nasal glucocorticoids
  - ▼ Coexisting persistent asthma and/or recurrent sinusitis/otitis
  - ▼ Occupational rhinitis
- Serum tests for allergy: Serum immunoassays for specific IgE antibodies are better alternates to SPTs for screening. These specific IgE tests are useful for testing-specific allergens that are not available for skin tests or when skin tests cannot be performed because a patient is taking treatment (e.g., histamine) that suppresses the cutaneous response.
- Allergen challenge tests: A nasal challenge can be used to test specific as well as nonspecific reactivity. It is clinically impractical and rarely performed.
- Other tests: Nasal cytology is performed by some to help differentiate rhinitis due to allergy from that due to infection. Wright stain of nasal secretions usually, but not always, reveals predominance of eosinophils in cases of allergic rhinitis. The presence of neutrophils suggests an infectious process. Other diagnostic testing assays, cytotoxic testing, provocation neutralization

13

testing, and specific or nonspecific IgG determinations are unproven and inappropriate.

▼ Component-resolved diagnosis (CRD) is also known as molecular allergy diagnosis, in which individual allergen molecules are used to characterize a patient's IgE specificity. This offered either as panels of selected allergens that can be used as serum (ImmunoCAP) assays or microarray-based assay of more than 100 molecules. CRDs are available in Europe and used only as a research tool in the United States.

Suggested Readings

Gentile D, Bartholow A, Valovirta E, et al. Current and future directions in pediatric allergic rhinitis. *J Allergy Clin Immunol: In Practice.* 2013;1:214–226.

Ng ML, Warlow RS, Chrishanthan N, et al. Preliminary criteria for the definition of allergic rhinitis: a systemic evaluation of clinical parameters in a disease cohort (I). *Clin Exp Allergy.* 2000;30:1314.

Ng ML, Warlow RS, Chrishanthan N, et al. Preliminary criteria for the definition of allergic rhinitis: a systemic evaluation of clinical parameters in a disease cohort (II). *Clin Exp Allergy.* 2000;30:1417.

ACID–BASE DISORDERS

❏ Definition

Acid–base balance disorders are usually encountered in acutely ill or complicated medical and surgical patients. The plasma concentration of hydrogen ion (pH^+) is very low (approximately 40 nmol/L), and it is constantly maintained within a narrow range by

- Excretion of CO_2 by the lungs
- Excretion of H^+ by the kidneys

Everyday approximately 15,000 mmol of CO_2 is produced by endogenous metabolism and then excreted by the lungs. Similarly, normal diet generates 50–100 mmol of H^+ per day, derived mostly from metabolism of sulfur-containing amino acids. The maintenance of stable H^+ level is required for normal cellular function, since small fluctuations in the H^+ concentrations have important effects on the activity of cellular enzymes. There is a relatively narrow range of extracellular H^+ concentration (16–160 nmol/L: pH 7.8–6.8) that is compatible with life. Changes in H^+ are nonlinear; hence, measuring pH masks the magnitude of acid–base disorders.

BUFFER SYSTEMS (BICARBONATE–CARBONIC ACID)

- This buffer is at highest concentration in the blood, and it is also plays an important role in acid–base regulation. Carbonic acid (CO_2) is a volatile acidic gas and is soluble in water. It readily diffuses from cells to blood, where it combines with water to produce carbonic acid, which immediately dissociates in to bicarbonate and hydrogen ions.
- pH, HCO_3^-, and pCO_2 are related by the equation:

$$pH = pK - [HCO_3^- / (0.03 \times pCO_2)]$$

where pK is defined as the pH at which HCO_3^- and H_2CO_3 (0.03% pCO_2) are in equal concentrations.

- Normal concentrations of HCO_3^- and H_2CO_3 in the blood are in the ratio of 20:1 and with a pK of 6.1. This excess base HCO_3^-, along with volatility of CO_2, gives ability to prevent overaccumulation of acid. The lungs through the loss of CO_2 provide the ultimate buffering capacity. Bicarbonate is regulated by the kidneys and CO_2 is regulated by the lungs and the ratio of HCO_3^- to H_2CO_3 that determines the pH.
- Laboratories measure pH and pCO_2 directly and calculate HCO_3 using the Henderson-Hasselbalch equation:

$$\text{Arterial pH} = 6.1 + \log[(HCO_3) + (0.03 \times pCO_2)],$$

where 6.1 is the dissociation constant for CO_2 in aqueous solution and 0.03 is a constant for the solubility of CO_2 in plasma at 37°C.

RESPIRATORY AND METABOLIC SYSTEMS IN ACID–BASE REGULATION

❏ Respiratory System

- Arterial CO_2 is influenced by ventilatory rate; pCO_2 is considered the respiratory component of the bicarbonate–CO_2 buffer system. Because CO_2 is the end product of aerobic metabolism, continuous buffering CO_2 is required for the regulation of pH.
- The arterial pCO_2 represents a balance between tissue production of CO_2 and pulmonary removal of CO_2. An elevated pCO_2 usually indicates hyperventilation. This leads to respiratory acidosis (hypoventilation) or respiratory alkalosis (hyperventilation).
- The respiratory rate can alter arterial pH in minutes.

❏ Metabolic (Renal) System

- When H^+ levels deviated from normal, the kidneys respond by reabsorbing or secreting hydrogen, bicarbonate, and other ions to regulate the blood pH. Metabolic acidosis may develop; either H^+ accumulates or bicarbonate ions are lost. Metabolic alkalosis may develop from either loss of H^+ or increase in bicarbonate.
- Unlike the respiratory system, the renal system requires hours to days to significantly affect pH by altering the excretion of bicarbonate.

13

ANALYZING ACID–BASE DISORDERS (TABLE 13-2)

- When analyzing acid–base disorders, several points should be kept in mind:
- Determination of pH and blood gases should be performed preferentially on arterial blood. Venous blood is useless for judging oxygenation or if perfusion is not adequate, but it offers an estimate of acid–base status. Venous pH is

TABLE 13–2. Metabolic and Respiratory Acid–Base Changes in Blood

	pH	pCO$_2$	HCO$_3^-$
Acidosis			
Acute metabolic	D	N	D
Compensated metabolic	N	D	D
Acute respiratory	D	I	N
Compensated respiratory	N	I	I
Alkalosis			
Acute metabolic	I	N	I
Chronic metabolic	I	I	I
Acute respiratory	I	D	N
Compensated respiratory	N	D	D

D = decreased; I = increased; N = normal.

approximately 0.03–0.04 lower than in arterial blood, and CO$_2$ pressure (pCO$_2$) is normally approximately 3–4 mm higher.

- Blood specimens should be packed in ice immediately; a delay of even a few minutes will cause erroneous results, especially if the WBC count is high.
- Determination of electrolytes, pH, and blood gases should be performed on blood specimens obtained simultaneously, since the acid–base situation may be very labile (Table 13-3).
- Repeated determinations are often indicated because of the development of complications, the effect of therapy, and other factors.
- Acid–base disorders are often mixed rather than in the pure form. These mixed disorders may represent simultaneously occurring diseases, complications superimposed on the primary condition, or the effect of treatment.
- Changes in chronic forms may be notably different from those in the acute forms.
- For judging hypoxemia, it is also necessary to know the patient's Hb or Hct and whether the patient was breathing room air or oxygen when the specimen was drawn.
- ABGs cannot be interpreted without clinical information about the patient.
- Renal compensation for a respiratory disturbance is slower (3–7 days) but more successful than respiratory compensation for a metabolic disturbance, but it cannot completely compensate for arterial CO$_2$ pressure (PaCO$_2$) >65 mm Hg, unless another stimulus for HCO$_3$ retention is present. The respiratory mechanism responds quickly but can only eliminate sufficient CO$_2$ to balance the mildest metabolic acidosis (Table 13-4).
- A normal pH does not ensure the absence of an acid–base disturbance if the pCO$_2$ is not known.
- An abnormal HCO$_3$ indicates a metabolic rather than a respiratory problem (Table 13-5; Figures 13-2 and 13-3).
- Decreased HCO$_3^-$ indicates metabolic acidosis.
- Increased HCO$_3^-$ indicates metabolic alkalosis.

TABLE 13–3. Illustrative Serum Electrolyte Values in Various Conditions

Condition	pH	HCO₃⁻(mEq/L)	Potassium (mEq/L)	Sodium (mEq/L)	Chloride (mEq/L)
Normal	7.35–7.45	24–26	3.5–5.0	136–145	100–106
Metabolic acidosis					
Diabetic acidosis	7.2	10	5.6	122	80
Fasting	7.2	16	5.2	142	100
Severe diarrhea	7.2	12	3.2	128	96
Hyperchloremic acidosis	7.2	12	5.2	142	116
Addison disease	7.2	22	6.5	111	72
Nephritis	7.2	8	4.0	129	90
Nephrosis	7.2	20	5.5	138	113
Metabolic alkalosis					
Vomiting	7.6	38	3.2	150	94
Pyloric obstruction	7.6	58	3.2	132	42
Duodenal obstruction	7.6	42	3.2	138	49
Respiratory acidosis	7.1	30	5.5	142	80
Respiratory alkalosis	7.6	14	5.5	136	112

TABLE 13–4. Summary of Pure and Mixed Acid–Base Disorders

	Decreased pH	Normal pH	Increased pH
Increased pCO₂	Respiratory acidosis with or without incompletely compensated metabolic alkalosis or coexisting metabolic acidosis	Respiratory acidosis and compensated metabolic alkalosis	Metabolic alkalosis with incompletely compensated respiratory acidosis or coexisting respiratory acidosis
Normal pCO₂	Metabolic acidosis	Normal	Metabolic alkalosis
Decreased pCO₂	Metabolic acidosis with incompletely compensated respiratory alkalosis or coexisting respiratory alkalosis	Respiratory alkalosis and compensated metabolic acidosis	Respiratory alkalosis with or without incompletely compensated metabolic acidosis or coexisting metabolic alkalosis

Data from Friedman HH. *Problem-Oriented Medical Diagnosis*, 3rd ed. Boston, MA: Little, Brown; 1983.

- Respiratory acidosis is associated with a pCO₂ >45 mm Hg.
- Respiratory alkalosis is associated with a pCO₂ <35 mm Hg.
- Therefore, mixed metabolic and respiratory acidosis is characterized by low pH, low HCO_3^-, and high pCO₂.
- Mixed metabolic and respiratory alkalosis is characterized by high pH, high HCO_3^-, and low pCO₂.
- In severe metabolic acidosis, respiratory compensation is limited by inability to hyperventilate pCO₂ to less than approximately15 mm Hg; beyond that, small increments of the H⁺ produce disastrous changes in pH and prognosis; therefore, patients with lung disorders (e.g., COPD, neuromuscular

TABLE 13–5. Immediate and Delayed Compensatory Response to Acid–Base Disturbances

Acid–Base Abnormality	Immediate Response (By the Lungs)	Delayed Response (By the Kidneys)
Respiratory alkalosis	↑pCO_2 by decreasing ventilation	↓HCO_3^- excretion ↓Acid excretion
Respiratory acidosis	↓pCO_2 by increasing ventilation	↑HCO_3^- retention ↑Acid excretion
Metabolic alkalosis	↑pCO_2 by decreasing ventilation	↓HCO_3^- excretion ↓Acid excretion
Metabolic acidosis	↓pCO_2 by increasing ventilation	↑HCO_3^- retention ↑Acid excretion

↑, increases; ↓, decreases.

weakness) are very vulnerable because they cannot compensate by hyperventilation. In metabolic alkalosis, respiratory compensation is limited by CO_2 retention, which rarely causes pCO_2 >50–60 mm Hg (because increased CO_2 and hypoxemia stimulate respiration very strongly); consequently, pH is not returned to normal (Table 13-6).

- *Base excess (BE)*
- BE hypothetically "corrects" pH to 7.40 by first "adjusting" pCO_2 to 40 mm Hg, thereby allowing comparison of resultant HCO_3^- with normal value at that pH (24 mmol/L). Normal = –2 to +2 mmol/L.
- BE can be calculated by determined values for pH and HCO_3^- by this formula:

$$BE \ (mmol/L) = HCO_3^- + 10 \ (7.40 - pH) - 24$$

- Negative BE indicates depletion of HCO_3^-. It does not distinguish primary from compensatory derangement.

RESPIRATORY ALKALOSIS

- Respiratory alkalosis is defined as a decreased pCO_2 of <38 mm Hg.

❑ **Caused by Hyperventilation**
- CNS disorders (e.g., infection, tumor, trauma, CVA, anxiety–hyperventilation)
- Hypoxia (e.g., high altitudes, ventilation–perfusion imbalance, PE)
- Cardiovascular (e.g., CHF, hypotension)
- Pulmonary disease (e.g., pneumonia, pulmonary emboli, asthma, pneumothorax)
- Drugs (e.g., salicylate intoxication, methylxanthines, β-adrenergic agonists)
- Metabolic (e.g., acidosis [diabetic, renal, lactic], Cirrhosis, liver failure)
- Others (e.g., fever, pregnancy, gram-negative sepsis, pain)
- Mechanical overventilation, cardiopulmonary bypass

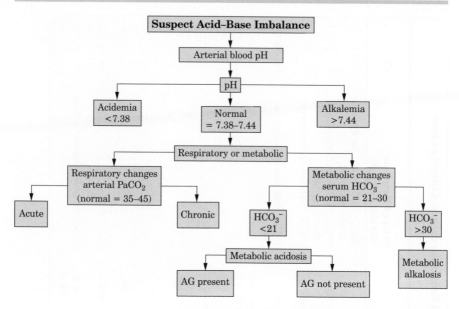

Figure 13-2 *Algorithm for acid–base imbalance and anion gap (AG).*

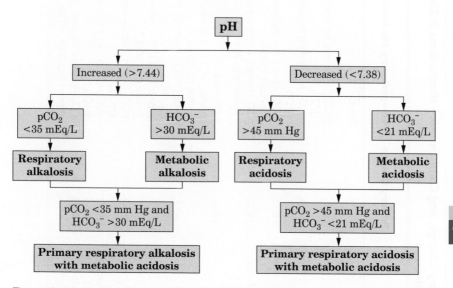

Figure 13-3 *Algorithm illustrating effects of metabolic and respiratory acid–base changes in blood.*

❑ **Diagnostic Findings**

- Acute hypocapnia: Usually only a modest decrease in plasma HCO_3^- concentrations due to conversion to CO_2 and marked alkalosis
- Chronic hypocapnia: Usually only a slight alkaline pH (not usually >7.55)

TABLE 13–6. Primary Change, and Compensatory Mechanisms in Delayed Response to, and Chloride Level in Acid–Base Disturbances

	Primary Change	Compensatory Mechanism	Delayed Response (By the Kidneys)	Cl^-
Respiratory alkalosis	$\downarrow pCO_2$	None	$\downarrow HCO_3^-$ 3–5 mmol/L for every 10 mm Hg $\uparrow pCO_2$	↑
Respiratory acidosis	$\uparrow pCO_2$	$\uparrow HCO_3^-$ 1 mmol/L for every 10 mm Hg $\uparrow pCO_2$	$\uparrow HCO_3^-$ 3–5 mmol/L for every 10 mm Hg $\uparrow pCO_2$	→
Metabolic alkalosis	$\uparrow HCO_3^-$	$\uparrow pCO_2$ 3–5 mm Hg for every 10 mmol/L $\uparrow HCO_3^-$	$\downarrow HCO_3^-$ excretion $\downarrow$ acid excretion	→
Metabolic acidosis with increased anion gap	$\downarrow HCO_3^-$	$\downarrow pCO_2$ 1.0–1.3 mm Hg mmol/L for every 1 mmol/L $\uparrow HCO_3^-$	$\uparrow HCO_3^-$ retention $\uparrow$ acid excretion	No change
Metabolic acidosis normal anion gap	$\downarrow HCO_3^-$	pCO_2 changes 2 for every pH change after decimal (e.g., if pH = 7.25, $pCO_2 = 25 \pm 2$)		↑
Respiratory alkalosis	$\downarrow pCO_2$	*Acute:* none *Chronic:* $\downarrow HCO_3^-$ 3–5 mmol/L for every 10 mm Hg $\uparrow pCO_2$		↑
Respiratory acidosis	$\uparrow pCO_2$	*Acute:* $\uparrow HCO_3^-$ 1 mmol/L for every 10 mm Hg $\uparrow pCO_2$ *Chronic:* $\uparrow HCO_3^-$ 3–5 mmol/L for every 10 mm Hg $\uparrow pCO_2$		→
Metabolic alkalosis	$\uparrow HCO_3^-$	$\uparrow pCO_2$ 3–5 mm Hg for every 10 mmol/L $\uparrow HCO_3^-$		→
Metabolic acidosis with increased anion gap	$\downarrow HCO_3^-$	$\downarrow pCO_2$ 1.0–1.3 mm Hg for every 1 mmol/L $\downarrow HCO_3^-$		No change
Metabolic acidosis with normal anion gap	$\downarrow HCO_3^-$	pCO_2 changes 2 for every pH change after decimal (e.g., if pH = 7.25, $pCO_2 = 25 \pm 2$)	Hyperchloremic metabolic acidosis	↑

↑, increased; ↓, decreased.

RESPIRATORY ACIDOSIS

- Laboratory findings differ in acute and chronic conditions.

❑ **Acute Respiratory Acidosis**

- Caused by decreased alveolar ventilation impairing CO_2 excretion:
- Cardiopulmonary (e.g., pneumonia, pneumothorax, pulmonary edema, foreign body aspiration, laryngospasm, bronchospasm, mechanical ventilation, cardiac arrest).
- CNS depression (e.g., general anesthesia, drugs, brain injury, infection).
- Neuromuscular (e.g., Guillain-Barré syndrome, hypokalemia, myasthenic crisis).
- Acidosis is severe (pH 7.05–7.10), but HCO_3^- concentration is only 29–30 mmol/L.
- Severe mixed acidosis is common in cardiac arrest, when respiratory and circulatory failure causes marked respiratory acidosis and severe lactic acidosis.

❑ **Chronic Respiratory Acidosis**

- Caused by chronic obstructive or restrictive conditions:
- Nerve disease (e.g., poliomyelitis).
- Muscle disease (e.g., myopathy).
- CNS disorder (e.g., brain tumor).
- Restriction of thorax (e.g., musculoskeletal, scleroderma, pickwickian syndrome).
- Pulmonary disease (e.g., prolonged pneumonia, primary alveolar hypoventilation).
- Acidosis is not usually severe.
- Beware of commonly occurring mixed acid–base disturbances (e.g., chronic respiratory acidosis with superimposed acute hypercapnia resulting from acute infection, such as bronchitis or pneumonia).
- Superimposed metabolic alkalosis (e.g., due to diuretics or vomiting) may exacerbate the hypercapnia.

METABOLIC ALKALOSIS

Complex disorder: The main event is either loss of H^+ or gain of HCO_3^-. Alkalosis will quickly be corrected by compensatory mechanisms unless some factors are acting to maintain the alkalosis.

❑ **Causes**

- Loss of acid:
- Vomiting, gastric suction, gastrocolic fistula
- Diarrhea in mucoviscidosis (rarely)
- Villous adenoma of colon
- Aciduria secondary to potassium depletion
- Excess of base caused by administration of
- Absorbable antacids (e.g., sodium bicarbonate; milk-alkali syndrome)
- Salts of weak acids (e.g., sodium lactate, sodium or potassium citrate)
- Some vegetarian diets
- Citrate due to massive blood transfusions

13

- Potassium depletion (causing sodium and H⁺ to enter the cells):
- GI loss (e.g., chronic diarrhea)
- Lack of potassium intake (e.g., anorexia nervosa, IV fluids without potassium supplements for treatment of vomiting or postoperatively)
- Diuresis (e.g., mercurials, thiazides, osmotic diuresis)
- Extracellular volume depletion and chloride depletion
- Dehydration, reducing intracellular volume, thereby stimulating aldosterone, causing excretion of potassium and H⁺
- All forms of mineralocorticoid excess (e.g., primary aldosteronism, Cushing syndrome, administration of steroids, large amounts of licorice) causing excretion of potassium and H⁺
- Glycogen deposition
- Chronic alkalosis
- Potassium-losing nephropathy
- Hypoproteinemia per se may cause a nonrespiratory alkalosis. Decreased albumin of 1 g/dL causes an average increase in standard bicarbonate of 3.4 mmol/L, an apparent base excess of +3.7 mmol/L, and a decrease in AG of approximately 3 mmol/L.

❑ **Diagnostic Findings**

- Serum pH is increased (>7.60 in severe alkalemia).
- Total plasma CO_2 is increased (bicarbonate >30 mmol/L).
- pCO_2 is normal or slightly increased.
- Serum pH and bicarbonate above those predicted by the pCO_2 (by nomogram).
- Hypokalemia is an almost constant feature and is the chief danger in metabolic alkalosis.
- Decreased serum chloride is relatively lower than sodium.
- BUN may be increased.
- Urine pH is >7.0 (≤7.9) if potassium depletion is not severe and concomitant sodium deficiency (e.g., vomiting) is not present. With severe hypokalemia (<2.0 mmol/L), urine may be acid in presence of systemic alkalosis.
- Metabolic alkalosis patients may be volume depleted and chloride responsive or have volume expansion and be chloride resistant.
- When the urine chloride is low (<10 mmol/L) and the patient responds to chloride treatment, the cause is more likely loss of gastric juice, diuretic therapy, or rapid relief of chronic hypercapnia. Chloride replacement is completed when urine chloride remains >40 mmol/L.
- When the urine chloride is high (20 mmol/L) and the patient does not respond to NaCl treatment, the cause is more likely hyperadrenalism or severe potassium deficiency.
- Acid–base maps (Figure 13-4) are a graphic solution of the Henderson-Hasselbalch equation, which predicts the HCO_3^- value for each set of pH/pCO_2 coordinates. They also allow a check of the consistency of ABG and automated analyzer determinations, since these may determine the total CO_2 content, of which 95% is HCO_3^-.
- These maps contain bands that show the 95% probability range of values for each disorder. If the pH/pCO_2 coordinate is outside the 95% confidence band, then the patient has at least two acid–base disturbances.

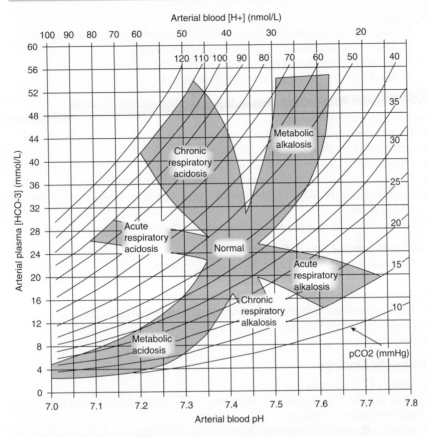

Figure 13–4 *Acid–base map. The values demarcated for each disorder represent a 95% probability range for each pure disorder. Coordinates lying outside these zones suggest mixed acid–base disorders.*

- These maps are of particular use when one of the acid–base disturbances is not suspected clinically. If the coordinates lie within a band, it is not a guarantee of a simple acid–base disturbance.

13

METABOLIC ACIDOSIS

❑ With Increased Anion Gap (AG >15 mmol/L)

- Lactic acidosis—most common cause of metabolic acidosis with increased AG (frequently >25 mmol/L) (see following section "Lactic Acidosis")
- Renal failure (AG <25 mmol/L)
- Ketoacidosis
  - ▼ DM (AG frequently >25 mmol/L)
  - ▼ Associated with alcohol abuse (AG frequently 20–25 mmol/L)
  - ▼ Starvation (AG usually 5–10 mmol/L)

- Drugs
  - ▼ Salicylate poisoning (AG frequently 5–10 mmol/L; higher in children)
  - ▼ Methanol poisoning (AG frequently >20 mmol/L)
  - ▼ Ethylene glycol poisoning (AG frequently >20 mmol/L)
  - ▼ Paraldehyde (AG frequently >20 mmol/L)

❏ **With Normal Anion Gap: Hyperchloremic Metabolic Acidosis**
Decreased Serum Potassium
- Renal tubular acidosis (RTA)
- Acquired (e.g., drugs, hypercalcemia)
- Inherited (e.g., cystinosis, Wilson disease)
- Carbonic anhydrase inhibitors (e.g., acetazolamide, mafenide)
- Increased loss of alkaline body fluids (e.g., diarrhea, loss of pancreatic or biliary fluids)
- Ureteral diversion (e.g., ileal bladder or ureter, ureterosigmoidostomy)

Normal or Increased Serum Potassium
- Hydronephrosis
- Early renal failure
- Administration of HCl (e.g., ammonium chloride)
- Hypoadrenalism (diffuse, zona glomerulosa, or hyporeninemia)
- Renal aldosterone resistance
- Sulfur toxicity

❏ **Diagnostic Findings**
- Serum pH is decreased (<7.3).
- Total plasma CO_2 content is decreased; <15 mmol/L almost certainly rules out respiratory alkalosis.
- Serum potassium is frequently increased; it is decreased in RTA, diarrhea, or carbonic anhydrase inhibition; also, increased serum chloride.
- Azotemia suggests metabolic acidosis due to renal failure.
- Urine is strongly acid (pH 4.5–5.2) if renal function is normal.
- In evaluating acid–base disorders, calculate the AG (see earlier discussion).

LACTIC ACIDOSIS

- Indicates acute hypoperfusion and tissue hypoxia.
- Should be considered in any metabolic acidosis with increased AG (>15 mmol/L).
- Diagnosis is confirmed by exclusion of other causes of metabolic acidosis and serum lactate ≥5 mmol/L (upper limit of normal = 1.6 for plasma and 1.4 for whole blood). There is considerable variation in the literature in limits of serum lactate and pH to define lactic acidosis.
- In lactic acidosis, the increase in AG is usually greater than the decrease in HCO_3^-, in contrast to DKA, in which the increase in AG is identical to the decrease in HCO_3^-.
- Exclusion of other causes by
- Normal serum creatinine and BUN (increased acetoacetic acid [but not beta-hydroxybutyric acid] will cause false increase of creatinine by colorimetric assay).

- Osmolar gap <10 mOsm/L.
- Negative nitroprusside reaction (nitroprusside test for ketoacidosis measures acetoacetic acid but not β-hydroxybutyric acid; thus, the blood ketone test may be negative in DKA).
- Urine negative for calcium oxalate crystals.
- No known ingestion of toxic substances.
- Laboratory findings due to underlying diseases (e.g., DM, renal insufficiency).
- Laboratory tests for monitoring therapy:
- Arterial pH, pCO_2, HCO_3^-, serum electrolytes every 1–2 hours until the patient is stable
- Urine electrolytes every 6 hours
- Associated or compensatory metabolic or respiratory disturbances (e.g., hyperventilation or respiratory alkalosis) may result in normal pH
- Type A caused by tissue hypoxia (e.g., acute hemorrhage, severe anemia, shock, asphyxia), marathon running, seizures
- Type B without tissue hypoxia caused by
- Common disorders (e.g., DM, uremia, liver disease, infections, malignancies, alkaloses).
- Drugs and toxins (e.g., ethanol, methanol, ethylene glycol, salicylates, metformin).
- Hereditary enzyme defects (e.g., methylmalonic acidemia, propionic acid-uria, defects of fatty acid oxidation, pyruvate dehydrogenase deficiency, pyruvate carboxylase deficiency, multiple carboxylase deficiency, glycogen storage disease type I).
- Others (e.g., starvation, short bowel syndrome).
- With a typical clinical picture (acute onset following nausea and vomiting, altered state of consciousness, hyperventilation, high mortality).
- Decreased serum bicarbonate.
- Low serum pH, usually 6.98–7.25.
- Increased serum potassium, often 6–7 mmol/L.
- Serum chloride normal or low with increased AG.
- Increased serum phosphorus. Phosphorus-to-creatinine ratio >3 indicates lactic acidosis either alone or as a component of other metabolic acidosis.
- WBC count is increased (occasionally to leukemoid levels).
- Increased serum uric acid is frequent (up to 25 mg/dL in lactic acidosis).
- Increased serum AST, LD, and phosphorus levels.

MIXED ACID–BASE DISTURBANCES

13

- Mixed acid–base disturbances must always be interpreted with clinical data and other laboratory findings.

❑ **Respiratory Acidosis with Metabolic Acidosis**
- Acidemia may be extreme with
- pH <7.0 (H^+ >100 mmol/L).
- HCO_3^- <26 mmol/L. Failure of HCO_3^- to increase ≥3 mmol/L for each 10 mm Hg rise in pCO_2 suggests metabolic acidosis with respiratory acidosis.
- Examples: Acute pulmonary edema, cardiopulmonary arrest (lactic acidosis due to tissue anoxia and CO_2 retention due to alveolar hypoventilation).

- Mild metabolic acidosis superimposed on chronic hypercapnia causing partial suppression of HCO_3^- may be indistinguishable from adaptation to hypercapnia alone.

❏ **Respiratory Acidosis with Metabolic Alkalosis**

- Decreased or absent urine chloride indicates that chloride-responsive metabolic alkalosis is a part of the picture.
- In clinical setting of respiratory acidosis but with normal blood pH and/or HCO_3^- higher than predicted, complicating metabolic alkalosis may be present.
- Examples: chronic pulmonary disease with CO_2 retention developing metabolic alkalosis due to administration of diuretics, severe vomiting, or sudden improvement in ventilation ("posthypercapnic" metabolic alkalosis).

❏ **Metabolic Acidosis with Respiratory Alkalosis**

- pH may be normal or decreased.
- Hypocapnia remains inappropriate to decreased HCO_3^- for several hours or more.
- Examples: Rapid correction of severe metabolic acidosis, salicylate intoxication, gram-negative septicemia, initial respiratory alkalosis with subsequent development of metabolic acidosis. Primary metabolic acidosis with primary respiratory alkalosis with an increased AG is characteristic of salicylate intoxication in the absence of uremia and DKA.

❏ **Metabolic Alkalosis with Respiratory Alkalosis**

- Marked alkalemia with decreased pCO_2 and increased HCO_3^- is diagnostic.
- Examples: Hepatic insufficiency with hyperventilation plus administration of diuretics or severe vomiting; metabolic alkalosis with stimulation of ventilation (e.g., sepsis, pulmonary embolism, mechanical ventilation), which causes respiratory alkalosis.

❏ **Acute and Chronic Respiratory Acidosis**

- May be suspected when HCO_3^- is in intermediate range between acute and chronic respiratory acidosis (similar findings in chronic respiratory acidosis with superimposed metabolic acidosis or acute respiratory acidosis with superimposed metabolic alkalosis)
- Examples: Chronic hypercapnia with acute deterioration of pulmonary function causing further rise of pCO_2

❏ **Coexistence of Metabolic Acidosis of Hyperchloremic Type and Increased Anion Gap**

- May be suspected by plasma HCO_3^- that is lower than is explained by the increase in anions (e.g., AG = 16 mmol/L and HCO_3^- = 5 mmol/L)
- Examples: Uremia and proximal RTA, lactic acidosis with diarrhea, excessive administration of NaCl to a patient with organic acidosis

❏ **Coexistence of Metabolic Alkalosis and Metabolic Acidosis**

- May be suspected by acid–base values that are too normal for clinical picture
- Examples: Vomiting causing alkalosis plus bicarbonate-losing diarrhea causing acidosis

PEARLS

- *Pulmonary embolus*: Mild to moderate respiratory alkalosis is present unless sudden death occurs. The degree of hypoxia often correlates with the size and extent of the pulmonary embolus. pO_2 >90 mm Hg when breathing room air virtually excludes a lung problem.

- *Acute pulmonary edema*: Hypoxemia is usual. CO_2 is not increased unless the situation is grave.

- *Asthma*: Hypoxia occurs even during a mild episode and increases as the attack becomes worse. As hyperventilation occurs, the pCO_2 falls (usually <35 mm Hg); a normal pCO_2 (>40 mm Hg) implies impending respiratory failure; increased pCO_2 in a true asthmatic (not bronchitis or emphysema) indicates impending disaster and the need to consider intubation and ventilation assistance.

- *Chronic obstructive pulmonary disease* (bronchitis and emphysema) may show two patterns—"pink puffers," with mild hypoxia and normal pH and pCO_2 and "blue bloaters," with hypoxia and increased pCO_2; normal pH suggests compensation and decreased pH suggests decompensation.

- *Neurologic and neuromuscular disorders* (e.g., drug overdose, Guillain-Barré syndrome, myasthenia gravis, trauma, succinylcholine): Acute alveolar hypoventilation causes uncompensated respiratory acidosis with high pCO_2, low pH, and normal HCO_3^-. Acidosis appears before significant hypoxemia, and rising CO_2 indicates rapid deterioration and need for mechanical assistance.

- *Sepsis*: Unexplained respiratory alkalosis may be the earliest sign of sepsis. It may progress to cause metabolic acidosis, and the mixed picture may produce a normal pH; low HCO_3^- is useful for recognizing this. With deterioration and worsening of metabolic acidosis, the pH falls.

- *Salicylate poisoning* characteristically shows poor correlation between serum salicylate level and presence or degree of acidemia (because as pH drops from 7.4 to 7.2, the proportion of nonionized to ionized salicylate doubles and the nonionized form leaves the serum and is sequestered in the brain and other organs, where it interferes with function at a cellular level without changing blood levels of glucose, and so on). Salicylate poisoning in adults typically causes respiratory alkalosis, but in children, this progresses rapidly to mixed respiratory alkalosis/metabolic acidosis and then to metabolic acidosis (in adults, metabolic acidosis is said to be rare and a near-terminal event).

- *Isopropyl* (rubbing) alcohol poisoning produces enough circulating acetone to produce a positive nitroprusside test (it, therefore, may be mistaken for DKA; consequently, insulin should not be given until the blood glucose is known). In the absence of a history, positive serum ketone test associated with normal AG, normal serum HCO_3^-, and normal blood glucose suggests rubbing alcohol intoxication.

- *A change in chloride concentration independent of*, or out of proportion to, changes in sodium usually indicates an acid–base disorder.

13

CHAPTER 14

Toxicology and Therapeutic Drug Monitoring

Amanda J. Jenkins

Toxicology is the study of the adverse effects of chemicals on living organisms. Clinical toxicology is a subspecialty with emphasis on management of a poisoned patient. The application is focused on human beings but may be equally applied in veterinary medicine. The principles of clinical toxicology are applied to two main areas—emergency toxicology and therapeutic drug monitoring. Emerging fields include addiction medicine and pain management.

EMERGENCY TOXICOLOGY

❏ Purpose

The majority of poisoned patients enter the health care system in the emergency department. Treatment is often based on exposure history and signs and symptoms of poisoning based on physical examination. Laboratory testing may be performed to confirm the physician's diagnosis or to identify a toxin in the absence of a differential diagnosis.

Knowledge of toxidromes is important as a starting point for patient evaluation (Table 14-1). These consist of a collection of signs and symptoms that are typically produced by specific toxins.

❏ Application

Testing offered by clinical toxicology laboratories consists of screening and confirmation.

❏ Screening Methods and Limitations

Screening tests are usually conducted on urine. These require little or no sample preparation and are frequently immunoassay based. These tests have high sensitivity; however, they have limitations due to moderate specificity. Many commercially available tests cross-react with multiple drugs within a class due to choice of target drug. They may also be sensitive to adulterants. Clinicians must be aware of the

TABLE 14–1. Signs and Symptoms of Common Toxidromes

Toxidrome	Causal Agents	Signs and Symptoms
Opioid	Opioids, clonidine, phenothiazines	Hypothermia, bradypnea, lethargy, miosis, altered mental status
Sympathomimetic	Sympathomimetic amphetamines, cocaine, caffeine, salicylates	Hyperthermia, tachycardia, agitation, hypertension, tremor, restlessness, insomnia
Sedative–hypnotic	Barbiturates, benzodiazepines, ethanol	Hypothermia, lethargy, confusion, sedation, ataxia
Anticholinergic	Antipsychotics, atropine antihistamines (e.g., diphenhydramine)	Hyperthermia, mydriasis, tachycardia, dry flushed skin, decreased bowel sounds
Cholinergic	Organophosphates, physostigmine	Bradycardia/tachycardia, salivation, lacrimation, urination, diarrhea, emesis

commercial tests utilized in their laboratory, as cross-reactivities differ between manufacturers and within manufacturers over time.

These tests are typically performed on automated chemistry analyzers. Although individual drug–drug classes are available, many hospital laboratories offer these tests as panels and are available as "stat" tests.

Immunoassay testing may be based on

- Radioimmunoassay (RIA)
- Enzyme multiplied immunoassay technique (EMIT)
- Enzyme-linked immunosorbent assay (ELISA)
- Fluorescence polarization immunoassay (FPIA)
- Kinetic interaction of particles (KIMS)
- Cloned enzyme donor immunoassay (CEDIA)

Immunoassays are typically qualitative assays, although semiquantitative results are possible with some kits. For qualitative testing, the instrument is calibrated at one concentration, called the cutoff concentration. For example, when utilizing EMIT, all specimens that have absorbance values equivalent to this cutoff calibrator or greater will be reported as positive. Manufacturers provide this calibrator, so the laboratory has no choice in this concentration unless they alter the kit provided (e.g., dilution, to obtain alternate/user-defined cutoffs).

Cutoff concentrations for these kits have historically been decided with reference to the DHHS SAMSHA–mandated cutoffs for federal workplace drug testing, the so-called NIDA5 drugs/classes (PCP, opiates, cannabinoids [marijuana], cocaine metabolite, amphetamines). These cutoff concentrations are not generally appropriate for clinical use, since the cutoff values for several drug–drug classes are fairly high (see Table 14-2). This decreases the likelihood of false-positive results. The detection of drug abuse rather than legitimate drug use is targeted (see Forensic Toxicology).

Practitioners should also be aware of the relative cross-reactivities of the tests ordered. For example, immunoassays for opiates target morphine and typically do not produce positive results with samples containing synthetic and semisynthetic opioids such as oxycodone, fentanyl, propoxyphene, and tramadol.

TABLE 14-2. U.S. DHHS Cutoff Concentrations for Urine

Drug (Class)	Immunoassay Screening	Confirmation, ng/mL
6-Acetylmorphine	10	10 6-acetylmorphine
Amphetamines	500	250 amphetamine; 250 methamphetamine
Cannabinoids	50	15 THC-COOH
Cocaine metabolite	150	100 benzoylecgonine
MDMA	500	250 MDMA; 250 MDA; 250 MDEA
Opiates	2,000	2,000 morphine; 2,000 codeine; 10 6-AM
Phencyclidine	25	25 phencyclidine

Table 14-3 lists the detection time of several drugs in urine. Note variables that must be considered include dose, frequency and route of administration, formulation, and patient-related factors (e.g., disease, other drugs, genetic polymorphisms).

❑ **Confirmation Methods and Limitations**

Confirmation tests are typically performed following a positive screening result. Confirmatory tests are ordered if it is necessary to identify a specific drug, obtain a quantitative result, or make a determination for legal purposes. For example, a positive opiate immunoassay result will not establish the identity of the opiate. A more specific test is required. These are typically chromatography based and are not performed on a "stat" basis. Chromatography is a separation process based on the differential distribution of sample constituents between a moving mobile

TABLE 14-3. Approximate Detection Times in Urine of Some Drugs of Abuse

Drug	Detection Time
Heroin (as morphine)	1–2 d
Cocaine (as metabolites)	3 d
Morphine	1–2 d
Amphetamine 3,4-methylenedioxymethamphetamine (MDMA)	1–2 d
Methadone (as metabolites)	3–7 d
Volatiles	<1 d
Oxycodone	1–2 d
Gamma-hydroxybutyrate (GHB)	12–24 h
Phencyclidine (PCP)	1–2 wk
11-Nor-delta 9-tetrahydrocannabinol-9-carboxylic acid (THCA) (marijuana metabolite) (single use)	2–7 d
Barbiturates	
All except phenobarbital	2 d
Phenobarbital	1–2 wk
Benzodiazepines	
All except flunitrazepam	5–7 d
Flunitrazepam (as metabolites)	<3 d

and a stationary phase. Chromatography is a separation technique not identification. Mass spectrometry provides identification, since it provides mass and charge information unique to individual drugs. Identification may not be necessary in therapeutic drug monitoring (TDM). Sample pretreatment, extraction, and complex instrumental analysis are required. Common methods used for confirmation tests are

Gas chromatography (GC)
High-performance liquid chromatography (HPLC)
GC/mass spectrometry (GC/MS, GC/MS/MS)
Liquid chromatography/mass spectrometry (LC/MS, LC/MS/MS)

❏ Interpretation of Quantitative Results in Urine

Drug concentrations in urine are not reflective of the dose of drug administered or a specific dosing regimen. Semiquantitative results provided by immunoassays may reflect contributions from more than one drug. For example, a presumptive positive immunoassay screen for opiates may be due to the presence of morphine, heroin, 6-acetylmorphine, and codeine in the specimen. Confirmation testing should provide identification of each drug present and may also provide quantitative results for each specific drug. In these instances, the laboratory may report total or free drug levels, that is, drug present that may be conjugated or unconjugated.

The concentration of drug present in a random urine specimen is the result of the drug delivery system, acute or chronic drug administration, the time of specimen collection, the hydration status of the individual, renal and hepatic function, urine pH, the presence of other drugs resulting in drug interactions, individual pharmacokinetics, and pharmacogenetic polymorphisms. Urine drug/creatinine ratios may be calculated in order to minimize effects on drug concentrations due to changes in the fluid intake of the patient. Monitoring over time may assist in the determination between abstinence and renewed drug use.

❏ Specimen Validity and Drug Testing Background

Specimen validity is an important but often overlooked aspect of laboratory testing. Validity refers to the correct specimen identity (i.e., a urine sample is in fact human urine). The collectors of samples in physician offices and other sites have the responsibility of ensuring that adequate specimens are collected from patients. The validity of a specimen may be questioned if the sample is substituted or adulterated.

- A *substituted* sample is a substance provided in place of the donor's specimen. This may be drug-free urine (from another individual) or another liquid such as water.
- An *adulterated* sample is a specimen to which substance(s) have been added to destroy the drug in the sample or interfere with the analytical tests utilized to detect drugs. Common additives include vinegar, bleach, liquid hand soap, lemon juice, and household cleaners. In the last several years, commercial products have become available to subvert drug tests. These products have been found to contain substances that include glutaraldehyde, sodium chloride, chromate, nitrite, surfactant, and peroxide/peroxidase.

In addition, specimens may be *diluted* by adding liquids to the urine at the time of collection to decrease the concentration of drug in the sample below the cutoff concentration used for the test. In vivo dilution involves the ingestion of diuretics

14

and other substances to remove the drugs from the body or dilute the urine, for example, drinking an excessive quantity of water before a drug test.

Minimizing Specimen Validity Issues at the Collection Site

In many industries where urine is collected for drug testing for nonmedical purposes, for example, preemployment screening, specimens are collected under chain of custody and also several physical procedures are in place to minimize the likelihood of specimen substitution or adulteration. These procedures include witnessing the collection, not providing access to water in the bathroom, and coloring toilet bowl water. In addition, donors may not be permitted to wear loose clothing in which a substituted specimen could be hidden. Before the specimen is sealed in the collection container with tamper-resistant tape, the collector may record the temperature of the specimen (normal range for validity testing considered 90–100°F) as well as the urine color.

Urine Characteristics

Physical, chemical, or DNA tests may be used to assure the validity of a specimen. These tests are most frequently requested in connection with urine drug testing, especially for drugs of abuse such as cannabinoids (marijuana), heroin, and cocaine.

Creatinine, specific gravity, and pH are tests performed to assess whether a specimen is consistent with normal human urine. The U.S. Department of Health and Human Services Mandatory Guidelines specify acceptable ranges for these tests (for federally regulated drug testing specimens), and clinical laboratories and other providers have tended to adopt these values, some with slight modifications.

Creatinine is formed as a result of creatine metabolism in skeletal muscle, and the amount produced is relatively constant within an individual. This parameter is utilized clinically to assess renal function. A level ≥20 mg/dL in human urine is considered normal. Diluted and substituted (with water) specimens will have creatinine concentrations <20 mg/dL.

Specific gravity for liquids is the ratio of the density of a substance (urine) to the density of water at the same temperature. Hence, it is a measurement of the concentration of dissolved solids in the urine. The specific gravity of normal human urine ranges between 1.003 and 1.030. High values may be caused by disease (kidney disease, glucosuria, liver disease, dehydration, adrenal insufficiency, and proteinuria), whereas low values may be caused by diabetes insipidus (DI). Dilution and adulteration (e.g., with the organic solvents methanol and ethanol) results in a value <1.000.

The pH of normal human urine is typically between 5.0 and 8.0. The reference range is 4.5–9.0. This parameter can be affected by diet, medications, and disease. Acidic urine may be caused by acidosis (respiratory and metabolic), uremia, severe diarrhea, starvation, and diets with a large intake of acid-containing fruit. In contrast, an alkaline urine may be attributed to alkalosis, urinary tract infections, high-vegetable diets, and sodium bicarbonate. Individuals with dietary or disease causes of acidic or alkaline urine will be consistently in this range, rather than a random urine high or low due to adulteration or substitution. If lemon juice or vinegar is added to urine, the pH is lowered. A high urine pH results from the addition of bleach or soap.

Methodology

Tests should be conducted as soon as possible after urine collection. Creatinine may be determined by dipstick or automated clinical chemistry analyzer based on a chemical reaction that produces a color result. The specific gravity may be measured by refractometry in which the refractive index of the urine is determined. Alternatively, the dipstick method is based on ionic strength. A procedure available for automated clinical chemistry analyzers utilizes urine chloride ion concentration and spectrophotometry. pH is measured using a pH meter or colorimetrically manually or using an automated clinical chemistry analyzer.

Laboratories also offer tests for common adulterants. These include specific tests for nitrite and glutaraldehyde, typically using colorimetric assays, or generalized tests for oxidants. The latter detects compounds that exert their action by oxidation and include chromate and peroxidase. The method as performed on an automated clinical chemistry analyzer evaluates the reaction between a substrate and oxidant in the sample producing color that can be measured at a specific wavelength.

Specimen Requirements

A random urine specimen should be refrigerated after collection and sent to the laboratory as soon as possible. Urine samples suspected of bacterial contamination will produce invalid pH results. Sodium azide should not be used as a preservative, as this may cause interference with the Oxidant test. Table 14-4 presents reference ranges.

 # THERAPEUTIC DRUG MONITORING

❑ Purpose

Therapeutic drug monitoring (TDM) is the determination of drug levels in blood. The purpose of such measurement is to optimize the dose in order to achieve maximum clinical effect. TDM is typically performed on drugs with a low therapeutic index.

Indications

- Signs of toxicity.
- Therapeutic effect not obtained.
- Suspected noncompliance.
- Drug has narrow therapeutic range.
- To provide or confirm an optimal dosing schedule.

14

TABLE 14–4. Reference Ranges for Urine Specimens	
Component	**Range**
pH	4.5–9.0
Creatinine	≥20 mg/dL
Specific gravity	1.003–1.040
Oxidants	<200 mcg/mL

- To confirm cause of organ toxicity (e.g., abnormal liver or kidney function tests).
- Other diseases or conditions exist that affect drug utilization.
- Drug interactions that have altered desired or previously achieved therapeutic concentration are suspected.
- Drug shows large variations in utilization or metabolism between individuals.
- Need medicolegal verification of treatment, cause of death or injury (e.g., suicide, homicide, accident investigation), or to detect use of forbidden drugs (e.g., steroids in athletes, narcotics).
- Differential diagnosis of coma.

❑ **Applications**

- The clinician must be aware of the various influences on pharmacokinetics—factors such as half-life, time to peak and to steady state, protein binding, and excretion.
- The route of administration and sampling time after last dose of drug must be known for proper interpretation. For some drugs (e.g., quinidine), different assay methods produce different values, and the clinician must know the normal range for the test method used for the patient.
- In general, peak concentrations alone are useful when testing for toxicity, and trough concentrations alone are useful for demonstrating a satisfactory therapeutic concentration. Trough concentrations are commonly used with such drugs as lithium, theophylline, phenytoin, carbamazepine, quinidine, tricyclic antidepressants, valproic acid, and digoxin. Trough concentrations can usually be drawn at the time the next dose is administered (*this does not apply to digoxin*). Both peak and trough concentrations are used to avoid toxicity but ensure bactericidal efficacy (e.g., gentamicin, tobramycin, vancomycin).
- IV and IM administration should usually be sampled 30 minutes to 1 hour after administration is ended to determine peak concentrations (meant only as a general guide; the laboratory performing the tests should supply its own values).
- Blood should be drawn at a time specified by that laboratory (e.g., 1 hour before the next dose is due to be administered). This trough concentration should ideally be greater than the minimum effective serum concentration.
- If a drug is administered by IV infusion, blood should be drawn from the opposite arm.
- The drug should have been administered at a constant rate for at least 4–5 half-lives before blood samples are drawn.
- Unexpected test results may be due to interference by complementary and alternative medicines (e.g., high digoxin levels may result from interference from danshen, Chan Su, or ginseng).

Criteria

- Available methodology must be specific and reliable.
- Blood concentration must correlate with therapeutic and toxic effects.
- Therapeutic window is narrow with danger of toxicity on therapeutic doses.
- Correlation between blood concentration and dose is poor.
- Clinical effect of drug is not easily determined.

❏ Drugs for Which Drug Monitoring May Be Useful

- Antiepileptic drugs (e.g., phenobarbital, phenytoin)
- Theophylline
- Antimicrobials (aminoglycosides [gentamicin, tobramycin, amikacin], chloramphenicol, vancomycin, flucytosine [5-fluorocytosine])
- Antipsychotic drugs
- Antianxiety drugs
- Cyclic antidepressants
- Lithium
- Cardiac glycosides, antiarrhythmics, antianginal, antihypertensive drugs
- Antineoplastic drugs
- Immunosuppressant drugs
- Anti-inflammatory drugs (e.g., NSAIDs, steroids)
- Drugs of abuse: addiction treatment, pain management
- Athletic performance enhancement drugs (e.g., androgenic anabolic steroids, erythropoietin)

❏ Pharmacokinetics

Pharmacokinetics (PK) is the study of the time course of drugs in the body. PK seeks to relate the concentration of drug in a specimen to the amount of drug administered (dose). PK investigates

- Absorption
- Distribution
- Metabolism
- Excretion or elimination

Changes in these parameters affect drug concentrations.

Absorption

Absorption describes the process in which the drug or xenobiotic enters the bloodstream. For intravenous/intra-arterial administration, there is no absorption. Other common routes of administration include oral, intramuscular, subcutaneous, inhalation, rectal, intrathecal, oral mucosa, dermal, and intranasal. The following factors affect the bioavailability (amount absorbed compared with amount administered):

- Surface area
- Solubility
- Blood supply
- Concentration
- pH
- Molecular size and shape
- Degree of ionization

Distribution

This describes the transfer of the drug from site of administration throughout the body. This is generally movement from the bloodstream to tissues. Therefore, it is a function of the blood supply to the tissues. A drug may rapidly be distributed to highly perfused tissues such as brain, heart, liver, and kidney, whereas slower distribution will occur for muscle, fat, and bone. Factors affecting drug absorption are also relevant to distribution. Plasma protein binding is an additional factor to consider.

14

Metabolism

Drugs are chemically altered to facilitate removal from the body. This process is performed mainly in the liver by enzymes. Other sites of enzyme activity include the GI tract, blood, kidney, and lung. Phase I metabolism describes transformation of functional groups on the drug molecule. Phase II are known as conjugation reactions and involve addition of endogenous substances to render the compound more water soluble. The most common conjugation reaction involves the addition of uridine diphosphate-glucuronic acid with hydroxyl or amino groups to form glucuronides. Opiates and benzodiazepines are highly glucuronidated prior to excretion.

Excretion

Removal of drug from the body typically occurs in urine from the kidney, feces from the liver, and breath from the lung. Drugs are also eliminated in sweat, breast milk, and sebum. Removal of drug by the liver, clearance, depends on blood flow to the liver, which may be increased in the presence of food, the presence of phenobarbital, and decreased during exercise, dehydration, disease (cirrhosis, CHF), and the presence of anesthetics. Removal of drug also depends on the ability of the liver to extract drug from the bloodstream. This includes diffusion and carrier systems. Renal excretion is a function of filtration, secretion, and reabsorption. Again the processes that affect transfer across biologic membranes must be considered.

❏ Conclusions

In general, increases in serum/plasma drug concentrations may be observed in

1. Overdose
2. Coingestion of drugs that compete for metabolic enzymes
3. Liver and renal failure/insufficiency
4. Age-related increases due to loss in enzyme activity, decreases in absorption, blood flow, intestinal motility
5. Genetic polymorphisms—slow metabolizers
6. Movement of drugs from tissue depots

In general, decreases in serum/plasma drug concentrations may be observed in

1. Decreased oral bioavailability
2. Increased metabolism due to coingestion of drugs that induce metabolic enzymes such as phenobarbital, phenytoin
3. Increased renal clearance
4. Increases in plasma proteins (results in decreases in observed serum drug concentrations, since most tests measure unbound or free drug concentrations)

❏ Alternate Matrices

Drugs may be detected in nontraditional matrices

- Meconium
- Oral fluid (saliva)
- Sweat
- Hair

The majority of hospital laboratories do not offer testing in these specimens. Sample pretreatment prior to testing is often required and, therefore, are not offered on a "stat" basis. Special sample collection devices are available for sweat and oral fluid. Hair testing provides a longer detection window for drugs than does serum or urine and is generally reflective of chronic exposure.

❏ **Units**

Drugs concentrations are reported using several concentration units.

- ng/mL, which are equivalent to mcg/L

Note that "mcg" are used throughout this text because "ug" or "μg" are prohibited abbreviations. When handwritten the "u" may be misread as "m."

- mcg/mL, which are equivalent to mg/L

Note that ethanol concentrations in the clinical setting are typically reported in mg/dL. Conversion to g% (g/dL) is often requested; for example, 80 mg/dL is equivalent to 0.08 g/dL. To convert mg/dL to g/dL, divide by 1,000. Conversely, to convert g/dL to mg/dL, multiply by 1,000.

 ADDICTION MEDICINE

❏ **Purpose**

Provision of professional health care services to treat a diagnosed substance use disorder

❏ **Application**

Drug testing during treatment to assess and monitor the clinical status of an individual. Testing should be limited to that which is medically necessary. Testing is appropriate in inpatient and outpatient settings and is especially important at the beginning of treatment. Periodic random drug testing in this population may act as a deterrent to substance use and aids in identifying lapses in treatment. In addition, such testing may identify compounds that have potential drug interactions with a prescribed medication.

❏ **Screening Methods and Limitations**

- Point of care or laboratory immunoassay tests are the most common screening tests utilized.
- Urine, serum, oral fluid, and hair are all potentially useful specimens to monitor drug abstinence or compliance with prescribed medications.
- Oral fluid and serum are the preferred specimens in assessing impairment.
- Specialized laboratory services are usually required for drug testing in oral fluid and hair.
- Positive screening results should be confirmed before any adverse action is taken against an individual.
- A typical drug testing panel for addiction medicine includes
  - ▼ *Urine*:
    - Opiates—morphine, codeine, 6-acetylmorphine
    - Opioids—buprenorphine, methadone, oxycodone, oxymorphone, hydrocodone, hydromorphone

- Benzodiazepines
- Cannabinoids
- Cocaine (mtb)
- Amphetamine/methamphetamine/MDMA
- Phencyclidine
- Cotinine

▼ *Serum*:
- Ethanol

❑ Confirmation Methods and Limitations

- Confirmation methods are chromatographic and generally require 24–48 hours to provide results.
- Urinary quantitative results of a prescribed medication may be useful under some circumstances (e.g., to assist in differentiating active smoking from passive exposure to nicotine), but in general, qualitative identification of the drug is sufficient.
- Quantitative serum ethanol results are useful in assessing the degree of impairment.

 PAIN MANAGEMENT

❑ Purpose
Use of opioids and other medications (nonopioid analgesics, benzodiazepines, antidepressants, anticonvulsants, muscle relaxants) to treat pain of noncancer origin

❑ Application
Urine drug monitoring to ensure safe and effective therapy. This includes continued effectiveness for pain relief; assessment of the potential for misuse, addiction, or diversion.

Drug testing in this population does not mirror the traditional DOA testing. The testing requirements are dependent upon

- Patient population
- Specific drug(s) of interest
- Specimen
- Sensitivity
- Specificity
- Requirement for quantitative results

The objectives of periodic urine drug tests are

- To detect drug use
  ▼ Verify adherence to prescribed medications
  ▼ Identify use of undisclosed drugs
- To discourage drug misuse
  ▼ Decrease potential of abuse
  ▼ Decrease potential for diversion

❏ Screening Methods and Limitations

- May be point of care (POC) or laboratory immunoassay tests or high-resolution mass spectrometric techniques. Results obtained will depend upon screening method. Variables include sensitivity and specificity.
- IA tests with low cross-reactivity to a class of compounds have a high probability of false-negative results, and therefore, consideration should be given to confirm these drugs regardless of screening result, for example, opioids and benzodiazepines.
- A typical urine drug testing panel for pain management includes
  - ▼ Opiates—morphine, codeine, 6-acetylmorphine
  - ▼ Opioids—fentanyl, buprenorphine, methadone, tramadol, oxycodone, oxymorphone, hydrocodone, hydromorphone, meperidine, tapentadol
  - ▼ Benzodiazepines
  - ▼ Muscle relaxants—carisoprodol
  - ▼ Cannabinoids
  - ▼ Cocaine (mtb)
  - ▼ Amphetamine/methamphetamine/MDMA
  - ▼ Barbiturates—phenobarbital, butalbital
  - ▼ Phencyclidine

❏ Confirmation Methods and Limitations

- The decision-making process of whether to order confirmation testing should include the following:
  - ▼ Are the screen results inconsistent with clinical expectations?
  - ▼ Does the screening test detect the drug(s) of interest?
  - ▼ Are quantitative results required?
- Drug levels in urine cannot be used to estimate dose.
- The presence of opioid process impurities may explain apparent inconsistent results.

❏ Interpretation

- Drug not detected due to
  - ▼ Drug not taken/administered
  - ▼ Drug taken incorrectly (decreased dose or frequency)
  - ▼ Variable drug delivery—drug not absorbed
  - ▼ Accelerated metabolism, elimination
  - ▼ Drug–drug interaction
  - ▼ Specimen collected outside detection window
  - ▼ Specimen dilute, substituted, adulterated
  - ▼ Test not designed to detect drug
  - ▼ Clinic or laboratory error
- Drug detected due to
  - ▼ Drug was taken/administered.
  - ▼ Drug detected is a process impurity.
  - ▼ Drug detected is an expected metabolite of a prescribed drug.
  - ▼ Incorrect prescription filled.
  - ▼ Drug obtained elsewhere.
  - ▼ Drug added to specimen.

14

▼ Result is a false positive (for IA screens).
▼ Clinic or laboratory error.
■ Knowledge of drug metabolic profiles is important.
  ▼ For many drugs, parent drug and metabolite should be present. For example, buprenorphine and norbuprenorphine would be expected to be present in a patient taking buprenorphine. The presence of norbuprenorphine is indicative of metabolism.
■ Knowledge of the pharmacokinetic characteristics of drugs is important.
  ▼ Drug absorption rates vary based on different formulations and routes of administration.
  ▼ Serum/plasma half-lives and urinary elimination half-lives assist in assessing drug detection times and therefore the likelihood that a test on a specimen collected at a specified time after drug administration will be positive.
■ Quantitative urine levels may be useful to identify
  ▼ Minor metabolic pathways
  ▼ Low levels of allowable process impurities in pharmaceutical preparations
  ▼ Possible specimen adulteration

 ## FORENSIC TOXICOLOGY

❏ Purpose

The discipline of clinical toxicology involves treating the poisoned patient, monitoring compliance with medications, or drug abstinence and monitoring drug concentrations in order to optimize dosing. The purpose is to treat patients. The discipline of forensic toxicology, however, involves the application of toxicology for legal purposes. Therefore, results from forensic toxicologic analysis may be used in courts of law. The level of proof is greater in forensic cases. As a result, specimen integrity is essential, and a chain of custody is utilized. Screening results are confirmed by a more specific and usually more sensitive technique. Forensic toxicology is broadly divided into three categories:

■ Medicolegal death investigation
  ▼ Toxicologic analysis used to assist coroners and medical examiners in determining the cause and manner of death. Specimen types that may be included in this testing are blood from two sites, urine, vitreous humor, bile, cerebrospinal fluid, and tissues such as liver and brain.
■ Drug testing
  ▼ Typically utilizing urine to test for drugs of abuse. Individuals may be subject to drug testing programs in the workplace, probation/parole (criminal justice system), sports, and in schools.
■ Human performance
  ▼ Assessing the effects of drugs on human behavior to include operating a vehicle under the influence of ethanol and other drugs. Whole blood, serum/plasma, and urine are commonly used for this testing.

❏ Application

Although similar drugs may be detected and similar analytical techniques utilized in both clinical and forensic toxicology, the purpose of the testing is different, and interpretation of the findings is often dissimilar. Since laboratories may perform both types of testing, the practitioner should be aware of potential differences. One important difference is that immunoassay screening cutoff concentrations may vary between clinical and forensic applications. For example, clinical laboratories typically use a cutoff of 300 ng/mL for the qualitative screening opiate immunoassay. However, in the forensic application of workplace, drug testing 2,000 ng/mL is typically used. If a laboratory is conducting testing under the national laboratory certification program, utilized for testing federal employees, it is mandated by law to use this cutoff. However, a cutoff of 2,000 ng/mL for opiates is inappropriate for clinical applications due to the potential for significant false-negative results. Table 14-2 summarizes the screening and confirmation cutoff concentrations for laboratories accredited through the U.S. Department of Health and Human Services.

Suggested Readings

Burtis CA, Ashwood ER, Bruns DE, eds. *TIETZ Fundamentals of Clinical Chemistry*. St. Louis, MI: Saunders Elsevier, 2008.

Crumpton SD, Sutheimer CA. Specimen adulteration and substitution in workplace drug testing. *Forensic Sci Rev.* 2007;19(1):1–27.

Jenkins AJ, ed. *Drug Testing in Alternate Biological Specimens*. Totowa, NJ: Humana Press, 2008.

Karch SB, ed. *Drug Abuse Handbook*. Boca Raton, FL: CRC Press, 2007.

Mozayani A, Raymon L, eds. *Handbook of Drug Interactions A clinical and forensic guide*, 2nd ed. New York, NY: Humana Press Springer, 2012.

Paul BD, Dunkley CS. Specimen validity testing. *Forensic Sci Rev.* 2007;19(1):29–47.

Ropero-Miller JD, Goldberger BA, eds. *Handbook of workplace drug testing*, 2nd ed. Washington, DC: AACC Press, 2009.

Shaw LM, ed. *The Clinical Toxicology Laboratory Contemporary Practice of Poisoning Evaluation*. Washington, DC: AACC, Inc., 2001.

Wu A. Urine adulteration before testing for drugs of abuse. In: Shaw LM, ed. *The Clinical Toxicology Laboratory Contemporary Practice of Poisoning Evaluation*. Washington, DC: AACC Press, 2001.

CHAPTER 15

Transfusion Medicine

Vishesh Chhibber

INTRODUCTION

The purpose of this chapter is to provide some basic information about transfusion medicine (TM). In order to provide care to patients, training and/or experience in TM is necessary. Please refer to the suggested reading for additional information. Purposefully omitted in this chapter is a discussion of blood collection and donor as well as therapeutic apheresis.

PRETRANSFUSION TESTING

The decision to transfuse blood must be conveyed to a blood bank as a written or electronic order by a physician. In emergent situations, a verbal request for blood may be appropriate, but this should be documented and followed by a written or electronic order as soon as possible. In order to provide compatible blood to a patient, a pretransfusion sample is required for blood bank testing. The sample must be labeled with the patient's name as well as a second unique identifier such as the patient's date of birth (DOB) or a medical record number. Most institutions also require additional information on the specimen such as the identity of the phlebotomist and the date that the sample was drawn. Due to the potentially lethal consequences of incorrect patient identification during sample acquisition or errors during testing, it is preferred that two blood bank specimens be drawn and tested from a patient at different times. The results of the testing should also be compared to any historical blood bank data available for the patient.

Pretransfusion testing needs to be performed using the patient's red blood cells (RBC) and either plasma or serum. Usually, hemolyzed or lipemic samples are not accepted by blood banks as testing such samples may yield inaccurate results. Once an appropriate specimen is received, testing is performed to determine the patient's ABO group and Rh (D) type followed by screening of the patient's plasma for unexpected red cell antibodies. After the testing is completed, a suitable unit of donor blood is selected for the patient and checked for compatibility by performing a crossmatch.

AGGLUTINATION (DAT AND IAT)

The majority of testing performed in blood banks involves checking for the presence of agglutination of patient, donor, or reagent red cells. The goal of this testing is to predict compatibility of blood products upon transfusion. Agglutination is "clumping" of red cells caused by the binding of antibody to antigens on the red cell membrane. This usually occurs in two phases: (1) sensitization of the red cells by the antibody binding to antigens and (2) lattice formation that results in macroscopic agglutination. Centrifugation is usually necessary to bring red cells in close proximity for agglutination as there is a net negative charge on the surface of red cells that prevents their aggregation and agglutination. Additionally, as it is possible for IgG antibodies to result in red cell sensitization without agglutination, it is often necessary to add a secondary antibody to cause lattice formation. The secondary antibody required is an antibody to human globulins, specifically IgG and complement. This antihuman globulin (AHG) or Coombs reagent can be used to perform a direct antiglobulin test (DAT) as well as an indirect antiglobulin test (IAT). When performing a DAT, AHG is added to a patient's RBCs that are suspected to be sensitized. This is unlike an IAT where AHG is added to a suspension of reagent (or donor) red cells and the patient's plasma that is suspected to contain an antibody to the reagent (or donor) red cells. In either test, the addition of AHG will result in agglutination if the red cells are sensitized by the antibody. Although many institutions perform pretransfusion testing as described above in small test tubes, some larger institutions are performing some (or most) of their testing using newer technology (gel columns and solid-phase testing).

PERFORMING A TYPE AND SCREEN

Prior to transfusion of blood, a patient's ABO and Rh type must be determined and the patient's plasma should be checked for expected and unexpected antibodies. The blood typing usually begins with the forward ABO grouping performed by testing a patient's red cells for the presence of A and B antigens using commercially available anti-A and anti-B antibodies. Subsequently, a reverse grouping is

TABLE 15–1. Antigens and Antibodies Present in Each ABO Blood Group

ABO Blood Group	Antigens	Antibodies
A	A	Anti-B
B	B	Anti-A
AB	A, B	None
O	None	Anti-A, anti-B

performed by checking the patient's plasma for anti-A and anti-B antibodies using reagent group A and group B red cells. With rare exception, patients who lack A or B antigens on their red cells should have an antibody to the antigen that is not present (see Table 15-1). Any discrepancy in the forward and reverse ABO grouping must be resolved prior to transfusion of blood products and if urgent transfusion is necessary, group O red cells and group AB plasma should be provided prior to the resolution of this discrepancy.

In order to determine a patient's blood type, the patient's red cells must also be tested with anti-D to determine whether the patient expresses the D antigen on his or her red cells. If the patient's red cells do not agglutinate with the anti-D reagent antibody, some institutions may perform weak D testing by adding AHG. Weak D testing will detect patients who have a quantitative or qualitative difference in the D antigen expressed on their red cells. Patients who have a weak D phenotype do not have enough D antigen on their red cells to result in direct agglutination, and agglutination is seen only after the addition of AHG. Patients who have a partial D phenotype have a qualitative difference in the D antigen that also requires AHG for agglutination. Although some institutions will perform weak D typing on patients, it is not necessary to do so as weak D and partial D patients will otherwise be considered Rh negative and will receive D-negative blood products. The same holds true for pregnant patients; while it is not necessary to perform weak D testing, some institutions choose to do so. If a pregnant patient with a weak D phenotype is typed as D negative (because the institution does not perform weak D testing on patients), she will be treated with Rh immune globulin unnecessarily (as she is not able to be immunized to the D antigen), but this will likely not result in any harm to the patient (also see discussion on prenatal testing in this chapter). However, blood donors must be typed for the weak D antigen because red cells from a weak D donor can immunize Rh-negative patients to the D antigen.

Once the patient's blood type (ABO and Rh) is determined, their plasma or serum must be checked for unexpected antibodies to non-ABO red cell antigens. The goal of the antibody screen is to detect clinically significant antibodies to red cell antigens that can cause hemolytic transfusion reactions (HTR) and hemolytic disease of the fetus and newborn (HDFN). Antibodies that bind to red cells at body temperature (37°C) and are detected using AHG are more likely to be clinically significant than cold reactive antibodies that do not result in agglutination at 37°C or the AHG phase of testing. Some of the more commonly encountered clinically significant antibodies include antibodies to D, C, E, c, e, S, s, K, k, Fy^a, Fy^b, Jk^a, Jk^b. Reagent red cells must be able to detect these antibodies as well as antibodies to M, N, P1, Le^a, Le^b.

CROSSMATCH

After a type and screen is completed, an appropriate blood product can be selected to transfuse the patient. Ideally, ABO identical blood products should be transfused, but due to inventory management constraints, often ABO compatible (but not ABO identical) products are issued for transfusion. Table 15-2 reviews the type of red cells and plasma that are compatible with each of the ABO blood groups.

Plasma, platelets, and cryoprecipitate can be transfused without a crossmatch. However, for RBC transfusion, each unit of red cells should be crossmatched with the recipient's plasma prior to transfusion. The type of crossmatch necessary depends on whether the patient's antibody screen is positive or negative.

If the patient's antibody screen is negative, generally an immediate spin crossmatch is performed by simply mixing the red cells selected for transfusion with the patient's plasma and checking for agglutination after centrifugation. An immediate spin crossmatch is essentially a second check of the donor and recipient's ABO compatibility as agglutination will be seen if the patient's plasma has ABO antibodies to cognate antigens on the red cells selected for transfusion. In some institutions, patients who have a negative antibody screen may be eligible for an "electronic crossmatch" if the institution has validated the blood bank information/computer system to not allow an incompatible blood product to be issued to the patient. If the patient had a positive antibody screen, a complete crossmatch using AHG is appropriate. Many clinically significant non-ABO alloantibodies are IgG antibodies and will not result in agglutination unless AHG is added to the suspension of red cells and plasma. Thus, patients who have a positive antibody screen should have the crossmatch performed by incubating the patient's plasma and donor red cells at body temperature followed by addition of AHG.

The sample of blood used to perform the crossmatch (as well as the type and screen) must be recently acquired from the patient if the patient has been recently transfused or pregnant. This is necessary because the patient may produce an antibody to a RBC antigen within a few days after being exposed to allogeneic red cells. Generally, a sample should not be more than 3 days old if the patient has been recently transfused or pregnant, but a sample drawn up to 2 weeks prior to transfusion is acceptable if the patient has not had any recent exposure to blood. It is also important to review the blood bank history to prevent the transfusion of RBCs that may have antigens that the patient previously had antibodies to. In these patients, the antibody titer may decrease in strength to below detectable levels, but

TABLE 15-2. Blood Products That are Compatible with Each ABO Blood Group

Blood Group	Compatible Red Cells	Compatible Plasma
A	A, O	A, AB
B	B, O	B, AB
AB	A, B, AB, O	AB
O	O	O, A, B, AB

subsequent exposure to the antigen can result in brisk antibody production and a delayed hemolytic transfusion reaction. Unlike RBC transfusion, transfusion of other blood products does not require a recent sample because selection is based on the patient's blood type, and a crossmatch does not need to be performed.

 # TRANSFUSION OF BLOOD PRODUCTS

Transfusion of blood products carries significant risks. Thus, prior to any transfusions, the risks and benefits should be carefully assessed and blood products should be provided to the patient only if the benefits outweigh the risks. Today, transfusion of whole blood is exceedingly rare in the United States. Patients are usually transfused with the specific blood component that is required (e.g., packed red cells, plasma, platelets, or cryoprecipitate).

RED CELL TRANSFUSION

The goal of red cell transfusion is to increase oxygen delivery to tissues when necessary. Red cell transfusion is appropriate for the treatment of anemia if it will ameliorate symptoms of anemia or aid in correcting or preventing the adverse physiologic consequences of anemia. Most patients will tolerate a loss of approximately 50% of their circulating hemoglobin before they start to experience significant consequences due to acute anemia. In acute blood loss, symptoms due to hypovolemia are usually seen before symptoms due to anemia. In chronically anemic patients (patients who become anemic over weeks or months), compensatory mechanisms allow patients to tolerate lower hemoglobin levels than patients who become acutely anemic. Considering the many variables involved, it is often challenging to determine whether tissue ischemia exists and whether it will be alleviated with red cell transfusion.

❑ Who Should Be Suspected?

There is a significant variation in RBC transfusion practices between institutions. Most studies that have audited transfusion of blood products have reported that there was unnecessary transfusion of patients and there is a trend toward more conservative hemoglobin transfusion triggers. Authorities in TM agree that most patients with a hemoglobin of <6 g/dL will need red cell transfusion and most patients with a hemoglobin of >10 g/dL will not require red cell transfusion. There is also general agreement that within this range, the transfusion of blood products needs to be individualized to the patient. At the author's institution, a trigger of a hemoglobin of 7 g/dL is used for most hospitalized patients with the notable exception of patients with unstable cardiac disease (see Table 15-3).

PLASMA TRANSFUSION

The previous practice of using plasma as a volume expander has largely become extinct. Today, plasma is almost always transfused to patients due to a deficiency of one or more proteins present in normal plasma. The proteins that are most

TABLE 15–3. Common Indications for Blood Product Transfusion and Special Processing

Red blood cells (after bleeding has stopped, one unit of packed RBC increases Hb 1 g/dL in an average sized adult)

Active blood loss

Hct ≤21% or Hb ≤7 g/dL

Hct ≤24% or Hb ≤8 g/dL and symptomatic

Hct ≤25% or Hb ≤8.3 g/dL and acute coronary syndrome

Platelets

Platelets ≤10,000/μL

Platelets ≤20,000/μL and sepsis, multisystem failure or high risk for outpatient hemorrhage

Platelets ≤50,000/μL with surgery or active bleeding

Platelet function defect and symptomatic or impending surgery/invasive procedure

Intraoperative hemostatic defect

Plasma

Prolonged prothrombin time (e.g., liver disease) and symptomatic or invasive procedure planned

Factor XI or XIII deficiency

Thrombotic microangiopathy

C1 esterase inhibitor deficiency (hereditary angioedema) and symptomatic

Intraoperative hemostatic defect

Overdose of oral vitamin K antagonist with evidence of bleeding

Cryoprecipitate (contains fibrinogen, factors VIII and XIII, von Willebrand factor, and fibronectin)

Mild factor VIII deficiency and symptomatic or with surgery/invasive procedure (if factor VIII concentrate not available)

von Willebrand disease and symptomatic or with surgery/invasive procedure (if von Willebrand factor concentrate not available)

Hypofibrinogenemia and symptomatic or with surgery/invasive procedure

Intraoperative hemostatic defect

Factor XIII deficiency

Special blood product processing (not routinely needed)

Irradiated blood products

Directed donor product from blood relative (to avoid graft versus host disease)

Intensive chemotherapy with marrow suppression

Stem cell transplant candidate or recipient

Newborn, prematurity, intrauterine transfusion

Washed blood cell products

Congenital IgA deficiency with anti-IgA antibodies

Repeated severe hypersensitivity transfusion reactions despite appropriate medication

Leukocyte-reduced blood products

≥2 documented febrile transfusion reactions

Chronically transfusion dependent

Transplant candidate or recipient

High cytomegalovirus risk

Patient is a pregnant woman

Newborn, premature, intrauterine transfusion

Patient undergoing splenectomy

Patient with congenital immune deficiency

15

commonly repleted are coagulation factors. Other deficient proteins that may be repleted with plasma transfusion include ADAMTS 13 in patients with TTP and complement factors in patients with HUS.

❏ Who Should Be Suspected?

Despite the most common indication for plasma transfusion being the treatment of coagulopathy, there are no clear guidelines for the appropriate use of plasma in this setting. Thus, very often plasma is transfused unnecessarily to patients who do not benefit from it.

A more proactive approach in regard to plasma transfusion is appropriate in bleeding patients who require massive transfusion of blood products. In such patients, if coagulopathy develops, it may result in excessive bleeding that can be life threatening and it may be extremely difficult to correct a severe coagulopathy. These patients have multiple factors contributing to the coagulopathy including dysfunction of the enzymes of the coagulation cascade (due to hypothermia and acidosis) and consumption of coagulation factors due to DIC.

❏ Considerations

Several types of plasma products are available for transfusion. These include fresh frozen plasma (FFP), frozen plasma 24 (FP24), and thawed plasma (TP). FFP is plasma that has been separated from a whole blood collection and put into a freezer within 8 hours of collection. FP 24 is plasma that has been placed in the freezer within 24 hours of collection. Both of these products can be kept frozen up to 1 year; however, once thawed, they must be used within 24 hours. Thawed plasma is FFP or FP24 that has been relabeled as "thawed plasma" and now can be used for up to 5 days after thawing. The concentration of the majority of coagulation factors does not vary significantly among FFP, FP24, and TP with the exception of factor V and factor VIII. FP24 and TP have lower concentrations of factor V and factor VIII as these two factors have the shortest in vitro half-life. However, factor 5 deficiency is rare, and factor 8 is an acute-phase reactant that is often elevated in patients requiring plasma transfusion. Most often, the vitamin K–dependent factors (II, VII, IX, and X) are the factors that need to be replaced in order to correct coagulopathy. These factors are stable at refrigerator temperatures and not significantly decreased in FP24 or TP.

❏ Laboratory Findings

When assessing a patient for coagulopathy (usually an acquired coagulopathy), the most common laboratory tests ordered are a prothrombin time (PT)/international normalized ratio (INR) and an activated partial thromboplastin time (aPTT). The PT is very sensitive and will be abnormal before coagulopathy will result in bleeding. Generally, an increase in bleeding is not usually seen until the PT is >1.3 times the upper limit of the normal range (which usually corresponds to an INR of approximately 2). In nonbleeding patients with an elevated INR due to warfarin use, vitamin K can be used to correct the coagulopathy (over 6–24 hours) without plasma transfusion. It is also important to note that plasma transfusion is significantly more effective in decreasing a patient's INR when the INR is significantly elevated. As the patient's INR gets closer to or below 2, a large amount of plasma will result in a much smaller decrease in the INR than the same volume of plasma given to the same patient at a higher INR. Another important consideration when transfusing plasma, especially prior to an invasive/surgical intervention, is that the plasma should be transfused within a few hours of the intervention. The in vivo half-life of some of the coagulation factors that need correction (such as factor 7) is a few hours and correcting the coagulopathy with plasma transfusion >8 hours prior to transfusion will likely be of little benefit. Additionally, the use of plasma for warfarin reversal will likely decrease significantly with the recent approval of four factor prothrombin complex concentrate (PCC) in the United States.

CRYOPRECIPITATED AHF TRANSFUSION

A unit of cryoprecipitated AHF (also known as cryoprecipitate) is prepared from a unit of plasma. When frozen plasma is placed in a refrigerator and starts to thaw, there is precipitation of some proteins. This precipitate contains a significant proportion of the factor VIII, von Willebrand factor, fibrinogen, fibronectin, and factor XIII that is present in the unit of plasma. Subsequently, the unit is centrifuged to separate the precipitate from the supernatant plasma. The cryoprecipitate is then frozen until it is necessary to transfuse.

❏ Who Should Be Suspected?
In the past, cryoprecipitate was used to treat patients who had hemophilia A. But due to safer alternatives, cryoprecipitate is no longer used for this purpose in the United States. The primary use for cryoprecipitate today is to replete fibrinogen in patients with hypofibrinogenemia or disfibrinogenemia (e.g., patients with DIC, patients requiring massive transfusion).

❏ Laboratory Findings
Fibrinogen levels between 50 and 100 mg/dL are generally adequate in patients to achieve hemostasis. However, levels <100 mg/dL may cause in vitro laboratory testing abnormalities. The volume of a unit of cryoprecipitate is approximately 15 mL, and for transfusions in adults, generally 10 units are pooled for an adequate dose. However, it is possible to calculate the exact number of units needed to reach a specific fibrinogen level if the patient's fibrinogen level is known. Occasionally, cryoprecipitate is also used in uremic patients and in patients with von Willebrand disease as a source of von Willebrand factor.

PLATELET TRANSFUSION

Platelet transfusion is generally performed to correct an abnormality of platelet function or platelet count in order to prevent bleeding or treat active bleeding. The most common indication for platelet transfusion is prophylaxis in thrombocytopenic patients. Although there are no well-accepted guidelines in regard to prophylactic platelet transfusion, some consensus has been achieved and many institutions follow similar practices.

15

❏ Laboratory Findings
In patients who are severely thrombocytopenic and do not have additional risk factors for bleeding, a threshold platelet count of 10,000/μL is commonly accepted. In patients who are having an invasive CNS, ophthalmologic, or possibly a pulmonary

procedure, a count of 100,000/µL is often targeted. Even though most experts agree that this count is higher than needed to achieve hemostasis, it is still considered a reasonable target because it protects against a precipitous drop in platelet count that can result in bleeding into these organs causing serious morbidity or mortality. For other invasive or surgical procedures, most authorities concur that platelet counts above 50,000/µL are generally adequate.

❑ Considerations

Some of the causes of qualitative defects of platelet function include congenital diseases (e.g., Glanzmann thrombasthenia, Bernard-Soulier disease), medications (e.g., aspirin, clopidogrel), and dysfunction due to medical device interaction (e.g., cardiopulmonary bypass). In these patients, the platelet counts may be normal, but due to abnormal platelet function, transfusion of one unit of apheresis platelets (or an equivalent dose of whole blood–derived platelets) is often appropriate. In patients on antiplatelet medications who present with acute bleeding, especially bleeding into the central nervous system, two apheresis platelets (or equivalent) are often transfused.

Platelet products can be collected using apheresis technology or can be produced by separation from whole blood collections. For adult patients, 4–8 units of whole blood–derived platelets must be pooled for one transfusion dose or alternatively a single apheresis unit collected from one donor can be transfused. Both types of platelet products are commonly used, and each one has some advantages and disadvantages. One significant advantage of apheresis platelet products is that they are collected from a single donor and can be used to transfuse patients who require HLA-selected platelet products.

❑ Who Should Be Suspected?

Patients who get immunized to HLA antigens due to pregnancy, organ transplantation, or previous exposure to blood products may not respond adequately to platelet transfusion. Platelets have HLA class 1 (A and B) antigens on their surface, and if the recipient has antibodies to the HLA antigens of the donor, there may be no increment in platelet count posttransfusion. The most effective way to prevent immunization to HLA antigens is by leukoreduction of blood products. However, if a patient is already immunized to HLA antigens, there are several strategies that can be employed to transfuse these refractory patients. These include platelet crossmatching, HLA matching, and selection of platelet products from donors who lack the cognate HLA antigens to which the patient has antibodies. However, prior to attaining HLA-selected platelet units, it might be reasonable to transfuse fresh ABO identical apheresis platelets as ABO incompatibility and older age of transfused platelets have been reported to decrease posttransfusion platelet increments.

Platelet crossmatching is performed by mixing a sample of the patient's plasma with platelet products that may potentially be transfused and checking for a reaction between them. If reactivity is present, the crossmatch is interpreted as positive and the platelet product is not transfused to the patient. If necessary, additional platelet products can be crossmatched with the patient until a product that does not have reactivity with the patient's plasma is procured. One substantial benefit to HLA crossmatching is that it is possible to find compatible platelet products without determining the patient or the donors HLA type. However, HLA crossmatching can only be performed on platelet products that are ABO compatible, and the data available comparing HLA crossmatching with HLA matching show that platelet crossmatching is likely an inferior strategy.

HLA matching is performed by HLA typing patients as well as platelet donors. Once HLA typing data are available, platelet products that either completely match or are very similar for HLA class 1 (A and B) antigens are selected for transfusion. The HLA match of the recipient to the donor can be rated from A (all four antigens match) to D (two or more antigen mismatch). HLA matching of platelets is effective in achieving good count increments when the donors are very well matched (A or B level matches) to the patient. However, if a patient is widely immunized and the platelet product is not well matched (C or D level matches), the patient will likely not respond to the platelet transfusion. Additionally, HLA matching may be difficult in smaller institutions that do not have HLA laboratories or large platelet inventories.

A third strategy that is as successful as HLA matching and likely superior to crossmatching is selection of platelet products that avoids HLA antibodies present in the patient. In order to use this strategy, the patient must be tested for HLA antibodies. Once the specificity of the HLA antibodies in the patient is determined, platelet products from donors that lack cognate HLA antigens are selected for transfusion. This strategy can be very effective for patients who are refractory, even if an institution has a limited platelet inventory. However, if the patient is widely immunized to HLA antigens, donors with compatible HLA types will need to be recruited or compatible apheresis platelet products will need to be brought in from large blood centers with extensive inventories of platelets. This strategy has the additional benefit of determining whether the patient is refractory due to the presence of HLA antibodies or other causes. It is also important to reassess the patient every few weeks to check for any changes in the HLA antibodies present.

Another less common immunologic cause for platelet refractoriness is antibodies to antigens present on platelets other than HLA. Patients with these platelet-specific antibodies will require platelet products from rare donors that lack these antigens. The most commonly encountered antibody to a platelet-specific antigen is anti–HPA-1a (anti-Pl^{A1}).

In addition to these immunologic causes, there are many nonimmune causes for an inadequate response to platelet transfusion. These include fever, sepsis, disseminated intravascular coagulation (DIC), splenomegaly, bleeding, as well as treatment with certain medications. Most of these reasons for refractoriness may persist until the patient's underlying medical condition is adequately treated.

GRANULOCYTE TRANSFUSION

Granulocyte transfusion has decreased dramatically over the last two decades. Previously, granulocytes were frequently transfused to neutropenic patients undergoing chemotherapy or to patients with congenital neutrophil abnormalities (e.g., chronic granulomatous disease) who had infections.

❑ Who Should Be Suspected?
Due to advances in antimicrobial therapy, granulocytes are now only transfused to patients who are temporarily neutropenic and have a life-threatening bacterial or fungal infection that is unresponsive to antimicrobial therapy. Based on published literature,

it is not clear if the addition of granulocyte transfusion provides any benefit when compared to antimicrobial therapy alone. The published studies have had variable conclusions, but there appears to be a trend toward benefit in the studies that have transfused higher doses of granulocytes with each transfusion. If a decision is made to transfuse granulocytes, generally one product is transfused daily until the patient has an absolute neutrophil count above 500/μL.

Granulocytes are collected using an apheresis device from healthy volunteer donors. However, granulocyte transfusion carries significant risks. Some of the risks include CMV transmission, HLA immunization, and severe pulmonary reactions. Additionally, granulocytes must be transfused the same day that they are collected and thus are transfused prior to the completion of standard infectious disease testing performed on blood donors. Platelet donors who recently had negative infectious disease testing are often used as granulocyte donors, but there remains a risk of infectious disease transmission. As with any other blood product transfusion, the risk–benefit ratio must be carefully examined prior to the transfusion of granulocytes.

RISKS AND ADVERSE CONSEQUENCES RELATED TO BLOOD PRODUCT TRANSFUSION

Transfusion of blood products may be life saving but also carries a significant risk of adverse consequences for the recipient (Table 15-4). Some of the possible adverse consequences that have been well documented include infectious disease transmission, transfusion-associated immunomodulation, and transfusion reactions.

❏ Considerations
Transfusion of blood products has resulted in transmission of bacteria, viruses, parasites, and prions. In order to minimize the risk of transmission of these infectious agents, donors are screened using a donor history questionnaire. Subsequently, each donor is tested for several transmissible infectious diseases with each donation. If any of the infectious disease testing is positive, the blood product is discarded and the donor is deferred from subsequent donation as appropriate. The donor screening process and infectious disease testing have significantly decreased the risk of infectious disease transmission over the last three decades.

Other possible adverse consequences of blood product transfusion include transfusion reactions (TR). The most common transfusion reactions include allergic transfusion reactions (ATR) and febrile nonhemolytic transfusion reactions (FNHTR), while hemolytic transfusion reactions (HTR), transfusion-related acute lung injury (TRALI), and transfusion-associated circulatory overload (TACO) are the leading causes of morbidity and mortality related to transfusion.

ALLERGIC TRANSFUSION REACTIONS

ATRs are usually caused by the transfusion of foreign plasma proteins. The majority of allergic reactions are limited to skin manifestations such as urticaria, erythema, and pruritus. These reactions can be treated with antihistamines and/or corticosteroids. If allergic reactions prove to be recurrent, the patient can also be premedicated with these medications. A minority of patients may have more severe

TABLE 15–4. Adverse Effects of Blood Transfusions

Condition/Infection	Frequency or Risk/Unit Transfused
Immune mediated	
Acute	
Acute hemolytic transfusion reactions. Laboratory findings reflect acute intravascular hemolysis, acute renal failure, disseminated intravascular coagulation (DIC), and cardiovascular failure.	1 in 76,000 acute hemolytic reactions; 1 in 1.8 million incompatible units transfused are fatal
Febrile nonhemolytic transfusion reaction. Must exclude other causes of fever. May be accompanied by chills/rigors.	0.1–1% (with leukocyte-reduced blood products)
Transfusion-related acute lung injury (TRALI). Occurs during or up to 6 h after transfusion. Caused by activation of neutrophils in the patient's pulmonary vasculature resulting in diffuse bilateral lung infiltrates on chest radiography and acute respiratory distress. May be accompanied by fever, rigors, and hypotension.	May be as frequent as 1:1,200 transfusions
Allergic transfusion reaction	13%
Acute anaphylaxis (shock, hypotension, angioedema, respiratory distress); occurs a few seconds to a few minutes into transfusion.	1:20,000–1:50,000
Chronic (delayed)	
Alloimmunization to red cell antigens	1%
Alloimmunization to HLA antigens (may lead to platelet refractoriness)	10%
Delayed hemolytic transfusion reaction. Anamnestic antibody response, commonly due to previous sensitization of RBCs against minor (non-ABO) blood group antibodies; results in delayed (2–10 d) transfusion reaction with extravascular hemolysis. Mild clinical and laboratory findings. Rarely, it can be severe, even fatal, especially in patients with sickle cell anemia.	1 in 6,000
Graft versus host disease* (transfusion associated).	Rare
Posttransfusion purpura: thrombocytopenia 5–10 d after blood transfusion containing platelets	Rare
Nonimmune mediated	
Acute (immediate)	
Volume overload	<1%
Nonimmune hemolysis (heat, cold, osmotic, mechanical)	Infrequent
Electrolyte imbalance (K^+, Mg^2, Ca^{2+}). Not common in transfusion of small volumes, but common in massive transfusion situations if appropriate precautions not taken. May be related to the citrate used as anticoagulant.	Unknown
Coagulopathy (e.g., with massive transfusions)	Unknown
Chronic (delayed)	
Transfusional hemosiderosis (e.g., multiple transfusions in aplastic anemia, MDS, sickle cell anemia, thalassemia major)	Unknown

15

(Continued)

TABLE 15–4. Adverse Effects of Blood Transfusions (*Continued*)

Infections

Viral

Hepatitis A	1:1,000,000†
Hepatitis B	1:50,000–1:170,000†
Hepatitis C	1:1–2,000,000
HIV	<1:2,000,000†
HTLV types I and II	1:19,000–1:80,000†
Cytomegalovirus	3–12 in 100; infrequent with leukocyte-reduced components
Parvovirus B19	1:10,000† (more common with plasma-derived products)
RBV	Rare
Human herpes virus 8	3.2% seroprevalence
West Nile, other arboviruses	23 confirmed cases in the United States by 2002
Dengue fever	2 cases confirmed

Prion caused

Classic and variant Creutzfeldt-Jakob disease and bovine spongiform encephalopathy	4 probable cases reported in the United Kingdom

Bacterial

Bacterial contamination per RBC unit transfused in the United States	1:500,000
Bacterial contamination per platelet unit	1:5,000
Syphilis	Rare
Chlamydia pneumonia	Likely, but no definitive evidence
Rocky Mountain spotted fever (*Rickettsia rickettsii*), *Rickettsia*	Unknown

Parasitic

Plasmodium	1:4,000,000
Babesia	>20 reported cases
Trypanosoma cruzi (Chagas disease)	Unknown
Leishmania	<1:20,000

Transfusion-associated graft versus host disease (TA-GVHD) occurs when immunocompetent T lymphocytes are transfused into a patient who cannot reject them, and they engraft in the recipient, proliferate, and mount an immune attack against the host tissues. TA-GVHD occurs 4–30 d after transfusion of any cellular blood component. It may occur in a nonimmunocompetent recipient or in an immunocompetent recipient who receives histocompatible donor lymphocytes, especially from blood relatives, which can recognize a different HLA haplotype in the recipient. There are molecular techniques to diagnosis TA-GVHD. Mortality is nearly 90% in the full-blown syndrome. Irradiation of blood products virtually eliminates the risk of this complication.

†Estimates published by the British Committee for Standards in Haematology.

ATRs that may involve the patient's airway (e.g., laryngeal edema). On rare occasion, it is also possible that a patient may have an anaphylactic reaction, which presents with hemodynamic instability in addition to the symptoms seen in a severe allergic reaction. In these patients, beta-adrenergics and aggressive supportive care may be necessary.

☐ Who Should Be Suspected?

Although the cause of anaphylactic transfusion reactions is often unknown, classically they have been described in IgA-deficient patients with anti-IgA antibodies shortly after initiation of a blood product transfusion. If additional transfusion is required in patients with a history of severe allergic or anaphylactic transfusion reactions, red cells and platelets should be washed to reduce their plasma content. Plasma should only be transfused in these patients if it is lifesaving and should be from IgA-deficient donors if the patient is IgA deficient.

FEBRILE NONHEMOLYTIC TRANSFUSION REACTIONS (FNHTR)

FNHTRs present as reactions where a rise of ≥1°C is seen, possibly with associated chills/rigors. These reactions are usually self-limited and may be mitigated by treatment with antipyretics. Prior to the reaction being declared an FNHTR, investigation to exclude other causes is imperative as fever may be a component of other types of transfusion reactions (such as HTRs).

HEMOLYTIC TRANSFUSION REACTIONS (HTR)

HTRs result from the transfusion of incompatible blood products. The most common cause of HTRs is transfusion of incompatible red cells. The alloantibody causing the HTR can be to ABO antigens or other blood group antigens. The incompatible transfusion may have been caused by an error in patient identification (during sample acquisition or blood product transfusion), an error when performing the type and screen (or crossmatch), or an error when issuing the blood product.

☐ Who Should Be Suspected?

Acute HTR can be life threatening and classically present with fever, flank pain, red/dark urine, pain at infusion site, nausea/vomiting, diarrhea, hypotension, and a feeling of impending doom. The severity of the reaction in these cases is often related to the dose of incompatible RBCs transfused. Thus, whenever a transfusion reaction is suspected, the transfusion should be terminated immediately and a posttransfusion specimen should be sent to the blood bank for workup. If the patient appears to be having a severe HTR, the patient will need supportive care, possibly in an ICU setting. In order to prevent acute tubular necrosis, it is critical to maintain renal blood flow and urinary flow by administering intravenous fluids and diuretics. Additionally, intravenous immunoglobulin (IVIG) may be of benefit in some patients.

In many instances, if the hemolysis is due to a non-ABO blood group antibody, the patient will present with a delayed HTR, which is characterized by a drop in hematocrit, a rise in bilirubin, and the presence of a previously undetected antibody. These patients may be completely asymptomatic or may present with jaundice, dark urine, and/or symptoms of anemia. It is important to note that in addition to any acute management, the serologic workup of the patient is critical as the patient will likely require subsequent transfusion. If the incompatibility is not discovered, the patient may have another HTR that may be more severe than the previous.

15

TRANSFUSION-RELATED ACUTE LUNG INJURY (TRALI)

TRALI is one of the leading causes of mortality related to blood product transfusion and is caused by activation of the recipient's neutrophils in the pulmonary vasculature. This results in increased vascular permeability in the pulmonary capillaries and extravasation of serum into the alveolar spaces. The neutrophils of the recipient are activated by HLA antibodies, antineutrophil antibodies, or lipid activators in the blood product transfused.

❑ Who Should Be Suspected?
The classic presentation of TRALI is a patient who develops acute respiratory distress either during or within 6 hours of transfusion of a blood product that contains plasma. Patients may also have fever, chills, hypotension, and diffuse bilateral lung infiltrates on chest radiography. The treatment for TRALI is mainly providing supportive care that may include oxygenation and possibly ventilatory support. Although corticosteroids have been used in patients with TRALI, it is not clear if there is any benefit to their use. As TRALI is caused by the blood products donated by a particular donor, the patient can be transfused with additional blood products if necessary. However, the donor implicated in the reaction should be removed from the donor pool.

TRANSFUSION-ASSOCIATED CIRCULATORY OVERLOAD (TACO)

❑ Who Should Be Suspected?
In clinical practice, it is often difficult to differentiate TRALI from TACO. Some features that differ between TACO and TRALI include (1) hypertension in TACO (vs. hypotension in TRALI), (2) fever is not seen in TACO, (3) the B-type natriuretic peptide is significantly elevated in TACO, and (4) brisk response to diuresis may be seen in TACO. A history of cardiac dysfunction or excessive/rapid volume infusion also suggests TACO as the likely etiology of the reaction.

 # MANIPULATION OF BLOOD PRODUCTS

Blood component therapy is significantly safer and superior to the transfusion of whole blood as a patient is transfused with only the blood component that is necessary. Additional blood product manipulation (other than component separation) may also be necessary for a small minority of patients. Some of the possible manipulations include leukoreduction, irradiation, and washing of blood components.

Leukoreduction is usually performed during component preparation by filtration. Some of the benefits of leukoreduction include a reduced risk of febrile transfusion reactions, immunomodulation, CMV transmission, and HLA immunization. Previously, leukoreduction was performed only for a select group of patients (e.g., oncology patients, other chronically transfused patients). However, due to the multiple benefits of leukoreduction and increased availability of prestorage filtration, many institutions now provide leukoreduced blood products for all patients.

Irradiation of blood products is performed to reduce the risk of transfusion-associated graft versus host disease (TA-GVHD) in patients susceptible to this almost uniformly fatal condition. TA-GVHD occurs due to engraftment of viable lymphocytes that are transfused with a cellular blood product resulting in an immune response against the recipient's tissues. This condition is similar to conventional GVHD with one important exception. Unlike patients with conventional GVHD, patients with TA-GVHD also have destruction of the hematopoietic cells in the patient's bone marrow. This results in irreversible pancytopenia and patients usually succumb to infection or bleeding.

❑ **Considerations**

Gamma irradiation of cellular blood products prevents TA-GVHD. The indications for transfusion of irradiated blood products include (but is not limited to) (1) hematologic malignancies and some solid neoplasms, (2) hematopoietic progenitor cell transplantation, (3) intrauterine transfusions, (4) premature/low birth weight infants, (5) newborns with erythroblastosis, (6) congenital immunodeficiencies, (7) treatment with purine analogues and related drugs, (8) treatment with alemtuzumab and related drugs, (9) granulocyte transfusions, and (10) transfusion from a genetically similar donor (includes family members/relatives, HLA-selected donors, genetically homogeneous populations). Irradiation of blood products is not necessary for patients with HIV infection. Please see the suggested reading for a more comprehensive discussion of TA-GVHD and irradiation of blood products.

Washing of RBCs and platelets is occasionally necessary in patients who have severe or recurrent allergic transfusion reactions. The allergen causing the reaction is usually a protein that is present in the donor's plasma. Plasma is present in packed RBC as well as whole blood–derived and apheresis platelets, and washing these products using saline in a device designed to do so will remove almost all of the plasma in the product. Since washing the blood component will result in loss of some of the red cells and platelets in the product, washing should only be performed for patients who require it.

 PERINATAL TRANSFUSION PRACTICE

HEMOLYTIC DISEASE OF THE FETUS AND NEWBORN (HDFN)

HDFN is caused by maternal alloantibodies to fetal red cell antigens and is an important cause of fetal morbidity and mortality. If untreated, HDFN can result in fetal anemia, high-output cardiac failure, and hydrops fetalis. The TM service plays an important role in the diagnosis and treatment of HDFN.

❑ **Who Should Be Suspected?**

Currently in the United States, HDFN is seen most commonly in group O women who have a non–group O fetus. Although common, the HDFN seen in these patients is usually mild. However, if an Rh-negative mother has anti-D and the fetus is D positive, this fetus is at a very high risk of HDFN. Due to the use of Rh immune globulin (RhIg), a commercially available antibody to the D antigen, the prevalence of HDFN has substantially decreased in developed countries. Other commonly implicated antibodies in HDFN include K, c, C, and Fy^a.

15

In order to prevent or initiate early treatment of HDFN, all pregnant patients should have a type and screen performed at their first prenatal visit, and their medical history should be reviewed for any previous transfusion or alloimmunization due to pregnancy or transfusion. The alloantibodies implicated in HDFN are usually IgG antibodies that cross the placenta and result in hemolysis and anemia of the fetus.

If the patient has any clinically significant antibodies, titers of the antibody should be performed and repeated monthly. If the titer rises to 16 or higher (may vary by institution) with AHG, there is a significant risk of HDFN, and the risk to the fetus can be further assessed by determining whether the cognate antigen is present on the red cells of the fetus. The phenotype of the fetus can be determined by checking the father's red cell phenotype and/or by amniocentesis/cordocentesis. If necessary, the patient should be referred to an experienced high-risk obstetrician who will closely follow the pregnancy and assess the fetus for anemia using color Doppler ultrasound of the middle cerebral artery blood flow. If the fetus is significantly anemic, intrauterine transfusion of the fetus can be considered. After delivery of a fetus at risk of HDFN, the cord blood should be evaluated. If the neonate has a positive DAT and significant hemolysis resulting in anemia and/or hyperbilirubinemia, an exchange transfusion of the neonate must be considered. For transfusing the neonate (as well as intrauterine transfusion if necessary), group O, Rh-negative, irradiated red cells that are crossmatch compatible with the mother are generally preferred.

❏ Considerations

The maternal alloantibodies to red cell antigens that cause HDFN may be produced because of prior exposure to blood due to transfusion or pregnancy. When alloimmunization occurs due to pregnancy, it is usually at the time of delivery or late in the pregnancy. Thus, it is unlikely that HDFN would occur during the first pregnancy if the patient has no history of transfusion of blood products.

Rh PROPHYLAXIS

Prior to the use of RhIg, anti-D was the most common cause of HDFN as the D antigen is very immunogenic. If appropriately used, RhIg can prevent almost all cases of alloimmunization to the D antigen in Rh-negative pregnant patients. However, if the patient has already been immunized to the D antigen and made the anti-D alloantibody, administration of RhIg does not provide any benefit and is not indicated. Generally, a single 300-µg vial of RhIg (which will cover 30 mL of fetal whole blood or 15 mL of fetal red cells) is given prophylactically at 28 weeks if the patient is D negative. A subsequent dose is then administered shortly after (but must be within 72 hours of) delivery if the neonate is D positive. The amount of RhIg to be given after delivery is determined by testing the mother's blood for the presence of fetal red cells. Often the initial screening test for maternal–fetal hemorrhage is the rosette test, which is performed by adding anti-D to maternal blood, followed by indicator D-positive red cells. This results in "rosettes" or agglutination of red cells surrounding the D-positive fetal red cells. The rosette test will be positive if the volume of fetal blood in maternal circulation is >30 mL. If the rosette test is negative, one vial of RhIg is administered to cover the small amount of fetal blood in the maternal circulation that may be present. If the rosette test is positive, the amount of fetal red cells in the maternal circulation can be quantitated using flow cytometry or the Kleihauer-Betke (acid/elution) test. The Kleihauer-Betke is performed by treating maternal red cells on a thin slide smear with acid and then counterstaining the slide. Fetal hemoglobin is resistant to acid treatment so maternal cells will appear as "ghosts" while fetal cells will be pink. Usually, 2,000 cells are counted, and the percentage of fetal red cells is determined and multiplied by the maternal blood volume to determine the volume of fetal blood in the maternal circulation. The maternal blood volume can be calculated using the mother's height and weight or alternatively 5,000 mL is occasionally used as an estimate of the blood volume of postpartum women. Alternatively, flow cytometry can also be used to determine the amount of fetal–maternal hemorrhage. The amount of RhIg to be given to the mother is then determined using the estimated volume of fetal blood in circulation that must be covered by RhIg. The volume of fetal–maternal hemorrhage is then divided by 30 mL (that each 300 µg vial of RhIg will cover) to determine the number of vials necessary. The result of the calculation is rounded to the closest whole number and then one additional vial is added to allow for an error in the estimation/calculation. Additional doses of RhIg may also be necessary in Rh-negative women if the patient has any events that may have introduced fetal blood into the maternal circulation such as trauma, version, abortion, or amniocentesis (please refer to the suggested reading for additional discussion).

 CONCLUSION

Over the last 100 years, there have been significant advances in the field of transfusion medicine. All of the major blood groups have been identified and techniques for serologic testing have been developed. Today, almost all hospitals have blood banks that are able to provide blood products to patients who require them. Although transfusion can be life saving, there are significant risks associated with blood product transfusion. Thus, blood products should only be transfused if necessary.

Suggested Readings

Roback J, Grossman B, Harris T, et al., eds. *Technical Manual*, 17th ed. Bethesda, MD: AABB Press; 2011.

Simon T, Snyder E, Solheim B, et al., eds. *Rossi's Principles of Transfusion Medicine*, 4th ed. Bethesda, MD: Blackwell Publishing; 2009.

15

LAB TESTS

SECTION 2

LAB TESTS

CHAPTER 16

Laboratory Tests

Lokinendi V. Rao and Liberto Pechet

16

16

This chapter presents the most commonly ordered serum, plasma, and whole blood laboratory tests arranged in alphabetical order. Each entry is titled using the most common naming convention existing in the United States. When appropriate, alternate name(s), definition, reference ranges, clinical use, interpretation, limitations, and suggested readings are given. Microbiology tests such as laboratory cultures have been organized into a separate chapter, Infectious Disease Assays (p. 1203). The basis of current molecular assays is reviewed in the chapter on Hereditary and Genetic Diseases (p. 473).

It is important to note that many of these tests are available by point-of-care testing (POCT). The main advantage of POCT is immediate turnaround time. However, it is also necessary to consider the disadvantages of POCT, such as reliability of interpretation due to lower assay sensitivity and susceptibility to interfering substances. Other issues include ensuring personnel proficiency, quality assurance, data management, and cost.

1,5-ANHYDROGLUCITOL (1,5-AG)

❏ **Definition**

- 1,5-Anhydroglucitol (1,5-AG), sometimes known as GlycoMark, is a monosaccharide that shows a structural similarity to glucose. Its main source in humans is dietary ingestion, particularly meats and cereals. In addition, 10% of 1,5-AG is derived from endogenous synthesis. It is generally not metabolized, and in healthy subjects, it achieves a stable plasma concentration that reflects a steady balance between ingestion and urinary excretion.
- **Normal range:** 10.7–32.0 µg/mL in males; 6.8–29.3 µg/mL in females.

❏ **Use**

- Used clinically to monitor short-term glycemic control in patients with diabetes (1–2 weeks)
- Useful marker for postprandial hyperglycemia
- Performs better than hemoglobin A_{1C} for monitoring glucose profile in pregnancies complicated by type 1 diabetes

❏ **Interpretation**

Increased In

- 1,5-AG may be increased during IV hyperalimentation.

Decreased In

- Individuals with renal glucose thresholds that are markedly different from 180 mg/dL (e.g., chronic renal failure, pregnancy, and dialysis) and in those undergoing steroid therapy.
- α-Glucosidase inhibitors can decrease 1,5-AG by interfering with its intestinal absorption.

❏ **Limitations**

- In patients with poorly controlled DM, 1,5-AG is less sensitive to modest changes in glycemic control because of continuous glycosuria.
- Levels can be influenced by factors such as dairy product, races, uric acid, triglycerides, liver disease, gastrectomy state, and cystic fibrosis.

11-DEOXYCORTISOL

❑ **Definition**

- 11-Deoxycortisol, also known as cortodoxone, corticosterone, and compound S, is a steroid and an immediate precursor to the production of cortisol. It can be synthesized from 17-hydroxyprogesterone. Excretion in urine is included in 17-ketogenic steroid (17-KGS) and Porter-Silber 17-OHKS measurements, which were originally used to provide some measure of cortisol production. The direct measurement of cortisol has replaced determinations of 17-KS and 17-OHKS.
- **Normal range:** <50 ng/dL in males; <33 ng/dL in females.

❑ **Use**

- Diagnosis of and monitoring therapeutic response in CAH due to 11β-hydroxylase deficiency
- Assessment of adrenal response in the metyrapone test; result after metyrapone stimulation is >8,000 ng/dL

❑ **Interpretation**
Increased In

- Values are increased in CAH (P450cII deficiency) and following metyrapone administration in normal persons.

Decreased In

- Values are decreased in adrenal insufficiency.

❑ **Limitations**

- Patients with myxedema, some pregnant patients, and those on oral contraceptives respond poorly during the test.

17α-HYDROXYPROGESTERONE

❑ **Definition**

- 17α-Hydroxyprogesterone, also known as hydroxyprogesterone, is a 21-carbon steroid produced in the adrenals—and also in the ovaries, testes, and placenta—that serves as a biosynthetic precursor to cortisol.
- **Normal range:** 18–469 ng/dL (see Table 16.1).

TABLE 16–1. Range of Normal Values for 17α-Hydroxyprogesterone

Patient Group	Median (ng/dL)	Range (ng/dL)
Male (20–59 y)	143	60–342
Female		
Follicular phase	67	19–182
Luteal phase	210	22–469
Taking oral contraceptives	79	18–251
Postmenopausal	46	20–172

16

❏ Use

- Diagnosis and management of congenital adrenal hyperplasia, hirsutism, and infertility

❏ Interpretation
Increased In

- The luteal phase of menstruating women and pregnancy, during which it rises.
- When defective 21-alpha hydroxylase and 11-beta hydroxylase are present.
- The most common form of CAH, where deficiency of the enzyme 21-hydroxylase blocks normal synthesis of cortisol, leading to a compensatory increase of ACTH secretion; this results in increased levels.

❏ Limitations

- Circulating normally exhibits a diurnal pattern similar to that of cortisol, with higher values in the early morning than in the late afternoon. Hence, the time of collection should be standardized.
- Spuriously elevated levels are sometimes seen in premature and sick newborns due to interference with other steroid metabolites. 17α-Hydroxypregnenolone sulfate (percent cross-reactivity: 3.8%) has been identified as the most significant interferent in direct assays.
- 17α-Hydroxyprogesterone values for women with late-onset CAH have been found to overlap with those encountered in hirsute, oligomenorrheic women who do not have the disorder. Accordingly, it is important to determine ACTH-stimulated 17α-hydroxyprogesterone levels in women suspected of having late-onset CAH.

17-KETOSTEROIDS, URINE (17-KS)

❏ Definition

- 17-Ketosteroids, urine (17-KS), are breakdown products of androgens and are an adrenal function test. Examples of 17-KS include androstenedione, androsterone, estrone, and dehydroepiandrosterone. An alternative and more specific test for adrenal androgen function is dehydroepiandrosterone sulfate in serum.
- **Normal range:** depends on sex and age (Table 16.2).

❏ Use

- Evaluation of glucocorticoid production and neuroendocrine function
- Evaluation of androgenic adrenal and testicular function in normal male individuals and primarily adrenal androgenic secretion in normal female individuals

❏ Interpretation
Increased In

- Adrenal tumor
- Congenital adrenal hyperplasia (very rare)
- Cushing syndrome
- Ovarian cancer
- Testicular cancer
- Ovarian dysfunction (polycystic ovarian disease)

TABLE 16–2. Normal Ranges for 17-Ketosteroids in the Urine

Age	Value (mg/d)
Male	
0–11 mo	0.0–1.0
1–5 y	1.0–2.0
6–10 y	1.0–4.4
11–12 y	1.3–8.5
13–16 y	3.4–9.8
17–50 y	5.3–17.6
≥51 y	4.1–12.1
Female	
0–11 mo	0.0–1.0
1–5 y	1.0–2.0
6–10 y	1.4–3.9
11–12 y	3.8–9.5
13–16 y	4.5–17.1
17–50 y	4.4–14.2
≥51 y	3.2–10.6

Decreased In
- Addison disease
- Castration
- Hypopituitarism
- Myxedema
- Nephrosis

❑ **Limitations**
- A large number of substances may interfere with this test.
- Decreases may be caused by carbamazepine, cephaloridine, cephalothin, chlormerodrin, digoxin, glucose, metyrapone, promazine, propoxyphene, reserpine, and others.
- Increases may be caused by acetone, acetophenide, ascorbic acid, chloramphenicol, chlorothiazide, chlorpromazine, cloxacillin, dexamethasone, erythromycin, ethinamate, etryptamine, methicillin, methyprylon, morphine, oleandomycin, oxacillin, penicillin, phenaglycodol, phenazopyridine, phenothiazine, piperidine, quinidine, secobarbital, spironolactone, and others.

5,10-METHYLENETETRAHYDROFOLATE REDUCTASE (MTHFR) MOLECULAR ASSAY*

❑ **Definition**
- Mutations, C677T and A1298C, in the 5,10-methylenetetrahydrofolate reductase (*MTHFR*) gene increase the risk of thrombosis (OMIM# 188050) and other cardiovascular disorders as a result of an elevated plasma homocysteine concentration (OMIM# 236250).
- **Normal values:** negative or no mutations are found.

16

*Submitted by Edward Ginns, MD and Marzena M. Galdzicka, PhD.

❑ **Use**

■ Suspected coronary artery disease, homocystinuria, neural tube defects, spontaneous abortion, or MTHFR deficiency

❑ **Limitations**

■ The results of a genetic test may be affected by DNA rearrangements, blood transfusion, bone marrow transplantation, or rare sequence variations.

5-HYDROXYINDOLEACETIC ACID (5-HIAA) URINE

❑ **Definition**

■ 5-Hydroxyindoleacetic acid (5-HIAA), also known as serotonin metabolite, is the major urinary metabolite of serotonin.
■ **Normal range:** 0.0–15.0 mg/day (24-hour urine); 0.0–14.0 mg/g creatinine.

❑ **Use**

■ Helps diagnose and monitor treatment for serotonin-secreting carcinoid tumors

❑ **Interpretation**

Increased In

■ Whipple disease
■ Nontropical sprue
■ Small increases possible in pregnancy, ovulation, and postsurgical stress
■ Various food ingestions (e.g., pineapples, kiwi, bananas, eggplant, plums, tomatoes, avocados, plantains, walnuts, pecans, hickory nuts, coffee)
■ Use of certain drugs (e.g., acetanilid, acetaminophen, acetophenetidin, caffeine, coumaric acid, diazepam [Valium], ephedrine, fluorouracil, glyceryl guaiacolate [guaifenesin], heparin, melphalan [Alkeran], mephenesin, methamphetamine, methocarbamol, naproxen, nicotine, Lugol solution, promethazine, phenothiazine, hydroxyl tryptophan)

Decreased In

■ Use of certain drugs (e.g., chlorpromazine, promazine, imipramine, isoniazid, monoamine oxidase inhibitors, methenamine, methyldopa, phenothiazines, promethazine)
■ Renal insufficiency (possible)

❑ **Limitations**

■ Foods rich in serotonin and medications, over-the-counter drugs, and herbal remedies that may affect metabolism of serotonin must be avoided at least 72 hours before and during collection of urine for 5-HIAA.
■ Twenty-four–hour collections are generally recommended, but random collections may be used. Refrigeration is the most important aspect of specimen preservation.
■ Urinary 5-HIAA is increased with malabsorption, in 75% of cases, usually when a carcinoid tumor is far advanced (with large liver metastases, often 300–1,000 mg/day), but may not be increased despite massive metastases.

- Sensitivity is 73%.
- The test is useful in the diagnosis of only 5–7% of patients with carcinoid tumors but in approximately 45% of those with liver metastases.
- Disease extent and prognosis correlate generally with urine 5-HIAA excretion, and the level becomes normal after successful surgery. If urine HIAA is normal, the blood level of serotonin or a precursor, 5-hydroxytryptophan should be checked.

5′-NUCLEOTIDASE (5′-RIBONUCLEOTIDEPHOSPHOHYDROLASE, 5′-NT)

❑ Definition

- This membrane-bound enzyme of the liver is increased in diseases of the liver, particularly if the hepatobiliary tract is involved. The appearance of 5′-NT in serum is due to cholestasis, and its significance is similar to that of ALP and GGT. However, 5′-NT is not as subject to drug induction as GGT and ALP, and it is not subject to confusion with alternate sources of the enzyme, as is seen with ALP.
- **Normal range:** 2.0–8.0 U/L.

❑ Use

- Determining cholestatic liver disease, particularly when GGT and ALP could be falsely elevated due to drug induction
- Better test for secondary tumors and lymphomas of the liver than ALP

❑ Interpretation
Increased In

- 5′-NT is increased in the following conditions:
  - ▼ Hepatobiliary disease with intrahepatic or extrahepatic biliary obstruction
  - ▼ Hepatic carcinoma
  - ▼ Early biliary cirrhosis
  - ▼ Pregnancy (third semester)
  - ▼ Inflammatory arthritis

❑ Limitations

- 5′-NT can be elevated in hyperammonemia due to analytical interference.
- Normal in pregnancy and postpartum period (in contrast to serum leucine aminopeptidase and ALP).

ACETAMINOPHEN (*N*-ACETYL-*p*-AMINOPHENOL; APAP)

❑ Definition

- Nonopioid analgesic, antipyretic

❑ Use

- Relief of pain, such as headaches and toothaches
- Reduction of fever

16

❑ **Interpretation**

- Screen of urine: indication of exposure
- Screen of serum: used to assess potential toxicity
- **Normal range:** 5–20 µg/mL serum
- **Potentially toxic:** >150 µg/mL measured 4 hours postdose

❑ **Limitations**

- Screening
  - ▼ Serum/urine: colorimetric or immunoassay on automated chemistry analyzers
    - High bilirubin concentrations [>50 µg/mL] may cause false-positive results with immunoassay-based tests.
    - Plasma may be tested in place of serum. Anticoagulants such as EDTA and heparin do not generally interfere with the assay.
    - Do not use whole blood.
- Confirmation:
  - ▼ Serum/urine–HPLC or GC/MC
  - ▼ APAP is highly conjugated by glucuronidation and sulfation.
  - ▼ An assay that includes a hydrolysis step provides total APAP levels, which are not useful for assessing toxicity.

ACETYLSALICYLIC ACID

See Salicylates (Aspirin).

ACID PHOSPHATASE

❑ **Definition**

- Acid phosphatase is a hydrolytic enzyme secreted by various cells, and it has five isoenzymes. The greatest amount per gram of tissue is found in semen (prostate); it is also detectable in bone, liver, spleen, kidney, RBCs, and platelets. The acid phosphatase test is also known as prostatic acid phosphatase (PAP), the serum acid phosphatase test, and the tartrate-resistant acid phosphatase (TRAP) test.
- **Normal range:** 0–0.8 U/L.

❑ **Use**

- Predicts recurrence after radical prostatectomy for clinically localized prostate cancer and following response to androgen ablation therapy, when used in conjunction with PSA

❑ **Interpretation**

Increased In

- Acid phosphatase is increased in the following conditions:
  - ▼ Prostate cancer
  - ▼ Gaucher disease and Niemann-Pick disease
  - ▼ One day to 2 days after prostatic surgery or biopsy
  - ▼ Prostatic manipulation or catheterization
  - ▼ Benign prostatic hyperplasia, prostatitis, prostate infarct
  - ▼ Vaginal swabs from rape victims.

❏ Limitations

- PAP is no longer used to screen for or to stage prostate cancer. In most instances, serum PSA is used instead.
- PAP measurement must not be regarded as an absolute test for malignancy, since other factors including benign prostatic hyperplasia, prostatic infarction, and manipulation of the prostate gland may result in elevated serum PAP concentrations.
- PAP measurements provide little additional information beyond that provided by PSA measurements.

Suggested Reading

Moul JW, Connelly RR, Perahia B, et al. The contemporary value of pretreatment prostatic acid phosphatase to predict pathological stage and recurrence in radical prostatectomy cases. *J Urol.* 1998;159:935–940.

ACTH STIMULATION (COSYNTROPIN) TEST

❏ Definition

- Cosyntropin is synthetic ACTH (1–24), which has the full biologic potency of native ACTH (1–39). It is a rapid stimulator of cortisol and aldosterone secretion.

❏ Use

- This is the initial test used to distinguish primary from secondary adrenal insufficiency.
- It is not helpful in the diagnosis of Cushing syndrome. Several protocols are used to assess the response to exogenous ACTH administration (see below).

Low-Dose ACTH Stimulation Test

- This test involves physiologic plasma concentrations of ACTH and provides a more sensitive index of adrenocortical responsiveness.
- It is performed by measuring serum cortisol immediately before and 30 minutes after IV injection of cosyntropin in a dose of either 1 μg/1.73 m^2 or 0.5 μg/1.73 m^2.
- There is no commercially available preparation of "low-dose" cosyntropin. The vials of cosyntropin currently available contain 250 μg and come with sterile normal saline to be used as a diluent. One prepares the low-dose solution of cosyntropin locally.

High-Dose ACTH Stimulation Test

- This test consists of measuring serum cortisol immediately before and 30 and 60 minutes after IV injection of 250 μg of cosyntropin. This dose of cosyntropin results in pharmacologic plasma ACTH concentrations for the 60-minute duration of the test.
- The advantage of the high-dose test is that the cosyntropin can be injected using the IM route, because pharmacologic plasma ACTH concentrations are still achieved.
- Salivary cortisol can also be measured during this test. Salivary cortisol increases to 19 ± 0.8 ng/mL (range: 8.7–36 ng/mL) 1 hour after injection.

16

Eight-Hour ACTH Stimulation Test

- The 8-hour test, which is now rarely performed, consists of infusing 250 μg of cosyntropin continuously over 8 hours in 500 mL of isotonic saline. A 24-hour urine specimen is collected the day before and the day of the infusion for cortisol or 17-hydroxycorticoid and creatinine determination, and serum cortisol is determined at the end of the infusion. Plasma ACTH concentrations are supraphysiologic throughout the infusion.
- The 24-hour urinary excretion of 17-hydroxycorticoid should increase three- to fivefold over baseline on the day of ACTH infusion.

Two-Day ACTH Infusion Test

- The 2-day ACTH infusion test is similar to the 8-hour infusion test, except that the same dose of ACTH is infused for 8 hours on 2 consecutive days.
- This test may be helpful in distinguishing secondary from tertiary adrenal insufficiency. The 1-day 8-hour test is too short for this purpose, whereas longer tests add little further useful information.
- Urinary excretion of 17-hydroxycorticoid should exceed 27 mg during the first 24 hours of infusion and 47 mg during the second 48 hours.

❑ **Interpretation**

- Low-dose stimulation test: A value of 18 μg/dL or more, before or after ACTH injection, is indicative of normal adrenal function.
- High-dose stimulation test: A serum cortisol value of 20 μg/dL or more at any time during the test, including before injection, is indicative of normal adrenal function.
- Eight-hour stimulation test: Serum cortisol should reach 20 μg/dL in 30–60 minutes after the infusion is begun and exceed 25 μg/mL after 6–8 hours.
- Two-day infusion test: Serum cortisol should reach 20 μg/mL in 30–60 minutes after the ACTH infusion is begun and exceed 25 μg/mL after 6–8 hours. Both serum and urinary steroid values increase progressively thereafter, but the ranges of normal are not well defined.

❑ **Limitations**

- In healthy individuals, cortisol responses are greatest in the morning, but in patients with adrenal insufficiency, the response to cosyntropin is the same in the morning and afternoon. Therefore, ACTH stimulation tests should be done in the morning to minimize the risk of misdiagnosis in a normal individual.
- The criteria for a minimal normal cortisol response of 18–20 μg/dL are derived from the responses of healthy volunteers. However, in some studies, higher cutoff points for the diagnosis of adrenal insufficiency are based on the ACTH test responses of patients known to have an abnormal response to insulin.
- Variability in cortisol assays creates an additional problem with setting criteria for a normal response to ACTH that apply to all centers. Studies comparing cortisol results obtained with different assays showed a positive bias of Radioimmunoassays (RIA) and EIAs of 10–50% compared to a reference value obtained using isotope dilution GC/MS.
- In women, the response to ACTH is affected by the use of oral contraceptives, which increase cortisol-binding globulin levels.

- The response to ACTH varies with the underlying disorder. If the patient has hypopituitarism with deficient ACTH secretion and secondary adrenal insufficiency, then the intrinsically normal adrenal gland should respond to maximally stimulating concentrations of exogenous ACTH if given for a sufficiently long time. The response may be less than that in normal subjects and initially sluggish due to adrenal atrophy resulting from chronically low stimulation by endogenous ACTH. If, on the other hand, the patient has primary adrenal insufficiency, endogenous ACTH secretion is already elevated, and there should be little or no adrenal response to exogenous ACTH.
- A clearly subnormal response to the low-dose or high-dose ACTH stimulation test is diagnostic of primary or secondary adrenal insufficiency, whereas a normal response excludes both disorders.
- Cortisol values between 18.0 and 25.4 µg/dL represent a range of uncertainty in which patients may have discordant responses to ACTH, insulin, and/or metyrapone. Higher concentrations represent a normal response in the non-ICU setting.
- The low-dose test is not valid if there has been recent pituitary injury, and it supports the conclusion that a 30-minute serum cortisol concentration <18 µg/dL indicates impaired adrenocortical reserve. In addition, the low-dose test does not reliably indicate hypothalamic–pituitary–adrenal axis suppression in preterm infants whose mothers received dexamethasone for <2 weeks before delivery to hasten fetal lung development. The CRH test should be used in this situation.

ACTIVATED CLOTTING TIME (ACT)*

❑ **Definition**

- Activated clotting time (ACT) is a rapid point-of-care standardized clotting time, performed by automated well-calibrated instruments, such as the Medtronic automated coagulation timer (ACT). A baseline ACT has to be established in each POCT area after induction of anesthesia and opening the chest for cardiopulmonary bypass surgery, because surgery and anesthesia shorten it. The ACT may also vary slightly with the lot number of the control cartridge.
- **Normal range in the absence of heparin (with Medtronic coagulometer):** 74–125 seconds.

❑ **Use**

- ACT is the most widely used measure of anticoagulation with heparin (and neutralization of heparin with protamine) during extracorporeal circulation. After the initial dose of heparin, the ACT is maintained at >275 seconds for off-pump coronary procedures and >350 seconds for on-pump procedures by periodic administration of heparin.

❑ **Interpretation**

- There is some controversy concerning whether monitoring heparinization by ACT alone ensures optimal heparin and protamine doses. A poor correlation

16

---

*Submitted By Liberto Pechet, MD.

was found between ACT and heparin measurements using anti-Xa assays. Nevertheless, experience has shown that institution of anticoagulation and monitoring under ACT guidance and reversal improves hemostasis, limits blood loss, and reduces the need for transfusions.

❏ **Limitations**

- The response of ACT to heparin varies from individual to individual and with heparin potency.
- Underlying coagulopathies (antithrombin III deficiency, clotting factor deficiencies, DIC) must be excluded.
- Medications that inhibit platelet function (aspirin, NSAIDs) may affect ACT.
- Preanalytical errors (sample dilution or contamination with heparin, blood activation) must be avoided. It is particularly important to avoid the use of blood samples contaminated by heparin flushes.

ACTIVATED PROTEIN C RESISTANCE (APCR)*

❏ **Definition**

- APCR reflects resistance to proteolysis of activated factor V by activated protein C (APC). Ninety-five percent of APCR cases are due to factor V Leiden, a genetic mutation in factor V that predisposes to venous thromboembolism (5–10 times greater risk in heterozygotes and 50–100 times greater risk in homozygote carriers). The remaining 5% are found in pregnancy, malignancy, and the antiphospholipid antibody syndrome. Ratios are generated either from a modified PTT or, more recently, by activating protein C with southern copperhead venom, using dilute Russell viper venom as the clotting reagent. The test is performed in the presence of added APC, where in normal individuals, there is an elongation due to delayed generation of fibrin when factor V is lysed; in the absence of APC, where factor V remains intact, there is no elongation. Patients with APCR have a lesser prolongation of clotting in the presence of APC than controls.
- **Normal value: >1.8.**

❏ **Use**

- APCR is one of the assays recommended to investigate the etiology of venous thrombophilia. The congenital form, factor V Leiden, is present in 5% of individuals of European descent and in a high proportion of patients with unprovoked venous thromboembolism. It is virtually absent in patients of pure African ancestry.

❏ **Limitations**

- Protein C levels <50% and initial anticoagulation with vitamin K antagonists may give falsely low ratios. In these situations, the genetic test for factor V Leiden is recommended. The APCR assay is valid in patients stabilized on vitamin K antagonists or heparin.

---

*Submitted By Liberto Pechet, MD.

TABLE 16–3. Normal Range of Adiponectin

Body Mass Index (kg/m²)	Male (µg/mL)	Female (µg/mL)
<25	4–26	5–37
25–30	4–20	5–28
>30	2–20	4–22

- The assay is invalid in clotted specimens, as well as in lipemic, hemolyzed, or icteric samples. The assay is also invalid if blood is drawn with the wrong anticoagulant or the tubes are not filled appropriately.

ADIPONECTIN

❑ **Definition**

- Adiponectin, a hormone secreted exclusively by adipose tissue, has an important role in the regulation of tissue inflammation and insulin sensitivity. Perturbations in adiponectin concentration have been associated with obesity and the metabolic syndrome. Levels of the hormone are inversely correlated with body fat percentage in adults, whereas the association in infants and young children is more unclear.
- **Normal range:** see Table 16.3.

❑ **Use**

- Higher adiponectin levels are associated with a lower risk of type 2 diabetes across diverse populations, consistent with a dose–response relationship.

❑ **Interpretation**

Increased In

- Twofold before a meal and decreases to trough levels within 1 hour after eating
- More than twofold in hemodialysis patients

Decreased In

- Type 2 diabetes mellitus
- Obesity and metabolic syndrome

❑ **Limitations**

- Adiponectin exerts some of its weight reduction effects via the brain. This is similar to the action of leptin, but the two hormones perform complementary actions and can have additive effects.
- Due to its important cardiometabolic actions, adiponectin represents a biologic molecule worth being studied as a new emerging biomarker of disease and also as a target for pharmacologic treatments.

Suggested Reading

Li S, Shin HJ, Ding EL, et al. Adiponectin levels and risk of type 2 diabetes: a systematic review and meta-analysis. *JAMA.* 2009;302(2):179–188.

16

ADRENOCORTICOTROPIC HORMONE (ACTH)

❏ **Definition**

- ACTH is a polypeptide hormone produced by the anterior pituitary gland that exists principally as a chain of 39 amino acids, with a molecular mass of approximately 4,500 Da. Its biologic function is to stimulate cortisol secretion by the adrenal cortex. ACTH secretion is in turn controlled by the hypothalamic hormone CRF and by negative feedback from cortisol.
- **Normal range:** <46 pg/mL.

❏ **Use**

- Diagnosis of Addison disease, CAH, Cushing syndrome, adrenal carcinoma, and ectopic ACTH syndrome

❏ **Interpretation**

Increased In

- Addison disease
- CAH
- Pituitary-dependent Cushing disease
- Ectopic ACTH–producing tumors
- Nelson syndrome

Decreased In

- Secondary adrenocortical insufficiency
- Adrenal carcinoma
- Adenoma
- Hypopituitarism

❏ **Limitations**

- Plasma levels of ACTH exhibit a significant diurnal variation. ACTH is normally highest in the early morning (6–8 AM) and lowest in the evening (6–11 PM). Cortisol levels are frequently measured at the same time as ACTH.
- Because ACTH is released in bursts, its levels in the blood can vary from minute to minute.
- ACTH is unstable in blood, and proper handling of specimen is important.
- Most commercial RIAs are insensitive and nonspecific, measuring intact ACTH as well as precursors and fragments. Highly sensitive IRMAs measure intact ACTH only.
- RIAs are recommended for investigating ectopic ACTH–producing tumors, because some of the tumors secrete ACTH precursors and fragments. IRMAs are more sensitive than RIAs and are useful for investigating disorders of the hypothalamic–pituitary–adrenal system.

- Patients taking glucocorticoids may have suppressed levels of ACTH with an apparent high level of cortisol.
- Pregnancy, menstruation, and stress increase secretion.

ALLERGEN TESTS, SPECIFIC IMMUNOGLOBULIN E (IgE)

❑ Definition

- Allergic diseases are manifested as hyperresponsiveness in the target organ, whether the skin, nose, lung, or GI tract. Most tests for "allergy" are actually tests for allergic sensitization, or the presence of allergen-specific IgE.
- Most patients who experience symptoms upon exposure to an allergen have demonstrable IgE that specifically recognizes that allergen, making these tests essential tools in the diagnosis of allergic disorders.
- *In vitro* testing for allergy has certain advantages:
  - ▼ It poses no risk to the patient of an allergic reaction.
  - ▼ It is not affected by medications (antihistamines, etc.) the patient may be taking.
  - ▼ It is not reliant upon skin integrity or affected by skin disease.
  - ▼ It can be more convenient for the patient. In vitro testing requires submitting a blood sample and does not necessitate a separate visit for skin testing.
- Clinical performance of specific IgE-based serum allergen tests typically has sensitivity ranging from 84% to 95% and specificity ranging from 85% to 94%.
- Various types of specific panels, mixes, as well as specific allergen tests currently performed at various labs and contact your lab for details.

Normal range:

kU_A/L	Class	Level of Allergen-Specific IgE Antibody
0.35	0	Absent
0.35–0.69	I	Low
0.70–3.49	II	Medium
3.50–17.49	III	High
17.5–49.99	IV	Very high
50.0–100	V	Very high
>100	VI	Very high

❑ Use

- To establish the diagnosis of an allergic disease and to define the allergens responsible for eliciting signs and symptoms
- To identify allergens that may be responsible for allergic disease and/or anaphylactic episode and to confirm sensitization to particular allergens prior to beginning immunotherapy

16

- To investigate the specificity of allergic reactions to insect venom allergens, drugs, or chemical allergens

❑ Interpretation

Increased In

- Detection of IgE antibodies in serum (Class 1 or greater) indicates an increased likelihood of allergic disease as opposed to other etiologies and defines the allergens that may be responsible for eliciting signs and symptoms.

Decreased In

- NA.

❑ Limitations

- The demonstration of sensitization is not sufficient to diagnose an allergy, however, because a sensitized individual may be entirely asymptomatic upon exposure to the allergen in question. Thus, allergy tests must be interpreted in the context of the patient's specific clinical history, and the diagnosis of an allergic disorder cannot be based solely on a laboratory result.
- If the result is markedly positive (e.g., a Class VI result), the history suggests a past reaction to the allergen, and the allergen is well characterized, then the diagnosis of an allergy can usually be made without further evaluation. If the result is weakly positive, then further evaluation is usually needed.
- A negative immunoassay result in the setting of a strongly suggestive history does not exclude allergy. In this situation, a skin prick test should be considered (if not contraindicated).
- False-positive results of allergen-specific IgE can theoretically occur in patients with extremely elevated total IgE levels.
- Tests used largely in research settings include immunoblotting, basophil histamine or leukotriene release tests, basophil activation, and levels of eosinophil mediators, etc., are not standardized, and are generally not superior to skin testing, and cannot be recommended for routine clinical use.
- Allergen-specific IgG and IgG4 tests, which are believed to correlate with normal immunologic responses to foreign substances, are not useful in the diagnosis of IgE-mediated allergy, with the exception of venom allergy. Unreliable testing methods include provocation/neutralization tests, kinesiology, cytotoxic tests, and electrodermal testing.
- In food allergy, circulating IgE antibodies may remain undetectable despite a convincing clinical history because these antibodies may be directed toward allergens that are revealed or altered during industrial processing, cooking, or digestion and therefore do not exist in the original food for which the patient is tested.
- Identical results for different allergens may not be associated with clinically equivalent manifestations, due to differences in patient sensitivities.

ALBUMIN, SERUM

❑ **Definition**

- Albumin is the most important protein and constitutes 55–65% of total plasma protein. Approximately 300–500 g of albumin is distributed in the body fluids, and the average adult liver synthesizes approximately 15 g/day. Albumin's half-life is approximately 20 days, with 4% of the total albumin pool being degraded daily. The serum albumin concentration reflects the rate of synthesis, the degradation, and the volume of distribution. Albumin synthesis is regulated by a variety of influences, including nutritional status, serum oncotic pressure, cytokines, and hormones.
- **Normal range:**
  - ▼ 0–4 months: 2.0–4.5 g/dL
  - ▼ 4 months–16 years: 3.2–5.2 g/dL
  - ▼ >16 years: 3.5–4.8 g/dL

❑ **Use**

- Assess nutritional status
- Evaluate chronic illness
- Evaluate liver disease

❑ **Interpretation**

Increased In

- Dehydration
- High-protein diet

Decreased In

- Decreased synthesis by the liver:
  - ▼ Acute and chronic liver disease (e.g., alcoholism, cirrhosis, hepatitis)
  - ▼ Malabsorption and malnutrition
  - ▼ Fasting, protein–calorie malnutrition
  - ▼ Amyloidosis
  - ▼ Chronic illness
  - ▼ DM
  - ▼ Decreased growth hormone levels
  - ▼ Hypothyroidism
  - ▼ Hypoadrenalism
  - ▼ Genetic analbuminemia
- Acute-phase reaction, inflammation, and chronic diseases:
  - ▼ Bacterial infections
  - ▼ Monoclonal gammopathies and other neoplasms
  - ▼ Parasitic infestations
  - ▼ Peptic ulcer
  - ▼ Prolonged immobilization
  - ▼ Rheumatic diseases
  - ▼ Severe skin disease
- Increased loss over body surface:
  - ▼ Burns

16

- ▼ Enteropathies related to sensitivity to ingested substances (e.g., gluten sensitivity, Crohn disease, ulcerative colitis)
- ▼ Fistula (gastrointestinal or lymphatic)
- ▼ Hemorrhage
- ▼ Kidney disease
- ▼ Rapid hydration or overhydration
- ▼ Repeated thoracentesis or paracentesis
- ▼ Trauma and crush injuries
- ■ Increased catabolism:
  - ▼ Fever
  - ▼ Cushing disease
  - ▼ Preeclampsia
  - ▼ Thyroid dysfunction
- ■ Plasma volume expansion:
  - ▼ CHF
  - ▼ Oral contraceptives
  - ▼ Pregnancy

❑ Limitations

- ■ In clinical practice, one of the two dye-binding assays—bromocresol green (BCG) and bromocresol purple (BCP)—is used for measuring albumin levels, and systematic differences between these methods have long been recognized.
- ■ BCG methods are subject to nonspecific interference from binding to nonalbumin proteins, whereas BCP is more specific. BCP has been shown to underestimate serum albumin in pediatric patients on hemodialysis and patients in chronic renal failure. Chronic dialysis units often have little influence over the method.
- ■ Antialbumin antibodies are commonly found with hepatic dysfunction and are typically of IgA type.
- ■ Ischemia-modified albumin, in which the metal-binding capacity of albumin has decreased due to exposure to ischemic events, is a biologic marker of myocardial ischemia.

ALCOHOLS (VOLATILES, SOLVENTS)*

❑ Definition

- ■ Alcohols are organic compounds that contain the –OH group, including methanol (CH_3OH), ethanol (ethyl alcohol; C_2H_5OH), isopropanol (rubbing alcohol), and methanol (wood alcohol). Although acetone (CH_3COCH_3) is a ketone, not an alcohol, it is included in this group, because it is often detected in the same testing methodology.
- ■ **Normal range:**
  - ▼ Ethanol: <10 mg/dL.
    - ● 50 mg/dL: decreased inhibition, slight incoordination
    - ● 100 mg/dL: slow reaction time; altered sensory ability

---

*Submitted By Amanda J. Jenkins, PhD.

- 150 mg/dL: altered thought processes; personality, behavior changes
- 200 mg/dL: staggering gait, nausea, vomiting, mental confusion
- 300 mg/dL: slurred speech, sensory loss, visual disturbance
- 400 mg/dL: hypothermia, hypoglycemia, poor muscle control, seizures
- 700 mg/dL: unconsciousness, decreased reflexes, respiratory failure (may also occur at lower concentrations)
  - ▼ Isopropanol (isopropyl alcohol): <10 mg/dL (normal); toxic effects generally seen at 50–100 mg/dL.
  - ▼ Methanol: <10 mg/dL (normal); levels >25 mg/dL are generally considered toxic.
  - ▼ Acetone: <10 mg/dL; effects are said to be similar to ethanol for similar blood levels, but the anesthetic potency is greater.

❏ **Use**

- Beverage (ethanol)
- Solvent and reagent
- Vehicle in chemical and pharmaceutical industries
- Antiseptic (isopropyl alcohol)

❏ **Limitations**

- Immunoassay testing for ethanol may have cross-reactivity <1% with isopropanol alcohol, methanol, ethylene glycol, and acetaldehyde; <15% with *n*-propanol.
- Elevated concentrations of acetone are detected in specimens during diabetic ketoacidosis and fasting ketoacidosis and may range from 10 to 70 mg/dL.
- In many headspace gas chromatographic methods, acetonitrile coelutes with acetone, leading to a false-positive result. Acetonitrile may be a component in cosmetic nail remover.
- A positive urine ethanol due to the presence of yeast in the patient's urine has been described. In these cases, glucose was also present in the urine.

ALDOSTERONE

❏ **Definition**

- Primary mineralocorticoid secreted by the adrenal zona glomerulosa. The role of aldosterone in metabolism is the control of sodium and potassium. Regulating sodium ion concentration, in turn, regulates fluid volume. Aldosterone acts to decrease excretion of sodium and increase the excretion of potassium at the kidney, sweat glands, and salivary glands.
- **Normal range:**
  - ▼ 8:00–10:00 AM (sitting): 3–34 ng/dL
  - ▼ 8:00–10:00 AM (supine): 2–19 ng/dL
  - ▼ 4:00–6:00 PM (sitting): 2–23 ng/dL

❏ **Use**

- Diagnosis of primary hyperaldosteronism
- Differential diagnosis of fluid and electrolyte disorders
- Assessment of adrenal aldosterone production

16

❏ **Interpretation**

Increased In

- Primary aldosteronism
- Secondary aldosteronism
- Barter syndrome
- Pregnancy
- Very low–sodium diet
- Urine aldosterone also increased in nephrosis

Decreased In

- Hyporeninemic hypoaldosteronism (Cushing syndrome)
- CAH
- Congenital deficiency of aldosterone synthetase
- Addison disease
- Very high–sodium diet

❏ **Limitations**

- Many physiologic factors affect plasma aldosterone. Posture, salt intake, use of antihypertensive drugs, use of steroids, oral contraceptives, age, stress, exercise, menstrual cycle, and pregnancy can all have a strong influence on aldosterone results.
- Licorice may mimic aldosterone effects and should be avoided 2 weeks before the test.

ALKALINE PHOSPHATASE (ALP)

❏ **Definition**

- ALP refers to a family of enzymes that catalyze hydrolysis of phosphate esters at an alkaline pH. There are at least five isoenzymes derived from the liver (sinusoidal and bile canalicular surface of hepatocytes), bone, intestine (brush border of mucosal cells), placenta, and tumor-associated tissues separated by electrophoresis. Placenta and tumor-associated ALP are the most heat resistant to inactivation. More than 95% of total ALP activity comes from the bone and liver (approximately 1:1 ratio). The half-life of ALP is 7–10 days.
- Normal range:
  ▼ 0–1 year: 150–350 IU/L
  ▼ 1–16 years: 30–300 IU/L
  ▼ >16 years: 30–115 IU/L

❏ **Use**

- Diagnosis and treatment of the liver, bone, intestinal, and parathyroid diseases

❏ **Interpretation**

Increased In

- Increased bone formation
- Bone diseases (metastatic carcinoma of the bone, myeloma, Paget disease)
- Renal disease (renal rickets due to vitamin D–resistant rickets associated with secondary hyperparathyroidism)

- Liver disease (e.g., infectious mononucleosis, uncomplicated extrahepatic biliary obstruction, liver abscess)
- Miscellaneous (extrahepatic sepsis, ulcerative colitis, pancreatitis, phenytoin, and alcohol use)
- Bone origin—increased deposition of calcium
  - ▾ Hyperparathyroidism
  - ▾ Paget disease (osteitis deformans) (highest reported values 10–20 times normal). Marked elevation in the absence of liver disease is most suggestive of Paget disease of bone or metastatic carcinoma from the prostate.
  - ▾ Increase in cases of metastases to bone is marked only in prostate carcinoma.
  - ▾ Osteoblastic bone tumors (osteogenic sarcoma, metastatic carcinoma).
  - ▾ Osteogenesis imperfecta (due to healing fractures).
  - ▾ Familial osteoectasia.
  - ▾ Osteomalacia, rickets.
  - ▾ Polyostotic fibrous dysplasia.
  - ▾ Osteomyelitis.
  - ▾ Late pregnancy; reverts to normal level by 20th day postpartum.
  - ▾ Children <10 years of age and again during prepubertal growth spurt may have three to four times adult values; adult values are attained by age 20.
  - ▾ Administration of ergosterol.
  - ▾ Hyperthyroidism.
  - ▾ Transient hyperphosphatasemia of infancy
  - ▾ Hodgkin disease.
  - ▾ Healing of extensive fractures (slightly).
- Liver disease
  - ▾ Any obstruction of the biliary system (e.g., stone, carcinoma, primary biliary cirrhosis) is a sensitive indicator of intrahepatic or extrahepatic cholestasis. Whenever the ALP is elevated, a simultaneous elevation of 5′-nucleotidase (5′-N) establishes biliary disease as the cause of the elevated ALP. If the 5′-N is not increased, the cause of the elevated ALP must be found elsewhere (e.g., bone disease).
    - Liver infiltrates (e.g., amyloid or leukemia)
    - Cholangiolar obstruction in hepatitis (e.g., infectious, toxic)
    - Hepatic congestion due to heart disease
    - Adverse reaction to therapeutic drug (e.g., chlorpropamide) (progressive elevation of serum ALP may be first indication that drug therapy should be halted); may be 2–20 times normal
    - Increased synthesis of ALP in the liver
  - ▾ Diabetes mellitus—44% of diabetic patients have 40% increase of ALP.
  - ▾ Parenteral hyperalimentation of glucose.
- Liver diseases with increased ALP
  - ▾ Less than three to four times increase lacks specificity and may be present in all forms of liver disease.
  - ▾ Two times increase: acute hepatitis (viral, toxic, alcoholic), acute fatty liver, cirrhosis.
  - ▾ Two to ten times increase: nodules in the liver (metastatic or primary tumor, abscess, cyst, parasite, TB, sarcoid); is a sensitive indicator of a hepatic infiltrate.

▼ Increase more than two times the upper limit of normal in patients with primary breast or lung tumor with osteolytic metastases is more likely caused by liver than by bone metastases.

▼ Five times increase: infectious mononucleosis, postnecrotic cirrhosis.

▼ Ten times increase: carcinoma of the head of the pancreas, choledocholithiasis, and drug cholestatic hepatitis.

▼ Fifteen to twenty times increase: primary biliary cirrhosis, primary or metastatic carcinoma. The GGT-to-ALP ratio >2.5 is highly suggestive of alcohol abuse.

▼ Chronic therapeutic use of anticonvulsant drugs (e.g., phenobarbital, phenytoin).

■ Placental origin: appears at 16th–20th week of normal pregnancy, increases progressively to two times normal up to onset of labor, and disappears 3–6 days after delivery of placenta. ALP may be increased during complications of pregnancy (e.g., hypertension, preeclampsia, eclampsia, threatened abortion) but is difficult to interpret without serial determinations. It is lower in diabetic than in nondiabetic pregnancy.

■ Intestinal origin: is a component in approximately 25% of normal sera; increases 2 hours after eating in persons with blood type B or O who are secretors of the H blood group. ALP has been reported to be increased in cirrhosis, various ulcerative diseases of the GI tract, severe malabsorption, chronic hemodialysis, and acute infarction of the intestine.

▼ Benign familial hyperphosphatasemia.

▼ Ectopic production by neoplasm (Regan isoenzyme) without involvement of the liver or bone (e.g., Hodgkin disease; cancer of the lung, breast, colon, or pancreas; highest incidence in ovary and cervical cancers).

▼ Vascular endothelium origin—some patients with myocardial, pulmonary, renal (one third of cases), or splenic infarction, usually after 7 days during the phase of organization.

▼ Hyperphosphatasia (liver and bone isoenzymes).

▼ Hyperthyroidism (liver and bone isoenzymes). Increased ALP alone in a chemical profile, especially with a decreased serum cholesterol and lymphocytosis, should suggest excess thyroid medication or hyperthyroidism.

▼ Primary hypophosphatemia (often increased).

▼ ALP isoenzyme determinations are not widely used clinically; heat inactivation may be more useful to distinguish bone from liver source of increased ALP (extremely Ninety percent heat-labile: bone, vascular endothelium, reticuloendothelial system; extremely 90% heat-stable: placenta, neoplasms; intermediate 60–80% heat stable: liver, intestine). Also differentiate by chemical inhibition (e.g., L-phenylalanine) or use serum GGT, leucine aminopeptidase.

▼ Children—mostly bone; little or no liver or intestine.

▼ Adults—liver with little or no bone or intestine; after age 50, increasing amounts of bone.

Decreased In

■ Hypothyroidism

■ Gross anemia

■ Hypophosphatemia

- Vitamin B$_{12}$ deficiency
- Nutritional deficiency of zinc or magnesium
- Excess vitamin D ingestion
- Milk-alkali (Burnett) syndrome
- Congenital hypophosphatasia (enzymopathy of liver, bone, kidney isoenzymes)
- Achondroplasia
- Hypothyroidism, cretinism
- Pernicious anemia (one third of patients)
- Celiac disease
- Malnutrition
- Scurvy
- Postmenopausal women with osteoporosis taking estrogen replacement therapy
- Therapeutic agents (e.g., corticosteroids, trifluoperazine, antilipemic agents, some hyperalimentation)
- Cardiac surgery with cardiopulmonary bypass pump

Normal In

- Inherited metabolic diseases (Dubin-Johnson, Rotor, Gilbert, and Crigler-Najjar syndromes; type I–V glycogenoses, mucopolysaccharidoses; increased in Wilson disease and hemochromatosis related to hepatic fibrosis).
- Consumption of alcohol by healthy persons (in contrast to GGT); may be normal even in alcoholic hepatitis.
- In acute icteric viral hepatitis, the increase is less than two times normal in 90% of cases, but when ALP is high and serum bilirubin is normal, infectious mononucleosis should be ruled out as a cause of hepatitis.

❏ Limitations

- The elevation in ALP tends to be more marked (more than threefold) in extrahepatic biliary obstruction (e.g., by stone or by cancer of the head of the pancreas) than in intrahepatic obstruction, and it is greater the more complete the obstruction. Serum enzyme activities may reach 10–12 times the upper limit of normal, returning to normal on surgical removal of the obstruction.
- Day-to-day variation is 5–10%.
- Recent food ingestion can increase as much as 30 U/L.
- ALP is 15% and 10% higher in African American men and women, respectively, compared to other racial/ethnic groups.
- Twenty-five percent higher with increased body mass index, 10% higher with smoking, 20% lower with the use of oral contraceptives.
- Common drugs, including penicillin derivatives, antiepileptic drugs, antihistamines, cardiovascular drugs, etc., can increase blood levels.

ALPHA$_1$-ANTITRYPSIN (AAT, ALPHA-1 TRYPSIN INHIBITOR, ALPHA-1 PROTEINASE INHIBITOR)

❏ Definition

- AAT is a member of the serpin family of protease inhibitors, produced mostly in the liver. It protects the lungs from damage caused by the proteolytic enzyme, neutrophil elastase. The normal AAT allele is the M allele. Over

16

100 allelic variants have been described, of which the most common severely deficient variants are the S and Z alleles. It is normally the major constituent of the alpha-1 band on routine serum electrophoresis. AAT deficiency is severely underrecognized, with long intervals between the first symptom and diagnosis. Clinical manifestations of severe deficiency of AAT typically involve the lung (e.g., early-onset emphysema with a basilar predominant pattern on imaging), the liver (e.g., cirrhosis), and, rarely, the skin (e.g., panniculitis).

■ **Normal range:** 88–174 mg/dL.

❑ **Use**

■ Workup of individuals with suspected disorders such as familial chronic obstructive lung disease, emphysema, asthma, bronchiectasis
■ Diagnosis of AAT deficiency
■ Diagnosis of juvenile and adult cirrhosis of the liver

❑ **Interpretation**
Increased In

■ Inflammation (acute-phase reacting protein)
■ Infection, tissue injury or necrosis, rheumatic disease, and some malignancies
■ Estrogen administration (oral contraceptives, pregnancy, especially third semester)

Decreased In

■ Deficiency states (hereditary)
■ Hepatic disease (hepatitis, cholestasis, cirrhosis, or hepatic cancer)
■ Pulmonary emphysema, COPD

❑ **Limitations**

■ Phenotypic studies are recommended to confirm a suspected hereditary deficiency.
■ False-positive results can occur if rheumatoid factor present.

α-FETOPROTEIN (AFP) TUMOR MARKER, SERUM

❑ **Definition**

■ AFP is a glycoprotein that is normally produced during gestation by the fetal liver and yolk sac, the serum concentration of which is often elevated in patients with hepatocellular carcinoma (HCC). It is also found in some patients with cancer of the testes and ovaries.
■ **Normal range:** 0.6–6.60 ng/mL.

❑ **Use**

■ Marker for hepatocellular and germ cell (nonseminoma) carcinoma.
■ Follow-up management of patients undergoing cancer therapy, especially for testicular and ovarian tumors and for hepatocellular carcinoma. The measurement of AFP in serum, in conjunction with serum human chorionic

gonadotropin, is an established regimen for monitoring patients with non-seminomatous testicular cancer. In addition, monitoring the rate of AFP clearance from serum after treatment is an indicator of the effectiveness of therapy. Conversely, the growth rate of progressive cancer can be monitored by serially measuring serum AFP concentration over time.

- Serial serum AFP testing is a useful adjunctive test for managing nonseminomatous testicular cancer.

❑ **Interpretation**

- *AFP is increased in the following disorders:*
  - ▼ Ataxia telangiectasia
  - ▼ Hereditary tyrosinemia
  - ▼ Primary hepatocellular carcinoma
  - ▼ Teratocarcinoma
  - ▼ Gastrointestinal tract cancers with and without liver metastases
  - ▼ Benign hepatic conditions such as acute viral hepatitis, chronic active hepatitis, and cirrhosis

❑ **Limitations**

- AFP is not recommended as a screening procedure to detect cancer in the general population. This assay is intended only as an adjunct in the diagnosis and monitoring of AFP-producing tumors. The diagnosis should be confirmed by other tests or procedures.
- Serum levels of AFP do not correlate well with other clinical features of HCC, such as size, stage, or prognosis.
- A case–control study evaluated the diagnostic characteristics of the serum AFP in screening for HCC in patients with different types of chronic liver disease. The following sensitivities and specificities were observed:
  - ▼ AFP cutoff 16 µg/L (sensitivity 62%, specificity 89%)
  - ▼ AFP cutoff 20 µg/L (sensitivity 60%, specificity 91%)
  - ▼ AFP cutoff 100 µg/L (sensitivity 31%, specificity 99%)
  - ▼ AFP cutoff 200 µg/L (sensitivity 22%, specificity 99%)
- False-positive elevations can occur with tumors of the GI tract or with liver damage (e.g., cirrhosis, hepatitis, or drug or alcohol abuse) and pregnancy.
- Failure of the AFP value to return to normal by approximately 1 month after surgery suggests the presence of residual tumor.
- Elevation of AFP after remission suggests tumor recurrence; however, tumors originally producing AFP may recur without an increase in AFP.
- Fucosylated form of serum AFP that is most closely associated with HCC is recognized by a lectin from the common lentil (AFP-L3). AFP-L3 is most useful in the differential diagnosis of individuals with total serum AFP ≤200 ng/mL.

Suggested Reading

Trevisani F, D'Intino PE, Morselli-Labate AM, et al. Serum alpha-fetoprotein for diagnosis of hepatocellular carcinoma in patients with chronic liver disease: influence of HBsAg and anti-HCV status. *J Hepatol.* 2001;34(4):570–575.

16

AMINOTRANSFERASES (AST, ALT)

❑ **Definition**

- Aspartate aminotransferase (AST) and Alanine aminotransferase (ALT) are members of the transaminase family of enzymes, widely distributed in cells throughout the body. AST is primarily found in the heart, liver, skeletal muscle, and kidney, whereas ALT is found primarily in the liver and kidney, with lesser amounts in the heart and skeletal muscle. AST and ALT activities in the liver are about 7,000 and 3,000 times serum activities, respectively.
- **Normal range:**
  ▼ AST:
    - Less than or equal to 1 year: 30–80 U/L
    - Greater than 1 year: 10–40 U/L
  ▼ ALT:
    - Less than or equal to 1 year: 5–50 U/L
    - Greater than 1 year: 10–40 U/L

❑ **Use**

- Most sensitive tests for acute hepatocellular injury (e.g., viral, drug); precedes increase in serum bilirubin by approximately 1 week

❑ **Interpretation**

Increased In

- Hepatocellular damage, liver cell necrosis, or injury of any cause.
- Alcoholic hepatitis (AST > ALT).
- Viral and chronic hepatitis (ALT > AST).
- Early acute hepatitis: AST is usually higher initially, but by 48 hours, ALT is usually higher.
- AST levels of 500 U/L suggest acute hepatocellular injury; seldom >500 U/L in obstructive jaundice, cirrhosis, viral hepatitis, AIDS, alcoholic liver disease.
- Acute fulminant viral hepatitis: Abrupt AST rise may be seen (rarely >4,000 IU/L) and declines more slowly; positive serologic tests and acute chemical injury.
- Congestive heart failure, arrhythmia, sepsis, and GI hemorrhage AST levels reach to a peak of 1,000–9,000 U/L, declining by 50% within 3 days and to <100 U/L within a week, suggesting shock liver with centrolobular necrosis. Serum bilirubin and ALP reflect underlying disease.
- Trauma to skeletal or heart muscle.
- Acute heart failure (AST > ALT).
- Severe exercise, burns, heat stroke.
- Hypothyroidism.
- Drug-induced injury to the liver.
- Acute bile duct obstruction due to a stone: Rapid rise of AST and ALT to very high levels (e.g., >600 U/L and often >2,000 U/L) followed by a sharp fall in 12–72 hours is said to be typical.

Decreased In

- Azotemia
- Chronic renal dialysis
- Pyridoxal phosphate deficiency states (e.g., malnutrition, pregnancy, alcoholic liver disease)

❑ Limitations

- Half-life of AST is 18 hours and that of ALT is 48 hours.
- The patient is rarely asymptomatic with ALT and AST levels >1,000 U/L.
- AST >10 times normal indicates acute hepatocellular injury, but lesser increases are nonspecific and may occur with virtually any form of liver injury.
- Increases ≤8 times upper limit of normal are nonspecific; may be found in any liver disorder.
- Rarely increased >500 U/L (usually <200 U/L) in posthepatic jaundice, AIDS, cirrhosis, and viral hepatitis.
- Usually <50 U/L in fatty liver.
- Less than 100 U/L in alcoholic cirrhosis; ALT is normal in 50%, and AST is normal in 25% of these cases.
- Less than 150 U/L in alcoholic hepatitis (may be higher if the patient has delirium tremens).
- Less than 200 U/L in approximately 50% of patients with cirrhosis, metastatic liver disease, lymphoma, and leukemia.
- Normal values may not rule out liver disease: ALT is normal in 50%, and AST is normal in 25% of cases of alcoholic cirrhosis.
- Degree of increase has a poor prognostic value.
- Serial determinations reflect clinical activity of liver disease. Persistent increase may indicate chronic hepatitis.
- Mild increase of AST and ALT (usually <500 U/L) with ALP increased greater than three times normal indicates cholestatic jaundice, but more marked increase of AST and ALT (especially >1,000 U/L) with ALP increased less than three times normal indicates hepatocellular jaundice.
- Rapid decline in AST and ALT is a sign of recovery from disease but in acute fulminant hepatitis may represent loss of hepatocytes and poor prognosis.
- Poor correlation of increased concentration with extent of liver cell necrosis and has a little prognostic value.
- Although AST, ALT, and bilirubin are most characteristic of acute hepatitis, they are unreliable markers of severity of injury.
- ALT has 45% variation during the day; highest in afternoon and lowest at night. Both AST and ALT exhibit 10–30% variation from 1 day to next. AST levels are 15% higher in African American men.

AMMONIA (BLOOD NH$_3$, NH$_3$, NH$_4$)

❑ Definition

- Ammonia is derived mostly from protein degradation. Most of the ammonia in the blood comes from the intestine, where colonic bacteria use ureases to breakdown urea to ammonia and CO_2. Eight-five percent of blood from the intestine is carried directly to the liver via the portal vein and 85% of ammonia is converted back to urea and excreted by the kidneys and colon. *Helicobacter pylori* in the stomach appears to be an important source of ammonia in patients with cirrhosis.
- **Normal range:** <50 µmol/L.

16

❑ **Use**

- In the diagnosis of hepatic encephalopathy and hepatic coma in the terminal stages of liver cirrhosis, hepatic failure, acute and subacute necrosis, and Reye syndrome. Hyperammonemia in infants may be an indicator of inherited deficiencies of the urea cycle metabolic pathway.
- Should be measured in cases of unexplained lethargy and vomiting, encephalopathy, or any neonate with unexplained neurologic deterioration.
- Not useful to assess the degree of dysfunction (e.g., in Reye syndrome, hepatic function improves and the ammonia level falls, even in patients who finally die of these disorders).

❑ **Interpretation**

Increased In

- Certain inborn errors of metabolism (e.g., defects in urea cycle, organic acid defects).
- Transient hyperammonemia in newborn; unknown etiology; may be life threatening in the first 48 hours.
- May occur in any patient with severe liver disease (e.g., acute hepatic necrosis, terminal cirrhosis, and after portacaval anastomosis). Increased in most cases of hepatic coma but correlates poorly with degree of encephalopathy. Not useful in known liver disease but may be useful in encephalopathy of unknown cause.
- Moribund children: Moderate increases (≤300 μmol/L) without being diagnostic of a specific disease.
- GU tract infection with distention and stasis.
- Ureterosigmoidostomy.
- Some hematologic disorders, including acute leukemia and after bone marrow transplantation.
- Total parenteral nutrition.
- Smoking, exercise, valproic acid therapy.

Decreased In

- Hyperornithinemia (deficiency of ornithine aminotransaminase activity) with gyrate atrophy of the choroid and retina

❑ **Limitations**

- Atmospheric ammonia may cause falsely elevated results.
- The presence of ammonium ions in anticoagulants may produce falsely elevated results.
- Ammonia levels are not always high in all patients with urea cycle disorders.
- High-protein diet may cause increased levels.
- Ammonia levels may also be elevated with GI hemorrhage.
- Ammonia increases due to cellular metabolism: 20% in 1 hour and 100% by 2 hours.
- Prolonged tourniquet application can falsely raise blood ammonia levels.

AMNIOCENTESIS

See Prenatal Screening.

AMPHETAMINES*

❑ **Definition**

- Sympathomimetic amines with central nervous system stimulant activity.
- Other names: amphetamine (Adderall, Dexedrine, Benzedrine, "bennies"), methamphetamine (Desoxyn, "ice," "speed," "meth"), ecstasy (3,4-methylene-dioxymethamphetamine; MDMA), 3,4-methylenedioxyamphetamine (MDA), 3,4-methylenedioxyethylamphetamine (MDEA, MDE, "Eve"), pseudoephedrine (Sudafed), ephedrine, phentermine (Adipex), and methylphenidate (Ritalin).
- Other psychotropic amines include 4-bromo-2,5-dimethoxyamphetamine, p-methoxyamphetamine (PMA), and p-methoxymethamphetamine (PMMA). These are not generally detected in screening tests and may not be reported in confirmation tests unless specifically requested.
- Other drugs that are metabolized to methamphetamine/amphetamine: benzphetamine, clobenzorex, famprofazone, fenethylline, and fenproporex.

❑ **Use**

- Appetite suppressants
- Mood enhancers (psychotropics)
- Treatment of attention deficit hyperactivity disorder
- Nasal decongestants, bronchodilators

❑ **Limitations**

- Screen [urine]: immunoassay on automated chemistry analyzers
    - ▼ Amphetamine: Generally do not give positive results for L-amphetamine, MDA, MDMA, ephedrine, phentermine.
    - ▼ Ecstasy: The target analyte of most immunoassays is MDMA. Screen will not give positive results with D/L-amphetamine, D/L-methamphetamine, phentermine, ephedrine, pseudoephedrine, PMA, PMMA.
- Screen [serum]: ELISA
    - ▼ Target analyte: D-amphetamine. Will not give positive results with L-amphetamine, L-methamphetamine, phenylpropanolamine, MDMA, MDE.
    - ▼ May produce positive results with MDA.
- Confirmation [serum/urine]:
    - ▼ Confirmation techniques do not typically differentiate between D and L forms of amphetamine and methamphetamine.

AMYLASE

❑ **Definition**

- Amylases are a group of hydrolases that degrade complex carbohydrates into fragments. Amylase is produced by the exocrine pancreas and the salivary glands to aid in the digestion of starch. It is also produced by the small intestine mucosa, ovaries, placenta, liver, and fallopian tubes.
- **Normal range:** 5–125 U/L.

16

---

*Submitted By Amanda J. Jenkins, PhD.

❏ **Use**

- To diagnose and monitor pancreatitis or other pancreatic diseases
- In the workup of any intra-abdominal inflammatory event

❏ **Interpretation**

Increased In

- Acute pancreatitis (e.g., alcoholic, autoimmune). Urine levels reflect serum changes by a time lag of 6–10 hours.
- Acute exacerbation of chronic pancreatitis.
- Drug-induced acute pancreatitis (e.g., aminosalicylic acid, azathioprine, corticosteroids, dexamethasone, ethacrynic acid, ethanol, furosemide, thiazides, mercaptopurine, phenformin, triamcinolone).
- Drug-induced methodologic interference (e.g., pancreozymin [contains amylase], chloride and fluoride salts [enhance amylase activity], lipemic serum [turbidimetric methods]).
- Obstruction of pancreatic duct by
  ▼ Stone or carcinoma
    ● Drug-induced spasm of the sphincter of Oddi (e.g., opiates, codeine, methyl choline, cholinergics, chlorothiazide) to levels 2–15 times normal
    ● Partial obstruction + drug stimulation
  ▼ Biliary tract disease
  ▼ Common bile duct obstruction
  ▼ Acute cholecystitis
- Complications of pancreatitis (pseudocyst, ascites, abscess).
- Pancreatic trauma (abdominal injury; following ERCP).
- Altered GI tract permeability:
  ▼ Ischemic bowel disease or frank perforation
  ▼ Esophageal rupture
  ▼ Perforated or penetrating peptic ulcer
  ▼ Postoperative upper abdominal surgery, especially partial gastrectomy (≤2 times normal in one third of patients)
- Acute alcohol ingestion or poisoning.
- Salivary gland disease (mumps, suppurative inflammation, duct obstruction due to calculus, radiation).
- Malignant tumors (especially pancreas, lung, ovary, esophagus; also breast, colon); usually >25 times upper reference limit, which is rarely seen in pancreatitis.
- Advanced renal insufficiency; often increased even without pancreatitis.
- Macroamylasemia.
- Others, such as chronic liver disease (e.g., cirrhosis; ≤2 times normal), burns, pregnancy (including ruptured tubal pregnancy), ovarian cyst, diabetic ketoacidosis, recent thoracic surgery, myoglobinuria, presence of myeloma proteins, some cases of intracranial bleeding (unknown mechanism), splenic rupture, and dissecting aneurysm.
- It has been suggested that a level >1,000 Somogyi units is usually due to surgically correctable lesions (most frequently stones in biliary tree), the pancreas being negative or showing only edema; but 200–500 U is usually associated

with pancreatic lesions that are not surgically correctable (e.g., hemorrhagic pancreatitis, necrosis of pancreas).

- Increased serum amylase with low urine amylase may be seen in renal insufficiency and macroamylasemia. Serum amylase ≤4 times normal in renal disease only when creatinine clearance is <50 mL/minute due to pancreatic or salivary isoamylase; but rarely more than four times normal in the absence of acute pancreatitis.

Decreased In

- Extensive marked destruction of the pancreas (e.g., acute fulminant pancreatitis, advanced chronic pancreatitis, advanced cystic fibrosis). Decreased levels are clinically significant only in occasional cases of fulminant pancreatitis.
- Severe liver damage (e.g., hepatitis, poisoning, toxemia of pregnancy, severe thyrotoxicosis, severe burns).
- Methodologic interference by drugs (e.g., citrate and oxalate decrease activity by binding calcium ions)
  ▼ Normal: 1–5%
  ▼ Macroamylasemia: <1%; very useful for this diagnosis
  ▼ Acute pancreatitis: >5%; use is presently discouraged for this diagnosis
- Amylase-to-creatinine clearance ratio = (urine amylase/serum amylase) (serum creatinine/urine creatinine) × 100

Normal In

- Relapsing chronic pancreatitis
- Patients with hypertriglyceridemia (technical interference with test)
- Frequently normal in acute alcoholic pancreatitis

❏ Limitations

- Composed of pancreatic and salivary types of isoamylases distinguished by various methodologies; nonpancreatic etiologies are almost always salivary; both types may be increased in renal insufficiency.
- An elevation of total serum α-amylase does not specifically indicate a pancreatic disorder, since the enzyme is produced by the salivary glands, mucosa of the small intestine, ovaries, placenta, liver, and the lining of the fallopian tubes.
- Pancreatic amylase results may be elevated in patients with macroamylase. This elevated pancreatic amylase is not diagnostic for pancreatitis. By utilizing serum lipase and urinary amylase values, the presence or absence of macroamylase may be determined.

AMYLASE, URINE (AMYLASE/CREATININE CLEARANCE RATIO [ALCR])

❏ Definition

- The ratio between amylase and creatinine in serum and urine. Also referred as fractional excreted of amylase. ALCR is calculated as:

$$\frac{\text{urine amylase}}{\text{serum amylase}} \times \frac{\text{serum creatinine}}{\text{urine creatinine}} \times 100$$

16

- **Normal range:**
  - ▼ Amylase urine: 1–17 U/hour
  - ▼ ALCR: 1–4%

❑ **Use**

- Differential diagnosis of pancreatitis
- Diagnosis of pseudocyst of the pancreas, where the urine amylase may remain elevated for weeks after the serum amylase has returned to normal, after a bout of acute pancreatitis.

❑ **Interpretation**

Increased In

- Pancreatitis (>6%)
- DKA
- Renal insufficiency
- Duodenal perforation
- Large doses of corticosteroids
- Pancreatic cancer
- Myeloma and light chain disease

Decreased In

- Macroamylasemia

❑ **Limitations**

- Macroamylasemia is characterized by high serum amylase but normal urine amylase. The ALCR remains useful for the diagnosis of macroamylasemia. In macroamylasemia, the clearance is very low.

ANDROSTENEDIONE, SERUM

❑ **Definition**

- Androstenedione, also known as 4-androstenedione, is a 19-carbon steroid hormone produced in the adrenal glands and the gonads (testes as well as ovaries) as an intermediate step in the biochemical pathway that produces the androgen testosterone and the estrogens estrone and estradiol. It is a major adrenal androgen in serum.
- **Normal range:** 0.0–4.4 ng/mL (see Table 16.4).

❑ **Use**

- Diagnosis of virilism and hirsutism
- Suspicion of anabolic steroid abuse

❑ **Interpretation**

Increased In

- CAH caused by 21-hydroxylase deficiency; marked increase is suppressed to normal levels by adequate glucocorticoid therapy.
  - ▼ Suppressed level reflects adequacy of therapeutic control.

TABLE 16–4. Normal Ranges for Serum Androstenedione

Age/Tanner Stage	Female (ng/mL)	Male (ng/mL)
7–9 y	0.0–0.9	0.0–0.8
10–11 y	0.0–3.0	0.0–1.3
12–13 y	0.4–3.4	0.0–1.6
14–15 y	0.7–4.3	0.4–2.9
16–17 y	0.9–4.1	1.1–3.1
18–40 y	0.5–4.3	0.9–2.9
≥41 y	0.4–2.7	0.8–2.2
Postmenopausal women	<1.0	
Tanner stage I	<1.6	<0.9
Tanner stage II	<2.2	<1.4
Tanner stage III	0.6–4.4	<2.6
Tanner stage IV–V	0.9–3.8	1.0–3.0

▼ Androstenedione may be better than 17-hydroxyprogesterone for monitoring therapy because it shows minimal diurnal variation, better correlation with urinary 17-KS excretion, and plasma levels that are not immediately affected by a dose of glucocorticoid.
- Adrenal tumors
- Cushing disease
- Polycystic ovarian disease

Decreased In
- Addison disease
- Any condition that causes partial or complete adrenal or gonadal failure

ANGIOTENSIN II

❏ Definition
- Angiotensin II is the biologically active product of renin–angiotensin system. It is an oligopeptide of eight amino acids and very strong physiologic vasoconstrictor. The concentration of ACE is highest in the lung, and it had been thought that most angiotensin II formation occurred in the pulmonary circulation. It is now clear, however, that ACE is produced in the vascular endothelium of many tissues; therefore, angiotensin II can be synthesized at a variety of sites, including the kidney, vascular endothelium, adrenal gland, and brain.
- Alternative enzymatic pathways not involving ACE may contribute to angiotensin II production. Angiotensin II binds to its specific receptors and exerts its effects in the brain, kidney, adrenal, vascular wall, and the heart. The actions of circulating angiotensin II contribute to hypertension. This may indirectly influence cardiac function, irrespective of any direct effect on the heart and myocardium.
- Circulating angiotensin II promotes sodium and water reabsorption, increasing intravascular fluid volume, which in turn increases cardiac preload and, therefore, stroke volume. Circulating angiotensin II causes systemic arteriolar vasoconstriction, thereby increasing vascular resistance and cardiac afterload.

16

Angiotensin II also affects the autonomic nervous system, stimulating the sympathetic nervous system and reducing vagal activity. These actions are oriented toward maintaining the blood pressure when the renin–angiotensin system is activated by effective volume depletion.
- **Normal range:** 10–60 pg/mL.

❏ **Use**
- Evaluating hypertension

❏ **Interpretation**

Increased In
- Hypertension
- Renin-secreting juxtaglomerular renal tumor
- Volume depletion
- CHF

Decreased In
- Anephric patients
- Primary aldosteronism
- Cushing syndrome

❏ **Limitations**
- Patient should be on normal-sodium diet and be recumbent for 30 minutes before specimen collection.
- Short lived in plasma (half-life is 5 minutes) degraded into inactive peptides, plasma should be separated and frozen immediately.

ANGIOTENSIN-CONVERTING ENZYME (ACE, KINASE II)

❏ **Definition**
- ACE production occurs mainly in the epithelial cells of the pulmonary bed. Smaller amounts are found in blood vessels and renal tissue, where ACE converts angiotensin I to angiotensin II; this conversion helps regulate arterial blood pressure. Angiotensin II stimulates the adrenal cortex to produce aldosterone. Aldosterone helps the kidneys maintains water balance by retaining sodium and promoting the excretion of potassium.
- **Normal range:** 8–53 U/L.

❏ **Use**
- Evaluation of patients with suspected sarcoidosis
- Evaluate the severity and activity of sarcoidosis
- Evaluation of hypertension
- Evaluation of Gaucher disease

❏ **Interpretation**

Increased In
- Active pulmonary sarcoidosis (50–75% of patients but only 11% with inactive disease)

- Gaucher disease (100%)
- DM (>24%)
- Hyperthyroidism (81%)
- Leprosy (53%)
- Chronic renal disease
- Cirrhosis (25%)
- Silicosis (>20%)
- Berylliosis (75%)
- Amyloidosis
- TB infection
- Connective tissue diseases
- Fungal disease, histoplasmosis

Decreased In
- Far-advanced lung neoplasms
- Anorexia nervosa associated with hypothyroidism
- COPD, emphysema, lung cancer, cystic fibrosis
- Starvation

❏ **Limitations**
- False-positive rate equals 2–4%.
- Levels may be normal in lymphoma and lung cancer.
- Serum ACE is significantly reduced in patients on ACE inhibitors (e.g., enalapril and captopril).
- The reference interval for children and adolescents may be as much as 50% higher than specimens from adults.
- Serum ACE abnormality has been reported in 20–30% of α1-antitrypsin variants (MZ, ZZ, and MS Pi types) but in only about 1% of individuals with normal MM Pi type. There is evidence that paraquat poisoning (because of its effect on pulmonary capillary endothelium) is associated with elevated serum ACE.

ANION GAP (AG)

❏ **Definition**
- The AG is an arithmetic approximation of difference between routinely measured serum anions (23) and cations (11) = 12 mmol/L.
- Unmeasured ions include proteins (mostly albumin) = 15 mmol/L, organic acids = 5 mmol/L, phosphates = 2 mmol/L, sulfates = 1 mmol/L; total = 23 mmol/L.
- Unmeasured cations include calcium = 5 mmol/L, potassium = 4.5 mmol/L, magnesium = 1.5 mmol/L; total = 11 mmol/L.
- Calculated as $Na^+ - (Cl^- + HCO_3^-)$; **typical normal values** = 8–16 mmol/L; **if K^+ is included, normal** = 10–20 mmol/L; reference interval varies considerably depending on instrumentation and between individuals. Increased AG reflects amount of organic (e.g., lactic acid, ketoacids) and fixed acids present.
- AG initially began as a measure of quality assurance.

16

❏ **Use**

- Identify cause of a metabolic acidosis
- Supplement to laboratory quality control, along with its components

❏ **Interpretation**

Increased In

- Organic (e.g., lactic acidosis, ketoacidosis)
- Inorganic (e.g., administration of phosphate, sulfate)
- Protein (e.g., hyperalbuminemia, transient)
- Exogenous (e.g., salicylate, formate, paraldehyde, nitrate, penicillin, carbenicillin)
- Not completely identified (e.g., hyperosmolar hyperglycemic nonketotic coma, uremia, poisoning by ethylene glycol, methanol)
- Artifactual
  - ▼ Falsely increased serum sodium
  - ▼ Falsely decreased serum chloride or bicarbonate
- When AG >12–14 mmol/L, diabetic ketoacidosis is the most common cause, uremic acidosis is the second most common cause, and drug ingestion (e.g., salicylates, methyl alcohol, ethylene glycol, ethyl alcohol) is the third most common cause; lactic acidosis should always be considered when these three causes are ruled out. In small children, rule out inborn errors of metabolism.

Decreased In

- Hypoalbuminemia (most common cause), hypocalcemia, hypomagnesemia.
- Artifactual (laboratory error, most frequent cause).
- "Hyperchloremia" in bromide intoxication (if chloride determination by colorimetric method).
- False increase in serum chloride or HCO_3^-.
- False decrease in serum sodium (e.g., hyperlipidemia, hyperviscosity)
  - ▼ Increased unmeasured cations
  - ▼ Hyperkalemia, hypercalcemia, hypermagnesemia
- Increased proteins in multiple myeloma, paraproteinemias, polyclonal gammopathies (these abnormal proteins are positively charged and lower the AG).
- Lithium and bromide overdose.
- Simultaneous changes in ions may cancel each other out, leaving AG unchanged (e.g., increased Cl^- and decreased HCO_3^-). The change in AG should equal change in HCO_3^-; otherwise a mixed, rather than simple, acid–base disturbance is present.

ANTIARRHYTHMIC DRUGS

See Cardiovascular Drugs.

ANTIBIOTICS

❏ **Definition**

- Antibiotics are substances that destroy or inhibit the growth of microorganisms. Antibiotics consist of chemical groups such as β-lactams, polyenes, macrolides, tetracyclines, aminoglycosides, and sulfonamides. Names include amikacin, chloramphenicol, gentamicin, kanamycin, streptomycin, tobramycin, and vancomycin.

- **Normal therapeutic (and toxic) levels:** see Table 16.5.

❑ **Use**

- Prevention and treatment of infections caused by bacteria

❑ **Limitations**

- Testing must be performed on serum or plasma.
- Peak concentrations: collect specimen 30–120 minutes after completion of infusion (drug and route dependent).
- Trough concentrations: collect specimen 5–90 minutes before next infusion (drug dependent).
- Testing methodologies: immunoassay (e.g., fluorescence polarization) or HPLC.
- *Specimens must be frozen* for streptomycin and amphotericin B.
- Specimens must be protected from light for trimethoprim and amphotericin.

TABLE 16–5. Therapeutic and Toxic Serum Concentrations for Antibiotics

	Therapeutic Concentration (µg/mL)	Potentially Toxic Level (µg/mL)
Amikacin		
Peak	15–25	>30
Trough	2–5	>8
Chloramphenicol		
Peak	10–20	25
Trough	5–10	15
Gentamicin		
Peak	5–10	12
Trough	0.5–2	>2
Kanamycin		
Peak	20–25	
Trough	5–10	
Netilmicin		
Peak	4–8	8
Trough	1–2	2
Streptomycin		
Peak	5–20	40
Trough	<5	40
Tobramycin		
Peak	5–10	12
Trough	0.5–2	>2
TMP/SMX		
Peak (TMP)	4–8	8
Peak (SMX)	1–2	>2
Vancomycin		
Peak (not recommended)	30–40	>80
Trough	5–10	>20

16

- Unacceptable specimens:
  ▼ Hemolyzed
  ▼ Collection tubes with additives such as serum separator, citrate, oxalate, or fluoride
- Trimethoprim may be detected in urine in general toxicology screens utilizing GC/MS.

ANTICARDIOLIPIN ANTIBODIES (ACAs)

❑ **Definition**

- Cardiolipins, and other related phospholipids, are lipid molecules found in cell membranes and platelets. They play an important role in the blood clotting process. When antibodies are formed against cardiolipins (ACAs against IgG, IgM, and IgA), they increase an affected patient's risk of developing recurrent inappropriate blood clots (thrombi) in both arteries and veins.
- Other names include antiphospholipid antibodies.
- **Normal range:** see Table 16.6.

❑ **Use**

- Evaluation of suspected cases of antiphospholipid antibody syndrome (APS).
- Unexplained blood clot.
- Recurrent miscarriages.
- ACAs are present in APS, SLE, acute infections, HIV, and certain cancers and with some drug (e.g., phenytoin, penicillin, procainamide). They occur in the general population, with the prevalence increasing with age.

❑ **Interpretation**

- APS is present if at least one of the clinical criteria and one of the laboratory criteria that follow are met.
  ▼ Clinical criteria
    ● Vascular thrombosis
    ● One or more clinical episodes of arterial, venous, or small vessel thrombosis, in any tissue or organ. Thrombosis must be confirmed by objective validated criteria (i.e., unequivocal findings of appropriate imaging studies or histopathology). For histopathologic confirmation, thrombosis should be present without significant evidence of inflammation in the vessel wall.
  ▼ Pregnancy morbidity
    a. One or more unexplained deaths of a morphologically normal fetus at or beyond the 10th week of gestation, with normal fetal morphology documented by ultrasound or by direct examination of the fetus.

TABLE 16–6. Normal Levels of ACAs

	Negative	Indeterminate	Positive	Strong Positive
IgG antibody	<15 GPL	15–19 GPL	20–80 GPL	>80 GPL
IgM antibody	<15 MPL	17–19 MPL	20–80 MPL	>80 MPL
IgA antibody	<12 APL	12–19 APL	20–80 APL	>80 APL

   b. One or more premature births of a morphologically normal neonate before the 34th week of gestation because of (i) eclampsia or severe preeclampsia defined according to standard definitions or (ii) recognized features of placental insufficiency.
   c. Three or more unexplained consecutive spontaneous abortions before the 10th week of gestation, with maternal anatomic or hormonal abnormalities and paternal and maternal chromosomal causes excluded.
   d. In studies of populations of patients who have more than one type of pregnancy morbidity, investigators are strongly encouraged to stratify groups of subjects according to a, b, or c above.
■ **Laboratory criteria.** (Investigators are strongly advised to classify APS patients in studies into one of the following categories: I, more than one laboratory criteria present [any combination]; IIa, LA present alone; IIb, aCL antibody present alone; IIc, anti-β_2 glycoprotein-I antibody present alone.)
   ▼ LAs present in plasma, on two or more occasions at least 12 weeks apart, detected according to the guidelines of the International Society on Thrombosis and Haemostasis (Scientific Subcommittee on LAs/phospholipid-dependent antibodies).
   ▼ ACA of IgG and/or IgM isotype in serum or plasma, present in medium or high titer (i.e., >40 GPL or MPL, or greater than the 99th percentile), on two or more occasions, at least 12 weeks apart, measured by a standardized ELISA.
   ▼ Anti-β_2 glycoprotein-I antibody of IgG and/or IgM isotype in serum or plasma (in titer >99th percentile), present on two or more occasions, at least 12 weeks apart, measured by a standardized ELISA, according to recommended procedures.

❏ Limitations

■ The cardiolipin IgA isotype is usually detected with either IgG or IgM isotypes in patients with APS; however, agreement among patients grouped according to cardiolipin titers for IgA seems lower than those for the other types. In patients with collagen disease, IgA associates with thrombocytopenia, skin ulcers, and vasculitis, indicating a patient subgroup at risk for specific clinical manifestations, and it is highly prevalent in African American patients with SLE. Hence, this isotype appears to identify patient subgroups rather than adding diagnostic power.
■ A negative result means only that the cardiolipin antibody class tested (IgG, IgM, and/or IgA) is not present at this time. Because cardiolipin antibodies are the most common of the antiphospholipid antibodies, it is not unusual to find them emerging, temporarily due to an infection or drug, or asymptomatically as a person ages. The low to moderate concentrations of antibody seen in these situations are frequently not significant, but they must be examined in conjunction with a patient's symptoms and other clinical information.

Suggested Reading

Miyakis S, Lockshin MD, Atsumi T, et al. International consensus statement on an update of the classification criteria for definite antiphospholipid syndrome (APS). *J Thromb Haemost.* 2006;4:295–306.

16

ANTICOAGULANTS, CIRCULATING*

❏ **Definition**

- Circulating anticoagulants are antibodies that inhibit the function of specific coagulation factors, most commonly factor VIII or IX. They may be acquired following multiple transfusions in hemophiliacs (alloantibodies) or spontaneous (autoantibodies)—most commonly against factor VIII. Lupus anticoagulants (LA) are sometimes clinically associated with circulating anticoagulants

❏ **Use**

- A circulating anticoagulant is suspected under two conditions:
  - ▼ A patient with hemophilia A or B who has had multiple transfusions and whose bleeding does not stop on infusion of the missing factor
  - ▼ A middle-aged person, especially if diagnosed with lymphoma, or a postpartum patient who develops unprovoked hemorrhages

❏ **Interpretation**

- In a patient with hemophilia A or less commonly B, serial determinations of factor A or B show no elevations following infusions.
- In a patient with no previous bleeding history, the finding of a prolonged PTT should raise the suspicion of an acquired circulating anticoagulant. If incubation at 37°C of half normal plasma with half patient's plasma for 1–2 hours does not correct the prolonged PTT, a circulating anticoagulant is diagnosed (unless the patient is receiving unfractionated heparin, or the sample is contaminated with heparin).
- Specific titration of the inhibitor's potency is performed for either factor VIII or IX inhibitors, and the results are reported in Bethesda Inhibitory Units.

ANTICOAGULATION DNA PANEL†

❏ **Definition**

- The anticoagulation DNA panel tests for genetic variants in the *CYP2C9* and *VKORC1* genes that account for >50% of variation in warfarin response. Genotyping may reduce the need for INR surveillance as genotype-based dosing regimens are established.
- Variants tested by the anticoagulation panel include
  - ▼ *CYP2C9* *1 (normal)
  - ▼ *CYP2C9* *2 (c.430C>T; Arg144Cys)
  - ▼ *CYP2C9* *3 (c.1075A>C; Ile359Leu)
  - ▼ *VKORC1* *1 (normal)
  - ▼ *VKORC1* *2 promoter variant (c.−1639G>A)
- **Normal values:**
  - ▼ *CYP2C9* *1/*1
  - ▼ *VKORC1* *1/*1

---

*Submitted By Liberto Pechet, MD.
†Submitted by Edward Ginns, MD and Marzena M. Galdzicka, PhD.

❏ Use

- Initiating warfarin (Coumadin) therapy
- Optimizing dosing for warfarin

❏ Limitations

- The results of a genetic test may be affected by DNA rearrangements, blood transfusion, bone marrow transplantation, or rare sequence variations.

ANTICONVULSANTS*

❏ Definition

- A compound used to prevent or treat seizures
- Classic agents: carbamazepine (Tegretol), phenobarbital (Luminal), phenytoin (Dilantin), ethosuximide (Zarontin), valproic acid (Depakene, Depakote). Newer agents gabapentin (Neurontin), lamotrigine (Lamictal), oxcarbazepine (Trileptal), vigabatrin (Sabril), topiramate (Topamax), zonisamide (Zonegran)

❏ Use

- Treatment of seizure disorders
- **Normal therapeutic levels:** see Table 16.7

❏ Limitations

- Phenobarbital may be detected by immunoassay-based screening tests for barbiturates in urine and serum.
- Immunoassay tests are available for semiquantitative analysis in serum of topiramate, valproic acid, phenytoin, phenobarbital (may demonstrate significant cross-reactivity with other barbiturates), and zonisamide.
- Lamotrigine, breakdown products or artifacts of topiramate, carbamazepine, 10-OH-carbazepine, and phenytoin may be detected in general drug screens

TABLE 16–7. Normal Therapeutic Levels of Anticonvulsants

Drug	Level (μg/L Serum/Plasma)
Carbamazepine	6.0–12
10,11-Epoxide	0.2–2.0
Phenobarbital	15–40
Phenytoin	10–20
Ethosuximide	40–100
Valproic acid	50–100
Gabapentin	2.2–6.1
Lamotrigine	0.4–9.0
Oxcarbazepine	0.5–1.2
10-Hydroxycarbazepine	3.7–37
Vigabatrin	18–77
Topiramate	1.7–8.0
Zonisamide	2.9–28

16

*Submitted By Amanda J. Jenkins, PhD.

in urine or serum that utilize alkaline or weakly acidic liquid- or solid-phase extractions followed by gas chromatography or GC/MS analysis.

■ For the majority of anticonvulsants, specific tests are required.

ANTIDEPRESSANTS*

❏ **Definition**

■ Multicyclic compounds that inhibit the reuptake of neurotransmitters or block their metabolism, resulting in an increase concentration of monamines in the synapse.

■ Tricyclic antidepressants (TCAs): amitriptyline (Elavil), nortriptyline, doxepin, imipramine (Tofranil), desipramine, trimipramine, protriptyline, clomipramine (Anafranil)

■ Selective serotonin reuptake inhibitors (SSRIs): fluoxetine (Prozac), sertraline (Zoloft), fluvoxamine (Luvox), citalopram (Celexa), paroxetine (Paxil)

■ Other agents:
  ▼ Amoxapine (Moxadil), maprotiline, trazodone (Desyrel), bupropion (Wellbutrin)
  ▼ Venlafaxine (Effexor), mirtazapine (Remeron), nefazodone (Serzone), duloxetine (Cymbalta)

■ **Normal range:** see Table 16.8; not established for all drugs in this class

❏ **Use**

■ Treatment of mood disorders and depression

❏ **Limitations**

■ Immunoassay screening of serum/plasma/urine for TCAs does not detect other antidepressants (e.g., SSRIs).

TABLE 16–8. Normal Therapeutic Levels for Antidepressants*

Drug/Drug Combination	Normal Level (ng/mL)	Potentially Toxic Level (ng/mL)
Amitriptyline + nortriptyline	95–250	>500
Nortriptyline	50–150	>500
Imipramine + desipramine	150–300	>500
Desipramine	100–300	>500
Doxepin + nordoxepin	100–300	>400
Protriptyline	70–240	>400
Bupropion	50–100	
Trazodone	800–1,600	
Fluoxetine	50–480, with 20–60 mg/d	
Norfluoxetine	50–450, with 20–60 mg/d	
Clomipramine + norclomipramine	220–500	>900†

*Not established for all drugs in this class.
†When used as an antidepressant, therapeutic range not well established when prescribed for obsessive–compulsive disorder.

*Submitted By Amanda J. Jenkins, PhD.

- Target analytes: imipramine, nortriptyline.
- Cutoff concentrations:
  - ▼ 10–50 ng/mL ELISA
  - ▼ 300 or 500 ng/mL EIA qualitative
  - ▼ 150 ng/mL EIA semiquantitative
- Variable cross-reactivity with other TCAs, metabolites: consult the manufacturer's package insert.
- Will not detect SSRIs and newer antidepressants.
- No SSRI-specific immunoassays are currently available.
- General drug screens comprising alkaline liquid–liquid extraction or solid-phase extraction followed by GC/MS or gas chromatography analysis detect TCAs, SSRIs, trazodone, bupropion, venlafaxine, mirtazapine, and amoxapine with limit of detection ranging from 20 to 250 ng/mL.

ANTIDIURETIC HORMONE

❏ **Definition**

- Antidiuretic hormone (ADH), also known as vasopressin or arginine vasopressin, is a hormone secreted by the posterior pituitary. It regulates the water permeability of renal collecting ducts and urine concentrating ability by increasing water reabsorption, which is mediated by transcellular water channels (aquaporins).
- **Normal range:** <1.5 pg/mL (see Table 16.9 for effect of plasma osmolality on ADH levels).

❏ **Use**

- Diagnosis and differential diagnosis of DI and psychogenic polyuria
- Diagnosis of SIADH
- Differential diagnosis of hyponatremias

❏ **Interpretation**
Increased In

- Nephrogenic DI (partial or complete): high ADH and low osmolality
- Primary psychogenic polydipsia
- SIADH inappropriately increased for degree of plasma osmolality (i.e., normal ADH relative to osmolality)
- Ectopic ADH syndrome
- Certain drugs (e.g., chlorpropamide, phenothiazine, Tegretol)

TABLE 16–9. Plasma Osmolality Influences on ADH Levels	
Values in mOsm/kg	**Values in pg/mL**
270–280	<1.5
280–285	<2.5
285–290	1–5
290–295	2–7
295–300	4–12

16

Decreased In

- Central DI (partial or complete): decreased for level of plasma osmolality
- Psychogenic polydipsia
- Nephrotic syndrome

❏ **Limitations**

- Higher secretion occurs at night; in erect posture; with pain, stress, or exercise; and with increased plasma osmolality.
- Lower secretion occurs in recumbency, hypoosmolality, volume expansion, and hypertension.
- Plasma sample should not be left at room temperature.

ANTIHYPERTENSIVES

See Cardiovascular Drugs.

ANTI-INFLAMMATORIES

See Acetaminophen, Salicylates.

ANTINEOPLASTICS

See Methotrexate.

ANTIMITOCHONDRIAL ANTIBODIES

❏ **Definition**

- Mitochondrial antibodies are found in a variety of liver diseases and have been characterized to react with at least nine different mitochondrial antigens (M1–M9). M2, M1, and M7 are antigens on the inner mitochondrial membranes while the M3, M4, M5, M6, M8, and M9 antigens are present on the outer membranes. Antibodies to the M2, M4, M8, and M9 antigens are found in patients with PBC. About 95% of patients with PBC will be positive for anti-M2. When M4 and M9 are also present, the patient usually has a more rapidly progressive disease course. Some PBC patients (<5%) may only have anti-M9. These patients are usually early in the disease course and may have a more limited disease.
- Normal range:
  - ▼ Immunofluorescence assay (IFA): negative, if positive, results are tittered, ELISA: <1:40 titer.
  - ▼ AMA titers >1:40 are significant.

❏ **Use**

- Diagnosis of primary biliary cirrhosis (PBC)

❏ **Interpretation**

Increased In

- Ninety-five percent of PBC cases

Decreased In
- NA

❑ **Limitations**
- Quantitative measurements of AMA do not reflect on the progression of the disease.
- Five to ten percent of cases of PBC do not have detectable levels of AMA.
- Some individuals with host versus graft disease have measurable levels.
- Although AMAs serve as highly sensitive markers for the diagnosis of PBC, AMAs can frequently be detected in patients with other diseases, such as primary systemic sclerosis, Sjögren syndrome, rheumatoid arthritis, and autoimmune hepatitis.
- The M2, M4, and M8 staining patterns are indistinguishable by immunofluorescence, so specific EIA assays must be used to determine which of these antibodies are present in a positive serum. Anti-M9 antibodies can only be detected by EIA assay.

ANTI–SMOOTH MUSCLE ANTIBODIES (ASM)

❑ **Definition**
- Smooth muscle antibodies are directed toward actin, myosin, and occasionally against other contractile proteins in muscle cells. Smooth muscle antibodies can present in a variety of liver disease states. Smooth muscle antibodies can be useful in differentiating liver disease when used in conjunction with other laboratory results and the patient's clinical symptoms.
- **Normal range:**
  - ▼ IFA: negative; if positive, results are tittered, ELISA: <1:40 titer.
  - ▼ ASM titers >1:40 are significant.

❑ **Use**
- Aids in the diagnosis of chronic active hepatitis
- Differential diagnosis of liver disease
- Rule out SLE (test usually negative in SLE)

❑ **Interpretation**
Increased In
- Chronic active hepatitis
- Autoimmune hepatitis type 1
- Hepatitis B
- Hepatitis C
- Primary biliary cirrhosis
- Primary sclerosing cholangitis
- Overlap syndromes

Decreased In
- NA

16

❑ **Limitations**

- A positive test is not diagnostic for any one disease state.
- Low titers are seen in acute viral hepatitis, PBC, infection mononucleosis, malignant myeloma, and ovarian carcinoma.

ANTI–PARIETAL CELL ANTIBODIES (APC)

❑ **Definition**

- Antibodies to gastric parietal cells that react with the cell membrane, cytoplasmic antigens, or gastric intrinsic factor are present in essentially all (>90%) of individuals with pernicious anemia. In 70% of patients, antibodies reactive with the vitamin B_{12}–binding site of intrinsic factor are present, and in 50% of patients, additional antibodies are present, which react with a second antigenic site on the 44,000-Da intrinsic factor protein molecule. These autoantibodies lead to a pathologic immune process termed "chronic autoimmune gastritis," which may slowly progress for 10–20 years and finally terminate in gastric atrophy. The gastric atrophy results in a lack of absorption of vitamin B_{12} and leads to megaloblastic anemia in patients with anti–parietal cell antibodies. Pernicious anemia is associated with a variety of other autoimmune diseases including thyrotoxicosis, Hashimoto thyroiditis, insulin-dependent DM, primary Addison disease of the adrenals, primary ovarian failure, primary hypoparathyroidism, vitiligo, Myasthenia gravis, and the Lambert-Eaton syndrome.
- **Normal range:**
  - ▼ IFA: negative; if positive, results are tittered, ELISA: <1:40 titer.
  - ▼ APC titers greater than 1:40 are significant.

❑ **Use**

- Aids in the evaluation of patients suspected of having pernicious anemia
- Evaluation of immune-mediated deficiency of vitamin B_{12} with or without megaloblastic anemia

❑ **Interpretation**
Increased In

- Pernicious anemia
- Atrophic gastritis
- Diabetes
- Gastric ulcer
- Thyroid disease

Decreased In

- NA

❑ **Limitations**

- High blood levels are also seen in people with inflammation of the lining of the stomach, stomach ulcers, and stomach cancer.
- APC antibodies may occur with increased frequency in unaffected family members, a small percentage of healthy individuals, and patients with other autoimmune diseases, such as autoimmune thyroiditis.

ANTINEUTROPHIL CYTOPLASMIC ANTIBODY (ANCA)

❏ **Definition**

- ANCA testing plays a critical role in the diagnosis and classification of vasculitides. It is associated with a number of vasculitides, including Wegener granulomatosis (WG), Churg-Strauss syndrome (CSS), microscopic polyangiitis (MPA), and idiopathic necrotizing and crescentic glomerulonephritis.
- Two types of ANCA assays are currently in wide use: IFA and ELISA. Of these two techniques, IFA is more sensitive, and ELISA is more specific. The optimal approach to clinical testing for ANCA is, therefore, to screen with IFA and confirm all positive results with ELISAs directed against the vasculitis-specific target antigens proteinase 3 (PR3) and myeloperoxidase antibodies (MPOs).
- When the sera of patients with ANCA-associated vasculitis are incubated with ethanol-fixed human neutrophils, two major IFA patterns are observed: the cytoplasmic neutrophil antibody (cANCA) and perinuclear antineutrophil cytoplasmic antibody (pANCA) patterns. Other staining patterns have been described and are generally noted as "atypical."
- Specific immunochemical assays demonstrate that cANCAs comprise mainly antibodies to PR3 and pANCA antibodies to MPO.
- The PR3-ANCA pattern has been predominantly associated with cases of active WG and CSS, but many also be seen in MPA.
- MPO-ANCA has been primarily in MPA, CSS, and rarely in WG.
- pANCA pattern variations not associated with MPO (atypical) patterns may be observed on IFA testing in patients with immune-mediated conditions other than systemic vasculitis (e.g., connective tissue disorders, inflammatory bowel disease, infections, and autoimmune hepatitis).
- **Normal value:** negative.

❏ **Use**

- Evaluation of patients suspected of having WG or systemic vasculitis, especially patients with renal disease, pulmonary disease, or unexplained multiorgan disease possibly due to vasculitis

❏ **Interpretation**

Increased In

- c-ANCA (PR3 positive):
  - ▼ Systemic necrotizing vasculitis
    - Common: WG
    - CSS
    - May also be seen in systemic necrotizing vasculitis of polyarteritis group, pauci-immune type of idiopathic crescentic glomerulonephritis.
  - ▼ Propylthiouracil drug
- pANCA (MPO positive):
  - ▼ Systemic necrotizing vasculitis
    - Common: microscopic polyarteritis
    - CSS
    - Uncommon in WG
  - ▼ Hydralazine, minocycline, propylthiouracil

16

- pANCA (to various antigens, MPO negative):
  ▼ Connective tissue disease
    - Antiphospholipid antibody syndrome
    - Juvenile chronic arthritis
    - Polymyositis/dermatomyositis
    - Relapsing polychondritis
    - RA
    - Sjögren syndrome
    - SLE
  ▼ Inflammatory bowel disease
    - Ulcerative colitis (60–85%)
    - Crohn disease (10–40%)
    - Bacterial enteritis (rare)
  ▼ Autoimmune liver diseases
    - Primary sclerosing cholangitis
    - Autoimmune hepatitis
  ▼ Infections
    - Chromomycosis
    - HIV-1
    - Acute malaria
- Five percent healthy controls

❑ **Limitations**

- There is a subjective component to the interpretation of IFA, because the tests are based on visual interpretation of the IF pattern, which is not straightforward. It depends on the experience of the individual who performs the assay.
- ANCA testing is not standardized; the sensitivity and specificity will vary with the laboratory. The cANCA pattern has a greater specificity than the pANCA pattern for vasculitis. However, even positive cANCA IFA results were associated with vasculitis in only 50% of patients.
- Antibodies to a host of azurophilic granule proteins can cause a pANCA staining pattern; these include antibodies directed against lactoferrin, elastase, cathepsin G, bactericidal permeability inhibitor, catalase, lysozyme, β-glucuronidase, and others. A positive pANCA IFA staining pattern may also be detected in a wide variety of inflammatory illnesses and has a low specificity for vasculitis.
- Individuals with ANA frequently have "false-positive" results on ANCA testing by IFA.
- Certain medications may induce forms of vasculitis associated with ANCA. The strongest links between medications and ANCA-associated vasculitis are with drugs employed in the treatment of hyperthyroidism: propylthiouracil, methimazole, and carbimazole. Hydralazine and minocycline are less commonly associated with the induction of ANCA-associated vasculitis. Other implicated drugs include penicillamine, allopurinol, procainamide, thiamazole, clozapine, phenytoin, rifampicin, cefotaxime, isoniazid, and indomethacin.
- Using IFA and ELISA testing in a sequential fashion substantially increases the positive predictive value of an ANCA assay.

- Elevations in the titers of ANCA do *not* predict disease flares in a timely manner. If a patient was ANCA positive during a period of active disease, a persistently ANCA-negative status is consistent with, but not absolutely a proof of, remission.
- ANCA testing should not be used to screen nonselected patient groups where the prevalence of vasculitis is low. These tests are most valuable when selectively ordered in clinical situations where some forms of ANCA-associated vasculitis are seriously considered.
- A negative ANCA result should not be used to exclude disease.

ANTINUCLEAR ANTIBODY (ANA)

❑ **Definition**

- ANAs refer to a diverse group of antibodies that target nuclear and cytoplasmic antigens. ANAs have been detected in the serum of patients with many rheumatic and nonrheumatic diseases as well as in patients with no definable clinical syndrome. The strong association of ANA with SLE is well established, and this finding satisfies the 1 of 11 criteria available for diagnosis.
- These autoantibodies may be useful as an aid in the diagnosis of systemic rheumatic diseases such as SLE, mixed connective tissue disease (MCTD), undifferentiated connective tissue disease, Sjögren syndrome, scleroderma (systemic sclerosis), polymyositis, and others. The diagnosis of a systemic rheumatic disease is based primarily on the presence of compatible clinical signs and symptoms. The results of tests for autoantibodies, including ANA and specific autoantibodies, are ancillary.
- **Normal range:** negative.

❑ **Use**

- Evaluating patients suspected of having a systemic rheumatic disease

❑ **Interpretation**
Increased In

- SLE
- Drug-induced SLE
- Lupoid hepatitis
- MCTD
- Polymyositis
- Progressive systemic sclerosis
- RA
- Sjögren syndrome

❑ **Limitations**

- Some patients without clinical evidence of an autoimmune disease or a systemic rheumatic disease may have a detectable level of ANA. This finding is more common in women than in men, and the frequency of a detectable ANA in healthy women >40 years old may approach 15–20%. ANA may also be detectable following viral illnesses, in chronic infections, or in patients treated with many different medications.

16

■ The traditional tool used to detect ANAs is IFA, which is a labor-intensive microscopic technique. Test interpretation is operator dependent. This assay is considered the gold standard for ANA testing with greater sensitivity. The IFA testing is currently performed using Hep-2 cells, and they contain approximately 100–150 possible antigens, and most of them are not well defined and/or characterized. When performed with a history and physical examination, it identifies almost all patients with SLE (95% sensitivity), although the specificity of this assay is only 57%. In addition, ANA by IFA has the sensitivity of 85% for systemic sclerosis, 61% for polymyositis/dermatomyositis (PM-DM), 48% for Sjögren syndrome, 57% for juvenile idiopathic arthritis, 100% for drug-induced lupus, 100% for MCTD, and autoimmune hepatitis (60%), as well as being important in monitoring and assessing prognosis in individuals with the Raynaud phenomenon.

■ Multiplex immunoassay (MIA) tests have been recently developed for use in clinical laboratory. They utilize individually identifiable, fluorescence microspheres (beads), each coupled with a different antigen or antigen mixture to test for multiple antibodies simultaneously in the same tube. This multiplex ANA screen is intended for qualitative screening of specific ANAs, the quantitative detection of dsDNA antibodies, and semiquantitative detection of 10 separate antibody assays (chromatin, ribosomal-P, SSA, SSB, Sm, SmRNP, RNP [ribonucleoprotein], Scl-70 [topoisomerase I], Jo-1, and centromere-B). This ANA by MIA screen detects the presence of clinically relevant circulating autoantibodies in serum. These assays are specific compared to IFA, and they are not as sensitive as IFA, because it is not looking at 100–150 possible antigens in the Hep-2 cells, rather specifically looking at 11 specific targeted antibodies. These assays have typical sensitivities of 66–94% for SLE, 94% for Sjögren, 68% for systemic sclerosis, and 48% for PM-DM. They are specific compared to IFA for detecting specific targeted connective tissue disorders. In persons with no connective disease, the specificity of MIA ranged from 77 to 91%, and in apparently healthy individuals, it is at 93%.

■ Disorders associated with a positive ANA titer include chronic infectious diseases, such as mononucleosis, hepatitis C infection, subacute bacterial endocarditis, TB, and HIV, and some lymphoproliferative diseases.

■ The presence of ANAs is rarely associated with malignancy, with the exception of dermatomyositis, in which both may be present. ANAs have also been identified in up to 50% of patients taking certain drugs; however, most of these patients do not develop drug-induced lupus.

Drugs that may cause positive results include carbamazepine, chlorpromazine, ethosuximide, hydralazine, isoniazid, mephenytoin, methyldopa, penicillins, phenytoin, primidone, procainamide, and quinidine.

■ **Antibodies to double-stranded DNA (dsDNA)**
   ▼ Moderate to high titers of antibodies directed against dsDNA are very specific (97%) for SLE, making them very useful for diagnosis. Anti-dsDNA have also been found at low frequency (<5%), and usually in low titer and with low avidity, in patients with RA, Sjögren syndrome, scleroderma, Raynaud phenomenon, MCTD, discoid lupus, myositis, uveitis, juvenile arthritis, antiphospholipid syndrome, Grave disease, Alzheimer disease, and autoimmune hepatitis.

▼ Titers of anti-dsDNA antibodies often fluctuate with disease activity and are, therefore, useful in many patients for following the course of SLE.

▼ There is a well-recognized association of high titers of IgG anti-dsDNA titers, especially for high avidity antibodies, with active GN; there also appear to be highly enriched amounts of anti-dsDNA antibodies in the glomerular deposits of immune complexes found in patients with lupus nephritis. These observations have led many investigators to believe that anti-dsDNA antibodies are of primary importance in the pathogenesis of lupus nephritis.

▼ Anti-dsDNA antibodies have also been reported in patients receiving minocycline, etanercept, infliximab, and penicillamine.

▼ An increased frequency of these antibodies has also been noted in some otherwise normal individuals, particularly first-degree relatives of patients with lupus and some laboratory workers.

- **Antibodies to chromatin**
  ▼ Chromatin refers to the complex of histones and DNA. Assaying for the presence of antichromatin (antinucleosome) antibodies may be more clinically relevant than testing for individual antihistone antibodies. Antichromatin antibodies are present in 69% of those with SLE but in 10% or less of patients with Sjögren syndrome, scleroderma, or antiphospholipid syndrome. Among those with SLE, the prevalence of antichromatin antibodies is twofold higher in those with renal disease (58% vs. 29%).

- **Anti-Smith antibodies and anti-RNP antibodies**
  ▼ The anti-Smith (anti-Sm) and anti-ribonucleoprotein (anti-RNP) systems are considered together, since they coexist in many patients with SLE and bind to related but distinct antigens.

  ▼ Anti-Sm antibodies occur more frequently in African Americans and Asians than in Caucasians with SLE.

  ▼ Anti-Sm antibodies generally remain positive when titers of anti-DNA antibodies have fallen into the normal range and clinical activity of SLE has waned. Therefore, measurement of anti-Sm titers may be useful diagnostically, particularly at a time when DNA antibodies are undetectable.

  ▼ Anti-RNP antibodies bind to antigens that are different from but related to Sm antigens. These antibodies bind to proteins containing only U1-RNA. Anti-RNP antibodies are found in 3–69% of patients with SLE but are a defining feature in the related syndrome, MCTD. The antibody is present in lower titers in several other rheumatic diseases, including primary Raynaud phenomenon, RA, and scleroderma.

- **Ro/SSA and La/SSB antibodies**
  ▼ Anti-Ro/SSA and anti-La/SSB antibodies have been detected with high frequency in patients with Sjögren syndrome. They also have diagnostic usefulness in patients with SLE. They are infrequently seen in other connective tissue diseases such as scleroderma, polymyositis, MCTD, and RA.

  ▼ Anti-Ro/SSA antibodies have been associated with photosensitivity, a rash known as subacute cutaneous lupus, cutaneous vasculitis (palpable purpura), interstitial lung disease, neonatal lupus, and congenital heart block connective tissue disease. A minority evolve into a well-defined disorder.

  ▼ Anti-La/SSB antibodies are found in the following circumstances:

16

- It is very unusual to encounter sera that contain anti-La/SSB activity without demonstrable antibodies to Ro/SSA in patients with SLE or Sjögren syndrome.
- Isolated anti-La/SSB antibody activity has been seen in some patients with primary biliary cirrhosis and autoimmune hepatitis.
- Antibodies to the La/SSB antigen are present in 70–95% of patients with primary Sjögren syndrome, and in 10–35% of patients with SLE, and are occasionally seen in patients with cutaneous LE, scleroderma disorders, and RA.
- Antibodies to topoisomerase I (Scl-70)
■ Antibodies to Scl-70, proteins associated with the centromere (CEN-A, CEN-B), U3-ribonucleoprotein (U-3 RNP), and RNA polymerases I and III. These antibodies are highly specific for systemic sclerosis and are associated with a higher risk of interstitial lung disease. When present in high titers, they are associated with more extensive skin involvement and disease activity.

■ **Antibodies to Ribo-P**
▼ The reported incidence of antiribosomal P protein antibodies among patients with SLE is variable. These antibodies were initially detected in 10–20% of patients with SLE; however, several authors (particularly those studying Asian populations and children) have reported higher incidence rates (40–50%). Some clinical data suggest that the presence of antiribosomal P protein antibodies among patients with lupus is associated with lupus cerebritis. The presence of antibodies to ribosomal P protein has an overall sensitivity and specificity for neuropsychiatric lupus of 26% and 80%, respectively. The test characteristics were similar for psychosis, mood disorder, or both (sensitivity 27%, specificity 80%). These antibodies may also be found among patients with lupus hepatitis and/or nephritis.

■ **Antibodies to Jo-1**
▼ Antibodies to the Jo-1 antigen (histidyl-tRNA synthetase) are found in approximately 30% of adult patients with myositis (including polymyositis, dermatomyositis, and overlap syndromes) and are particularly common (approximately 60%) in patients with both myositis and interstitial lung disease (cryptogenic fibrosing alveolitis or pulmonary interstitial fibrosis). Jo-1 antibodies are most commonly found in patients with the antisynthetase syndrome, which is characterized by acute onset, steroid-responsive myositis with interstitial lung disease, fever, symmetrical arthritis, Raynaud phenomenon, and mechanic's hands. The presence of Jo-1 antibodies in idiopathic polymyositis patients is usually accompanied by severe disease, tendency to relapse, and poor prognosis.

ANTIPSYCHOTICS*

❑ **Definition**
■ Antipsychotics are neuroleptic drugs in the following groups: phenothiazines, thioxanthenes, dibenzoxazepines, dihydroindoles, butyrophenones,

*Submitted By Amanda J. Jenkins, PhD.

TABLE 16–10. Normal Levels of Antipsychotics

	Normal Range	Toxic Level
Lithium	0.4–1.0 mEq/L (serum trough—12 h postdose)	>1.5 mEq/L
Haloperidol	2.0–15.0 ng/mL	
Olanzapine	5–75 ng/mL	
Clozapine	100–700 ng/mL	
Fluphenazine	0.2–2.0 ng/mL	
Chlorpromazine	Adult therapeutic: 50–300 ng/mL	Adult: >500 ng/mL
	Child therapeutic: 30–80 ng/mL	Child: >200 ng/mL

and diphenylbutylpiperidine and alkali metal. Typical antipsychotics: chlorpromazine (Thorazine), fluphenazine (Permitil), thioridazine (Mellaril), thioxanthene, haloperidol (Haldol), and loxapine (Loxitane). Atypical antipsychotics: clozapine (Clozaril), olanzapine (Zyprexa), quetiapine (Seroquel), and risperidone (Risperdal).
- Other agent: lithium (Lithobid).
- **Normal range:** see Table 16.10.

❏ **Use**
- Treatment of psychoses, schizophrenia, mania, Tourette syndrome (haloperidol)

❏ **Limitations**
- Immunoassay: RIA—nonspecific, semiquantitative due to varying cross-reactivity with parent drug and metabolites.
- Fluorometry: nonspecific, semiquantitative due to interferences from metabolites.
- Hemolyzed specimens are unacceptable. Remove serum from clot as soon as possible.
- Lithium: Lithium heparin and sodium fluoride/potassium oxalate tubes are unacceptable.

ANTISPERM AUTOANTIBODIES–IMMUNOBEAD BINDING TEST*

❏ **Definition**
- The immunobead binding test for antisperm antibodies identifies antibodies on sperm cells by immunoglobulin class and general specificity (head, midpiece, and tail) by means of their ability to agglutinate polyacrylamide beads coated with anti-Ig class–specific antibodies.
- **Reference range:** ≤20% of sperm cells bound to immunobeads.

❏ **Use**
- Confirmation of sperm autoimmunity, as suggested by the presence of agglutinated sperm and/or reduced motility in a semen analysis. Only the IgG and IgA classes of such antibodies are clinically significant.

16

*Submitted by Charles R. Kiefer, PhD.

❑ Interpretation

Increased In	Decreased In
▪ Sperm autoimmunity (clinically significant if >50% sperm are coated and other evidence of impaired fertilizing capacity is present)	▪ No lower limit defined

❑ Limitations

- Minimum specimen volume for microscopic analysis is 0.1 mL.

Suggested Reading

Bohring C, Krause W. Immune infertility: towards a better understanding of sperm (auto)-immunity. The value of proteomic analysis. *Hum Reprod.* 2003;18:915–924.

ANTITHROMBIN (AT)*

❑ Definition

- AT, also known as antithrombin III, is a natural inhibitor of thrombin and of other clotting factors essential in the coagulation cascade. It is synthesized in the liver. In the presence of heparin, the activity of AT is enhanced approximately 1,000 times.
- **Normal range (for functional activity):** 75–125%. The functional assay can be performed in a clot detection system or in a chromogenic one. The antigen normal range is the same as for the functional assay, but the assay is rarely necessary in clinical practice.

❑ Use

- Because deficiency of AT may result in a thrombophilic syndrome, determination of AT is indicated in cases suspected of congenital thrombophilia. It is also of help in determining the prognosis in disseminated intravascular coagulation (DIC) because levels become markedly decreased in severe cases.

❑ Interpretation

- Acquired deficiencies have been reported in severe liver disease, some malignancies, use of oral contraceptives, nephrotic syndrome, and severe infections, especially if associated with DIC (the assay is useful in determining the severity of DIC: it decreases in parallel with increasing severity of the syndrome).
- AT is not affected by deficiency in vitamin K or by vitamin K antagonists.
  - ▼ It decreases during heparin therapy.
  - ▼ Severe deficiency may result in diminished anticoagulant effect of heparin.

❑ Limitations

- Clotted specimen, incomplete filling of test tubes, severe lipemia, icteric samples, and hemolysis produce unreliable results.

---

*Submitted By Liberto Pechet, MD.

- Heparin therapy interferes with the coagulant assay but not with the chromogenic one.
- AT results are affected by the use of thrombin inhibitors such as hirudin (or its congeners) or argatroban and the newer antithrombin drugs.

APOLIPOPROTEINS (APO) A-1 AND B

❑ **Definition**
- An apolipoprotein is a protein component of lipoprotein, whose main function is to transport lipids. Apolipoproteins play an important role in maintaining structural integrity and solubility of lipoproteins and play an important role in lipoprotein receptor recognition and regulation of certain enzymes in lipoprotein metabolism. Apolipoprotein A (apo-A; also known as Apo A-1) is the major protein (90%) of HDL. Apolipoprotein B (apo B) is major protein component of low-density lipoprotein and is important in regulating cholesterol synthesis and metabolism.
- **Normal range:**
  - ▼ Apo A-1
    - Male: 94–178 mg/dL
    - Female: 101–199 mg/dL
  - ▼ Apo B
    - Male: 55–140 mg/dL
    - Female: 55–125 mg/dL
  - ▼ Apo B/A-1 ratio
    - One half risk
    - Male: 0.4
    - Female: 0.3
  - ▼ Average risk:
    - Male: 1.0
    - Female: 0.9
  - ▼ Twice average risk:
    - Male: 1.6
    - Female: 1.5

❑ **Use**
- To evaluate the risk of CAD: Levels of apo A-1 are inversely associated with premature cardiovascular disease and peripheral vascular disease. The ratio of apo A to apo B has greater sensitivity and specificity for CAD than individual lipid or lipoproteins.
- To evaluate atherosclerotic disease.
- To detect Tangier disease.

❑ **Interpretation**
Apo A-1 Increased In
- Familial hyperalphalipoproteinemia (a rare genetic disorder)

Apo A-1 Decreased In
- Nephrosis and chronic renal failure
- Familial hypoalphalipoproteinemia (rare genetic disorder)

16

- Uncontrolled diabetes
- Apo C-II deficiency
- Apo A-1 melano disease
- Apo A-1-C-III deficiency
- Hepatocellular disease
- Parkinson disease

Apo-B Disorders Increased In
- Hepatic disease
- Hyperlipoproteinemia IIa, IIb, and V
- Cushing syndrome
- Porphyria
- Werner syndrome
- Diabetes
- Familial combined hyperlipidemia
- Hypothyroidism
- Nephrotic syndrome, renal failure

Apo B Decreased In
- Tangier disease
- Hyperthyroidism
- Hypobetalipoproteinemia
- Apo C-II deficiency
- Malnutrition
- Reye syndrome
- Severe illness
- Surgery
- Abetalipoproteinemia
- Cirrhosis

❏ **Limitations**
- Drugs that affect apo A-1:
  - ▼ Increased: carbamazepine, estrogens, ethanol, lovastatin, niacin, oral contraceptives, phenobarbital, pravastatin, simvastatin
  - ▼ Decreased: androgens, beta blockers, diuretics, and progestins
- Other factors that affect apo A-1:
  - ▼ Increased: exercise
  - ▼ Decreased: smoking, pregnancy, diet high in polyunsaturated fats, and weight reduction
- Drugs that affect apo B:
  - ▼ Increased: androgens, beta blockers, diuretics, progestins
  - ▼ Decreased: estrogen, lovastatin, simvastatin, niacin, and thyroxine
- Other factors that affect apo B:
  - ▼ Increased: pregnancy
  - ▼ Decreased: diet high in polyunsaturated fats and low cholesterol, weight reduction
- Other: apo A-1 and apo B are acute-phase reactants and thus should not measured in sick patients.

BENZODIAZEPINES*

❑ **Definition**

- A class of drugs with a three-ringed chemical structure consisting of a benzene ring, a seven-member diazepine ring, and a phenyl ring attached to the 5-position of the diazepine ring. The CNS depressant activity of these drugs is mediated through the neurotransmitter, GABA.
- Specific agents: alprazolam (Xanax), chlordiazepoxide (Librium), diazepam (Valium), temazepam (Restoril), oxazepam (Serax), flunitrazepam (Rohypnol), lorazepam (Ativan), midazolam (Versed), clonazepam (Klonopin), and triazolam (Halcion).
- **Normal range:** see Table 16.11.

❑ **Use**

- Assistance in the treatment of panic attacks, panic disorders, and agoraphobia (alprazolam, clonazepam)
- Treatment of anxiety (diazepam, lorazepam)
- Treatment of seizures (diazepam, clonazepam)
- Treatment of insomnia (temazepam, triazolam)
- Preoperative sedation and to assist in induction of surgical anesthesia (midazolam, diazepam, lorazepam)
- Muscle relaxant (diazepam)
- Treatment of alcohol dependence (chlordiazepoxide, diazepam)

❑ **Interpretation**

- When evaluating concentrations in plasma/serum, effect of multiple active moieties must be considered. When evaluating concentrations in urine, metabolite rather than parent may be detected. Active metabolites are
  - ▼ Alprazolam: alpha-hydroxy alprazolam
  - ▼ Flunitrazepam: 7-aminoflunitrazepam
  - ▼ Midazolam: alphahydroxy and 4-hydroxy midazolam
  - ▼ Triazolam: alphahydroxy and 4-hydroxy triazolam

TABLE 16–11. Reference Ranges of Benzodiazepines

	Normal Range (serum/plasma; ng/mL)
Alprazolam	10–100
Chlordiazepoxide	500–2,500
Clonazepam	5–75
Diazepam	100–1,500 (may be higher to control alcohol withdrawal and in schizophrenic patients)
Flunitrazepam	10–20
Lorazepam	5–240
Midazolam	8–150 (higher for surgical anesthesia; may be >1,000)
Oxazepam	300–1,500
Temazepam	200–1,200
Triazolam	2–10

16

*Submitted By Amanda J. Jenkins, PhD.

▼ Diazepam: nordiazepam, temazepam, oxazepam
▼ Chlordiazepoxide: demoxepam, norchlordiazepoxide, nordiazepam, oxazepam
▼ Temazepam: oxazepam

❑ **Limitations**

■ Testing: screening by immunoassay for urine and serum
  ▼ ELISA (serum)
    ● Target analyte: temazepam
    ● Cutoff concentration: 10 ng/mL
    ● No cross-reactivity with clonazepam, flunitrazepam, lorazepam and metabolites, and oxazepam
  ▼ EMIT (serum/urine)
    ● Target analyte: nitrazepam (urine), diazepam (serum)
    ● Cutoff concentration: 200 or 300 ng/mL urine, 50 ng/mL serum
    ● Due to low cross-reactivity, will *not* detect flunitrazepam, clonazepam, lorazepam (urine); low cross-reactivity with chlordiazepoxide and demoxepam (serum)
    ● Cross-reactivity with alprazolam manufacturer (vendor) dependent

■ Confirmation for urine and serum
  ▼ Sample pretreatment necessary
  ▼ Derivatization may be necessary for metabolite detection.
  ▼ Hydrolysis of urine samples increases detectability.
  ▼ Gas chromatography (GC).
  ▼ HPLC.
  ▼ Low-dose benzodiazepines may not be measurable by GC and HPLC (triazolam, flunitrazepam).
  ▼ GC/MS [MS].
  ▼ LC/MS/[MS].
  ▼ Target drug: parent drug and metabolites.
  ▼ Limit of quantitation: typically 5–20 ng/mL.

BETA-2 MICROGLOBULIN, SERUM, URINE, CEREBROSPINAL FLUID

❑ **Definition**

■ β_2-Microglobulin is a cell membrane–associated 100-amino-acid peptide, a component of the lymphocyte HLA complex. Because it is present on all nucleated cells and is almost totally reabsorbed and catabolized by the proximal tubules, it serves as a marker of immune activation and proximal tubular function. It is found in nearly all body fluids.

■ **Normal range:**
  ▼ Serum: males: 0.60–2.28 mg/L; females: 0.60–2.45 mg/L
  ▼ Urine: 0–300 µg/L
  ▼ CSF: 1.5 + 0.2 mg/L

❑ **Use**

■ Prognostic marker for some lymphoproliferative disorders (adult acute lymphocytic leukemia, AIDS).

- Prognosis assessment of multiple myeloma (as a tumor marker, it reflects burden of tumor cells).
- Evaluation of renal tubular disorders, index of GFR.
- CSF β_2-microglobulin levels have been used as a disease indicator of a variety of conditions, including multiple sclerosis, neuro-Behçet disease, sarcoidosis, AIDS–dementia complex, and meningeal metastases, especially meningeal dissemination of acute leukemia and malignant lymphoma.

❑ **Interpretation**
Increased In
- AIDS
- Aminoglycoside toxicity
- Amyloidosis
- Autoimmune disorders
- Breast cancer
- Crohn disease
- Felty syndrome
- Hepatitis
- Hepatoma
- Hyperthyroidism
- Inflammation of all types
- Leukemia (chronic lymphocytic)
- Lung cancer
- Lymphoma
- Multiple myeloma
- Poisoning with heavy metals, such as mercury or cadmium
- Renal dialysis
- Renal disease (glomerular): serum only; renal disease (tubular): urine only
- Sarcoidosis
- SLE
- Vasculitis
- Viral infections (e.g., CMV)

Decreased In
- Renal disease (glomerular): urine only; renal disease (tubular): serum only
- Response to zidovudine (AZT)

❑ **Limitations**
- Drugs and proteins that may increase serum β_2-microglobulin levels include cefuroxime, cyclosporin A, gentamicin, interferon-α, pentoxifylline, tumor necrosis factor, lithium, and radiographic contrast media.
- Drugs that may decrease serum β_2-microglobulin levels include zidovudine.
- Drugs that may increase urine β_2-microglobulin levels include azathioprine, cisplatin, cyclosporin A, furosemide, gentamicin, mannitol, nifedipine, sisomicin, and tobramycin.
- Drugs that may decrease urine β_2-microglobulin levels include cilostazol.

16

BICARBONATE (HCO$_3^-$), BLOOD

❏ **Definition**

■ Bicarbonate is an indicator of the buffering capacity of the blood. Low bicarbonate indicates that a larger pH change will occur for a given amount of acid or base produced.

■ Bicarbonate in the blood is calculated from the pH and PCO$_2$ using the Henderson-Hasselbalch equation.

■ **Normal range:**
▼ Arterial: 21–28 mEq/L
▼ Venous: 22–29 mEq/L

❏ **Use**

■ Significant indicator of electrolyte dispersion and anion deficit.

■ Together with pH determination, bicarbonate measurements are used in the diagnosis and treatment of numerous potentially serious disorders associated with acid–base imbalance in the respiratory and metabolic systems. Some of these conditions are diarrhea, renal tubular acidosis, carbonic anhydrase inhibitors, hyperkalemic acidosis, renal failure, and ketoacidosis.

❏ **Interpretation**

Increased In

■ Primary metabolic alkalosis
■ Primary respiratory acidosis
■ Severe vomiting
■ Lung disease (COPD)
■ Cushing syndrome
■ Diuretics
■ Primary hyperaldosteronism
■ Laxative abuse

Decreased In

■ Primary metabolic acidosis
■ Primary respiratory alkalosis
■ Addison disease
■ Ethylene glycol or methanol poisoning
■ Chronic diarrhea
■ Salicylate overdose

❏ **Limitations**

■ Bicarbonate can be determined by titration, but this is rarely done.

■ HCO$_3^-$ is the largest fraction contributing to the total CO$_2$. Therefore, both parameters usually change in the same direction.

■ The standard HCO$_3^-$ is the concentration of HCO$_3^-$ in whole blood at 38°C equilibrated at a PCO$_2$ of 40 mm Hg with the blood Hb fully oxygenated.

TABLE 16–12. Normal Range of Bilirubin		
Total Bilirubin		
From Age	**Reference Range**	**Critical Range**
0–1 d	0.0–6.0 mg/dL	>15 mg/dL
1–2 d	0.0–8.0 mg/dL	>15 mg/dL
2–5 d	0.0–12.0 mg/dL	>15 mg/dL
5 d–4 mo	0.3–1.2 mg/dL	>15 mg/dL
>4 mo–	0.3–1.2 mg/dL	None
Direct bilirubin	0.0–0.4 mg/dL	None

BILIRUBIN; TOTAL, DIRECT, AND INDIRECT

❏ **Definition**

- These assays are commonly used tests to assess liver function. Daily production of unconjugated bilirubin is mainly from senescent erythrocytes. The half-life of unconjugated bilirubin is <5 minutes. UDP-glucuronyl transferase catalyzes rapid conjugation of bilirubin to the liver; conjugated bilirubin is excreted in bile and is essentially absent from the blood of the normal individuals. Delta bilirubin (bili protein) is produced by reaction of conjugated bilirubin with albumin, and its half-life is 17–20 days. Bilirubin is typically measured in two assays for "total" and "direct"; subtracting direct from total gives "indirect bilirubin." The direct bilirubin measures the majority of delta and conjugated bilirubin and a small percentage of unconjugated bilirubin.
- **Normal range:** age dependent (see Table 16.12).

❏ **Use**

- Assessing liver function
- Evaluating a wide range of diseases affecting the production, uptake, storage, metabolism, or excretion of bilirubin
- Monitoring the efficacy of neonatal phototherapy

❏ **Interpretation**

Increased In

- Hepatocellular damage
- Biliary obstruction
- Hemolytic diseases
- Neonatal physiologic jaundice
- Gilbert disease, Crigler-Najjar syndrome
- Hypothyroidism
- Dubin-Johnson syndrome
- Increased conjugated (direct) bilirubin in
  - ▼ Hereditary disorders (e.g., Dubin-Johnson syndrome, rotor syndrome).
  - ▼ Hepatic cellular damage (e.g., viral, toxic, alcohol, drugs). Increased conjugated bilirubin may be associated with normal total bilirubin in up to one third of patients with liver diseases.
  - ▼ Biliary duct obstruction (extrahepatic or intrahepatic).

16

▼ Infiltrations, space-occupying lesions (e.g., metastases, abscess, granulomas, amyloidosis).
▼ Direct bilirubin:
  ● Twenty to forty percent of total: more suggestive of hepatic than of posthepatic jaundice
  ● Forty to sixty percent of 1: occurs in either hepatic or in posthepatic jaundice
  ● Greater than 50% of total: more suggestive of posthepatic than of hepatic jaundice
▼ Total serum bilirubin >40 mg/dL indicates hepatocellular rather than extrahepatic obstruction.
■ Increased unconjugated (indirect) bilirubin in (conjugated, 20% of total)
  ▼ Increased bilirubin production.
  ▼ Hemolytic diseases (e.g., hemoglobinopathies, RBC enzyme deficiencies, DIC, autoimmune hemolysis).
  ▼ Ineffective erythropoiesis (e.g., pernicious anemia).
  ▼ Blood transfusions.
  ▼ Hematomas.
  ▼ Hereditary disorders (e.g., Gilbert disease, Crigler-Najjar syndrome).
  ▼ Drugs (e.g., causing hemolysis).

Decreased In
■ Drugs (e.g., barbiturates)

❏ Limitations
■ Specimens should be protected from light and analyzed as soon as possible.
■ Compounds that compete for binding sites on serum albumin contribute to lower serum bilirubin levels (e.g., penicillin, sulfisoxazole, acetylsalicylic acid).
■ Day-to-day variations are 15–30% and increase an average of one- to twofold with fasting up to 48 hours.
■ Total bilirubin is 33% and 15% lower in African American men and women, respectively, compared to other racial/ethnic groups.
■ Light exposure can decrease total bilirubin up to 50% per hour.
■ Total serum bilirubin not a sensitive indicator of hepatic dysfunction; it may not reflect degree of liver damage. Must exceed 2.5 mg/dL to produce clinical jaundice; >5 mg/dL seldom occurs in uncomplicated hemolysis unless hepatobiliary disease is also present.
■ Total bilirubin is generally less markedly increased in hepatocellular jaundice (<10 mg/dL) than in neoplastic obstructions (≤20 mg/dL) or intrahepatic cholestasis.
■ In extrahepatic biliary obstruction, bilirubin may rise progressively to a plateau of 30–40 mg/dL (due in part to balance between renal excretion and diversion of bilirubin to other metabolites). Such a plateau tends not to occur in hepatocellular jaundice, and bilirubin may exceed 50 mg/dL (partly due to concomitant renal insufficiency and hemolysis).
■ Concentrations are generally higher in obstruction due to carcinoma than due to stones.

- In viral hepatitis, higher serum bilirubin suggests more liver damage and longer clinical course.
- In acute alcoholic hepatitis, >5 mg/dL suggests a poor prognosis.
- Increased serum bilirubin with normal ALP suggests constitutional hyperbilirubinemias or hemolytic states.
- Due to renal excretion, maximum bilirubin is 10–35 mg/dL; if renal disease is present, it may reach 75 mg/dL.
- Conjugated bilirubin >1.0 mg/dL in an infant always indicates disease.
- Serum bilirubin (conjugated-to-total):
  - ▼ Less than 20% conjugated: constitutional (e.g., Gilbert disease, Crigler-Najjar syndrome)
- Hemolytic states:
  - ▼ Twenty to forty percent conjugated: favors hepatocellular disease rather than extrahepatic obstruction; disorders of bilirubin metabolism (e.g., Dubin-Johnson, Rotor syndromes)
  - ▼ Forty to sixty percent conjugated: occurs in either hepatocellular or extrahepatic type
  - ▼ Greater than 50% conjugated: favors extrahepatic obstruction rather than hepatocellular disease

Suggested Readings

Dufour DR, Lott JA, Nolte FS, et al. Diagnosis and monitoring of hepatic injury. I. Performance characteristics of laboratory tests. *Clin Chem.* 2000;46:2027–2049.
Stevenson DK, Wong RJ, Vreman HJ. Reduction in hospital readmission rates for hyperbilirubinemia is associated with use of transcutaneous bilirubin measurements. *Clin Chem.* 2005;51:481–482.

BLEEDING TIME (BT)*

❏ Definition

- BT is a functional test for primary hemostasis (platelets and small vessels), infrequently performed nowadays (see below under limitations).
- **Normal range:** 4–7 minutes (slightly longer in women).

❏ Use

- The method of Ivy as modified by Mielke, using a commercially available template, is the best standardized way to perform BT. A blood pressure cuff on the upper arm is inflated to 40 mm Hg, two small skin incisions are made through the template on the volar surface of the forearm, and cessation of bleeding is counted every 30 seconds.
- BT may be used when better standardized equipment is not available for:
  - ▼ Workup of patients with the suspected diagnosis of a platelet defect or von Willebrand disease. Note the extreme variability of BT in patients with von Willebrand disease.
  - ▼ Monitoring hemostatic therapy for patients diagnosed with bleeding associated with von Willebrand disease, a thrombocytopathy, or uremia (creatinine >1.1 mg/L impairs hemostasis).
  - ▼ Prior to kidney biopsy in patients with uremia.

16

---

*Submitted By Liberto Pechet, MD.

❏ **Interpretation**

- BT is not proven to be of value in the following conditions:
  - ▼ Patients with liver disease
  - ▼ Patients prior to general surgery, coronary bypass, or coronary stent insertion
  - ▼ Patients prior to orthopedic, ear–nose–throat, or neurosurgery
  - ▼ In the follow-up of patients receiving ASA, NSAIDs, or antiplatelet drugs (clopidogrel, prasugrel)
  - ▼ Patients with myeloproliferative neoplasms or myelodysplastic syndromes
- BT is contraindicated when platelet counts are <50,000 cells/µL because it may be difficult to arrest bleeding at the incision site and the test may be noncontributory.
- BT is not prolonged in coagulation disorders such as the hemophilias.

❏ **Limitations**

- These include the operator's variability in technique, limited precision, accuracy, reproducibility, and also variability in the same patients at different times. "In vitro" BT equipment, such as platelet function analyzer (PFA 100), is better standardized and has better reproducibility.
- *Many health care organizations have discontinued the use of BT entirely.*

BLOOD GAS, pH

❏ **Definition**

- pH is the negative logarithm of the hydrogen ion concentration and is an index of acidity and alkalinity of the blood. It changes nonlinearly masking magnitude of acid–base disorders. The hydrogen ion concentration is dictated by the ratio of two quantities: the HCO_3^- concentration, which is regulated by the kidneys, and the PCO_2, which is controlled by the lungs.
- **Normal range:**
  - ▼ Arterial: 7.35–7.45
  - ▼ Venous: 7.31–7.41

❏ **Use**

- To evaluate acid–base disorders

❏ **Interpretation**

Increased In

- Metabolic alkalosis (plasma bicarbonate excess)
- Excessive alkali administration
- Potassium depletion (GI loss, lack of potassium intake, diuresis)
  - ▼ Excess adrenal steroids (Cushing disease, primary aldosteronism)
  - ▼ Chronic alkalosis
  - ▼ Potassium-losing nephropathy
- Respiratory alkalosis (decreased dissolved CO_2)
  - ▼ Hysteria
  - ▼ Stimulation of respiratory center by increased intracranial pressure
  - ▼ Hypoxia with normal overall alveolar diffusion of CO_2

▼ Fever
▼ Salicylate poisoning (early)
▼ Excessive artificial ventilation

Decreased In
- Metabolic acidosis (bicarbonate deficit)
- Increased formation of acids
  ▼ Ketosis (DM, starvation, hyperthyroidism, high-fat low-carbohydrate diet, after trauma)
  ▼ Cellular hypoxia including lactic acidosis
- Decreased excretion of H^+
  ▼ Renal failure (prerenal, renal, and postrenal)
  ▼ Renal tubular acidosis
  ▼ Fanconi syndrome
  ▼ Acquired (drugs, hypercalcemia)
  ▼ Inherited (cystinosis, Wilson disease)
  ▼ Addison disease
- Respiratory acidosis
  ▼ Emphysema, pneumonia, and pulmonary edema
  ▼ Bronchoconstriction, plugs, and drugs depressing the respiratory center
  ▼ Obstructive or restrictive pulmonary disease

❏ Limitations
- The pH of freshly drawn blood decreases on standing at a rate of 0.04–0.08 pH U/hour at 37°C, by approximately 0.03 U/hour at 25°C, but only 0.008 U/hour at 4°C.

BLOOD UREA NITROGEN (BUN)

❏ Definition
- Protein and nucleic acid catabolism results in the formation of urea and ammonia. Urea is synthesized mainly in the liver, and >90% is excreted through the kidneys.
- **Normal range:** 7–23 mg/dL.

❏ Use
- Most widely used screening test for the evaluation of kidney function.
- Along with the serum creatinine, BUN levels aid in the differential diagnosis of prerenal, renal, and postrenal hyperuremia.
- Diagnosis of renal insufficiency: filtered freely in the glomerulus; ≤50% is reabsorbed.
- Assessment of glomerular function: A BUN of 10–20 mg/dL almost always indicates normal glomerular function.
- In chronic renal disease, BUN correlates better with symptoms of uremia than does serum creatinine.
- Provides evidence of hemorrhage into the upper GI tract.
- Assessment of patients requiring nutritional support for excess catabolism, for example, burns, cancer.

16

❏ Interpretation

Increased In

- Impaired kidney function: A BUN of 50–150 mg/dL implies serious impairment of renal function. A markedly increased BUN (150–250 mg/dL) is virtually conclusive evidence of severely impaired glomerular function.
- Prerenal azotemia—any cause of reduced renal blood flow:
  - ▼ CHF
  - ▼ Salt and water depletion (vomiting, diarrhea, diuresis, sweating)
  - ▼ Shock
- Postrenal azotemia—any obstruction of urinary tract (increased BUN-to-creatinine ratio).
- Increased protein catabolism (serum creatinine remains normal):
  - ▼ Hemorrhage into the GI tract
  - ▼ AMI
  - ▼ Stress

Decreased In

- Diuresis (e.g., with overhydration, often associated with low protein catabolism).
- Severe liver damage (e.g., drugs, poisoning, hepatitis). A low BUN of 6–8 mg/dL is frequently associated with states of overhydration or liver disease.
  - ▼ Increased utilization of protein for synthesis (e.g., late pregnancy, infancy, acromegaly, malnutrition, anabolic hormones)
  - ▼ Diet (e.g., low-protein and high-carbohydrate, IV feedings only, impaired absorption [celiac disease], malnutrition)
  - ▼ Nephrotic syndrome (some patients)
  - ▼ SIADH
  - ▼ Inherited hyperammonemias (urea is virtually absent in blood)

❏ Limitations

- Urea levels increase with age and protein content of the diet.
- Corticosteroids, tetracyclines, and drugs causing nephrotoxicity frequently increase BUN.
- The presence of ammonium ions in anticoagulants may produce falsely elevated results.

BONE MARROW ANALYSIS*

❏ Definition

- Bone marrow analysis refers to studies of an *aspirate* or/and a *biopsy* with the objective of obtaining marrow samples. The bone marrow is usually obtained from the posterior iliac crest. The test is indicated when abnormalities in the peripheral blood are found that require additional etiologic, classification and prognostic details. The procedure can be performed at the bedside or in the office.
- **Normal range:** Cellularity-to-fat ratio is 100% at birth and declines ≈10% each decade; 9:1 in young children; 2:1 in young adults; 1:1 in middle-aged adults; gradually decreases to 1:9 in the elderly. Differential distribution

---

*Submitted By Liberto Pechet, MD.

tables of the various hematopoietic lineages can be found in hematology and pathology textbooks.

❑ **Use**

- Bone marrow aspirates are used for their excellent cellular morphologic maturation and definition of cellular abnormalities, cytochemistry, cytogenetic studies, molecular studies, flow cytometry, microbial culture and identification, occasionally electron microscopic studies, and tissue culture. Aspirates can also be used for bone marrow transplantation, where large amounts of marrow need to be collected. (Concentrated peripheral blood stem cells are now used in most cases for this purpose.)
- Bone marrow biopsies are useful for examination of intact marrow tissue and overall cellularity, histochemistry, and immunohistochemistry, as well as for certain molecular diagnostic tests. Biopsies are excellent for evaluating iron stores, fibrosis, granulomas, abscesses, metastases, and vascular lesions.
- Bone marrow is studied to diagnose or follow-up various conditions that may affect it or infiltrate it.
  - ▼ For the diagnosis of anemia of iron deficiency bone marrow iron stains are the gold standard; also helpful in some cases of iron overload
  - ▼ Neoplasms that originate in or infiltrate the marrow: leukemias, myeloproliferative neoplasms, myelodysplastic syndromes, plasmacytic neoplasms, metastases; amyloidosis
  - ▼ Staging of Hodgkin and other lymphomas
  - ▼ Tumors and infections (e.g., TB) that invade the marrow and result in leukoerythroblastic peripheral blood picture (myelophthisic anemia)
  - ▼ Aplastic anemia, agranulocytosis, cytopenias
  - ▼ Unexplained anemia, splenomegaly, lymphadenopathy
  - ▼ Megaloblastic anemias (rarely necessary)
  - ▼ Exposure to drugs resulting in bone marrow damage
  - ▼ Follow-up therapy for leukemias, lymphoma (in cases that present with bone marrow infiltration), myelodysplastic and myeloproliferative neoplasms
  - ▼ Monitoring recovery following stem cell transplantation and marrow-ablative therapy
  - ▼ Infectious diseases and fever of unknown etiology (cultures, organism identification)

❑ **Limitations**

- Bone marrow aspirate may be diluted with peripheral blood and contain too few cellular elements.
- Bone marrow biopsy may have insufficient tissue for accurate diagnosis; the underlying condition may result in patchy infiltrations of the marrow (e.g., myelomas), and the pathology may be missed.

BRAIN NATRIURETIC PEPTIDE (BNP)

❑ **Definition**

- Other names include B-type natriuretic peptide, N-terminal pro b-type natriuretic peptide, and NT-proBNP. BNP is a hormone secreted by myocytes in the ventricles (left ventricle) in response to pressure overload/myocyte

16

stretch, with potent diuretic, natriuretic, and vascular smooth muscle relaxing effects. The heart normally produces low levels of a precursor protein, pro-BNP, which is cleaved to release the active hormone, BNP, and an inactive fragment, NT-proBNP.

- **Normal range:**
  - ▼ BNP: <100 pg/mL
  - ▼ NT-proBNP: 0–74 years of age: ≤124 pg/mL; 75 years of age and older: ≤449 pg/mL

❑ Use

- Screening and diagnosis of CHF: BNP and NT-proBNP levels in the blood may be useful to establish prognosis in heart failure because both markers are typically higher in patients with worse outcome.
- Reading >480 pg/mL = 51% chance of cardiac/noncardiac events in next 6 months.
- Reading <230 pg/mL = 2.5% chance of cardiac/noncardiac events in next 6 months.
- Reading >130 pg/mL = 19% chance of sudden death.
- Reading <130 pg/mL = 1% chance of sudden death.
- Differential diagnosis of dyspnea: Readings <100 pg/mL rule out CHF as cause of dyspnea, and readings >400 pg/mL indicate a 95% likelihood of CHF. Readings between 100 and 400 pg/mL warrant further workup.
- Determination of severity of CHF: Higher values correlate with increasing New York Heart Association classes I–IV. BNP is a prognostic tool for classes III and IV.
- Diagnosis of left ventricular dysfunction: Routine testing is not recommended for screening asymptomatic patient populations for left ventricular dysfunction. Increase in BNP in right heart failure is less than in left ventricular dysfunction.
- At appropriate cutoff values, BNP and NT-proBNP have similar S/S = 70%/70% and NPV = 80%.
- Greater increases predict worse adverse outcomes in patients with CHF.
- Increased values after acute myocardial infarction predict poorer prognosis.
- BNP increases with arrhythmias that are less marked.
- BNP and NT-proBNP can be increased in renal failure, especially if dialysis is needed.
- Abnormal echocardiogram without symptoms: mean value = 300 pg/mL.

❑ Interpretation

Increased In

- Heart failure
- Left ventricular dysfunction
- Renal impairment
- Coronary artery disease
- Valvular disease
- Arrhythmias
- Brain injury
- Anemia (BNP)
- Sepsis and shock (NT-proBNP)

❑ Limitations

- Routine blood BNP or NT-proBNP testing is not justified for determining specific therapy for patients with chronic or acute heart failure.
- Nesiritide (human recombinant BNP) increases BNP. Studies indicate a minimal effect on NT-proBNP.
- Age and exercise also increase BNP.
- Obesity decreases BNP.
- Intraindividual variation (approximately 50% and 60%, respectively, for BNP and NT-proBNP from week to week) indicates altered cardiac status.

Suggested Readings

Apple FS, Wu HB, Jaffe AS, et al. National Academy of Clinical Biochemistry and IFCC Committee for Standardization of Markers of Cardiac Damage Laboratory Medicine Practice Guidelines: Analytical issues for biomarkers of heart failure. *Circulation*. 2007;226:e95–e98.

Steiner J, Guglin M. BNP or NTproBNP? A clinician's perspective. *Int J Cardiol*. 2008;129(1):5–14.

Tang WH, Francis GS, Morrow DA, et al. National Academy of Clinical Biochemistry Laboratory Medicine: National Academy of Clinical Biochemistry Laboratory Medicine Practice Guidelines: clinical utilization of cardiac biomarker testing in heart failure. *Circulation*. 2007;116(5): e99–e109.

BRONCHODILATORS

See Theophylline (1,3-Dimethylxanthine).

β-TRACE PROTEIN

❑ Definition

- β-Trace protein is also known as BTP or lipocalin-type prostaglandin D synthase. This test is currently not widely available in commercial laboratories. Research use only test. BTP, a low molecular weight glycoprotein freely filtered through the glomerular basement membrane and with minimal nonrenal elimination, is an ideal marker for GFR. BTP has been shown to be a more sensitive marker of GFR than creatinine in patients with chronic kidney disease, in kidney transplant recipients, and in children.
- **Normal range:** 0.40–0.74 mg/L.

❑ Use

- Alternative marker for GFR in children as well as in DM and various renal diseases.
- The early diagnosis of fistulas leaking CSF is an accurate marker of CSF leakage (CSF rhinorrhea).

❑ Limitations

- Patients with renal insufficiency and bacterial meningitis have increase serum and decreased CSF levels.
- There are no clear cut and accurate cutoff values available, which is a major determinant of diagnostic significance.

16

Suggested Reading

Pöge U, Gerhardt TM, Stoffel-Wagner B, et al. β-Trace protein is an alternative marker for GFR in renal transplantation patients. *Clin Chem.* 2005;51:1531.

BUN-TO-CREATININE RATIO

❑ **Definition and Use**

- The BUN-to-creatinine ratio is used to differentiate prerenal and postrenal azotemia from renal azotemia. Because of considerable variability, it should be used only as a rough guide.
- **Normal range** (usual range for most people on normal diet: 12–16).

❑ **Interpretation**

Increased Ratio (>10:1) with Normal Creatinine In

- Prerenal azotemia (e.g., heart failure, salt depletion, dehydration, blood loss) due to decreased GFR
- Catabolic states with increased tissue breakdown
- GI hemorrhage; a ratio ≥36 is reported to distinguish upper from lower GI hemorrhage in patients with negative gastric aspirate.
- High protein intake
- Impaired renal function plus
  - ▼ Excess protein intake or production or tissue breakdown (e.g., GI bleeding, thyrotoxicosis, infection, Cushing syndrome, high-protein diet, surgery, burns, cachexia, high fever)
  - ▼ Urine reabsorption (e.g., ureterocolostomy)
  - ▼ Patients with reduced muscle mass (subnormal creatinine production)
- Certain drugs (e.g., tetracycline, glucocorticoids)
- Selective increase in plasma urea (diuretic-induced azotemia) during use of loop diuretics

Increased Ratio (>10:1) with Elevated Creatinine In

- Postrenal azotemia (BUN rises disproportionately more than creatinine) (e.g., obstructive uropathy)
- Prerenal azotemia superimposed on renal disease

Decreased Ratio (<10:1) with Decreased BUN In

- Acute tubular necrosis
- Low-protein diet, starvation, severe liver disease, and other causes of decreased urea synthesis
- Repeated dialysis (urea rather than creatinine diffuses out of extracellular fluid)
- Inherited deficiency of urea cycle enzymes (e.g., hyperammonemias—urea is virtually absent in blood)
- SIADH (due to tubular secretion of urea)
- Pregnancy

Decreased Ratio (<10:1) with Increased Creatinine In

- Phenacemide therapy (accelerates conversion of creatine to creatinine)

- Rhabdomyolysis (releases muscle creatinine)
- Muscular patients who develop renal failure

❏ **Limitations**
- DKA (acetoacetate causes false increase in creatinine with certain methodologies, resulting in normal or decreased ratio when dehydration should produce an increased ratio)
- Cephalosporin therapy (interferes with creatinine measurement)

CALCITONIN

❏ **Definition**
- Calcitonin, also known as thyrocalcitonin, is a polypeptide hormone secreted by parafollicular C cells of thyroid. It acts directly on osteoclasts to decrease bone-resorbing activity and to cause decreased serum calcium.
- **Normal range:**
  ▼ Older children and adults: <12 pg/mL in males; <5 pg/mL in females
  ▼ Infants and young children: <40 pg/mL in children <6 months; <15 pg/mL in children 6 months to 3 years (Basuyau)

❏ **Use**
- Serum calcitonin is determined to diagnose recurrence of medullary carcinoma or metastases after the primary tumor has been removed or to confirm complete removal of the tumor if basal calcitonin has been previously increased.
- Measurement of serum calcitonin has not been a part of the routine evaluation of patients with thyroid nodules in the United States. The high frequency of falsely high serum calcitonin values and the accuracy of fine needle aspiration biopsy argue against a change in this recommendation. Furthermore, occasional patients with locoregional metastases or locally invasive medullary thyroid carcinoma (MTC) have normal unstimulated serum calcitonin concentrations.

❏ **Interpretation**
Increased Values
- Carcinoma of the lung, breast, islet cell, or ovary and carcinoid due to ectopic production and in myeloproliferative disorders
- Hypercalcemia of any etiology, stimulating calcitonin production
- Zollinger-Ellison syndrome
- C-cell hyperplasia
- Pernicious anemia
- Acute or chronic thyroiditis
- Chronic renal failure

Decreased Values
- Following surgical therapy for MTC
  ▼ In cases of complete cures, serum calcitonin levels fall into the undetectable range over a variable period of several weeks.

16

▼ A rise in previously undetectable or very low postoperative serum calcitonin levels is highly suggestive of disease recurrence or spread and should trigger further diagnostic evaluations.

❏ **Limitations**

■ Basal fasting level may be increased in patients with MTC, even when there is no palpable mass in the thyroid.

  ▼ Values follow a circadian pattern, with a peak after lunchtime.

  ▼ Basal level is normal in approximately one third of cases of MTC.

■ Levels of >2,000 pg/mL are almost always associated with MTC, with rare cases due to obvious renal failure or ectopic production of calcitonin.

■ Levels of 500–2,000 pg/mL generally indicate medullary carcinoma, renal failure, or ectopic production of calcitonin.

■ Levels of 100–500 pg/mL should be interpreted cautiously with repeat assays and provocative tests. If repeat tests in 1–2 months are still abnormal, some authors recommend total thyroidectomy.

■ This test is not useful for evaluating calcium metabolic diseases.

■ Falsely elevated values may occur in serum from patients who have developed human antimouse antibodies or heterophilic antibodies.

Suggested Readings

Basuyau JP, Mallet E, Leroy M, et al. Reference intervals for serum calcitonin in men, women, and children. *Clin Chem.* 2004;50:1828–1830.

Saad MF, Ordonez NG, Rashid RK, et al. Medullary carcinoma of the thyroid. A study of the clinical features and prognostic factors in 161 patients. *Medicine (Baltimore).* 1984;63: 319–342.

CALCIUM, IONIZED

❏ **Definition**

■ Ionized calcium is the physiologically active form of calcium. Ionized calcium homeostasis is regulated by the parathyroid glands, bone, kidney, and intestine. It is most frequently used in ICUs and operating rooms.

■ **Normal range:** 4.6–5.3 mg/dL.

■ **Critical range:** <4.1 or >5.9 mg/dL.

❏ **Use**

■ In patients with hypocalcemia or hypercalcemia with borderline serum calcium and altered serum proteins.

■ Approximately 50% of calcium is ionized; 40–45% is bound to albumin; 5–10% is bound to other anions (e.g., sulfate, phosphate, lactate, and citrate); only the ionized fraction is physiologically active. Total calcium values may be deceiving, because they may be unchanged even if ionized calcium values are changed (e.g., increased blood pH increases protein-bound calcium and decreases ionized calcium, and PTH has the opposite effect) (blood pH should always be performed with ionized calcium, which is increased in acidosis and decreased in alkalosis). However, in critically ill patients, elevated total serum calcium usually indicates ionized hypercalcemia, and normal total serum calcium is evidence against ionized hypocalcemia.

- Ionized calcium is the preferred measurement rather than total calcium, because it is physiologically active and can be rapidly measured, which may be essential in certain situations (e.g., liver transplantation and rapid or large transfusion of citrated blood make interpretation of total calcium nearly impossible).
- Life-threatening complications are frequent when serum ionized calcium <2 mg/dL.
- With multiple blood transfusions, ionized calcium <3 mg/dL may be an indication to administer calcium.

❏ **Interpretation**
Increased In
- Normal total serum calcium associated with hypoalbuminemia may indicate ionized hypercalcemia.
- About 25% of patients with hyperparathyroidism have normal total but increased ionized calcium levels.
- Acidosis
- Metastatic bone tumor
- Milk-alkali syndrome
- Multiple myeloma
- Paget disease
- Sarcoidosis
- Tumors producing a PTH-like substance
- Vitamin D intoxication

Decreased In
- Alkalosis (e.g., hyperventilation, to control increased intracranial pressure) (total serum calcium may be normal), administration of bicarbonate to control metabolic acidosis
- Increased serum free fatty acids (increased calcium binding to albumin) due to
  - ▼ Certain drugs (e.g., heparin, IV lipids, epinephrine, norepinephrine, isoproterenol, alcohol)
  - ▼ Severe stress (e.g., acute pancreatitis, DKA, sepsis, AMI)
  - ▼ Hemodialysis
- Hypoparathyroidism (primary, secondary)
- Vitamin D deficiency
- Toxic shock syndrome
- Fat embolism
- Hypokalemia protects the patient from hypocalcemic tetany; correction of hypokalemia without correction of hypocalcemia may provoke tetany
- Malabsorption
- Osteomalacia
- Pancreatitis
- Renal failure
- Rickets

16

❑ Limitations

- Differences in specimen preparation and electrode selectivity are probably responsible for differences in reported reference ranges. Heparin itself causes 0.04 mg/dL decrease for each unit added per milliliter of blood.
- Adjusting the pH of the specimen to 7.4 at the time of measurement is not necessary if the specimen is collected anaerobically.
- Various formulas are available for calculating ionized calcium using total calcium, albumin, and total protein. However, these formulas may not apply in some situations; their use is discouraged.
- Hypomagnesemia or hypermagnesemia; patients respond to serum magnesium that becomes normal but not to calcium therapy. Serum magnesium should always be measured in any patient with hypocalcemia.
- Increase of ions to which calcium is bound:
  - ▼ Phosphate (e.g., phosphorus administration in treatment of DKA, chemotherapy causing tumor lysis syndrome, rhabdomyolysis)
  - ▼ Bicarbonate
  - ▼ Citrate (e.g., during blood transfusion)
  - ▼ Radiographic contrast media containing calcium chelators

CALCIUM, TOTAL

❑ Definition

- Ninety-nine percent of the body's calcium is in bone. Of the remainder (of 1%) in blood, about 50% is ionized (free), about 10% is bound to anions (e.g., phosphate, bicarbonate), and about 40% (of 1%) in blood is bound to plasma proteins, (80–40%) of that to albumin.
- **Normal range:** 8.7–10.7 mg/dL.
- **Critical values:** <6.6 or >12.9 mg/dL.

❑ Use

- Diagnosis and monitoring of a wide range of disorders, including disorders of protein and vitamin D, and diseases of the bone, kidney, parathyroid gland, or GI tract.

❑ Interpretation
Increased In

- Hyperparathyroidism, primary and secondary
- Acute and chronic renal failure
- Following renal transplantation
- Osteomalacia with malabsorption
- Aluminum-associated osteomalacia
- Malignant tumors (especially breast, lung, kidney; 2% of patients with Hodgkin or non-Hodgkin lymphoma)
  - ▼ Direct bone metastases (up to 30% of these patients) (e.g., breast cancer, Hodgkin and non-Hodgkin lymphoma, leukemia, pancreatic cancer, lung cancer)
  - ▼ Osteoclastic activating factor (e.g., multiple myeloma, Burkitt lymphoma; may be markedly increased in human T-cell leukemia virus-I–associated lymphoma

▼ Humoral hypercalcemia of malignancy
▼ Ectopic production of 1,25-dihydroxyvitamin D_3 (e.g., Hodgkin and non-Hodgkin lymphoma)
■ Granulomatous disease (e.g., uncommon in sarcoidosis, TB, leprosy; more uncommon in mycoses, berylliosis, silicone granulomas, Crohn disease, eosinophilic granuloma, catscratch fever)
■ Effect of drugs
▼ Vitamin D and A intoxication
▼ Milk-alkali (Burnett) syndrome (rare)
▼ Diuretics (e.g., thiazides)
▼ Others (estrogens, androgens, progestins, tamoxifen, lithium, thyroid hormone, parenteral nutrition)
■ Renal failure, acute or chronic
■ Other endocrine conditions
▼ Thyrotoxicosis (in 20–40% of patients; usually <14 mg/dL)
▼ More uncommon: Some patients with hypothyroidism, Cushing syndrome, adrenal insufficiency, acromegaly, pheochromocytoma (rare), VIPoma syndrome
▼ Multiple endocrine neoplasia
■ Acute osteoporosis (e.g., immobilization of young patients or in Paget disease)
■ Miscellaneous
▼ Familial hypocalciuric hypercalcemia
▼ Rhabdomyolysis causing acute renal failure
▼ Porphyria
▼ Dehydration with hyperproteinemia
▼ Hypophosphatasia
▼ Idiopathic hypercalcemia of infancy
■ Concomitant hypokalemia is not infrequent in hypercalcemia. Concomitant dehydration is almost always present because hypercalcemia causes nephrogenic diabetes insipidus.

Decreased In (Tables 16.13 and 16.14)

■ Hypoparathyroidism
▼ Surgical
▼ Idiopathic infiltration of parathyroids (e.g., sarcoid, amyloid, hemochromatosis, tumor)

TABLE 16–13. Serum Phosphate, PTH, and Vitamin D Levels in Various Hypocalcemic Disorders

Hypocalcemic Disorders	Serum PO_4	PTH	25(OH)D	1,25(OH)$_2$D
Hypoparathyroidism	I	D	N	D
Pseudohypoparathyroidism	I	I	N	D
Vitamin D deficiency	D	I	D	Low N
1α-Hydroxylase deficiency	D	I	N	D
1,25(OH)$_2$D resistance	D	I	N	I

PO_4, phosphate; N, normal; I, increased; D, decreased.

16

TABLE 16–14. Variations of Various Serum and Urine Analytes in Association with Hypocalcemic Disorders

Hypocalcemia Associated with	Increased	Decreased
Serum PTH	Pseudohypoparathyroidism Renal failure, acute/chronic Malabsorption Vitamin D deficiency Phosphate administration	Hypoparathyroidism Acute pancreatitis Magnesium deficiency
Serum phosphorus	Hypoparathyroidism Pseudohypoparathyroidism Renal failure, acute (oliguric phase)/chronic Phosphate administration	Vitamin D deficiency Acute pancreatitis Renal failure, acute (diuretic phase) Malabsorption
Serum bicarbonate and pH	Hypoparathyroidism	
Serum Mg	Renal failure, acute/chronic	Magnesium deficiency Acute pancreatitis Renal failure, acute (diuretic phase)
Urine calcium	Hypoparathyroidism	Other causes of hypocalcemia
Urine phosphate	Renal failure, chronic Vitamin D deficiency Malabsorption Phosphate administration	Hypoparathyroidism Pseudohypoparathyroidism Magnesium deficiency
Urine cAMP	Renal failure, chronic Vitamin D deficiency Malabsorption	Hypoparathyroidism Pseudohypoparathyroidism

- ▼ Hereditary (e.g., DiGeorge syndrome)
- ▼ Pseudohypoparathyroidism
- ▼ Chronic renal disease with uremia and phosphate retention, Fanconi syndromes, renal tubular acidosis
- ▼ Malabsorption of calcium and vitamin D, obstructive jaundice
- ▼ Insufficient calcium, phosphorus, and vitamin D ingestion
- ▼ Bone disease (osteomalacia, rickets)
- ▼ Starvation
- ▼ Late pregnancy
- ■ Altered bound calcium citrate
  - ▼ Multiple citrated blood transfusions
  - ▼ Dialysis with citrate anticoagulation
- ■ Hyperphosphatemia (e.g., phosphate enema/infusion)
- ■ Rhabdomyolysis
- ■ Tumor lysis syndrome
- ■ Acute severe illness (e.g., pancreatitis with extensive fat necrosis, sepsis, burns)
- ■ Respiratory alkalosis
- ■ Certain drugs
  - ▼ Cancer chemotherapy drugs (e.g., cisplatin, mithramycin, cytosine arabinoside)
  - ▼ Fluoride intoxication

▼ Antibiotics (e.g., gentamicin, pentamidine, ketoconazole)
▼ Chronic therapeutic use of anticonvulsant drugs (e.g., phenobarbital, phenytoin)
▼ Loop-active diuretics
▼ Calcitonin
▼ Gadolinium-based magnetic resonance (MR) imaging contrast agents.
- Osteoblastic tumor metastases
- Neonates born of complicated pregnancies
  ▼ Hyperbilirubinemia
  ▼ Respiratory distress, asphyxia
  ▼ Cerebral injuries
  ▼ Infants of diabetic mothers
  ▼ Prematurity
  ▼ Maternal hypoparathyroidism
- Hypermagnesemia (e.g., magnesium for treatment of toxemia of pregnancy)
- Magnesium deficiency
- Toxic shock syndrome

Temporary hypocalcemia after subtotal thyroidectomy in >40% of patients; >20% are symptomatic.

❑ **Limitations**

- Total serum protein and albumin should always be measured simultaneously for proper interpretation of serum calcium levels, since 0.8 mg of calcium is bound to 1.0 g of albumin in serum; to correct, add 0.8 mg/dL for every 1.0 g/dL that serum albumin falls below 4.0 g/dL; binding to globulin only affects total calcium if globulin >6 g/dL.
- Serum levels increased by
  ▼ Hyperalbuminemia (e.g., multiple myeloma, Waldenström macroglobulinemia)
  ▼ Dehydration
  ▼ Venous stasis during blood collection by prolonged application of tourniquet
  ▼ Use of cork-stoppered test tubes
  ▼ Hyponatremia (<120 mEq/L), which increases the protein-bound fraction of calcium, thereby slightly increasing the total calcium (opposite effect in hypernatremia)
- Serum levels decreased by
  ▼ Hypomagnesemia (e.g., due to cisplatin chemotherapy)
  ▼ Hyperphosphatemia (e.g., laxatives, phosphate enemas, chemotherapy of leukemia or lymphoma, rhabdomyolysis)
  ▼ Hypoalbuminemia
  ▼ Hemodilution

CALCIUM, URINE

❑ **Definition**

- Urinary calcium levels reflects intake, rates of intestinal calcium absorption, bone resorption, and renal loss. Hypercalcemia of any cause raises

16

urinary calcium excretion, and its measurement adds little to the differential diagnosis of hypercalcemia. Fasting calcium excretion is useful when assessing the contribution of abnormal renal tubular handling of calcium to disorders of calcium homeostasis.

- **Normal range:**
  - ▼ Twenty-four–hour urine: 100–300 mg/day
  - ▼ Random urine:
    - Males: 12–244 mg/g creatinine
    - Females: 9–328 mg/g creatinine

❑ Use

- Evaluation of patients with disorders of bone disease, calcium metabolism, and renal stones
- Follow-up of patients on calcium therapy for osteopenia
- Best test of calcium excretion in the investigation of possible familial benign hypocalciuric hypercalcemia

❑ Interpretation

Increased In

- Primary hyperparathyroidism
- Humoral hypercalcemia of malignancy
- Vitamin D excess
- Sarcoidosis
- Fanconi syndrome
- Osteolytic bone metastases
- Myeloma
- Osteoporosis
- Distal renal tubular acidosis
- Idiopathic hypercalciuria
- Thyrotoxicosis
- Paget disease
- Malignant neoplasm of breast or bladder

Decreased In

- Familial hypocalciuric hypercalcemia
- Hypoparathyroidism
- Pseudohypoparathyroidism
- Rickets and osteomalacia
- Hypothyroidism
- Celiac sprue
- Steatorrhea

❑ Limitations

- Calcium and protein intake and phosphorus excretion alter urinary calcium excretion.
- Decreases late in normal pregnancy.
- About one third of hyperparathyroid patients have normal urine output.

CALPROTECTIN, STOOL

❑ **Definition**

- Calprotectin is a major calcium-binding protein found predominantly in neutrophils with antimicrobial and antiproliferative activities. When inflammatory processes occur, calprotectin is released due to the degranulation of neutrophil granulocytes. In bowel inflammation, calprotectin may be detected in the stool. An increased calprotectin concentration in stool is the direct consequence of neutrophil degranulation due to mucosal damage. Calprotectin levels are higher in feces than in plasma and significantly elevated in IBD patients (ulcerative colitis and Crohn disease) and in indeterminate colitis. Similar sensitivity and specificity as of fecal lactoferrin assay.
- **Normal range:** negative.

❑ **Use**

- Diagnose inflammatory bowel disease (IBD), including Crohn disease and ulcerative colitis
- Differentiate IBD from irritable bowel syndrome (IBS)
- Monitor IBD activity and predict relapse

❑ **Interpretation**

Increased In
- Screening for inflammation in patients presenting with abdominal pain and diarrhea
- Distinguish patients with active IBD from noninflammatory IBS
- Monitor IBD activity

Decreased In
- NA

❑ **Limitations**

- Presence of GI infections and colorectal cancer may falsely elevate levels.
- Does not differentiate among inflammatory bowel pathologies.
- False negatives are more common in children and teenagers than in adults.
- Fecal calprotectin levels increase after use of nonsteroidal anti-inflammatory drugs, that levels may change with age.
- Bleeding (e.g., nasal or menstrual) may cause an elevated fecal calprotectin level.

CANCER ANTIGEN 15-3 (CA 15-3)

❑ **Definition**

- This glycoprotein is a mucinous carbohydrate antigen product of the MUC1 gene expressed on various adenocarcinomas, especially breast. It is a high molecular weight (300–450 kDa) 1 polymorphic epithelial mucin.
- **Normal value:** <38 U/mL.

16

❑ Use

- Marker for breast carcinoma. United States Food and Drug Administration (USFDA) approval is only for detection of breast carcinoma recurrence before symptoms and to monitor response to treatment. Significant change is ±25%.
- Not approved for screening, although increased values may occur ≤9 months before clinical evidence of disease.

❑ Interpretation

Increased In

- Approximately 80% metastatic breast cancer
- Pancreas, lung, ovarian, colorectal, and liver cancers with less specificity

❑ Limitations

- CA 15-3 should not be used to diagnose breast cancer.
- Clinical sensitivity is 0.60, the specificity is 0.87, and the PPV is 0.91.
- It is considered equivalent to cancer antigen 27.29 mucin marker.

Suggested Reading

Duffy MJ, Duggan C, Keane R, et al. High preoperative CA 15-3 concentrations predict adverse outcome in node-negative and node-positive breast cancer: study of 600 patients with histologically confirmed breast cancer. *Clin Chem.* 2004;50:559–563.

CANCER ANTIGEN 19-9 (CA 19-9)

❑ Definition

- CA 19-9 is a modified Lewis(a) blood group antigen and has been used as a tumor marker. It is shown to be elevated in sera of some patients with GI tumors.
- **Normal value:** <35 U/mL.

❑ Use

- Detection, diagnosis, and prognosis of pancreatic cancer
- Monitor response to therapy (e.g., postsurgical recurrence correlates with increased concentrations)
- May be a useful adjunct to CEA for diagnosis and to detect early recurrence of certain cancers
- May indicate development of cholangiocarcinoma in patients with primary sclerosing cholangitis

❑ Interpretation

Increased In

- Carcinoma of the pancreas (80%).
- Pancreatitis—concentrations are usually <75 U/mL but are much higher in pancreatic cancer.
- Hepatobiliary cancer (22–51%).
- Gastric cancer (42%).
- Colon cancer (20%) is associated with very poor prognosis.
- Noncancerous conditions that may elevate include cirrhosis, cholangitis, hepatitis, pancreatitis, and nonmalignant GI diseases.
- Can be considered as a marker of MTC dedifferentiation and diseases aggressiveness.

Decreased In
❑ **Limitations**

- Individuals with blood group antigen Le a-b- do not synthesize CA 19-9 (5–10% of population).
- No value in screening because its PPV <1%. However, levels of >1,000 U/mL have 97% PPV.
- The CA 19-9 levels in a given specimen determined with assays from different manufacturers can vary due to differences in assay methods and reagent specificity and cannot be used interchangeably. If, in the course of monitoring a patient, the assay method used is changed, additional sequential testing should be carried out to confirm baseline values.

CANCER ANTIGEN 27.29 (CA 27.29)

❑ **Definition**

- Monoclonal antibody to a glycoprotein (Muc-1) that is present on the apical surface of normal epithelial cells. Tumor marker similar to cancer antigen 15-3
- **Normal value:** <38.6 U/mL

❑ **Use**

- As an aid in monitoring patients previously treated for stage II or III breast cancer.

❑ **Interpretation**
Increased In

- One third of early stage I and II breast cancers and two thirds of later stage III and IV breast cancers
- Associated malignancies: colon, gastric, hepatic, lung, pancreatic, ovarian, and prostate cancers
- Benign conditions: breast, liver, and kidney disorders; ovarian cysts, tuberculosis, sarcoidosis, endometriosis, SLE, lactation, and pregnancy

❑ **Limitations**

- Lacks predictive value in early-stage breast cancer and thus has no role in screening for or diagnosis of the malignancy.
- The concentration of CA 27.29 in a given specimen can vary because of differences in assay methods and reagent specificity. Values obtained with different assay methods should not be used interchangeably.
- Levels of CA 27.29 should not be interpreted as absolute evidence of the presence or the absence of malignant disease. Measurements of CA 27.29 should always be used in conjunction with other diagnostic procedures.

CANCER ANTIGEN-125 (CA-125), SERUM

❑ **Definition**

- CA-125 is a large glycoprotein (200–1,000 kDa) found on the surface of many ovarian cancer cells and in some normal tissues. It is a product of the *MUC16* gene.
- **Normal range:** 0–35 U/mL.

16

❑ **Use**

- CA-125 is recommended, together with transvaginal ultrasound, for early detection of ovarian cancer in women with hereditary syndromes because early intervention may be beneficial in these women. It is also recommended as an adjunct in distinguishing benign from malignant suspicious pelvic masses, particularly in postmenopausal women.
- It is not suggested for screening asymptomatic women.
- Measurements may also be used to monitor response to chemotherapeutic response.

❑ **Interpretation**

Increased Values
- Malignant disease
  - ▼ Fallopian tube tumors (100%), nonmucinous epithelial ovarian carcinoma (85%), cervical adenocarcinoma (83%), endometrial adenocarcinoma (50%), and squamous cell carcinomas of vulva or cervix (<15%)
  - ▼ Trophoblastic tumors (45%)
  - ▼ Non-Hodgkin lymphoma (40%) with pleuropericardial or peritoneal involvement
  - ▼ Cancers of the pancreas, liver, and lung
- Conditions that affect the endometrium
  - ▼ Pregnancy (27%)
  - ▼ Menstruation, endometriosis
- Pleural effusion or inflammation (e.g., cancer, congestive heart failure)
- Peritoneal effusion or inflammation (e.g., pelvic inflammatory disease) and especially in bacterial peritonitis in which the ascitic concentration is greater than the serum concentration
- Some nonmalignant conditions
  - ▼ Cirrhosis, severe liver necrosis (66%)
  - ▼ Other diseases and disorders of the GI tract, liver, and pancreas
  - ▼ Renal failure
- Healthy persons (1%)

Decreased Values
- Postmenopausal women
- African American and Asian women, for whom normal values are lower

❑ **Limitations**

- Human antimurine or heterophile antibodies.
- The CA-125 level is not increased in mucinous adenocarcinoma.
- Different assays do not produce equivalent values and should not be used interchangeably.
- Most of the commercially available assays quote the upper reference limit of 35 IU/mL; some studies have shown that the detection of disease can be significantly improved by lowering the cutoff value.

- Normal concentration of CA-125 does not exclude tumor.
- CA-125 is not useful for distinguishing benign from malignant pelvic masses, even at high concentrations.
- Although CA-125 may be increased ≤12 months before clinical evidence of disease, it is not recommended for screening women for serous carcinoma of the ovary because it is not increased in 20% of cases at the time of diagnosis and in <10% of stage I and II cases (low sensitivity and specificity; high false-positive rate).
  - ▼ There is little benefit to early detection of late-stage cancers.
- Postoperative monitoring for persistent or recurrent disease; poorer prognosis if elevated 3–6 weeks after surgery.
  - ▼ Lower levels in patients with no residual tumor or <2 cm of residual tumor.
  - ▼ Concentration >35 U/mL detects residual cancer in 95% of patients, but a negative test does not exclude residual disease.
- Rising level of CA-125 during chemotherapy is associated with tumor progression, and fall to normal is associated with response. It remains elevated in stable or progressive serous carcinoma of the ovary.
- Rising concentrations may precede clinical recurrence by many months and may be indication for second-look operation, but lack of increased values does not indicate the absence of persistent or recurrent tumor.
- Greater concentration is roughly related to poorer survival; >35 U/mL is highly predictive of tumor recurrence.
  - ▼ With values >65 U/mL, 90% of women have cancer involving the peritoneum.
  - ▼ Higher levels are also seen in serous cystadenocarcinoma.
- Sequential determinations are more useful than a single test, because levels in benign disease do not show significant change but progressive rise occurs in malignant disease.
- CA-125 is positive in 80% of cases of common epithelial tumors (50% of early-stage disease). It should be noted that 0.6% of normal women older than 50 years of age have increased levels of CA-125.
- Prognosis may be better if
  - ▼ There is a 50% decline in concentration within 5 days after surgery.
  - ▼ A postoperative-to-preoperative concentration ratio of 0.1 generally occurs within 4 weeks.
  - ▼ People with a postoperative-to-preoperative concentration ratio of >0.1 to <0.5 may benefit from chemotherapy, but the recurrence rate is high.
  - ▼ Patients with a postoperative-to-preoperative concentration ratio of >0.8 should consider alternative therapy (e.g., radiation, different chemotherapy combinations).

Suggested Reading

Fritsche HA, Bast RC. CA 125 in ovarian cancer: advances and controversy. *Clin Chem.* 1998;44:1379–1380.

CANNABIS SATIVA*

❑ **Definition**

- An aromatic annual plant with origins in central Asia. The plant is known to contain 61 cannabinoids, including delta-9-tetrahydrocannabinol (delta-9-THC) and cannabidiol.
- Other names: marijuana, hashish, hash, sinsemilla, pot, grass.

❑ **Use**

- No federally recognized medical use (schedule I, Controlled Substances Act)
- Self-administered for its mood-altering properties—stimulant/depressant at low doses; CNS depressant at high doses

❑ **Limitations**

- Screening assays are commonly immunoassay based.
  - ▼ ELISA for blood, serum, plasma
    - Target analyte: delta-9-THC
    - Cutoff concentration–variable 2–5 ng/mL
    - May exhibit significant cross-reactivity with 11-hydroxy-THC, carboxy-THC [THC-COOH]
    - Low cross-reactivity with cannabidiol, cannabinol, delta-8-THC
  - ▼ EIA for urine
    - Target analyte: THC-COOH (metabolite)
    - Cutoff concentration: 20 ng/mL, 50 ng/mL
    - Approximately 50% cross-reactivity with cannabinol, 11-OH-THC
- Confirmation assays are commonly chromatography based regardless of specimen
  - ▼ Highly glucuronidated–hydrolysis recommended for analysis of urine
  - ▼ Urine confirmation assays typically target *only* THC-COOH; limit of detection/quantitation is 5–15 ng/mL
  - ▼ GC/MS: selected ion -monitoring mode for quantitative analysis of serum, plasma for THC, 11-OH-THC, THC-COOH; limits of quantitation: 1–5 ng/mL.
  - ▼ LC/MSn (multiple MS).
    - Multiple reaction–monitoring mode for qualitative or quantitative analysis of THC, 11-OH-THC, THC-COOH
    - Limits of detection/quantitation: 0.5–5 ng/mL

CARBON DIOXIDE, TOTAL

❑ **Definition**

- Total carbon dioxide consists of carbon dioxide (CO_2) in solution or bound to proteins, bicarbonate (HCO_3^-), carbonate (CO_3^{2-}), and carbonic acid (H_2CO_3). In practice, 80–90% is present as HCO_3^- and is a general guide to the body's buffering capacity. It is usually measured with electrolytes as a panel.

---

*Submitted By Amanda J. Jenkins, PhD.

- **Normal range:**
  - ▼ 0–2 years: 20–25 mmol/L
  - ▼ 2–16 years: 22–28 mmol/L
  - ▼ >16 years: 24–32 mmol/L

❏ **Use**

- To evaluate the total CO_3^{2-} buffering system in the body as well as the acid–base balance

❏ **Interpretation**

Increased In

- Respiratory acidosis with CO_2 retention
- Metabolic alkalosis (e.g., prolonged vomiting)
- Airway obstruction
- Alcoholism
- Aldosteronism
- Cardiac disorders
- Emphysema
- Fat embolism
- Pulmonary dysfunction
- Renal disorders

Decreased In

- Respiratory alkalosis, as in hyperventilation
- Metabolic acidosis (e.g., diabetes with ketoacidosis)
- Alcoholic ketosis
- Dehydration
- Diarrhea
- Head trauma
- High fever
- Hepatic disorders
- Hyperventilation
- Malabsorption syndromes
- Starvation and uremia

❏ **Limitations**

- Antacids, corticotrophin, mercurial and thiazide diuretics, and sodium bicarbonate increase blood levels.
- Acetazolamide, ammonium chloride, aspirin, chlorothiazide diuretics, methicillin, paraldehyde, and tetracycline decrease blood levels.
- High altitudes decrease values.
- Hyperthermia increases blood levels.

CARBOXYHEMOGLOBIN (CARBON MONOXIDE, COHB, HBCO)

❏ **Definition**

- COHB is Hb with carbon monoxide (CO) instead of the normal oxygen bound to it. CO has a much great affinity than oxygen for Hb. The source of the CO may be exhaust (such as from a car, truck, boat, or generator), smoke from a fire, or tobacco smoke. COHB is formed in CO poisoning. The

COHB level is useful in judging the extent of CO toxicity and in considering the effect of smoking on the patient. A direct correlation has been claimed between CO level and symptoms of atherosclerotic diseases, angina, and MI. Physiologically, COHB levels increase due to hemolysis. CO is a natural by-product of the breakdown of protoporphyrin to bilirubin.

■ **Normal range:**
  ▼ Nonsmokers: 0.5–1.5% saturation of Hb
  ▼ Smokers (1–2 packs/day): 4–5%
  ▼ Heavy smokers (>2 packs/day): 8–9%

❏ **Use**
  ■ Verifying CO toxicity in cases of suspected exposure

❏ **Interpretation**
Increased In
  ■ CO poisoning
  ■ Hemolytic disease
  ■ Blood in the intestine
  ■ Reactions of intestinal bacteria
  ■ Calorie reduction
  ■ Following exercise
  ■ Methylene chloride toxicity (found in paint removers)

❏ **Limitations**
  ■ COHB diminishes at a rate of about 15% per hour when the patient is removed from the contaminated environment.
  ■ The most common cause of CO toxicity is exposure to automobile exhaust fumes. Significant levels of COHB can also be observed in heavy smokers. Victims of fires often show elevated levels from inhaling CO generated during combustion.
  ■ Susceptibility to CO poisoning is increased in anemic persons.

CARCINOEMBRYONIC ANTIGEN (CEA)

❏ **Definition**
  ■ CEA is a glycoprotein normally produced only during early fetal life and rapid multiplication of epithelial cells, especially those of the digestive system. CEA also appears in the blood of chronic smokers. Less than 25% of patients with disease confined to the colon have elevated CEA. Sensitivity is increased with advancing tumor stage. CEA levels should be ordered only after malignancy has been confirmed. CEA levels typically return to normal within 4–6 weeks after surgical resection. Major role is in following patients for relapse after intended curative treatment. The American Society of Clinical Oncology recommends monitoring CEA levels every 2–3 months for at least 2 years in patients with stage II and III disease.
  ■ **Normal values:** <2.5 ng/mL in nonsmokers; <5 ng/mL in smokers.

❏ **Use**
  ■ Monitoring colorectal cancer and selected other cancers such as medullary thyroid carcinoma, cancers of the rectum, lung, pancreas, stomach, and ovaries

- May be useful in assessing the effectiveness of chemotherapy or radiation treatment
- Diagnosis of malignant pleural effusion
- Not useful in screening the general population for undetected cancers

❑ **Interpretation**

Increased In

- Cancer. There is a wide overlap in values between benign and malignant disease. Increased concentrations are suggestive but not diagnostic of cancer.
  - ▼ Seventy-five percent of patients with carcinoma of endodermal origin (colon, stomach, pancreas, lung) have CEA titers >2.5 ng/mL, and two thirds of these titers are >5 ng/mL. CEA is increased in about one third of patients with small cell carcinoma of the lung and in about two thirds with non–small cell carcinoma of the lung.
  - ▼ Fifty percent of patients with carcinoma of nonentodermal origin (especially cancer of the breast, head and neck, ovary) have CEA titers >2.5 ng/mL, and 50% of the titers are >5 ng/mL. Titers are increased in >50% of cases of breast cancer with metastases and 25% without metastases, but they are not associated with benign lesions.
  - ▼ Forty percent of patients with noncarcinomatous malignant disease have increased CEA concentrations, usually 2.5–5.0 ng/mL.
  - ▼ Increased in 90% of all patients with solid tissue tumors, especially with metastases to the liver or lung, but they are increased in only 50% of patients with local disease or only intra-abdominal metastases.
  - ▼ May be increased in effusion fluid due to these cancers. Active nonmalignant inflammatory diseases (especially of the GI tract [e.g., ulcerative colitis, regional enteritis, diverticulitis, peptic ulcer, chronic pancreatitis]) frequently have elevated concentrations that decline when the disease is in remission.
- Liver disease (alcoholic, cirrhosis, chronic active hepatitis, obstructive jaundice) because metabolized by the liver.
- Other disorders:
  - ▼ Renal failure
  - ▼ Fibrocystic disease of the breast

❑ **Limitations**

- When an abnormal level is found, the test should be repeated. If confirmed, the patient should undergo imaging of potential reoccurrence sites.
- Same methodology should be used to monitor an individual patient. A significant change in plasma concentration is +25%.
- After complete removal of colon cancer, CEA should fall to normal in 6–12 weeks. Failure to decline to normal concentrations postoperatively suggests incomplete resection. Immunohistochemistry of resected specimen is used to identify 20% of these cancers that do not express CEA for whom monitoring is misleading. In such cases, may use serum ALP and diagnostic imaging.
- Prognosis is related to serum concentration at time of diagnosis (stage of disease and likelihood of recurrence). CEA concentrations <5 ng/mL before therapy suggest localized disease and a favorable prognosis, but a concentration >10 ng/mL suggests extensive disease and a poor prognosis; >80% of colon carcinoma patients with values >20 ng/mL have recurrence within 14 months

16

after surgery. Plasma CEA >20 ng/mL correlates with tumor volume in breast and colon cancer and is usually associated with metastatic disease or with a few types of cancer (e.g., cancer of the colon or pancreas); however, metastases may occur with concentrations <20 ng/mL. Values <2.5 ng/mL do not rule out primary, metastatic, or recurrent cancer. Increased values in node-negative colon cancer may identify poorer-risk patients who may benefit from chemotherapy.

- Patterns of CEA change during chemotherapy.
  - ▼ Uninterrupted increase indicating failure to respond.
  - ▼ Decrease indicating response to therapy.
  - ▼ Surge in CEA for weeks followed by a decrease indicating response.
  - ▼ Immediate, sustained decrease followed by an increase indicating lack of response to therapy.
  - ▼ Significant is 25–35% change from baseline of equal or increased values during the first 2 months of therapy.
  - ▼ Survival is significantly longer if titer decreases below this baseline.

CARDIOVASCULAR DRUGS (SEE DIGOXIN)*

❏ **Definition**
- Cardiovascular drugs include the antiarrhythmics, the anticoagulant warfarin, and antihypertensives, as well as the β-adrenergic antagonist propranolol and the drug digoxin (see p. 925).
- **Normal therapeutic values:** see Table 16.15.

❏ **Use**
- To treat arrhythmia, hypertension, blood clotting, and angina.
- The majority of these drugs are not routinely monitored as clinical effects do not generally correlate with serum or plasma levels. Notable exceptions are digoxin and procainamide.
- Where concentrations are required, specific gas chromatography and HPLC procedures have been developed (e.g., procainamide/N-acetylprocainamide [NAPA], quinidine, mexiletine, diltiazem, verapamil, amiodarone, and metabolite, warfarin). Limits of quantitation vary according to the drug and methodology.
- Immunoassay tests (e.g., FPIA) are available for procainamide, quinidine.
- In addition, lidocaine, diltiazem, verapamil, and quinidine are qualitatively detectable in urine with a simple alkaline liquid–liquid or solid-phase extraction followed by GC/MS analysis. Limits of detection range from 50 to 250 ng/mL.

❏ **Interpretation**
- Rifampin may decrease verapamil serum concentrations.

❏ **Limitations**
- With procainamide, separate cells from plasma as soon as possible to prevent loss of drug during storage.
- Hemolyzed samples are unacceptable.

---

*Submitted By Amanda J. Jenkins, PhD.

TABLE 16–15. Cardiovascular Drugs

| Drug Name | | | Therapeutic | Potential Toxic |
Generic	Brand	Used to Treat	Level	Level*
Antiarrhythmics				
Amiodarone	Cordarone	Supraventricular and ventricular arrhythmias[†]	1.5–2.5 µg/mL	≥3.0 µg/mL
Flecainide	Tambocor	Ventricular arrhythmias	0.2–1.0 µg/mL [trough]	>1.0 µg/mL
Lidocaine	Xylocaine	Ventricular arrhythmias (also prevention)	1.4–6.0 µg/mL	>6.0 µg/mL
Mexiletine	Mexitil	Arrhythmias	0.5–2.0 µg/mL [trough]	>1.5 µg/mL
Procainamide (active metabolite: NAPA) NAPA: 6–20 µg/mL	Pronestyl Procainamide: ≥12 µg/mL	Supraventricular and ventricular arrhythmias	Procainamide: 4–10 µg/mL	NAPA: >30 µg/mL
Quinidine	Duraquin	Supraventricular and ventricular arrhythmias	1.5–4.5 µg/mL	>10.0 µg/mL
Verapamil (calcium channel blocker)	Calan	Supraventricular dysrhythmias, angina pectoris, and hypertension	50–200 ng/mL [peak serum]	≥400 ng/mL [peak serum]
Anticoagulant				
Warfarin	Coumadin	Blood clotting; drug, a synthetic vitamin K antagonist, is an anticoagulant[‡]	7 mg/L	10 mg/L
Antihypertensives				
Diltiazem (calcium channel blocker)	Cardizem	Angina pectoris and hypertension[§]	40–200 ng/mL	
Nifedipine	Procardia	Angina pectoris and hypertension[¶]	25–100 ng/mL	>100 ng/mL
Beta–adrenergic Antagonist				
Propranolol	Inderal	Arrhythmias and hypertension	30–250 ng/mL	

*Toxic concentrations have not been established.
[†]Monitor TSH and T_4 values during therapy.
[‡]Prothrombin time is used to assess efficacy as target INR: 2.0–3.0. Consider long-term, low-intensity (INR 1.5–2.0), or standard-intensity (INR 2–3) warfarin therapy for patients with idiopathic events.
[§]Effect on platelets may increase bleeding time.
[¶]Decreased glucose tolerance.

16

CATECHOLAMINES, SERUM

❏ **Definition**

- The catecholamines (epinephrine, norepinephrine, and dopamine) are found in the adrenal medulla, neurons, and brain. All three catecholamines are derived from tyrosine and are important neurotransmitters in the CNS and also play a crucial role in the autonomic regulation of many homeostatic functions. Other names: adrenaline, catecholamine fractionation, unconjugated dopamine, epinephrine, noradrenaline, and norepinephrine.
- **Normal range:** see Table 16.16.

❏ **Use**

- Diagnosis of pheochromocytoma and paraganglioma, as an auxiliary test to fractionated plasma and urine metanephrine measurements.
- Diagnosis and follow-up of patients with neuroblastoma and related tumors, as an auxiliary test to urine VMA and homovanillic acid (HVA) measurements.
- Evaluation of patients with autonomic dysfunction/failure or autonomic neuropathy.

❏ **Interpretation**

Increased In (Epinephrine)

- Anger, exercise, fear, burns
- Ganglioblastoma and ganglioneuroma
- Hypoglycemia
- Hypotension

TABLE 16–16. Normal Range for Catecholamines

Age	Value in pg/mL
Epinephrine	
2–10 d	36–400
11 d–3 mo	55–200
4–11 mo	55–440
12–23 mo	36–640
24–35 mo	18–440
3–17 y	18–460
≥18 y	10–200
Norepinephrine	
2–10 d	170–1,180
11 d–3 mo	370–2,080
4–11 mo	270–1,120
12–23 mo	68–1,810
24–35 mo	170–1,470
3–17 y	85–1,250
≥18 y	80–520
Dopamine	
≥2 d	0–20

- Hypothyroidism
- DKA
- Neuroblastoma
- Paragangliomas
- Pheochromocytoma

Decreased In
- Norepinephrine: anorexia nervosa
- Autonomous nervous system dysfunction
- Orthostatic hypotension
- Dopamine: possibly decreased in Parkinson disease

❑ Limitations
- Most assays measure only free catecholamines, but a few measure both free and conjugated types. Free amines are more closely associated with tumor load than conjugated ones.
- Physiologic stimuli, drugs, or improper specimen collection slightly increases the levels. Patients should not eat, use tobacco, or drink caffeinated beverages for at least 4 hours before collection. Measurement of plasma or urine fractionated metanephrines provides better diagnostic sensitivity than measurement of catecholamines.
- Plasma levels drop quickly within 5 minutes if RBCs are not separated from plasma once collected.
- Amphetamines and amphetamine-like compounds, appetite suppressants, bromocriptine, buspirone, caffeine, carbidopa–levodopa, clonidine, dexamethasone, diuretics (in doses sufficient to deplete sodium), ethanol, isoproterenol, labetalol, methyldopa, MAO inhibitors, nicotine, nose drops, propafenone (Rythmol), reserpine, theophylline, tricyclic antidepressants, and vasodilators may interfere with this test, and the results may not be predictable.
- Children under 2 years of age show elevated response to stress.
- For accurate results, patient should be in supine for 30 minutes prior to collection.

CELL COUNT, BODY FLUID ANALYSIS*

❑ Introduction
- This section focuses on the microscopic evaluation of fluids accumulated in body cavities: cerebrospinal, pleural, pericardial, and peritoneal (ascites). Synovial fluids are described below under "Other Body Fluids." Aspiration followed by chemical, microscopic, cytologic, microbiologic, and, if indicated, flow cytometry examinations should help determine the etiology of accumulated pathologic fluids by providing important information regarding infection, hemorrhage, inflammation, or malignant infiltration. Total cell counts are performed using undiluted (or in the case of very high counts, diluted) body fluids with a hemocytometer. Differential counts are done using a smear following centrifugation (Cytospin) and staining with

16

---

*Submitted By Liberto Pechet, MD.

Wright-Giemsa stain. Bacterial identification and cultures and the chemistry of body fluids are described separately.

CEREBROSPINAL FLUID (CSF)*

❑ **Definition**

- CSF is produced by the choroid plexus in the lateral third and fourth ventricles of the brain. In normal adults, the total CSF volume is 90–150 mL. Eighty percent of the CSF is contained in the arachnoid space in the cranium and spinal cord, where a small amount can be extracted for examination, most commonly through a lumbar puncture. CSF pressure is measured by a manometer.
- **Normal values:**
  - ▼ Appearance: clear, colorless
  - ▼ Normal opening adult pressure: 90–180 mL of water in an adult in the lateral decubitus position with the legs and neck in a neutral position
  - ▼ Cell count and differential (Table 16.17):
    - ● Adults: WBC 0–5 cells/mm^3, RBC 0/mm^3
    - ● Newborns: WBC 0–30/mm^3, RBC 0/mm^3

❑ **Use**

- Examination of CSF is required when CNS involvement by inflammatory, infectious, neoplastic, or neurologic complications are suspected. Up to 20 mL of fluid can be removed in the adult.
- CSF is divided into three sterile tubes:
  - ▼ Chemistry and immunology studies
  - ▼ Microbiology examinations
  - ▼ Cell count, differential, and cytology (if indicated)

❑ **Interpretation**

- Increased number or red blood cells: either hemorrhagic tap or subarachnoid hemorrhage
- Increased number of neutrophils: bacterial or early viral CNS infection, early CNS TB, CNS syphilis, fungal infection, contamination with peripheral blood through traumatic tap, CNS hemorrhage
- Increased number of lymphocytes: viral infection of the CNS, CNS TB, acute lymphocytic leukemia or lymphoma of the CNS, cryptococcal infection of

TABLE 16–17. Differential Counts for CSF (Mean ± SD)

Type of Cells	Adults	Neonates
Lymphocytes	62% ± 34	20% ± 18
Mononuclear cells and monocytes	36% ± 20	72% ± 22
Neutrophils	2% ± 5	3% ± 5
Histiocytes	Rare	Rare
Eosinophils	Rare	Rare

*Submitted By Liberto Pechet, MD.

the CNS, fungal infection of the CNS, CNS syphilis, parasitic disease infecting the CNS, Guillain-Barré syndrome
- Increased eosinophils: parasitic infection of the CNS, fungal infection of the CNS, viral infection of the CNS, CNS syphilis, allergic reaction
- Increased basophils: chronic myelogenous leukemia
- Tumor cells: primary or metastatic tumors of the CNS
- Xanthochromia (yellowish discoloration): marker of previous intracerebral bleeding

OTHER BODY FLUIDS: PLEURAL, PERICARDIAL, AND PERITONEAL SPACES

❑ **Definition**
- Under normal conditions, a very small amount of fluid (up to 50 mL) is present. This facilitates movement of membranes against each other. Abnormal fluid accumulation is called a serous effusion. In the presence of effusions, fluid can be aspirated from the affected cavity, either for diagnosis or for relief of pressure, commonly both. Finding substantial amounts of fluid always reflects a pathologic process.

❑ **Interpretation**
- Pleural fluid
  - ▼ Appearance
    - Cloudiness: neutrophils present, indicating infection
    - Milkiness: chylous effusion
    - Bloody: traumatic tap, malignancy, pneumonia, trauma, status postmyocardial infarction, or pulmonary infarction
  - ▼ Cell counts and differentials
    - WBC count $>1 \times 10^9$/L with lymphocytes >50%: TB, cancer, lymphoma, CLL
    - WBC count $>1 \times 10^{10}$/L with approximately 80% neutrophils: effusions associated with bacterial pneumonia
    - WBC with eosinophilia: postpneumothorax, trauma, hypersensitivity reactions, CHF, fungal and parasitic infections, SLE, Hodgkin lymphoma
- Pericardial fluid
  - ▼ Appearance
    - Bloody: pericarditis, status postmyocardial infarction, TB, RA, SLE, carcinoma, aspiration of blood from the cardiac cavity
  - ▼ Cell counts and differential
    - WBC count 1×10^9/L with increased lymphocytes: pericardial tuberculosis
    - WBC count 1×10^9/L with increased neutrophils: bacterial or viral pericarditis
- Peritoneal fluid
  - ▼ Appearance
    - Cloudy or turbid: appendicitis, pancreatitis, intestinal volvulus, ruptured bowel, sepsis
    - Bile-stained: perforated duodenal ulcer, perforated intestine, gallbladder disease or perforation, acute pancreatitis

16

- Milky: chylous effusion
- Bloody: traumatic tap, intra-abdominal injury

▼ Cell counts and differential on lavage fluid

- RBC count >1 × 10^{11}/L: intra-abdominal injury
- WBC count 0.5 × 10^9/L: possible peritonitis

▼ Cell counts and differential on undiluted ascitic fluid

- WBC count 0.3 × 10^9/L: bacterial peritonitis if >50% neutrophils, cirrhosis of the liver if <25% neutrophils
- Increased lymphocytes: tuberculous peritonitis
- Increased eosinophils: CHF, hypereosinophilic syndrome, eosinophilic gastroenteritis, chronic peritoneal dialysis, abdominal lymphoma, ruptured hydatid cyst, vasculitis

❏ Limitations

- All cell counts should be performed promptly to prevent cell deterioration; distorted or degenerated cells should not be counted.
- Specimens with large clots cannot be processed.

CERULOPLASMIN

❏ Definition

- Major copper-carrying protein in the blood. An α-2 globulin, it plays a role in both iron and copper metabolism. Other names: CP, ferroxidase, iron(II):oxygen oxidoreductase.
- **Normal range: 22–58 mg/dL.**

❏ Use

- Evaluation of acute-phase response
- Assessment of possible Wilson disease
- Assessment of Menkes kinky hair syndrome, aceruloplasminemia

❏ Interpretation

Increased In

- Inflammation, infection (acute and chronic), tissue injury
- Cardiovascular disease
- Pregnancy (double the baseline values in third trimester)
- Cancer
- Cirrhosis
- Estrogen supplementation and oral contraceptives
- RA
- Primary sclerosing cholangitis
- Alzheimer disease
- Use of birth control pills

Decreased In

- Hepatolenticular degeneration (Wilson disease)
- Autosomal recessive disease involving copper metabolism
- Kwashiorkor, malabsorption

- Nephrosis, nephritic syndrome
- Menkes kinky hair syndrome
- Aceruloplasminemia

❑ **Limitations**

- Anticonvulsant therapy, methadone, tamoxifen, oral contraceptives, and smoking increase serum levels.

CHLORIDE

❑ **Definition**

- Chloride is the major extracellular anion; it is not actively regulated normally. It reflects changes in sodium; if it changes independent of sodium, this is usually due to an acid–base disorder.
- **Normal range: 97–110 mmol/L.**

❑ **Use**

- With sodium, potassium, and carbon dioxide to assess electrolyte, acid–base, and water balance. Chloride usually changes in the same direction as sodium except in metabolic acidosis with bicarbonate depletion and metabolic alkalosis with bicarbonate excess, when serum sodium levels may be normal.

❑ **Interpretation**

Increased In

- Metabolic acidosis associated with prolonged diarrhea with loss of sodium bicarbonate
- Renal tubular diseases with decreased excretion of hydrogen ions and decreased reabsorption of bicarbonate ("hyperchloremic metabolic acidosis")
- Respiratory alkalosis (e.g., hyperventilation, severe CNS damage)
- Drugs
- Excessive administration of certain drugs (e.g., ammonium chloride, IV saline, salicylate intoxication, acetazolamide therapy)
- False (methodologic) increase due to bromides or other halogens
- Retention of salt and water (e.g., corticosteroids, guanethidine, phenylbutazone)
- Some cases of hyperparathyroidism
- Diabetes insipidus, dehydration
- Sodium loss > chloride loss (e.g., diarrhea, intestinal fistulas)
- Ureterosigmoidostomy

Decreased In

- Prolonged vomiting or suction (loss of hydrochloric acid)
- Metabolic acidosis with accumulation of organic anions
- Chronic respiratory acidosis
- Salt-losing renal diseases
- Adrenocortical insufficiency
- Primary aldosteronism
- Expansion of extracellular fluid (e.g., SIADH, hyponatremia, water intoxication, CHF)

16

- Burns
- Drugs
- Alkalosis (e.g., bicarbonates, aldosterone, corticosteroids)
- Diuretic effect (e.g., ethacrynic acid, furosemide, thiazides)
- Other loss (e.g., chronic laxative abuse)

❏ **Limitations**

- Direct ISE (ion-selective electrode) measurements do not give the volume displacement error in specimens with high lipid or protein content, as indirect ISE and flame measurements do.
- May be slightly decreased after meals; fasting specimen collection is recommended.

CHLORIDE, URINE

❏ **Definition**

- Chloride is reabsorbed with sodium throughout the nephron. Because of its relationship with other electrolytes, urinary chloride results can be used to help assess volume status, salt intake, and causes of hypokalemia and to aid in the diagnosis of renal tubular acidosis (RTA). Approximately 30% of hypovolemic patients have >15 mmol/L difference between urine sodium and chloride concentrations. This is due to the excretion of sodium with another anion (such as bicarbonate, HCO_3^-) or to the excretion of chloride with another cation (such as ammonium, NH_4^+). The normal response to acidemia is to increase urinary acid excretion, primarily NH_4^+. When urine NH_4^+ levels are high, the urine anion gap [(Na + K) – Cl] will have a negative value, since chloride levels will exceed that of Na and K by the approximate amount of NH_4^+ in the urine. Therefore, the urine chloride concentration may be inappropriately high in diarrhea-induced hypovolemia because of the need to maintain the electroneutrality as NH_4^+ excretion is enhanced.
- **Normal range:** see Table 16.18.

❏ **Use**

- Assess volume status, salt intake, and causes of hypokalemia. It is helpful to measure urine chloride concentration in a patient who seems to be volume depleted but has a somewhat elevated urine sodium concentration.
- Aid in the diagnosis of RTA.
- Evaluate electrolyte composition of urine and acid–base balance studies. It is helpful to measure urine chloride in patients with a normal anion gap metabolic acidosis. In the absence of renal failure, this may be due to diarrhea or one of the forms of RTA.

❏ **Interpretation**
Increased In

- Postmenstrual diuresis
- Massive diuresis from any cause
- Salt-losing nephritis
- Potassium depletion

TABLE 16–18. Normal Values for Urine Chloride	
24-h Urine	**mmol/d**
Male	
<10 y	36–110
10–14 y	64–176
>14 y	110–250
>60 y	95–195
Female	
<10 y	18–74
10–14 y	36–173
>14 y	110–250
>60 y	95–195
Random urine	**mmol/g creatinine**
Male	25–253
Female	39–348

- Adrenocortical insufficiency
- Tubulointerstitial disease
- Batter syndrome

Decreased In
- Premenstrual salt and water retention
- Excessive extrarenal chloride loss
- Adrenocortical hyperfunction
- Postoperative chloride retention

❑ **Limitations**
- Urine chloride excretion approximates the dietary intake.
- Bromides can cause falsely elevated results.

CHOLESTEROL, HIGH-DENSITY LIPOPROTEIN (HDL)

❑ **Definition**
- HDL, also known as HDL-C, is produced by the liver and consists of mostly cholesterol, protein, and phospholipid. It carries cholesterol in the bloodstream from the tissues to the liver (reverse cholesterol transport). HDL is termed the "good cholesterol," because its levels are inversely related to CHD, and it is an independent risk factor.
- **Normal range:** see Table 16.19.

❑ **Use**
- Assessment of risk of heart disease and atherosclerosis
- Ordered in combination with total cholesterol, LDL, and triglycerides as a lipid profile

❑ **Interpretation**
Increased In
- Hyperalphalipoproteinemia

TABLE 16–19. Reference Values for HDL Cholesterol

HDL Cholesterol Level	Comments
<40 mg/dL	Major risk factor for heart disease
40–59 mg/dL	"The higher, the better"
≥60 mg/dL	Considered protective against heart disease

- Regular physical activity or exercise
- Weight loss
- Chronic liver disease

Decreased In
- Uncontrolled diabetes
- Hepatocellular disease
- Chronic renal failure, nephrosis, uremia
- Cholestasis
- Abetalipoproteinemia
- Familial hyper-α-lipoproteinemia (Tangier disease)
- Deficiency of apo A-I and apo C-III

❑ **Limitations**
- HDL is increased due to moderate ethanol consumption, estrogens, and insulin.
- HDL is decreased due to starvation; stress and recent illness; smoking; obesity and lack of exercise; drugs such as steroids, thiazide diuretics, and beta blockers; hypertriglyceridemia (>1,700 mg/dL); and elevated serum immunoglobulin levels.
- Other factors that may also increase cholesterol include cigarette smoking, age, hypertension, family history of premature heart disease, preexisting heart disease, and DM.
- Low levels of HDL-C (with or without associated co-lipid abnormalities) are seen in Asians than in non-Asians. This is a distinct phenotype associated with increased risk for CHD.

Suggested Reading

National Institutes of Health, National Heart Lung and Blood Institute's National Cholesterol Education Program. http://www.nhlbi.nih.gov/about/ncep/. Accessed November 18, 2010.

CHOLESTEROL, LOW-DENSITY LIPOPROTEIN (LDL)

❑ **Definition**
- LDL cholesterol, also known as LDL-C, is produced by the metabolism of VLDL cholesterol and consists of mostly cholesterol, protein, and phospholipids that carry cholesterol in the bloodstream from the liver to the peripheral tissues. LDL-C is termed the "bad cholesterol," and LDL-C levels are associated with atherosclerosis and coronary heart disease.
- Normal range: see Table 16.20.

TABLE 16–20. Reference Intervals for LDL Cholesterol

LDL Cholesterol Level	Category
<100 mg/dL	Optimal
100–129 mg/dL	Near optimal/above optimal
130–159 mg/dL	Borderline high
160–189 mg/dL	High
≥190 mg/dL	Very high

❑ **Use**

- To determine risk of heart disease and atherosclerosis. LDL-C is calculated when ordered in combination with total cholesterol, HDL cholesterol, and triglycerides as a lipid profile.

❑ **Interpretation**

Increased In

- Familial hypercholesterolemia
- Nephrotic syndrome
- Hepatic disease
- Hepatic obstruction
- Chronic renal failure
- Hyperlipidemia types II and III
- DM

Decreased In

- Abetalipoproteinemia
- Hyperthyroidism
- Tangier disease
- Hypolipoproteinemia
- Chronic anemia
- Lecithin cholesterol acyltransferase deficiency
- Apo C-II deficiency
- Hyperlipidemia type I

❑ **Limitations**

- LDL-C values may be high because of a diet high in saturated fats and cholesterol, pregnancy, or use of steroids.
- LDL values should be measured only on fasting samples.
- LDL cholesterol may be decreased because of acute stress, recent illness, and estrogens.
- Other factors that may affect LDL-C values: cigarette smoking, hypertension (blood pressure >140/90 mm Hg or taking antihypertensive medication), family history of premature CHD (CHD in male first-degree relative <55 years; CHD in female first-degree relative <65 years), and age (men >45 years; women >55 years). See Table 16.21 for additional information.
- At this time, there are no specific recommendations on the routine measurement of LDL particle size and number.

16

TABLE 16–21. Adult Treatment Panel III LDL-C Goals and Cutoff Points for Therapy

Risk Category	LDL-C Goal	Initiate TLC	Consider Drug Therapy[1]
High risk: CHD[2] or CHD risk equivalents[3] (10-y risk >20%)	<100 mg/dL (optional goal: <70 mg/dL)[4]	≥100 mg/dL[5]	≥100 mg/dL[6] (<100 mg/dL: consider drug options)[1]
Moderately high risk: 2+ risk factors[7] (10-y risk 10–20%)[8]	<130 mg/dL[9]	≥130 mg/dL[5]	≥130 mg/dL (100–129 mg/dL: consider drug options)[10]
Moderate risk: 2+ risk factors[7] (10-y risk <10%)[8]	<130 mg/dL	≥130 mg/dL	≥160 mg/dL
Lower risk: 0–1 risk factor[11]	<160 mg/dL	≥160 mg/dL	≥190 mg/dL (160–189 mg/dL: LDL-C–lowering drug optional)

[1]When LDL-lowering drug therapy is employed, it is advised that intensity of therapy be sufficient to achieve at least a 30–40% reduction in LDL-C levels.

[2]Coronary heart disease (CHD) includes history of myocardial infarction, unstable angina, stable angina, coronary artery procedures (angioplasty or bypass surgery), or evidence of clinically significant myocardial ischemia.

[3]CHD risk equivalents include clinical manifestations of noncoronary forms of atherosclerotic disease (peripheral arterial disease, abdominal aortic aneurysm, and carotid artery disease [transient ischemic attacks or stroke of carotid origin or >50% obstruction of a carotid artery]), diabetes, and 2+ risk factors with 10-y risk for hard CHD >20%.

[4]Very high risk favors the optional LDL-C goal of <70 mg/dL, and in patients with high triglycerides, non–HDL-C <100 mg/dL.

[5]Any person at high risk or moderately high risk who has lifestyle-related risk factors (e.g., obesity, physical inactivity, elevated triglyceride, low HDL-C, or metabolic syndrome) is a candidate for therapeutic lifestyle changes to modify these risk factors regardless of LDL-C level.

[6]If baseline LDL-C is <100 mg/dL, institution of an LDL-lowering drug is a therapeutic option on the basis of available clinical trial results. If a high-risk person has high triglycerides or low HDL-C, combining a fibrate or nicotinic acid with an LDL-lowering drug can be considered.

[7]Risk factors include cigarette smoking, hypertension (BP >140/90 mm Hg or on antihypertensive medication), low HDL-C (<40 mg/dL), family history of premature CHD (CHD in male first-degree relative <55 y of age; CHD in female first-degree relative <65 y of age), and age (men ≥45 y; women ≥55 y).

[8]Electronic 10-y risk calculators are available at www.nhlbi.nih.gov/guidelines/cholesterol.

[9]Optional LDL-C goal <100 mg/dL.

[10]For moderately high-risk persons, when LDL-C level is 100–129 mg/dL, at baseline or on lifestyle therapy, initiation of an LDL-lowering drug to achieve an LDL-C level <100 mg/dL is a therapeutic option on the basis of available clinical trial results.

[11]Almost all people with zero or 1 risk factor have a 10-y risk <10%, and 10-y risk assessment in people with zero or 1 risk factor is thus not necessary.

❏ **Other Considerations**

▪ The lipid profile does not measure LDL level directly but rather estimates it using the Friedewald equation:

$$LDL - C(mg / dL) = total\,cholesterol\\ -HDL\,cholesterol - (0.20 \times triglycerides)$$

▪ Note: The formula is only valid from a fasting specimen, and triglycerides must be <400 mg/dL.
▪ LDL-C can be measured directly when the triglycerides are elevated.

Suggested Reading

National Institutes of Health, National Heart Lung and Blood Institute's National Cholesterol Education Program. http://www.nhlbi.nih.gov/about/ncep/. Accessed November 18, 2010.

CHOLESTEROL, TOTAL, SERUM

❏ **Definition**

▪ A steroid, carried in the bloodstream as a lipoprotein. It is necessary for cell membrane functioning and as a precursor to bile acids, progesterone, vitamin D, estrogens, glucocorticoids, and mineralocorticoids.
▪ **Normal range:** see Table 16.22.

❏ **Use**

▪ Assessment of risk of heart disease and atherosclerosis
▪ Ordered in combination with HDL, LDL, and triglycerides as a lipid profile

❏ **Interpretation**

Increased In

▪ Pregnancy
▪ Drugs: beta blockers, anabolic steroids, vitamin D, oral contraceptives, and epinephrine
▪ Obesity
▪ Smoking
▪ Alcohol
▪ Diet high in cholesterol and fats

TABLE 16–22. Initial Classification Based on Total Cholesterol and HDL Cholesterol

Total Cholesterol Level	Category
<200 mg/dL	Desirable level that puts a person at a lower risk of coronary heart disease. A cholesterol level of ≥200 mg/dL raises the risk
200–239 mg/dL	Borderline high
≥240 mg/dL	High blood cholesterol. A person with this level has more than twice the risk of CHD as someone whose cholesterol is <200 mg/dL

16

- Renal failure
- Hypothyroidism
- Glycogen storage disease (i.e., von Gierke and Werner diseases)
- Familial hypercholesterolemia
- DM
- Biliary cirrhosis, hepatocellular disease
- Hyperlipoproteinemia types I, IV, V
- Prostate and pancreatic neoplasms

Decreased In
- Acute illness such as a heart attack
- Malnutrition
- Liver disease
- Myeloproliferative diseases
- Chronic anemias
- Infection
- Hyperthyroidism
- Stress
- Primary lipoproteinemias
- Tangier disease (familial alphalipoprotein deficiency)

❏ **Limitations**
- Intraindividual variation may be up to 10%.
- Seasonal variation is 8% higher in the winter than in summer.
- Positional variation is 5% and 10–15% lower when phlebotomized sitting or recumbent, respectively, as opposed to standing.
- Other factors that may also increase cholesterol include cigarette smoking, age, hypertension, family history of premature heart disease, preexisting heart disease, and DM.

Suggested Reading

American Heart Association. Cholesterol. http://www.heart.org/HEARTORG/Conditions/Cholesterol/CholestrolATH_UCM_001089_SubHomePage.jsp. Accessed November 18, 2010.

CHOLINESTERASE (PSEUDOCHOLINESTERASE) AND DIBUCAINE INHIBITION

❏ **Definition**
- Cholinesterase is an enzyme that catalyzes the hydrolysis of the neurotransmitter Ach into choline and acetic acid, a reaction necessary to allow a cholinergic neuron to return to its resting state after activation.
- Serum cholinesterase, often called pseudocholinesterase or PChE, is distinguished from acetylcholinesterase (AChE or "true cholinesterase") by both location and substrate.
  - ▼ PChE is found primarily in the liver.
  - ▼ AChE, also known as RBC cholinesterase, erythrocyte cholinesterase, or Ach acetylhydrolase, is found primarily in the blood and neural synapses.

- The difference between the two types of cholinesterase has to do with their respective preferences for substrates: AChE hydrolyzes Ach more quickly, and PChE hydrolyzes butyrylcholine more quickly.
- Phenotype interpretation is based on the total PChE activity and the percent of inhibition caused by dibucaine. Although there are >25 different phenotypes, most are extremely rare. Patients with unusual phenotypes cannot metabolize succinylcholine or mivacurium in the normal fashion; therefore, these patients can have prolonged paralysis following the use of these drugs.
- Other names: choline esterase II, SChE, Ach acylhydrolase, butyrylcholinesterase (BChE), dibucaine inhibition, and plasma cholinesterase.
- **Normal range:**
  - ▼ Pseudocholinesterase, total: 2,900–7,100 U/L
  - ▼ Dibucaine inhibition: 70–90% (congenital deficiency 18–20%)

❑ Use

- Monitoring exposure to organophosphorus insecticides
- Monitoring patients with liver disease, particularly those undergoing liver transplantation
- Identifying patients who are homozygous for the atypical gene and have low levels of PChE that are not inhibited by dibucaine
- Identifying patients, who are heterozygous for the atypical gene and have lower than normal levels of PChE and varying levels of inhibition with dibucaine

❑ Interpretation
Increased In
- Type IV hyperlipoproteinemia
- DM
- Hyperthyroidism
- Insecticide exposure (organophosphates)
- Nephritic syndrome
- Psychosis
- Breast cancer

Decreased In
- Genetic PChE variants
- Severe pernicious anemia (PA), aplastic anemia
- Cirrhosis
- CHF (causing liver disease)
- Hepatic carcinoma
- Malnutrition
- Acute infections and burns
- AMI, pulmonary embolism
- Muscular dystrophy
- After surgery
- Chronic renal disease

❑ Limitations
- PChE levels are not to be confused with AChE levels. PChE levels are earlier indicators than AChE levels of organophosphate exposure.

16

- Patients with normal PChE activity show 70–90% inhibition by dibucaine, whereas patients homozygous for the abnormal allele show little or no inhibition (0–20%) and usually low levels of enzyme. Heterozygous patients have intermediate PChE levels and response to inhibitors.
- Dibucaine inhibition is no value over total PChE, for the diagnosis of organophosphorus pesticide exposure.
- Anabolic steroids, carbamates, cyclophosphamide, estrogens, glucocorticoids, lithium, neuromuscular relaxants, oral contraceptives, organophosphorus insecticides, and radiographic agents decrease the circulating levels.
- Serum separator tubes, citrate anticoagulants, detergents, and heavy metals also decrease the serum levels.

CHORIONIC VILLUS SAMPLING

See Prenatal Screening.

CHROMOGRANIN A, PLASMA

❑ **Definition**

- Chromogranin, also known as CGA and parathyroid secretory protein 1, is a member of the chromogranin/secretogranin (granins) family of neuroendocrine secretory proteins. It is a precursor to several functional peptides, including vasostatin, pancreastatin, catestatin, and parastatin. These peptides negatively modulate the neuroendocrine function of the releasing cell (autocrine) or nearby cells (paracrine). Chromogranin A is cleaved by an endogenous prohormone convertase to produce several peptide fragments. Peptides derived from chromogranin A with uncertain function include chromostatin, WE-14, and GE-25. The method of measurement is EIA.
- **Normal range: 0–50 ng/mL.**

❑ **Use**

- As an indicator for pancreas and prostate cancer
- Aid in diagnosis of functioning neuroendocrine tumors; predicts response to treatment
- Aid in diagnosis of nonfunctioning neuroendocrine tumors (e.g., thyroid carcinoma, small cell lung cancer, anterior pituitary adenoma)

❑ **Interpretation**
Disorders with Increased Values

- Functioning neuroendocrine tumors and hyperplasia
- Pheochromocytoma, aortic, and carotid body tumors
- Neural tumors (e.g., neuroblastoma, ganglioneuroma, paraganglioma, medulloblastoma)
- Carcinoid tumors in various locations
- Gastroenteropancreatic tumors (e.g., gastrinoma, insulinoma, VIPoma)
- Parathyroid adenoma, carcinoma, hyperplasia
- Thyroid medullary carcinoma, hyperplasia

- Tumors with variable neuroendocrine differentiation (e.g., breast, prostate)— low sensitivity
- DM, kidney, liver, or heart failure; correlates with severity of the CHF

Disorders without Increased Values
- Tumors with possible neuroendocrine lineage (e.g., choriocarcinoma, thymoma, malignant melanoma, renal cell carcinoma)
- After adrenal-to-caudate autografting and schizophrenia

Disorders with Decreased Values
- CSF in Parkinson disease

❏ Limitations

- Chromogranin A may not distinguish neuroendocrine hyperplasia from tumor.
- EIA may have lower limit of detection than RIA. Results obtained with different assay methods or kits cannot be used interchangeably.

CLOT RETRACTION*

Clot retraction does not take place in the absence of functional platelets or of fibrinogen. Historically, it was the earliest test used in the discovery of thrombasthenia, but it is no longer in use.

CLOTTING FACTORS†

❏ Definition

- Clotting factors are circulating plasma proteins. The final coagulation product, the clot, results from the interaction of clotting factors through an enzymatic cascade. In vivo, many of these interactions take place on lipid surfaces, the most abundant of which are provided by platelets. In contrast, in vitro, the cascade can be dissected into three pathways: intrinsic, extrinsic, and common. Although to some extent artificial, this distinction remains useful for performing and understanding the tests of coagulation. For instance, PT reflects the extrinsic and common pathway, whereas PTT reflects the intrinsic and common pathway. Fibrinogen, the penultimate step in the generation of clots, is the target of the common pathway, being changed by thrombin into fibrin; finally, fibrin is consolidated by factor XIII to generate a stable clot, essential for achieving hemostasis through clotting. (Primary hemostasis through activation of platelets and the von Willebrand factor is discussed separately.)
- **Properties of individual clotting factors:**
  - ▼ **Factor II** (prothrombin): Synthesized in the liver; becomes active only after carboxylation by vitamin K. It is converted to thrombin (factor IIa). Its deficiency results in prolonged PT and PTT.
  - ▼ **Thrombin** (factor IIa): A major coagulant that converts fibrinogen into fibrin; has multiple functions, including as an anticoagulant, by binding

---

*Submitted By Liberto Pechet, MD.
†Submitted By Liberto Pechet, MD.

16

to thrombomodulin on endothelial cell surfaces to convert protein C into its active form.

▼ **Factor V:** Synthesized in the liver; 20% is released from platelets. Cofactor in the conversion of factor II to IIa. Vitamin K has no effect on its activity. Proteolyzed by the protein C/S complex.

▼ **Factor VII:** Synthesized in the liver. Becomes activated in a complex with tissue factor. Factor VII requires carboxylation by vitamin K for its activity. Shortest half-life of all clotting factors (4 hours) reflected in the initial rapid elongation in PT (elevation of INR) in patients started on vitamin K antagonists. Recombinant factor VIIa is used therapeutically.

▼ **Factor VIII** (antihemophilic factor): Synthesized in the liver and endothelial cells of others organs (principally the spleen). It is unaffected by liver failure or vitamin K deficiency. Principal cofactor in the intrinsic pathway of coagulation. PT (INR) not affected by deficiency of factor VIII. PTT becomes prolonged when factor VIII decreases to <40%. Serves as substrate for proteolysis by the protein C/S complex. Purified or recombinant factor VIII preparations are used therapeutically.

▼ **Factor IX** (also known as Christmas factor): Synthesized in the liver. Requires vitamin K to become active in coagulation. Principal factor in the intrinsic pathway of coagulation. PT (INR) not affected by deficiency of factor IX. PTT becomes prolonged when factor IX decreases to <40%. Purified and recombinant factor IX are used therapeutically.

▼ **Factor X:** Synthesized in the liver. Requires vitamin K to become active in coagulation. Principal factor in the common pathway of coagulation where it converts factor II into IIA (thrombin). Both PT (INR) and PTT affected in marked deficiencies.

▼ **Factor XI:** Synthesized in the liver and megakaryocytes. Activates factors XII and IX in the intrinsic pathway. If markedly decreased, it may prolong PTT but not PT.

▼ **Factor XII** (Hageman factor): Synthesized in the liver. Activated by collagen, disrupted basement membranes, activated platelets, and high molecular weight kininogen and prekallikrein in conjunction with factor XI. PTT (but not PT) is prolonged in severe deficiency. No bleeding diathesis associated with its congenital deficiency.

▼ **High molecular weight kininogen and prekallikrein** (Fletcher factor): Clotting factors that activate the early phase of the intrinsic pathway and the complement system. May prolong PTT (not PT) when decreased. No bleeding diathesis associated with their congenital deficiencies.

▼ **Factor XIII** (fibrin-stabilizing factor): Synthesized in the liver; also present in platelets. Stabilizes polymerized fibrin in the presence of calcium. Its deficiency does not affect PT (INR) or PTT. In its absence, clots are soluble in 5-molar urea.

▪ **Normal ranges:**
  ▼ *Factors based on PT reagent:*
  - Factor II: 70–120%
  - Factor V: 70–150%
  - Factor VII: 70–150%
  - Factor X: 70–150%

▼ *Factors based on PTT reagent:*
- Factor VIII: 70–150%
- Factor IX: 70–120%
- Factor XI: 60–120%
- Factor XII: 60–150%
- Prekallikrein: 55–207%
- High molecular weight kininogen: 59–135%

❏ Use

- Quantitation of clotting factors can be achieved through assays specific for each factor, whether chromogenic or, more commonly, automated clotting tests. A plasma deficient in each factor is purchased and used to find out whether it corrects the patient's plasma. When there is correction, the patient's defect has been identified and can be quantitated using a reference curve obtained with dilutions of normal pooled plasmas.
- A plasma deficient in any factor(s) active in the extrinsic and common pathway (VII, V, X, and II) results in a prolonged PT. These four factors are quantitated in assays that use PT reagents as activators. Plasma deficient in factors active in the intrinsic (and common) pathway (high molecular weight kininogen, prekallikrein, and factors XII, XI, IX, and VIII) prolongs the PTT and is assayed with PTT reagents.
- When to use clotting factor tests:
  - ▼ When a discrete congenital clotting deficiency (most commonly factors VIII and IX) is suspected
  - ▼ Occasionally, to separate the effect of oral anticoagulants (decrease in factors II, VII, IX, and X but not V or VIII) from liver disease (deficiencies of all these clotting factors, including factor V, but not factor VIII)
  - ▼ To measure blood heparin (factor Xa inhibition) and possibly when therapeutic inhibitors of factor X are used therapeutically

❏ Interpretation
Increased In
- **Factor II:** The genetic mutation *G20210A* predisposes to thromboembolism.
- **Factor VII:** Pregnancy and oral contraceptive use. An increase in factor VII has been linked to thrombophilia in some studies.
- **Factor VIII:** Acute-phase reactant (acute inflammatory conditions), pregnancy, and the use of oral contraceptives. If markedly increased, it may predispose to thromboembolism.
- **Factor IX:** Pregnancy and use of oral contraceptives. Very elevated values have been associated with a tendency to thromboembolism.
- **Factor X:** Pregnancy and use of oral contraceptives.

Decreased In
- **Factor II**
  - ▼ Congenital deficiency (recessive inheritance): Bleeding of various severities in homozygotes
  - ▼ Acquired deficiency: Liver disease, DIC, pathologic fibrinolysis, vitamin K deficiency, or warfarin therapy

16

- **Factor V**
  - ▼ Congenital: inherited autosomal deficiency; bleeding in homozygotes
  - ▼ Acquired: liver disease, DIC, or pathologic fibrinolysis
- **Factor VII**
  - ▼ Congenital deficiency: manifested by variable bleeding in homozygotes
  - ▼ Acquired: liver disease, vitamin K deficiency, vitamin K antagonist therapy
- **Factor VIII**
  - ▼ Congenital: hemophilia A in male patients and in some female carriers of the hemophilia gene (usually mild decrease); von Willebrand disease, especially if moderate to severe
  - ▼ Acquired: Acquired anti–factor VIII autoantibodies in previously unaffected individuals; acquired anti–factor VIII alloantibodies in multiply transfused hemophilia A patients; DIC and pathologic fibrinolysis
- **Factor IX**
  - ▼ Congenital: hemophilia B:X-linked transmission
  - ▼ Acquired: liver disease, vitamin K deficiency or use of vitamin K antagonists, nephrotic syndrome, amyloidosis, autoantibodies to factor IX in previously healthy individuals (extremely rare), alloantibodies in hemophilia B patients treated with factor IX infusions
- **Factor X**
  - ▼ Congenital: rare autosomal recessive defect. Homozygotes may have a bleeding diathesis.
  - ▼ Acquired: severe liver disease; vitamin K deficiency or use of vitamin K antagonists, DIC, amyloidosis
- **Factor XI**
  - ▼ Congenital: autosomal recessive inheritance; mild bleeding diathesis if markedly decreased
- **Factor XIII**
  - ▼ Congenital: severe bleeding in homozygous state; impaired wound healing
  - ▼ Acquired: liver disease; acute promyelocytic leukemia; autoantibodies against factor XIII

❏ **Limitations**

- Improperly filled test tubes or the use of different anticoagulants than recommended (3.2% sodium citrate as provided in blue top tubes).
- Improperly stored plasma.
- Hyperlipidemic, hemolyzed, or icteric blood may affect the results with some coagulation instruments.
- Contamination with heparin or dilution of the collected blood if indwelling catheters are used.

CLOTTING TIME (LEE-WHITE CLOTTING TIME)*

The clotting time is characterized by low sensitivity and poor standardization. It is of only historical interest and is no longer in use.

*Submitted By Liberto Pechet, MD.

COBALT

❑ **Definition**

- Cobalt is an essential trace element and an integral part of cyanocobalamin (vitamin B_{12}). It is also used industrially in the manufacture of high-strength alloys used for cutting/drilling tools, in the semiconductor industry, and as a pigment. Acutely toxic in large doses and in cumulative long-term low-level exposure from cobalt processing plants, hard metal industry, diamond polishing, and ceramic industry.
- Chronic exposure to inorganic cobalt salts, either by ingestion or by inhalation of dust, causes respiratory distress, dyspnea, and pneumoconiosis or can lead to cardiomyopathy. Inorganic cobalt can induce hemoglobin synthesis, as well as hypertriglyceridemia and hypercholesterolemia.
- Cobalt is quickly cleared through the kidneys, and urine cobalt measurements are a useful indicator of recent exposure.
- **Normal range:** Less than 1 µg/L.

❑ **Use**

- Assessing occupational and environmental cobalt exposure
- Detection of cobalt toxicity
- Monitoring metallic implants wear

❑ **Interpretation**

Increased In

- Renal patients receiving erythropoietin agents
- ESRD patients undergoing hemodialysis
- Very heavy drinkers of beer with added cobalt
- Individuals with deteriorating metal implants

Decreased In

- NA.

❑ **Limitations**

- Diet, medications, supplements (nutritional and mineral), B_{12}, or B-complex vitamins may interfere test results. Recommend avoid 3 days prior to testing.
- False-positive test results may occur from using noncertified trace element collection tubes.
- High concentrations of gadolinium and iodine are known to interfere (should wait 96 hours to clear).
- Analysis of cobalt concentration is of little use in the determination of vitamin B_{12} deficiency.
- To assess occupational exposure, sample should be collected at the end of the shift on the last day of workweek.

16

COCAINE*

❏ **Definition**

- This drug is an ester of benzoic acid and amino alcohol. Other names: benzoylmethylecgonine, ecgonine methyl ester benzoate. A therapeutic range has not been established when cocaine is used clinically as a local anesthetic in ophthalmic and otolaryngologic procedures. Cocaine is considered to be a drug of abuse and is controlled in schedule II of the U.S. Controlled Substances Act of 1970.

❏ **Use**

- Local anesthetic due to blockade of sodium channel conductance
- CNS stimulant: blocks reuptake of neurotransmitters norepinephrine, serotonin, dopamine

❏ **Interpretation**

- Cocaine is metabolized primarily to benzoylecgonine and ecgonine methyl ester. Further metabolism produces ecgonine and additional compounds. Coingestion of ethanol results in the formation of cocaethylene. Presence of these compounds is indicative of exposure but does not provide guidance as to the degree of intoxication or impairment. Clinical signs and symptoms must be used.
- The clinician should be aware of testing performed in the laboratory, especially the target analyte and whether the test is a screen or confirmation. The analyte present or absent may provide guidance to the time of exposure.

❏ **Limitations**

- Screening assays are commonly immunoassay based
  - ▼ ELISA for blood, serum, plasma
    - Target analyte: cocaine
    - Cutoff concentration: variable—20–50 ng/mL
    - Significant cross-reactivity with cocaethylene
    - Low cross-reactivity with ecgonine methyl ester, norcocaine, ecgonine
  - ▼ EIA for urine
    - Target analyte: benzoylecgonine (metabolite)
    - Cutoff concentration:
      - 150 ng/mL
      - 300 ng/mL
    - Approximately 50–60% cross-reactivity with cocaine and cocaethylene
    - Low cross-reactivity with EME, ecgonine
- Confirmation assays are commonly chromatography based regardless of the specimen.
  - ▼ GC/MS
    - Full scan mode for qualitative identification of cocaine, cocaethylene, and metabolites: limits of detection—20–50 ng/mL
    - Selected ion-monitoring mode for quantitative analysis of serum, plasma for cocaine, cocaethylene, and metabolites: limits of quantitation—5–20 ng/mL
  - ▼ LC/MSn (multiple MS)

*Submitted By Amanda J. Jenkins, PhD.

- Multiple reaction–monitoring mode for qualitative or quantitative analysis of cocaine, cocaethylene, and metabolites: limits of detection/quantitation—20–50 ng/mL

COLD AGGLUTININS

❑ Definition

- Autoantibodies with specificity against RBC determinants that react at low temperature but not at body temperature. (Reactions against i determinants are less common.) The cold-reactive agglutinins are of the IgM class immunoglobulins; very rarely IgG. The IgM autoantibodies bind at low temperature to complement on the RBC membrane.
- **Normal titer:** <1:32 (negative result).

❑ Use

- Hemolytic anemia, particularly in the presence of lymphoproliferative disorders
- When the clinical symptomatology suggests cold agglutinin disease

❑ Interpretation

- Cold agglutinin titers above 1:32 are diagnostic for the presence of cold agglutinin disease. The titer in affected patients may be >1,000.

❑ Limitations

- Blood must be collected, clotted, and the serum separated at 37°C, and in addition, the sample must be maintained at 37°C. Alternatively, it can be collected on EDTA at room temperature, but then, it must be warmed for at least 15 minutes at 37°C.
- The direct (Coombs) antiglobulin test is positive against C3d and C4d components of complement.
- Low levels may also found in healthy individuals and those with peripheral vascular disease or nonlymphoid neoplasm.
- Cold-reacting autoantibodies are mostly IgM, occasionally IgG, and rarely IgA. May be polyclonal, also can be monoclonal usually with kappa light chain.
- Refrigeration of blood at any time adversely affects the results, as does severely hemolyzed or lipemic specimens.

COMBINED FIRST-TRIMESTER AND SECOND-TRIMESTER SCREENING (INTEGRATED/SEQUENTIAL SCREENING)

See Prenatal Screening.

COMPLEMENT SYSTEM ASSAYS*

❑ Definition

- The complement system is a major component of innate and adaptive immunity; upon activation, the complement results in the formation of the membrane attack complex (MAC) that releases peptides called anaphylatoxins.

*Submitted by Liberto Pechet, MD.

About 90% of complement components are synthesized in the liver and are acute-phase proteins.

- There are three pathways of activation: Classical (antibody-sensitized cells), alternative (early defense against microorganisms), and mannose-binding lectin (MBL) (recognizes microorganisms in the absence of antibodies that are replaced by a lectin, such as mannose-binding protein [MBP]). MBL is formed in the liver. It belongs to a family of molecules called collectins. Many components of the complement system interact through cascading mechanisms. The nine components of the classical pathway are designated by the upper case letter C, followed by a number indicating the order of appearance during the cascading sequence (the only exception is C4, which acts before C2). The components of the alternate pathway are called factors and are designated by upper-case letters (example: factor H, factor D). For the MBL pathway, the components are referred to by the abbreviations of the proteins' names.
- All three pathways of complement activation converge at the activation of C3 and assembly of the membrane attack complex, which is formed by components C5–C9.

❑ Use

- Complement should be investigated in patients with recurrent pyogenic infections (but with normal white cell counts and immunoglobulins), recurrent angioedema, cryoglobulinemic vasculitis, and with multiple family members with recurrent neisserial infections. Patients with deficiencies in the alternate pathway factors D, B, P, H, and I, or the late complement components C3, C5–C9, are particularly susceptible to infections with *Neisseria meningitidis*.
- To determine the presence of deficiencies of individual components, and *whether the deficiency is acquired or inherited.*
- The total hemolytic complement assay (CH50 or THC) is a global test; it is decreased if any of the components of the classical pathway are deficient. The AH50 assay screens for abnormalities in the alternate pathway. The use of CH50 and AH50 assays allows identification of abnormalities in both pathways. When the CH50 is very low, the next step is to measure specific complement components.

❑ Normal Ranges

- Complement levels are determined by immunologic and functional assays.
- The most commonly used assays are C3, C4, CH50, and AH50 (see Complement Components in Plasma and Their Deficiencies table).

❑ Interpretation

Decreased in acquired conditions (see Complement Components in Plasma and Their Deficiencies table). Decreases in complement in acquired conditions are usually only partial and affect several components of the system. They are most commonly due to complement consumption.

Associated with arthritis

- Active systemic lupus erythematosus (SLE), especially if associated with renal disease. About 50% of patients with SLE have reductions in C3 and C4. Low complement levels correlate with more severe disease, especially with renal involvement. Normalization reflects good therapeutic results.

- Hepatitis B or C
- Essential mixed cryoglobulinemia
- Serum sickness

Associated with vasculitis

- Rheumatoid vasculitis
- Essential mixed cryoglobulinemia
- Sjögren syndrome
- Hypocomplementemic vasculitis

Associated with nephritis

- Acute poststreptococcal GN (transient decline in C3)
- IgA nephropathy
- Membranous nephropathy
- Types I and II membranoproliferative glomerulonephritis
- SLE nephritis;
- Tubulointerstitial nephritis
- Dense deposit disease: C3 and factor B levels are low, and C4 is normal
- Goodpasture syndrome

Associated with miscellaneous conditions

- The antiphospholipid antibody syndrome
- Bacterial endocarditis
- Cryoglobulinemia (decreased C2 and C4)
- Acquired angioedema due to C1 inhibitor deficiency in B-cell lymphoproliferative diseases
- Alcoholic liver disease: low C3 and C4 due to decreased synthesis
- Acquired deficiency of decay accelerating factor (DAF) and CD59—complement regulatory proteins that normally inhibit complement activation—develops in PNH, resulting in accelerated red cell hemolysis
- Evans syndrome

Synovial Fluid

- Depressed CH50 is found in the synovial fluid of joints in
  - ▼ Seronegative rheumatoid arthritis
  - ▼ SLE
  - ▼ Pseudogout and gout
  - ▼ Reiter syndrome
  - ▼ Gonococcal arthritis

Decreased in Inherited Conditions (see *Complement Components in Plasma and Their Deficiencies* table)

Inherited deficiencies are characterized by the absence of single complement component. Most inherited disorders of the classical pathway are transmitted as autosomal recessive traits and are symptomatic in the heterozygous. Exception is partial C4 deficiency that predisposes to SLE.

- Hereditary angioedema an autosomal dominant disease; patients have very low C4, but normal C3
- C1q deficiency: more than 90% develop SLE

16

- Deficiency of C1r or C1s as well as partial deficiency of C4 predispose to the development of SLE
- Deficiency of C4a or C4b is associated with the development of other diseases (scleroderma, IgA nephropathy, childhood diabetes, etc.)
- Familial Mediterranean fever (C5a inhibitor)
- Urticarial vasculitis and recurrent infections (C3)
- Severe combined immunodeficiency (C1q)
- X-linked hypogammaglobulinemia (C1q)
- Recurrent neisserial infections (C5, C6, C7, C8, C9, and the alternate pathway)
- Congenital deficiencies of C2 or C4 may present with lupus-like or other autoimmune disorder involving:
  - ▼ Arthritis
  - ▼ Nephritis
  - ▼ Rashes
  - ▼ Pneumococcal infections
- Heterozygous mutations in plasma factors H and I result in consumption of C3, predisposing patients to infections and glomerulonephritis.
- A genetic deficiency of complement regulatory proteins has been identified in 40–80% of cases of **atypical hemolytic uremic syndrome (aHUS)**, a rare syndrome of microangiopathic hemolysis, thrombocytopenia, and renal failure. A deficiency of factor H (the most frequent abnormality in aHUS), C3 mutations, and deficiencies of membrane cofactor protein, factor I, factor B, and thrombomodulin.
- Properdin (alternate pathway) deficiency is transmitted as an X-linked condition, and these males are affected by *Neisseria meningitidis*, often of unusual types.
- Lectin pathway deficiencies are rare: deficiencies of MBL, MBL-associated protease 2, and ficolin-3 are associated with pyogenic infections, especially with encapsulated bacteria.

Increased
In inflammatory conditions that increase acute-phase reactants.

- **Complement may be normal or increased in:**
  - ▼ Juvenile rheumatoid arthritis
  - ▼ Palindromic arthritis
  - ▼ Pseudogout and gout
  - ▼ Reiter syndrome
  - ▼ Gonococcal arthritis

❑ Pitfalls
Complement activity is unstable and heat-labile, and it is reduced after a few hours in samples kept at room temperature. Serum samples should not be kept at room temperature for more than 6 hours or refrigerated for more than 7 days prior to analysis.

- Specimens left to *clot* at refrigerated temperature lose activity because of complement activation.
- Complement components deteriorate in samples that are repeatedly thawed and frozen.
- Severe hemolysis, lipemia, or bilirubinemia may interfere with accurate measurement.

Complement Components in Plasma and Their Deficiencies*

Protein	Concentration in Plasma, mg/mL	Clinical Correlations
Global tests		
CH50: 60–144 CEA units		
AH50 (screens for abnormalities of the alternate pathway): 59% or greater CEA units		
Classical Pathway		
	150, 50, 50	GN, SLE
C4	300–600	Scleroderma, SLE, IgA nephropathy, membranous GN
C2	20	SLE, juvenile RA, GN
Alternative Pathway		
Factor B	200	*Neisseria meningitidis* infections
Factor D	2	Recurrent pyogenic infections
Properdin	25	Recurrent pyogenic infections, fulminant meningococcemia
MBL Pathway		
MBL	Per specialized labs	Recurrent infections
MASP-1	1.5–13	
MASP-2	Unknown	
Common to All Pathways		
C3	1,200–1,300	Recurrent pyogenic infections, GN
Membrane Attack Complex		
C5	80	Recurrent disseminated neisserial infections, SLE
C6	45	Recurrent disseminated neisserial infections
C7	90	Recurrent disseminated neisserial infections, Raynaud disease
C8	55	Recurrent disseminated neisserial infections
C9	60	None
Fluid-Phase Control Proteins		
C1-Inhibitor	240	Hereditary angioedema, autoimmune diseases
C4b	250	Angioedema, Behcet's-like syndrome
Factor I	35	Recurrent pyogenic infections
Factor H	300–450	Recurrent pyogenic infections, GN, age-related macular degeneration
Cell-Bound Proteins		
CR1		Anemia and SLE
CR3		Leukocyte adhesion deficiency-1, recurrent pyogenic infections, leukocytosis
DAF/CD59/HRF (acquired)		PNH

16

*Modified from Massey HD, McPherson RA. In: *Henry's Clinical Diagnosis and Management by Laboratory Methods,* Table 47-3, p.920, and Table 47-4, p.921 22nd ed. Saunders, 2011.

Suggested Readings

Botto M, Kirshfink M, Macor P, et al. Complement in human diseases: lessons from complement deficiencies. *Mol Immunol.* 2009;46:2774–2783.

Nester CM, Thomas CP. Atypical hemolytic uremic syndrome: what is it, how is it diagnosed, and how is it treated? *Hematology Am Soc Hematol Educ Program.* 2012;2012:617–625.

COMPLETE BLOOD COUNT (CBC)*

❑ Definition

- CBC is a numerical report of all blood elements, as well as a description of some of their major characteristics. Most laboratories use automated counters. The CBC reports include RBC count, WBC count, platelet count, Hb, Hct (volume of packed red cells), mean platelet volume, and other parameters (described under individual tests). The CBC may be ordered as a simple count of blood elements and RBC indices or as a test that includes a WBC differential.

❑ Use

- CBC is used for screening whenever abnormalities in RBCs, WBCs, or platelets are suspected.
- New analyzers may separate reticulocytes and platelets into young and mature populations that help detect bone marrow regeneration. Automated counters flag abnormalities in RBCs, WBCs, and platelets, triggering examination of the peripheral blood smear.

❑ Limitations

- Proper specimen collection is required for reliable and accurate reporting of the CBC. Misleading results occur if the specimens contain clots, if the blood is not properly mixed, or in the presence of agglutinated RBCs. Specific pitfalls are described under each lineage.

 COOMBS (ANTIGLOBULIN) TEST†

DIRECT COOMBS TEST (DAT)

❑ Definition

- The DAT is used to detect IgG antibodies or complement components on the RBC surface membrane by incubating Coombs (rabbit anti-human globulin [AHG]) reagent with the patient's washed RBCs. The Coombs reagent can selectively bind IgG or C3 or be polyspecific and contain both anti-IgG and anti-C3.

❑ Use

- DAT is useful in diagnosing autoimmune hemolysis [see p. 377]), hemolytic diseases of the newborn [see p. 380]), drug-induced hemolysis, and hemolytic transfusion reactions [see p. 757]).

*Submitted By Liberto Pechet, MD.
†Submitted By Vishesh Chhibber, MD.

- The DAT is often used whenever hemolysis of red cells is suspected as being caused by autoantibodies. The assay determines if red cells have been coated in vivo with immunoglobulins, complement, or both.

❑ **Interpretation**

Positive DAT

- The DAT is positive whenever the patient's red cells are coated with autoantibodies that developed against the patient's own red cells.
- Hemolytic disease of the newborn (erythroblastosis fetalis).
- Warm autoimmune hemolytic anemias.
  ▼ Idiopathic.
  ▼ Evan syndrome (ITP and hemolytic anemia).
- Cold autoimmune hemolytic anemia/cold agglutinin disease.
- It is also positive when alloantibodies in a recipient's circulation react with antigens on recently transfused red cells, as well as alloantibodies in maternal circulation, which cross the placenta and coat fetal red cells.
  ▼ Alloimmune (acute/delayed) hemolytic transfusion reactions.
  ▼ Hemolytic disease of the newborn.
  ▼ If the DAT is positive following recent transfusions, the antibodies can be eluted from RBCs and identified.
- Drug-induced reactions, such as
  ▼ Alpha-methyldopa
  ▼ L-Dopa
  ▼ High doses of penicillin
  ▼ Quinidine
- In patients who have not been transfused within the preceding 3 months, a positive DAT almost always reveals autoimmune antibodies.

Negative DAT

- Hemolytic anemias caused by an intrinsic RBC defect (e.g., G6PD [see p. 970], hemoglobinopathies [see p. 363])

❑ **Limitations**

- Finding of a positive DAT indicates the presence of red cell autoantibodies, alloantibodies following transfusions, or of coating of red cells with excess immunoglobulins. It requires additional workup to elucidate the etiology of the immunoglobulins by performing tests for antibody specificity: cold agglutinins (see p. 377 under hemolytic anemias), Donath-Landsteiner antibody (see p. 379), and also serum protein electrophoresis or immunofixation when a plasmacytic disease (see p. 432) is suspected. The administration of certain drugs (α-methyldopa, IV penicillin, or procainamide) and recent transfusions must also be excluded.
- False-positive results may occur in plasma cell myeloma and lymphoplasmacytic lymphoma.
- 1:10,000 normal blood donors have a positive DAT.
- A negative DAT can rarely be seen in patients with autoimmune hemolytic anemia if only a small amount of IgG is bound to the RBC membrane.
- A negative DAT does not rule out hemolysis. For instance, DAT is negative in some cases of drug-induced hemolytic anemias, hemoglobinopathies, hereditary spherocytosis, and other hereditary hemolytic anemias.

16

INDIRECT COOMBS TEST (IAT)

❏ **Definition**

- The IAT uses the patient's serum (or plasma), which is incubated with reagent or donor RBCs. Subsequently, this mixture is washed to remove unbound globulins and then incubated with Coombs reagent. Agglutination is seen if the patient's serum contains antibodies against the RBCs.
- In about 80% of patients with autoimmune hemolytic anemia, the autoantibodies are also present in serum.
- Alloantibodies to RBC antigens induced by previous blood transfusions or fetal–maternal incompatibility are also detected by this assay. These alloantibodies are usually present only in serum because they do not bind to the patient's RBCs, and the DAT is negative in these cases.

❏ **Use**

- The utility of the IAT in blood banking stems from its great sensitivity in detecting various IgG antibodies in a patient's serum. It is used to detect the presence of alloantibodies directed against non-ABO blood group antigens.
  - ▼ Antibody screening and cross-matching prior to blood transfusions.
  - ▼ Prenatal testing of pregnant women.
- In some cases of autoimmune hemolytic anemia, the IAT and the DAT may be positive because some autoantibody attaches to the RBCs and some (excess) antibody may not be bound to red cells and be present in the serum.

❏ **Interpretation**

- The IAT is positive in the presence of serum alloantibodies in patients previously transfused and immunized against non-self–red cell antigens.

❏ **Limitations**

- The IAT may be unable to detect low titer antibodies.
- A positive IAT requires further investigation to identify more precisely the offending antibody.

CO-OXIMETRY

❏ **Definition**

- Co-oximetry refers to the measurement of various forms of hemoglobin by dedicated multiwavelength spectrophotometry. It is a measure of the potential oxygen-carrying capacity of the blood.

❏ **Use**

- It usually measures concentrations of oxygenated hemoglobin (oxyHb), deoxygenated hemoglobin (deoxyHb or reduced Hb), COHB, and methemoglobin (MetHb) as a percentage of the total hemoglobin concentration in the blood sample.

❏ **Indications**

- History consistent with toxin exposure
- Hypoxia fails to improve with the administration of oxygen

- Existence of a discrepancy between the PaO_2 on a blood gas determination and the oxygen saturation on pulse oximetry (SpO_2)
- Suspected other dyshemoglobinemias such as methemoglobinemia or carboxyhemoglobinemia

Oxygen Saturation (SO₂)

- Calculated as O_2 Hb/O_2 Hb + HHB × 100%.
- The availability of oxygen to tissues is dependent not only on SO_2 but also on the affinity of O_2 to Hb. It is clinically useful in cyanosis and erythrocytosis. It may differentiate between diminished oxygenation of blood, as in pulmonary diseases and admixture of venous blood, as in an AV shunt.
- Percent saturation in newborns is 40–90% and thereafter 94–98%; values decrease with age.

Oxyhemoglobin

- This represents the fraction of oxygenated Hb in relation to the total Hb present, including non–oxygen-binding Hb. In healthy individuals, oxyhemoglobin and oxygen saturation are approximately equal. In the presence of dyshemoglobins, oxyhemoglobin can be considerably lower than oxygen saturation. Although the oxygen saturation often remains within the reference limits, the oxygen-carrying capacity of the blood may be severely decreased.
- **Normal range: 94–100%.**

Carboxyhemoglobin

- This is Hb that has carbon monoxide instead of the normal oxygen bound to it. Carbon monoxide (CO) has a much great affinity than oxygen for hemoglobin.
- Carboxyhemoglobin is formed in carbon monoxide poisoning. The source of the carbon monoxide may be exhaust (such as from a car, truck, boat, or generator), smoke from a fire, or tobacco smoke. The carboxyhemoglobin level is useful in judging the extent of CO toxicity and in considering the effect of smoking on the patient. A direct correlation has been claimed between CO level and symptoms of atherosclerotic diseases, angina, and MI.
  - ▼ Nonsmokers: 0.5–1.5% saturation of Hb
  - ▼ Smokers: 1–2 packs/day: 4–5%
  - ▼ Heavy smokers: >2 packs/day: 8–9%

Methemoglobin

- This is produced by the oxidation of the normal ferrous iron of Hb to ferric iron, making it chemically useless for respiration.
- A small amount of methemoglobin is normally present in blood, but the conversion of a larger fraction of hemoglobin into methemoglobin results in perceptible cyanosis. Methemoglobinemia may be acquired anytime in life by exposure to a number of different chemical agents, such as nitrites, or it may be congenital due a genetic condition.
- **Normal: 0.06–0.24 g/dL.**

COPPER

16

❏ Definition

- Copper is a metal component of various enzymes (e.g., cytochrome oxidase, superoxide dismutase, tyrosinase) involved in Hb synthesis, bone and

TABLE 16–23. Normal Levels of Serum Copper

Age	Male (µg/dL)	Female (µg/dL)
≤6 mo	20–70	20–70
7 mo–18 y	90–190	90–190
≥19 y	70–140	80–155

elastic tissue development, and CNS function. Copper test levels need to be evaluated and compared to ceruloplasmin levels.

- **Normal range:** see Table 16.23.

❑ Use

- Aids in the diagnosis of Wilson disease
- Assessment of primary biliary cirrhosis
- Assessment of primary sclerosing cholangitis

❑ Interpretation

Increased In

- Wilson disease (low to normal, total copper blood, high free serum, and urine copper)
- Anemias
  - ▼ PA
  - ▼ Megaloblastic anemia of pregnancy
  - ▼ Iron deficiency anemia
  - ▼ Aplastic anemia
- Leukemia and lymphoma
- Infection, acute and chronic
- Biliary cirrhosis and sclerosing cholangitis
- Hemochromatosis
- Collagen diseases (including SLE, RA, acute RF, GN)
- Hypothyroidism
- Hyperthyroidism
- Frequently associated with increased CRP
- Ingestion of oral contraceptives and estrogens
- Pregnancy

Decreased In

- Wilson disease: Mutation interferes with copper transport from intestinal mucosal cytoplasm to Golgi apparatus, where it becomes bound to protein
- Menkes kinky hair syndrome
- Nephrosis (ceruloplasmin lost in urine)
- Acute leukemia in remission
- Some iron deficiency anemias of childhood (that require copper as well as iron therapy)
- Kwashiorkor, chronic diarrhea
- ACTH and corticosteroids

❑ Limitations

- Serum copper may be elevated with infection, inflammation, stress, RA, with some cancers, medications such as carbamazepine and phenobarbital.

- Concentrations are 2–3 × normal in the third trimester of pregnancy.
- Copper may be lowered with corticosteroids, zinc, malnutrition, and malabsorption.
- Serum specimen should be collected in a trace element-free tube, such as royal blue sterile tube, to avoid contamination.
- High urinary copper levels support the diagnosis but are not unique to Wilson disease, as they can be sometimes observed in autoimmune hepatitis and cholestasis.

CORTICOTROPIN-RELEASING HORMONE (CRH)

❏ Definition

- CRH is a 41-amino-acid peptide hypothalamic factor that increases ACTH release from pituitary cells. CRH is synthesized by neurons in the parvocellular division of the hypothalamic paraventricular nuclei. The axons of the nuclei project to the median eminence, where CRH is secreted into the hypophyseal portal blood. The ACTH released by CRH stimulates the secretion of cortisol and other adrenal steroids, such as DHEA and, transiently, aldosterone. CRH circulates in human plasma bound to a high-affinity binding protein, which reduces its bioactivity and increases its clearance. In addition to being produced in the hypothalamus, CRH is also synthesized in peripheral tissues, such as T lymphocytes, and is highly expressed in the placenta. In the placenta, CRH is a marker that determines the length of gestation and the timing of parturition and delivery. Other names: corticoliberin, corticotropin-releasing factor (CRF).
- **Normal range:** up to 10 pg/mL.

❏ Use

- To exclude the possibility of an extrapituitary CRH-secreting tumor

❏ Interpretation

Increased In

- Cushing syndrome
- Ectopic tumors producing ACTH
- Third trimester of pregnancy

Decreased In

- Alzheimer disease
- Autosomal recessive hypothalamic corticotropin deficiency

❏ Limitations

- The patient should be fasting 10–12 hours and should not take any corticosteroid, ACTH, or estrogen medications, if possible, for at least 48 hours prior to collection of specimen. An AM specimen is preferred. This test is rarely used.
- A rapid increase in circulating levels of CRH occurs at the onset of parturition.
- Plasma CRH concentrations do not correlate with plasma ACTH or serum cortisol concentrations or with altered hypothalamic–pituitary–adrenal axis function (e.g., in primary adrenal insufficiency or Cushing syndrome, or

16

during insulin-induced hypoglycemia or metyrapone administration). Some investigators have reported a correlation between plasma CRH and plasma ACTH or serum cortisol in pregnancy, but others have not.

■ The contribution of hypothalamic CRH to peripheral plasma CRH concentrations is small; most of the plasma CRH presumably comes from nonhypothalamic sources.

■ However, under certain circumstances, such as insulin-induced hypoglycemia or during major surgery, small increments in plasma CRH concentrations may reflect hypothalamic CRH release.

CORTICOTROPIN-RELEASING HORMONE (CRH) STIMULATION TEST

❑ **Definition**

■ CRH is a 41-amino-acid peptide, secreted by the paraventricular nucleus of the hypothalamus in response to stress. It acts on the anterior lobes of the pituitary to release ACTH. There is considerable sequence homology of CRH among species; as a result, both ovine and human CRH can be used in testing. Also known as: CRH after low-dose dexamethasone test.

■ **Normal range:**
  ▼ CRH stimulation test:
    ● Most patients with Cushing disease respond with ACTH and cortisol increases within 45 minutes after CRH. However, the criteria for interpretation have varied at different centers.
    ● Basal plasma ACTH concentrations increase 35–9,005 (mean 400%) in normal subjects and reach a peak of 10–120 pg/mL, 10–30 minutes after CRH injection; serum cortisol concentrations increase 20–600% (mean 250%) to 13–36 μg/dL (mean 25 μg/dL), reaching a peak 30–60 minutes after CRH injection.
  ▼ CRH after low-dose dexamethasone test:
    ● Cortisol 1.4 μg/L is virtually 100% specific and 100% diagnostic for Cushing syndrome.

❑ **Use**

■ Objectives
  ▼ To evaluate the cause of ACTH-dependent Cushing syndrome (with or without vasopressin analogs)
  ▼ To discriminate between pseudo-Cushing and Cushing syndrome
  ▼ To discriminate between primary and central adrenal insufficiency

■ CRH stimulation test: The patient fasts for 4 hours or more, after which an intravenous access line is established and synthetic ovine CRH (1 μg/kg body weight or 100 μg total dose) is injected as an intravenous bolus. Blood samples for ACTH and cortisol are drawn 15 (or 5) and 0 minutes before and as often as 5, 10, 15, 30, 45, 60, 90, and 120 minutes after CRH injection. However, in Cushing syndrome, if one measures only the plasma ACTH response, the samples at −5, −0, 15, and 30 minutes are sufficient, and if one measures only the serum cortisol response, the samples at −15, 0, 45, and

60 minutes are sufficient. Normally both hormones should be measured, since the criteria for a positive response may include increases in either plasma ACTH or serum cortisol concentrations.

- CRH test after low-dose dexamethasone procedure: The patient takes 0.5 mg of dexamethasone every 6 hours for 2 days (a total of eight doses); 2 hours after the last dexamethasone dose is taken, 1 μg/kg of CRH is administered intravenously. Blood for a plasma cortisol measurement is drawn 15 minutes after the CRH injection.

❑ **Interpretation**
- Normal or exaggerated response: pituitary Cushing disease
- No response: ectopic ACTH-secreting tumor

❑ **Limitations**
- Responses to CRH are variable among subjects and from one time to another in the same subject.
- The increment in plasma ACTH is the same in the morning and evening; however, the peak value is greater in the morning in normal subjects when the basal plasma ACTH concentration is higher. In contrast, the peak serum cortisol value is similar at both times of day, but the increment is smaller in the morning when the basal value is higher. In patients with Cushing syndrome, in whom the normal circadian rhythm in ACTH secretion is absent, the CRH test can be performed at any time of day with similar results.
- The response to CRH depends on the cause of the hypoadrenalism.
  - ▼ Patients with primary pituitary ACTH deficiency (secondary adrenal insufficiency) have decreased plasma ACTH and serum cortisol responses to CRH.
  - ▼ Patients with hypothalamic disease (i.e., CRH deficiency) usually have exaggerated and prolonged plasma ACTH responses; the plasma cortisol responses are subnormal.
  - ▼ The CRH stimulation test is more reliable than the ACTH stimulation test in detecting pituitary–adrenal suppression in preterm infants whose mothers received a short course of dexamethasone before delivery to hasten fetal lung development.

CORTISOL FREE URINE, 24 HOURS

❑ **Definition**
- Cortisol free urine, 24-hour, or urinary free cortisol provides a direct and reliable practical index of cortisol secretion. It is an integrated measure of serum free cortisol level that is not affected by body weight.
- **Normal range:**
  - ▼ Males: <60 μg/day; <32 μg/g creatinine
  - ▼ Females: <45 μg/day; <45 μg/g creatinine

❑ **Use**
- Aids in the diagnosis of hypercortisolism caused by Cushing syndrome
- Adrenal insufficiency (limited usefulness)

16

- Assisting in diagnosing acquired or inherited abnormalities of 11β-hydroxy steroid dehydrogenase (cortisol-to-cortisone ratio)
- Diagnosis of pseudohyperaldosteronism due to excessive licorice consumption

❑ **Interpretation**

- Cortisol free urine, 24-hour, is increased in Cushing syndrome. The patient can be assumed to have Cushing syndrome if basal urinary cortisol excretion is more than 3 × the upper limit of normal and one other test is abnormal.
- This result is found in 95% of cases of Cushing syndrome. Values <100 μg/24 hours exclude the diagnosis, and values >300 μg/24 hours confirm the diagnosis. If values are intermediate, a dexamethasone suppression test is indicated.
- It is decreased in adrenal insufficiency.

❑ **Limitations**

- Urinary cortisol may be detected by antibody-based (immunoassays) or structurally based (HPLC-MS) tests, and the immunoassays may be less specific because antibodies may cross-react with similar steroids.
- An increase is the most useful screening test (best expressed as per gram creatine, which should vary by <10% daily; if variation is >10%, two more 24-hour specimens should be collected). Values should be measured in three consecutive 24-hour specimens to ensure proper collection and account for daily variability, even in Cushing syndrome.
- Increased values may occur in depression, chronic alcoholism, eating disorders, and polycystic ovary syndrome but do not exceed 300 μg/24 hours.
- Various drugs (e.g., carbamazepine, phenytoin, phenobarbital, primidone) will falsely elevate free cortisol levels.
- Acute and chronic illnesses can increase free cortisol levels.
- Renal disease due to decreased excretion may falsely lower the levels of free cortisol.

CORTISOL, SALIVA

❑ **Definition**

- Serum free cortisol freely diffuses into saliva. Therefore, measurements of salivary cortisol (hydrocortisone) more accurately reflect the serum free cortisol. The salivary cortisol concentration is independent of salivary flow rate.
- **Normal range:** varies diurnally, with concentrations about 5.6 ng/mL at 8:00–9:00 AM and about 1 ng/mL at 11:00 PM.

❑ **Use**

- Screening for Cushing syndrome.
- Diagnosis of Cushing syndrome in patients presenting with symptoms or signs suggestive of the disease.
- Assessing cortisol secretion serially in ambulatory patients. Measurements are helpful in patients with cyclical Cushing syndrome.

❑ **Interpretation**

- Late evening levels are increased in Cushing syndrome.
- Morning levels are decreased in adrenal insufficiency.

❑ Limitations

- Several factors influence analytical measurement and accuracy of salivary cortisol levels, including collection processes, devices, sample handling, processing and storage, and choice of analytical method.
- Changes in cortisol-binding globulin and albumin affect total cortisol levels but not free levels in serum and saliva.

CORTISOL, SERUM

❑ Definition

- Cortisol (hydrocortisone) is the major glucocorticoid produced and secreted by the adrenal cortex. It affects the metabolism of protein, fat, and carbohydrates; maintenance of muscle and myocardial integrity; and the suppression of inflammatory and allergic activities.
- **Normal range:**
  - ▼ AM cortisol: 8.7–22.4 µg/dL
  - ▼ PM cortisol: <10 µg/dL

❑ Use

- Discrimination between primary and secondary adrenal insufficiency
- Differential diagnosis of Cushing syndrome

❑ Interpretation

- The most common cause of increased plasma cortisol levels in women is a high circulating concentration of estrogen (e.g., estrogen therapy, pregnancy), resulting in increased concentration of cortisol-binding globulin.
- Patients with severe illness and sepsis have reduced cortisol-binding globulin and albumin levels, resulting in lowered cortisol levels.

❑ Limitations

- Bound cortisol circulates in an available but temporarily inactive state. The physiologic activity of cortisol depends on levels of the small fraction of circulating unbound cortisol.
- Acute stress (including hospitalization and surgery), alcoholism, depression, and many drugs (e.g., exogenous cortisones, anticonvulsants) can obliterate normal diurnal variation, affect response to suppression/stimulation tests, and cause elevated baseline levels.
- Patients taking prednisone may have falsely increased cortisol levels because prednisone is converted to prednisolone after ingestion, and prednisolone has a 41% cross-reactivity.
- Cortisol levels may be increased in pregnancy and with exogenous estrogens.
- Some patients with depressive disorders have a hyperactive hypothalamic–pituitary–adrenal axis, similar to Cushing syndrome.

16

C-PEPTIDE

❏ **Definition**

■ Human C-peptide is a 31-amino-acid chain with a molecular mass of approximately 3,020 Da. Metabolically inert, it originates in the pancreatic B cells as a by-product of the enzymatic cleavage of proinsulin to insulin. In this process, insulin and C-peptide are split from the prohormone and secreted into the portal circulation in equimolar concentrations. Within limits, C-peptide levels can serve as a valuable index to insulin secretion. Therefore, low C-peptide levels are to be expected where insulin secretion is diminished, as in insulin-dependent diabetes, or suppressed, as a normal response to exogenous insulin, whereas elevated C-peptide levels may result from the increased B-cell activity observed in insulinomas.

■ **Normal range:** 0.9–7.1 ng/mL.

❏ **Use**

■ For estimating insulin levels in the presence of antibodies to exogenous insulin

■ Diagnosis of factitious hypoglycemia due to surreptitious administration of insulin in which high serum insulin levels occur with low C-peptide levels

■ Evaluation of insulinoma

■ Monitoring pancreatic and islet cell transplant function

❏ **Interpretation**

Increased In

■ Insulinoma

■ Type 2 DM

Decreased In

■ Exogenous insulin administration (e.g., factitious hypoglycemia)

■ Type 1 DM

❏ **Limitations**

■ C-peptide serum levels correlate with insulin levels in blood, except in islet cell tumors and possibly in obese patients.

C-REACTIVE PROTEIN, HIGH SENSITIVITY

❏ **Definition**

■ High-sensitivity C-reactive protein (hs-CRP or cardiac CRP) is an acute-phase reactant produced by hepatocytes and induced by the release of interleukin 1 and 6. It reflects activation of systemic inflammation. Blood levels of CRP are known to rise rapidly from normal baseline levels to as high as 50 mg/dL as part of the body's nonspecific inflammatory response to infection or injury. The hs-CRP test is more sensitive than the standard CRP test.

■ **Normal range:** <0.3 mg/dL (see Table 16.24).

TABLE 16–24. Cardiovascular Risk Classification by CRP*

Risk Level	CRP (mg/L)
Low	<1.0
Average	1.0–3.0
High	>3.0

*Cardiovascular disease risk assessment guidelines for CRP recommended by the CDC and the American Heart Association (CDC/AHA).
Source: Pearson TA, Mensah GA, Alexander RW, et al. Markers of inflammation and cardiovascular disease. Application to clinical and public health practice. A Statement for Healthcare Professionals From the Centers for Disease Control and Prevention and the American Heart Association. *Circulation.* 2003;107:499–511.

❑ **Use**

- Performing risk assessment for cardiovascular disease: Cardiac disease is believed to be the end result of interplay between minor changes in the cardiovascular endothelium and the corresponding inflammatory response to these changes.
  - ▼ hs-CRP is an independent risk factor for cardiovascular disease, stroke, and peripheral vascular disease. It adds to the predictive value of total cholesterol and HDL cholesterol for future events.
  - ▼ hs-CRP may be useful as an independent marker of prognosis for recurrent events in patients with stable coronary disease or acute coronary syndrome. Recent evidence supporting this potential application has shown that high baseline values of CRP in individuals without a history of cardiac disease were associated with an increased incidence of subsequent cardiac events.
- Determining risk of hypotension: hs-CRP has been reported as a risk factor for hypotension.

❑ **Interpretation**

- hs-CRP appears within 24–48 hours, peaks at 72 hours, and becomes negative after 7 days; it correlates with peak CK-MB levels, but the CRP peak occurs 1–3 days later.
- Failure of CRP to return to normal indicates tissue damage in the heart or elsewhere. The absence of a CRP increase raises the question of necrosis in prior 2–10 days. CRP is usually normal in patients with unstable angina in the absence of tissue necrosis and a normal troponin T (<0.1 ng/mL).
- Peak hs-CRP correlates with peak CK-MB following AMI. CRP may remain increased for at least 3 months following AMI.

Increased In

- Acute or chronic inflammatory change
- Tissue injury or necrosis
- Ischemia or infarction of other tissues
- Infections, inflammation, tissue injury, or necrosis (possible)
- Metabolic syndrome
- Elevated blood pressure
- Malignant (but not benign) tumors, especially of the breast, lung, and GI tract
- Pancreatitis

16

- Postsurgery
- Burns, trauma
- Leukemia: fever, blast crisis, or cytotoxic drugs
- Cigarette smoking
- Hormone therapy, estrogen, and progesterone

Decreased In
- Exercise and weight loss
- Moderate alcohol consumption
- Drugs (e.g., statins, fibrates, niacin)

❏ Limitations
- Race and gender differences affect CRP levels. One study indicates that black patients have higher levels than white patients and women have higher levels than men.

Suggested Readings
Khera A, McGuire DK, Murphy, et al. Race and gender differences in C-reactive protein levels. *J Am Coll Cardiol.* 2005;46:464–469.

Pearson TA, George A, Mensah R, et al. Markers of inflammation and cardiovascular disease. Application to clinical and public health practice. A Statement for healthcare professionals from the Centers for Disease Control and Prevention and the American Heart Association. *Circulation.* 2003;107:499–511.

C-REACTIVE PROTEIN (CRP), SERUM

❏ Definition
- CRP is a cytokine-induced, acute-phase protein and is useful in the detection and evaluation of infection, tissue injury, and inflammatory disorders. Plasma levels begin increasing within 4–6 hours after initial tissue injury and continue to increase several hundred-folds within 24–48 hours. CRP remains elevated during the acute-phase response and returns to normal with restoration of tissue structure and function. The rise in CRP is exponential, doubling every 8–9 hours. The half-life is <24 hours.
- **Normal range:** Less than 10 mg/L.

❏ Use
- For evaluation of infection, tissue injury, and inflammatory disorders
- Provides information for the diagnosis, therapy, and monitoring of inflammatory disorders
- Independent risk factor for atherosclerosis, cardiac vascular events, hypertension, and MI

❏ Interpretation
Increased In
- Acute inflammation
- Rheumatoid arthritis, lupus
- Cardiovascular disease, atherosclerosis
- Oral contraceptives

- Inflammatory bowel disease
- Giant cell arteritis
- Osteomyelitis
- Cancer of the lymph nodes
- Pregnancy

Decreased In
- Patients treated with carboxypenicillins
- Liver failure

❏ **Limitations**
- Elevated C-reactive protein (CRP) values are nonspecific and should not be interpreted without a complete clinical history.
- Heterophile antibodies may falsely increase levels.
- Elevated levels of CRP are influenced by genetics, age, a sedentary lifestyle, stress, exposure to environmental toxins, and diet that specifically contains refined, processed, and manufactured foods.

CREATINE

❏ **Definition**
- Creatine is synthesized in the liver, taken up by muscle for stored energy as creatine phosphate, and broken down to creatinine; it then enters the circulation and is excreted by the kidneys.
- **Normal range:**
  ▾ Male: 0.2–0.7 mg/dL
  ▾ Female: 0.3–0.9 mg/dL

❏ **Use**
- Serum creatine levels may be significantly increased in amyotrophic lateral sclerosis, dermatomyositis, myasthenia gravis, starvation, muscular dystrophies, and trauma. Creatine synthesis is stimulated by methyltestosterone and may also be increased in hyperthyroidism, diabetic acidosis, and puerperium.
- This test is rarely used clinically.

❏ **Interpretation**
Increased In
- High dietary intake (meat)
- Destruction of muscle
- Hyperthyroidism (this diagnosis is almost excluded by normal serum creatine)
- Active RA
- Testosterone therapy

Decreased In
- Not clinically significant
- Drugs (e.g., TMP/SMX, cimetidine, cefoxitin)

❏ **Limitations**
- Artifactual decrease in DKA

16

CREATINE KINASE (CK), TOTAL*

❑ **Definition**

- CK is an enzyme that catalyzes the interconversion of ATP and creatine phosphate, controlling energy flow within cells, principally muscle. Its activity is greatest in striated muscle, heart tissue, and brain. The determination of CK activity is a proven tool in the investigation of skeletal muscle disease (muscular dystrophy) and is also useful in the diagnosis of myocardial infarction or stroke.
- **Normal range:**
  - ▼ Male: 49–348 IU/L
  - ▼ Female: 38–206 IU/L

❑ **Use**

- Marker for injury or diseases of cardiac muscle with good specificity
- Measurement of choice for striated muscle disorders

❑ **Interpretation**

Increased In

- Necrosis or inflammation of cardiac muscle: disorders listed under CK-MB (CK index usually >4%)
- Necrosis, inflammation, or acute atrophy of striated muscle
  - ▼ Disorders listed under CK-MB (CK index usually <4%)
  - ▼ Muscular dystrophy
  - ▼ Myotonic dystrophy
  - ▼ Amyotrophic lateral sclerosis (>40% of cases)
  - ▼ Polymyositis (70% of cases; average 20 × ULN)
  - ▼ Thermal and electrical burns (values usually higher than in AMI)
  - ▼ Rhabdomyolysis (especially with trauma and severe exertion); marked increase may be 1,000 times ULN
  - ▼ Severe or prolonged exercise as in marathon running (begins 3 hours after start of exercise; peaks after 8–16 hours; usually normal by 48 hours); smaller increases in well-conditioned athletes
  - ▼ Status epilepticus
  - ▼ Parturition and frequently the last few weeks of pregnancy
  - ▼ Malignant hyperthermia
  - ▼ Hypothermia
  - ▼ Familial hypokalemic periodic paralysis
  - ▼ McArdle disease
- Drugs and chemicals
  - ▼ Cocaine
  - ▼ Alcohol
  - ▼ Emetine (ipecac)—(e.g., bulimia)
  - ▼ Chemical toxicity; benzene ring compounds (e.g., xylene) depolarize the surface membrane and leach out low molecular weight enzymes, producing very high levels of total CK (100% fraction muscle [MM]) with increased LD) (3–5 × normal)

*Submitted By Craig S. Smith, MD.

- Half of patients with extensive brain infarction. Maximum levels are reached in 3 days; the increase may not appear before 2 days; levels are usually lower than in AMI and remain increased for a longer time; levels return to normal within 14 days; high mortality is associated with levels >300 IU. Elevated serum CK in brain infarction may obscure diagnosis of concomitant AMI.
- Some persons with large muscle mass (≤2 times normal) (e.g., football players).
- **Slight increase** (occasionally) in
  - ▼ Variable increase after IM injection to two to six times normal level; returns to normal 48 hours after cessation of injections; rarely affects CK-MB, LD-1 (lactate dehydrogenase-1), AST
  - ▼ Muscle spasms or convulsions in children
  - ▼ Healthy African Americans when compared to Caucasian/Hispanic populations
- Moderate hemolysis

Decreased In
- Decreased muscle mass (e.g., elderly, malnutrition, alcoholism)
- RA (about two thirds of patients)
- Untreated hyperthyroidism
- Cushing disease
- Connective tissue disease not associated with decreased physical activity
- Pregnancy level (8th–12th week) is said to be approximately 75% of non-pregnant level
- Various drugs (e.g., phenothiazine, prednisone, estrogens, tamoxifen, ethanol), toxins, and insecticides (e.g., aldrin, dieldrin)
- Metastatic tumor in the liver
- Multiple organ failure
- Intensive care patients with severe infection or septicemia

Normal In
- Pulmonary infarction
- Renal infarction
- Liver disease
- Biliary obstruction
- Some muscle disorders
  - ▼ Thyrotoxicosis myopathy
  - ▼ Steroid myopathy
  - ▼ Muscle atrophy of neurologic origin (e.g., old poliomyelitis, polyneuritis)
- PA
- Most malignancies
- Scleroderma
- Acrosclerosis
- Discoid lupus erythematosus

❏ Limitations
- Following MI, CK activity increases 4–8 hours after acute onset, activities peak at 12–36 hours, and usually returns to normal activities in 3–4 days. Although total CK has been used as a diagnostic tool for MI detection, along

with CK-MB, it has been predominantly replaced with troponin I or T due to lack of myocardial specificity.

- Exercise and muscle trauma (contact sports, traffic accidents, IM injections, surgery, convulsions, wasp or bee stings, and burns) can elevate serum CK values.
- To distinguish myoglobinuria from hemoglobinuria, serum CK and LD may be helpful. CK is normal with uncomplicated hemolysis, but LD and LD-1 usually are increased.

CREATINE KINASE ISOENZYMES (CK-BB, CK-MM, CK-MB)*

❑ **Definition**

- Creatine kinase is an enzyme consisting of three major isoenzymes, CK-BB (brain), CK-MB (heart) (see p. 901), and CK-MM (skeletal muscle). CK-BB is rarely present. It has been described as a marker for adenocarcinoma of the prostate, breast, ovary, colon, and GI tract, and for small cell anaplastic carcinoma of the lung. CK-BB has been reported with severe shock and/or hypothermia, infarction of bowel, brain injury, stroke, as a genetic marker in some families with malignant pyrexia, and with MB in alcoholic myopathy. CK-MM is found in normal serum.

❑ **Use**

- Detection of macroforms of creatine kinase (CK)
  - ▼ Diagnosing skeletal muscle disease, in conjunction with aldolase
  - ▼ CK isoenzymes are not widely used in clinical practice today due to the use of troponin and CK-MB mass assays but may be useful in differential diagnosis when CK elevated as well
- *The CK-BB isozyme is rarely encountered clinically.*

❑ **Interpretation**

Increased In

- Malignant hyperthermia, uremia, brain infarction or anoxia, Reyes syndrome, necrosis of the intestine, various metastatic neoplasms (especially prostate), biliary atresia

MACRO CK ISOENZYME†

❑ **Definition**

- This isoenzyme is a high molecular mass complex of a CK isoenzyme and immunoglobulin, most often CK-BB and monoclonal IgG and a kappa light chain. Macro CK type 2 is an oligomeric mitochondrial CK complex that migrates cathodically or close to CK-MM. It is found primarily in adults who are severely ill with malignancies or liver disease, or in children who have myocardial disease. It occurs transiently in about 1% of hospitalized patients and indicates a poor prognosis, except in children.

---

*Submitted By Craig S. Smith, MD.
† Submitted By Craig S. Smith, MD.

❑ Use

- Macroenzymes should be suspected when enzyme levels are persistently raised with relatively constant levels, and there is no obvious clinical explanation or other laboratory abnormality.

❑ Interpretation

- The clinical relevance of macro CK type 1 is not clearly established. It is not associated with a particular type of disease and has been observed in patients with various diseases, as well as in apparently healthy individuals. There are several reported disease associations, including hypothyroidism, neoplasia, autoimmune disease, myositis, and cardiovascular disease. The last two have the strongest reported associations and may support the diagnosis of an autoimmune process, but this may in part be explained by a higher frequency of requests for CK levels in these groups of patients. Myositis, including autoimmune myositis, polymyositis, malignancy-associated dermatomyositis, and drug-induced myositis, has been diagnosed in >50% of the patients with macro CK type.
- Atypical macro isoenzyme is found primarily in adults who are severely ill with malignancies or liver disease or in children who have myocardial disease. It occurs transiently in about 1% of hospitalized patients and indicates a poor prognosis, except in children.

❑ Limitations

- *Atypical macro isoenzyme may cause falsely high or low CK-MB results (depending on type of assay), resulting in an incorrect diagnosis of myocardial infarction (MI) or delayed recognition of an actual MI.* The atypical macro isoenzyme is discovered in <2% of all CK isoenzyme electrophoresis studies.

CREATINE KINASE MB (CK-MB)*

❑ Definition

- CK-MB is the myocardial fraction associated with MI and occurs in certain other states. MB can be used in estimation of infarct size. CK-MB, or CK-MB fraction, is an 84-kDa molecular weight enzyme that represents 40% of the CK present in myocardial tissue. As with total CK, CK-MB typically begins to rise 4–6 hours after the onset of infarction but is not elevated in all patients until about 12 hours. Elevations return to baseline within 36–48 hours, in contrast to elevations in serum troponin, which can persist for as long as 10–14 days. This means that CK-MB, unlike troponins, cannot be used for the late diagnosis of an acute MI but can be used to suggest infarct extension if levels rise again after declining. CK-MB generally comprises a lower fraction of total CK in skeletal muscle than in the heart. As a result, percentage criteria (4%) have been proposed to distinguish skeletal muscle damage from cardiac damage. However, these criteria are not recommended. They

*Submitted By Craig S. Smith, MD.

16

improve specificity but do so at the cost of sensitivity in patients who have both skeletal and cardiac injury.

■ Normal range:

	Reference Interval	
Analyte	Male	Female
CK-MB	<4.4 ng/mL	<4.4 ng/mL
CK-MB index	0.0–4.0	0.0–4.0

❏ **Use**

■ CK-MB is a widely used early marker for myocardial injury.

❏ **Interpretation**

Increased In

■ Necrosis or inflammation of cardiac muscle (CK index approximately 2.5%; in all other causes, CK index usually <2.5%):
  ▼ AMI.
  ▼ Cardiac contusion.
  ▼ After thoracic/open heart surgery, values return to baseline in 24–48 hours. AMI is difficult to diagnose in the first 24 postoperative hours.
  ▼ Resuscitation for cardiac arrest may increase CK and CK-MB in approximately 50% of patients, with peak at 24 hours, due to defibrillation (>400 J) and chest compression, but CK-MB/CK total ratio may not be increased, even with AMI.
  ▼ Percutaneous transluminal coronary angioplasty.
  ▼ Myocarditis.
  ▼ Prolonged supraventricular tachycardia.
  ▼ Cardiomyopathies (e.g., hypothyroid, alcohol).
  ▼ Collagen diseases involving the myocardium.
  ▼ Coronary angiography (transient).
■ Necrosis, inflammation, or acute atrophy of striated muscle:
  ▼ Exercise myopathy; slight to significant increases in 14–100% of persons after extreme exercise (e.g., marathons); smaller increases in well-conditioned athletes
  ▼ Skeletal muscle trauma with rhabdomyolysis, myoglobinuria
  ▼ Skeletal muscle diseases (e.g., myositis, muscular dystrophies, polymyositis, collagen vascular diseases [especially SLE])
  ▼ Familial hypokalemic periodic paralysis
  ▼ Electrical and thermal burns and trauma (approximately 50% of patients; but not supported by LD-1 > LD-2)
  ▼ Drugs (e.g., alcohol, cocaine, halothane [malignant hyperthermia], ipecac)
■ Endocrine disorders (e.g., hypoparathyroid, acromegaly, DKA; hypothyroidism—total CK four to eight times ULN in 60–80% of cases; becomes normal within 6 weeks of replacement therapy)

- Some infections:
  - ▼ Viral (e.g., HIV, EBV, influenza, picornaviruses, coxsackievirus, echovirus, adenoviruses)
  - ▼ Bacterial (e.g., *Staphylococcus*, *Streptococcus*, *Clostridium*, *Borrelia*)
  - ▼ Rocky Mountain spotted fever
  - ▼ Fungal
  - ▼ Parasitic (e.g., trichinosis, toxoplasmosis, schistosomiasis, cysticercosis)
- Others:
  - ▼ Malignant hyperthermia; hypothermia
  - ▼ Reye syndrome
  - ▼ Peripartum period for first day beginning within 30 minutes
  - ▼ Acute cholecystitis
  - ▼ Hyperthyroidism and chronic renal failure, which may cause persistent increase although the proportion of CK-MB remains low
  - ▼ Acute exacerbation of obstructive lung disease
  - ▼ Drugs (e.g., aspirin, tranquilizers)
  - ▼ Carbon monoxide poisoning
- Some neoplasms:
  - ▼ For example, prostate, breast
  - ▼ Ninety percent of patients following cryotherapy for prostate carcinoma with peak at 16 hours to about five times ULN; similar increase in total CK
- Percent activity distribution of CK isoenzymes in tissue

	CK-MB
Skeletal muscle	1
Myocardium	22
Brain	0

- A CK-MB >15–20% should raise the possibility of an atypical macro CK-MB.

Not Increased In

- Angina pectoris, exercise testing for CAD, or pericarditis. Elevation implies necrosis of cardiac muscle, even if a discrete infarct is not identified.
- Following diagnostic cardiac catheterization or cardiac pacemaker unless myocardial injury is sustained during the procedure.
- IM injections (total CK may be slightly increased).
- Seizures (total CK may be markedly increased).
- Brain infarction or injury (total CK may be increased).

❏ Limitations

- The presence of CK-MB is not unequivocally specific for myocardium, because it is found in patients with muscular dystrophies, polymyositis, hypothermia and hyperthermia, uremia, DKA, and septic shock. Renal failure, tissue damage following surgery, and cardiac contusion may also cause an elevation of CK-MB.
- Cardiac troponin is the preferred marker for the diagnosis of MI. CK-MB by mass assay is an acceptable alternative when cardiac troponin is not available.

16

Suggested Readings

Apple FS, Preese LM. Creatine kinase-MB: Detection of myocardial infarction and monitoring reperfusion. *J Clin Immunoassay.* 1994;17:24–29.

Gibler WB, Lewis LM, Erb RE, et al. Early detection of acute myocardial infarction in patients presenting with chest pain and nondiagnostic ECGs: Serial CK-MB sampling in the emergency department. *Ann Emerg Med.* 1990;19(12):1359–1366.

CREATININE CLEARANCE (CrCl)

❑ Definition

- This test compares the creatinine in a 24-hour sample of urine to the creatinine level in the blood to show how much blood the kidneys are filtering out each minute. It is calculated by the formula:

$$\frac{U_{Cr} \times 24\text{-hour volume}}{P_{Cr} \times 24 \times 60 \text{ minutes}}$$

where U_{Cr} is urine creatinine, P_{Cr} is plasma creatinine
- **Normal range:**
  - ▼ Male: 90–139 mL/minute
  - ▼ Female: 80–125 mL/minute

❑ Use

- Evaluate glomerular function
- Monitor effectiveness of treatment in renal disease

❑ Interpretation

- Acromegaly
- Acute tubular necrosis
- Carnivorous diets
- CHF
- Dehydration
- Diabetes
- Exercise
- Exposure to nephrotoxic drugs and chemicals
- Gigantism
- GN
- Hypothyroidism
- Infections
- Neoplasms (bilateral renal)
- Nephrosclerosis
- Polycystic kidney disease
- Pyelonephritis
- Renal artery atherosclerosis and obstruction
- Renal disease
- Renal vein thrombosis
- Shock and hypovolemia
- TB

Decreased In

- Acute or chronic GN
- Anemia
- Chronic bilateral pyelonephritis
- Hyperthyroidism
- Leukemia
- Muscle wasting diseases
- Paralysis
- Polycystic kidney disease
- Shock
- Urinary tract obstruction (e.g., from calculi)
- Vegetarian diets

❑ **Limitations**

- CrCl approximates GFR but overestimates it due to the fact that creatinine is secreted by the proximal tubule as well as filtered by the glomerulus.
- Measurement of CrCl should be considered in circumstances when the estimating equation based on serum creatinine is suspected to be inaccurate or for patients with estimated GFR >60 mL/minute/1.73 m² when a more accurate clearance measure is required for clinical decision making. Such circumstance may occur in people who are undergoing evaluation for kidney donation, treatment with drugs with significant toxicity that are excreted by the kidneys (e.g., high-dose methotrexate), or consideration for participation in research protocols.
- Indications for a clearance measurement because estimates based on serum creatinine may be inaccurate because of extremes of age and body size, severe malnutrition or obesity, disease of skeletal muscle, paraplegia or quadriplegia, a vegetarian diet, rapidly changing kidney function, or pregnancy.
- Drugs that may increase urine CrCl include enalapril, oral contraceptives, prednisone, and ramipril.
- Drugs that may decrease the urine CrCl include acetylsalicylic acid, amphotericin B, carbenoxolone, chlorthalidone, cimetidine, cisplatin, cyclosporine, guancydine, ibuprofen, indomethacin, mitomycin, oxyphenbutazone, paromomycin, probenecid (coadministered with digoxin), and thiazides.
- Excessive ketones in urine may cause falsely decreased values.
- Failure to follow proper technique in collecting 24-hour specimen may invalidate test results.
- Failure to refrigerate the specimen throughout the urine collection period allows decomposition of creatinine, causing falsely decreased values.
- Consumption of large amounts of meat, excessive exercise, and stress should be avoided for 24 hours before the test.

Suggested Reading

National Kidney Foundation KDOQI Clinical Practice Guidelines for Chronic Kidney Disease: Evaluation, Classification, and Stratification. http://www.kidney.org/professionals/kdoqi/guidelines_ckd/p5_lab_g4.htm. Accessed November 18, 2010.

16

CREATININE WITH ESTIMATED GLOMERULAR FILTRATION RATE (eGFR)

❏ **Definition**

- Creatinine is formed by the hydrolysis of creatine and phosphocreatine in muscle and by ingestion of meat. It is freely filtered at the glomerulus and secreted at the proximal tubule; some is resorbed. GFR is equal to the total of the filtration rates of the functioning nephrons in the kidney.
- **Normal range:**
  - ▼ **Creatinine**
    - 0–1 month: 0.00–1.00 mg/dL
    - 1 month–1 year: 0.10–0.80 mg/dL
    - 1–16 years: 0.20–1.00 mg/dL
    - >16 years, female: 0.50–1.20 mg/dL
    - >16 years, male: 0.60–1.30 mg/dL
  - ▼ **eGFR**
    - >16 years: >60 mL/minute/1.73 m²
    - Three equations are currently used for the calculation of GFR:
      - *IDMS-Traceable MDRD Study Equation for the calculation of GFR:*
        - GFR (mL/minute/1.73 m²) = $175 \times (S_{cr})^{-1.154} \times (age)^{-0.203} \times (0.742$ if female) $\times$ (1.212 if African American) (conventional units); where S_{cr} is serum creatinine.
        - (The equation has not been validated in children and will only be reported for patients >16 years of age. The equation is normalized for an average adult body surface area of 1.73 m²; weight and height adjustment is not necessary.)
      - Cockcroft-Gault formula
        - CrCl = {((140 − age) × weight)/(72 SCr)} × 0.85 if female
        - Where CrCl is expressed in milliliters per minute, age in years, weight in kilograms, and serum creatinine (SCr) in milligrams per deciliter.
      - The chronic kidney disease epidemiology collaboration (CKD-EPI) creatinine equation is based on the same four variables as the modification of diet in renal disease (MDRD) Study equation, but uses a two-slope spline to model the relationship between estimated GFR and serum creatinine, and a different relationship for age, sex, and race. The equation was reported to perform better and with less bias than the MDRD Study equation, especially in patients with higher GFR. This results in reduced misclassification of CKD.
        - GFR = $141 \times \min(Scr/\kappa,1)^{\alpha} \times \max(Scr/\kappa,1)^{-1.209} \times 0.993^{Age} \times 1.018$ [if female] $\times 1.159$ [if black]
        - Where Scr is serum creatinine (mg/dL), κ is 0.7 for females and 0.9 for males, α is −0.329 for females and −0.411 for males, min indicates the minimum of Scr/κ or 1, and max indicates the maximum of Scr/κ or 1.

❏ **Use**

▪ To diagnose renal insufficiency; more specific and sensitive indicator of renal disease than of BUN. Use of simultaneous BUN and creatinine determinations provides more information in conditions.

▪ Adjusting dosage of renally excreted medications.

▪ Monitoring renal transplant recipients.

▪ Serum creatinine levels are a proxy for reduced skeletal muscle mass.

▪ eGFR: Serum creatinine measurement is used in estimating GFR for people with CKD and those with risk factors for CKD (DM, hypertension, cardiovascular disease, and family history of kidney disease).

❏ **Interpretation**

Increased In

▪ Diet: ingestion of creatinine (roast meat).

▪ Muscle disease: gigantism, acromegaly.

▪ Pre- and postrenal azotemia.

▪ Impaired kidney function; 50% loss of renal function is needed to increase serum creatinine from 1.0 to 2.0 mg/dL. Therefore, the test is not sensitive for mild to moderate renal injury.

▪ An increase in serum creatinine occurs in 10–20% of patients taking aminoglycosides and ≤20% of patients taking penicillins (especially methicillin).

Decreased In

▪ Pregnancy: Normal value is 0.4–0.6 mg/dL. A value >0.8 mg/dL is abnormal and should alert the clinician to further diagnostic evaluation.

▪ Creatinine secretion is inhibited by certain drugs (e.g., cimetidine, trimethoprim).

▪ Proxy for reduced skeletal muscle mass.

❏ **Limitations**

▪ Artifactual decrease by:
  ▼ Marked increase of serum bilirubin
  ▼ Enzymatic reaction (glucose >100 mg/dL)

▪ Artifactual increase due to
  ▼ Reduction of alkaline picrate (e.g., glucose, ascorbate, uric acid). Ketoacidosis may substantially increase serum creatinine results with alkaline picrate reaction.
  ▼ Formation of colored complexes (e.g., acetoacetate, pyruvate, other ketoacids, certain cephalosporins).
  ▼ Enzymatic reaction: 5-Fluorocytosine may increase serum creatinine ≤0.6 mg/dL.
  ▼ Other methodologic interference (e.g., ascorbic acid, phenolsulfonphthalein, L-dopa).
  ▼ Some medications inhibit tubular secretion of creatinine, thereby decreasing creatinine clearance and increasing serum creatinine without a change in GFR. These medications include the following:
    ● Cephalosporin and aminoglycoside antibiotics
    ● Flucytosine

16

- Cisplatin
- Cimetidine
- Trimethoprim

▼ The Cockcroft-Gault equation estimates creatinine clearance and is not adjusted for body surface area. The CKD-EPI and MDRD Study equations estimate GFR adjusted for body surface area. GFR estimates from the CKD-EPI and MDRD Study equations can therefore be applied to determine level of kidney function, regardless of a patient's size. In contrast, estimates based on the Cockcroft-Gault equation can be used for drug dosage recommendations, whereas GFR estimates based on the MDRD Study should be "unadjusted" for body surface area.

▼ The Cockcroft-Gault equation appears to be less accurate than the MDRD Study equation, specifically in older and obese people.

▼ Modifications of the CKD-EPI and MDRD Study equations have been developed for Japanese and Chinese people. They have not yet been validated for Japanese or Chinese people living in other countries, including the United States. Studies in other ethnic groups have not yet been performed.

CREATININE, URINE

❑ **Definition**

■ Creatine is synthesized from amino acids in the kidney, liver, and pancreas. The creatine is then transported in the blood to other organs where it is synthesized into creatinine. In the absence of kidney disease, the urinary creatinine is excreted in rather constant amounts and represents glomerular filtration and active tubular excretion of the kidney. Because the creatinine is excreted from the body at a constant rate, there are expected values for creatinine in normal human urine. Specimen validity testing is the evaluation of the specimen to determine if it is consistent with normal human urine (creatinine values >20 mg/dL). Creatinine is made at a steady rate and is not affected by diet or by normal physical activities.

■ **Normal range:** see Table 16.25.

TABLE 16–25. Normal Values for Urine Creatinine

By Sex	Value
24-h urine	mg/d
Male	800–2,000
Female	600–1,800
Random urine	mg/dL
Male	
<40 y	24–392
>40 y	22–328
Female	
<40 y	16–327
>40 y	15–278

❑ **Use**

- Urinary creatinine, in conjunction with serum creatinine, is used to calculate the creatinine clearance, a measure of renal function.

❑ **Interpretation**

Increased In

- Exercise
- Acromegaly
- Gigantism
- DM
- Infections
- Hypothyroidism
- Animal meat diet

Decreased In

- Hyperthyroidism
- Anemia
- Muscular dystrophy
- Decreased muscle mass
- Advances renal disease
- Leukemia
- Vegetarian diets

❑ **Limitations**

- Urine creatinine is not ordered alone. Creatinine clearance, which requires a serum creatinine, offers useful renal function data. Serum creatinine alone is not an adequate index of glomerular filtration rate.
- Twenty-four–hour urine creatinine levels are used as an approximate check on the completeness of 24-hour urine collection.

CRYOFIBRINOGEN

❑ **Definition**

- Cryofibrinogen is an abnormal complex of proteins that precipitate out of plasma as it is cooled. These cold, insoluble protein complexes can be composed of fibrin, fibrinogen, and fibrin split products, in conjunction with other plasma proteins. If refrigerated serum and plasma both form a precipitate, then the precipitated proteins are referred to as cryoglobulins (see below). If, however, precipitation develops after refrigeration of plasma but does not occur in cold serum, the plasma precipitate is referred to as cryofibrinogen. Cryofibrinogenemia can be a primary (essential) condition or it may arise in association with an underlying condition, such as malignancy, infection, inflammation, diabetes, pregnancy, scleroderma, or oral contraceptives. A few familial cases have been reported. Skin biopsies may show leukocytoclastic vasculitis. Morbidity associated with cryofibrinogenemia occurs as the result of thrombotic occlusion of the small to medium arteries by insoluble protein complexes. Most individuals with cryofibrinogenemia are asymptomatic.

16

- **Normal range:**
  - ▼ Negative: No precipitate at 72 hours refrigerated; quantitation and immunotyping are not generally performed on positive cryofibrinogen.

❏ Use

- Patients with unexplained cutaneous ulcers, ischemia, or necrosis on cold-exposed areas
- Evaluating patients with vasculitis, glomerulonephritis, and lymphoproliferative diseases

❏ Interpretation

Increased In

- Vasculitis
- Hematologic and solid neoplasms
- Thromboembolic conditions
- Multiple myeloma
- Scleroderma
- Transient benign condition associated with infection
- Oral contraceptives

❏ Limitations

- If heparin is used as an anticoagulant in blood collection tubes, it may complex with fibrinogen, fibrin, and fibronectin and leads to falsely positive results. Therapeutically administered heparin may also produce false-positive results. Therefore, collected blood should be anticoagulated with EDTA, citrate, or oxalate and maintained at 37°C until the plasma is collected.
- Fasting specimen recommended. Proper collection and transport of specimen is critical to the outcome of the assay.
- May cause erroneous WBC count when performed on electronic cell counter.

Suggested Reading

Nash JW, Ross P Jr, Neil Crowson A, et al. The histopathologic spectrum of cryofibrinogenemia in four anatomic sites. Skin, lung, muscle, and kidney. *Am J Clin Pathol.* 2003;119: 114–122.

CRYOGLOBULINS

❏ Definition

- Cryoglobulins are abnormal serum proteins that precipitate at low temperatures and dissolve when temperature is raised. They cannot be identified by serum protein electrophoresis. Cryoglobulins are made up of monoclonal antibodies IgM or IgG, rarely IgA. IgM tends to precipitate at lower temperatures than does IgG cryoglobulin.
- Other names: cryocrit, cryoprotein.
- Cryoglobulins are classified as follows:
  - ▼ **Type I** (monoclonal immunoglobulin, especially IgM κ type)
    - Causes 25% of cases.

- Most commonly associated with multiple myeloma and Waldenström macroglobulinemia; other lymphoproliferative diseases with M components; occasionally it may be idiopathic.
- If present in large amounts (>5 mg/dL serum), blood may gel when drawn.
- Severe symptoms (e.g., Raynaud syndrome, gangrene without other causes).
- ▼ Type II (monoclonal immunoglobulin mixed with at least one other type of polyclonal immunoglobulin, most commonly IgM and polyclonal IgG; always with RF)
  - Causes up to 25% of cases
  - Associated most often with chronic hepatitis C virus (HCV) infection; less often with hepatitis B virus (HBV), EBV, bacterial and parasitic infections, autoimmune disorders, Sjögren syndrome, syndrome of essential mixed cryoglobulinemia, immune complex nephritis (e.g., membranoproliferative GN, vasculitis)
  - High titer RF without definite rheumatic disease
  - C4 levels decreased
- ▼ Type III (mixed polyclonal immunoglobulin, most commonly IgM–IgG combinations, usually with RF)
  - Causes approximately 50% of cases
  - Most commonly associated with lymphoproliferative disorders, connective tissue diseases (e.g., SLE), and persistent infections (e.g., HCV)
- ■ **Normal range:**
  - ▼ Usually present in small amounts (<1 mg/dL serum) in normal persons.
  - ▼ If positive, immunotyping of the cryoprecipitate is performed.

❏ Use

- ■ To assist in diagnosis of neoplastic diseases, acute and chronic infections, and collagen diseases
- ■ To detect cryoglobulinemia in patients with symptoms indicating or mimicking Raynaud disease, cyanosis, and skin ulceration
- ■ To monitor course of connective tissue disorders

❏ Interpretation

- ■ Cryoglobulins with a detected monoclonal protein normally prompt a clinical investigation to determine if an underlying disease exists.

❏ Limitations

- ■ Cryoglobulins are not to be confused with cryofibrinogen (see above section), which precipitates only in plasma, under cold conditions.
- ■ Failure to maintain sample at normal body temperature before centrifugation can affect results.
- ■ A recent fatty meal can increase turbidity of the blood.

Suggested Readings

Coblyn JS, McCluskey RT. Case records of the Massachusetts General Hospital. Weekly clinicopathological exercises. Case 3-2003: a 36-year-old man with renal failure, hypertension and neurologic abnormalities. *N Engl J Med.* 2003;348:333–342.

Kallemuchikkal U, Gorevic PD. Evaluation of cryoglobulins. *Arch Pathol Lab Med.* 1999;123:119–125.

CRYSTAL IDENTIFICATION, SYNOVIAL FLUID

❏ **Definition**

- Synovial fluid, often referred to as "joint fluid," is a viscous liquid found in the joint cavities. Synovial membranes line the joints, bursae, and tendon sheaths. The function of the synovial fluid is to lubricate the joint space and transport nutrients to the articular cartilage.
- The aspiration and analysis of synovial fluid may be done to determine the cause of joint disease, especially when accompanied by an abnormal accumulation of fluid in the joint (effusion). The joint disease may be crystal-induced, degenerative, inflammatory, or infectious. Morphologic analysis for cells and crystals, together with Gram stain and culture, help in the differentiation.
- Normal synovial fluid is a clear, pale yellow, viscous liquid that does not clot. When a synovial membrane is inflamed for any reason, the WBC count in the synovial fluid increases.
- In a rough fashion, one can classify this fluid into four groups.
  - ▼ Noninflammatory effusions (group I) occur when the WBC count is normal or minimally increased, as in traumatic arthritis or degenerative joint disease. Only rarely will such fluid have WBC counts of >2,000 cells/mm³.
  - ▼ Noninfectious mildly inflammatory effusions (group II) with WBC counts rarely >5,000 cells/mm³ occur in SLE and scleroderma.
  - ▼ In noninfectious acute inflammatory effusions (group III) characteristic of classic rheumatoid arthritis, gout, pseudogout, and rheumatic fever, the WBC count varies from 5,000 to 25,000 cells/mm³ but may exceed 50,000 or even 100,000 cells/mm³.
  - ▼ In the inflammatory effusions caused by infection (group IV), the WBC count commonly varies from 25,000 to >100,000 cells/mm³. As the WBC count becomes elevated, the percentage of polymorphonuclear leukocytes generally increases, the hyaluronate becomes degraded, and the synovial fluid sugar falls.
- Examination of synovial fluid for crystals is facilitated by having a microscope with polarizing filters and a quarter waveplate (also known as a "red compensator"). Birefringence is a term used to describe the optical property associated with certain transparent crystals in which the speed of propagation of light along the major and minor axes of the crystal differs, causing the plane of polarized light to be rotated.
- Detection of birefringent crystals is facilitated by use of two plane polarizing filters, one between the light source and the sample, and the other between the sample and the observer's eye. When the polarized filters are crossed, the background appears dark, and birefringent material, including a variety of crystals, appears brighter than the background.
- Several types of crystals have been found in synovial fluids (Table 16.26). The two most important are monosodium urate (MSU), characteristic of gouty effusions, and calcium pyrophosphate dihydrate (CPPD), characteristic of the effusions of pseudogout (crystal deposition disease). Other crystals such as calcium hydroxyapatite, calcium oxalate, cholesterol, and corticosteroid esters may also be associated with inflammatory effusions.

TABLE 16–26. Birefringent Materials in Synovial Fluid

Material	Usual Shape, Size	Birefringence	Cause	Location Within or Outside of PMNs, Macrophages
Crystals				
Monosodium urate	Needle, rod, parallel edges; 8–10 μm long	Strongly; −	Gout	Within or outside
Calcium pyrophosphate dihydrate	Rhomboid; may be rod, diamond, square, needle; <10 μm long	Weakly; +	Pseudogout	Only within
Calcium oxalate	Bipyramidal	Strong; 0	Long-term renal dialysis	Within or outside
Hydroxyapatite, other basic calcium phosphates	Aggregates only: small, (<1 μm), round, irregular	Weak; 0	Degenerating, calcifying joint (e.g., acute or chronic arthritis)	
Cholesterol	Flat, plate, corner notch; may be needle, rectangle; often >100 μm	Variable		
Cartilage, collagen	Irregular, rod-like	Strong; +		
Charcot-Leyden	Spindle; crystalloids of eosinophil membrane protein	Variable	Eosinophilic synovitis	
Steroids				
Betamethasone acetate	Rods; blunt ends; 10–20 μm	Strong; −	Injection into joint	
Cortisone acetate	Large rods	Strong; +		
Methyl prednisone acetate	Small, pleomorphic; tend to clump	Strong; 0		
Prednisone tebutate	Small, pleomorphic, branched, irregular	Strong; +		
Triamcinolone acetonide	Small, pleomorphic fragments; tend to clump	Strong; 0		
Triamcinolone hexacetonide	Large rods, blunt ends; 15–60 μm	Strong; 0		
Anticoagulants				
EDTA (dry)	Small, amorphous	Weak	Injection into joint	
Lithium heparin (not sodium)	May resemble pseudogout	Weak; +		
Other Materials				
Debris	Small, irregular, nonparallel	Variable edges		
Fat (cholesterol esters)	Globules	Strong; Maltese cross		
Starch granules	Round; size varies	Strong; Maltese cross		

+, positive birefringence; −, negative birefringence; 0, no axis.

Crystals are best seen in fresh, wet-mount preparations examined with polarizing light.

Hydroxyapatite complexes (diagnostic of apatite disease) and basic calcium phosphate complexes can be identified only by EM; most cases are suspected clinically but never confirmed.

EDTA, ethylenediaminetetraacetic acid; PMN, polymorphonuclear neutrophil.

Source: Judkins SW, Cornbleet PJ. Synovial fluid crystal analysis. *Lab Med.* 1997;28:774. With permission from American Society for Clinical Pathology and ASCP Press.

16

- Crystals that cause inflammation are usually 0.5 to approximately 20 μm in length, sparingly soluble in water, and capable of being phagocytized. At the peak of inflammation, most are intracellular.
- **Normal range:** absent (no crystals present).

❑ **Use**

- According to the American College of Radiology, synovial fluid analysis should be undertaken in the febrile patient with an acute flare of established arthritis (e.g., RA, osteoarthritis) to rule out superimposed septic arthritis.
- Repeated aspiration and synovial fluid analysis may be used to monitor the response of septic arthritis to treatment and may also be valuable for diagnosis of some cases of gout in which the initial aspirate does not have detectable crystals.

❑ **Interpretation**

- Positive identification of crystals provides a definitive diagnosis of joint disease.

❑ **Limitations**

- Powdered anticoagulants such as oxalate are themselves crystalline; their use may cause confusion, masking the presence of synovial fluid crystals definitive for the disease.
- Substantial variability has been noted among hospital laboratories in the ability to properly identify the presence or absence of MSU and CPPD crystals in synovial fluids. Studies of the performance of different hospital laboratories on the same synovial fluids suggest that MSU crystals are more easily detected than CPPD crystals.
- MSU crystals: reported sensitivity ranges from 63 to 78%; specificity from 93 to 100% (positive likelihood ratio of 14 for a diagnosis of gout).
- CPPD crystals: reported sensitivity ranges from 12 to 83%; specificity from 78 to 96% (positive likelihood ratio of 2.9 for a diagnosis of CPPD-associated arthritis).
- The stability of crystals in synovial fluids is studied by many at different temperatures. CPPD crystals dissolved significantly, and MSU crystals were detectable up to weeks but became smaller and less numerous. As storage time increased, new artificial crystals developed in the form of star-shaped arrays, plate-like structures, and positive birefringent Maltese crosses. Synovial fluid should be evaluated within 1 hour of collection.

CYCLIC CITRULLINATED PEPTIDE ANTIBODY, IgG

❑ **Definition**

- Antibodies to citrullinated proteins are markers of RA, especially for early diagnosis of the disease. In some cases, these antibodies may be detected many years before the onset of the first symptoms. Other names: CCP-IgG, citrullinated antibody, anticitrullinated antibody, anticitrullinated protein antibody (ACPA).

- **Normal range:**
  - ▼ Less than 20 U: negative
  - ▼ 20–39 U: weak positive
  - ▼ 40–59 U: moderate positive
  - ▼ ≥60 U: strong positive

❏ **Use**

- Evaluating patients suspected of having RA. The 2010 American College of Rheumatology guidelines recommend performing at least one serologic test (RF or CCP-IgG) and one acute-phase response measure (ESR or CRP) to classify a patient as having or not having definite RA in addition to a history of symptom duration and a thorough joint evaluation.
- Differentiating RA from other connective tissue diseases that may present with arthritis and may be positive for RF, such as HCV-associated cryoglobulinemia, undifferentiated polyarthritis, and Sjögren syndrome.
- Differential diagnosis of early polyarthritis.

❏ **Interpretation**

- Increased in RA (a positive result for CCP antibodies indicates a high likelihood of RA).

❏ **Limitations**

- The sensitivity of CCP-IgG for RA varies from about 50–75%, depending on the assay and study population, whereas specificity for RA is relatively high, usually >90%.
- Not all individuals with RA will have detectable anti-CCP antibodies, and elevated anti-CCP antibodies may be seen in individuals with no evidence of clinical disease.
- The use of anti-CCP antibody levels for monitoring the progression and/or remission of RA has not been established.
- The diagnostic value of anti-CCP antibodies has not been determined for juvenile arthritis.

Suggested Reading

Aletaha D, Neogi T, Silman A, et al. 2010 Rheumatoid arthritis classification criteria: an American College of Rheumatology/European League Against Rheumatism collaborative initiative. *Ann Rheum Dis.* 2010;69(9):1580–1588.

CYSTATIN C (CysC)

❏ **Definition**

- CysC is a 13-kDa, nonglycosylated basic protein that is produced by all nucleated cells. It is a cysteine protease inhibitor. Cystatin C is present in all investigated body fluids and is not affected by age, gender, muscle mass, or the inflammatory process. Cystatin C is removed from circulation by glomerular filtration and is completely reabsorbed and degraded in the tubules. Therefore, the plasma concentration of cystatin C is almost exclusively determined by the GFR, making cystatin C an excellent indicator of GFR.

16

- **Normal range:**
  - ▼ 0–3 months: 0.8–2.3 mg/L
  - ▼ 4–11 months: 0.7–1.5 mg/L
  - ▼ 1–3 years: 0.5–1.3 mg/L
  - ▼ 4–8 years: 0.5–1.3 mg/L
  - ▼ 9–17 years: 0.5–1.3 mg/L
  - ▼ ≥18 years: 0.5–1.0 mg/L

❏ **Use**

- New marker to estimate GFR independent of gender, age, and muscle mass, and cirrhosis; does not need to be corrected for height or weight. It is superior to serum creatinine.
- Sensitive marker of allograft function (although it may not be an optimal marker in patients receiving glucocorticoids).
- In the assessment of adverse cardiovascular events (CHF, ischemia, death) because kidney dysfunction is associated with such events.

❏ **Interpretation**

Increased In

- Glucocorticoid treatment
- May also be affected by thyroid disorders

❏ **Limitations**

- Due to immaturity of renal function in neonates, cystatin C levels are higher in those <3 months of age.
- Increased levels can be associated with higher levels of CRP or BMI and steroid use.
- In transplant patients, extrarenal elimination at higher levels and higher intraindividual variation compared to serum creatinine.

CYSTIC FIBROSIS (CF) MUTATION ASSAY*

❏ **Definition**

- CF assay identifies mutations in the cystic fibrosis transmembrane conductance regulator (*CFTR*) gene. To date, more than 1,700 mutations have been identified for CF (OMIM# 219700). Current guidelines, revised by the American College of Medical Genetics (ACMG) in 2004, recommend for routine screening a 23-mutation panel. CF screening also may identify the 5T/7T/9T variants in the CFTR gene. Complete analysis of the CFTR gene by DNA sequencing is appropriate for patients with a clinical diagnosis consistent with CF, patients with a family history of CF, males with congenital bilateral absence of the vas deferens, or newborns with a positive newborn screening result when mutation testing, using the standard 23-mutation panel, has a negative result.
- **Normal values:** negative or no mutations are found.

❏ **Use**

- Confirmatory diagnostic testing

*Submitted by Edward Ginns, MD and Marzena M. Galdzicka, PhD.

- Carrier testing (for the identification of heterozygotes)
- Prenatal diagnosis
- Available tests can be grouped as
  - ▼ Targeted mutation analysis tests.
    - 23-mutation panel recommended by the ACMG in 2004.
    - Panels testing for more than 23 mutations.
    - Reflex testing for the poly T variant (5T/7T/9T), a string of thymidine bases located in intron 8, is recommended for individuals having the *R117H* mutation or an adult male patient who is being evaluated for congenital absence of the vas deferens (CAVD). The 5T variant is thought to decrease the efficiency of intron 8 splicing.
  - ▼ Sequence analysis: Analysis of the entire coding region, promoter exon–intron boundaries, and specific intronic regions—testing to identify rare mutant alleles.
  - ▼ Deletion analysis: By MLPA (multiplex ligation–dependent probe amplification) or other molecular method.
  - ▼ Next-generation sequencing represents an integration of carrier screening and diagnostic testing in one lab test. Differentiation between CF screening and CF diagnostic testing occurs during the software analysis. CF screening software allows viewing of sequencing results according to a predetermined panel of clinically relevant CFTR mutations. CF diagnostic software allows one to see all variants found within the CFTR gene. The complexity of the interpretation of the results is much higher for the diagnostic test than for carrier screening test.

❏ **Limitations**

- The results of a genetic test may be affected by DNA rearrangements, blood transfusion, bone marrow transplantation, or rare sequence variations.

CYSTINE, URINE (CYSTINURIA PANEL)

❏ **Definition**

- Cystinuria is an autosomal recessive defect in reabsorptive transport of cystine and the dibasic amino acids ornithine, arginine, and lysine from the luminal fluid of the renal proximal tubule and small intestine. The only phenotypic manifestation of cystinuria is cystine urolithiasis, which often recurs throughout an affected individual's lifetime.
- The disorder is divided into three subtypes: Rosenberg I, II, and III. Cystinuria type I is the most common variant. Type I heterozygotes show normal aminoaciduria. Heterozygotes of types II and III often manifest cystinuria without cystine calculi and may be at increased risk for other types of urolithiasis. Type I heterozygotes are distinguished by normal levels of urinary cystine.
- Unlike type I and type II homozygotes, type III homozygotes show an increase in plasma cystine concentration after oral cystine administration.
- To classify cystinuria clinically, urinary cystine can be measured in each parent of a proband as phenotype I (recessive, urinary cystine level <100 μmol/g of creatinine), phenotype II (dominant, urinary cystine level >1,000 μmol/g of creatinine), and phenotype III (partially dominant, urinary cystine level

16

TABLE 16–27. Age-Based Reference Range for Cystine, Arginine, Lysine, and Ornithine

	0–5 mo µmol/g of Creatinine	6–11 mo µmol/g of Creatinine	1–3 y µmol/g of Creatinine	4–12 y µmol/g of Creatinine	13 y and older µmol/g of Creatinine
Arginine	0–124	0–97	0–80	0–62	0–44
Cystine	62–345	53–133	53–186	35–106	27–151
Lysine	133–1,761	115–699	89–611	89–602	62–513
Ornithine	0–168	0–71	0–71	0–62	0–44

100–1,000 µmol/g of creatinine). Cystinuria can also be classified based on the age at which symptoms first appear (i.e., infantile, juvenile, adolescent).
- **Normal range:** see Table 16.27.

❑ **Use**
- Diagnosis of cystinuria
- Monitoring of patients with cystinuria on therapy

❑ **Interpretation**
Increased In
- Cystinosis
- Cystinurias
- Cystinlysinuria
- Nephrolithiasis
- Nephrotoxicity due to heavy metals
- Renal tubular acidosis
- Wilson disease
- First semester of pregnancy

Decreased In
- Severely burned patients

❑ **Limitations**
- Urinary excretion is age dependent.
- Cystine excretion is normal in dibasic aminoaciduria.

CYTOGENETICS: FLUORESCENCE IN SITU HYBRIDIZATION (FISH), CHROMOSOME ANALYSIS, AND KARYOTYPING*

❑ **Definition**
- **FISH:** Molecular hybridization of a fluorescently labeled, cloned sequence of interest to a mitotic chromosome or interphase nucleus.
- **Chromosome analysis:** Microscopic visual inspection of banded mitotic chromosomes that assess the entire genome with the ability to detect chromosome aberrations larger than approximately 5–10 megabases.
- **Karyotyping:** An ordered pairing of chromosomes that aids in detecting chromosome anomalies.

*Submitted by Patricia Minehart Miron, PhD.

❏ **Use**

- **FISH**
  - ▼ Assessment of a specific region of the genome; allows detection of abnormalities that are too small to be visualized by conventional cytogenetics (e.g., microdeletions, microduplications)
  - ▼ Also may be performed on interphase (nondividing) cells, eliminating the necessity of cell culture and thereby allowing rapid turnaround times, and assessment of specimens that contain few or no dividing cells
- **Chromosome analysis:** used to identify abnormalities of chromosome number and structure that may be causal for mental retardation, congenital anomalies, pregnancy loss, infertility, and cancer
- **Karyotyping**
  - ▼ A tool in chromosome analysis.
  - ▼ Sometimes used (incorrectly) to mean chromosome analysis; a karyotype is not a stand-alone test.

❏ **Interpretation**

- **FISH**
  - ▼ **Normal** (two intact copies of sequence in a diploid cell)
  - ▼ **Abnormal:** examples include deletion of the genomic region, additional copies of region, and positional rearrangement of region
- **Chromosome analysis**
  - ▼ **Normal:** 46,XY (male) or 46,XX (female)
  - ▼ **Abnormal:**
    - ● Numeric: incorrect chromosome number (e.g., +21 in Down syndrome)
    - ● Structural: abnormal chromosome structure (e.g., deletion of the chromosome 5 short arm (5p–) in Wolf-Hirschhorn syndrome, translocation such as t(9;22) in CML)

❏ **Limitations**

- **FISH:** A targeted test, it cannot provide the total genomic assessment provided by conventional chromosome analysis.
- **Chromosome analysis:** requires *dividing cells*; therefore, all submitted specimens must contain viable cells that can be cultured in the laboratory.

D-DIMERS*

❏ **Definition**

- Plasma D-dimers are fibrin derivatives generated by the action of plasmin on cross-linked fibrin fragments D, indicating that the clotting mechanism had been activated and thrombin generated. Although it is a direct marker of active fibrinolysis, it is an indirect, but very useful, marker of ongoing coagulation.
- **Normal range:** <0.2 µg/mL for the latex assay; <1.1 mg/L for the ultrasensitive immunoturbidimetric test.

16

*Submitted By Liberto Pechet, MD.

❑ Use

- Two D-dimer assays are available, each with a different use.
  - ▼ The latex agglutination D-dimer has relatively low sensitivity; hence, it is not positive in single clots but elevated when multiple clots are generated. For this reason, it had been proven to be the most specific and sensitive test in the diagnosis of DIC.
  - ▼ The ultrasensitive D-dimer is performed by ELISA or immunoturbidimetric techniques that allow its precise quantitation. Because of its exquisite sensitivity, it becomes elevated in the presence of single clots.
    - ● Its main value is its high negative predictive ability, because a negative ultrasensitive D-dimer excludes thromboembolic events, with approaching 100% certitude (depending on methodology and equipment used). Although POC methods are available, they have slightly lower negative predictive values.
    - ● Elevated values are less useful, although persistent elevations after 3–6 months of anticoagulation following a thromboembolic event suggest a high probability of recurrent events.

❑ Interpretation

- The cutoff value for the ultrasensitive D-dimer is <1.1 mg/L (it varies with methods and equipment used). Any values below 1.1 mg/L are considered negative and are used in most diagnostic algorithms for the exclusion of deep vein thrombosis (DVT) or pulmonary embolism (PE) in low probability situations.
- The latex D-dimer is elevated in all situations with multiple clots, the prototype being DIC. The higher the titer, the more severe the DIC may be
- The ultrasensitive D-dimer is elevated in the following conditions:
  - ▼ DVT and PE
  - ▼ DIC
  - ▼ Renal, liver, or cardiac failure
  - ▼ Disseminated cancer and monoclonal gammopathies
  - ▼ Pregnancy
  - ▼ Major injury and surgery
  - ▼ Increasing age
  - ▼ Inflammatory conditions

❑ Limitations

- The ultrasensitive D-dimer may be falsely elevated or decreased in hyperlipidemic or very turbid blood samples and in patients treated with mouse monoclonal antibodies.
- RF may give false-positive results.

DEHYDROEPIANDROSTERONE SULFATE, SERUM (DHEA-SULFATE)

❑ Definition

- DHEA-S is produced by androgenic zone of the adrenal cortex. DHEA is the principal human C-19 steroid and has very low androgenic potency but serves as the major direct or indirect precursor for most sex steroids. The bulk of DHEA is secreted as a 3-sulfoconjugate (DHEA-S). Both hormones are

TABLE 16–28. Normal Ranges of DHES-S

Sex	Median (µg/dL)	(Central 95%) (µg/dL)
Female	170	35–430
Male	280	80–560

albumin bound, but binding of DHEA-S is much tighter. In gonads and several other tissues, most notably skin, steroid sulfatases can convert DHEA-S back to DHEA, which can then be metabolized to stronger androgens and to estrogens. During pregnancy, DHEA-S and its 16-hydroxylated metabolites are secreted by the fetal adrenal gland in large quantities. They serve as precursors for placental production of the dominant pregnancy estrogen, estriol.
- **Normal range:** see Table 16.28.

❑ **Use**
- Indicator of adrenal cortical function, especially for differential diagnosis of virilization, and investigations of hirsutism and alopecia in women. It is also of value in the assessment of adrenarche and delayed puberty.
- Differential diagnosis of Cushing syndrome.
- Replaces 17-KS urine excretion with which it correlates; shows no significant diurnal variation, thereby providing rapid test for abnormal androgen secretion.

❑ **Interpretation**
Increased In
- CAH: Markedly increased values can be suppressed by dexamethasone. Highest values occur in CAH due to deficiency of 3β-hydroxysteroid dehydrogenase.
- Adrenal carcinoma: Markedly increased levels cannot be suppressed by dexamethasone.
- Cushing syndrome caused by bilateral adrenal hyperplasia: Shows higher values than Cushing syndrome due to benign cortical adenoma, in which values may be normal or low.
- Cushing disease (pituitary etiology): Moderate increase in hypogonadotropic hypogonadism; DHEA-S is usually normal for chronologic age and high for bone age in contrast with idiopathic delayed puberty, in which DHEA-S is low relative to chronologic age and normal relative to bone age.
- First few days of life, especially in sick or premature infants.
- Polycystic ovary syndrome: Adrenal hyperandrogenism is a fairly typical facet of this syndrome.

Decreased In
- Addison disease
- Adrenal hypoplasia

❑ **Limitations**
- Extremely high levels (>700 or 800 µg/dL) in women are suggestive of a hormone-secreting adrenal tumor. By contrast, DHEA-SO_4 levels are typically normal in the presence of ovarian tumors.
- There are currently no established guidelines for DHEA-S replacement/supplementation therapy or its biochemical monitoring.

16

- Many drugs and hormones can result in changes in DHEA-S levels. In most cases, the drug-induced changes are not large enough to cause diagnostic confusion, but when interpreting mild abnormalities in DHEA-S levels, drug and hormone interactions should be taken into account. Examples of drugs/hormones that can reduce DHEA-S levels include insulin, oral contraceptive drugs, corticosteroids, CNS agents that induce hepatic enzymes (e.g., carbamazepine, clomipramine, imipramine, phenytoin), many antilipemic drugs (e.g., statins, cholestyramine), dopaminergic drugs (e.g., levodopa/dopamine, bromocriptine), fish oil, and vitamin E.
- Drugs that may increase DHEA-S levels include metformin, troglitazone, prolactin, danazol, calcium channel blockers (e.g., diltiazem, amlodipine), and nicotine.

DEHYDROEPIANDROSTERONE, SERUM (DHEA, DHEA UNCONJUGATED)

❑ **Definition**
- DHEA has very low androgenic potency but serves as the major direct or indirect precursor for most sex steroids. DHEA is secreted by the adrenal gland, and production is at least partly controlled by ACTH; the bulk of DHEA is secreted as a 3-sulfoconjugate DHEA-S. Both hormones are albumin bound, but DHEA-S binding is much tighter. As a result, circulating concentrations of DHEA-S are much higher (>100-fold) compared to DHEA. In most clinical situations, DHEA and DHEA-S results can be used interchangeably. In gonads and several other tissues, most notably skin, steroid sulfatases can convert DHEA-S back to DHEA, which can then be metabolized to stronger androgens and to estrogens. During pregnancy, DHEA/DHEA-S and their 16-hydroxylated metabolites are secreted by the fetal adrenal gland in large quantities. They serve as precursors for placental production of the dominant pregnancy estrogen, estriol. Within weeks after birth, DHEA/DHEA-S levels fall by 80% or more and remain low until the onset of adrenarche at age 7 or 8 in girls and age 8 or 9 in boys.
- **Normal range** (adults): male: 180–1,250 ng/dL; female: 130–980 ng/dL.

❑ **Use**
- Diagnosing and differential diagnosis of hyperandrogenism (in conjunction with measurements of other sex steroids).
- An adjunct in the diagnosis of CAH; DHEA/DHEA-S measurements play a secondary role to the measurements of cortisol/cortisone, 17α-hydroxyprogesterone, and androstenedione.
- Diagnosing and differential diagnosis of premature adrenarche.

❑ **Interpretation**
Increased In
- Hyperandrogenism
- Androgen-producing adrenal tumors
- CAH due to 3β-hydroxysteroid dehydrogenase deficiency

Decreased In
- With age in men and women, hyperlipidemia, psychosis, psoriasis

❏ **Limitations**
- DHEA levels increase until the age of 20 to a maximum roughly comparable to that observed at birth. Levels then decline over the next 40–60 years to around 20% of peak levels.
- Currently, the correlation of serum DHEA/DHEA-S level with disease risk factors has not been completely established. There are currently no established guidelines for DHEA replacement/supplementation therapy or its biochemical monitoring.

DEXAMETHASONE SUPPRESSION OF PITUITARY ACTH SECRETION TEST (DST)

❏ **Definition**
- Dexamethasone is a potent synthetic glucocorticoid not detected by serum, urine, and salivary cortisol assays. Dexamethasone should not fully suppress ACTH and, therefore, should not decrease adrenal secretion of cortisol. Dexamethasone suppression tests are used to assess the status of the HPA axis and for the differential diagnosis of adrenal hyperfunction.
- **Low-dose dexamethasone suppression tests** are good standard screening tests to differentiate patients with Cushing syndrome of any cause from patients who do not have Cushing syndrome. Principle: If the hypothalamic–pituitary axis is normal, any supraphysiologic dose of dexamethasone is sufficient to suppress pituitary ACTH secretion. This should lead to reductions in cortisol secretion and its concentration in serum and saliva, as well as in the 24-hour urine excretion. Two main protocols are used: overnight 1-mg screening test and standard 2-day, 2-mg test.
- **High-dose suppression** tests are based on the fact that ACTH secretion in Cushing disease is only relatively resistant to glucocorticoid negative feedback inhibition and does not suppress normally with either the overnight 1-mg or the 2-day low-dose test. By increasing the dose of dexamethasone four- to eightfold, ACTH secretion can be suppressed in most patients with Cushing disease. Therefore, this test is used to distinguish patients with Cushing disease (Cushing syndrome caused by pituitary hypersecretion of ACTH) from most patients with ectopic ACTH syndrome (Cushing syndrome caused by nonpituitary ACTH-secreting tumors).

LOW-DOSE TEST: OVERNIGHT 1-mg SCREENING TEST

❏ **Definition**
- Overnight screening test is a quick screening test for nonsuppressible cortisol production and subclinical or clinical Cushing syndrome and should not be used as the sole criterion for excluding the diagnosis of Cushing syndrome.

16

❑ **Use**

- Dexamethasone (1 mg) is taken orally between 11 PM and midnight, and a single blood sample is drawn at 8 AM the next morning for assay of serum cortisol.

❑ **Interpretation**

- The 2008 Endocrine Society Guidelines suggest a diagnostic serum cortisol criterion of 1.8 µg/dL.
- This test has a significant false-positive rate when sensitivity is maximized. Using a serum cortisol criterion of <3.6 µg/dL, the test has a 12–15% false-positive rate. If, however, the criterion for suppression of serum cortisol is increased to <7.2 µg/dL, the false-positive rate falls to 7%. This suggests that the multiple criteria may be useful in interpreting the test.
- The salivary cortisol concentration at 8 AM after 1 mg dexamethasone given at midnight was 0.8 ± 0.4 ng/mL (range 0.6–1.1 ng/mL) in 101 normal subjects, a sensitivity and specificity of 100%.

LOW-DOSE TEST: STANDARD 2-DAY (2-mg) TEST

❑ **Use**

- The 2-day test is used to assess suppressibility in patients with an equivocal overnight test or in patients who have not had an overnight test.
- Dexamethasone, 0.5 mg, is taken orally every 6 hours, usually at 8 AM, 2 PM, 8 PM, and 2 AM, for a total of eight doses.
- Blood is drawn 2 or 6 hours after the last dose for measurement of cortisol.

❑ **Interpretation**

- The normal response to the 2-day test consists of the following:
  - ▼ Urinary cortisol excretion should fall to <10 µg/24 hours on the 2nd day of dexamethasone administration.
  - ▼ Serum cortisol concentration is <5 µg/dL, a plasma ACTH concentration is <5 pg/mL, and a serum dexamethasone concentration is between 2.0 and 6.5 ng/mL.
  - ▼ In a recent meta-analysis, the 1-mg test and the 2-day 2-mg test were both accurate, but the 2-mg test had slightly less diagnostic accuracy.

HIGH-DOSE TEST: OVERNIGHT (8-mg) TEST

❑ **Use**

- Dexamethasone (8 mg) is taken orally between 11 PM and midnight, and a single blood sample is drawn at 8 AM the next day for measurement of serum cortisol.
- With this protocol, the 8 AM serum cortisol concentration is <5 µg/dL in most patients with Cushing disease (i.e., a pituitary tumor) and is usually undetectable in normals.

HIGH-DOSE TEST: STANDARD 2-DAY (8-mg) TEST

❑ **Use**

- The patient collects at least one baseline 24-hour urine, at 8 AM.
- The patient begins taking 2 mg of dexamethasone orally every 6 hours for a total of 8 doses, usually at 8 AM, 2 PM, 8 PM, and 2 AM, and the urine collections are continued.
- In practice, this test is often performed immediately after completing the low-dose dexamethasone suppression test (if the test is positive).
- The urine collections are assayed for urinary free cortisol and creatinine. In addition, a blood specimen can be collected 6 hours after the last dose of dexamethasone for measurement of cortisol, dexamethasone, and ACTH.
- This protocol leads to the following values in normal subjects:
  - ▼ Urinary free cortisol excretion is <5 μg/24 hours.
  - ▼ Serum cortisol and plasma ACTH are low and usually undetectable.
  - ▼ Serum dexamethasone ranges from about 8 to 20 ng/mL.

❑ **Limitations of All Tests**

- False-positive results may occur in acute and chronic illness, alcoholism, depression, and due to certain drugs (e.g., phenytoin, phenobarbital, primidone, carbamazepine, rifampicin, and spironolactone).
- Atypical or false-positive responses may occur also due to alcohol, estrogens, birth control pills, pregnancy, obesity, acute illness and stress, and severe depression.
- Not a good choice for patients in whom CBG levels may be abnormal.
- Noncompliance (check by measuring plasma dexamethasone).
- Some patients with large ACTH-producing pituitary adenomas have marked resistance to high-dose dexamethasone suppression. In long-standing cases, nodular hyperplasia of the adrenal may develop causing autonomous cortisol production and resistance to dexamethasone test.
- No suppression in 80% of cases in ectopic ACTH syndrome or nodular adrenal hyperplasia.
- Urine cortisol and plasma cortisol are not decreased after high or low doses of dexamethasone in adrenal adenoma or carcinoma or ectopic ACTH syndrome.
- Patients with psychiatric illness may be resistant and do not reproducibly suppress.

DIGOXIN*

❑ **Definition**

- Digoxin is an analogue of digitoxin.
- A cardiac glycoside derived from *Digitalis lanata* consisting of a steroid nucleus and a lactone coupled with sugar moieties.

16

*Submitted By Amanda J. Jenkins, PhD.

- Other name: Lanoxin.
- **Normal therapeutic range:** 0.8–2.0 ng/mL (1.2–2.6 nmol/L).

❑ Use

- Treatment of CHF and atrial fibrillation/flutter

❑ Interpretation

- **Toxic range:** >2.5 ng/mL, but 10% of patients may show toxicity at <2 ng/mL.
- Toxicity may be observed at a lower serum concentration in presence of hypokalemia, hypercalcemia, hypomagnesemia, hypoxia, and heart disease.
- Increased with coadministration of
  - ▼ Quinidine
  - ▼ Verapamil
  - ▼ Amiodarone
  - ▼ Indomethacin
  - ▼ Cyclosporin A

❑ Limitations

- Draw blood 6–8 hours (or 8–24 hours) after last oral dose after steady state has been achieved in 1–2 weeks.
- Pediatric toxic concentration may be higher; therapeutic index is very low (i.e., small difference between therapeutic and toxic blood concentration). However, approximately 10% of patients have serum concentration of 2–4 ng/mL without evidence of toxicity. On a dose of 0.25 mg/day, mean serum concentration is 1.2 ± 0.4 ng/mL; on a dose of 0.5 mg/day, mean serum concentration is 1.5 ± 0.4 ng/mL. A *Digitalis* leaf dose of 0.1 g/day produces the same serum concentration as 0.1 mg/day of crystalline digitoxin. There is ECG evidence of toxicity in one third to two thirds of patients, with no symptoms or signs.
- False low results may be due to spironolactone.
- Endogenous digoxin-like substances may produce positive test results in persons who have not received the drug, especially in
  - ▼ Uremia.
  - ▼ Severe agonal states and postmortem—therefore, a high postmortem concentration may not have been high before death and a normal postmortem concentration suggests that the antemortem concentration was not toxic.
- Because most methods measure both endogenous digoxin-like substances and inactive metabolites of digoxin, therapeutic monitoring should mostly be used to assess patient compliance and to confirm drug toxicity.
- Tests: bioassay, Na^+/K^+-ATPase receptor assay, colorimetry, fluorometry, HPLC, GC, enzyme assay, immunoassay, and LC/MS.
- Immunoassay is the most widely used methodology: RIA, FPIA, EIA, and chemiluminescence.
  - ▼ Confounders in analysis-low concentrations, steroid-like nucleus, endogenous digoxin-like immunoreactive factors (observed in patients with renal failure, liver disease, MI, newborns, pregnancy, hypertension, strenuous exercise, volume expansion), digoxin metabolites, presence of antidote (Fab).
  - ▼ Immunoassays exhibit <5% cross-reactivity with digitoxin and digoxigenin, and 80–100% with the metabolites digoxigenin bis- and monodigitoxoside.
  - ▼ Hb, lipid, and bilirubin do not typically interfere.

DILUTE RUSSELL VIPER VENOM (dRVVT) ASSAY*

❏ **Definition**

- The dRVVT assay detects the presence of LA. This test is helpful for the diagnosis of the antiphospholipid antibody syndrome and acquired thrombophilia.

❏ **Use**

- The dRVVT assay consists of three stages:
  ▼ The screening reagent initiates plasma clotting by directly activating factor X, thereby bypassing both the intrinsic and extrinsic pathways of coagulation. LA antibodies prolong the clotting time. If the clotting time is not prolonged in the presence of the dilute venom, LA is not present, and the second stage of the assay is omitted.
  ▼ If the clotting time is prolonged (>20% of the control), a PTT analysis on a 1:1 incubation of normal plasma with the patient's plasma to discriminate between an inhibitor or a clotting factor deficiency (correction of the clotting time to <44 seconds) is routinely done. If there is no correction, and the clotting time remains prolonged, an inhibitor has been demonstrated, and the laboratory proceeds with the next step.
  ▼ A "confirmation" reagent containing a high concentration of phospholipid is added to the plasma under study. If the clotting time in the first phase has been prolonged by LA antibodies, the reagent neutralizes the antibodies and the clotting time becomes shorter, similar to that of the control. If the clotting time elongation in the first stage is not due to LA but a different inhibitor, the clotting time in the presence of the confirmation reagent remains elongated. Additional studies to rule out other etiologies for the initially prolonged clotting time are then indicated.
- Results are expressed as a ratio: The clotting time of the screening reagent is divided by the clotting time of the confirmation tests.

❏ **Interpretation**

- Ratio >2.0: LA strongly present.
- Ratio of 1.6–2.0: LA moderately present.
- Ratio between 1.2 and 1.6: LA may be present, but in a low titer.

❏ **Limitations**

- LA antibodies may vary in their properties, and the results may be positive in the dRVVT assay but not in other assays. Because of that, at least two type of assays have been recommended for each patient.
- Heparin levels >1 U/mL prolong the first-stage assay.

Suggested Reading

Lambert M, Ferrard-Sasson G, Dubucquoi S, et al. Dilute Russell viper-venom time improves identification of antiphospholipid syndrome in a lupus anticoagulant-positive patient population. *Thromb Haemost.* 2009;101:577–581.

16

---

*Submitted By Liberto Pechet, MD.

DIRECT AND INDIRECT ANTIGLOBULIN TESTS (DAT AND IAT)*

❑ **Definition**

- Previously known as the direct and IATs, these assays play a major role in transfusion medicine as well as in the diagnosis of immune hemolytic anemias (see p. 377), because they detect antibodies either bound to RBCs (the DAT), or in serum (the indirect antiglobulin test, IAT). In patients that have not been transfused within the preceding 3 months, a positive DAT almost always reveals autoimmune antibodies.
- The IAT is used to demonstrate in vitro reactions between RBCs and antibodies that sensitize red cells that express the corresponding antigen. The patient's serum or plasma is incubated with red cells, which are then washed to remove unbound globulins. Agglutination that develops when the antiglobulin reagent is added indicates a reaction between serum antibodies (usually the result of immunization from previous transfusions) and red cells.
- The antiglobulin reagent consists in most cases of rabbit antibodies directed against human IgG. Other reagents used in the DAT assay are anticomplement (anti-C3dg) or a mixture of anti-IgG and anti-C3dg. If the DAT is positive following recent transfusions, the antibodies can be eluted from RBCs and the eluted antibodies must be identified.

❑ **Use**

- The DAT is used whenever hemolysis of red cells is suspected as being caused by autoantibodies. The assay determines if red cells have been coated in vivo with immunoglobulins, complement, or both.
- The utility of the IAT in blood banking stems from its great sensitivity in detecting various IgG antibodies in the recipient's serum prior to transfusions. It is part of the antibody screening test. It is used to detect the presence of alloantibodies directed against non-ABO blood group antigens.
- In cases of severe autoimmune hemolytic anemia, both the DAT and the IAT may be positive because the excess antibodies elute from the red cell membranes and spill out into serum.

❑ **Interpretation**

- Both the DAT and the IAT are reported and interpreted as either positive or negative.
- The DAT is positive whenever the patient's red cells are coated with autoantibodies that developed against the patient's own red cells. It is also positive when alloantibodies in a recipient's circulation react with antigens on recently transfused red cells, as well as alloantibodies in maternal circulation, which cross the placenta and coat fetal red cells. Antibodies directed against certain drugs may also bind to red cell membranes and result in a positive test.
- The IAT is positive in the presence of serum alloantibodies in patients previously transfused and immunized against non-self–red cell antigens.

---

*Submitted By Vishesh Chhibber, MD.

❑ Limitations

- Finding of a positive DAT indicates the presence of red cell autoantibodies, alloantibodies following transfusions, or of coating of red cells with excess immunoglobulins. It requires additional workup to elucidate the etiology of the immunoglobulins by performing tests for antibody specificity: cold agglutinins (see p. 377 under hemolytic anemias), Donath-Landsteiner antibody (see p. 379), and also serum protein electrophoresis or immunofixation when a plasmacytic disease (see p. 432) is suspected. The administration of certain drugs (α-methyldopa, IV penicillin, or procainamide) and recent transfusions must also be excluded.
- A negative DAT does not rule out hemolysis but only hemolysis of autoimmune etiology. For instance, DAT is negative in some cases of drug-induced hemolytic anemias, hemoglobinopathies, hereditary spherocytosis, and other hereditary hemolytic anemias.
- A positive IAT requires further investigation to identify more precisely the offending antigen(s).

ENZYME TESTS THAT DETECT CHOLESTASIS (ALP, 5′-NUCLEOTIDASE, GGT, LAP)

❑ Definition

- ALP refers to a group of enzymes that catalyze the hydrolysis of a large number of organic phosphate esters at an alkaline pH optimum. The major value of the serum ALP in the diagnosis of liver disorders is in the recognition of cholestatic disease. However, an elevation in the ALP concentration is a relatively common finding and does not always indicate the presence of hepatobiliary disease. The degree of elevation does not distinguish between intra- and extrahepatic cholestasis. Elevations in serum 5′-nucleotidase are seen in the same types of hepatobiliary diseases associated with an increased serum ALP. Most studies suggest that serum ALP and 5′-nucleotidase are equally valuable in demonstrating biliary obstruction or hepatic infiltrative and space-occupying lesions. Elevated serum levels of gamma-glutamyl transpeptidase (GGT) are found in diseases of the liver, biliary tract, and pancreas, and reflect the same spectrum of hepatobiliary disease as ALP, 5′-nucleotidase, and leucine aminopeptidase. Serum GGT and ALP correlate reasonably well. There are conflicting data as to whether serum GGT has better sensitivity for hepatobiliary disease than ALP or leucine aminopeptidase.

❑ Interpretation

- Increased ALP in liver diseases (due to increased synthesis from proliferating bile duct epithelium) is the best indicator of biliary obstruction but does not differentiate intrahepatic cholestasis from extrahepatic obstruction. In cholestasis, ALP level is increased out of proportion to other liver function tests.
- Increases before jaundice occurs.
- High values (greater than five times normal) favor obstruction and normal levels virtually exclude this diagnosis.
- Markedly increased in infants with congenital intrahepatic bile duct atresia but is much lower in extrahepatic atresia.

16

- **Increased 10 times normal:** carcinoma of the head of the pancreas, choledocholithiasis, and drug cholestatic hepatitis.
- **Fifteen to twenty times increase:** primary biliary cirrhosis, primary or metastatic carcinoma.
- Increase (3–10 times normal) with only slightly increased transaminases may be seen in biliary obstruction and converse in liver parenchymal disease (e.g., cirrhosis, hepatitis); increased greater than three times normal in <5% of acute hepatitis.
- Increased (2–10 times normal; usually 1.5–3 times increase) serum ALP and LD in early infiltrative (e.g., amyloid) and space-occupying diseases of the liver (e.g., tumor, granuloma, abscess).
- Increase less than three to four times normal is nonspecific and may occur in all types of liver diseases (e.g., congestive heart failure, infiltrative liver diseases, cirrhosis, acute [viral, toxic, alcoholic] or chronic hepatitis, acute fatty liver).
- **Increased five times normal:** infectious mononucleosis, postnecrotic cirrhosis.
- Increased ALP (of liver origin) and LD with normal serum bilirubin, AST, and ALT suggest obstruction of one hepatic duct or metastatic or infiltrative disease of the liver.
- GGT/ALP ratio >5 favors alcoholic liver disease.
- Isolated increase of GGT is a sensitive screening and monitoring test for alcoholism. Increased GGT due to alcohol or anticonvulsant drugs is not accompanied by increased ALP.
- Serum 5′-nucleotidase (5′-N) and LAP parallel the increase in ALP in obstructive type of hepatobiliary disease, but the 5′-N is increased only in the latter and is normal in pregnancy and bone disease, whereas the LAP is increased in pregnancy but is usually normal in bone disease. GGT is normal in bone disease and pregnancy. Therefore, these enzymes are useful in determining the source of increased serum ALP. Although serum 5′-N usually parallels ALP in liver disease, it may not increase proportionately in individual patients.

Serum Enzyme	Biliary Obstruction	Pregnancy	Childhood; Bone Disease
ALP	Increased	Increased	Increased
GGT	Increased	Normal	Normal
5′-N	Increased	Normal	Normal
LAP	Increased	Increased	Normal

- Bilirubin ("bile") in urine implies increased serum conjugated bilirubin and excludes hemolysis as the cause. Often precedes clinical icterus. May occur without jaundice in anicteric or early hepatitis, early obstruction, or liver metastases. (Tablets detect 0.05–0.1 mg/dL; dipsticks are less sensitive; test is negative in normal persons.)
- Complete absence of urine urobilinogen strongly suggests complete bile duct obstruction; is normal in incomplete obstruction and decreased in some phases of hepatic jaundice. Increased in hemolytic jaundice and subsiding

hepatitis. Increase may evidence hepatic damage even without clinical jaundice (e.g., some patients with cirrhosis, metastatic liver disease, congestive heart failure). Presence in viral hepatitis depends on the phase of disease (normal is <1 mg or 1 Ehrlich U/2-hour specimen).

ERYTHROCYTE SEDIMENTATION RATE (ESR)*

❑ **Definition**

- ESR is the distance in millimeters that erythrocytes fall during 1 hour in a sample of venous blood (Westergren principle). Newer techniques allow the test to be performed in 30 minutes, resulting in improved turnaround time.
- **Normal range:** 0–15 mm/hour in men and 0–20 mm/hour in women.

❑ **Use**

- ESR is not a good screening test because of its low sensitivity. CRP is superior to ESR because it is more sensitive and reflects a more rapid change in the patient's condition. ESR may be used as a screening test to detect the presence of a systemic disease; however, a normal test does not exclude malignancy or other serious disease, although it does rule out temporal arteritis or polymyalgia rheumatica.
- Finding a much accelerated ESR (>100 mm/hour) in patients with ill-defined symptoms directs the physician to search for a severe systemic disease, especially paraproteinemias, disseminated malignancies, connective tissue diseases, and severe infections such as bacterial endocarditis.
- Finding a normal ESR in patients with paraproteinemia suggests the development of hyperviscosity syndrome.
- ESR is also used to monitor the course or response to therapy of diseases if greatly accelerated initially.

❑ **Interpretation**

Increased In

- Infections
- Vasculitis, including temporal arteritis
- Inflammatory arthritis
- Renal disease
- Anemia
- Malignancies and plasma cell dyscrasias
- Acute allergy
- Tissue injury, including myocardial infarction
- Pregnancy (but not first trimester)
- Estrogen administration
- Aging

Decreased In

- Polycythemia vera
- Sickle cell anemia
- CHF

16

---

*Submitted By Liberto Pechet, MD.

- Typhoid and undulant fever, malarial paroxysm, trichinosis, pertussis, infectious mononucleosis, uncomplicated viral diseases
- Peptic ulcer
- Acute allergy

❏ **Limitations**

Causes of a Falsely Increased ESR
- Increased fibrinogen; increased gamma- and betaglobulins
- Drugs (dextran, penicillamine, theophylline, vitamin A, methyldopa, methysergide)
- Technical factors (e.g., hemolyzed sample, high temperature in the laboratory)
- Hypercholesterolemia

Causes of a Falsely Decreased ESR
- Abnormally shaped RBCs (sickle cells, spherocytes, acanthocytes)
- Microcytosis
- HbC disease
- Hypofibrinogenemia
- Technical factors (low temperature in the laboratory, clotted blood)
- Extreme leukocytosis
- Drugs (quinine, salicylates, high steroid levels, drugs that cause high glucose levels)

ESTRADIOL, UNCONJUGATED

❏ **Definition**
- Most active of endogenous estrogens, primarily produced in ovaries with additional amounts produced by adrenal glands and testes (in men).
- Other names: estradiol 17 beta, E_2.
- Normal range: see Table 16.29.

❏ **Use**
- Of value, together with gonadotropins, in evaluating menstrual and fertility problems in women
- In the evaluation of gynecomastia or feminization states due to estrogen-producing tumors, menstrual cycle irregularities, and sexual maturity in female patients and in monitoring of human menopausal gonadotropin (Pergonal) therapy

TABLE 16–29. Normal Range of Values for Estradiol, Unconjugated

Sex and Condition	Reference Range (pg/mL)
Males	<20–47
Postmenopausal females	<20–40
Nonpregnant females:	
Midfollicular	27–122
Periovulatory	95–433
Midluteal	49–291

❑ **Interpretation**

Increased In

- Feminization in children
- Estrogen-producing tumors
- Gynecomastia
- Hepatic cirrhosis
- Hyperthyroidism

Decreased In

- Primary and secondary hypogonadism
- PCOs
- Eating disorders, anorexia nervosa.

❑ **Limitations**

- Oral contraceptives inhibit physiologic increase.
- Estradiol values from pregnant females may be affected by high levels of estriol such as those present in the second and third trimesters of pregnancy.
- Current estradiol assays are sensitive for women of child-bearing age and induction of ovulation monitoring. In contrast, levels in postmenopausal women, men, and prepubertal children <20 pg/mL are not adequate.
- HPLC-MS methods are sensitive and specific compared to immunoassays, and lack of standardization and analytical variations makes test results need to be interpreted with caution.

ESTROGEN/PROGESTERONE RECEPTOR ASSAY

❑ **Definition**

- Estrogen and progesterone receptors play a role in hormone-directed transcriptional activation.
- Other names: estrogen receptor assay (ERA), progesterone receptor assay (PGRA), progesterone receptor protein (PRP), estrogen receptor protein (ERP).
- **Normal range (ERP, PRP):**
  ▼ Negative: <5% of nuclei staining
  ▼ Borderline: 5–19% of nuclei staining
  ▼ Positive: 20% of nuclei staining

❑ **Use**

- To identify patients with breast cancers likely to respond to either additive or ablative hormone therapies

❑ **Interpretation (Table 16.30)**

Limitations

- Assay is performed on paraffin-embedded, formalin-fixed tissue.
- Receptor status is influenced by age.
- The definition of positive and negative may vary from laboratory to laboratory due to tissue and antibody treatment and antibody specificity.

16

TABLE 16–30. Percentage of Patients Who Respond to Hormone Therapy Based on the Test Results of Estrogen and Progesterone Receptor Assay

Percent Response to Hormone Therapy	Estrogen Receptor Protein (ERP)	Progesterone Receptor Protein (PRP)
75–80	Positive	Positive
40–50	Positive	Negative
25–30	Negative	Positive
10	Negative	Negative

Suggested Reading

Ogawa Y, Moriya T, Kato Y, et al. Immunohistochemical assessment for estrogen receptor and progesterone receptor status in breast cancer: Analysis for a cut-off point as the predictor for endocrine therapy. *Breast Cancer.* 2004;11(3):267–275.

ESTROGENS (TOTAL), SERUM

❏ **Definition**

■ Estrogens are involved in development and maintenance of the female pheno-type, germ cell maturation, and pregnancy. They also are important for many other, non–gender-specific processes, including growth, nervous system matu-ration, bone metabolism/remodeling, and endothelial responsiveness. The two major biologically active estrogens in nonpregnant humans are estrone (E_1) and estradiol (E_2). A third bioactive estrogen, estriol (E_3), is the main preg-nancy estrogen but plays no significant role in nonpregnant women or men.

■ **Normal range:** see Table 16.31.

TABLE 16–31. Normal Ranges of Estrogens

Estradiol (Tandem Mass Spectrometry)

Reference Intervals: Children (pg/mL)

Tanner Stage	Male	Female
I	<8	<56
II	<10	2–133
III	1–35	12–277
IV and V	3–35	2–259
Age (y)	Male	Female
7–9	<7	<36
10–12	<11	1–87
13–15	1–36	9–249
16–17	3–34	2–266

Reference Intervals: Adults (pg/mL)

≥18 y	Male	Female
	10–42	**Premenopausal:** Early follicular: 30–100 Late follicular: 100–400 Luteal: 50–150 **Postmenopausal:** 2–21

TABLE 16–31. Normal Ranges of Estrogens (Continued)

Estrone (Tandem Mass Spectrometry)

Reference Intervals: Children (pg/mL)

Tanner Stage	Male	Female
I	<7	<27
II	<11	1–39
III	1–31	8–117
IV and V	2–30	4–109
Age (y)	Male	Female
7–9	<7	<20
10–12	<11	1–40
13–15	1–30	8–105
16–17	1–32	4–133

Reference Intervals: Adults (pg/mL)

	Male	Female
≥18 y	9–36	**Premenopausal:**
		Early follicular: <150
		Late follicular: 100–250
		Luteal: <200
		Postmenopausal:
		3–32 pg/mL

Estrogens, Total (By Calculation)

Reference Intervals: Children (pg/mL)

Tanner Stages:	Male	Female
I	1–11	1–86
II	1–19	3–169
III	3–61	23–351
IV and V	4–62	8–341
Age (y)	Male	Female
7–9	<10	1–48
10–12	1–19	2–116
13–15	3–62	15–333
16–17	4–64	6–354

Reference Intervals: Adults (pg/mL)

	Male	Female
18 y	19–69	**Premenopausal**
		Early follicular: 30–250
		Late follicular: 200–650
		Luteal: 50–350
		Postmenopausal
		5–52

Use

- Overall status of estrogens in females or males
- Must be interpreted according to phase of the menstrual cycle

❏ Interpretation

Increased In

- Estrogen-producing tumors (e.g., granulosa cell tumor, theca-cell tumor, luteoma), secondary to stimulation by hCG-producing tumors (e.g., teratoma, teratocarcinoma)

- Pregnancy
- Gynecomastia

Decreased In
- Ovarian failure
- Primary hypofunction of the ovary:
  - ▼ Autoimmune oophoritis is the most common cause; usually associated with other autoimmune endocrinopathies (e.g., Hashimoto thyroiditis, Addison disease, type 1 DM); may cause premature menopause
  - ▼ Resistant ovary syndrome
  - ▼ Toxic (e.g., irradiation, chemotherapy)
  - ▼ Infection (e.g., mumps)
  - ▼ Tumor (primary or secondary)
  - ▼ Mechanical (e.g., trauma, torsion, surgical excision)
  - ▼ Genetic (e.g., Turner syndrome)
  - ▼ Menopause
- Secondary hypofunction of the ovary: disorders of the hypothalamic–pituitary axis

ESTRONE

❑ **Definition**

- Estrone (E_1) is more potent than estriol (E_3) but is less potent than estradiol (E_2). Estrone is converted to estrone sulfate, and it acts as a reservoir that can be converted as needed to the more active estradiol. Estrone is the major circulating estrogen in postmenopausal women. In premenopausal women, estrone levels generally parallel those of estradiol, rising gradually during the follicular phase and peaking just prior to ovulation, with a secondary and smaller increase during the luteal phase. After menopause, estrone levels do not decline as dramatically as estradiol levels, possibly due to increased conversion of androstenedione to estrone.
- Normal range:
  - ▼ Children: see Table 16.32.
  - ▼ Adults: see Table 16.33.

TABLE 16–32. Reference Intervals for Estrone in Children

	Boys (pg/mL)	Girls (pg/mL)
Tanner Stage	<7	<27
I	<11	1–39
II	1–31	8–117
III	2–30	4–109
IV and V		
Age (y)	<7	<20
7–9	<11	1–40
10–12	1–30	8–105
13–15	1–32	4–133

TABLE 16–33. Reference Intervals for Estrone in Adults*

Female	Male

Premenopausal
  Early follicular: <150 pg/mL
  Late follicular: 100–250 pg/mL
  Luteal: <200 pg/mL
Postmenopausal: 3–32 pg/mL
	9–36 pg/mL

*Eighteen years of age and older.

❏ **Use**

- Diagnosis of precocious and delayed puberty
- Workup of suspected disorders of sex steroid metabolism
- In the fracture risk assessment of postmenopausal women

❏ **Interpretation**

Increased In

- Possibly in polycystic ovarian syndrome, androgen-producing tumors, or estrogen-producing tumors.
- Possibly increased in postmenopausal vaginal bleeding due to peripheral conversion of androgenic steroids. Increased estrone levels may be associated with increased levels of circulating androgens and their subsequent peripheral conversion.

Decreased In

- Inherited disorders of sex steroid metabolism
- Testicular feminization

❏ **Limitations**

- Significant diurnal variations in plasma levels
- Digoxin and estrogens increase in plasma levels

ETHYLENE GLYCOL*

❏ **Definition**

- A colorless, odorless, sweet tasting nonvolatile liquid found in antifreeze, coolants, deicers, brake fluids, detergents, paints, and inks
- Other name: 1,2-ethanediol
- **Normal range:** none; threshold limit value for occupational exposure: 100 mg/m³

❏ **Use**

- Antifreeze
- Softening agent and stabilizer
- Solvent

16

*Submitted By Amanda J. Jenkins, PhD.

❏ **Interpretation**

- Minimum lethal oral dose for adults is approximately 100 mL; toxicity possible at serum concentrations >250 mg/L

❏ **Limitations**

- Propylene glycol, a similar compound used in pharmaceutical preparations is less toxic.
- Ethylene glycol can cause severe metabolic acidosis with increased anion gap and osmolal gap.
- Ethylene glycol is metabolized to glycoaldehyde, glycolic acid, glyoxylic acid, oxalic acid, formic acid, and carbon dioxide. These acids may interfere with testing of ethylene glycol and cause elevation of some immunoassay tests for lactate/lactic acid, triglycerides.
- Avoid serum separator tubes and gels (may impact results).

FACTOR V LEIDEN MOLECULAR ASSAY*

❏ **Definition**

- Factor V Leiden results from a *R506Q* mutation in the *F5* gene encoding factor V and is associated with increased risk of thrombophilia (OMIM# 188050). Heterozygosity for the factor V Leiden *R506Q* mutation is associated with resistance to activated protein C and a 5- to 10-fold increased risk of venous thrombosis. Homozygosity for this mutation is associated with resistance to APC and an approximately 80-fold increased risk of venous thrombosis. Other factors can further increase the risk of thrombosis.
- **Normal values:** negative or no mutations are found.

❏ **Use**

- Factor V Leiden testing should be performed in the following cases:
  - ▼ A first occurrence of a venous thrombotic embolism (VTE) before age 50 years
  - ▼ A first unprovoked VTE at any age
  - ▼ A history of recurrent VTE
  - ▼ Venous thrombosis at unusual sites (e.g., cerebral, mesenteric, portal or hepatic veins)
  - ▼ VTE during pregnancy or the puerperium
  - ▼ VTE associated with use of oral contraceptives or hormone replacement therapy
  - ▼ A first VTE in an individual with a first-degree family member with VTE before age 50 years
  - ▼ Women with unexplained fetal loss occurring after 10 weeks of gestation
- Factor V Leiden testing may be considered in the following cases:
  - ▼ In women with unexplained severe preeclampsia, placental abruption, or a fetus with intrauterine growth retardation
  - ▼ A first VTE related to the use of tamoxifen or other selective estrogen receptor modulators

---

*Submitted by Edward Ginns, MD and Marzena M. Galdzicka, PhD.

▼ Female smokers younger than age 50 years with an MI or stroke
▼ Individuals older than age 50 years with a first provoked VTE in the absence of malignancy or an intravascular device
▼ Asymptomatic adult family members of a known factor V Leiden proband, especially those with a strong family history of VTE at a young age
▼ Asymptomatic female family members of probands with known factor V Leiden thrombophilia who are pregnant or who are considering oral contraceptive use or pregnancy
▼ Women with recurrent unexplained first-trimester pregnancy loss with or without second- or third-trimester pregnancy loss
▼ Children with arterial thrombosis

❑ **Limitations**

■ The results of a genetic test may be affected by DNA rearrangements, blood transfusion, bone marrow transplantation, or rare sequence variations.
■ F5 gene mutations, other than R506Q, are not evaluated by this assay.

FACTOR VIII (ANTIHEMOPHILIC FACTOR)*,†

❑ **Definition**

■ Factor VIII is synthesized in the liver and endothelial cells of other organs, including the spleen, which plays an important role in the synthesis of factor VIII. It is unaffected by liver failure or vitamin K deficiency.
■ It is the principal cofactor in the intrinsic pathway of coagulation and serves as a substrate for proteolysis by the proteins C/protein S complex.
■ PT (INR) is not affected by deficiency of factor VIII.
■ Most laboratories use a specific coagulant assay to measure factor VIII.
  ▼ Chromogenic assays are also available.
  ▼ Immunologic assays determine factor VIII antigen. The antigen is concordant to activity in most cases but may be normal occasionally in patients with a functional defect in the molecule.
■ **Normal range: 70–150%.**

❑ **Use**

■ Purified or recombinant factor VIII is used therapeutically for patients with hemophilia A.
■ Immunologic assays for factor VIII may be useful in the diagnosis of von Willebrand disease but are not necessary in the diagnosis of most cases of hemophilia.

❑ **Interpretation**
Decreased In

■ If factor VIII decreases below 40%, PTT becomes prolonged. In the presence of an inhibitor to factor VIII, PTT remains prolonged even after therapeutic infusions of factor VIII; mixing the patient's plasma with normal plasma in a 1:1 proportion does not correct the prolonged PTT and does not increase

16

---

*Submitted By Liberto Pechet, MD.
†Note: Similar concepts apply to the quantitation of factor IX and its inhibitors.

the original low factor VIII. Specific methodology can report the titer of the inhibitor in Bethesda inhibitory units.

- **Congenital disorders**
  - ▼ Hemophilia A: usually severe deficiency in male carriers and usually mild decrease in female carriers of the hemophilia gene
  - ▼ von Willebrand disease (see p. 454): especially if moderate to severe; more so in individuals with blood type B
- **Acquired disorders**
  - ▼ Acquired anti–factor VIII autoantibodies in previously unaffected individuals
  - ▼ Acquired anti–factor VIII alloantibodies in hemophilia A patients treated with multiple infusions of factor VIII
  - ▼ DIC and pathologic fibrinolysis

Increased In

- Acute-phase reactant (acute inflammatory conditions).
- Pregnancy and the use of oral contraceptives.
- If markedly increased, it may predispose to thromboembolism.

FACTOR XI*

❏ Definition

- Factor XI is synthesized in the liver and megakaryocytes. Factor XI is activated by factor XIIa and by thrombin, the preferred activator on platelet surface. In turn, factor XI activates factors XII and IX in the intrinsic pathway. Factor XI is not affected by vitamin K antagonists.
- **Normal range: 60–120%.**

❏ Use

- For the diagnosis of factor XI deficiency, a specific functional assay to quantitate the factor has to be performed.

❏ Interpretation

- If factor XI is decreased to <20–25%, PTT, but not PT, is prolonged. A normal PTT does not rule out a mild factor XI deficiency.
- Antibody inhibitors develop relatively often as a consequence of replacement therapy in factor XI–deficient patients.
- Decreased values are characteristic for patients with factor XI deficiency. Acquired low values occur in severe liver disease and DIC.
- High levels of factor XI have been recently shown to be a risk factor for venous thromboembolism.

FACTOR XII (HAGEMAN FACTOR)†

❏ Definition

- Factor XII is synthesized in the liver. It circulates in an inactive form. It is activated by collagen, disrupted basement membranes, and activated platelets, as

*Submitted By Liberto Pechet, MD.
†Submitted By Liberto Pechet, MD.

well as by high molecular weight kininogen and prekallikrein in conjunction with factor XI. It is unaffected by vitamin K antagonists.

- **Normal range: 60–150%.**

❑ **Use**

- Specific factor assay is needed for the diagnosis of factor XII deficiency and to distinguish the anomaly from factor XI or other intrinsic pathway initiating factors deficiencies.

❑ **Interpretation**

- PTT, but not PT, is prolonged in severe deficiency.
- Asian populations have lower factor XII levels than Caucasians (average, 44%).
- Factor XII levels are decreased in the neonate; they reach adult values at 2 weeks of age.
- Factor XII levels are increased in pregnancy.

❑ **Limitations**

- Factor XII may be artifactually decreased by the presence of LA.

FACTOR XIII*

❑ **Definition**

- Factor XIII is synthesized in the liver and also present in high concentrations in platelets. Factor XIII is a plasma transglutaminase proenzyme activated by thrombin in the presence of calcium. It promotes clot stability by forming intermolecular covalent bonds between fibrin monomers.
- **Normal range:** reported qualitatively as normal or decreased; quantitation performed in reference laboratories.

❑ **Use**

- Factor XIII values are decreased in factor XIII deficiency, which can be either inherited or acquired.

❑ **Interpretation**

Decreased In

- Inherited deficiency
- AML
- Liver disease
- Association with hypofibrinogenemia in obstetric complications such as DIC
- Presence of circulating inhibitors

FATTY ACIDS, FREE

❑ **Definition**

- Free fatty acids are formed by the breakdown of lipoprotein and triglycerides. All but 2–5% of the serum fatty acids are esterified. The "nonesterified" or "free" fatty acids are protein bound. Epinephrine, norepinephrine, glucagon,

16

---

*Submitted By Liberto Pechet, MD.

TSH, and ACTH release free fatty acids. Tumors producing such hormones cause release of excessive quantities of free fatty acids. Other names: non-esterified fatty acids (NEFA), FFA.

- **Normal range:**
  - ▼ Adults: 8–25 mg/dL or 0.28–0.89 mmol/L
  - ▼ Children (or obese adults): <31 mg/dL or <1.0 mmol/L

❏ **Use**

- Monitoring nutritional status in the presence of malabsorption, starvation, and long-term parenteral nutrition.
- Valuable for the differential diagnosis of polyneuropathy when Refsum disease is suspected. In this disease, the enzyme that degrades phytanic acid is lacking.
- Detection of pheochromocytoma and glucagon thyrotropin and adrenocorticotropin-secreting tumors.
- Diabetes management.

❏ **Interpretation**

Increased In

- Poorly controlled DM
- Pheochromocytoma
- Hyperthyroidism
- Huntington chorea
- von Gierke disease
- Alcoholism
- Acute myocardial infarction
- Reye syndrome
- Phytanic acid increased in:
  - ▼ Refsum disease
  - ▼ Zellweger syndrome
  - ▼ Neonatal adrenoleukodystrophy
  - ▼ β-Lipoproteinemia

Decreased In

- CF
- Malabsorption (acrodermatitis enteropathica)
- Zinc deficiency (arachidonic acid and linoleic acid low)

❏ **Limitations**

- Free fatty acids increase by 12–25% in 24 hours in refrigerated plasma.
- Strenuous exercise, anxiety, hypothermia, and long-term fasting elevate the levels.
- Long-term IV or parenteral nutrition therapy decrease the levels.
- Prolonged fasting or starvation affects levels (rise as much as three times normal).

FECAL FAT

❏ **Definition**

- Test for steatorrhea or excess fat in bowel movements due to fat. Helps to estimate the percentage of dietary fat that the body does not absorb
- **Normal range:** <7 g of fat per 24 hours

❑ Use

- Aids in the diagnosis of malabsorption
- As a follow-up to other stool tests and blood tests to investigate the cause of chronic diarrhea and loose, fatty, foul-smelling stools (steatorrhea)

❑ Interpretation

- A person who consumes 100 g of fat per day would have an average stool fat of <7 g/24 hours. Fecal excretion of more than 7 g of fat in a 24-hour period or more than 7% of the measured fat intake over a 3-day period is indicative of fat malabsorption or steatorrhea malabsorption.

Increased In

- The absence or significant decrease of the pancreatic enzymes, amylase, lipase, trypsin, and chymotrypsin limits fat, protein, and carbohydrate digestion, resulting in steatorrhea due to fat malabsorption.
- The underlying condition of steatorrhea includes
  - ▼ Celiac disease
  - ▼ Chronic pancreatitis
  - ▼ Crohn disease
  - ▼ Cystic fibrosis
  - ▼ Gallstones (cholelithiasis)
  - ▼ Pancreatic cancer
  - ▼ Pancreatitis

Decreased In

- NA

❑ Limitations

- For a 72-hour stool collection, 50–150 g of fat a day for 2–3 days prior to and during the stool collection period needs to be consumed. The fat should be long-chain triglycerides (such as corn or olive oil, not butter).
- False-positive results can occur due to mineral oil or castor oil present in the specimen.

FERRITIN

❑ Definition

- Ferritin is the cellular storage protein for iron, with 1 ng of ferritin per mL indicating 10 mg of total iron stores. It is a huge (440 kDa), 24-subunit protein consisting of light and heavy chains, which can store up to 4,500 atoms of iron. Ferritin is an acute-phase reactant, and, along with transferrin and its receptor, coordinates cellular defense against oxidative stress and inflammation. Ferritin measured clinically in plasma is usually apoferritin, a non–iron-containing molecule.
- **Normal range:**
  - ▼ Male: 23–336 ng/mL (in patients with normal iron stores, it should be >30 ng/mL)
  - ▼ Females: 11–306 ng/mL

16

❏ Use

- Predict and monitor iron deficiency
- Determine response to iron therapy or compliance with treatment
- Differentiate iron deficiency from chronic disease as cause of anemia
- Monitor iron status in patients with chronic renal disease with or without dialysis
- Detect iron overload states and monitor rate of iron accumulation and response to iron depletion therapy
- Population studies of iron levels and response to iron supplement

❏ Interpretation

Increased In

- Acute and chronic liver disease.
- Alcoholism (declines during abstinence).
- Malignancies (e.g., leukemia, Hodgkin disease).
- Infection and inflammation (e.g., arthritis).
- Hyperthyroidism, Gaucher disease, acute myocardial infarction.
- Iron overload (e.g., hemosiderosis, idiopathic hemochromatosis).
- Anemias other than iron deficiency (e.g., megaloblastic, hemolytic, sideroblastic, thalassemia major and minor, spherocytosis, porphyria cutanea tarda).
- Renal cell carcinoma due to hemorrhage within tumor.
- End-stage renal disease; values ≥1,000 μg/L are not uncommon. Values <200 μg/L are specific for iron deficiency in these patients.

Decreased In

- Iron deficiency
- Hemodialysis

❏ Limitations

- In hepatic, malignant, and inflammatory conditions, ferritin levels can be normal. In such cases, bone marrow stain of iron may be used to exclude iron deficiency.
- Transferrin saturation is more sensitive to detect early iron overload in hemochromatosis; serum ferritin is used to confirm diagnosis and as an indication to proceed with liver biopsy. Ratio of serum ferritin (in ng/mL) to ALT (in IU/L) >10 in iron-overloaded thalassemic patients but averages ≤2 in viral hepatitis; ratio decreases with successful iron chelation therapy.
- Increases with age, is higher in men than in women, in women who use oral contraceptives, and in persons who eat red meat compared to vegetarians.

FETAL BIOPSY

See Prenatal Screening.

FETAL BLOOD SAMPLING (PERCUTANEOUS UMBILICAL BLOOD SAMPLING [PUB], CORDOCENTESIS)

See Prenatal Screening.

FETAL LUNG MATURITY (FLM)–LAMELLAR BODY COUNTS (LBC)

❑ **Definition**
- Most common test currently use in the United States. LBCs are concentrically layered "packages" of phospholipids produced by type II pneumocytes. LBCs represent the storage form of surfactant. They are present in amniotic fluid in increasing quantities as gestation advances. They are similar in size as platelets and can be counted in most hematology analyzers.
- **Normal range:**
  - ▼ Mature fetal lungs: ≥50,000/µL
  - ▼ Borderline: 15,000–50,000/µL
  - ▼ Immature fetal lungs: ≤15,000/µL

❑ **Use**
- Predicting FLM and assessing the risk of developing neonatal respiratory distress syndrome, when performed during 32–39 weeks of gestation

❑ **Interpretation**
- Increased in mature fetal lungs
- Decreased in immature fetal lungs

❑ **Limitations**
- It is as accurate as TDM/FLEXII FPIA method (no longer available) surfactant/albumin ratio.
- LBCs not indicated >39 weeks of gestation.
- Amniotic fluid samples should be free of blood or meconium contamination.

FIBRINOGEN (FACTOR I)*

❑ **Definition**
- Fibrinogen is a glycoprotein synthesized in the liver. It is modified by thrombin to become fibrin, a visible clot. It is also an acute-phase reactant.
- **Normal range:** 150–400 mg/dL (most abundant circulating clotting factor).

❑ **Use**
- This test detects decreased or abnormal fibrinogen.
- It may be used to determine the severity and evolution of DIC by performing serial determinations.
- Because of the initial elevation of fibrinogen, its determination is not useful in the *diagnosis* of DIC.

❑ **Interpretation**
- Severe fibrinogen deficiency may prolong PT, PTT, and TT.

Increased In†
- Acute inflammatory/infectious processes
- Cancer

---

*Submitted By Liberto Pechet, MD.
†Increased fibrinogen thought to contribute to thrombophilia.

16

- Pregnancy and use of oral contraceptives
- Older age
- Early DIC

Decreased In

- Congenital afibrinogenemia or hypofibrinogenemia.
- Dysfibrinogenemia (congenital or acquired).
- DIC and pathologic fibrinolysis. Fibrinogen is consumed after initial elevation as an acute-phase reactant.
- Very advanced liver disease.

❑ Limitations

Preanalytic

- Clotted specimens or those obtained with the wrong anticoagulant
- Inappropriately filled test tubes
- Inappropriately stored blood
- Hyperlipidemic, icteric, or hemolyzed blood
- Hct >55%

FIBRINOGEN DEGRADATION PRODUCTS (FDPs)*

❑ Definition

- FDPs represent fragments D and E, major breakdown products of fibrinogen and fibrin. FDPs do not distinguish between fibrinolysis, fibrinogenolysis (the effect of pathologic or therapeutic fibrinolysis), or the combined effect of fibrinolysis plus thrombin generation, as seen in DIC.
- **Normal range:** <10 μg/mL.

❑ Use

- FDP, as performed in most laboratories, is a simple and rapid semiquantitative, latex-based test.
- It is used, in conjunction with other assays, to diagnose activated fibrinolysis or DIC in suspected patients.

❑ Interpretation

- Causes of increased results:
  - ▼ Pathologic and therapeutic fibrinolysis
  - ▼ DIC
  - ▼ Venous thromboembolism and pulmonary embolism
  - ▼ Myocardial infarction
  - ▼ Following trauma and surgery
  - ▼ Disseminated cancer
  - ▼ Complications of pregnancy
  - ▼ Small increase with exercise, severe liver disease

---

*Submitted By Liberto Pechet, MD.

❑ **Limitations**

- Because of its rather limited sensitivity, FDP may not be elevated in single, discrete clots, as seen in isolated deep vein thrombosis or in pulmonary embolism. In such situations, a sensitive D-dimer assay is recommended.
- The assay itself, if performed on serum obtained from firmly clotted blood (the designated test tubes contain a potent coagulant venom). If blood is drawn on tubes containing anticoagulant, the assay is invalid (newer tests that use plasma have been developed).
- In the presence of rheumatoid factor, the results may be falsely elevated.

FIBRONECTIN, FETAL (fFN)

❑ **Definition**

- This protein is located at the choriodecidual interface, between fetal membranes and the lining of the uterus. It acts as a kind of "glue" that binds the fetus to the mother. The fFN test measures the protein "leaked" through the cervix into the vagina in pregnancy's final stages, as the fetus prepares for the birth process.
- **Normal range:** negative.

❑ **Use**

- To predict the risk of preterm delivery in symptomatic patients, since identifying women with preterm contractions who will go on to deliver prematurely is an inexact process
- To identify asymptomatic women, usually in a high-risk group (e.g., previous preterm delivery, multiple gestation), who are most likely to deliver preterm

❑ **Interpretation**
Increased (Positive) In

- Up to 40% of women with signs and symptoms deliver within the next 7 days.
- A woman tested at 24 weeks is nearly 60 times more likely to deliver within the next 4 weeks compared with a woman with a normal fetal fibronectin test when taken between weeks 22 and 24. The test detects nearly two thirds of the preterm births that occur prior to 28 weeks.

Decreased (Negative) In

- 99.5% of women with signs and symptoms will not deliver within the next 7 days.
- Less than 1% of women with identified risk factors will deliver before 28 weeks if they have a normal fetal fibronectin test result at 22–24 weeks.

❑ **Limitations**

- fFN results should not be interpreted as absolute evidence for the presence or absence of a process that will result in delivery in <14 days from specimen collection in symptomatic women or delivery in ≤34 weeks, 6 days in asymptomatic women evaluated between 22 weeks, 0 days and 30 weeks, 6 days of gestation.

16

- A positive rapid fFN result may be observed for patients who have experienced cervical disruption caused by, but not limited to, events such as sexual intercourse, digital cervical examination, or vaginal probe ultrasound.
- The rapid fFN result should always be used in conjunction with information available from the clinical evaluation of the patient and other diagnostic procedures such as cervical examination of a cervical microbiologic culture, assessment of uterine activity, and evaluation of other risk factors.
- The assay has been optimized with specimens taken from the posterior fornix of the vagina or the ectocervical region of the external cervical os. Samples obtained from other locations should not be used.
- Assay interference from the douches, white blood cells, red blood cells, bacteria, and bilirubin has not been ruled out.
- Manipulation of the cervix may lead to false-positive results. Specimens should be obtained prior to digital examination or manipulation of the cervix.
- Care must be taken not to contaminate the swab or cervicovaginal secretions with lubricants, soaps, or disinfectants (e.g., K-Y Jelly lubricant, Betadine disinfectant, Monistat cream). These substances may interfere with absorption of the specimen by the swab.
- Patients with suspected or known placental abruption, placenta previa, or moderate or gross vaginal bleeding should not be tested for fFN.

FIRST-TRIMESTER SCREENING

See Prenatal Screening.

FLOW CYTOMETRY ANALYSIS IN THE CLINICAL EVALUATION OF HEMATOLOGIC DISEASES*

❑ **Definition and use**

- Flow cytometry is a powerful tool for detailed analysis of complex populations in a short period of time. It integrates fluidics, optics, electronics, computer, software, and laser technologies in a single platform. It uses the principles of light scattering, light excitation, and emission of fluorochrome molecules to generate specific multiparameter data from particles and cells. Parameters measured by flow cytometry include intrinsic properties, such as forward scatter and side scatter, and extrinsic properties. Flow cytometric analysis has become a routine test in the diagnosis of hematologic diseases, including leukemias, lymphomas, plasma cell neoplasms, myeloproliferative neoplasms, myelodysplastic syndromes, and paroxysmal nocturnal hemolysis. Flow cytometric analysis can also be utilized in immunology, DNA analysis, and evaluation of genetic disorders. In addition, flow cytometric analysis can be used not only for diagnosis but also for disease prognosis and disease follow-up. A variety of clinical samples can be analyzed by flow cytometry, and they include peripheral blood, bone marrow aspirate, serous cavity fluid, cerebrospinal fluid, urine, fine needle aspirate, and solid tissue.

*Submitted by Hongbo Yu, MD.

- It is important to know about the commonly used immunologic markers and the design and utilization of flow cytometric panels in a variety of hematologic diseases, such as acute myeloid leukemia, acute lymphocytic leukemia, B-cell lymphoma, T-cell lymphoma, plasma cell neoplasm, paroxysmal nocturnal hemolysis, and myelodysplastic syndrome. Panel design is a critical step in flow cytometric analysis, and flow cytometric panels are designed to discern cell lineage, level of cell differentiation, and in many cases subclassification of the neoplasm being studied. Below are two tables with commonly used flow cytometry immunologic markers, which can provide practical guidelines to effective use of flow cytometric technology in the clinical laboratory. For specific flow cytometric findings in particular diseases, please refer to Chapter of "Hematologic Diseases."

Useful Flow Cytometric Immunologic Markers in Hematologic Neoplasms

Markers Useful in B-Cell Neoplasms	Markers Useful in T-Cell Neoplasms	Markers Useful in Plasma Cell Neoplasms	Markers Useful in Myeloid/Monocytic Neoplasms
CD19	CD1a	CD38	CD13
CD20	CD2	CD138	CD33
CD22	CD3	CD56	CD117
CD79a	CD5	CD117	CD15
CD5	CD7	Kappa light chain	CD14
CD23	CD4	Lambda light chain	CD64
CD10	CD8	CD19	CD11b
CD11c	CD25	CD20	CD235a
CD103	CD16		CD41
CD25	CD56		CD61
FMC7	CD57		Myeloperoxidase
Kappa light chain	TdT		CD45
Lambda light chain	CD34		CD34
TdT			
CD34			

Commonly Used Cluster of Differentiation (CD) Antigens

Cluster	Synonyms	Family and Function	Normal Hematopoietic Cell Distribution
CD1a–e		Ig superfamily HLA class I–like Nonpeptide and glycolipid antigen presentation	Thymocytes dendritic cells, Langerhans cells, other antigen-presenting cells, some B cells
CD2	Leukocyte function antigen (LFA)-2	Ig superfamily T-cell activation regulation	Thymocytes T cells, NK cells, thymic B cells, B-cell subset
CD3		Ig superfamily TCR signal transduction	Thymocytes, T cells
CD4		Ig superfamily T-cell receptor costimulatory molecule, HIV receptor	Stem cells, thymocytes, T cells, monocytes/macrophages

(Continued)

Commonly Used Cluster of Differentiation (CD) Antigens (*Continued*)

Cluster	Synonyms	Family and Function	Normal Hematopoietic Cell Distribution
CD5		Scavenger receptor superfamily T-cell costimulatory molecule	Thymocytes, T cells, B-cell subsets
CD7		Ig superfamily Costimulatory molecule	Stem cells, thymocytes, T cells, NK cells
CD8		Ig superfamily Costimulatory molecule	Thymocytes, T cells, NK cells
CD10	Common acute lymphoblastic leukemia antigen (CALLA)	B-cell growth regulation Neutral endopeptidase	Pre-B cells, germinal center B cells, granulocytes
CD11b	Macrophage-1 antigen (Mac-1) α chain	CAM family Adhesion, chemotaxis, neutrophil activation, C3bi receptor	Granulocytes, monocytes, NK cells, T- and B-cell subsets
CD11c	Complement receptor (CR) 4 α chain	CAM family Adhesion, costimulation	Monocytes/macrophages, granulocytes, NK cells, T- and B-cell subsets, dendritic cells
CD13	Alanyl (membrane) aminopeptidase (ANPEP)	Zinc metallopeptidase Coronavirus receptor, CMV infection	Granulocyte and monocyte lineage
CD14	Lipopolysaccharide (LPS) receptor	Monocyte and granulocyte activation	Monocytes/macrophages, granulocytes
CD15	Lewis X	Adhesion cell rolling	Monocytes, granulocytes
CD16	FcγRIII	Ig superfamily IgG Fc receptor	NK cells, granulocytes, monocytes/macrophages, T-cell subsets
CD19		Ig superfamily Signal transduction for B-cell maturation, differentiation, and activation	B-cell lineage
CD20		Tetraspanin family B-cell activation, Ca^{++} channel and proliferation	B-cell lineage
CD21	Complement receptor (CR) 2	Regulator of complement activation (RCA) family Regulator of complement activation, Epstein-Barr virus receptor, B-cell activation	Mature resting B cells, mantle and marginal zone B cells, follicular dendritic cells, thymocyte subsets
CD22		Ig superfamily B-cell adhesion and costimulation	B-cell lineage
CD23	FcεRII	Sialoadhesion, Ig superfamily IgE synthesis regulation, low-affinity IgE Fc receptor	B cells, monocytes, dendritic cells
CD25		IL-2 receptor α chain, T-cell activation	Activated T cells, B cells, monocytes/macrophages

Cluster	Synonyms	Family and Function	Normal Hematopoietic Cell Distribution
CD30		TNF receptor superfamily Negative T-cell selection in thymus Involved in TCR-mediated cell death	Activated T, B, and NK cells, monocytes
CD33		Ig superfamily Carbohydrate binding/lectin	Myeloid and monocyte lineage including progenitors
CD34		Sialomucin family Cell–cell adhesion	Hematopoietic stem cells
CD38		Regulation of cell activation and proliferation Adhesion	Progenitor and activated hematopoietic cells, plasma cells
CD41	Glycoprotein IIb (GPIIb)	Integrin family Platelet aggregation	Platelets and megakaryocytes
CD45	Leukocyte common antigen (LCA)	T and B antigen receptor costimulatory molecule	Hematopoietic cells, differential isoform expression on T- and B-cell subsets
CD56	Neural cell adhesion molecule (NCAM)	Ig superfamily Cell–cell adhesion	NK cells, T-cell subsets
CD57		Unknown	NK cells, T-cell subsets
CD61	Glycoprotein IIIa (GPIIIa)	Integrin family Platelet activation and aggregation, cell–matrix adhesion	Platelets and megakaryocytes
CD68		Scavenger receptor family	Macrophages
CD71	Transferrin receptor	Iron uptake	Erythroid precursors
CD79a		Antigen receptor signal transduction	B-cell lineage and plasma cells
CD103		Type I transmembrane protein T-cell adhesion in intestinal epithelium	Intraepithelial lymphocytes, activated T cells, mast cells, monocytes
CD117	c-kit	Type III tyrosine kinase growth factor receptor family, Ig superfamily Stem cell factor binding and signaling	CD34+ stem cells, myeloblasts, promyelocytes, monoblasts, erythroblasts, megakaryoblasts, mast cells
CD123	IL-3Rβ	Type I cytokine receptor family Binding subunit for IL-3, growth, and differentiation of myeloid cells	Myeloid cells, progenitor cells, NK cells, B-cell subsets
CD138	Syndecan-1	Syndecan proteoglycan family Extracellular matrix adhesion	Pre-B cells, plasma cells

16

(*Continued*)

Commonly Used Cluster of Differentiation (CD) Antigens (*Continued*)

Cluster	Synonyms	Family and Function	Normal Hematopoietic Cell Distribution
CD158e,i,k	Killer cell immunoglobulin– like receptor (KIR) family	Ig superfamily Inhibition of NK lysis via MHC I binding	NK cells, T-cell subsets
CD163		Scavenger receptor superfamily Macrophage differentiation/ activation	Macrophages
CD235a	Glycophorin A	Type I transmembrane protein MN blood group determinant	Erythrocytes

FOLATE, SERUM AND ERYTHROCYTES (RBCs)

❑ **Definition**
- Folate refers to all derivatives of folic acid. Folate is an essential vitamin present in a wide variety of foods such as dark leafy vegetables, citrus fruits, yeast, beans, eggs, and milk. Folate is vital to normal cell growth and DNA synthesis. A folate deficiency can lead to megaloblastic anemia and ultimately to severe neurologic problems. Folate levels in both serum and RBCs are used to assess folate status. The serum folate level is an indicator of recent folate intake. RBC folate is the best indicator of long-term folate stores. A low RBC folate value may indicate a prolonged folate deficiency. Other names: vitamin B_9.
- **Normal range:**
  - ▼ Serum folate: >6.5 ng/mL
  - ▼ RBC folate: 280–903 ng/mL

❑ **Use**
- Evaluation of folate deficiency

❑ **Interpretation**
Increased In
- Blind loop syndrome
- Vegetarian diet
- Distal and small bowel disease
- PA

Decreased In
- Untreated folate deficiency, associated with megaloblastic anemia
- Infantile hyperthyroidism
- Alcoholism
- Malnutrition
- Scurvy

- Liver disease
- Vitamin B_{12} deficiency
- Dietary amino acid excess
- Chronic hemodialysis
- Celiac disease
- Disorders of glutathione metabolism
- Sideroblastic anemia
- Pregnancy
- Whipple disease
- Amyloidosis

❑ **Limitations**
- Serum folate is a relatively nonspecific test. Low serum folate levels may be seen in the absence of deficiency, and normal levels may be seen in patients with macrocytic anemia, dementia, neuropsychiatric disorders, and pregnancy disorders.
- Patients with low RBC folate or megaloblastic anemia should be evaluated for vitamin B_{12} deficiency. To distinguish between vitamin B_{12} and folate deficiency, determination of homocysteine (HCS) and methylmalonic acid (MMA) will help. In vitamin B_{12} deficiency, both HCS and MMA are elevated, whereas in folate deficiency, only HCS levels are elevated.

FOLLICULAR-STIMULATING HORMONE (FSH) AND LUTEINIZING HORMONE (LH), SERUM

❑ **Definition**
- These glycoproteins are produced by the anterior pituitary gland, regulated by hypothalamic gonadotropin-releasing hormone (GnRH) and feedback by gonadal steroid hormones. FSH stimulates follicular growth and stimulates seminiferous tubules and testicular growth. LH stimulates ovulation and production of estrogen and progesterone. LH controls production of testosterone by Leydig cells.
- **Normal range:** see Table 16.34.

❑ **Use**
- Diagnosis of gonadal, pituitary, hypothalamic disorders
- Diagnosis and management of infertility

❑ **Interpretation**
Increased In
- Primary hypogonadism (anorchia, testicular failure, menopause)
- Gonadotropin-secreting pituitary tumors
- Precocious puberty (secondary to a CNS lesion or idiopathic)
- Complete testicular feminization syndrome
- Luteal phase of menstrual cycle

16

TABLE 16–34. Normal Ranges of Human FSH and LH

	Males (mIU/mL)	Females (mIU/mL)			
		Midfollicular Phase	Midcycle Peak	Midluteal Phase	Postmenopausal
FSH					
Number	65	29	26	27	50
Mean	5.88	6.43	12.27	3.45	60.76
Range	1.27–19.26	3.85–8.78	4.54–22.51	1.79–5.12	16.74–113.59
LH					
Number	50	29	26	27	50
Mean	3.75	5.88	52.84	4.84	30.55
Range	1.24–8.62	2.12–10.89	19.18–103.03	1.20–12.86	10.87–58.64

Decreased In
- Secondary hypogonadism
- Kallmann syndrome (inherited X-linked or autosomal isolated deficiency of GnRH; occurs in both sexes) found in approximately 5% of patients with primary amenorrhea. Causes failure of both gametogenic function and sex steroid production (LH and FSH are "normal" or undetectable but rise in response to prolonged GnRH stimulation)
- Pituitary LH or FSH deficiency
- Gonadotropin deficiency

❏ Limitations
- Because of the episodic, circadian, and cyclic nature of its secretion, clinical evaluations may require determinations in pooled multiple serial specimens.

FRUCTOSAMINE, SERUM

❏ Definition
- Fructosamine describes serum proteins that have been glycated (i.e., derivatives of nonenzymatic reaction product of a sugar [glucose] with serum protein [albumin]). It reflects the mean glucose concentration in blood over recent period (2–3 weeks), whereas glycated Hb (HbA_{1c}) is indicative of blood glucose over intermediate to long term (4–8 weeks).
- **Normal range** (nondiabetic individuals): 170–285 µmol/L.

❏ Use
- To assess short-term glycemic control in diabetic patients.
- When glycated Hb cannot be used due to interferences (e.g., abnormal Hb), which invalidate HbA_{1c}.
- It should be compared with previous values in the same patient rather than reference range.

❏ Interpretation
Increased In
- Hyperglycemia in patients with poorly controlled DM

❏ Limitations
- Because the assay is nonspecific, color may be generated by compounds other than glycated proteins. Interferences are seen from ascorbic acid (vitamin C) and elevated bilirubin values. However, the second-generation assays have been shown to be highly specific for glycated proteins.
- Fasting blood glucose and HbA_{1c} are the usual and preferred means of monitoring glycemic control.
- Changes in fructosamine values correlate with significant changes in serum protein concentrations (e.g., liver disease, acute systemic illness). Abnormal values also occur during abnormal protein turnover (e.g., thyroid disease), even though patients are normoglycemic. It may be obviated by using fructose: albumin ratio.

16

- The within-subject variation for serum fructosamine is higher than that for HbA_{1C}; as a result, serum fructosamine concentrations must change more before a significant change can be said to have occurred.

GALACTOSE-1-PHOSPHATE URIDYLTRANSFERASE (GALT)

❏ **Definition**

- GALT is an enzyme responsible for converting ingested galactose to glucose. This measurement is used to identify in born errors of galactose metabolism, which can result in widespread tissue damage and abnormalities such as cataracts, liver disease, and renal disease. It also causes failure to thrive and mental retardation. The screening test should be done immediately to enable diet treatment if testing is positive.
- The deficiency of three enzymes, galactokinase (GALK), GALT or UDP, and galactose-4-epimerase (GALE), is clinically important and results in inborn errors of galactose metabolism.
  - ▼ GALT deficiency, referred to as classical galactosemia or GG genotype, is the most commonly occurring of the three disorders.
  - ▼ GALK deficiency is the second most common cause of galactosemia and results in a milder variant of galactosemia. GALK deficiency is very rare and usually is expressed by occurrence of juvenile cataracts in the absence of mental retardation (which occurs in transferase deficiency).
  - ▼ GALE deficiency is an extremely rare cause of galactosemia.
- Other names: GPT, galactokinase, and galactose-1-phosphate.
- **Normal range:** 14.7–25.4 U/g Hb.

❏ **Use**

- Diagnosis of GALT deficiency, the most common cause of galactosemia
- Confirmation of abnormal state newborn screening results

❏ **Interpretation**

- Decreased in galactosemia

❏ **Limitations**

- Enzyme activity only may not differentiate variant form of galactosemia or carriers. For a more accurate evaluation of patients suspected to have galactosemia, the preferred test is a genetic test to identify mutation.

GAMMA GLUTAMYL TRANSFERASE (GGT)

❏ **Definition**

- The activity of this membrane-bound enzyme comes primarily from the liver. GGT is responsible for the extracellular metabolism of glutathione, the main antioxidant in cells. It is slightly more sensitive than ALP in obstructive liver disease.
- **Normal range:**
  - ▼ 0–3 months: 4–120 IU/L
  - ▼ 3 months–1 year: 2–35 IU/L

▼ 1–16 years: 2–25 IU/L
▼ ≥16 years: 7–50 IU/L

❑ Use

- To diagnose and monitor hepatobiliary disease; most sensitive enzymatic indicator of liver disease
- To ascertain whether observed elevations of ALP are due to skeletal disease (normal GGT) or reflect the presence of hepatobiliary disease (elevated GGT)
- As a screening test for occult alcoholism
- To aid in diagnosis of liver disease in the presence of bone disease, pregnancy, or childhood, which increase serum ALP and LAP but not GGT

❑ Interpretation

Increased In

- DM, hyperthyroidism, RA, COPD.
- Drugs (phenytoin, carbamazepine, cimetidine, furosemide, heparin, methotrexate, oral contraceptives, and valproic acid).
- Liver disease—generally parallels changes in serum ALP, LAP, and 5′-NT but is more sensitive.
- Acute hepatitis. Elevation is less marked than that of other liver enzymes, but it is the last to return to normal and, therefore, is useful to indicate recovery.
- Chronic active hepatitis; increased (average more than seven times ULN) more than in acute hepatitis; more elevated than AST and ALT. In dormant stage, it may be the only enzyme elevated.
- Alcoholic hepatitis; average increase >3.5 times ULN.
- Alcohol abuse; a GGT/ALP ratio >2.5 is highly suggestive.
- Cirrhosis. In inactive cases, average values are lower (four times ULN) than in chronic hepatitis. Increases of more than 10–20 times normal in cirrhotic patients suggest superimposed primary carcinoma of the liver (average increase >21 times ULN).
- Primary biliary cirrhosis. Elevation is marked: average >13 times ULN.
- Fatty liver; elevation parallels that of AST and ALT but is greater.
- Obstructive jaundice. Increase is faster and greater than that of serum ALP and LAP; average increase more than five times ULN.
- Liver metastases; parallels ALP; elevation precedes positive liver scans. Average increase >14 times ULN.
- Cholestasis. In mechanical and viral cholestasis, GGT and LAP are increased about equally, but in drug-induced cholestasis, GGT is much more increased than LAP. Average increase more than six times ULN.
- Children; much more increased in biliary atresia than in neonatal hepatitis (300 IU/L is useful differentiating level). Children with α1-antitrypsin deficiency have higher levels than other patients with biliary atresia.
- Pancreatitis. The GGT level is always elevated in acute pancreatitis. In chronic pancreatitis, it is increased when there is involvement of the biliary tract or active inflammation.
- AMI; increased in 50% of patients. Elevation begins on the 4th to the 5th day, reaching a maximum at 8–12 days. With shock or acute right heart failure, an early peak may appear within 48 hours, with a rapid decline followed by a later rise.

16

- When increased, it is a risk factor for myocardial infarction and cardiac death.
- Heavy use of alcohol; the most sensitive indicator and a good screening test for alcoholism, because elevation exceeds that of other commonly assayed liver enzymes.
- Some cases of carcinoma of the prostate.
- Neoplasms, even in the absence of liver metastases; especially malignant melanoma, carcinoma of the breast and lung; highest levels seen in hypernephroma.
- Others (e.g., gross obesity [slight increase], renal disease, cardiac disease, postoperative state).

Decreased In
- Hypothyroidism

Normal In
- Pregnancy (in contrast to serum ALP, LAP) and children older than 3 months of age; therefore, may aid in differential diagnosis of hepatobiliary disease occurring during pregnancy and childhood
- Bone disease or patients with increased bone growth (children and adolescents); therefore, useful in distinguishing bone disease from liver disease as a cause of increased serum ALP
- Renal failure
- Strenuous exercise

❑ **Limitations**
- Half-life is about 7–10 days; in alcohol-associated liver injury, the half-life is increased to as much as 28 days, suggesting impaired clearance.
- Day-to-day variations are 10–15%; approximately double in African Americans.
- There is a 25–50% increase with higher body mass index.
- Values are 25% lower during early pregnancy.

GASTRIN

❑ **Definition**
- Gastrin is a hormone secreted by the G-cells of the antrum of the stomach and the pancreatic islet of Langerhans. Its secretion is stimulated by alkalinity, by distention of the stomach by the antrum, by vagal stimulation, and by the presence of peptides, amino acids, alcohol, or calcium in the stomach. Its secretion is inhibited by gastric acidity via negative feedback system.
- Principal forms of gastrin in the blood are G-34 (big gastrin), G-17 (little gastrin), and G-14 (mini gastrin). Each of these circulates in nonsulfated and sulfated forms.
- The gastric stimulation test after calcium infusion (15 mg of Ca/kg in 500 mL normal saline over 4 hours) is useful in patients with marked elevation

of gastrin levels. This test should be reserved for patients with a negative secretin test, gastric acid hypersecretion, and a strong suspicion of Z-E syndrome.

- **Normal range:**
  - ▼ Gastrin: 0–100 pg/mL
  - ▼ Gastrin stimulation test (after secretin): no response or slight suppression
  - ▼ Gastrin stimulation test (after calcium infusion): little or no increase over baseline

❏ **Use**

- Diagnosis of Z-E syndrome: The gastrin test after secretin (2–3 U/kg injected over 30 seconds) is preferred provocative test for patients suspected of having Z-E syndrome.
- Diagnosis of gastrinoma: Basal and secretin-stimulated serum gastrin measurements are the best laboratory tests for gastrinoma.
- Investigation of patients with achlorhydria or pernicious anemia.

❏ **Interpretation**

Increased In

- Increased serum gastrin without gastric acid hypersecretion
  - ▼ Atrophic gastritis, especially when associated with circulating parietal cell antibodies
  - ▼ PA in approximately 75% of patients
  - ▼ Some cases of carcinoma of the body of the stomach, a reflection of the atrophic gastritis that is present
  - ▼ Gastric acid inhibitor therapy
  - ▼ After vagotomy
- Increased serum gastrin with gastric acid hypersecretion
  - ▼ Z-E syndrome
  - ▼ Hyperplasia of antral gastrin cells
  - ▼ Isolated retained antrum (a condition of gastric acid hypersecretion and recurrent ulceration after antrectomy and gastrojejunostomy that occurs when the duodenal stump contains antral mucosa)
- Increased serum gastrin with gastric acid normal or slight hypersecretion
  - ▼ RA
  - ▼ DM
  - ▼ Pheochromocytoma
  - ▼ Vitiligo
  - ▼ Chronic renal failure with serum creatinine >3 mg/dL; occurs in 50% of patients
- Pyloric obstruction with gastric distention
- Short-bowel syndrome due to massive resection or extensive regional enteritis
- Incomplete vagotomy

Decreased In

- Antrectomy with vagotomy
- Hypothyroidism
- Drugs, including anticholinergics and tricyclic antidepressants

16

❑ **Limitations**

- Gastrin levels follow circadian rhythms (lowest in early morning and highest during the day).
- No consistent relationship has been established between *H. pylori* and gastric acid secretion or serum gastrin levels.

GAUCHER DISEASE MOLECULAR DNA ASSAY*

❑ **Definition**

- Gaucher disease (GD) molecular DNA testing identifies mutations in the acid β-glucosidase (*GBA*) gene in carriers and affected individuals. Glucosylceramidase enzyme activity is very low in affected individuals, but enzyme assay is not recommended for detection of *GBA* gene mutation carriers. Carrier testing should be accomplished through DNA testing of the *GBA* gene.
- **Normal values:** negative or no mutations are found.

❑ **Use**

- **Carrier testing for Ashkenazi Jewish individuals**
- **Carrier testing for at-risk family members of affected individuals**
- For carrier testing use:
  - ▼ Targeted mutation analysis:
    - A panel of four common mutations comprising (legacy mutation name in parenthesis):
      - *p.N409S (Asn370Ser), p.L483P (Leu444Pro), c.84dupG (84GG), c.115+1G>T, (IVS2+1G>A)*
      - More extended panels include additional less common mutations such as:
      - *p. V433L (Val394Leu), p.D448H (Asp409His), p.R502C (Arg463Cys), p.R535H (Arg496His), g.5879del55 (1263del55)*
- **Confirmatory diagnosis in symptomatic individuals use:**
  - ▼ GBA gene sequence analysis: Analysis of the entire coding region and exon–intron boundaries is useful for identifying rare mutant alleles associated with GD.
- **Prenatal diagnosis—when both parental mutations are known use:**
  - ▼ Mutation-specific testing for known familial mutations

❑ **Limitations**

- The results of a genetic test may be affected by DNA rearrangements, blood transfusion, bone marrow transplantation, or rare sequence variations.

GENETIC CARRIER TESTING

❑ **Definition**

- Parental testing performed to assess carrier status for a specific genetic abnormality. Typically performed on DNA from a blood specimen to test

*Submitted by Edward Ginns, MD and Marzena M. Galdzicka, PhD.

for targeted mutations, but testing also can include other modalities such as enzymatic testing and gel electrophoresis.

❑ **Use**

- Carrier testing for autosomal recessive disease (may be targeted to specific ethnic groups). Examples:
  - ▼ CF: DNA testing for common mutations
  - ▼ Spinal muscular atrophy: DNA testing for common mutation
  - ▼ Sickle cell anemia: presence of sickling; confirmed by Hb electrophoresis
  - ▼ Tay-Sachs disease: enzyme activity
  - ▼ α-Thalassemia and β-thalassemia: decreased mean corpuscular volume; confirmed by Hb electrophoresis
- Carrier testing for X-linked disease. Example:
  - ▼ Fragile X (DNA testing for premutation); not currently offered to general population

❑ **Limitations**

- DNA testing for common mutations does not eliminate the possibility that an individual carries a rare mutation not included in the screening panel. Therefore, even if testing is negative, a residual carrier risk remains. Residual risk depends on many factors, including disease prevalence, patient ethnicity, family history, and the number of mutations included in the screen.

GHRELIN

❑ **Definition and Use**

- Ghrelin is a 3.5-kDa protein of 28-amino-acid peptide that is the natural ligand for the growth hormone secretagogue receptor. Based on its structure, it is a member of the motilin family of peptides. When administered peripherally or into the CNS, ghrelin stimulates secretion of growth hormone, increases food intake, and produces weight gain. Ghrelin, which is produced by the stomach, increases during periods of fasting or under conditions associated with negative energy balance such as starvation or anorexia. In contrast, ghrelin levels are low after eating or with hyperglycemia and in obesity. Accumulating evidence indicates that ghrelin plays a central role in the neurohormonal regulation of food intake and energy homeostasis.
- **Normal range** (fasting plasma levels): approximately 550–650 pg/mL.

❑ **Interpretation**

Increased In
- Fasting
- Cachexia and anorexia

Decreased In
- After eating

❑ **Limitations**

- This test is not available routinely in many commercial clinical laboratories.

16

GLIADIN (DEAMIDATED) ANTIBODIES, IgG AND IgA

❏ **Definition**

- ▪ ELISA-based deamidated gliadin (DGP) antibody assay is a more useful test in the diagnosis of celiac disease than the native gliadin antibody assays. DGP assays seem to be equivalent to, but not better than, tissue transglutaminase–IgA (TTG-IgA); however, DGP assays may have additive benefits in celiac screening because the combination of the two tests can increase the sensitivity without actually lowering the specificity. The DGP test also may be beneficial in circumstances when the TTG results are indeterminate. In addition, among young children, it seems to appear before TTG and to resolve faster in the context of gluten withdrawal.
- ▪ Other names: DGP, gliadin IgA, and IgG.
- ▪ **Normal range:**
  - ▼ Negative: ≤19 U
  - ▼ Weak positive: 20–30 U
  - ▼ Positive: ≥31 U

❏ **Use**

- ▪ For initial evaluation for celiac disease in IgA-deficient population
- ▪ Monitoring response to dietary therapy
- ▪ When TTG-IgA is normal in patients with villous atrophy
- ▪ Patients with a high pretest probability of celiac disease but a negative TTG-IgA: guiding a decision regarding the need for endoscopy and biopsy

❏ **Interpretation**

Increased In

- ▪ Celiac disease
- ▪ Dermatitis herpetiformis

❏ **Limitations**

- ▪ Biopsy of the proximal small intestine is indicated to confirm the diagnosis of celiac disease in a patient with positive serologic test(s) for antibodies to TTG or deamidated gliadin. It is recommended that multiple tissue specimens be taken at biopsy to avoid false-negative histology in patients with focal disease.
- ▪ The levels of antibodies to TTG and deamidated gliadin peptides decline slowly in patients treated with a gluten-free diet, and serologic testing may be repeated to assess the response to treatment. In a typical patient, it may take up to 1 year for results to normalize. Persistently elevated results suggest poor adherence to the gluten-free diet.

GLUCAGON

❏ **Definition**

- ▪ Polypeptide hormone secreted by the islet alpha cells in the pancreas. Stimulates the production of glucose in the liver and the oxidation of fatty acids

- **Normal range** (by age):
  - ▼ Newborn (1–3 days): 0–1,750 pg/mL
  - ▼ Child (4–14 years): 0–148 pg/mL
  - ▼ Adult: 20–100 pg/mL

❏ **Interpretation**

Increased In
- Glucagonoma
- Diabetes mellitus
- Chronic renal failure
- Hyperlipoproteinemia types III and IV
- Severe stress, infections, trauma, burns, surgery, and acute hypoglycemia

Decreased In
- Cystic fibrosis
- Chronic pancreatitis

GLUCAGON STIMULATION TEST

❏ **Definition and Use**
- Failure of glucagon to increase after arginine stimulation is seen in glucagon deficiencies such as cystic fibrosis and chronic pancreatitis.
- This test is of rare clinical utility.
- After fasting overnight, an IV infusion of 0.5 g arginine/kg (not >30 g) should be given over 30 minutes. Fasting samples should be drawn at 15, 30, 45, and 60 minutes.
- Normal range: peak glucagon concentration at 30 minutes: 100–1,500 pg/mL.

❏ **Limitations**
- Arginine also stimulates insulin.
- There is an exaggerated response in diabetes, chronic renal failure, and liver failure.

GLUCOSE TOLERANCE TEST, ORAL (OGTT)

❏ **Definition and Use**
- OGTT should be reserved principally for patients with "borderline" fasting plasma glucose levels. It is necessary for the diagnosis of impaired fasting glucose and impaired glucose tolerance. All pregnant women should be tested for gestational DM with a 50-g dose at 24–28 weeks of pregnancy; if that is abnormal, OGTT should be performed for confirmation. OGTT is the gold standard, and currently, its chief use is in the diagnosis of gestational DM (GDM).
- **Normal range:** see Tables 16.35 and 16.36.

16

TABLE 16–35. Blood Test Levels for Diagnosis of Diabetes and Prediabetes			
	Hemoglobin A1c (%)	**Fasting Glucose (mg/dL)**	**2-Hour OGTT (mg/dL)**
Normal	≤5.6	≤99	≤139
Prediabetes	5.7–6.4	100–125	140–199
Diabetes	≥6.5	≥126	≥200

❏ **Interpretation**

■ Criteria for the diagnosis of DM (males and nonpregnant females) (*one* of the following) (Table 16.35):

▼ Symptoms of DM plus casual (random) plasma/serum glucose concentration ≥200 mg/dL. Casual is defined as any time of day without regard to time since the last meal.

▼ Fasting plasma glucose (FPG) ≥126 mg/dL. Fasting is defined as no caloric intake for at least 8 hours.

▼ A_{1C} ≥ 6.5%. Test should be performed in laboratory using a method NGSP certified and standardized to the DCCT assay.

▼ Two-hour postload glucose (PG) ≥200 mg/dL during an OGTT. The test should be performed using a 75-g glucose load.

● In the absence of unequivocal hyperglycemia with acute metabolic decompensation, these criteria should be confirmed by repeat testing on a separate day. The third measure (OGTT) is not recommended for routine clinical use.

● For diagnosis of DM in nonpregnant adults, at least two values of OGTT should be increased (or fasting serum glucose ≥140 mg/dL on more than one occasion) and other causes of transient glucose intolerance must be ruled out.

■ Criteria for the diagnosis of GDM (any degree of glucose intolerance with onset or first recognition during pregnancy), with the screening test for GDM:

▼ A fasting serum glucose level >126 mg/dL or a casual plasma glucose >200 mg/dL meets the threshold for the diagnosis of DM if confirmed on a subsequent day, and it precludes the need for any glucose challenge.

▼ In the absence of this degree of hyperglycemia, evaluation for GDM in women with average or high-risk characteristics should follow one of two approaches.

● One-step approach:

• Perform a diagnostic 75-g oral glucose tolerance test (OGTT) without prior plasma/serum glucose screening (Table 16.36).

• This approach may be cost-effective in high-risk patients or populations.

● Two-step approach:

• Perform an initial screening by measuring the plasma or serum glucose concentrations 1 hour after a 50-g oral glucose load (GCT) and perform a subsequent diagnostic OGTT on those women exceeding the glucose threshold value on the GCT.

• A value of ≥140 mg/dL 1 hour after the 50-g load indicates the need for a full diagnostic, 100-g load, 3-hour OGTT performed in the fasting state (Table 16.36).

TABLE 16–36. Screening and Diagnostic Scheme for GDM

One-Step (IADPSG*Consensus) 75-g OGTT

State	Plasma Glucose (mg/dL)
Fasting	≥92
1 h	≥180
2 h	≥153

Two-Step (NIH Consensus) 50-g GCT (First Step) and 100-g OGTT (Second Step)

		Plasma Glucose (mg/dL)	
		100-g OGTT	
State	50-g GCT	Carpenter/Coustan	NDDG†
Fasting		95	105
1 h	≥140‡	180	190
2 h		155	165
3 h		140	145

*International Association of Diabetes and Pregnancy Study Groups.
†National Diabetes Data Group.
‡American College of Obstetricians and Gynecologists recommend 135 mg/dL for high-risk ethnic minorities with higher prevalence of GDM.

- Two or more of the venous plasma concentrations must be met or exceeded for a positive diagnosis. The test should be done in the morning after an overnight fast of between 8 and 14 hours and after at least 3 days of unrestricted diet (≥150 g carbohydrate per day) and unlimited physical activity. The subject should remain seated and should not smoke throughout the test.
- With either approach, the diagnosis of GDM is based on OGTT.

❏ **Limitations**

- Prior diet of >150 g of carbohydrate daily, no alcohol, and unrestricted activity for 3 days before test.
- Test in morning after 10–16 hours of fasting. No medication, smoking, or exercise (remain seated) during test.
- Not to be done during recovery from acute illness, emotional stress, surgery, trauma, pregnancy, inactivity due to chronic illness; therefore, is of limited or no value in hospitalized patients.
- Certain drugs should be stopped several weeks before the test (e.g., oral diuretics, oral contraceptives, and phenytoin). Loading dose of glucose consumed within 5 minutes:
- OGTT is not indicated in
  ▼ Persistent fasting hyperglycemia (>140 mg/dL).
  ▼ Persistent fasting normoglycemia (<110 mg/dL).
  ▼ Patients with typical clinical findings of DM and random plasma glucose >200 mg/dL.
  ▼ Secondary diabetes (e.g., genetic hyperglycemic syndromes, following administration of certain hormones).
  ▼ OGTT should never be used for the evaluation of reactive hypoglycemia.
  ▼ OGTT is of limited value for the diagnosis of DM in children.

16

Suggested Reading

Standards of Medical Care in Diabetes—2014 position statement. *Diabetes Care*. 2014;37(1): S14–S80.

GLUCOSE, CEREBROSPINAL FLUID (CSF)

❏ **Definition**

- Glucose in the CSF is about two thirds of the serum glucose measured during the preceding 2–4 hours in normal adults. This ratio decreases with increasing serum glucose levels. CSF glucose levels generally do not go above 300 mg/dL regardless of serum levels. Critical values are <30 mg/dL. Glucose in the CSF of neonates varies much more than that in adults, and the CSF-to-serum ratio is generally higher than in adults.
- **Normal range:** 50–80 mg/dL.

❏ **Use**

- Diagnosis of tumors, infections, inflammation of the CNS, and other neurologic and medical conditions.

❏ **Interpretation**

Increased In

- Elevated levels of glucose in the blood
- CNS syphilis

Decreased In

- CNS infections (glucose levels are usually normal in viral infections)
- Chemical meningitis
- TB meningitis
- Cryptococcal meningitis
- Mumps
- Primary and metastatic tumors of meninges
- Sarcoidosis
- Inflammatory conditions
- Subarachnoid hemorrhage
- Hypoglycemia

❏ **Limitations**

- Normal glucose levels do not rule out infection because up to 50% of patients who have bacterial meningitis have normal CSF glucose levels.

GLUCOSE, URINE

❏ **Definition**

- Detection of glucose on a semiquantitative urine dipstick or Clinitest tablets is an insensitive means of screening for type 2 diabetes. The high rate of false-negative results suggests that the urine dipstick is not adequate as a screening test. In addition, not all patients with glucosuria have diabetes. Glucosuria can occur with defects in renal tubular function, as seen in type 2 (proximal)

TABLE 16–37. Normal Values for Urine Glucose

Specimen Type	Value
24-h urine	0.04–0.21 g/d
Random urine	In mg/g creatinine
Male	
<40 y	3–181
>40 y	19–339
Female	
<40 y	5–203
>40 y	8–331

renal tubular acidosis and in familial renal glucosuria, a genetic disorder associated with salt-wasting, polyuria, and volume depletion.

- **Normal range:** see Table 16.37.

❑ **Use**

- Aiding the evaluation of glucosuria and renal tubular defects
- Management of DM

❑ **Interpretation**

Increased In

- Any cause of increased blood glucose
- Endocrine disorders (DM, thyrotoxicosis, gigantism, acromegaly, Cushing syndrome)
- Major trauma
- Stroke
- Myocardial infarction
- Oral steroid therapy
- Burns, infections
- Pheochromocytoma

Decreased In

- Treatment with ascorbic acid, levodopa, or mercurial diuretics

❑ **Limitations**

- Prolonged exposure of urine sample to room temperature lower glucose results due to microbial contamination and glycolysis.
- Specific gravity >1.020 and increased pH cause reduced sensitivity and falsely low glucose levels.

GLUCOSE, WHOLE BLOOD, SERUM, PLASMA

❑ **Definition**

- A blood glucose test measures the amount of a type of sugar, called glucose. Glucose comes from carbohydrate foods and is the main source of energy used by the body. Glucose levels are regulated by insulin and glucagon.
- **Normal ranges:** see Table 16.38.

16

TABLE 16–38. Normal Ranges for Glucose

Age	Reference Range	Critical Range
0–4 mo	50–80 mg/dL	<35, >325 mg/dL
4 mo–1 y	50–80 mg/dL	<35, >325 mg/dL
>1 y	70–99 mg/dL	<45, >500 mg/dL

❏ **Use**

- Diagnosis of DM
- Control of DM
- Diagnosis of hypoglycemia
- Other carbohydrate metabolism disorders including gestational diabetes, neonatal hypoglycemia, idiopathic hypoglycemia, and pancreatic islet cell carcinoma
- Criteria for the diagnosis of DM (American Diabetes Association Expert Committee)
  - ▼ Four ways to diagnose diabetes are possible. Each must be confirmed on a subsequent day by any one of the four methods given above.
    - Symptoms of diabetes plus casual (random) plasma/serum glucose concentration ≥200 mg/dL (11.1 mmol/L). Casual is defined as any time of day without regard to time since the last meal.
    - FPG (fasting plasma glucose) ≥126 mg/dL (7.0 mmol/L). Fasting is defined as no caloric intake for at least 8 hours.
    - Two-hour PG (postload glucose) ≥200 mg/dL (11.1 mmol/L) during an OGTT. The test should be performed using a 75-g glucose load.
    - HbA_{1C} of >6.5%.
  - ▼ In the absence of unequivocal hyperglycemia with acute metabolic decompensation, these criteria should be confirmed by repeat testing on a separate day. The third measure (OGTT) is not recommended for routine clinical use.
  - ▼ The Expert Committee recognizes an intermediate group of subjects whose glucose levels, although not meeting the criteria for diabetes, are nevertheless too high to be considered altogether normal. This group is defined as having FPG levels >110 mg/dL but <126 mg/dL or 2-hour values in OGTT of >140 mg/dL but <200 mg/dL.

❏ **Interpretation**
Increased In

- DM, including:
  - ▼ Hemochromatosis
  - ▼ Cushing syndrome (with insulin-resistant diabetes)
  - ▼ Acromegaly and gigantism (with insulin-resistant diabetes in early stages, hypopituitarism later)
- Increased circulating epinephrine
  - ▼ Adrenalin injection
  - ▼ Pheochromocytoma
  - ▼ Stress (e.g., emotion, burns, shock, anesthesia)

- Acute pancreatitis
- Chronic pancreatitis (some patients)
- Wernicke encephalopathy (vitamin B_1 deficiency)
- Some CNS lesions (subarachnoid hemorrhage, convulsive states)
- Effect of drugs (e.g., corticosteroids, estrogens, alcohol, phenytoin, thiazides, propranolol, chronic hypervitaminosis A)

Decreased In

- Pancreatic disorders
  - Islet cell tumor, hyperplasia
  - Pancreatitis
  - Glucagon deficiency
- Extrapancreatic tumors
  - Carcinoma of the adrenal gland
  - Carcinoma of the stomach
  - Fibrosarcoma
  - Other
- Hepatic disease
  - Diffuse severe disease (e.g., poisoning, hepatitis, cirrhosis, primary or metastatic tumor)
- Endocrine disorders
  - Hypopituitarism*
  - Addison disease
  - Hypothyroidism
  - Adrenal medulla unresponsiveness
  - Early DM
- Functional disturbances
  - Postgastrectomy
  - Gastroenterostomy
  - Autonomic nervous system disorders
- Pediatric anomalies
  - Prematurity*
  - Infant of diabetic mother
  - Ketotic hypoglycemia
  - Zetterström syndrome
  - Idiopathic leucine sensitivity
  - Spontaneous hypoglycemia in infants
- Enzyme diseases
  - von Gierke disease*
  - Galactosemia*
  - Fructose intolerance*
  - Amino acid and organic acid defects*
- Methylmalonic acidemia*
- Glutaric acidemia, type II*
- Maple syrup urine disease*

---

*May cause neonatal hypoglycemia.

16

- 3-Hydroxy, 3-methyl glutaric acidemia*
  - ▼ Fatty acid metabolism defects*
- Acyl CoA dehydrogenase defects*
- Carnitine deficiencies*
- Other
  - ▼ Exogenous insulin (factitious)
  - ▼ Oral hypoglycemic medications (factitious)
  - ▼ Leucine sensitivity
  - ▼ Malnutrition
  - ▼ Hypothalamic lesions
  - ▼ Alcoholism

❑ **Limitations**

- Most glucose strips and meters quantify whole blood glucose, whereas most laboratories use plasma or serum, which reads 10–15% higher.
- In whole blood glucose determinations, hematocrit of >55% causes decreased result. Hematocrit of <35% causes increased result.
- Blood samples in which serum is not separated from blood cells show glucose values decreasing at rate of 3–5% per hour at room temperature.
- Postprandial capillary glucose is ≤36 mg/dL higher than venous glucose at peak of 1 hour postprandial; usually returns to negligible fasting difference within 4 hours, but in approximately 15% of patients, there may still be >20 mg/dL difference.
- Low oxygen content (e.g., venous blood, high altitudes >3,000 m) gives falsely increased values.
- Strenuous exercise, strong emotions, shock, burns, and infections can increase glucose physiologically.

Suggested Readings

American Diabetes Association Clinical Practice Recommendations: Executive Summary. Standards of Medical Care in Diabetes—2010. *Diabetes Care.* 2010;33(Suppl 1):S11–S69.
Sacks D, Bruns DE, Goldstein DE, et al. Guidelines and recommendations for laboratory analysis in the diagnosis and management of diabetes mellitus. *Clin Chem.* 2002;48(3):436–472.

GLUCOSE-6-PHOSPHATE DEHYDROGENASE (G6PD)

❑ **Definition**

- G6PD catalyzes the initial step in the hexose monophosphate shunt and is critical in protecting RBCs from oxidant injury. Deficiency of G6PD results in rigidity and lysis of RBCs, preferentially affecting older cells. G6PD deficiency is a hereditary (sex linked) abnormality.
- **Screening assay:** reported as normal or deficient.
- **Normal range (quantitative assay):** 7.0–20.5 U/g Hb.

❑ **Use**

- The G6PD assay is used when G6PD deficiency is suspected (abnormal red cell break down).

❏ **Interpretation**

Decreased In

- Hemolytic anemia
- All persons with favism (but not all persons with decreased G6PD have favism)

❏ **Limitation**

- This assay should not be used following a hemolytic crisis in African Americans who carry the A⁻ variant, because reticulocytes (elevated after acute hemolysis) may have sufficient enzyme to give erroneous normal results. Most individuals with G6PD deficiency as appropriate.

GROWTH HORMONE (GH)

❏ **Definition**

- GH is a polypeptide (191 amino acids) originating in the anterior pituitary. Its metabolic effects are primarily anabolic. It promotes protein conservation and engages a wide range of mechanisms for protein synthesis. It also enhances glucose transport and facilitates the buildup of glycogen stores. Testing is used in the diagnosis and treatment of various forms of inappropriate growth hormone secretion.

- **Normal range:**
  ▼ 0–7 years: 1–13.6 ng/mL
  ▼ 7–11 years: 1–16.4 ng/mL
  ▼ 11–15 years: 1–14.4 ng/mL
  ▼ 15–19 years: 1–13.4 ng/mL
  ▼ Adult male: 0–4 ng/mL
  ▼ Adult female: 0–18 ng/mL

❏ **Interpretation**

Increased In

- Pituitary gigantism
- Acromegaly
- Laron dwarfism (defective GH receptor)
- Ectopic GH secretion (neoplasm of the stomach and lung)
- Malnutrition
- Renal failure
- Cirrhosis
- Stress, exercise, prolonged fasting
- Uncontrolled diabetes mellitus
- Anorexia nervosa

Decreased In

- Pituitary dwarfism
- Hypopituitarism
- Adrenocortical hyperfunction

❏ **Limitations**

- Random levels provide little diagnostic information.

16

- GH levels vary throughout the day, making it difficult to define a reference range or to judge an individual's status based on single determination.
- Periods of sleep and wakefulness, exercise, stress, hypoglycemia, estrogens, corticosteroids, L-dopa, and factors influence the rate of growth hormone secretion.
- Because of its similarity to prolactin and placental lactogen, earlier GH immunoassays were often plagued with falsely high values in pregnant and lactating women.

GROWTH HORMONE–RELEASING HORMONE (GHRH, SOMATOCRININ)

❑ **Definition and Use**

- A 44-amino-acid peptide, secreted by the hypothalamus, stimulates the pituitary to release growth hormone. Useful in differentiating between a pituitary tumor and ectopic GHRH hypersecretion.
- **Normal range:** <50 pg/mL.

❑ **Interpretation**

Increased In

- One percent of cases of acromegaly caused by GHRH by hypothalamus or ectopic secretion by neoplasms (e.g., pancreatic islet, carcinoid of the thymus or bronchus, neuroendocrine tumors)

Normal In

- Most cases of acromegaly due to pituitary tumors

HALLUCINOGENS*

See Amphetamines, *Cannabis sativa*.

❑ **Definition**

- Drugs that are capable of altering perception of reality, also known as psychotomimetic drugs. Although many drugs (e.g., anticholinergics, cocaine) can induce delusions and/or hallucinations, this class has the capacity to reliably induce states of altered perception, feeling, and thought.
- Other names:
  - ▼ Ketamine: 2-(2-chlorophenyl)-2-(methyl-amino) cyclohexanone
  - ▼ Phencyclidine: PCP, 1-(1-phenylcyclohexyl) piperidine, angel dust, elephant tranquilizer, peace pill, Sherman, T
  - ▼ D-lysergic acid diethylamide (LSD): 9,10-d-*N*,*N*-diethyl-6-methylergoline-8b-carboxamide, microdots, window pane
- **Normal range:** ketamine: 500–2,000 ng/mL plasma [IV administration]; PCP/LSD: not available

*Submitted By Amanda J. Jenkins, PhD.

❑ **Use**

- Ketamine: induction of anesthesia
- Phencyclidine: no current medical use in the United States; abused as a hallucinogen
- LSD: no current medical use in the United States; abused as a hallucinogen

❑ **Limitations**

- LSD unstable in light, elevated temperature, and alkaline conditions and may irreversibly adsorb to containers.
- **Screening:** individual drug-specific tests required; immunoassay based on automated chemistry analyzers using blood/serum/urine
  ▼ **Ketamine**
  - No tests currently available by immunoassay
  - TLC procedures have a high limit of detection of approximately 1,000 ng/mL.
  - See confirmation: readily detected with alkaline liquid–liquid or solid-phase extraction followed by gas chromatography or GC/MS analysis.
  ▼ **PCP**
  - Tests available from multiple manufacturers
  - Target; PCP
  - Limit of quantitation: 25 ng/mL [urine]; 2–10 ng/mL [blood/serum]
  - Little to no cross-reactivity with PCP metabolites and varying cross-reactivity (20–90%) with PCP analogs [e.g., TCP-1-(1-thiophenecyclohexyl) piperidine]
  - May cross react with dextromethorphan
  ▼ **LSD**
  - Target: D-LSD
  - Limit of quantitation: 0.5 ng/mL
  - Low (<20%) cross-reactivity with metabolites, no cross-reactivity with lysergic acid
- **Confirmation:** chromatography based; sample pretreatment/extraction procedure often required
  ▼ **Ketamine** [blood/serum/urine]
  - Gas chromatography
  - HPLC
  - GC/MS
  - Target analyte: ketamine
  - Limit of quantitation: 25–50 ng/mL
  ▼ **PCP** [blood/serum/urine]
  - Gas chromatography
  - HPLC
  - GC/MS
  - Target analyte: PCP
  - Limit of quantitation: 10–50 ng/mL
  ▼ **LSD** [blood/serum/urine]
  - LC/MS
  - LC/MS/MS

16

- Target analytes; D-LSD, hydroxy-LSD, 2-oxo-LSD, 2-oxo-3-hydroxy-LSD, N-desmethyl-LSD
- Limit of quantitation: 0.5–2 ng/mL
- Multiple identified and unidentified metabolites formed, resulting in a low confirmation rate for LSD of positive-screened specimens

HAPTOGLOBIN

❑ **Definition**

- Haptoglobin is a glycoprotein synthesized mainly in the liver. It sequesters free Hb released from hemolyzed RBCs, which is transported by macrophages to the liver where the heme is broken down to bilirubin. The same function is served by hemopexin and especially albumin. Haptoglobin is also an acute-phase reactant.
- **Normal range: 36–195 mg/dL.**

❑ **Use**

- Most sensitive test for RBC destruction; absent when the rate of destruction is double that of normal
- Indicator of chronic hemolysis (e.g., hereditary spherocytosis, PK deficiency, sickle cell disease, thalassemia major, untreated PA).
- In the diagnosis of transfusion reaction by comparison of concentrations in pretransfusion and posttransfusion samples. In a posttransfusion reaction, the serum haptoglobin level decreases in 6–8 hours; at 24 hours, it is <40 mg/dL or <40% of pretransfusion level.
- In paternity studies, may aid by determination of haptoglobin phenotypes.
- Evaluate known or suspected disorders involving a diffuse inflammatory process or tissue destruction, as indicated by elevated levels.

❑ **Interpretation**

Increased In

- Conditions associated with increased ESR and α-2 globulin (infections, inflammation, trauma, necrosis of tissue, hepatitis, scurvy, amyloidosis, nephrotic syndrome, disseminated neoplasms such as lymphomas and leukemias, collagen diseases such as rheumatic fever, RA, and dermatomyositis). Therefore, these conditions may mask the presence of concomitant hemolysis.
- One third of patients with obstructive biliary disease.
- Therapy with steroids or androgens.
- Aplastic anemia (normal to very high).
- DM.
- Smoking.
- Aging.
- Red cell membrane or metabolic defects (G6PD deficiency, hereditary spherocytosis, paroxysmal nocturnal hemoglobinuria).

Decreased In

- Hemoglobinemia (related to the duration and severity of hemolysis) due to

▼ Intravascular hemolysis (e.g., hereditary spherocytosis with marked hemolysis, PK deficiency, autoimmune hemolytic anemia, some transfusion reactions)
▼ Extravascular hemolysis (e.g., large retroperitoneal hemorrhage)
▼ Intramedullary hemolysis (e.g., thalassemia, megaloblastic anemias, sideroblastic anemias)
▼ Genetically absent in 1% of white population and 4–10% of the US blacks.
▼ Parenchymatous liver disease (especially cirrhosis)
▼ Protein loss via the kidney, GI tract, skin
▼ Infancy, pregnancy
▼ Malnutrition

❑ **Limitations**

■ Low haptoglobin is normal for the first 3–6 months of life. Haptoglobin is an acute-phase reactant and increases with inflammation or tissue necrosis.
■ Three main phenotypes of haptoglobin are known: Hp 1-1, 2-1, and 2-2. Hp 1-1 circulates as a monomer, and Hp 2-1 and 2-2 are polymers.
■ Significant interlaboratory variations are observed from the sera of healthy individuals.

HEAVY METALS*

❑ **Definition**

■ Elements in the periodic table that form cations due to electron loss when ionized. Metals with a high relative atomic mass and a density >5 g/cm³, which include aluminum, arsenic, lead (see p. 1028), mercury, cadmium, copper, selenium, thallium, and zinc
■ **Normal range:**
▼ Aluminum: <10 ng/mL (serum)
▼ Arsenic: <13 ng/mL (blood)
▼ Cadmium: <5 ng/mL (blood)
▼ Copper: <10 ng/mL (serum/plasma)
▼ Lead: <10 μg/dL (blood); <5 μg/dL (blood) for children under 6 years
▼ Mercury: <10 ng/mL blood
▼ Selenium: 58–234 ng/mL blood
▼ Thallium: <10 ng/mL serum
▼ Zinc: 0.6–1.2 μg/mL plasma

❑ **Use**

■ Many are naturally occurring in the environment (soil, air, water) and human body.
■ Depending on the metal, heavy metals have widespread use in consumer products such as cooking utensils, cosmetics, pharmaceutical products, packing materials, insecticides, wood products, batteries, computer chips, semiconductor industry, military, barometers, gauges, wiring, paint, fungicides,

*Submitted By Amanda J. Jenkins, PhD.

preservatives, canning industry, glass, plastic, ceramics, smelting, and refining and construction industries.

❏ **Limitations**

- Typically, whole blood, free of clots, is tested. (Note exceptions above under normal range.)
- Specimen must be collected using a procedure that minimizes environmental contamination. Specimen container must be trace-element free (e.g., royal blue sodium EDTA tube).

HEMATOCRIT (Hct)*

❏ **Definition and Use**

- Hct is the ratio of spun RBCs to plasma, reflecting the volume of packed RBCs. It may be performed manually following centrifugation or calculated in automated counters as the product of MCV and the RBC count. It is expressed as a percentage.
- **Normal range** (adults): 37–47% for women and 42–52% for men.

❏ **Interpretation**

- Abnormalities in Hct levels parallel those for Hb.

❏ **Limitations**

- Errors may occur in patients with polycythemia vera, as well as in those with very high WBC counts because of an elevated buffy coat, with RBC agglutination, and with large platelets. These errors are more marked in the manual methods.
- Errors in both methodologies may also occur in patients with abnormal plasma osmotic pressure. Such errors are minimized with the current generation machines.
- Technical errors in blood preparation may also result in false values (see "Hemoglobin" below). In blood kept at room temperature for more than 6 hours, the Hct and MCV are elevated due to swelling of RBCs, whereas cell counts and indices are stable for 24 hours.

HEMOGLOBIN (Hb)†

❏ **Definition**

- Hb is the respiratory protein of RBCs, consisting of 3.8% heme and 96.2% globin. There are more than 800 variants due to mutations in the globin molecule.
- **Normal range** (adults): 12–16 g/dL in women and 14–18 g/dL in men.

---

*Submitted By Liberto Pechet, MD.
†Submitted By Liberto Pechet, MD.

❑ Use

- Hb is of great utility in detecting anemias or erythrocytosis.

❑ Interpretation

Decreased In

- Hb is reduced in all anemias, in most cases as a consequence of another underlying disease or a deficiency (iron, folate, vitamin B_{12}).

Increased In

- Hb is higher as a physiologic response to high altitude due to low oxygen tension or in advanced lung or cardiac disease.
- Certain myeloproliferative neoplasms, especially polycythemia vera, present with inappropriate elevation of Hb.

HEMOGLOBIN (Hb) VARIANT ANALYSIS*

❑ Definition

- Hb variant analysis is a separation process used to identify normal and abnormal forms of Hb. HbA is the main form of Hb in the normal adult. HbF (fetal) is the major Hb in the fetus, and the remainder is HbA_2. Approximately 800 mutant forms of hemoglobin have been identified. Some are asymptomatic, especially in heterozygotes. Some may cause major morbid effects, especially in homozygotes. Globins found in different hemoglobins during fetal and adult life are indicated by Greek characters: α, β, γ, and δ. Variations in the amino acid composition of the globin chains cause the hemoglobinopathies.
- **Normal range:** In healthy adults, 95–98% of the total Hb is HbA (α2 β2), 2–3% is HbA_2 (α2 δ2), and 0.8–2.0% is fetal Hb (HbF) (α2 γ2). Note that the reference range is different in individuals younger than age 1. See Table 16.39.

❑ Use

- Evaluate a positive sickle cell screening test to differentiate sickle cell trait from sickle cell disease.
- Once there is a high clinical suspicion and the preliminary hematologic and genetic information point toward a hemoglobinopathy, an investigation for definitive diagnosis of an abnormal Hb is warranted. Such a diagnosis will
  - ▼ Assist in the diagnosis of thalassemia, especially in patients with a family history positive for the disorder
  - ▼ Evaluate Coombs negative hemolytic anemia of unknown etiology
- Measurement of HbA_2 and HbF has great clinical value in the diagnosis as well as in characterization of some Hb structural variants and other hemoglobinopathies.
- Increase in the HbA_2 level is considered the most characteristic diagnostic feature of β-thalassemia trait and represents an essential test in the screening programs for β-thalassemia prevention.

16

---

*Submitted By Liberto Pechet, MD.

TABLE 16–39. Normal Values for Hemoglobin Variants by Age

Age	HbF (%)	HbA$_2$ (%)	HbA (%)
0–30 d	61–81	<1.3	19–39
1 mo	46–67	<1.3	33–54
2 mo	29–61	<1.9	39–71
3 mo	15–56	<3.0	44–85
4 mo	9.4–29	2.0–2.8	68–89
5 mo	2.3–22	2.1–3.1	75–96
6 mo	2.7–13	2.1–3.1	84–96
8 mo	2.3–12	1.9–3.5	84–96
10 mo	1.5–5.0	2.0–3.3	92–97
12 mo	1.3–5.0	2.0–3.3	92–97
>1 y	<2%	1.5–3.5	96–100

- Hemoglobin A$_2$ prime is a delta chain variant Hb occurring in a small percentage of individuals of African ancestry. On HPLC, Hb A$_2$ prime falls in the Hb S window, but its retention time differs from that of Hb S. When quantifying Hb A$_2$ for the diagnosis of β-thalassemia heterozygosity, it is essential to add together the A$_2$ and A$_2$ prime to obtain a "total Hb A$_2$."
- There are two methods in use to screen for Hb variants:
  ▼ HPLC is used as the primary screening tool because it readily quantitates HbA, HbA$_2$, and HbF; in addition, it presumptively identifies three of the most common Hb variants seen in North America: HbS, HbC, and HbD. All other abnormal variants will be flagged and need to be identified by hemoglobin electrophoresis (HE).
  ▼ Alkaline and acid HE is used to investigate the whole array of Hb variants. A practical method for HE is cellulose acetate at alkaline pH. Hb molecules in an alkaline solution have a net negative charge and move toward the anode. The method separates HbA, HbA$_2$, HbS, HbF, and HbC. Citrate agar gel electrophoresis at an acid pH separates hemoglobin variants that migrate together on cellulose acetate: HbS from HbD and HbG, HbC from HbE and HbO. Many of the hemoglobin forms that are difficult to differentiate by gel HE can be differentiated by HPLC. For instance, on gel electrophoresis, HbA$_2$ is difficult to distinguish from HbC because they migrate together. Testing by HPLC allows the quantification of HbA$_2$ in the presence of HbC. The two methods complement each other.
  ▼ All Hb variants that are not diagnosed by these two methods require further testing with mass spectroscopy, capillary isoelectric focusing, or sequencing of DNA fragments generated by PCR.

❑ **Interpretation**
Increases
- HbA$_2$: megaloblastic anemia, β-thalassemias
- HbF: acquired aplastic anemia, hereditary persistence of fetal Hb, hyperthyroidism, leakage of fetal blood into maternal circulation, leukemia (acute

or chronic), myeloproliferative neoplasms, sickle cell disease, thalassemias, β chain substitutions
- HbC (second most common variant in the United States)
- HbD (hemoglobinopathy that may also be found in combination with HbS or thalassemia)
- HbE
- HbS (sickle trait or disease)

Decreases In HbA₂

Decreases In HbA$_2$
- α-Thalassemia
- Erythroleukemia
- Iron deficiency anemia (untreated)
- Sideroblastic anemia

❏ Limitations

- HbA$_2$ and HbF levels should be considered in conjunction with family history plus laboratory data, including serum iron, TIBC, ferritin, red cell morphology, hemoglobin, Hct, and MCV.
- Blood transfusions may temporarily obscure or dilute abnormal Hb.
- When using HPLC, when HbA$_2$ exceeds 10%, the presence of HbE or other Hb with similar resolution should be investigated.
- Quantitation of hemoglobins is performed optimally after 1 year of age.
- Hb Lepore arises from an unequal crossing-over and recombination event between adjacent δ and β globin genes. The resulting Hb has the mobility of HbS on alkaline electrophoresis and HbA on acid electrophoresis.
- HbH is composed of a tetramer of normal β chains, resulting in a markedly reduced production of α chains. HbH has mobility much faster at alkaline pH than HbA. (HbH disease is a severe form of α-thalassemia with only one α chain.)

HEMOGLOBIN A$_{1c}$

❏ Definition

- Glucose combines with Hb continuously and nearly irreversibly during the life span of RBC (120 days). Therefore, glycosylated Hb (GHb) will be proportional to mean plasma glucose level during previous 6–12 weeks. May be reported as HbA$_{1c}$ or as total of A$_{1b}$, A$_{1a}$, or A$_{1c}$.

Values may not be comparable with different methodologies and even different laboratories using same methodology.

- **Normal range** (ADA 2010 recommendations):
  - ▼ <5.6%
  - ▼ 5.7–6.4% increased risk for diabetes
  - ▼ >6.5% diabetic range
- The interpretation of HbA$_{1c}$ levels is not intuitively obvious to many patients with DM, who are accustomed to thinking in terms of blood glucose levels. The American Diabetes Association (ADA) has called for laboratories to express HbA$_{1c}$ results as estimated average blood glucose (eAG). ADA

16

believes that eAG will be easier for patients to understand and will lead to improved management of DM.

■ The formula recommended to calculate eAG is

$$eAG(mg / dL) = 28.7 \times hemoglobin A1c - 46.7$$

❑ **Use**

■ Monitoring compliance and long-term blood glucose level control in patients with diabetes.
■ Index of diabetic control (direct relationship between poor control and development of complications).
■ Predicting development and progression of diabetic microvascular complications.
■ Possibly for diagnosis of DM. Usefulness is still to be determined.

❑ **Interpretation**

■ A_{1C} test should be performed at least two times a year in patients who are meeting treatment goals (and who have stable glycemic control).
■ A_{1C} test should be performed quarterly in patients whose therapy has changed or who are not meeting glycemic goals.
■ Lowering A_{1C} to below or around 7% has been shown to reduce microvascular and neuropathic complications of type 1 and type 2 diabetes. Therefore, for microvascular disease prevention, the A_{1c} goal for nonpregnant adults in general is <7%.
■ Dietary preparation or fasting is not required.
■ An increase almost certainly means DM if other factors (see below) are absent (>3 SD above the mean has S/S = 99%/48%), but a normal value does not rule out impaired glucose tolerance. Values less than the normal mean are not seen in untreated DM.
■ May rise within 1 week after rise in blood glucose due to stopping therapy but may not fall for 2–4 weeks after blood glucose decrease when therapy is resumed.
■ Mean blood glucose in first 30 days (days 0–30) before sampling GHb contributes approximately 50% to final GHb value, whereas days 90–120 contribute only approximately 10%. Time to reach a new steady state is approximately 30–35 days.
■ When fasting blood glucose is <110 mg/dL, HbA_{1c} is normal in >96% of cases.
■ When fasting blood glucose is 110–125 mg/dL, HbA_{1c} is normal in >80% of cases.
■ When fasting blood glucose is >126 mg/dL, HbA_{1c} is normal in >60% of cases.
■ One percent increase in GHb is related to approximately 30 mg/dL increase in glucose.
■ When mean annual HbA_{1c} is <1.1 times ULN, renal and retinal complications are rare, but complications occur in >70% of cases when HbA_{1c} is >1.7 times ULN.

Increased In

- Fetal Hb above normal or 0.5% (e.g., heterozygous or homozygous persistence of HbF, fetomaternal transfusion during pregnancy)
- Chronic renal failure with or without hemodialysis
- Iron deficiency anemia
- Splenectomy
- Increased serum triglycerides
- Alcohol ingestion
- Lead and opiate toxicity
- Salicylate treatment

Decreased In

- Shortened RBC life span (e.g., hemolytic anemias, blood loss)
- Following transfusions
- Pregnancy
- Ingestion of large amounts (>1 g/day) of vitamin C or vitamin E
- Hemoglobinopathies (e.g., spherocytes), which produce variable increase or decrease depending on assay method.

HEPARIN ANTI-XA (LOW MOLECULAR WEIGHT HEPARIN)*

❑ **Definition**

- The a-Xa assay measures the functional plasma level of various heparins used for the prevention or therapy of thromboembolic events. It is not a direct measurement of heparin. The assay measures heparin's effectiveness when bound to antithrombin in interfering with the physiologic effect of factor Xa on factor II.

❑ **Use**

- The effectiveness of therapy with unfractionated heparin (UH) and its various derivatives (low molecular weight heparins [LMWH], fondaparinux) and new anti–factor Xa anticoagulants such as rivaroxaban. The quantitative effects of each of these agents are useful tools for determining the efficacy of the therapy. In most laboratories, a chromogenic assay is being used. While the assay in general is applicable to all the drugs mentioned above, specific calibrators are needed for each type of drug separately, to allow the production of specific curves on which the activity is determined precisely. Calibrators for rivaroxaban are presently being developed.
- The assay is not generally used for monitoring UH therapy, because the routinely used PTT is highly sensitive to the activity of this drug, and evidence-based guidelines have established its use. In the presence of a baseline prolonged PTT (such as in patients with lupus anticoagulant, "contact factor" deficiency), the a-Xa assay may replace the use of PTT.

16

*Submitted By Liberto Pechet, MD.

Similarly, in patients with very high levels of factor VIII, the PTT may underestimate the degree of anticoagulation produced by UH, and the plasma a-Xa will provide a more accurate measurement of the degree of anticoagulation.

- Since UH is used intravenously in most cases, once a steady infusion has been established, the time of obtaining the sample is not relevant.
- Obtaining a-Xa assay is not necessary in most cases when using LMWH, since fixed doses are given for either prophylactic or therapeutic use, based on body weight. There are situation when monitoring with this assay is necessary, because the body weight is not entirely representative of the drug's distribution or efficacy: in patients with impaired renal function, pregnancy, obesity, cachexia, infants, and burns (rapid body fluids shifts).

❏ **Interpretation**

- Reference ranges for a-Xa levels depend on the heparin type, dose, schedule, and indications. In the absence of heparin therapy, the a-Xa concentrations should be undetectable.

Therapeutic Ranges for Adults

- Intravenous infusion of UH: 0.30–0.70 IU/mL.
- LMWH: 0.40–1.10 a-XaU/mL for twice daily dosing or 1.00–2.00 a-FXaU/mL for once daily dosing. Blood should be drawn as a "peak" test, about 4 hours following the subcutaneous injection. Random or "through" a-Xa tests may be performed when there is concern of LMWH accumulation in patients with impaired renal function.
- *Prophylactic use* of LMWH: 0.20–0.50 a-XaU/mL.

❏ **Limitations**

- Great attention must be paid in preparing the plasma to be tested in order to eliminate platelet contamination (platelets when activated release platelet factor 4, a potent antiheparin protein). Careful and adequate centrifugation is necessary.
- Spuriously low results may be seen in patients with antithrombin deficiency.

HEPARIN-INDUCED THROMBOCYTOPENIA (HIT) ASSAYS*

❏ **Definition**

- HIT refers to thrombocytopenia that develops during or following the administration of heparin. There are various assays in use, none entirely satisfactory.
- There are two groups of assays:
  - ▼ Immunologic: ELISA assays: use specific IgG antibodies; these assays have a high negative and positive predictive value.

---

*Submitted By Liberto Pechet, MD.

▼ Functional: Serotonin release assay, the gold standard for diagnosing HIT. An alternative functional assay is platelet aggregation standardized to use heparin as the aggregating agent.

- **Normal values**
  - ▼ ELISA: negative if <0.4 optical density
  - ▼ Serotonin release assay (depends on the laboratory's own methodology): negative or positive

❑ **Use**

- An HIT assay should be performed whenever HIT is clinically suspected.

❑ **Limitations**

- ELISA requires well-trained, experienced technologists for accurate performance.
- Serotonin release requires the use of radioactive materials. It is performed in only a few reference laboratories.

HEREDITARY HEMOCHROMATOSIS MUTATION ASSAY*

❑ **Definition**

- Hereditary hemochromatosis (HH; OMIM# 235200) testing identifies mutations in the *HFE* gene. *HFE* mutations exhibit incomplete penetrance; therefore, the HFE genotype cannot be used as the sole diagnostic criterion for disease. The majority (approximately 80–90%) of HH patients are homozygous for the *C282Y* mutation. Less than 2% of all *C282Y/H63D* compound heterozygotes will develop HH. Other reported genotypes associated with a clinical diagnosis of HH include compound heterozygosity for *C282Y/S65C* and homozygosity for *H63D*.
- **Normal values:** negative or no mutations are found.

❑ **Use**

- Confirmatory diagnostic testing
- Predictive testing for at-risk relatives
- Carrier testing (for the identification of heterozygotes)
- Prenatal diagnosis (rarely performed)
- Two groups of tests are available:
  - ▼ Targeted mutation panels test for only two: *p.C282Y* (*c.845G>A*) and *p.H63D* (*c.187C>G*), or three mutations including *p.S65C* (*c.193A>T*)
  - ▼ HFE gene sequence analysis: analysis of the entire coding region—testing to identify rare mutant alleles

❑ **Limitations**

- The results of a genetic test may be affected by DNA rearrangements, blood transfusion, bone marrow transplantation, or rare sequence variations.

*Submitted by Edward Ginns, MD and Marzena M. Galdzicka, PhD.

16

HIGH MOLECULAR WEIGHT KININOGEN AND PREKALLIKREIN (FLETCHER FACTOR)*

❏ **Definition**

■ These clotting proteins activate the early phase of the intrinsic pathway and the complement system. When decreased, they may prolong PTT but not PT. They do not depend on vitamin K carboxylation.

■ **Normal ranges:**
  ▼ High molecular weight kininogen: 59–135%
  ▼ Prekallikrein: 55–207%

❏ **Interpretation**

Decreased In

■ Extremely rare congenital deficiencies
■ No bleeding diathesis associated with deficiencies; reflected in prolonged PTT

HOMOCYSTEINE (Hcy)†

❏ **Definition**

■ Total Hcy is a thiol-containing amino acid, produced by the intracellular demethylation of methionine to cysteine. Elevated tHcy has primary athero-genic and prothrombotic properties. Elevations in plasma homocysteine may be the result of genetic defects; nutritional deficiencies of vitamin B_6 (pyri-doxine), vitamin B_{12}, and folic acid; some chronic medical conditions such as chronic renal insufficiency; and certain drugs. The most common form of genetic hyperhomocysteinemia results from the production of a thermolabile variant of methylene tetrahydrofolate reductase (MTHFR). Homozygosity for this form of MTHFR is a relatively common cause of elevated total Hcy (tHcy) in the general population (5–14%). Highly elevated levels of tHcy are found in patients with homocystinuria (hyperhomocysteinemia), a rare genetic disorder of enzymes involved in homocysteine metabolism. These patients exhibit arterial and venous thromboembolism, severe early arteriosclerosis, mental retardation, osteoporosis, and ocular abnormalities. Moderately ele-vated levels of tHcy are associated with less severe genetic defects. Moderate hyperhomocysteinemia is an independent risk factor for venous and arterial thromboembolism but less profound than other well-established risk factors. Because of that, population screening for total Hcy level is not recommended.

■ **Normal range:** 5.0–15 μmol/L.

❏ **Use**

■ Elevated levels of tHcy may be used to exclude or confirm deficiencies of vitamin B_{12} or folate.
  ▼ It is recommended to test in patients using medications that interfere with folate status (methotrexate, antiepileptics), vegetarians without B_{12}

---

*Submitted By Liberto Pechet, MD.
†Submitted By Craig S. Smith, MD.

supplementation, unexplained anemia, peripheral neuropathy or myleopathy, recurrent spontaneous abortions or infertility.

▼ Testing also recommended for patients 40 years of age with coronary artery disease to exclude homocystinuria.

■ Elevations in tHcy levels have also been used as an independent risk factor of coronary or cerebral vascular disease. Treatment of moderate hyperhomocystinemia with folic acid supplementation for primary and secondary cardiovascular protection has met with inconsistent results and at present cannot be routinely recommended.

❑ **Interpretation**

■ Hyperhomocystinemia has been classified as follows:
   ▼ Moderate: 15–30 μmol/L
   ▼ Intermediate: 30–100 μmol/L
   ▼ Severe: >100 μmol/L

Increased In
■ Vitamin B_{12}, vitamin B_6, or folate deficiency
■ Hypothyroidism
■ Chronic renal failure
■ Coronary heart disease

Decreased In
■ Down syndrome
■ Pregnancy
■ Hyperthyroidism
■ Early diabetes

❑ **Limitations**

■ The plasma (or serum) must be separated immediately on collection to avoid continuous synthesis of Hcy by red cells.
■ Samples must be immediately stored on ice and serum centrifuged immediately, before a complete clot is formed, to prevent erroneous results due to the presence of fibrin.
■ Certain drugs, such as anticonvulsants, methotrexate, or nitrous oxide, may interfere with the assay.
■ Cigarette smoking and coffee consumption increase tHcy levels.
■ Intraindividual variability is approximately 8%; it can be as much as 25% in patients with hyperhomocystinemia.
■ Generally, a single measurement of tHcy is considered adequate.

Suggested Readings

Clarke R, Daly L, Robinson K, et al. Hyperhomocysteinemia: An independent risk factor for vascular disease. *N Engl J Med.* 1991;324:1149–1155.

Kluijtmans LA, Young IS, Boreham CA, et al. Genetic and nutritional factors contributing to hyperhomocysteinemia in young adults. *Blood.* 2003;101:2483–2488.

Refsum H, Smith AD, Ueland PM, et al. Facts and recommendations about total homocysteine determinations: An expert opinion. *Clin Chem.* 2004;50:3–32.

Wierzbodi AS. Homocysteine and cardiovascular disease: A review of the evidence. *Diab Vasc Dis.* 2007;4:143–149.

16

HOMOVANILLIC ACID, URINE (HVA)

❏ **Definition**

- HVA is the main terminal metabolite of catecholamine neurotransmitter, dopamine. For the diagnosis of neuroblastoma, it is important to carry out simultaneous determinations of HVA and VMA because either or both elevated.
- **Normal range:** 0.0–15.0 mg/day.

❏ **Use**

- Assist in the diagnosis of pheochromocytoma, neuroblastoma, and ganglioblastoma
- Monitor the course of therapy
- Screening for catecholamine-secreting tumors in children when accompanied by VMA
- Evaluating patients with possible inborn errors of catecholamine metabolism

❏ **Interpretation**

Increased In
- Neuroblastoma
- Pheochromocytoma
- Paraganglioma
- Riley-Day syndrome

Decreased In
- Schizotypal personality disorders

❏ **Limitations**

- Preferred specimen is 24-hour urine, because of intermittent excretion.
- Moderately elevated HVA may be caused by a variety of factors such as essential hypertension, intense anxiety, intense physical exercise, and numerous drug interactions (including some over-the-counter medications and herbal products).
- Medications that may interfere include amphetamines and amphetamine-like compounds, appetite suppressants, bactrim, bromocriptine, buspirone, caffeine, chlorpromazine, clonidine, disulfiram, diuretics (in doses sufficient to deplete sodium), epinephrine, glucagon, guanethidine, histamine, hydrazine derivatives, imipramine, levodopa (L-dopa, Sinemet), lithium, MAO inhibitors, melatonin, methyldopa (Aldomet), morphine, nitroglycerin, nose drops, propafenone (Rythmol), radiographic agents, rauwolfia alkaloids (Reserpine), and vasodilators. The effects of some drugs on catecholamine metabolite results may not be predictable.

HUMAN CHORIONIC GONADOTROPIN (hCG)

❏ **Definition**

- Glycoprotein hormone, which is also known as β-hCG and chorionic gonadotropin, is produced by the placenta, with structural similarity to the pituitary hormones FSH, TSH, and LH. The hCG test is widely used to detect pregnancy. It is also used as tumor marker for choriocarcinoma and some germ cell tumors.

TABLE 16–40. Representative Ranges in Human Chorionic Gonadotropin (hCG) During Normal Pregnancy

Approximate Gestational Age (weeks postconception)	Approximate hCG Range (mIU/mL)
0.2–1	5–50
1–2	50–500
2–3	100–5,000
3–4	500–10,000
4–5	1,000–50,000
5–6	10,000–100,000
6–8	15,000–200,000
8–12	10,000–100,000

- **Normal range:** ≥ 5.0 mIU/mL (generally indicative of pregnancy; Table 16.40).

❑ **Use**

- Diagnosis of pregnancy
- Investigation of suspected ectopic pregnancy
- Monitoring in vitro fertilization patients

❑ **Interpretation**

Increased In

- Normal pregnancy
- Recent termination of pregnancy
- Gestational trophoblastic disease
- Choriocarcinoma and some germ cell tumors
- Hydatiform mole

Decreased In

- Threatened abortion; microabortion
- Ectopic pregnancy

❑ **Limitations**

- False elevations (phantom hCG) may occur with patients who have human antianimal or heterophilic antibodies.
- Patients who have been exposed to animal antigens, either in the environment or as part of treatment or an imaging procedure, may have circulating antianimal antibodies present. These antibodies may interfere with the assay reagents to produce unreliable results.

HUMAN LEUKOCYTE ANTIGEN (HLA) TESTING*

❑ **Introduction**

- The human leukocyte antigen (HLA) system, located on the short arm of chromosome 6 at position 6p21.3, is the major histocompatibility complex

16

---

*Contributed by Neng Yu, MD.

(MHC) in humans containing a cluster of genes related to immune system. The classical HLA spans 3.6 Mb and is subdivided into three regions: class I, class II, and class III. Each region contains numerous gene loci, including expressed genes, transcripts, and pseudogenes. Many HLA loci are among the most polymorphic genes within the human genome.

- The class I region contains the genes encoding the "classical" class I HLA antigens, HLA-A, HLA-B, and HLA-C. Class I antigens, made up of an alpha chain and a beta chain (beta-2 microglobulin encoded on chromosome 15), are expressed on almost all cells of the body at varying density except erythrocytes and trophoblasts. This region also contains other HLA class I genes such as HLA-E, HLA-F, and HLA-G; MHC class I chain–related (MIC-A and MIC-B) genes; and a variety of other genes, not all of which are immune related.

- The class II region contains the genes encoding the "classical" class II molecules, HLA-DR, HLA-DQ, and HLA-DP. Class II antigens are only expressed on B cells, dendritic cells, and monocytes and can be induced during inflammation on many other cell types that normally have little or no expression. The class II molecules also consist of an alpha and a beta chain both are encoded by genes within the MHC.

- Between class I and class II is the class III region. This region does not contain any of the HLA genes. It does, however, contain many genes of importance in the immune response, for example, complement, tumor necrosis factor, and heat shock protein.

- Clinical applications of HLA are associated with, but not limited to, the following: solid organ transplantation, stem cell transplantation, platelet transfusion, disease association, and drug sensitivity.

❑ Testing Methods

HLA Typing

- HLA typing was originally performed by serology. Due to the limited accuracy, the serologic HLA typing has largely been replaced by DNA PCR–based methods. Sequence-specific oligonucleotide probing (PCR-SSOP), sequence-specific primer amplification (PCR-SSP), and sequence-based typing (SBT) are commonly used in clinical HLA laboratories.

  ▼ **PCR-SSP:** Multiple pairs of PCR primers, designed to anneal within DNA regions present in certain alleles or groups of alleles, are used for PCR amplification. If the corresponding alleles are present, their specific amplicons can be detected by gel electrophoresis. The size of the PCR products needs to be known for interpretation, and the electrophoresis migration must be run longer to separate all PCR fragments.

  ▼ **PCR-SSOP:** Locus-specific PCR primers were selected to amplify the HLA locus of interest followed by the hybridization using sequence-specific oligonucleotide probes. The HLA genotype was assigned on oligonucleotide positive reactions. Currently, the Luminex platform is the most commonly used PCR-SSOP method. Oligonucleotide probes, covalently linked to a set of polystyrene carboxylated microbeads, are designed to specifically detect the nucleotide sequences at the polymorphic sites of the HLA specificities.

▼ **SBT:** This is the only technique that directly detects the nucleotide sequences of an allele, thus allowing exact assignment. Sequence analysis software generates final allele assignment by comparing the nucleotide sequence obtained with a database of all known alleles.

HLA Antibody Analysis

■ The deleterious role of HLA antibodies has become more apparent with the development of sensitive assays identifying previously undetectable antibody specificities in the last few years, replacing the less sensitive lymphocyte target–based complement-dependent cytotoxicity (CDC) assays. Depending upon the clinical application needs, HLA antibody analysis by CDC, ELISA, flow cytometry, and Luminex platform can all be utilized, either individually or in combination, to characterize the HLA antibody.

T- and B-cell crossmatch

■ The crossmatch is used to determine if the recipient has antibodies against the potential donor. The test is performed between the patient's serum and the potential donor's T and B cells. Complement-dependent cytotoxicity (CDC), anti–human globulin–enhanced CDC (AHG-CDC), and flow cytometric crossmatches are commonly used in the lab. The sensitivity of the crossmatch methods varies a lot; CDC as the least sensitive and flow as the most sensitive. A positive crossmatch is a strong indication of HLA incompatibility.

Engraftment Monitoring

■ To provide clinicians with accurate information of the engraftment status by quantitatively determining the proportion of donor- and recipient-derived cells in the patient posttransplant. Short tandem repeats (STRs) are the most commonly used markers for this assay. STRs, also referred to as microsatellites, are short sequences of DNA, distributed throughout the genome that is repeated in tandem variable number of times. The number of repeats of different STR markers varies between individuals, giving a highly polymorphic system that can be used to uniquely identify donor-derived DNA from patient-derived DNA. With the exception of monozygotic twins, careful selection of a number of STR markers will enable most patient-derived DNA to be distinguished from donor-derived DNA.

Suggested Reading

Bontadini A. HLA techniques: Typing and antibody detection in the laboratory of immunogenetics. *Methods*. 2012;56;471–476.

HLA TESTING AND DISEASE ASSOCIATIONS/DRUG HYPERSENSITIVITY REACTIONS

❏ **Definition**

■ The proteins encoded by HLA class I and class II genes in the major histocompatibility complex (MHC) are highly polymorphic and essential in

16

self versus nonself immune recognition. HLA variation is a crucial determinant of transplant rejection and susceptibility to a large number of infectious and autoimmune diseases. In addition, linkage disequilibrium extends across multiple HLA and non-HLA genes in the MHC. The identification of disease-specific susceptibility (risk) and protective markers can be used in immunogenetic profiling, risk assessment, and therapeutic decisions. Known HLA predisposition genes and their association with autoimmunity, infectious diseases, and drug sensitivities/side effects are constantly being refined; new associations are constantly emerging in light of expanded knowledge of the HLA genetic map.

❏ **Use**

■ The evolving use of various HLA typing methods has introduced confusion to the interpretation of disease associations. For example, many early studies, using serologic typing methods, identified an association with DR4 for RA. Because DR4 has many different alleles, some of which are RA associated while some are not, the associations were generally weaker than when precise alleles were subsequently investigated. Later studies using DNA-based methods have consistently shown that, in Caucasians, the alleles *DRB1*04:01, *04:04, *04:05,* and **04:08* are highly associated with RA. Another example is ankylosing spondylitis (AS) and HLA-B27. HLA-B27 is estimated to contribute only 16–50% of the total genetic risk. The strongest association with AS is with *HLA-B*27:05* among the Japanese and *HLA-B*27:04* in the Chinese. There are less frequent associations with the alleles HLA-B*27:01, *27:02, *27:03, *27:04, *27:07, *27:08,* and **27:10.*

■ Variations at individual amino acid sites have also shown promising results in understanding disease associations. In RA, for example, investigators were able to demonstrate that many of the HLA associations with RA are best explained by differences in the specific amino acids that occur at positions 11, 71, and 74 in HLA-DRB1; position 9 in HLA-B; and position 9 in HLA-DPB1, which are all located in peptide-binding grooves. These amino acid differences account for many of the MHC associations to RA risk. These sites may modulate differential binding to key antigens involved in autoimmunity.

■ Ethnic differences must also be taken into account. The frequency of a particular allele in one population can be very different from that in another population. For example, DR4 was shown not to be associated with RA in Israeli Jews because their most common DR4 allele, *DRB1*04:02,* is not associated with the disease. For the same reason, in disease association studies, the control group with which the patient group is compared must be ethnically matched for the results to be valid. Variations between patient populations are also responsible for some differences among studies.

- A sizable fraction of HLA alleles are in linkage disequilibrium (LD), the non-random association of alleles at two or more loci. This is very important when interpreting association studies. For example, the ancestral 8.1 haplotype spans the MHC region and includes *A*01:01-C*07:01-B*08:01-DRB1*03:01-DRB3*01:01-DQA1*05:01-DQB1*02:01*. Because all of these alleles can be associated and can occur together, it is therefore difficult to interpret which locus is primarily responsible for the disease risk in such cases.

- One limitation of population studies is that the results cannot be easily transferred to an individual patient. The alleles that have been shown to be associated with diseases are susceptibility alleles and are identical to genes that are present among normal individuals, albeit with a lower frequency. One can use the calculation of relative risk (RR) to determine the probability that the disease will occur among individuals positive for the allele when compared with individuals negative for the allele. RR is the ratio of the probability of the event occurring in the exposed group versus a nonexposed group.

- How do HLA antigens confer disease susceptibility? Data regarding the relationship of HLA antigens to disease susceptibility remain at the level of associations, not disease mechanisms. Nevertheless, HLA associations that are reproducible and robust provide important clues about the development of certain rheumatic diseases. A variety of models have been postulated to explain these associations functionally. These include the importance of HLA polymorphisms in:
  - ▼ Shaping the T-cell repertoire during development
  - ▼ Shaping the peripheral T-cell repertoire
  - ▼ Determining which antigenic peptides are bound and, therefore, presented to the immune system for recognition
  - ▼ Generating molecular mimicry between self antigens and either the HLA molecule itself or peptides that it recognizes
  - ▼ Affecting HLA protein presentation of either foreign or self-antigenic peptides to autoreactive T cells
  - ▼ Influencing how infection, exogenous agents, or "molecular mimicry" may reactivate silenced T cells in autoimmune diseases
  - ▼ Affecting immune suppression and cancer development in important ways through the loss of HLA gene expression because of viral infection, somatic mutations, or other causes
  - ▼ Influencing antigen processing and presentation

- Identification of the mechanistic basis of these disease associations may lead to novel and specific treatments, as well as preventive strategies.

- *Listed* below *are some of the current known disease associations based on various publications*:
  - ▼ **Ankylosing spondylitis:** *HLA-B*27* (especially *HLA-B*27:05*)
  - ▼ **Celiac disease:** *HLA-DQA1*05-DQB1*02:01, DQA1*03-DQB1*03:02*
  - ▼ **Uveitis:**
    - ● Acute anterior uveitis: *HLA-B*27* (especially *HLA-B*27:05*).
    - ● Behçet disease: *HLA-B*51*, RR is only 6–10.
    - ● Birdshot chorioretinopathy: *HLA-A*29* (especially with *HLA-A*29:02*).

▼ Idiopathic membranous glomerulonephritis insulin-dependent (type 1) diabetes mellitus:
  ● *H L A - D R B 1 * 0 3 : 0 1 - D Q A 1 * 0 5 : 0 1 - D Q B 1 * 0 2 : 0 1;* *HLA-DRB1*04:01/04:02/04:05-DQA1*03-DQB1*03:02*
▼ **Narcolepsy:** *HLA-DQB1*06:02* allele on the *DRB1*15:01-DQA1*01:02-DQB1*06:02* haplotype. Individuals homozygous for *HLA-DQB1*06:02* have a higher risk of acquiring narcolepsy than individuals heterozygous for this allele. Heterozygous with *HLA-DQB1*03:01,* *HLA-DQB1*05:01,* and *-DQB1*06:01* are thought to be protective.
▼ **Rheumatoid arthritis:**
  ● *HLA-DRB1*04:01/04:04/04:05/04:08,* *-DRB1*01:01* Caucasian; *HLA-DRB1*04:05* Japanese; *HLA-DRB1*14:02* American Indian
■ *HLA and drug sensitivities/side effects*:
  ▼ The reverse transcriptase inhibitor, **abacavir** and *HLA-B*57:01*, the gout prophylactic, **allopurinol** and *HLA-B*58:01*, and the antiepileptic, **carbamazepine** and *HLA-B*15:02*

Suggested Readings

Bharadwaj M, Illing P, Kostenko L. Personalized medicine for HLA-associated drug-hypersensitivity reactions. *Pers Med.* 2010;7(5):495–516.
de Bakker PIW, McVean G, Sabeti PC, et al. A high-resolution HLA and SNP haplotype map for disease association studies in the extended human MHC. *Nat Genet.* 2006;38(10):1166–1172.
HLA Association of autoimmunity and infectious diseases Poster by Texas BioGene, 2008.
http://www.uptodate.com/contents/human-leukocyte-antigens-hla-a-roadmap
Raychaudhuri S, Sandor C, Stahl EA, et al. Five amino acids in three HLA proteins explain most of the association between MHC and seropositive rheumatoid arthritis. *Nat Genet.* 2012;44:291.
Shiina T, Inoko H, Kulski JK. An update of the HLA genomic region, locus information and disease associations: 2004. *Tissue Antigens.* 2004;64:631.

HLA AND STEM CELL TRANSPLANT

❏ **Definition**

■ Allogeneic hematopoietic stem cell transplantation (HSCT) has been established as the top treatment of choice for hematologic malignancies and other hematologic or immune disorders. HSCT is also emerging as the most common cell-based immunotherapy to treat solid tumors. Since human leukocyte antigen (HLA), the major histocompatibility complex (MHC) in humans, can elicit an immune response either by presentation of variable peptides or by recognition of polymorphic fragments of foreign HLA molecules, selection of an HLA identical or near-identical donor is preferred. HLA disparity has been associated with graft failure, delayed immune reconstitution, graft versus host disease (GVHD), and mortality.

■ HLA is one of the most polymorphic gene systems in the human genome. Consequently, many patients lack HLA-matched donors. In recent years, advances in HLA testing and matching, extensive research on the role of each HLA locus mismatch on clinical outcome, and further knowledge of donor selection factors have made it easier to search for and select a partially matched donor. While the role of donor-specific HLA antibodies (DSA) in solid organ transplantation is well established, their importance in HSCT is only recently emerging. HLA antibody assessment should be incorporated into the HSCT donor selection process.

❏ **Use**
- The requirements for HLA testing can be very different based on various transplant protocols and conditioning regimens. A joint agreement, between the transplant program and the HLA lab, detailing the testing algorithm, which is customized to meet the needs of different programs and patient cohorts, is very important. Based on the requirements of ASHI, AABB, CAP, and FACT, a recommended testing algorithm is listed below:
  ▼ New transplant candidates:
    - High-resolution typing of HLA-A, HLA-B, HLA-C, HLA-DRB1, and HLA-DQB1 loci and intermediate-resolution typing of HLA-DQA1 and -DRB345 loci
    - HLA antibody screen and specificity identification using a highly sensitive method, for example, Luminex single antigen–bead (SAB) assay.
    - If a patient is identified as having strong DPB1 antibodies at the time of evaluation by Luminex SAB assay, the patient and potential donors should be typed for DPB1 to confirm DPB1 antibody specificity and avoid selecting donors with corresponding DPB1 antigens. Matching DPB1 can also improve the transplant outcome.
    - Recent transfusions should be documented. At least 2–3 weeks should pass prior to collecting a new sample for HLA antibody analysis after sensitizing events.
  ▼ Related donor typing
    - Intermediate-resolution typing of HLA-A, HLA-B, and HLA-DRB1 loci
    - If matched with the recipient, high-resolution typing of HLA-A, HLA-B, HLA-C, HLA-DRB1, and HLA-DQB1 loci and intermediate-resolution typing of HLA-DQA1 and HLA-DRB345 loci.
    - Identity confirmation by intermediate-resolution typing of HLA-A, HLA-B, and HLA-DRB1 loci with a new sample
  ▼ Unrelated donor search and typing
    - If a suitable matched related donor cannot be found, an unrelated donor search will be initiated. Transplant physicians, coordinators, and HLA lab staff will be involved in the donor search and selection. NMDP, BMDW, and individual donor registries will be searched using the patient's high-resolution typing data.
    - High-resolution typing of HLA-A, HLA-B, HLA-C, HLA-DRB1, and HLA-DQB1 loci and intermediate-resolution typing of HLA-DQA1 and HLA-DRB345 loci are performed for selected unrelated donors. Additional DPB1 matching can improve transplant outcome.
    - A 10/10 allele-matched unrelated donor is preferred. Mismatched donors will be evaluated on a case-by-case basis. If the patient has HLA antibodies, especially the class II antibodies, a final T- and B-cell crossmatch with the unrelated donor may be necessary. The most current patient serum on file is preferred for the final crossmatch.

16

▼ Cord blood search and typing
  ● If a suitable matched related donor cannot be found, a cord blood unit search will be initiated. NMDP, BMDW, and individual cord blood registries will be searched using the patient's high-resolution typing data.
    • High-resolution typing of HLA-A, HLA-B, HLA-C, HLA-DRB1, and HLA-DQB1 loci and intermediate-resolution typing of HLA-DQA1 and -DRB345 loci on the selected cord(s), attached segments preferred if available, cord bag can be used as well for retrospect typing. If resources are limited, whether financial or sample material, only high-resolution typing of HLA-A, B, and DRB1 loci will be performed.
  ● When a suitable family donor is not available, the choice of an unrelated donor or cord blood will depend on the degree of HLA match, cell dose of the cord blood unit, the urgency of the transplant, and other variables (donor age, sex, ABO incompatibility, HLA antibody, etc.) that may affect the transplant outcome.
▼ Patient and donor identity confirmation
  ● *Repeat HLA typing of recipient* using a new sample such that the individual's HLA typing is confirmed prior to final donor selection for related or unrelated transplantation.
  ● *Repeat HLA typing of a related or unrelated stem cell donor* using a new sample such that the donor's HLA typing is confirmed prior to stem cell collection. For unrelated donors, registry data are acceptable as the first of these two samples.
  ● *Identity typing* can be performed by intermediate-resolution HLA-A, HLA-B and HLA-DRB1 typing by PCR-SSOP.
  ● *Transplant program coordinators* are responsible for requesting the second sample for identity typing before final donor selection is made. For donors, the registry typing will be considered as the first typing and the extended high-resolution typing will be considered as the second typing.
  ● To ensure maximum accuracy:
    • Two sample collections on different dates, the second date should be prior to the final donor selection for related or unrelated donors or cords.
    • Two sample types (blood and buccal swab) if the first sample is blood. Buccal swabs are acceptable as the first or second or both collections. Buccal swab is recommended for patients with any acute diagnosis, for example, AML and ALL with blasts.
    • Two testing methods, PCR-SSOP/SSP or SBT
▼ KIR typing
  ● HSCT for leukemia can play a major role in reducing the risk of relapse by inducing a graft versus leukemia (GVL) effect. The effectiveness of mismatching inhibitory killer cell immunoglobulin–like receptors (KIR) on donor natural killer (NK) cells as a mechanism for GVL is being studied extensively. Together, the gene content of KIR, the T-cell and NK cell components of the graft, the graft source, the conditioning regimen, and mechanisms to reduce graft versus host disease (GVHD), will improve the overall benefit of HSCT.

- Generic KIR typing, to detect the presence/absence of the inhibitory KIR genes, can be performed on selected patients and donors. The ligand matching information and the B-haplotype content can provide assistance in selecting the best possible donors/cords. The matching and mismatching of inhibitory KIR in the graft verse host direction can be determined based on the patient HLA ligand and donor inhibitory KIR.
- ▼ Null allele typing
  - Alleles that have been shown not to be expressed, "null" alleles, have been given the suffix "N." Based upon regulations required by the American Society of Histocompatibility and Immunogenetics (ASHI) and the National Marrow Donor Program (NMDP), guidelines for null allele typing have been established. The HLA lab is required to test for the following null alleles when alleles and/or haplotypes that have been associated with the specific null alleles exist. Additional CWD null alleles are constantly being updated and incorporated into the required typing list.

Null Allele	Common Related Expressed Type	Associated Types Present When Resolution May Be Required
A*24:09N	A*24:02	B*40 or B*27
B*51:11N	B*51:01	A*02, C*15, and DRB1*04 (A*02:01, C*15, and DRB1*04:02)
C*04:09N	C*04:01	B*44, more specifically, B*44:03
DRB4*01:03N	DRB4:01	DRB1*07 and DQB1*03 (DRB1*07:01 and DQB1*03:03)
DRB5*01:08N	DRB5*01:02	DRB1*15 or, more specifically, DRB1*15:02

- ▼ Engraftment monitoring (EM) testing
  - Following HSCT, patients are monitored closely for early engraftment, evidence of graft rejection, or recurrence of the original disease. HSCT creates a donor/recipient chimerism in the patient, which can be quantitatively measured through short tandem repeat (STR) analysis of peripheral whole blood, lineage-specific subsets, whole marrow, or CD34 progenitor cells in the marrow to determine the percent chimerism.
  - The pretransplant samples used in the EM assay can be the samples used for HLA typing. No additional pretransplant samples from the patient or the donor are necessary. The most common postsamples are, whole blood, T cells (CD3), B cells (CD19/20), myeloid cells (CD15/CD33/CD66b), NK cells (CD56), whole marrow, and CD34 marrow.
  - Results are commonly reported as the percentage of donor chimerism within the post-HSCT samples. The assay sensitivity is a key element and has to be considered in results interpretation and reporting, for example, for a postsample with no patient DNA detected and assay sensitivity is 3%, the result should be reported as more than 97% donor DNA, no patient DNA detected, full engraftment.

16

Suggested Readings

Brand A, Doxiadis IN, Roelen DL. On the role of HLA antibodies in hematopoietic stem cell transplantation. *Tissue Antigens.* 2013;81(1):1–11.

Cooley S, Weisdorf DJ, Guethlein LA, et al. Donor selection for natural killer cell receptor genes leads to superior survival after unrelated transplantation for acute myelogenous leukemia. *Blood.* 2010;116:2411–2419.

Fleischhauer K, Shaw BE, Gooley T, et al. Effect of T-cell-epitope matching at HLA-DPB1 in recipients of unrelated-donor haemopoietic-cell transplantation: A retrospective study. *Lancet Oncol.* 2012;13(4):366–374.

Park M, Seo JJ. Role of HLA in hematopoietic stem cell transplantation. *Bone Marrow Res.* 2012;2012:680841.

Pegram HJ, Ritchie DS, Smyth MJ, et al. Alloreactive natural killer cells in hematopoietic stem cell transplantation. *Leuk Res.* 2011;35(1):14–21.

Nowak J. Role of HLA in hematopoietic SCT. *Bone Marrow Transplant.* 2008;42:S71–S76.

HYDROXYBUTYRATE BETA (BHB)

❏ Definition

- In DKA, three ketone bodies are produced: BHB, acetoacetic acid, and acetone. BHB is present in the greatest concentration and accounts for approximately 75% of the three ketone bodies. During periods of ketosis, BHB increases even more than acetoacetate and acetone and has been shown to be a better indicator of ketoacidosis, including subclinical ketosis. Other names for this test include 3-hydroxybutyric acid and ketones. Testing for ketones is generally performed with nitroprusside (Acetest) tablets or reagent sticks. A 4+ reaction with serum diluted 1:1 is strongly suggestive of ketoacidosis. Nitroprusside reacts with acetoacetate and acetone but not with BHB. This is important because BHB is the predominant ketone, particularly in severe DKA. It is, therefore, possible to have a negative serum nitroprusside reaction in the presence of severe ketosis.
- **Normal range:** 0.02–0.27 mmol/L.

❏ Use

- Monitoring therapy for DKA.
- Investigating the differential diagnosis of any patient presenting to the emergency department with hypoglycemia, acidosis, suspected alcohol ingestion, or an unexplained increase in the AG.
- In pediatric patients, the presence or absence of ketonemia/urea is an essential component in the differential diagnosis of inborn errors of metabolism.
- Key parameter monitored during controlled 24-hour fasts.

❏ Interpretation

Increased In

- Alcoholic ketoacidosis
- Lactic acidosis (shock, renal failure)
- Liver disease
- Infections
- Phenformin and salicylate poisoning

❏ **Limitations**
  ▪ Not detectable by common tests for ketone bodies
  ▪ The nitroprusside test (Acetest) may give false-negative readings because it does not detect BHB.

IMMUNOGLOBULIN A (IgA)

❏ **Definition**
  ▪ IgA makes up the majority of immunoglobulin in mucosal secretions, including nasal and pulmonary secretions, saliva and intestinal fluids, tears, and secretions of the genitourinary tract. IgA is important in preventing attachment or penetration of the body surfaces by microorganisms, and in protection against respiratory, GI, and GU infections. IgA cannot cross the placenta. It can be produced by infants, and their secretions tend to be typically low. IgA is the second most frequent type of monoclonal immunoglobulin identified in multiple myeloma.
  ▪ **Normal ranges:** see Table 16.41.

❏ **Use**
  ▪ Detection or monitoring of monoclonal gammopathies and immune deficiencies
  ▪ Assist in the diagnosis of multiple myeloma
  ▪ Monitor therapy for multiple myeloma
  ▪ Evaluate patients suspected of IgA deficiency prior to transfusion
  ▪ Evaluate anaphylaxis associated with the transfusion of blood and blood products (anti-IgA antibodies may develop in patients with low levels of IgA, possibly resulting in anaphylaxis when donated blood is transfused)

TABLE 16–41. Normal Ranges for IgA by Age	
Age	Range (mg/dL)
0–30 d	1–7
1 mo	1–53
2 mo	3–47
3 mo	5–46
4 mo	4–72
5 mo	8–83
6 mo	8–67
7–8 mo	11–89
9–11 mo	16–83
1 y	14–105
2 y	14–122
3 y	22–157
4 y	25–152
5–7 y	33–200
8–9 y	45–234
10–17 y	68–378
≥18 y	82–453

16

❑ Interpretation

Increased In

- Polyclonal:
  - ▼ Cirrhosis of the liver
  - ▼ Chronic infections
  - ▼ Chronic inflammatory diseases
  - ▼ Inflammatory bowel disease
  - ▼ RA with high titers of RF
  - ▼ SLE (some patients)
  - ▼ Mixed connective tissue diseases
  - ▼ Sarcoidosis (some patients)
  - ▼ Wiskott-Aldrich syndrome
- Monoclonal:
  - ▼ IgA myeloma (M component)
  - ▼ Solitary plasmacytoma
  - ▼ Alpha-heavy chain disease
  - ▼ MGUS
  - ▼ Lymphoma
  - ▼ Chronic lymphocytic leukemia

Decreased In

- Normal persons (1:700)
- Hereditary telangiectasia (80% of patients)
- Type III dysgammaglobulinemia
- Malabsorption (some patients)
- SLE (occasionally)
- Cirrhosis of the liver (occasionally)
- Still disease (occasionally)
- Recurrent otitis media (occasionally)
- Non-IgA myeloma
- Waldenström macroglobulinemia
- Acquired immunodeficiency
- Gastric carcinoma

❑ Limitations

- Immunochemical methods do not distinguish between polyclonal and monoclonal levels. Serum protein electrophoresis and immunofixation need to be performed for quantification of M-proteins.

IMMUNOGLOBULIN D (IgD)

❑ Definition

- IgD is mainly found on the surface of B cells and may help regulate B-cell function. IgD likely serves as an early B-cell antigen receptor; however, the function of the circulating IgD is largely unknown. IgD functions to activate some lymphocytes.
- Normal value: ≤15.3 mg/dL.

❑ **Use**

■ Diagnosis of rare IgD myelomas (greatly increased)

❑ **Interpretation**

Increased In

■ Monoclonal
▼ IgD multiple myeloma
▼ MGUS
■ Polyclonal
▼ Chronic infection (moderately)
▼ Autoimmune disease
▼ Acute viral hepatitis
▼ COPD
▼ After allogeneic bone marrow transplantation

Decreased In

■ Hereditary deficiencies
■ Acquired immunodeficiency
■ Non-IgD myeloma
■ Infancy, early childhood

❑ **Limitations**

■ An elevated IgD need to be identified as monoclonal or polyclonal by immunofixation method.

IMMUNOGLOBULIN E (IgE)

❑ **Definition**

■ IgE mediates allergic and hypersensitivity reactions. There is a significant overlap in total IgE between allergic and nonallergic individuals. Measurement of total IgE is not very useful as a standalone screen for allergy disease.
■ **Normal values:** see Table 16.42.

TABLE 16–42. Normal Values for IgE by Age	
Age (y)	**Value (kU/L)**
0–2	<53
2	<93
3	<120
4	<160
5	<192
6	<224
7	<248
8	<260
9	<304
10	<328
18	<127

16

❏ Use

- For allergy testing; IgE antibodies and skin tests are essentially interchangeable.
- Indicates various parasitic diseases.
- Diagnosis of E-myeloma.
- Diagnosis of bronchopulmonary aspergillosis; a normal serum IgE level excludes the diagnosis.

❏ Interpretation
Increased In

- Atopic diseases
  - ▼ Exogenous asthma in approximately 60% of patients
  - ▼ Hay fever in approximately 30% of patients
  - ▼ Atopic eczema
- Influenced by type of allergen, duration of stimulation, presence of symptoms, and hyposensitization treatment
- Parasitic diseases (e.g., ascariasis, visceral larva migrans, hookworm disease, schistosomiasis, *Echinococcus* infestation)
- Monoclonal IgE myeloma

Decreased In

- Hereditary deficiencies
- Acquired immunodeficiency
- Ataxia–telangiectasia
- Non-IgE myeloma

Normal In

- Asthma

❏ Limitations

- A normal level of IgE in serum does not eliminate the possibility of allergic disease.

IMMUNOGLOBULIN G (IgG)

❏ Definition

- IgG activates complement and fights infection. IgG represents 70–80% of the total serum immunoglobulins in the normal adults. It exists in four subclasses (IgG1, IgG2, IgG3, and IgG4). IgG1 predominates as 65% of the total IgG. IgG of maternal origin provides passive immunity to the neonate. It is transported across the placenta.
- **Normal ranges:** see Table 16.43.

❏ Use

- Diagnosis of IgG myeloma
- Diagnosis of hereditary and acquired IgG immunodeficiencies
- Serologic diagnosis of infectious diseases and immunity

❏ Interpretation
Increased In

- Monoclonal
  - ▼ Multiple myeloma

TABLE 16–43. Normal Ranges for IgG by Age

Age	Range (mg/dL)
0–30 d	611–1,542
1 m	241–870
2 mo	198–577
3 mo	169–558
4 mo	188–536
5 mo	165–781
6 mo	206–676
7–8 mo	208–868
9–11 mo	282–1,026
1 y	331–1,164
2 y	407–1,009
3 y	423–1,090
4 y	444–1,187
5–7 y	608–1,229
8–9 y	584–1,509
≥10 y	768–1,632

- ▼ Solitary plasmacytoma
- ▼ MGUS
- ▼ Lymphoma
- ▼ CLL
- Polyclonal
  - ▼ Sarcoidosis
  - ▼ Chronic liver disease (e.g., cirrhosis)
  - ▼ Autoimmune diseases
  - ▼ Parasitic diseases
  - ▼ Chronic infection
  - ▼ Intrauterine contraceptive diseases

Decreased In

- Protein-losing syndromes
- Pregnancy
- Non-IgG myeloma
- Waldenström macroglobulinemia
- Primary immunodeficiency states
- Combined with other immunoglobulin decreases:
  - ▼ Agammaglobulinemia
    - Acquired
    - Primary
    - Secondary (e.g., multiple myeloma, leukemia, nephrotic syndrome, protein-losing enteropathy)
    - Congenital
    - Hereditary thymic aplasia
    - Type I dysgammaglobulinemia (decreased IgG and IgA and increased IgM)
    - Type II dysgammaglobulinemia (absent IgA and IgM and normal levels of IgG)
    - Infancy, early childhood

IgG-to-ALBUMIN RATIO, CSF

❏ **Definition**

- The two most commonly used diagnostic laboratory tests for multiple sclerosis are the CSF index and oligoclonal banding. The CSF index is the IgG-to-albumin ratio in CSF compared to the IgG-to-albumin ratio in serum. The CSF index is, therefore, an indicator of the relative amount of CSF IgG compared to serum, and any increase in the index is a reflection of IgG production in the CNS. The IgG synthesis rate is a mathematical manipulation of the CSF index data and can also be used as a marker for CNS inflammatory diseases. The index is independent of the activity of the demyelinating process.
- **Normal range:**
  - ▼ IgG, CSF: 0.0–6.0 mg/dL
  - ▼ Albumin, CSF: 0–35 mg/dL
  - ▼ IgG-to-albumin ratio, CSF: 0.09–0.25

❏ **Use**

- Diagnosis of individuals with multiple sclerosis

❏ **Interpretation**

Increased In

- Multiple sclerosis.
- High normal values may indicate degenerative diseases such as cerebral or cerebellar atrophy, amyotrophic sclerosis, or brain tumor.

❏ **Limitations**

- The CSF index can be elevated in other inflammatory demyelinating diseases such as neurosyphilis, acute inflammatory polyradiculoneuropathy, and subacute sclerosing panencephalitis.
- Oligoclonal banding in the CSF is slightly more sensitive (85%) than the CSF index. The use of CSF index plus oligoclonal banding has been reported to increase the sensitivity to >90%.
- Normal levels can occur in incomplete obstruction of the spinal canal.
- Increase in albumin alone can be a result of a lesion in the choroid plexus or a blockage in the flow of CSF.
- Determination of myelin basic protein in CSF may be of use in diagnosis of multiple sclerosis or other active demyelinating processes.

IMMUNOGLOBULIN M (IgM)

❏ **Definition**

- IgM is the first antibody to appear in response to antigen. It can be produced by the fetus and cannot be crossed by the placenta.
- **Normal range:** see Table 16.44.

❏ **Use**

- Diagnosis of hereditary and acquired IgM immunodeficiencies
- Diagnosis of Waldenström macroglobulinemia
- Earliest Ig serologic diagnosis of infectious disease

TABLE 16–44. Normal Ranges for IgM by Age	
Age	**Range (mg/dL)**
0–30 d	0–24
1 mo	19–83
2 mo	16–100
3 mo	23–85
4 mo	26–96
5 mo	31–103
6 mo	33–97
7–8 mo	32–120
9–11 mo	39–142
1 y	41–164
2 y	46–160
3 y	45–190
4 y	41–186
5–7 y	46–197
8–9 y	49–230
≥10 y	60–263

❏ **Interpretation**

Increased In

- Polyclonal
  - ▼ Liver disease
  - ▼ Chronic infections
  - ▼ Secondary to nephritic syndrome
  - ▼ Hyper IgM syndrome
- Monoclonal
  - ▼ Waldenström macroglobulinemia
  - ▼ Lymphoma
  - ▼ CLL
  - ▼ Multiple myeloma (rare)
  - ▼ Schnitzler syndrome
  - ▼ Cold IgM antibody agglutinin
  - ▼ MGUS

Decreased In

- Protein-losing syndromes
- Non-IgM myeloma
- Infancy, early childhood

❏ **Limitations**

- Selective deficiency of IgM is a rare immune disorder in association with infection and normal levels of other immunoglobulin isotypes.

IMMUNOGLOBULINS, FREE LIGHT CHAINS, SERUM

❏ **Definition**

- Plasma cells do not produce complete immunoglobulin molecules. Instead, they produce the heavy and light chain components separately and then

16

assemble them before secretion into the bloodstream. Because plasma cells usually make slightly more light chain components, there are usually some leftover light chains that are secreted in the blood without being bound to a heavy chain. These are known as serum free light chains (FLCs). Normally, there are only very low levels of free light chains in the blood (serum).

- The Freelite, free kappa and free lambda light chain assays, are a new, highly sensitive aid in the diagnosis and monitoring of patients with multiple myeloma and related plasma cell disorders. The Freelite serum free kappa and free lambda light chain assays are run on serum and not on urine with increased sensitivity over current electrophoretic assays.
- Recent studies have shown that Freelite serum free kappa and lambda light chain assays:
  - ▼ Detect up to 82% of nonsecretory myeloma
  - ▼ Detect and monitor AL amyloid patients, including those with no monoclonal protein by immunofixation (IFE)
  - ▼ Detect and assess response to treatment in >95% of patients with light chain and intact Ig multiple myeloma
  - ▼ Detect up to 96% of intact immunoglobulin myeloma patients
  - ▼ Provide an earlier marker of therapeutic response or resistance, compared to whole immunoglobulin/M spike assays
  - ▼ Evaluate risk of progression to myeloma in patients with monoclonal gammopathy of undetermined significance (MGUS)
  - ▼ In combination with serum protein electrophoresis or IFE alone, provide the optimal detection rate for all paraproteins
- **Normal range:**
  - ▼ Free kappa: 3.30–19.40 mg/L
  - ▼ Free lambda: 5.71–26.30 mg/L
  - ▼ Kappa/lambda ratio: 0.26–1.65

❏ Use

- Diagnosis and monitoring progress of patients with nonsecretory myeloma and oligosecretory (<1 g/dL monoclonal protein in the serum and <200 mg/day monoclonal protein in the urine) myeloma
- Diagnosis and monitoring progress of patients with light chain myeloma as well as primary systemic amyloidosis, in whom the underlying clonal plasma cell disorder may otherwise be difficult to detect and monitor
- Predicting risk of progression of MGUS
- Predicting risk of progression of solitary bone plasmacytoma
- Diagnosis, monitoring during and after treatment, and perhaps prognosis of patients with multiple myeloma and an intact immunoglobulin

❏ Interpretation (Table 16.45)
Increased In (see Limitations)

- Multiple myeloma
- Lymphocytic neoplasms

TABLE 16–45. Interpretation of Serum Free Light Chain Assays in Serum

Kappa	Lambda	K/L Ratio	Interpretation
N	N	N	Normal serum
L	L	N	BM suppression without monoclonal gammopathy
L	L	H	Monoclonal gammopathy
L	L	L	Monoclonal gammopathy
L	N	N	Normal serum
L	N	L	Monoclonal gammopathy
L	H	L	Monoclonal gammopathy
N	L	H	Monoclonal gammopathy
N	L	N	Normal serum
N	N	H	Monoclonal gammopathy
N	N	L	Monoclonal gammopathy
N	H	N	Polyclonal Ig increase or renal impairment
N	H	L	Monoclonal gammopathy
H	L	H	Monoclonal gammopathy
H	N	H	Monoclonal gammopathy
H	N	N	Polyclonal Ig increase or renal impairment
H	H	N	Polyclonal Ig increase or renal impairment
H	H	H	Monoclonal gammopathy with renal impairment
H	H	L	Monoclonal gammopathy with renal impairment

- Waldenström macroglobulinemia
- Amyloidosis
- Light chain deposition disease
- Connective tissue diseases such as SLE
- Renal impairment (common)
- Overproduction of polyclonal free light chains (FLCs) from inflammatory conditions (common)
- Biclonal gammopathies of different FLC types (rare)

Decreased In
- Bone marrow function impairment

❑ Limitations

- Elevated kappa and lambda FLC may occur due to polyclonal hypergammaglobulinemia or impaired renal clearance. A specific increase in FLC (e.g., FLC kappa/lambda ratio) must be demonstrated for diagnostic purposes.

Suggested Readings

Bradwell AR. *Serum Free Light Chain Analysis*, 2nd ed. Birmingham, UK: The Binding Site Ltd; 2005:13–21.

Katzmann JA, Clark RJ, Abraham RS, et al. Serum reference intervals and diagnostic ranges for free κ and free λ immunoglobulin light chains: Relative sensitivity for detection of monoclonal light chains. *Clin Chem.* 2002;48:1437–1444.

16

IMMUNOSUPPRESSANTS*

❏ **Definition**

■ Cyclosporin A is a cyclic polypeptide containing 11 amino acids. It is produced by the fungus *Tolypocladium inflatum*.

■ Sirolimus is a macrocyclic triene antibiotic that is produced by fermentation of *Streptomyces hygroscopicus*. Sirolimus was discovered from a soil sample collected in Rapa Nui, which is also known as Easter Island. Structurally, sirolimus resembles tacrolimus and binds to the same intracellular binding protein or immunophilin known as FKBP-12.

■ Tacrolimus is a macrolide antibiotic produced by *Streptomyces tsukubaensis*.

■ Other names: cyclosporine (Sandimmune, Neoral); sirolimus (Rapamycin, Rapamune), and tacrolimus (FK-506, Prograf).

■ **Normal range:** see Table 16.46.

❏ **Use**

■ Cyclosporine is a drug that suppresses the immune system and is used to prevent organ rejection and marrow transplant. It is used in combination with other immunosuppressants or corticosteroids.

■ Although sirolimus was originally developed as an antifungal agent, it was later found to have immunosuppressive and antiproliferative properties.

■ Tacrolimus is an immunosuppressive drug that has been shown to be effective for the treatment of rejection following transplantation. Tacrolimus has been

TABLE 16–46. Normal Ranges of Immunosuppressants Following Transplantation

Drug	Type of Transplant	Therapeutic Concentration (ng/mL) 12 h Postdose
Cyclosporin A		
	Renal	100–200
	Cardiac	150–250
	Hepatic	100–400
	Bone marrow	100–300
		Toxicity at >400
Sirolimus		4–20 (trough)
	Kidney	4–12
	Liver	12–20
Tacrolimus		5–20 (12-h trough level)
	Kidney and liver	
	0–2 mo posttransplant	10.0–15.0
	3 mo and older	5.0–10.0
	Heart	
	0–2 mo posttransplant	10.0–18.0
	3 mo and older	8.0–15.0
		Toxicity at ≥26

---

*Submitted By Amanda J. Jenkins, PhD.

used for therapy of the following disorders: adult RA, as a single agent or in combination with methotrexate, adult refractory myositis, systemic sclerosis, Crohn disease, autoimmune chronic hepatitis, pediatric autoimmune enteropathy, uveitis, steroid-resistant nephrotic syndrome (severe), recalcitrant chronic plaque psoriasis, and atopic dermatitis (administered as ointment).

❏ **Limitations**

- Testing performed on whole-blood samples.
- Clotted and/or frozen specimens unacceptable.
- Testing performed by immunoassay or LC/MSn (multiple MS) technology.
  - ▼ Immunoassay (e.g., MEIA, EMIT, FPIA, RIA): FPIA demonstrates more cross-reactivity with cyclosporine metabolites than EMIT. Therefore, EMIT concentration may be 70% of FPIA concentration. Note that cross-reactivity of immunoassays may change over time, so consult the manufacturer's package insert for current information.
  - ▼ LC/MS concentrations are generally lower than immunoassay due to cross-reactivity of the immunoassay with metabolites.

INHIBINS A AND B, SERUM

❏ **Definition**

- Polypeptide hormones that belong to transforming growth factor family; these are secreted by granulosa cells of the ovary and Sertoli cells of the testis. Inhibit pituitary production of FSH. Secreted by the placenta during pregnancy. Inhibins are heterodimers and hence have two forms: alpha-beta A (inhibin A) and alpha-beta B (inhibin B).
- **Normal ranges:** see Tables 16.47 and 16.48.

❏ **Use**

- **Females:**
  - ▼ Inhibin A is mostly produced by the corpus luteum.
    - ● Undetectable before puberty.

TABLE 16–47. Normal Ranges for Inhibin A	
Age/Phase	**Inhibin A (Dimer) (pg/mL)**
Normal cycling females	
Early follicular phase (−14 to −10)	1.8–17.3
Mid-follicular phase (−9 to −4)	3.5–31.7
Late follicular phase (−3 to −1)	9.8–90.3
Midcycle (day 0)	16.9–91.8
Early luteal (1–3)	16.1–97.5
Mid-luteal (4–11)	3.9–87.7
Late luteal (12–14)	2.7–47.1
IVF-peak levels	354.2–1,690.0
PCOS–ovulatory	5.7–16.0
Postmenopausal	<7.9
Normal males	<2.1

16

TABLE 16–48. Normal Range for Inhibin B by Sex and Age

Male	Female
<3 y: no range established	<3 y: no range established
3–9 y: <162 pg/mL	3–9 y: <30 pg/mL
10–13 y: 42–339 pg/mL	10–13 y: < 93 pg/mL
14–17 y: 68–300 pg/mL	14–17 y: <140 pg/mL
≥18 y: <305 pg/mL	Premenopausal: <255 pg/mL
	Postmenopausal: <30 pg/mL

- Very low levels in postmenopausal state due to absent follicular secretions.
- During pregnancy is secreted by the placenta. Inhibin A peaks at 8–10 weeks, declines until 20 weeks, and then increases gradually to term.
- Also used as an effective marker for Down syndrome pregnancies.
▼ Inhibin B is produced by granulosa cells of small developing antral follicles.
  - Rises to peak in early puberty; constant level thereafter.
  - Gradually declines after age 40. In early menopause, follicular-phase inhibin B declines, whereas inhibin A and estradiol are still within normal range.
  - May indicate low ovarian reserve in perimenopausal women and transition to menopause; useful for assisted reproduction. Measured on days 3–5 of menstrual cycle.
▼ After menopause, inhibins A and B fall to very low levels.
▼ May be useful to screen for preeclampsia.
▼ As an aid in the diagnosis of patients with granulose cell tumors of the ovary, when used in combination with inhibin B.
- **Males:**
  ▼ Inhibin B is predominant in males and supports spermatogenesis by negative feedback of FSH.
  ▼ Inhibin A is not significant in males (normal values <480 pg/mL); values remain fairly constant.
  ▼ May be decreased in male infertility.

❑ Interpretation
Increased In
- Inhibin A: elevated during normal pregnancy
- Preeclampsia, Down syndrome, and some cancers
  ▼ Seventy percent of patients with granulose cell tumors
  ▼ Twenty percent of patients with epithelial ovarian tumors

Decreased In
- Ovarian aging

❑ Limitations
- Inhibin levels fluctuate during menstrual cycle.

INSULIN

❑ **Definition**

- This peptide hormone is enzymatically processed from proinsulin in pancreatic secretory granules of beta cells. Approximately 50% is removed from the blood during initial passage through the liver. Its half-life is 4–9 minutes. Secretion is regulated primarily by blood glucose levels; therefore, it should always be measured with concomitant blood glucose. Insulin deficiency is the crucial factor in the pathogenesis of type 1 DM.
- **Normal range: 6–27 μIU/mL.**

❑ **Use**

- Diagnosis of insulinoma
- Diagnosis of fasting hypoglycemia
- Not clinically useful for diagnosis of DM

❑ **Interpretation**

Increased In

- Insulinoma. Fasting blood insulin level >50 μU/mL in the presence of low or normal blood glucose level. Administration of tolbutamide or leucine causes a rapid rise of blood insulin to very high levels within a few minutes, with a rapid return to normal.
- Factitious hypoglycemia in the presence of normal blood glucose.
- Insulin autoimmune syndrome.
- Untreated mild DM in obese individuals. The fasting blood level is often increased.
- Cirrhosis due to insufficient clearance from blood.
- Acromegaly (especially with active disease) after ingestion of glucose.
- Reactive hypoglycemia after glucose ingestion, particularly with the diabetic type of glucose tolerance curve.

Decreased In

- Type 1 DM.
- Hypopituitarism.
- Severe DM with ketosis and weight loss, which may result in an absence of insulin. In less severe cases, insulin is frequently present but only at lower glucose concentrations.

❑ **Limitations**

- Insulin values are normal in
  - ▼ Hypoglycemia associated with nonpancreatic tumors
  - ▼ Idiopathic hypoglycemia of childhood, except after administration of leucine
- Circulating anti-insulin antibodies are often found in patients who have been treated with nonhuman forms of insulin. If present, these antibodies may interfere with the assay.
- For individuals who are significantly overweight, fasting insulin levels are typically somewhat higher than for adults of normal weight.

16

■ Heterophilic antibodies in human serum can react with the immunoglobulins included in the assay components, causing interference with in vitro immunoassays. Samples from patients routinely exposed to animals or animal serum products can demonstrate this type of interference, potentially causing an anomalous result.

INSULIN TOLERANCE TEST

❏ Definition

■ Insulin is administered, 0.1 U/kg body weight IV. A smaller dose should be used if hypopituitarism is suspected. IV glucose should be kept available to prevent severe reaction. Blood is obtained for serum glucose and cortisol assays (and for growth hormone [GH], if indicated) immediately before insulin is injected and 30 and 45 minutes thereafter. All patients, in whom adequate hypoglycemia is achieved, defined as 35 mg/dL or less should have some symptoms of hypoglycemia, either of sympathetic discharge or of CNS glucose deprivation, such as simply falling asleep.

❏ Use

■ Assessing syndromes of extreme insulin resistance
■ Crude classification of insulin sensitivity
■ Assessing GH deficiency

❏ Interpretation

■ Blood glucose normally falls to 50% of fasting level within 20–30 minutes and returns to fasting level within 90–120 minutes.
■ Blood glucose that falls <25% and returns rapidly to fasting level represents an increased tolerance to insulin.

Increased In

■ Hypothyroidism
■ Acromegaly
■ Cushing syndrome (peak cortisol response <18–20 µg/dL and change over baseline <7 µg/dL indicate glucocorticoid deficiency)
■ DM (some patients; especially older, obese ones)

Decreased In

■ Increased sensitivity to insulin (excessive fall of blood glucose)
  ▼ Hypoglycemic nonresponsiveness (lack of response by glycogenolysis)
  ▼ Pancreatic islet cell tumor
  ▼ Adrenocortical insufficiency
  ▼ Adrenocortical insufficiency secondary to hypopituitarism
  ▼ Hypothyroidism
    ● von Gierke disease (some patients)
    ● Starvation (depletion of liver glycogen)

❏ Limitations

■ In premenopausal women, the test can be performed at any phase of the menstrual cycle, because there are no cycle effects on the hypothalamic–pituitary–adrenal axis response to insulin-induced hypoglycemia.

- Almost all patients have some degree of perspiration. If the patient does not perspire, the adequacy of the stress stimulus must remain suspect irrespective of the serum glucose concentration.
- Most patients also have a hyperactive precordium (but not tachycardia or hypotension, because they are supine) and feelings of hunger, drowsiness, detachment, or anxiety. The last is common and sometimes severe, and many patients find this an unpleasant experience.
- Patients with primary or secondary adrenal insufficiency or long-standing DM have an impaired compensatory response to hypoglycemia.
- The criteria for a normal serum cortisol response ranged from 18 to about 22 μg/dL in multiple studies. Ideally, reference ranges would be determined locally, but this is rarely done in practice. If serum cortisol reaches this level, it is unimportant whether hypoglycemia was adequate. On the other hand, failure to reach this level is indicative of an inadequate response only if the serum glucose fell to 35 mg/dL or less. If this was not achieved, the stimulus was inadequate and the test must be repeated. It is the serum cortisol concentration that is achieved rather than the increment that is important.

INSULIN-LIKE GROWTH FACTOR–BINDING PROTEIN-3 (IGFBP-3)

❑ **Definition**

- This 264-amino-acid peptide (molecular weight, 29 kDa) is produced by the liver. It is the most abundant of a group of IGFBPs that transport and control bioavailability and half-life of insulin-like growth factors (IGFs), in particular IGF-I. In addition to its IGF-binding function, IGFBP-3 also exhibits intrinsic growth-regulating effects that are not yet fully understood but have evoked interest with regard to a possible role of IGFBP-3 as a prognostic tumor marker. Other name: somatomedin C–binding protein.
- **Normal range:** see Table 16.49.

❑ **Use**

- Diagnosing growth disorders
- Diagnosing adult growth hormone deficiency
- Monitoring of recombinant human growth hormone treatment
- Possible adjunct to IGF-I and growth hormone in the diagnosis and follow-up of acromegaly and gigantism

❑ **Interpretation**

Increased In

- Overproduction of GH
- Excessive rhGH therapy
- Chronic renal failure

Decreased In

- GH deficiency
- GH resistance
- Fasting/chronic malnutrition

16

TABLE 16–49. Normal Ranges for IGFBP-3

Age (in years Unless Otherwise Specified)	Reference Range (µg/mL)
0–15 d	0.5–1.4
1	0.7–3.6
2	0.8–3.9
3	0.9–4.3
4	1.0–4.7
5	1.1–5.2
6	1.3–5.6
7	1.4–6.1
8	1.6–6.5
9	1.8–7.1
10	2.1–7.7
11	2.4–8.4
12	2.7–8.9
13	3.1–9.5
14	3.3–10
15	3.5–10
16	3.4–9.5
17	3.2–8.7
18	3.1–7.9
19	2.9–7.3
20	2.9–7.2
21–25	3.4–7.8
26–30	3.5–7.6
31–35	3.5–7.0
36–40	3.4–6.7
41–45	3.3–6.6
46–50	3.3–6.7
51–55	3.4–6.8
56–60	3.4–6.9
61–65	3.2–6.6
66–70	3.0–6.2
71–75	2.8–5.7
76–80	2.5–5.1
81–85	2.2–4.5

- Hepatic failure
- Diabetes mellitus

❑ **Limitations**

- IGF-I and IGFBP-3 reference ranges are highly age dependent, and results must always be interpreted within the context of the patient's age.
- Discrepant IGFBP-3 and IGF-I results can sometimes occur due to liver and kidney diseases; however, this is uncommon, and such results should alert laboratories and physicians to the possible occurrence of a preanalytic or analytic error.
- At this time, IGFBP-3 cannot be reliably used as a prognostic marker in breast, colon, prostate, or lung cancer.
- IGFBP-3 assays exhibit significant variability among platforms and manufacturers. Direct comparison of results obtained by different assays is problematic. Rebaselining of patients is preferred if assays are changed.

INSULIN-LIKE GROWTH FACTOR-I (IGF-I)

❏ **Definition**

■ IGF-I is secreted by hypothalamus; release is mediated by growth hormone (GH) in many tissues, especially hepatocytes. It is a single polypeptide chain with 70-amino-acid residues with a molecular mass of 7,649 Da. It is structurally homologous to IGF-II and insulin. IGF-I circulates primarily in a high molecular weight tertiary complex with IGF-binding protein-3 (IGFBP-3) and acid-labile subunit. Plasma IGF-I levels are barely detectable at birth, rise gradually during childhood, peak during mid-puberty until approximately 40 years of age, and then decline gradually. Maternal plasma levels increase during pregnancy.

■ **Normal range:** see Table 16.50; 0–7 days: <26 ng/mL; 8–15 days: <41 ng/mL.

TABLE 16–50. Normal Range of IGF-I

Age (y)	Central 95% Range
16 d to 1 y	55–327
2	51–303
3	49–289
4	49–283
5	50–286
6	52–297
7	57–316
8	64–345
9	74–388
10	88–452
11	111–551
12	143–693
13	183–850
14	220–972
15	237–996
16	226–903
17	193–731
18	163–584
19	141–483
20	127–424
21–25	116–358
26–30	117–329
31–35	115–307
36–40	109–284
41–45	101–267
46–50	94–252
51–55	87–238
56–60	81–225
61–65	75–212
66–70	69–200
71–75	64–188
76–80	59–177
81–85	55–166

16

❑ Use

- Diagnosis of acromegaly and pituitary deficiency; preferable to GH because it is constant after eating and during the day
- Help determine optimum dosage of GH
- Screening other growth disorders
- Assessing nutritional status
- Monitoring effectiveness of nutritional repletion; a more sensitive indicator than prealbumin, transferrin index, or retinol-binding protein

❑ Interpretation

Increased In

- Acromegaly and gigantism
- Pregnancy (2–3 times nonpregnant values)

Decreased In

- Pituitary deficiency
- Laron dwarfism
- Anorexia or malnutrition
- Acute illness
- Hepatic failure
- Hypothyroidism
- DM
- Normal aging

INSULIN-LIKE GROWTH FACTOR-II

❑ Definition

- IGF-II is a 7.5 kDa, 67-amino-acid peptide that is thought to mediate some of the actions of growth hormone (GH). IGF-II peptide is structurally homologous to IGF-I and proinsulin. IGF-II is secreted by the liver and other tissue and is postulated to have mitogenic and metabolic actions at or near the sites of synthesis. IGF-II also appears in the peripheral circulation, where it circulates primarily in a high molecular weight tertiary complex with IGF-binding protein-3 (IGFBP-3) and acid-labile subunit. The proportion of unbound IGF-II in the circulation has been estimated at >5%. Plasma levels of IGF-II are dependent on adequate levels of GH and other factors, including adequate nutrition. The actions of IGF-II are mediated by binding to specific cell surface receptors. Although its specific physiologic role has not been defined, it has been postulated that the interplay of IGF-I and IGF-II with the different cell surface receptors and circulating binding proteins modulates tissue growth.
- **Normal ranges:**
  - ▼ Child, prepubertal: 334–642 ng/mL
  - ▼ Child, pubertal: 245–737 ng/mL
  - ▼ Adult: 288–736 ng/mL
  - ▼ GH deficiency: 51–299 ng/mL

❑ Use

- IGF-II is an adjunct to IGF-I in the clinical evaluation of GH-related disorders.

❑ **Interpretation**

Increased In

- Hypoglycemia associated with non–islet cell tumors
- Hepatoma
- Wilms tumor

Decreased In

- GH deficiency

INSULIN–TO–C-PEPTIDE RATIO

❑ **Definition**

- Insulin and C-peptide are secreted into portal vein in equimolar amounts, but serum ratio = 1:5 to 1:15 due to removal of approximately 50% of insulin from blood during initial passage through the liver. C-peptide half-life = approximately 30 minutes.
- **Normal range:** fasting molar ratio insulin to C-peptide = 1.0.

❑ **Use**

- To differentiate insulinoma from factitious hypoglycemia due to insulin

❑ **Interpretation**

- **Less than 1.0 in molarity units (or >47.17 µg/ng in conventional units)**
  - ▼ Increased endogenous insulin secretion (e.g., insulinoma, sulfonylurea administration)
  - ▼ Renal failure
- **Greater than 1.0 in molarity units (or <47.17 µg/ng in conventional units)**
  - ▼ Exogenous insulin administration
  - ▼ Cirrhosis

❑ **Limitations**

- There are ethnic differences in insulin/C-peptide ratio in both fasting and glucose-stimulated conditions in normal young nondiabetic pregnant women. Compared with their Caucasian and Hispanic counterparts, African American women had indices suggestive of lower insulin production and greater insulin resistance (i.e., a lower C-peptide concentration, a lower C/I ratio, and elevations in insulin and the I/G ratio).

INTRINSIC FACTOR ANTIBODY

❑ **Definition**

- Intrinsic factor (IF), or anti-intrinsic factor, intrinsic factor–blocking antibody, type 1 intrinsic factor antibody, IFAB, is a glycoprotein produced by the gastric parietal cells. It binds to, transports, and facilitates absorption from the terminal ileum of the very small amount of vitamin B_{12} in the diet. If there are antibodies to the parietal cells, the B_{12}-binding site of IF, or the binding site of IF to the ileum, the patient's ability to absorb dietary B_{12} by

the IF route will be reduced. Over time, the presence of these antibodies leads to a reduction in B$_{12}$ stores and ultimately to vitamin B$_{12}$ deficiency, the consequences of which vary. The presence of circulating autoantibodies to IF is a very specific indicator of PA. Antibodies against IF are found in approximately 50% of cases but rarely in other conditions.
■ **Normal range:** negative.

❑ **Use**
- Diagnosis of PA
- Evaluation of patients with decreased vitamin B$_{12}$ levels

❑ **Interpretation**
- Increased in PA

❑ **Limitations**
- Cyanocobalamin may give a false-positive test result.
- Methotrexate and folic acid may give false-positive test results.
- Negative or inconclusive test results do not exclude the diagnosis of PA.
- Some patients with other autoimmune diseases may have positive test results, particularly in patients with autoimmune thyroid disease or type 1 DM.

IODINE EXCRETION, URINE 24 HOURS

❑ **Definition**
- Iodine is an essential component of T$_4$ and T$_3$, and it must be provided in the diet. Inadequate iodine intake leads to inadequate thyroid hormone production, and all the consequences of iodine deficiency stem from the associated hypothyroidism. However, iodide excess can also cause thyroid dysfunction. Goiter is the most obvious manifestation of iodine deficiency. Low iodine intake leads to reduced T$_4$ and T$_3$ production, which results in increased thyrotropin (TSH) secretion in an attempt to restore T$_4$ and T$_3$ production to normal.
- **Normal range:**
  - ▼ International groups recommend the following median urinary iodine concentration as the best single indicator of iodine nutrition in populations:
    - Severe deficiency: 0–0.15 μmol/L (0–19 μg/L)
    - Moderate deficiency: 0.16–0.38 μmol/L (20–49 μg/L)
    - Mild deficiency: 0.40–0.78 μmol/L (50–99 μg/L)
    - Optimal iodine nutrition: 0.79–1.56 μmol/L (100–199 μg/L)
    - More than adequate iodine intake: 1.57–2.36 μmol/L (200–299 μg/L)
    - Excessive iodine intake: 2.37 μmol/L (300 μg/L)
  - ▼ The range in which the median falls is more important than the precise number.

❑ **Use**
- Diagnosis of transient thyroid dysfunction and iodine-induced hyperthyrosis
- Biochemical indicator for the assessment of iodine status
- Monitoring iodine excretion rate as an index of daily iodine replacement therapy
- Correlating total body iodine load with ^{131}I uptake studies in assessing thyroid function

❑ Interpretation

Increased In

- ▪ Dietary excess
- ▪ Recent drug or contrast media exposure

Decreased In

- ▪ Dietary deficiency

❑ Limitations

- ▪ Urinary iodine levels are influenced by gender, age, sociocultural and dietary factors, drug interferences, geographic location, and season.
- ▪ In most instances, it provides little useful information on long-term iodine status of the individual, since the results obtained merely reflect the dietary iodine intake.
- ▪ Administration of iodine-based contrast media and drugs containing iodine, such as amiodarone, will yield elevated results.
- ▪ High concentrations of gadolinium are known to interfere with most metals tests. If gadolinium-containing contrast media has been administered, a specimen should not be collected for 48 hours.
- ▪ Frozen specimens sometimes result in falsely lowered results.

Suggested Reading

International Council for the Control of Iodine Deficiency Disorders. WHO. UNICEF. *Assessment of Iodine Deficiency Disorders and Monitoring their Elimination. A Guide for Programme Managers*, 2nd ed. Geneva, Switzerland: World Health Organization; 2001.

IRON (Fe)

❑ Definition

- ▪ Iron exists in the body in many forms: hemoglobin in circulating red cells and developing erythroblasts, iron-containing proteins such as myoglobin and cytochromes, and bound to transferrin and storage in the form of ferritin and hemosiderin. Iron homeostasis is regulated strictly at the level of intestinal absorption and release of iron from macrophages. The serum iron level reflects Fe^{3+} bound to transferrin, not free Hb in serum.
- ▪ **Normal range:**
  - ▼ Female: 28–170 μg/dL
  - ▼ Male: 45–182 μg/dL

❑ Use

- ▪ Diagnosis of blood loss
- ▪ Differential diagnosis of anemias
- ▪ Diagnosis of hemochromatosis and hemosiderosis
- ▪ Evaluation of iron deficiency; should always be measured with TIBC
- ▪ Diagnosis of acute iron toxicity, especially in children
- ▪ Evaluation of thalassemia and sideroblastic anemia
- ▪ Monitor response to treatment for anemia

16

Increased In
- Idiopathic hemochromatosis
- Hemosiderosis of excessive iron intake (e.g., repeated blood transfusions, iron therapy, iron-containing vitamins) (may be >300 µg/dL)
- Decreased formation of RBCs (e.g., thalassemia, pyridoxine deficiency anemia, PA in relapse)
- Increased destruction of RBCs (e.g., hemolytic anemias)
- Acute liver damage (degree of increase parallels the amount of hepatic necrosis) (may be >1,000 µg/dL); some cases of chronic liver disease
- Progesterone birth control pills (may be >200 µg/dL) and pregnancy
- Premenstrual elevation by 10–30%
- Acute iron toxicity; serum iron-to-TIBC ratio is not useful for this diagnosis
- Repeated transfusions
- Lead poisoning
- Acute hepatitis
- Vitamin B$_6$ deficiency

Decreased In
- Iron deficiency anemia
- Normochromic (normocytic or microcytic) anemias of infection and chronic diseases (e.g., neoplasms, active collagen diseases)
- Acute and chronic infection
- Carcinoma
- Hypothyroidism
- Postoperative state and kwashiorkor
- Nephrosis (because of loss of iron-binding protein in urine)
- PA at onset of remission
- Menstruation (decreased by 10–30%)

❑ **Limitations**
- Serum iron is not reliable as the primary test to identify iron deficiency or screening for hemochromatosis and other iron overload diseases. For these conditions, a serum TIBC, percent transferrin saturation, and ferritin assay are recommended.
- Diurnal variation—normal values in midmorning, low values in midafternoon, very low values (approximately 10 µg/dL) near midnight. Diurnal variation disappears at levels <45 µg/dL.
- Iron dextran administration causes increase for several weeks (may be >1,000 µg/dL).
- Ingestion of oral contraceptives will elevate iron and/or total iron-binding capacity values.
- Not recommended for patients undergoing treatment with deferoxamine or other iron-chelating compounds.
- Ingestion of iron (including iron-fortified vitamins or supplements) may cause transient elevated iron levels.

IRON-BINDING CAPACITY, TOTAL (TIBC)

❑ **Definition**
- TIBC measures the blood's capacity to bind iron with transferrin (TRF). One milligram of TRF binds to 1.25 µg of iron, and, therefore, a serum TRF

level of 300 mg/dL is equal to TIBC of (300 × 1.25) 375 µg/dL. TIBC is an indirect way of assessing TRF level. TIBC correlates with serum TRF, but the relationship is not linear over the wide range of TRF values and is disrupted in diseases affecting transferrin-binding capacity and iron-binding proteins. TIBC should not be confused with unsaturated binding capacity (UIBC), where UIBC = TIBC minus serum iron (µg/dL).

- **Normal range: 255–450 µg/dL.**

❏ Use

- Differential diagnosis of anemias
- Should always be performed whenever serum iron is done to calculate percent saturation for diagnosis of iron deficiency
- Screening for iron overload
- Acute hepatitis
- Late pregnancy

❏ Interpretation

Increased In

- Iron deficiency
- Acute and chronic blood loss
- Acute liver damage
- Late pregnancy
- Progesterone birth control pills

Decreased In

- Hemochromatosis
- Cirrhosis of the liver
- Thalassemia
- Anemias of infection and chronic diseases (e.g., uremia, RA, some neoplasms)
- Nephrosis
- Hyperthyroidism

❏ Limitations

- Estrogens and oral contraceptives increase TIBC levels.
- Asparaginase, chloramphenicol, corticotropin, cortisone, and testosterone decrease the TIBC levels.

IRON SATURATION

❏ Definition

- This number represents the amount of iron-binding sites that are occupied. Iron saturation is a better index of iron stores than serum iron alone. Iron saturation is calculated as
  - ▼ **% Saturation = Serum iron/TIBC × 100**
- **Normal range: 20–50%.**

❏ Use

- Differential diagnosis of anemias
- Screening for hereditary hemochromatosis

16

❑ **Interpretation**

Increased In
- Hemochromatosis
- Hemosiderosis
- Thalassemia
- Birth control pills (≤75%)
- Ingestion of iron (≤100%)
- Iron dextran administration causes increase for several weeks (may be >100%)
- Vitamin B_6 deficiency
- Aplastic anemias

Decreased In
- Iron deficiency anemia (usually <10% in established deficiency)
- Anemias of infection and chronic diseases (e.g., uremia, RA, some neoplasms)
- Malignancy of the stomach and small intestine

ISLET AUTOANTIBODIES (IAA)

❑ **Definition**
- Diabetes-related (islet) autoantibody testing is primarily ordered to help distinguish between autoimmune type 1 DM and DM due to other causes (e.g., diabetes resulting from obesity and insulin resistance). In conjunction with family history, HLA typing, and measurement of other islet cell auto-antibodies, insulin autoantibody measurements are useful in predicting the future development of type 1 DM in asymptomatic children, adolescent, and young adults. If IAA, glutamic acid decarboxylase autoantibodies, or insulinoma-2–associated autoantibodies are present in an individual with DM, the diagnosis of type 1 DM has been established.
- **Normal range:** negative.

❑ **Use**
- Differential diagnosis of type 1 versus type 2 DM.
- Evaluating diabetics with insulin resistance.
- Investigation of hypoglycemia in nondiabetic subjects.
- Marker for type 1 DM. In 95% of cases of new-onset type 1 DM, ≤1 of 4 is positive (see Table 16.51).

TABLE 16–51. Autoimmune Antibodies in Type 1 DM

Islet Antibody	Frequency of Occurrence
Glutamic acid decarboxylase autoantibodies*	70–80%
Islet cell cytoplasmic autoantibodies	70–80%
Insulin autoantibodies	Adults <10%; children ~50% to ~60%
Insulinoma-2–associated autoantibodies (IA-2A)	(>60%)

*Recommended because it is most persistent islet autoantibody after onset of autoimmune DM.

❑ **Limitations**

- IAA testing must be performed before insulin therapy is initiated.
- Children at onset of type 1 DM are more commonly IAA positive than adults. Up to 80% of new–onset type 1 DM patients before the age of 5 years have IAA compared with only approximately 30% for adults.

JANUS KINASE-2 (JAK2) DNA MUTATION ASSAY*

❑ **Definition**

- The *V617F* mutation in the *JAK-2* gene is associated with myeloproliferative disorders (MPDs). This mutation was found in more than 80% (up to 97%) of patients with polycythemia vera, in approximately 50% of patients with idiopathic myelofibrosis (IMF), 30–50% of patients with essential thrombocythemia (ET), and also in other rare MPDs.
- **Normal values:** an individual is negative for the *JAK-2* gene mutation when the frequency of wild-type and mutant alleles is 100% and 0%, respectively.

❑ **Use**

- Suspected polycythemia vera (PV; OMIM# 263300), idiopathic myelofibrosis (IMF; OMIM# 254450), or essential thrombocythemia (ET)

❑ **Limitations**

- The results of a genetic test may be affected by DNA rearrangements, blood transfusion, bone marrow transplantation, or rare sequence variations.
- Genetic causes of MPDs, other than the *V617F* mutation, will not be detected.

KLEIHAUER-BETKE TEST†

❑ **Definition**

- The Kleihauer-Betke test was developed to quantify fetal RBCs in maternal blood in order to determine the amount of Rh immune globulin that needs to be administered.
- The test is performed by treating maternal red cells on a thin slide smear with acid and then counterstaining the slide. Fetal hemoglobin is resistant to acid treatment so maternal cells will appear as "ghosts" while fetal cells will be pink.
- After counting 2,000 red cells, the results are reported as a percentage of fetal red cells present in the maternal circulation. This result can be multiplied by the maternal blood volume in order to determine the volume of fetal blood (mL) present in the maternal circulation.
- **Normal range** (adult RBCs): <1% fetal Hb.

❑ **Interpretation**

- The presence of fetal RBCs in maternal blood indicates fetal–maternal hemorrhage.

16

*Submitted by Edward Ginns, MD and Marzena M. Galdzicka, PhD.
†Submitted By Vishesh Chhibber, MD.

❏ Limitations
False-Positive Results
- Fetal Hb–containing RBCs may be found in approximately 50% of pregnant women (but in only 1% of pregnancies is the infant anemic).
- Certain hematologic disorders in adults, such as leukemias or myelodysplastic syndromes, may increase the level of fetal-type hemoglobin.
- Lymphocytes may take up stain in varying degrees.

False-Negative Results
- A major blood group incompatibility between mother and infant can cause elimination of fetal RBCs due to hemolysis.

LACTATE DEHYDROGENASE

❏ Definition
- LD occurs in the cytoplasm of all cells; there are five isoenzymes. The highest concentrations are found in the heart, liver, skeletal muscle, kidney, and the RBCs, with lesser amounts in the lung, smooth muscle, and brain. LD catalyzes the interconversion of lactate and pyruvate.
- **Normal range: 110–240 IU/L.**

❏ Use
- To monitor tumor activity involving anemias and lung cancer
- Liver and renal disease
- After AMI (the use of LDH for MI detection has been replaced by cardiac troponins.)
- Marker for hemolysis, in vivo (e.g., hemolytic anemias) or in vitro (artifactual)

❏ Interpretation
Increased In
- Cardiac diseases
  - ▼ AMI. Increases in 10–12 hours, peaks in 48–72 hours (approximately three times normal). Prolonged elevation over 10–14 days was formerly used for late diagnosis of AMI; now replaced by C-troponins. An LD reading >2,000 IU suggests a poorer prognosis. An LD-1/LD-2 ratio >1 ("flipped" LD) may also occur in acute renal infarction, hemolysis, some muscle disorders, pregnancy, and some neoplasms.
  - ▼ CHF: LD isoenzymes are normal, or LD-5 may be increased due to liver congestion.
  - ▼ Insertion of intracardiac prosthetic valves consistently causes chronic hemolysis, with increase of total LD, LD-1, and LD-2. This is also often present before surgery in patients with severe hemodynamic abnormalities of cardiac valves.
  - ▼ Cardiovascular surgery: LD is increased ≤2 times normal without cardiopulmonary bypass and returns to normal in 3–4 days; with extracorporeal circulation, it may increase ≤4–6 times normal; this increase is more marked when the transfused blood is older.
  - ▼ Increases have been described in acute myocarditis and RF.

- **Liver diseases**
  - ▼ Cirrhosis, obstructive jaundice, and acute viral hepatitis show moderate increases.
  - ▼ Hepatitis—most marked increase is of LD-5, which occurs during prodromal stage and is greatest at time of onset of jaundice; total LD is also increased in 50% of the cases. LD increase is isomorphic in infectious mononucleosis. An ALT-to-LD or AST-to-LD ratio within 24 hours of admission ≥1.5 favors acute hepatitis over acetaminophen or ischemic injury.
  - ▼ Acute and subacute hepatic necrosis: LD-5 is also increased with other causes of liver damage (e.g., chlorpromazine hepatitis, carbon tetrachloride poisoning, exacerbation of cirrhosis, or biliary obstruction) even when total LD is normal.
  - ▼ Metastatic carcinoma to the liver may show marked increases. It has been reported that an LD-4–to–LD-5 ratio <1.05 favors diagnosis of hepatocellular carcinoma, compared to a ratio >1.05, which favors liver metastases in >90% of cases.
  - ▼ If liver disease is suspected but total LD is very high and isoenzyme pattern is isomorphic, rule out cancer.
  - ▼ Liver disease, per se, does not produce marked increase of total LD or LD-5.
  - ▼ Various inborn metabolic disorders affecting the liver (e.g., hemochromatosis, Dubin-Johnson syndrome, hepatolenticular degeneration, Gaucher disease, McArdle disease).
- **Hematologic diseases**
  - ▼ Untreated PA and folic acid deficiency show some of the greatest increases, chiefly in LD-1, which is >LD-2 ("flipped"), especially with Hb <8 g/dL.
  - ▼ Increased in all hemolytic anemias, which can probably be ruled out if LD-1 and LD-2 are not increased in an anemic patient; normal in aplastic anemia and iron deficiency anemia, even when the anemia is very severe.
- **Diseases of the lung**
  - ▼ Pulmonary embolus and infarction—pattern of moderately increased LD with increased LD-3 and normal AST 24–48 hours after onset of chest pain
  - ▼ Sarcoidosis
- **Malignant tumors**
  - ▼ Increased in approximately 50% of patients with various solid carcinomas, especially in advanced stages.
  - ▼ In patients with cancer, a higher LD level generally indicates a poorer prognosis. Whenever the total LD is increased and the isoenzyme pattern is nonspecific or cannot be explained by obvious clinical findings (e.g., MI, hemolytic anemia), cancer should always be ruled out. LD is moderately increased in approximately 60% of patients with lymphomas and lymphocytic leukemias and approximately 90% of patients with acute leukemia; degree of increase is not correlated with WBC counts; levels are relatively low in lymphatic types of leukemia. LD is increased in 95% of patients with chronic myelogenous leukemia, especially LD-3.

16

- Diseases of muscle
  - ▼ Marked increase of LD-5, likely due to anoxic injury of striated muscle
  - ▼ Electrical and thermal burns and trauma; marked increase of total LD (about the same as in MI) and LD-5
- **Renal diseases**
  - ▼ Renal cortical infarction may mimic pattern of AMI. Rule out renal infarction if LD-1 (>LD-2) is increased in the absence of MI or anemia or if increased LD is out of proportion to AST and ALP levels.
  - ▼ May be slightly increased (LD-4 and LD-5) in nephrotic syndrome. LD-1 and LD-2 may be increased in nephritis.
- **Miscellaneous conditions**
- These conditions may be related to hemolysis, involvement of the liver, striated muscle, or heart
  - ▼ Various infectious and parasitic diseases
  - ▼ Hypothyroidism, subacute thyroiditis
  - ▼ Collagen vascular diseases
  - ▼ Acute pancreatitis
  - ▼ Intestinal obstruction
  - ▼ Sarcoidosis
  - ▼ Various CNS conditions (e.g., bacterial meningitis, cerebral hemorrhage, or thrombosis)
  - ▼ Drugs

Decreased In

- Irradiation
- Genetic deficiency of subunits

❏ Limitations

- RBCs contain much more LD than serum. A hemolyzed specimen is not acceptable.
- LD activity is one of the most sensitive indicators of in vitro hemolysis. Causes can include transportation via pneumatic tube, vigorous mixing, or traumatic venipuncture.

LACTATE DEHYDROGENASE ISOENZYMES

❏ Definition

- LD is a tetrameric cytoplasmic enzyme. The most usual designation of the isoenzyme is LD-1 (H[4]), LD-2 (H[3]M), LD-3 (H[2]M[2]), LD-4 (HM[3]), and LD-5 (M[4]). The tissue specificity is derived from the fact that there is tissue-specific synthesis of subunits in well-defined ratios. Most notably, heart muscle cells preferentially synthesize H subunits, whereas liver cells synthesize M subunits nearly exclusively. Skeletal muscle also synthesizes largely M subunits so that LD(5) is both a liver and skeletal muscle form of LD. The LD-1 and LD-5 forms are ones most often used to indicate heart or liver pathology, respectively. LD isoenzyme patterns cannot be interpreted without the knowledge of clinical history (see Table 16.52).

TABLE 16–52. Percent Activity Distribution of LD Isoenzymes in Tissue

Organ	LD Activity				
	LD-1	**LD-2**	**LD-3**	**LD-4**	**LD-5**
Heart	60	30	5	3	2
Liver	0.2	0.8	1	4	94
Kidney	28	34	21	11	6
Cerebrum	28	32	19	16	5
Skeletal muscle	3	4	8	9	76
Lung	10	18	28	23	21
Spleen	5	15	31	31	18
RBCs	40	30	15	10	5
Skin	0	0	4	17	79

❏ **Use**

- LD is useful in the investigation of a variety of diseases involving the heart, liver, muscle, kidney, lung, and blood; and differentiating heart-synthesized LD from liver and other sources of LD.
- Isoenzymes are used by many clinicians in the diagnosis of MI in combination with total CK and CK-MB.
- Investigating unexplained causes of LD elevations.
- Detection of macro-LD.

❏ **Interpretation**
See Table 16.53.

- Macroenzymes, high molecular weight complexes, occur with LD as well as with CK and other enzymes. LD isoenzymes may complex to IgA or IgG. Such LD macroenzymes are characterized by abnormal position of isoenzyme bands, broadening or abnormal motility of a band, and otherwise unexplained increase of total serum LD. Some of these patients have abnormal ANA results and IgG complexes. Some have abnormalities of light chains but not in amounts that are useful for diagnosis. Treatment with streptokinase was found to produce an LD-streptokinase complex, which was seen as a band at the origin in electrophoresis.
- Increased total LD with normal distribution of isoenzymes may be seen in myocardial infarction, arteriosclerotic heart disease with chronic heart failure, and various combinations of acute and chronic diseases (this may represent a general stress reaction).
- About 50% of patients with malignant tumors have altered LD patterns. This change often is nonspecific and of no diagnostic value. Solid tumors, especially those of germ cell origin, may increase LD-1.
- In megaloblastic anemia, hemolysis, renal cortical infarction, and some patients with cancer, the isoenzyme pattern may mimic that of MI, but the time to peak value and the increase help to differentiate these conditions.
- An isoenzyme band cathodal to LD-5 has been called LD-6. It is not an immunoglobulin complex. It has occurred in subjects with liver disease and is said to indicate a grave prognosis.

16

TABLE 16–53. LD Isoenzyme Patterns in Various Disease Conditions

Condition	LD Isoenzyme(s) Increased
AMI	LD-1 more so than LD-2
Acute renal cortical infarction	LD-1 more so than LD-2
PA	LD-1
Sickle cell crisis	LD-1 and LD-2
Electrical and thermal burn, trauma	LD-5
Mother carrying erythroblastotic child	LD-4 and v5
AMI with acute congestion of the liver	LD-1 and LD-5
Early hepatitis	LD-5 (may become normal, even when ALT is still rising)
Malignant lymphoma	LD-3 and LD-4 (LD-2 may also increase) (reflects effect of chemotherapy)
Active chronic granulocytic leukemia	LD-3 increased in >90% of cases but normal during remission
Carcinoma of the prostate	5; 5:1 ratio >1
Dermatomyositis	5
SLE	3 and 4
Collagen disorders	2, 3, and 4
Pulmonary embolus and infarction	2, 3, and 4
Pulmonary embolus with acute cor pulmonale causing acute congestion of liver	3 and 5
Congestive heart failure	2, 3, and 4
Viral infections	2, 3, and 4
Various neoplasms	2, 3, and 4
Strenuous physical activity	4 and 5
Leptomeningeal carcinomatosis	5

❑ Limitations

- A hemolyzed specimen is not acceptable as RBCs contain much more LD than serum. Causes can include transportation via pneumatic tube, vigorous mixing, or traumatic venipuncture. Tubes should be void of air bubbles to prevent minor hemolysis.
- LD activity is one of the most sensitive indicators of in vitro hemolysis.
- Hemolysis causes anomalous elevation of LD-1 such that any ex vivo hemolysis must be strictly avoided.
- Freezing or prolonged storage at 4°C (>12 hours) causes LD-5 to be lost.
- Elevations of intermediate forms (LD-2–LD-4) of LD are rarely used to define a tissue of origin, and such reports are largely anecdotal.
- Although increases in serum LD also are seen following an MI, the test has been replaced by the determination of troponins.

LACTATE, BLOOD

❑ Definition

- Blood lactate, also known as 2-hydroxypropanoic acid, lactic acid, or L-lactate, is an end product of anaerobic glycolysis as an alternative to pyruvate entering the Krebs cycle, enabling metabolism of glucose. Major sites of production are skeletal muscle, brain, and erythrocytes. Lactate is metabolized by the liver.

- **Normal range:** 0.3–2.4 mmol/L.
- **Critical value:** >5 mmol/L.

❑ **Use**

- Monitoring of metabolic acidosis, lactic acidosis

❑ **Interpretation**

Increased In

- Hypoperfusion: CHF, shock
- Decrease oxygen content: hypoxemia, severe anemia, carbon monoxide poisoning
- Sepsis
- DKA
- Drugs and toxins (e.g., Ringer lactate solution, biguanides, retroviral therapy, isoniazid, acetaminophen, ethanol, ethylene glycol, and others)
- Strenuous exercise
- Seizures
- Liver failure
- Kidney failure
- D-Lactate acidosis (due to short bowel syndrome or other forms of malabsorption)
- Inborn errors of metabolism (e.g., pyruvate dehydrogenase deficiency, glycogen storage disease)

❑ **Limitations**

- No identified limitation.
- Methodologic interference (e.g., ascorbic acid).
- Proper specimen collection and processing techniques are critical for reliable results. Use of tourniquet or clenching hands increases lactate.
- This test does not measure D-lactate, an uncommon, often undiagnosed cause of lactic acidosis.
- A lactate/pyruvate ratio may be used to differentiate between causes of lactic acidosis. Certain congenital disorders in which pyruvate is not converted to lactate, for example, pyruvate dehydrogenase deficiency. In this case, pyruvate will accumulate, blood levels will be high, and the lactate/pyruvate ratio will be low.

LACTOFERRIN, STOOL

❑ **Definition**

- Glycoprotein, expressed by activated neutrophils. It is a sensitive and specific marker for detecting inflammation on chronic IBD. The lactoferrin stool assay offers a safe noninvasive, accurate method of differentiating IBD from IBS, once infectious causes of inflammation and colorectal cancer are ruled out. This assay is 86% sensitive and 100% specific in distinguishing IBD from

IBS, making this an important diagnostic tool. Patients with IBD oscillate between active and inactive disease states, and fecal lactoferrin increases 2–3 weeks prior to onset of clinical symptoms. During remission and effective treatment, fecal lactoferrin decreases significantly.
- **Normal range:** negative.

❑ Use

- Screening for inflammation in patients presenting with abdominal pain and diarrhea
- Distinguish patients with active IBD from noninflammatory IBS
- Monitor IBD activity

❑ Interpretation

Increased In
- Intestinal inflammation.
- Marked increase in active IBD.
- Moderately elevated levels of fecal lactoferrin may be found with red cells and leukocytes, in association with inflammatory diarrhea caused by entero-invasive pathogens.

Decreased In
- NA

❑ Limitations

- Test results should be interpreted in conjunction with breast-feeding status. Breast milk is naturally high in lactoferrin, and stool samples from breast-fed infants may cause a false positive with this assay.
- This test may not be appropriate for immunocompromised persons.
- Negative test does not exclude the presence of intestinal inflammation.

LEAD (Pb)

❑ Definition

- An element with four stable isotopes (204, 206, 207, and 208) found naturally in minerals; in man-made products such as paint, gasoline, cigarette smoke, solder in cans, and ceramics; and as a contaminant in soil and water.
- Normal range: <10 µg/dL (<0.48 mmol/L).

❑ Use

- Lead is malleable, ductile, and a poor conductor of electricity; therefore, it is used in building construction, bullets, lead–acid batteries, pewter, and radiation shields.

❑ Interpretation

- Refer to current local state or federal (CDC) guidelines regarding treatment at specific blood lead concentrations. Note that thresholds for treatment vary for adults, children, and pregnant women.
- See discussion of lead poisoning in Chapter 14.

❑ **Limitations**

- Whole blood free of clots.
- Specimen must be collected using a procedure that minimizes environmental contamination.
- Specimen container must be lead free.
- POC testing devices:
  - ▼ Electrochemical methodology
  - ▼ One-step sample pretreatment
  - ▼ Limit of quantitation: 3–5 µg/dL
  - ▼ Results available in <5 minutes
  - ▼ Results may agree within ±20% ICP-MS
- Laboratory-based instrumentation
  - ▼ Atomic absorption
    - Target analyte: nonionized atomic lead
    - Limit of quantitation: 1 µg/dL
  - ▼ Anodic stripping
    - Target analyte: oxidized lead
    - Limit of quantitation: 1–2 µg/dL
    - Requires sample pretreatment
  - ▼ Inductively coupled plasma MS
    - Target analyte: ions at mass/charge ratio of natural isotopes of Pb
    - Limit of quantitation: <1 µg/dL
    - Expensive technology

LECITHIN-TO-SPHINGOMYELIN (L:S) RATIO

❑ **Definition**

- The L:S ratio is based on the observation that there is outward flow of pulmonary secretions from the lungs into the AF, and this changes the phospholipid composition of AF, thereby enabling indirect assessment of fetal lung maturity. The concentrations of L and S in AF are approximately equal until 32–33 weeks of gestation, at which time the concentration of L begins to increase significantly, whereas the S concentration remains about the same. The measurement of S serves as a constant comparison for control of the relative increases in L because the volume of amniotic fluid cannot be accurately measured clinically. This technique involves TLC after organic solvent extraction. It is a difficult test to perform and interpret. The presence of blood or meconium can interfere with test interpretation. Empirically, the risk of respiratory distress syndrome (RDS) is exceedingly low when the L:S ratio is >2.0.
- **Normal range:** see Table 16.54.

❑ **Use**

- Traditional biochemical test to measure fetal lung maturity

❑ **Interpretation**

- Increased in mature fetal lungs (see Limitations and Table 16.54 for high ratios)
- Decreased in immature fetal lungs

16

TABLE 16–54. Values of L:S Ratio and Lung Maturity

L:S Ratio	Values in Some Laboratories	Lung Maturity
<1	<2.0	Very immature lungs (up to 30th wk of gestation); severe RDS is expected; lung maturity may require many weeks; do not resample before 2 wk
1.0–1.49		Immature lungs; moderate to severe RDS is expected; lung maturity may occur in 2 wk; resample in 1 wk
1.5–1.9	2.0–3.0	Lungs on threshold of maturity (within 14 d); mild to moderate RDS may occur. Test should be repeated in 1 wk
≥2	>3.0	Mature lungs (35th week of gestation); low incidence of RDS even if phosphatidylglycerol is absent. S/S = 80–85%
Abundant lecithin with trace or no sphingomyelin		Postmature lungs

❏ **Limitations**

- Labor-intensive test offered by few laboratories
- Offers no advantage over fluorescence polarization
- Sensitivity of >95%, specificity of 70%
- Blood and meconium contamination can affect result
- Definite exceptions to prediction of pulmonary maturity with L:S ratio >2.0
  - ▼ Infant of a diabetic mother (L:S ratio >2.0 has been frequently seen in cases in which RDS developed)
  - ▼ Erythroblastosis fetalis
- Possible exceptions
  - ▼ Intrauterine growth retardation
  - ▼ Toxemia of pregnancy
  - ▼ Hydrops fetalis
  - ▼ Placental disease
  - ▼ Abruptio placentae
  - ▼ Foam (shake) test

LEPTIN

❏ **Definition**

- Serum leptin level is associated with appetite and energy expenditure in healthy individuals. Leptin is produced primarily in fat cells and also in the placenta and probably in the stomach. Serum leptin concentrations are highly correlated with body fat content. These processes are stimulated by insulin, glucocorticoids, and tumor necrosis factor–alpha, another product of adipocytes. These observations suggest that leptin signals the brain about the quantity of stored fat.

- **Normal range:**
  - ▼ Male: 0.5–12.7 ng/mL
  - ▼ Female: 3.9–30.0 ng/mL

❏ **Use**

- Biomarker for body fat metabolism

❏ **Interpretation**

Increased In

- Obesity
- Pregnant women

Decreased In

- Fasting
- Very low–calorie diet

❏ **Limitations**

- Serum leptin concentrations increase with progressive obesity. The concentrations are higher in women than in men, for any measure of obesity, and they decrease with age in both women and men.
- Pregnant women have higher serum leptin concentrations than nonpregnant women.
- Serum leptin concentrations increase during childhood, with the highest concentrations in children who gain the most weight; higher serum leptin concentrations are associated with an earlier onset of puberty.
- The concentrations are similar in normal subjects and patients of the same weight with type 2 DM.
- There is a diurnal rhythm of serum leptin concentrations, the values being 20–40% higher in the middle of the night as compared with daytime. The peak shifts in parallel with shifts in the timing of meals.
- Leptin production is strongly influenced by nutritional state. Overeating increases serum leptin concentrations by nearly 40% within 12 hours, long before any changes in body fat stores. Conversely, in both normal-weight and obese subjects, fasting reduces serum leptin concentrations by 60–70% in 48 hours.

LEUCINE AMINOPEPTIDASE

❏ **Definition**

- LAP is a proteolytic enzyme widely distributed in bacteria, plants, and animals with high activity in the duodenum, kidney, and liver.
- **Normal range:** 1.0–3.3 U/mL.

❏ **Use**

- As a marker of hepatic and pancreatic carcinoma.
- As a marker of early tubular (renal) injury in diabetes and as an indicator of SLE activity.

16

- Parallels serum ALP except that
  - ▼ LAP is usually normal in the presence of bone disease or malabsorption syndrome.
  - ▼ LAP is a more sensitive indicator of choledocholithiasis and of liver metastases in anicteric patients.
- When serum LAP is increased, urine LAP is almost always increased, but when urine LAP is increased, serum LAP may have already returned to normal.

❏ Interpretation
Increased In
- Obstructive, space-occupying, or infiltrative lesions of the liver
- SLE, in correlation with disease activity
- Various neoplasms (even without liver metastases) (e.g., breast, endometrium, and germ cell tumors)
- Preeclampsia, between 33 and 39 weeks of pregnancy

❏ Limitations
- Testing serum LAP is generally not as sensitive or as convenient as testing other liver enzymes to detect some liver problems. ALT, AST, ALP, LDH, and GGT are more commonly measured for the same purpose. Unlike other liver enzymes, LAP can be measured in the urine.
- Elevated LAP activity in serum usually indicates diseases of liver and bile ducts, and this elevation is less affected by damage of liver parenchyma than by active participation of biliary tract in the process.

LEUKOCYTE ALKALINE PHOSPHATASE (LAP)*

❏ Definition
- LAP, or neutrophil alkaline phosphatase, refers to a staining reaction of peripheral blood smears. It reflects the presence of LAP in neutrophils and their precursors. Normally, about 20% of mature neutrophils show stainable leukocyte LAP activity.
- **Normal range:** score of 11–95. The scoring is based on counting 100 neutrophils and grading the stained granules from 0 to 4 on the basis of the intensity and appearance of the precipitated dye in the cytoplasm.

❏ Use
- LAP stain helps differentiate a severe neutrophilia (leukemoid reaction) and myeloproliferative neoplasms, where it is increased, from chronic myeloid leukemia, in which case it is decreased or absent.
- With the advent of modern diagnostic technologies, the use of LAP stains has diminished.

❏ Interpretation
Increased In
- Leukemoid reaction

---

*Submitted By Liberto Pechet, MD.

- Polycythemia vera and essential thrombocythemia (occasionally it may be normal)
- Idiopathic myelofibrosis
- Pregnancy
- Trisomy 21 and Klinefelter syndrome

Decreased In
- Chronic myeloid leukemia
- PNH and pernicious anemia
- Congenital hypophosphatasia

❏ Limitations
- Blood that is not processed soon after drawing may cause low LAP scores.
- There is observer-dependent variability.

LIPASE

❏ Definition
- Glycoprotein enzyme filtered by glomeruli and completely reabsorbed by proximal tubules; method should always include colipase in reagent
- **Normal range:** 0–50 U/L

❏ Use
- Investigating pancreatic disorders, usually pancreatitis
- More specific for pancreatitis than is for serum amylase; diagnosis of peritonitis, strangulated or infarcted bowel, pancreatic cyst

❏ Interpretation
Increased In
- Acute pancreatitis
- Perforated or penetrating peptic ulcer, especially with involvement of the pancreas
- Obstruction of pancreatic duct by
  - ▼ Stone
  - ▼ Drug-induced spasm of sphincter of Oddi (e.g., codeine, morphine, meperidine, methacholine, cholinergics) to levels 2–15 times normal
  - ▼ Partial obstruction plus drug stimulation
- Chronic pancreatitis
- Acute cholecystitis
- Small bowel obstruction
- Intestinal infarction
- Acute and chronic renal failure (increased two to three times in 80% of patients and five times in 5% of patients)
- Organ transplant (kidney, liver, heart), especially with complications (e.g., organ rejection, CMV infection, cyclosporin toxicity)
- Alcoholism
- DKA
- After ERCP

16

- Some cases of intracranial bleeding (unknown mechanism)
- Macro forms in lymphoma, cirrhosis
- Drugs
  - ▼ Induced acute pancreatitis (see preceding section on serum amylase)
  - ▼ Cholestatic effect (e.g., indomethacin)
  - ▼ Methodologic interference (e.g., pancreozymin [contains lipase], deoxycholate, glycocholate, taurocholate [prevent inactivation of enzyme], bilirubin [turbidimetric methods])
- Chronic liver disease (e.g., cirrhosis) (usually ≤2 times normal)

Decreased In
- Methodologic interference (e.g., presence of Hb, quinine, heavy metals, calcium ions)

Normal In
- Mumps
- Macroamylasemia
- Lower value in neonates

❏ Limitations
- Certain drugs such as cholinergics and opiates may elevate serum lipase.
- Renal disease may elevate the serum lipase.

LIPOPROTEIN-ASSOCIATED PHOSPHOLIPASE A$_2$ (Lp-PLA$_2$)*

❏ Definition
- Lipoprotein-associated phospholipase A$_2$ (Lp-PLA$_2$) is a 45-kDa protein enzyme produced by inflammatory cells and activated endothelial cells. It travels in the blood mainly with LDLs. Lp-PLA$_2$ hydrolyzes oxidized phospholipids in LDLs, resulting in formation of oxidized free fatty acids and lysophosphatidylcholine, which is proatherogenic. Alternate name is platelet-activating factor acetylhydrolase (PAF-AH).

❏ Use
- Lp-PLA$_2$ is considered a risk marker rather than a risk factor for cardiac heart disease.
  - ▼ In conjunction with hsCRP assay can reliably stratify low-, intermediate-, and high-risk populations.
    - Increased Lp-PLA$_2$ with low LDL-C increases risk of heart disease two times.
    - Increased Lp-PLA$_2$ with high CRP increases risk of heart disease three times.
  - ▼ Consensus panel recommendations are for Lp-PLA$_2$ assessment in moderate-risk individuals for CHD either independently or in conjunction with hsCRP.

---

*Submitted By Craig S. Smith, MD.

❑ Interpretation

- Concentrations ≥235 ng/mL are associated with increased risk of cardiovascular events, including myocardial infarction and ischemic stroke, and are predictive of short-term mortality in myocardial infarction patients.
- Elevated Lp-PLA$_2$ has been found to be associated with ischemic stroke and may be useful in risk assessment.

❑ Limitations

- Smoking increases Lp-PLA$_2$ measurements.

Suggested Reading

Corson MA, Jones PH, Davidson MH. Review of the evidence for the clinical utility of lipoprotein-associated phospholipase A2 as a cardiovascular risk marker. *Am J Cardiol.* 2008;101(12A):41F–50F.

LUPUS ANTICOAGULANT (LA)*

❑ Definition

- LAs are heterogeneous IgG or IgM autoantibodies that inhibit phospholipid-dependent assays of blood coagulation. Because phospholipid is essential for several steps in the coagulation cascade, the presence of LAs can prolong various phospholipid-dependent clotting times, such as PTT, PT, and the dilute Russell viper venom time (dRVVT, see p. 927).

❑ Use

- None of the tests mentioned in the Definition discussion is sufficiently sensitive to detect all LAs; therefore, *two screening tests* are required before LA can be excluded.
- The most commonly used screening tests are PT (1:100 diluted) and dRVVT. (Kaolin or micronized silica clotting time is no longer in use.) A positive screening test (prolonged dilute PT or dRVVT) requires confirmation by adding excess phospholipids in the test.

❑ Interpretation

- A normalization of the clotting time in either test confirms the presence of LA but requires that the tests be repeated in 12 weeks, because frequently the LA is a temporary phenomenon (Fig. 16.1).

❑ Limitations

- There is considerable interlaboratory variation with the performance of the LA assays, especially dRVVT. In recent surveys, there was a false-positive detection of LAs in 24% of samples and a false-negative result of 18.5% in participating centers.
  - ▾ One of the factors that may contribute to a false-positive result is contamination with heparin.
  - ▾ Preanalytical variables, such as improper plasma preparation, may lead to false-negative results because of contamination with platelets.

16

---

*Submitted By Liberto Pechet, MD.

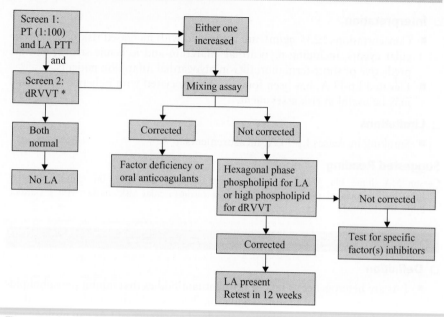

Figure 16–1 *Algorithm for testing lupus anticoagulant antibodies.*

- It is recommended that assessment for LA not be undertaken while the patient is on oral anticoagulants, if at all possible (see Fig. 16.1).

Suggested Readings

Giannakopoulos B, Passam F, Ioannou Y, et al. How we diagnose the antiphospholipid antibody syndrome. *Blood.* 2009;113:985–994.
Moffat KA, Ledford-Kraemer MR, Plumhoff EA, et al. Are laboratories following published recommendations for lupus anticoagulant testing? *Thromb Haemost.* 2009;101:178–184.

LUTEINIZING HORMONE (LH)

See Follicular-Stimulating Hormone (FSH) and Luteinizing Hormone (LH), Serum.

MAGNESIUM (Mg)

❑ **Definition**

- Mg is primarily an intracellular ion associated with GI absorption and renal excretion. At least 65–70% of Mg is in ionized state, and approximately 35% serum Mg is protein bound.
- **Normal range:** 1.6–2.4 mg/dL.
- **Critical values:** <1.0 and >4.9 mg/dL.

❑ **Use**

- Diagnosis and monitoring of hypomagnesemia and hypermagnesemia, especially in renal failure or GI disorders

- To monitor preeclampsia patients being treated with magnesium sulfate, although in most cases, monitoring clinical signs (respiratory rate and deep tendon reflexes) is adequate, and blood magnesium levels are not required

❏ **Interpretation**

Increased In

- Iatrogenic (is usual cause; most often with impaired renal function).
  - ▼ Diuretics (e.g., furosemide >80 mg/day, thiazides)
  - ▼ Antacids or enemas containing Mg
  - ▼ Laxative and cathartic abuse
  - ▼ Parenteral nutrition
  - ▼ Mg for eclampsia or premature labor
  - ▼ Lithium carbonate intoxication
- Renal failure (when GFR approaches 30 mL/minutes); in chronic renal failure, hypermagnesemia is inversely related to residual renal function. Increase is rarely observed with normal renal function.
- Dehydration with diabetic coma before treatment
- Hypothyroidism
- Addison disease and after adrenalectomy
- Controlled DM in older patients
- Accidental ingestion of large amount of sea water

Decreased In

- Almost always GI or renal disturbance; chronic Mg deficiency produces hypocalcemia secondary to decreased production and effectiveness of PTH.
  - ▼ GI disease
    - Malabsorption (e.g., sprue, small bowel resection, biliary and intestinal fistulas, abdominal irradiation, celiac disease, and other causes of steatorrhea; familial Mg malabsorption)
    - Abnormal loss of GI fluids (chronic ulcerative colitis, Crohn disease, villous adenoma, carcinoma of the colon, laxative abuse, prolonged aspiration of GI tract contents, vomiting)
  - ▼ Renal disease: a level >2 mEq/day in urine during hypomagnesemia indicates excessive renal loss.
    - Chronic GN
    - Chronic pyelonephritis
    - Renal tubular acidosis
    - Diuretic phase of acute tubular necrosis
    - Postobstructive diuresis
    - Drug injury
- Diuretics (e.g., mercurials, ammonium chloride, thiazides, furosemide)
- Antibiotics (e.g., aminoglycosides, gentamicin, tobramycin, carbenicillin, ticarcillin, amphotericin B)
- *Digitalis* (in 20% of patients taking *Digitalis*)
- Antineoplastic (e.g., cisplatin)
- Cyclosporine: tubular losses due to ions or nutrients
- Hypercalcemia
- Diuresis caused by glucose, urea, or mannitol

16

- Phosphate depletion
- Extracellular fluid volume expansion
- Primary renal Mg wasting
- Nutritional
  - ▼ Prolonged parenteral fluid administration without Mg (usually >3 weeks)
  - ▼ Acute and chronic alcoholism and alcoholic cirrhosis
  - ▼ Starvation with metabolic acidosis
  - ▼ Kwashiorkor, protein–calorie malnutrition
- Endocrine
  - ▼ Hyperthyroidism
  - ▼ Aldosteronism (primary and secondary)
  - ▼ Hyperparathyroidism and other causes of hypercalcemia
  - ▼ Hypoparathyroidism
  - ▼ DM (in ≤39% of patients; caused by osmotic diuresis)
- Metabolic
  - ▼ Excessive lactation
  - ▼ Third trimester of pregnancy
  - ▼ Insulin treatment of diabetic coma
- Other
  - ▼ Toxemia of pregnancy or eclampsia
  - ▼ Lytic tumors of bone
  - ▼ Active Paget disease of bone; caused by increased uptake by bone
  - ▼ Acute pancreatitis
  - ▼ Transfusion of citrated blood
  - ▼ Severe burns
  - ▼ Sweating
  - ▼ Sepsis
  - ▼ Hypothermia
- Mg deficiency frequently coexists with other electrolyte abnormalities; it may cause apparently unexplained hypocalcemia and hypokalemia and should always be measured in such cases. About 40% of patients have coexisting hypokalemia.
- About 90% of patients with high or low serum Mg levels are not clinically recognized; therefore, routine inclusion of Mg with electrolyte measurements has been suggested.
- *Digitalis* sensitivity and toxicity frequently occur with hypomagnesemia.
- Ionized Mg is decreased in only approximately 70% of critically ill patients with decreased total Mg.
- Because deficiency can exist with normal or borderline serum Mg levels, a 24-hour urine test may be indicated by frequent concomitant disorders (coexist with other electrolyte abnormalities).
- A 24-hour urine level <25 mg suggests Mg deficiency (in the absence of conditions or agents that promote magnesium excretion). If caused by renal loss, urine Mg should be >3.65–6 mg/day.
- If level is <2.4 mg/day, collect a 24-hour urine sample during IV administration of 72 mg of $MgCl_2$. Some 60–80% of the load is excreted by patients with normal Mg stores; <50% excretion suggests nonrenal Mg depletion.

❑ Limitations
- Serum magnesium levels may remain normal even when total body stores of magnesium are depleted up to 20%.
- Phylate, fatty acids, and an excess of phosphate impair Mg absorption
- Hemolysis yields elevated results because levels in erythrocytes are two to three times higher than in serum.

Suggested Reading
Lum G. Clinical utility of magnesium measurement. *Lab Med.* 2004;35:106.

MAGNESIUM, URINE

❑ Definition
- Magnesium is an important but commonly neglected electrolyte. Magnesium deficiency is often inadequately documented by serum magnesium levels. Urinary magnesium analyses have been advocated before and after therapeutic magnesium administration to further investigate the significance of apparent low serum magnesium. Abnormal levels of magnesium are most frequently seen in conditions or diseases that cause impaired or excessive excretion of magnesium by the kidneys or that cause impaired absorption in the intestines. Magnesium levels may be checked as part of an evaluation of the severity of kidney problems and/or of uncontrolled diabetes and may help in the diagnosis of GI disorders. Renal magnesium wasting occurs in renal transplant recipients who are on cyclosporine and prednisone. Renal conservation of magnesium is diminished by hypercalciuria, salt-losing conditions, and the SIADH.
- **Normal range:**
  - ▼ Twenty-four–hour urine: 72–120 mg/day
  - ▼ Random urine:
    - Male: 18–110 mg/g creatinine
    - Female: 14–139 mg/g creatinine

❑ Use
- Investigate chronic pancreas inflammation
- Decreased blood magnesium

❑ Interpretation
Increased In
- Alcohol
- Diuretics
- Bartter syndrome
- Corticosteroids
- Cisplatin therapy
- Aldosterone

Decreased In
- Insufficient magnesium intake
- Extrarenal loss

16

❑ Limitations

- Magnesium forms insoluble complexes with normal urine constituents that precipitate as soon as urine is passed. Acidification is not required.
- Urine concentration is diet dependent.
- Magnesium depletion could be common condition found in 26% of hospitalized patients.
- High concentrations of gadolinium are known to interfere with most metals tests.

MATERNAL SCREENING

See Prenatal Screening.

MEAN CORPUSCULAR HEMOGLOBIN (MCH)*

❑ Definition and Use

- MCH is the Hb concentration per RBC count. It has limited value in classifying anemias.
- Normal range: 27–34 pg per red cell.

❑ Interpretation
Increased In
- Macrocytic anemias and infants as well as newborns

Decreased In
- Microcytic and normocytic anemias

MEAN CORPUSCULAR HEMOGLOBIN CONCENTRATION (MCHC)†

❑ Definition and Use

- MCHC is the Hct divided by Hb. It has limited value in classifying anemias, although it may identify hypochromasia better than MCH.
- Normal range: 31.5–36 g.

❑ Interpretation
Decreased In
- Microcytic and normocytic anemias

Increased In
- Macrocytic anemias and hereditary spherocytosis
- Infants and newborns

---

*Submitted By Liberto Pechet, MD.
†Submitted By Liberto Pechet, MD.

MEAN CORPUSCULAR VOLUME (MCV)*

❏ **Definition**

- MCV represents the average measurement of RBC volume. It is measured directly by automated instruments but calculated as Hct divided by RBC count with manual methods.
- **Normal range: 82.0–101.0 fL.**

❏ **Use**

- MCV is helpful in the classification of anemias.

❏ **Interpretation**

Increased In
- Macrocytic anemias
- Myelodysplastic syndromes
- Alcoholism
- Liver diseases
- Hypothyroidism
- Hemolysis with high reticulocyte count
- Infants and newborns

Decreased In
- Iron deficiency anemias
- Thalassemias
- Hereditary sideroblastic anemia
- Lead poisoning
- Anemia of chronic disease and other hemoglobinopathies (may be decreased or normal)

❏ **Limitations**

- MCV may be artificially increased with marked leukocytosis, numerous large platelets, cold agglutinins, methanol poisoning, marked hyperglycemia, and marked reticulocytosis.
- MCV may be falsely decreased with in vitro hemolysis or fragmentation of RBCs.

MEAN PLATELET VOLUME (MPV)†

❏ **Definition**

- MPV reflects the frequency distribution of platelet volumes.
- **Normal range: 7.8–11.0 fL.**

❏ **Use**

- MPV is used to evaluate variations in platelet size as related to various platelet abnormalities.

---

*Submitted By Liberto Pechet, MD.
†Submitted By Liberto Pechet, MD.

16

❏ Interpretation

Increased In

- Hypothyroidism
- Myeloproliferative neoplasms
- All cases of accelerated bone marrow production of platelets (immune thrombocytopenias, postchemotherapy)
- Bernard-Soulier syndrome

Decreased In

- Disorders associated with decreased platelet production
- In some patients with sepsis
- In some patients with inherited thrombocytopenias, such as Wiskott-Aldrich syndrome

❏ Limitations

- Reference values appear to vary with the platelet count. MPV is affected by numerous variables related to specimen collection, the anticoagulant used, temperature, and duration of storage.

METANEPHRINES, URINE

❏ Definition

- Metanephrine and normetanephrine are metabolic products of epinephrine and norepinephrine, the adrenal medullary hormones secreted by pheochromocytomas. Fractionated tests provide higher diagnostic sensitivity than assays for total catecholamines.
- Normal range: see Table 16.55.

TABLE 16–55. Normal Range for Urine Metanephrines

Age	Reference Interval (μg/g Creatinine)
Metanephrine	
0–3 mo	0–700
4–6 mo	0–650
7–11 mo	0–650
1 y	0–530
2–5 y	0–500
6–17 y	0–320
≥18 y	0–300
Normetanephrine	
0–3 mo	0–3,400
4–6 mo	0–2,200
7–11 mo	0–1,100
1 y	0–1,300
2–5 y	0–610
6–17 y	0–450
≥18 y	0–400

❏ **Use**

- Confirmation of elevated plasma catecholamine levels
- Diagnosis of pheochromocytoma and paraganglioma
- Diagnosis and follow-up of patients with neuroblastoma and related tumors
- First line of test in patients with lower suspicion of pheochromocytoma (patients with resistant hypertension, hyper adrenergic spells, incidentally discovered adrenal mass that does not have imaging characteristics consistent with pheochromocytoma).

❏ **Interpretation**

- Increases occur with catecholamine-secreting neurochromatin tumors such as pheochromocytoma, paraganglioma, and neuroblastoma.

❏ **Limitations**

- No caffeine intake should occur before or during collection. MAO inhibitors should be discontinued at least 1 week prior to beginning collection.
- Methylglucamine in x-ray contrast medium can cause false-negative test results.
- False positives can be caused by stress and drugs, which includes amphetamines and amphetamine-like compounds, appetite suppressants, bromocriptine, buspirone, caffeine, carbidopa–levodopa (Sinemet), clonidine, dexamethasone, diuretics, methyldopa (Aldomet), nose drops, propafenone (Rythmol), tricyclic antidepressants, and vasodilators. The effects of some drugs on catecholamine metabolite results may not be predictable.

METHOTREXATE*

❏ **Definition**

- Folic acid antagonist. Other names: Folex, Mexate, Trexall.
- **Normal range:** TDM generally performed to ensure plasma/serum concentration <1 µmol/L at 48 hours postinfusion and <0.1 µmol/L at 72 hours postdose

❏ **Use**

- Methotrexate is an antineoplastic drug used solely or in combination with other antineoplastic drugs for the treatment of leukemia and other diseases.
- Severe psoriasis, sarcoidosis, and granulomatosis have been treated with methotrexate in relatively low doses.
- High-dose methotrexate (greater than approximately 20 mg/kg body weight) with citrovorum factor rescue have been used with favorable results in the treatment of osteogenic sarcoma, leukemia, non-Hodgkin lymphoma, lung cancer, carcinoma of the head and neck, and breast cancer.
- The efficacy of methotrexate in the treatment of other tumors such as prostate cancer is being investigated.

16

*Submitted By Amanda J. Jenkins, PhD.

❏ **Interpretation**

- Potential toxicity: Reported therapeutic and toxic ranges are dependent on dose and the time the sample is drawn postdose. Consult protocol to assess toxicity.
  - ▼ 24 hours: >10 µmol/L
  - ▼ 48 hours: >1.0 µmol/L
  - ▼ 72 hours: >0.1 µmol/L

❏ **Limitations**

- Immunoassay-based tests (EMIT, FPIA) for serum/plasma
- Serum must be collected in tubes without serum separator gel.
- Cells must be separated as soon as possible after collection.
- Heparinized, EDTA, and fluoridated collection tubes for plasma are acceptable.
- This assay measures the total (protein bound and free) levels of methotrexate in serum and plasma.
- It is known that aminopterin and APA (a metabolite of methotrexate) cross-react significantly with the EMIT assay and less so with the FPIA.
- Patients should be rebaselined when changing the methodology.
- Samples are stable for up to 24 hours when refrigerated and protected from light..

METHYLMALONIC ACID

❏ **Definition**

- Methylmalonic acid (MMA) is an intermediate in the propionate degradation pathway. Deficient activity of the enzyme responsible for the conversion of methylmalonyl CoA to succinyl CoA (methylmalonyl CoA mutase) results in the organic aciduria known as methylmalonic aciduria, with a classical presentation of neonatal onset metabolic acidosis, hyperammonemia, and poor outcome if untreated. The concentrations of the metabolic markers MMA and homocysteine (Hcy) are considered to be more sensitive indicators of vitamin B_{12} status. Both MMA and Hcy increase in vitamin B_{12} deficiency. However, Hcy has been shown to have low specificity, being influenced by lifestyle factors such as smoking and alcohol intake and increasing in patients with folate deficiency and renal impairment.
- **Normal range:** 0.00–0.40 µmol/L.

❏ **Use**

- Evaluation of methylmalonic academia in children.
- Evaluation of megaloblastic anemia (cobalamin deficiency). Serum MMA may be a more reliable marker of cobalamin deficiency than direct cobalamin determination.

❑ **Interpretation**

Increased In

- Vitamin B$_{12}$ deficiency
- Pregnancy
- Cobalamin genetic defects
- Methylmalonic acidemia

❑ **Limitations**

- Serum and urine levels are more reliable markers of cobalamine deficiency than direct cobalamine determination.
- Diet, nutritional status, and age should be considered in the evaluation of serum MMA level.

METYRAPONE TEST

❑ **Definition**

- The metyrapone stimulation test is based on the principle that decreasing serum cortisol concentrations is expected to produce an increase in ACTH secretion.

❑ **Use**

- The utilization of the metyrapone test has become less frequent as a result of the larger availability of plasma ACTH assays. The limited accessibility to metyrapone in certain countries, as well as the limited number of clinical laboratories who have maintained the urinary 17-hydroxycorticosteroid (17-OHCS) and serum 11-deoxycortisol tests, have also further limited the use of the metyrapone test.
- Metyrapone blocks the conversion of 11-deoxycortisol to cortisol by CYP11B1 (11-beta-hydroxylase, P-450c11), the last step in the synthesis of cortisol. It induces a rapid fall of cortisol and an increase of 11-deoxycortisol in serum.
- The metyrapone test can be performed as an overnight single-dose test or as a 2- or 3-day test. It cannot be performed in a patient who is taking any glucocorticoid.
  - ▼ The 2-day test is used primarily in the differential diagnosis of hypercortisolism.
    - The 2-day test is a slight variation on the standard 3-day test: 24-hour urine and 8 AM blood specimens are collected during and at the end of a baseline day and during and at the end of the day during which the patient takes 750 mg of metyrapone by mouth every 4 hours for six doses.
    - Urinary 17-OHCS excretion and serum 11-deoxycortisol are measured.
  - ▼ The 3-day test is used mainly for the evaluation of adrenal insufficiency.
    - The 3-day test is begun by obtaining a baseline 24-hour urine collection. Immediately after completing this collection, the patient begins taking metyrapone (750 mg orally every 4 hours for six doses) with a glass of milk or a small snack to minimize GI symptoms.

16

- Subsequent 24-hour urine specimens are collected the day of and the day after metyrapone administration for measurement of urinary 17-OHCS and creatinine excretion. Serum 11-deoxycortisol, cortisol, and plasma ACTH can also be measured 4 hours after the last dose of metyrapone.
▼ The single-dose overnight test can be used for both indications.
    - The single-dose test is performed by oral administration of metyrapone (30 mg/kg body weight, or 2 g for <70 kg, 2.5 g for 70–90 kg, and 3 g for >90 kg body weight) at midnight with a glass of milk or a small snack.
    - Serum 11-deoxycortisol and cortisol are measured between 7:30 and 9:30 AM the next morning; plasma ACTH can also be measured.

❏ **Interpretation**

Standard 3-Day Metyrapone Test

■ The increase in serum 11-deoxycortisol is used as a criterion of response as in the single-dose overnight test. Measuring serum cortisol and plasma ACTH is important, as a fall in serum cortisol confirms the metyrapone-induced biosynthetic blockade and an increase in plasma ACTH confirms that the changes in steroid levels are ACTH dependent.
■ A normal response is a two- to threefold increase above the baseline 24-hour urinary 17-OHCS excretion on either the day of or, more often, the day after metyrapone administration. The serum cortisol concentration should decrease to <5 μg/dL. The plasma ACTH concentration should exceed 75 pg/mL, with a mean of about 200 pg/mL 4 hours after the last metyrapone dose. An increase in serum 11-deoxycortisol to 7–22 μg/dL or more at 8 AM, 4 hours after the last dose of metyrapone.

Two-Day Metyrapone Test

■ A normal response to the 2-day test has not been defined. In the differential diagnosis of ACTH-dependent Cushing syndrome, however, a clear rise in plasma ACTH concentration indicates that the ACTH-secreting tumor responds to falling serum cortisol concentrations. In one large study, as an example, a positive response was defined as a >70% increase in urinary 17-OHCS excretion and/or more than a fourfold increase in serum 11-deoxycortisol concentrations.

Overnight Single-Dose Metyrapone Test

■ A normal response is 8 AM serum 11-deoxycortisol concentration of 7–22 μg/dL. A serum cortisol concentration at 8 AM of <5 μg/dL confirms adequate metyrapone blockade and thereby documents compliance and normal metabolism of metyrapone. Serum 11-deoxycortisol concentrations <7 μg/dL with concomitantly suppressed cortisol values indicate adrenal insufficiency.
■ The ACTH response to metyrapone can distinguish between primary and secondary insufficiency. In general, patients with secondary adrenal insufficiency have ACTH responses from 10 to 200 pg/mL, whereas patients with primary adrenal insufficiency have higher responses. However, healthy individuals have an ACTH response of 42–690 pg/mL. Because of this overlap, the ACTH response alone cannot be used to distinguish between healthy individuals and those with adrenal insufficiency.

❑ **Limitations**

- Adrenal tumor with excess cortisol production: no increase or fall in urinary 17-KS. The test is positive in 100% of patients with adrenal hyperplasias without tumor, 50% of those with adrenal adenomas, and 25% of those with adrenal carcinomas.
- Ectopic ACTH syndrome: It may not be accurate in this condition.
- Metyrapone administration may result in hypotension, nausea, and vomiting in patients with adrenal insufficiency; as a result, the 2- and 3-day tests should not be performed outside of the hospital in patients suspected of having this disorder.
- Acute or chronic ingestion of synthetic glucocorticoids can result in a subnormal response as a result of suppression of the corticotropes.
- One of the more common causes of a false-positive result is unusually rapid clearance of metyrapone from the plasma, resulting in inadequate blockade of cortisol biosynthesis. This is manifested by a serum cortisol concentration >7.5 µg/dL in the sample drawn at 8 AM in the overnight test, by a serum cortisol concentration >5 µg/dL 4 hours after the last dose of metyrapone, or by urinary cortisol excretion >20 µg/24 hours the day metyrapone was administered in the standard 2-day test.

MICROALBUMIN, URINE

❑ **Definition**

- The urine dipstick is a relatively insensitive marker for proteinuria, not becoming positive until protein excretion exceeds 300–500 mg/day. The normal rate of albumin excretion is <20 mg/day (15 µg/minute); persistent albumin excretion between 30 and 300 mg/day (20 and 200 µg/minute) is called microalbuminuria. Albumin excretion >300 mg/day (200 µg/minute) is considered to represent overt or dipstick positive proteinuria (also called macroalbuminuria).
- In type 1 and 2 DM, the presence of microalbuminuria on repeat specimens collected in the basal state may signify early diabetic nephropathy. It is a marker, in patients with or without diabetes, for cardiovascular mortality. For a definition of microalbuminuria, see Table 16.56.
- Measurement of the urine albumin-to-creatinine ratio in an untimed urinary sample is the preferred screening strategy for microalbuminuria. This test has several advantages: it does not require early morning or timed collections, it gives a quantitative result that correlates with the 24-hour urine values over a wide range of protein excretion, it is simple to perform and inexpensive,

TABLE 16–56. American Diabetes Association Definition of Microalbuminuria

Category	24-Hour Collection	Timed Collection	Spot Collection
Normal	<30 mg/24 h	<20 µg/min	<30 µg/mg creatinine
Microalbuminuria	30–300 mg/24 h	20–200 µg/min	30–300 µg/mg creatinine
Clinical albuminuria	>300 mg/24 h	>200 µg/min	>300 µg/mg creatinine

16

and repeat values can be easily obtained to ascertain that microalbuminuria, if present, is persistent.

- Other name: albumin/creatinine ratio.
- **Normal range:**
  - ▼ Albumin/creatinine ratio (random urine): <30.0 μg/mg creatinine
  - ▼ Microalbumin excretion (24-hour urine): 0–29.9 mg/day

❑ **Use**

- Diagnosis of kidney dysfunction.
- Recommended by the American Diabetes Association to screen for microalbuminuria.
- Medications that act on the renin–angiotensin system may delay onset of renal and cardiovascular disease, making screening for microalbumin important in the care of diabetic patients.

❑ **Interpretation**

- Increased excretion of albumin (microalbuminuria) is a predictor of future development of clinical renal disease in patients with hypertension or DM.

❑ **Limitations**

- Microalbuminuria may be seen transiently during pregnancy, after exercise, and with protein loading, hyperglycemia, fever, and urinary tract infections. There is also day-to-day, as well as diurnal, variation in albumin excretion. Hence, it is important to base treatment on the results of several tests.
- Vigorous exercise can cause a transient increase in albumin excretion. Patients should refrain from vigorous exercise in the 24 hours prior to the test.
- The optimal time to measure the urine albumin-to-creatinine ratio is not clearly defined. The first-morning void specimen is preferred.
- The accuracy of the urine albumin-to-creatinine ratio will be diminished if creatinine excretion is substantially different from the expected value; this is particularly important in patients with borderline values. Albumin excretion will be underestimated in a muscular man with a high rate of creatinine excretion and overestimated in a cachectic patient in whom muscle mass and creatinine excretion are markedly reduced.

Suggested Reading

American Diabetes Association. Standards of medical care in diabetes. *Diabetes Care.* 2004;27(Suppl 1):S79.

MÜLLERIAN INHIBITING SUBSTANCE

❑ **Definition**

- The primary function of müllerian inhibiting substance (MIS) is to initiate regression of müllerian structures in males as a part of normal sexual development. Secreted by the Sertoli cells of the testes during embryogenesis of the male fetus. It is also expressed by granulose cells of the ovary

TABLE 16–57. Normal Ranges for Müllerian-Inhibiting Substance	
Age	Range (ng/mL)
Male	
0–13 d	15.5–48.7
14 d–11 mo	39.1–91.1
12 mo–6 y	48.0–83.2
7–8 y	33.8–60.2
9 y to adult	3.0–5.4
Female	
0–8 y	0.0–7.1
9 y to adult	0.0–6.9

during reproductive years and controls the primary follicles by inhibiting the excessive follicular development by FSH. Other names: anti-müllerian hormone, müllerian inhibiting hormone.
- **Normal range:** see Table 16.57.

❏ **Use**

- Specific and sensitive marker for the presence of testicular tissue in boys with cryptorchidism.
- When measured either alone or in tandem with measurement of hCG-stimulated testosterone, MIS levels can be used to guide the treatment of these patients.
- Evaluation of the presence of any functioning testicular tissue in infants and children with ambiguous genitalia.
- Early detection of recurrence in patients with ovarian granulosa cell tumors.
- Assess the condition of PCO and premature ovarian failure.
- Assess ovarian reserve.

❏ **Interpretation**
Increased In
- PCOS (polycystic ovarian syndrome)

Decreased In
- Anorchia
- Abnormal or absence of testis
- Pseudohermaphroditism
- Syndrome of persistent müllerian ducts, despite the presence of structurally normal testes

❏ **Limitations**

- Compared with white women, average MIS values were lower among black (25.2% lower) and Hispanic (24.6% lower) women.
- Menopausal women or women with premature ovarian failure have very low levels.
- Not well-standardized test and not specific for malignancy. Interpretation needs to be in conjunction with clinical symptoms.

16

MULTIGENE CARRIER PANELS*

❏ **Definition**

- Universal Carrier Test provided by Counsyl is a noninvasive, saliva-based assay for more than 100 mostly autosomal recessive, Mendelian diseases offered to individuals or couples. InheriGen, GenPath tests for 164 autosomal recessive and X-linked inherited diseases, including Ashkenazi Jewish Diseases. InheriGen Plus, GenPath includes these 164 diseases and also screens for fragile X, spinal muscular atrophy, and cystic fibrosis carrier status.

❏ **Use**

- Carrier testing

❏ **Limitations**

- The results of a genetic test may be affected by DNA rearrangements, blood transfusion, bone marrow transplantation, or rare sequence variations.
- Results are provided for diseases and mutations tested on the panel. Diseases caused by repeat expansions (such as fragile X), sporadic deletions/duplications (such as Duchenne muscular dystrophy) may not included in the panel.

MYELOPEROXIDASE (MPO), PLASMA†

❏ **Definition**

- MPO is an enzyme stored in granules of PMNs and macrophages with primary anti-infective functions. It is released in plasma in inflammatory conditions and is thought to potentially play a role in CHD by oxidizing LDL and contributing to atherosclerotic plaque instability. MPO is elevated in angiographically proven CAD, acute coronary syndromes, and correlates with functional class in systolic heart failure.
- **Normal range:** <539 pm in healthy individuals.

❏ **Use**

- Marker of inflammation when elevated in plasma. MPO may be used for the evaluation of patients presenting with acute chest pain, in conjunction with ECG and cardiac biomarkers.

❏ **Interpretation**

- An initial increase independently predicts risk of myocardial infarction and adverse cardiac events and predicts sudden death in the next 1–6 months, even in the absence of signs of ischemic necrosis or of increase in other inflammatory markers, such as CRP. A low MPO improves the negative predictive value of normal troponins in unstable angina. At present, there is conflicting evidence for the additive diagnostic utility of MPO above established

*Submitted By Edward Ginns, MD and Marzena M. Galdzicka, PhD.
†Submitted By Craig S. Smith, MD.

cardiac biomarkers in acute chest pain patients, and it is not recommended for routine triage of ACS.

- Elevated plasma MPO concentration is associated with a more advanced cardiovascular risk profile; however, plasma MPO does not predict mortality independent of other cardiovascular risk factors in patients with stable coronary artery disease.

❏ Limitations

- It has been demonstrated that elevations of MPO can occur with the administration of heparin products, potentially confounding its accuracy.
- Elevated in rheumatoid arthritis.

Suggested Readings

Baldus S, Rudolph V, Roiss R, et al. Heparins increase endothelial nitric oxide bioavailability by liberating vessel-immobilized myeloperoxidase. *Circulation* 2006;113:1871–1878.

Peacock WF, Nagurney J, et al. Myeloperoxidase in the diagnosis of acute coronary syndromes: The importance of spectrum. *Am Heart J.* 2011;162:893–899.

Stefanescua A, Braun S, Ndrepepa G, et al. Prognostic value of plasma myeloperoxidase concentration in patients with stable coronary artery disease. *Am Heart J.* 2008;155(2):356–360.

MYOGLOBIN*

❏ Definition

- Myoglobin is the primary oxygen-carrying protein of muscle tissues found only in skeletal and cardiac muscle. It is a small-sized molecule that is rapidly released from damaged tissue and is not protein bound and rapidly excreted in urine. Plasma half-life is 9 minutes. It is linked in a reversible manner with oxygen, playing an important part in cellular aerobic metabolism.
- **Normal range** (may be wide): 6–90 ng/mL.
  - ▼ Male: 28–72 ng/mL
  - ▼ Female: 25–58 ng/mL

❏ Use

- A cardiac biomarker, myoglobin is the one of the earliest markers for myocardial necrosis.
- Myoglobin levels start to rise within 2–3 hours of myocardial infarction, reach their highest levels within 8–12 hours, and generally fall back to normal within 1 day.
- A negative myoglobin result effectively rules out a heart attack, but a positive result must be confirmed by testing for troponin or another biomarker.
- Sensitivity is >95% within 6 hours of onset of symptoms.
- Myoglobin may precede release of CK-MB by 2–5 hours.

❏ Interpretation

- Within 1–3 hours in >85% of patients with AMI, myoglobin peaks in about 8–12 hours (may peak within 1 hour) to about 10 times the upper reference

16

---

*Submitted By Craig S. Smith, MD.

limit and becomes normal in about 24–36 hours or less; reperfusion causes a peak 4–6 hours earlier.

■ It is also increased in

▼ Renal failure (high levels of urine myoglobin indicate an increased risk of kidney damage.)

▼ Shock

▼ Open heart surgery

▼ Carriers of progressive muscular dystrophy

▼ Extensive trauma

▼ Myocarditis

▼ Acute infectious diseases

● Seizure

● Toxin exposure: cocaine, narcotics, sea snake venom

● Malignant hypertension

❑ Limitations

■ With high-sensitivity troponins and 99% sensitivity cutoffs now currently used in MI diagnosis, myoglobin has been replaced by troponin as the preferred cardiac biomarker. Exceptions may be in rapid ACS protocols if local laboratory point-of-care troponin is unreliable. Nevertheless, myoglobin should not be the solitary biomarker used for diagnosis.

■ Increased values may occur with skeletal muscle damage, exhaustive exercise, or heavy alcohol abuse.

■ The myoglobin test displays a low specificity for AMI. Myoglobin may come from either heart or skeletal muscle, so an increase in serum myoglobin is not specific for damage to the heart.

■ Blood samples should be drawn every 2–3 hours for the first several hours after experiencing chest pain (myoglobin may be released in multiple short bursts) for accurate measurements.

■ Values are usually much higher in patients with uremia and muscle trauma compared to AMI.

■ Myoglobin should not be used for the diagnosis of MI but may be useful in conjunction with other biomarkers for prognosis postrevascularization.

Suggested Readings

deLemos JA, Morrow DA, Gibson CM, et al. The prognostic value of serum myoglobin in patients with non-ST-segment elevation acute coronary syndromes: Results from the TIMI 11B and TACTICS-TIMI 18 studies. *JACC.* 2002;40:238.

Ordway GA, Garry DJ. Myoglobin: An essential hemoprotein in striated muscle. *J Exp Biol.* 2004;207:3441–3446.

NEURON-SPECIFIC ENOLASE (NSE)

❑ Definition

■ Specific serum marker for the family of neuroendocrine tumors of amine precursor uptake and decarboxylation series, which includes neuroblastoma, retinoblastoma, medullary carcinoma of thyroid, carcinoid, pancreatic cell carcinoma, pheochromocytoma, and small cell carcinoma of the lung (SCLC)

■ **Normal range:** 3.7–8.9 µg/L

❑ **Use**

- A follow-up marker in patients with NSE-secreting tumors of any type
- An auxiliary test in the diagnosis of SCLC
- An auxiliary test in the diagnosis of carcinoids, islet cell tumors, and neuroblastomas
- An auxiliary tool in the assessment of comatose patients

❑ **Interpretation**

- NSE in both serum and CSF is a sensitive and specific marker of neuronal injury in various neurologic disorders.
- NSE is increased in neuroblastoma and SCLC.
- Useful in the differentiated diagnosis of Creutzfeldt-Jakob disease for other dementing disease.

❑ **Limitations**

- All NSE test results must be considered in the clinical context, and interferences or artifactual elevations should be suspected if the clinical NSE test results are at odds with the clinical picture or other tests. Not a screening test.
- Hemolysis can lead to significant artifactual NSE elevations, because erythrocytes contain NSE.
- Proton pump inhibitor treatment, hemolytic anemia, hepatic failure, and end-stage renal failure can also result in artifactual NSE elevations.
- When performing NSE testing for tumor diagnosis or follow-up, epileptic seizure, brain injury, encephalitis, stroke, and rapidly progressive dementia might result in false-positive results. On the other hand, when NSE testing is performed to assist in neurologic diagnosis, NSE-secreting tumors can represent a source of false-positive results.
- NSE values can vary significantly between methods/assays. Serial follow-up should be performed with the same assay. If assays are changed, patients should be rebaselined.

NEUTROPHIL TESTS FOR DYSFUNCTION*

❑ **Definition**

- Inherited or acquired disorders affecting neutrophils (and other leukocytes) may result in abnormal function and a predisposition to recurrent bacterial infections. Acquired neutrophil dysfunction may be the result of disorders of immunoglobulins, complement, or T cells; in such cases, the underlying disease should be characterized before specific assays for neutrophil dysfunction are undertaken.

❑ **Use**

- Neutrophil function tests are used to evaluate neutrophil dysfunction in patients with recurrent bacterial infections, especially in patients with a family history suggestive of a neutrophil dysfunction syndrome. The functions

16

*Submitted By Liberto Pechet, MD.

> **TABLE 16–58. Assays for Suspected Congenital Neutrophil Dysfunction Syndromes**
>
> | Assay | Abnormal in |
> |---|---|
> | NBT slide test: abnormal (negative test) | Chronic granulomatous disease |
> | Decreased chemotaxis (and giant granules) | Chediak-Higashi syndrome |
> | Mo-1, chemotaxis, and bacterial killing are markedly reduced; can be tested also by flow cytometry | Leukocyte adhesion deficiency |
> | Myeloperoxidase (for neutrophils) and lysozyme (for monocytes) | Primary myeloperoxidase deficiency (MYD) |
> | Chemotaxis and antilactoferrin stain of polymorphonuclear neutrophils are markedly reduced | Specific granule deficiency |
> | Chemotaxis and bacterial killing are markedly decreased | Neutrophil actin dysfunction, a genetic disorder |

used to investigate neutrophil dysfunction are adherence, locomotion, phagocytosis, and secretion (see Table 16.58). Morphologic studies are performed in parallel with the functional assays.

▪ Because of the rarity of these conditions, only a limited number are mentioned (see Table 16.58).

NICOTINE/COTININE*

❏ **Definition**

▪ Nicotine is a hygroscopic alkaloid obtained from tobacco. Cotinine is the major metabolite of nicotine.

▪ **Normal range** (serum): Cotinine
  ▼ Nonsmokers: <6 ng/mL
  ▼ Cigarette smokers: 10–50 ng/mL

❏ **Use**

▪ Insecticide and fumigant
▪ Constituent of tobacco products
▪ Constituent of smoking cessation products

❏ **Interpretation**

▪ Serum cotinine concentrations may be up to 10 times greater than corresponding nicotine level in smokers.
▪ Urine nicotine and cotinine concentrations in smokers are typically >1,000 ng/mL.

❏ **Limitations**

▪ Screening tests are immunoassay based typically target cotinine with a cutoff concentration of 100–500 ng/mL (for urine). Test may cross-react with 3-hydroxy cotinine.

*Submitted By Amanda J. Jenkins, PhD.

NONINVASIVE PRENATAL TESTING (NIPT)

See Prenatal Screening, Noninvasive.

OCCULT BLOOD, STOOL

❑ **Definition**

- Occult bleeding refers to the initial presentation of a positive fecal occult blood test (FOBT) result and/or iron deficiency anemia, when there is no evidence of visible blood loss to the patient or physician. The differential diagnosis for occult GI bleeding is broad. Some of the more common causes include colon cancer, esophagitis, peptic ulcers, gastritis, inflammatory bowel disease, vascular ectasias, portal hypertensive gastropathy, and gastric antral vascular ectasias. However, less common causes such as gastroesophageal cancers, hemosuccus pancreaticus, hemobilia, and infections also need to be considered. Non-GI sources of blood loss such as hemoptysis and epistaxis can also cause a positive FOBT. FOBT falls into two primary categories based on the detected analyte: guaiac based (gFOBT) and immunoassay based (FIT). gFOBT are the most common stool blood tests in use for colorectal cancer screening, and they detect blood in the stool through the pseudoperoxidase activity of heme or hemoglobin, whereas immunochemical-based tests react to human globin.
- **Normal range:** negative.

❑ **Use**

- Screens for carcinomas (particularly colon) and polyps of the GI tract
- Identifies GI bleeding related to upper GI bleeding (gastric ulcer)
- Screens for diverticulitis and colitis

❑ **Interpretation**

Increased In

- GI malignancies (colon)
- Diverticular disease
- GI polyps
- Ischemic bowel disease
- Inflammatory lesions (ulcerative colitis, Crohn disease, shigellosis, amebiasis)
- Trauma, bleeding diatheses
- Vasculitis (polyarteriosis nodosa, Henoch purpura, Schönlein purpura)
- Amyloidosis
- Hiatal hernia
- Neurofibromatosis
- Kaposi sarcoma
- Hematobilia

❑ **Limitations**

- If using guaiac-based test, individuals should be instructed to avoid aspirin and other NSAIDs, vitamin C, red meat, poultry, fish, and some raw

16

vegetables because of diet–test interactions that can increase the risk of both false-positive and false-negative (specifically, vitamin C) results.

▪ The sensitivity and specificity of a gFOBT has been shown to be highly variable and varies based on the brand or variant of the test; specimen collection technique; number of samples collected per test; whether or not the stool specimen is rehydrated; and variations in interpretation, screening interval, and other factors.

▪ A gFOBT test must be performed properly with three stool samples obtained at home. A single-stool sample FOBT collected after digital rectal examination in the office is not an acceptable screening test, and it is not recommended.

▪ FIT has several technologic advantages when compared with gFOBT. FIT detects Hb; therefore, it is more specific for human blood than guaiac-based tests are. In addition, because globin is degraded by digestive enzymes in the upper GI tract, FIT also are more specific for lower GI bleeding, thus improving their specificity for colorectal cancer. At this time, the optimal number of FIT stool samples is not established, but two samples may be superior to one.

▪ Drugs causing intestinal bleeding (e.g., aspirin, corticosteroids, and NSAIDs) and drugs causing colitis (e.g., methyldopa and a variety of antibiotics) can cause positive test results.

Suggested Reading

Levin B, Lieberman DA, McFarland B, et al. Screening and Surveillance for the Early Detection of Colorectal Cancer and Adenomatous Polyps, 2008: A Joint Guideline from the American Cancer Society, the US Multi-Society Task Force on Colorectal Cancer, and the American College of Radiology. *CA Cancer J Clin.* 2008;58:130–160.

OPIATES

See opioids.

OPIOIDS*

❑ Definition

▪ Opioids are natural and semisynthetic alkaloids prepared from opium and synthetic compounds whose pharmacologic properties, rather than structure, mimic morphine.

▪ Specific names: heroin, codeine, morphine, oxycodone, oxymorphone, hydrocodone, hydromorphone, buprenorphine, methadone, meperidine, propoxyphene (withdrawn from the US market), nalbuphine, fentanyl, levorphanol, butorphanol, pentazocine, tapentadol, tramadol.

▪ There is no single test that will screen for/confirm all the opioids listed.

▪ **Normal range:** drug and use dependent.

❑ Use

▪ Treatment of pain, usually moderate to severe
▪ Preoperative sedation

---

*Submitted By Amanda J. Jenkins, PhD.

- Postoperative analgesia and surgical and medical emergencies including myocardial infarction, trauma, burns, orthopedic pain
- Management of chronic pain associated with cancer
- Antitussive and antidiarrheal agent
- Detoxification and maintenance therapy of opiate addicts

❑ **Limitations**

- Screening
  - ▼ Typically performed in urine
  - ▼ Immunoassay-based technology performed on automated chemistry analyzers
    - EIA (KIMS, CEDIA), EMIT, RIA, FPIA
    - Qualitative
    - Target: morphine, morphine–glucuronide
      - These "opiate" assays *do not detect* the semi/synthetic opioids, which include buprenorphine, methadone, meperidine, propoxyphene, nalbuphine, fentanyl, levorphanol, butorphanol, pentazocine, tapentadol, and tramadol.
      - These "opiate" assays have variable cross-reactivity with oxycodone, oxymorphone, hydrocodone, and hydromorphone.
      - Cutoff concentration—user defined.
        - ○ 300 ng/mL
        - ○ 2,000 ng/mL
  - ▼ Specific immunoassays are available for individual synthetic compounds.
    - **Oxycodone:** cutoff concentration 100 ng/mL; depending on the manufacturer, may exhibit approximately 100% cross-reactivity with oxymorphone
    - **Methadone:** cutoff concentration 300 ng/mL; depending on the manufacturer, may exhibit approximately 40% cross-reactivity with methadol
    - **Buprenorphine:** cutoff concentration 5 ng/mL; typically do not exhibit cross-reactivity with norbuprenorphine
    - **Propoxyphene:** cutoff concentration 300 ng/mL; depending on the manufacturer, may exhibit approximately 60% cross-reactivity with norpropoxyphene
    - Variable cross-reactivity with opioid metabolites
  - ▼ Several vendors offer assays in semiquantitative mode.
  - ▼ Immunoassay available specifically for heroin metabolite-6-acetylmorphine: cutoff concentration 10 ng/mL; <1% cross reactivity with morphine, codeine, and synthetic opioids
- Screening in blood, serum
  - ▼ Immunoassay-based technology (FPIA, ELISA, RIA)
  - ▼ Opioid specific except for general "opiates," which targets morphine with a cutoff concentration typically of 10 ng/mL
  - ▼ Target (cutoff concentration)
    - Fentanyl <1 ng/mL
    - Methadone 10–50 ng/mL; <5% cross-reactivity with methadol
    - Oxycodone 10–50 ng/mL; >50% cross-reactivity with oxymorphone
    - D-Propoxyphene 10–50 ng/mL; >400% cross-reactivity with norpropoxyphene

16

- Confirmation/quantitation in serum, urine
  - ▼ Confirmation of urine samples often includes hydrolysis to cleave the glucuronide bond. In this case, the concentration provided is total drug (compared with free or unbound drug).
  - ▼ Common opioid confirmation profiles will include 6-acetylmorphine, morphine, codeine, oxycodone, oxymorphone, hydrocodone, and hydromorphone with limit of quantitation drug dependent but ranging 5–25 ng/mL.
  - ▼ Most synthetic opioids require individual specific tests for confirmation and quantitation; for potent low-dose synthetic opioids such as buprenorphine and fentanyl, the limit of quantitation is ≤1 ng/mL.
  - ▼ Sample preparation required: liquid–liquid or solid-phase extraction.
  - ▼ Testing methodologies: gas chromatography, HPLC, GC/MS, LC/MSn (multiple Sn).

OSMOLAL GAP

❏ Definition

- The osmolal gap is a mathematical concept similar to the AG that is used to detect concentration changes in osmotically active solutes rather than ion changes. The osmolal gap is calculated by subtracting the calculated osmolality from the measured osmolality.
- **Normal range: <10 mOsm/kg.**

❏ Use

- Osmolal gap has been used to estimate the blood alcohol. Serum osmolality increases 22 mOsm/kg for every 100 mg/dL of ethanol; therefore, estimated blood alcohol (mg/dL) = osmolal gap × 100 ÷ 22.

❏ Interpretation
Increased In

- Decreased serum water content:
  - ▼ Hyperlipidemia (serum will appear lipemic)
  - ▼ Hyperproteinemia (total protein >10 g/dL)
- Additional low molecular weight substances in the serum (measured osmolality is >300 mOsm/kg water).
- Ethanol; an especially large osmolal gap with a low or only moderately elevated ethanol level should raise the possibility of another low molecular weight toxin (e.g., methanol).
  - ▼ Methanol
  - ▼ Isopropyl alcohol
  - ▼ Mannitol (osmolal gap can be used to detect accumulation of infused mannitol in serum)
  - ▼ Ethylene glycol, acetone, ketoacidosis, and paraldehyde result in relatively small osmolal gaps, even at lethal levels
- Severely ill patients, especially those in shock, acidosis (lactic, diabetic, alcoholic), renal failure.

❑ **Limitations**
- Laboratory analytic error
  ▼ Random error from all measurements could add or subtract ≤15 mOsm/kg
  ▼ Use of incorrect blood collection tubes

OSMOLALITY, SERUM AND URINE

❑ **Definition**
- Osmolality refers to the osmotic concentration of a fluid. The osmolality of serum, urine, or any other body fluid depends on the number of active ions or molecules in a solution and yield important information about a patient's ability to maintain a normal fluid balance status. Osmolality is measured with an osmometer by freezing point depression or vapor pressure elevation techniques, or it can be calculated from a formula.
- Osmolarity is the osmotic concentration of solution expressed as osmoles of solute per liter of solution or the property of solution that depends on the concentration of solute per unit of total volume of solvent.
- Serum osmolality measures the amount of chemicals dissolved in the blood. Chemicals that affect serum osmolality include sodium, chloride, bicarbonate, proteins, and glucose. A serum osmolality test is done to evaluate electrolyte and water balance. Serum osmolality is controlled partly by ADH or vasopressin. ADH is produced by the hypothalamus and is released by the pituitary gland into the blood.
- Urine osmolality reflects the total number of osmotically active particles in the urine, without regard to the size or weight of the particles. Substances such as glucose, proteins, or dyes increase the urine specific gravity. Therefore, urine osmolality is a more accurate measurement of urine concentration than specific gravity, and urine osmolality can be compared with the serum osmolality to obtain an accurate picture of a patient's fluid balance.
- **Normal range:** see Table 16.59.

❑ **Use**
- Evaluate the balance between the water and the chemicals dissolved in blood.
- Determine whether severe dehydration or overhydration is present.
- Help determine if the hypothalamus is producing ADH normally.
- Help determine the cause of seizures or coma. In severe cases, an imbalance between water and electrolytes in the body can cause seizures or coma.
- Screen for the ingestion of certain poisons, such as isopropanol, methanol, or ethylene glycol.
- Evaluate concentrating ability of the kidneys.

TABLE 16–59. Normal Ranges for Osmolality		
	Reference Range (mOsm/kg)	**Critical Range (mOsm/kg)**
Serum or plasma	279–295	<250, >295
Urine	500–800	None

16

- Evaluate electrolyte and water balance.
- Used in workup for renal disease, SIADH, and diabetes insipidus.
- May be used with urinalysis when patient has had radiopaque substances, has glycosuria, or proteinuria
- Evaluate dehydration, amyloidosis. Osmolality is desirable in examination of neonatal urine when protein or glucose is present.

❏ **Interpretation**

Increased In

- Hyperglycemia
- DKA (osmolality should be determined routinely in grossly unbalanced diabetic patients)
- Nonketotic hyperglycemic coma
- Hypernatremia with dehydration
  - ▼ Diarrhea, vomiting, fever, hyperventilation, inadequate water intake
  - ▼ Diabetes insipidus—central
  - ▼ Nephrogenic diabetes insipidus—congenital or acquired (e.g., hypercalcemia, hypokalemia, chronic renal disease, sickle cell disease, effect of some drugs)
  - ▼ Osmotic diuresis—hyperglycemia, administration of urea or mannitol
- Hypernatremia with normal hydration—caused by hypothalamic disorders
  - ▼ Insensitivity of osmoreceptors (essential hypernatremia)—water loading does not return serum osmolality to normal; chlorpropamide may lower serum sodium toward normal
  - ▼ Defect in thirst (hypodipsia)—forced water intake returns serum osmolality to normal
- Hypernatremia with overhydration—iatrogenic or accidental (e.g., infants given feedings with high sodium concentrations or given $NaHCO_3$ for respiratory distress or cardiopulmonary arrest)
- Alcohol ingestion, which is the most common cause of hyperosmolar state and of coexisting coma and hyperosmolar state

Decreased In

- Hyponatremia with hypovolemia (urine sodium is usually >20 mmol/L)
  - ▼ Adrenal insufficiency (e.g., salt-losing form of CAH, congenital adrenal hypoplasia, hemorrhage into adrenals, inadequate replacement of corticosteroids, inappropriate tapering of steroids)
  - ▼ Renal losses (e.g., osmotic diuresis; proximal RTA; salt-losing nephropathies, usually tubulointerstitial diseases such as GU tract obstruction; pyelonephritis; medullary cystic disease; polycystic kidneys)
  - ▼ GI tract loss (e.g., vomiting, diarrhea)
  - ▼ Other losses (e.g., burns, peritonitis, pancreatitis)
- Hyponatremia with normal volume or hypervolemia (dilutional syndromes)
  - ▼ CHF, cirrhosis, nephrotic syndrome
  - ▼ SIADH

❏ **Limitations**

Variations in the urine osmolality play a central role in the regulation of the plasma osmolality and Na+ concentration. This response is mediated by osmoreceptors in the hypothalamus that influence both thirst and the secretion of ADH.

TABLE 16–60. The Relationship Between Serum and Urine Osmolality and the Clinical Significance of Laboratory Values

Serum Osmolality	Urine Osmolality	Clinical Significance
Normal values: 282–295 mOsm	Normal values: 500–800 mOsm	
Normal or increased	Increased	Fluid volume deficit
Decreased	Decreased	Fluid volume excess
Normal	Decreased	Increased fluid intake or diuretics
Increased or normal	Decreased (with no increase in fluid intake)	Kidneys unable to concentrate urine or lack of ADH (diabetes insipidus)
Decreased	Increased	SIADH

The relationship between serum and urine osmolality and the clinical significance of laboratory values are shown in Table 16.60.

$$(1.86 \times \text{serum Na}) + (\text{serum glucose} \div 18) + (\text{BUN} \div 28) + 9 (\text{in mg} / \text{dL})$$

or

in SI units: $= (1.86 \times \text{serum Na}) + \text{serum glucose (mmol/L)} + \text{BUN (mmol/L)} + 9$

- More simply: $NA^+ + K^+ + (BUN \div 28) + (\text{glucose} \div 18)$. Because K^+ is relatively small, and BUN has no influence on water distribution, the formula can be simplified to $2Na^+ + (\text{glucose} \div 18)$.

OSMOLALITY, STOOL

❑ **Definition**

- Measurement of osmolality of stool samples is helpful in evaluating patients with diarrhea. In normal stool, most small molecular weight substances are totally absorbed (except for electrolytes); thus, most of the osmotic activity of stool comes from electrolytes. A stool osmotic gap has been defined as the difference between the measured osmolality and a calculated osmolality (determined as two times the sum of Na and K ions in stool)
- **Normal range:**
  ▼ **0–16 years: 271–296 mOsm/kg**
  ▼ **17 years and older: 280–303 mOsm/kg**

❑ **Use**

- Determines if chronic diarrhea is osmotic or secretory in nature.

❑ **Interpretation**

- A fecal sodium >90 mmol/L and an osmolal gap <50 mOsm/kg suggests secretory diarrhea or osmotic diarrhea due to sodium-containing laxatives.
- A fecal sodium <60 mmol/L and an osmolal gap >100 mOsm/kg suggests osmotic diarrhea.
- Fecal sodium >150 mmol/L and osmolality >400 mOsm/kg suggests contamination with concentrated urine.

16

- Fecal osmolality <250 mOsm/kg suggests contamination with hypoosmotic urine or water.

Increased In
- Causes of osmotic diarrhea include:
  ▼ Bile salt deficiency
  ▼ Pancreatic insufficiency
  ▼ Celiac/tropical sprue
  ▼ Whipple disease
  ▼ Intestinal lymphoma
  ▼ Medications
  ▼ Lactose intolerance

Decreased In
- NA

❏ Limitations
- Formed stool is not a suitable specimen.

PARATHYROID HORMONE (PTH)

❏ Definition
- Peptide hormone secreted by parathyroid gland chief cells that controls ionized calcium levels in blood and body fluids by increasing 1,25-dihydroxyvitamin D_3 (by the kidney), mobilizing calcium from bone (due to increased osteoclast activity), increasing renal tubular resorption of calcium, and reducing renal clearance of calcium, increasing intestinal calcium absorption. The half-life of PTH is <5 minutes. Ionized calcium in blood inhibits PTH secretion. Biologic activity resides in the first 34 terminal amino acids. The intact hormone has 84 amino acids but can be quickly cleaved by proteolysis into smaller less-active fragments. Assay for the intact PTH has largely superseded tests for various PTH fragments. It is important that the PTH assay not cross-react with PTH (7-84) lacking the 6-N-terminal, which has been shown to be a weak antagonist to PTH activity and may lower serum and plasma calcium levels.
- **Normal range: 12–65 pg/mL.**

❏ Use
- Differential diagnosis of hyperparathyroidism and hypoparathyroidism.
- Very sensitive in detecting PTH suppression by 1,25-dihydroxyvitamin D; therefore, used for monitoring that treatment of chronic renal failure.
- Intraoperative PTH assay to determine removal of abnormally secreting tissue; may replace routine frozen section; can replace traditional four-gland explorations and distinguishes single from multiglandular disease.
- Preoperative and 10–20 minutes postresection assay; this causes 50–75% reduction, indicating successful resection of parathyroid adenoma.

❏ Interpretation
Increased In
- Primary and secondary hyperparathyroidism

- Pseudohypoparathyroidism
- Hereditary vitamin D dependency types 1 and 2, vitamin D deficiency
- Z-E syndrome
- Familial medullary thyroid carcinoma
- MEN types I, IIa, and IIb

Decreased In
- Autoimmune hypoparathyroidism
- Sarcoidosis
- Nonparathyroid hypercalcemia in the absence of renal failure
- Hyperthyroidism
- Hypomagnesemia
- Transient neonatal hypocalcemia
- DiGeorge syndrome

❑ **Limitations**
- At this time, there are significant intermethod variations in PTH results for different manufacturer assays. This is mainly due to cross-reactivity with various PTH fragments of the assay.
- The finding of a persistently high-normal calcium accompanied by a high-normal PTH (alternatively, a low-normal calcium accompanied by a low-normal PTH) warrants further investigation; for the PTH, although itself within normal limits, may still be inappropriately high (or inappropriately low) relative to the circulating calcium level.
- Because of a pronounced nocturnal rise in intact PTH levels observed in a small experimental male population, sampling after 10 AM for optimum discrimination between normals and those with mild primary hyperparathyroidism has been suggested.
- Sedative–hypnotic drug propofol (Diprivan) may give falsely low PTH values.
- High concentrations of hemolysis, lipemia, and bilirubin should be avoided.
- Rapid intraoperative PTH that declines ≥50% from the highest baseline in 10 minutes after resection indicates successful total excision.

PARATHYROID HORMONE–RELATED PEPTIDE (PTHrP)

❑ **Definition**
- PTHrP is a protein secreted by some cancer cells leading to humoral hypercalcemia of malignancy (HHM). It shares the same 13 N-terminal amino acids as PTH; however, the remaining structure is different. PTHrP is larger than PTH and contains 139–173 amino acids compared to 84 for PTH. PTHrP shares many actions with PTH leading to increased calcium release from bone, reduced renal calcium excretion, and reduced renal phosphate reabsorption. However, PTHrP does not produce the normal anion gap metabolic acidosis commonly found with hyperparathyroidism. See Tables 16.61–16.63 and Figures 16.2 and 16.3.
- **Normal value:** <1.3 pmol/L.

16

> ### TABLE 16–61. Serum Calcium and PTH in Various Conditions
>
> | | PTH Increased | PTH Not Increased |
> |---|---|---|
> | **Serum calcium decreased*** | Secondary hyperparathyroidism (chronic renal disease) | Hypoparathyroidism (surgical, autoimmunity, hormone resistance, magnesium deficiency) |
> | **Serum calcium increased†** | Primary hyperparathyroidism, familial hypocalciuric hypercalcemia, lithium-induced hypercalcemia, tertiary hyperparathyroidism | HHM, milk-alkali syndrome, thiazide diuretics, vitamin D or A intoxication, granulomatous diseases (sarcoidosis, TB), multiple myeloma, thyrotoxicosis, immobilization |
> | **Serum calcium normal** | Pregnancy nephrolithiasis, secondary hyperparathyroidism (chronic renal disease) | Normal |

HHM, humoral hypercalcemia of malignancy; PTH, parathyroid hormone.
*PTH may be normal or increased in hypocalcemic patients due to renal failure, acute pancreatitis, vitamin D deficiency.
†PTH may be normal or increased in hypercalcemic patients due to acromegaly, vitamin A intoxication, MEN type IIA, RTA, chronic renal failure.

❏ Use

- PTHrP is useful clinically in differentiating primary hyperthyroidism from HHM. Also useful as a marker in the management of patients with tumor-associated hypercalcemia.
- The usual pattern of HHM is elevated total and ionized calcium, low PTH in the absence of other causes of hypercalcemia (e.g., excessive vitamin D, sarcoid, TB). If the presence of a malignancy is uncertain, or there are several possible causes for hypercalcemia, measurement of PTHrP can be of assistance.
- HHM occurs in patients with cancer (typically squamous, transitional cell, renal, ovarian), 5–20% who have no bone metastases compared to patients with widespread bone metastases (myeloma, lymphoma, breast cancer).
- HHM occurs in approximately 20–35% of patients with breast cancer, approximately 10–15% of cases with lung cancer, approximately 70% of cases with multiple myeloma, and rare in lymphoma and leukemia.
- Rarely hypercalcemia may occur in association with benign tumors (e.g., pheochromocytoma, dermoid cyst of the ovary) ("humoral hypercalcemia of benignancy").
- Very high serum calcium (e.g., >14.5 mg/dL) is much more suggestive of HHM than primary HPT; less marked increase with renal tumors. Less than or equal to 5% of hypercalcemia patients have simultaneous HPT and HHM.

❏ Interpretation

Increased In

- Increased serum PTHrP (>2.6 pmol/L) can make a positive diagnosis in most cases of HHM, but approximately 20% of cancer patients with hypercalcemia have only local osteolytic changes with no increased PTHrP.
- PTHrP is also increased in (>2.6 pmol/L)
  - ▼ Greater than 80% of hypercalcemic patients with solid tumors with or without bone metastasis.

TABLE 16–62. Laboratory Findings in Various Diseases of Calcium and Phosphorus Metabolism

Disease	Serum Calcium*	Serum Phosphorus	Serum ALP	Urine Calcium†	Urine Phosphorus	Serum PTH	Serum 1,25-Dihydroxyvitamin D
Primary hyperparathyroidism	I	D (<3 mg/dL in 50%)	I slightly in 50% (N if no bone disease)	I in two thirds	I	I	I
Humoral hypercalcemia of malignancy	I; frequently marked	D in 50%	Frequently I	I	I	D	D
Familial hypocalciuric hypercalcemia	Mild I	N or slightly D	N	D or low; N		I or inappropriately N	Proportional to PTH
Hypoparathyroidism	D	I	N	D	D‡	D	D
Pseudohypoparathyroidism	D	I	N; occasionally D	D	D‡	N or I	D
Pseudohypoparathyroidism	N	N	N	N	N	N	
Secondary hyperparathyroidism (renal rickets)	D or N	I	I or N	D or I	D	I	D
Vitamin D excess	I	N	D	I	I	D	I
Rickets and osteomalacia	D or N	D or N	I	D	D	I	D
Osteoporosis	N	N	N or I	N or I	N		
Polyostotic fibrous dysplasia	N	N	I	N or I	N		
Paget disease	N or I	N or I	N or I	V			
Metastatic neoplasm to bone	N or I	V	N or I	N or I	N or I		
Multiple myeloma	N or I	V	N or I	N or I	N or I		I
Sarcoidosis	N or I	N or I	N or I	I	I		
Fanconi syndrome or renal loss of fixed base	D or N	D	I	D or I	I	D	D
Histiocytosis X (Letterer-Siwe disease, Hand-Schüller-Christian disease, eosinophilic granuloma)	N	N	N or I	N or I	N		
Hypercalcemia and excess intake of alkali (Burnett syndrome)	I	I or N	N	N	N		
Solitary bone cyst	N	N	N	N	N		N

D, decreased; I, increased; N, normal; V, variable.
*Serum calcium. Repeated determinations may be required to demonstrate abnormalities. Serum total protein level should always be known. See also response to cortisone.
†Urine calcium. The patient should be on a low-calcium diet (e.g., Bauer-Aub).
‡See Ellsworth-Howard test.

TABLE 16–63. Comparison of Primary Hyperparathyroidism (HPT) and Humoral Hypercalcemia of Malignancy (HHM)

	HHM	HPT
Etiology	Squamous or large cell carcinoma of the bronchus, hypernephroma of the kidney, cancer of the ovary, colon, others	Primary hyperplasia, adenoma, carcinoma of the parathyroids
Serum calcium	Very high: >14 mg/dL in 75% of patients Suppressed by cortisone in 25–50% of patients	Moderately high: >14 mg/dL in 25% of patients Suppressed by cortisone in 50% of cases with and 23% of cases without osteitis fibrosa
Serum PTH	Decreased	Increased
Serum PTHRP	Increased	Not increased
Serum chloride	Low: <99 mEq/L	High: >102 mEq/L
Serum chloride phosphorus ratio	<30	>33
Serum bicarbonate	Increased or normal	Normal or low
pH	Alkalosis	Acidosis
Serum ALP	Increased in 50% of patients, even without bone disease	Seldom increased unless bone disease is present
Serum phosphorus	Increased, normal, or low	Normal or low
Urine calcium	Often >400 mg/24 h	Usually <400 mg/24 h
Serum 1,25-dihydroxyvitamin D	Decreased	Increased
Urine cAMP	Increased in HHM but not due to bone metastases only	Increased in 90% of cases
ESR	Usually increased	Normal
Anemia	May be present	Absent
Serum albumin	Often decreased	Usually normal
Renal stones	Absent	Common
Pancreatitis	Rare	Occurs
Radiographic changes in hand bones	Absent	May be present

▼ Some patients with hypercalcemia and hematologic cancers.
▼ Approximately 10% of cancers without hypercalcemia; PTHrP becomes normal when hypercalcemia is corrected by treatment of cancer.
■ May be increased in nonmalignant pheochromocytoma.

Normal In
■ Healthy persons: values <1.0 pmol/L.
■ Other causes of hypercalcemia (e.g., sarcoidosis, vitamin D intoxication).
■ Low-normal or suppressed intact PTH (<20 pg/mL) excludes hyperparathyroidism.
■ Serum 1,25-dihydroxyvitamin D is usually decreased or low-normal in HHM but is increased in HPT.

❏ Limitations
■ Production of PTHrP by the fetoplacental unit can cause transient increase during pregnancy, especially in the third semester.

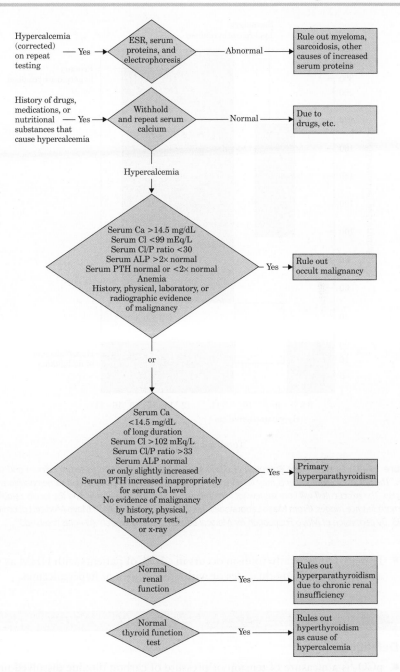

Figure 16–2 *Algorithm for diagnosis of hypercalcemia. (ESR, erythrocyte sedimentation rate; PTH, parathyroid hormone.) (Data from Wong ET, Freier EF. The differential diagnosis of hypercalcemia: an algorithm for more effective use of laboratory tests. JAMA. 1982;247:75 and Johnson KR, Howarth AT. Differential laboratory diagnosis of hypercalcemia. CRC Crit Rev Clin La Sci. 1984;21:51.)*

16

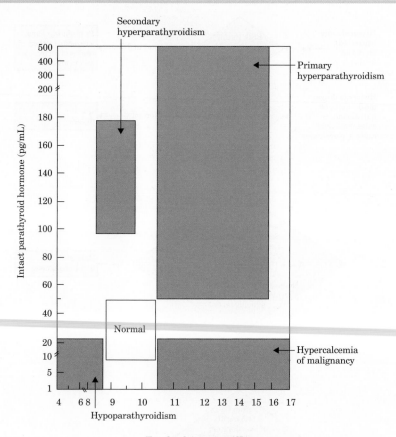

Figure 16–3 *Diagrammatic illustration of distribution of patients according to serum calcium and serum PTH. The values of some patients may lie outside the exact boundaries indicated, and some conditions may overlap. The exact cutoff will vary somewhat with the assays used, the patient mix, and the locally established normal reference ranges. (From* Mayo Laboratories Test Catalog. *Rochester, MN: Mayo Medical Laboratories; 1995. By permission of Mayo Foundation for Medical Education and Research. All rights reserved.)*

- Primary hyperparathyroidism occurs in ≤10% of patients with HHM as well as in those receiving thiazides or with other causes of hypercalcemia.

PARTIAL PRESSURE OF CARBON DIOXIDE (pCO₂), BLOOD

❏ Definition

- pCO_2 is a measure of tension or pressure of carbon dioxide dissolved in the blood. The pCO_2 of blood represents the balance between cellular production of CO_2 and ventilatory removal of CO_2. A normal, steady pCO_2 indicates that the lungs are removing CO_2 at about same rate as tissues producing CO_2. A change on pCO_2 indicates an alteration in this balance, usually due to the change in ventilatory status.

- **Normal range:**
  - ▼ Arterial: 35–45 mm Hg
  - ▼ Venous: 41–51 mm Hg

❏ **Interpretation**

Increased In

- Acute respiratory acidosis
  - ▼ Depression of respiratory center
  - ▼ Suppressed neuromuscular system
  - ▼ Pulmonary disorders
  - ▼ Inadequate mechanical ventilation
- Chronic respiratory acidosis
  - ▼ Decreased alveolar ventilation
  - ▼ Hypoventilation
- Compensation in metabolic alkalosis

Decreased In

- Respiratory alkalosis
  - ▼ Increased stimulation of respiratory center
  - ▼ Hypermetabolic states
  - ▼ Mechanical hyperventilation
- Compensation in metabolic acidosis

❏ **Limitations**

- Respiratory conditions will primarily affect pCO_2, whereas metabolic disturbances are first reflected in the HCO_3^-.
- Values are slightly lower in supine position.
- Difference between arterial blood and venous blood varies considerably, depending on the skin temperature, length of stasis, and muscular activity.

PARTIAL PRESSURE OF OXYGEN (pO₂), BLOOD

❏ **Definition**

- The partial pressure of oxygen (pO_2) is a measure of the tension or pressure of oxygen dissolved in the blood. The pO_2 of arterial blood is primarily related to the ability of the lungs to oxygenate blood from alveolar air.
- **Normal range:**
  - ▼ Arterial: >80–95 mm Hg (see Table 16.64)
  - ▼ Venous: 35–40 mm Hg

TABLE 16–64. Arterial pO₂	
Age (years)	**Range (mm Hg)**
0–14	>95
15–30	>96
31–50	>91
51–70	>85
71–110	>80

16

❏ **Use**

- ▪ To evaluate patients with pulmonary or acid–base disturbances
- ▪ To monitor patients with carbon monoxide poisoning, methemoglobinemia, or hemoglobin variant for O_2 saturation
- ▪ To manage patients on mechanical respirators
- ▪ Prior to thoracic or general surgery

❏ **Interpretation**

Increased In

- ▪ Decreased ventilation
  - ▼ Airway obstruction
  - ▼ Drug overdose
  - ▼ Metabolic disorders (e.g., myxedema, hypokalemia)
  - ▼ Neurologic disorders (e.g., Guillain-Barré syndrome, multiple sclerosis)
  - ▼ Muscle disorders (e.g., muscular dystrophy, polymyositis)
  - ▼ Chest wall abnormalities (e.g., scoliosis)
- ▪ Increased dead space in the lungs (perfusion decreased more than ventilation decreased)
  - ▼ Lung diseases (e.g., COPD, asthma, pulmonary fibrosis, mucoviscidosis)
  - ▼ Chest wall changes affecting lung parenchyma (e.g., scoliosis)
- ▪ Increased production (e.g., sepsis, fever, seizures, excess carbohydrate loads)

Decreased In

- ▪ Hypoventilation (e.g., chronic airflow obstruction): caused by increased alveolar CO_2 that displaces O_2.
- ▪ Alveolar hypoxia (e.g., high altitude, gaseous inhalation).
- ▪ Pulmonary diffusion abnormalities (e.g., interstitial lung disease): Supplemental oxygen usually improves pO_2.
- ▪ Right-to-left shunt: Supplemental oxygen has no effect; requires positive end-expiratory pressure.
  - ▼ Congenital anomalies of the heart and great vessels
  - ▼ Acquired (e.g., ARDS)
- ▪ Ventilation—perfusion mismatch: Supplemental O_2 usually improves pO_2.
  - ▼ Airflow obstruction (e.g., COPD, asthma)
  - ▼ Interstitial inflammation (e.g., pneumonia, sarcoidosis)
  - ▼ Vascular obstruction (e.g., PE)
- ▪ Decreased venous oxygenation (e.g., anemia).
- ▪ Cyanosis is clearly visible at pO_2 <40 mm Hg; may be seen at 50 mm Hg depending on skin pigmentation.

❏ **Limitations**

- ▪ Capillary blood is not suitable for estimation of high arterial pO_2 values.
- ▪ Values measured at 37°C must be corrected to the actual temperature of the patient.
- ▪ Drugs causing respiratory depression, for example, barbiturates, diazepam, heron, meperidine, and midazolam, cause decrease in pO_2.

PARTIAL THROMBOPLASTIN TIME (PTT, aPTT)*

❑ **Definition**

- The PTT assesses the coagulation activity of the intrinsic and common pathways of coagulation. It is the best *screening* test for the diagnosis of disorders of coagulation that do not involve factor VII (extrinsic pathway) or platelet function. The conventional prefix "activated" is obsolete; there is no nonactivated PTT in use. The "activation" reflects a technical aspect of the assay because the reagents contain a negatively charged surface that accelerates the rate of the reaction.
- **Normal range:** 22.3–34.0 seconds (varies slightly from lot to lot of reagent, type of the commercial reagent used, and equipment).

❑ **Use**

- Screening for hemophilia A and B and other possible coagulopathies (except factors VII and XIII). PTT is not affected by single clotting factor defects above 40% of normal.
- Detection of clotting inhibitors: This is best performed by mixing studies once an otherwise unexplained prolonged PTT is found. **Mixing equal parts of patient and normal plasma (1:1) for 1–2 hours at 37°C** normalizes the prolonged PTT if it is caused by a coagulation factor deficiency but *not if it is caused by an inhibitor.* The inhibitor is commonly a factor VIII inhibitor; LA can also prolong the PTT if LA-sensitive reagents are used.
- Monitoring of therapy with unfractionated heparin. It is not useful in monitoring low molecular weight heparins or fondaparinux; these anticoagulants can be monitored with anti-Xa assay.
- Not recommended for preoperative screening in patients without a personal or immediate family history of unprovoked bleeding.

❑ **Interpretation**

Increased (>36 seconds) In

- Single clotting factor deficiencies, the most common being factor VIII deficiency
- Inhibitors
- Therapy with unfractionated heparin
- Therapy with warfarin (variable response)
- Therapy with antithrombin agents such as hirudin and its derivatives, argatroban, and newer antithrombin (e.g., dabigatran), as well as anti-Xa agents (e.g., rivaroxaban)
- High-titer LA
- Moderate to severe von Willebrand disease

Decreased (<22 seconds) In

- Excessive generation of thrombin. No clinical correlation with a predisposition to thromboembolism has been definitely demonstrated.

16

*Submitted By Liberto Pechet, MD.

Normal In
- Thrombocytopenias and thrombocytopathies without associated clotting defects
- Majority of cases of mild von Willebrand disease
- Isolated defects of factor VII or XIII

❏ Limitations
Preanalytic Pitfalls
- Partial clotting of sample due to insufficient mixture with anticoagulant
- Overfilling or underfilling the test tube, thereby changing the 9 (blood)-to-1 (anticoagulant) ratio
- Use of wrong anticoagulant rather than the recommended 3.2% sodium citrate (currently used in blue top tubes)

Analytic Pitfalls
- Hemolyzed, severely icteric, or hyperlipemic blood may affect results (modern equipment may override icteric or hyperlipidemic blood)

Other Limitations: Drugs
- Short values may be seen with estrogen therapy or oral contraceptives.
- Prolonged values may result from diphenylhydantoin, naloxone, and radiographic contrast agents.

PERIPHERAL BLOOD SMEARS (PBS)*

❏ Definition
- The primary purpose of studying PBS is to obtain differential counts of WBC and to study blood cell morphology.

❏ Use
- Blood collected for CBC is prepared manually (or by automated equipment), smearing a thin layer of blood on a glass slide, and then staining with special dyes for microscopic examinations. They are most helpful for the rapid identification of anemias, leukemias, and platelet abnormalities. PBS are also studied for the presence of organisms. When malaria is suspected, the PBS (thin smear) is most useful in finding and identifying parasites (thick film: a concentrated technique by which a large amount of blood is placed in a small area; it is used in cases with sparse parasites).
- Special stains may be added to provide additional diagnostic information:
  - ▼ Leukocyte (neutrophil) alkaline phosphatase: normal range is 11–95. It is an absolute value derived for counting the leukocyte granules at the microscope. It is used primarily to differentiate between CML and leukocytosis of other etiologies. It is decreased in myeloid cells of CML patients and in some cases of myelodysplastic syndrome, as well as in pernicious anemia and PNH. It is increased in leukemoid reactions and myeloproliferative neoplasms.

---

*Submitted By Liberto Pechet, MD.

▼ Myeloperoxidase: Stains primary granules of neutrophils and secondary granules of eosinophils, identifying myeloid lineage (helpful for blast lineage identification in leukemias).

▼ Specific (naphthol AS-D chloroacetate esterase) identifies cells of myeloid series but not monocytes or lymphocytes.

▼ Nonspecific (α-naphthyl butyrate or α-naphthyl acetate) esterase identifies monocytic cells but does not stain granulocytes or eosinophils. These two stains may be used to identify leukemic lineage.

▼ Iron stain (used as Prussian blue reaction). It identifies iron in nucleated red cells (either as siderocytes or as ringed sideroblasts [myelodysplastic syndromes]); it also identifies Pappenheimer bodies in erythrocytes (RBCs, Table 16.73).

▼ Periodic acid–Schiff (PAS): Detects intracellular glycogen and neutral mucosubstances, which are found in most hematopoietic cells. It is helpful in the diagnosis of erythroleukemia because of the intensity of its diffuse staining in primitive erythroid cells.

❑ Limitations

■ Poorly prepared smears may be difficult to evaluate accurately.

PHOSPHATE, BLOOD

❑ Definition

■ Phosphate is used in the synthesis of phosphorylated compounds. It accompanies glucose into cells. The total body content in normal adults is approximately 700–800 g. About 80–85% of phosphate is contained in bones; the remaining 15–20% is in ICF in tissue as organic phosphates (phospholipids, nucleic acids, NADP, ATP). Only 0.1% is in the ECF as inorganic phosphate, and only this fraction of phosphorus is measured in routine clinical settings.

■ **Normal range:** see Table 16.65.

❑ Use

■ Monitoring of blood phosphate level in renal, endocrine, and GI disorders

❑ Interpretation

Increased In

■ Acute or chronic renal failure (most common cause) with decreased GFR
■ Most causes of hypocalcemia (except vitamin D deficiency, in which it is usually decreased)

TABLE 16–65. Normal Ranges for Phosphate

Age	Reference Range	Critical Range
0–28 d	4.2–9.0 mg/dL	<1.2 mg/dL
28 d–2 y	3.8–6.2 mg/dL	<1.2 or >8.9 mg/dL
2–16 y	3.5–5.9 mg/dL	<1.2 or >8.9 mg/dL
>16 y	2.5–4.5 mg/dL	<1.2 or >8.9 mg/dL

16

- Increased tubular reabsorption or decreased glomerular filtration of phosphate
  - ▼ Hypoparathyroidism (idiopathic, surgical, irradiation)
  - ▼ Secondary hyperparathyroidism (renal rickets)
  - ▼ Pseudohypoparathyroidism types I and II
  - ▼ Other endocrine disorders (e.g., Addison disease, acromegaly, hyperthyroidism)
  - ▼ Sickle cell anemia
- Increased cellular release of phosphate
  - ▼ Neoplasms (e.g., myelogenous leukemia, lymphomas)
  - ▼ Excessive breakdown of tissue (e.g., chemotherapy for neoplasms, rhabdomyolysis, malignant hyperthermia, lactic acidosis, acute yellow atrophy, thyrotoxicosis)
  - ▼ Bone disease (e.g., healing fractures, multiple myeloma [some patients], Paget disease [some patients], osteolytic metastatic tumor in bone [some patients])
  - ▼ Childhood
- Increased phosphate load: exogenous phosphate (oral or IV) form
- Phosphate enemas, laxatives or infusions
- Excess vitamin D intake
- IV therapy for hypophosphatemia or hypercalcemia
- Milk-alkali (Burnett) syndrome (some patients)
- Massive blood transfusions
- Hemolysis of blood
- Miscellaneous
  - ▼ High intestinal obstruction
  - ▼ Sarcoidosis (some patients)

Decreased In

- Primary hypophosphatemia
- Decreased GI absorption
  - ▼ Decreased dietary intake
  - ▼ Decreased intestinal absorption, for example, malabsorption, steatorrhea, secretory diarrhea, vomiting, vitamin D deficiency, drugs (antacids, alcohol, glucocorticoids)
- Decreased renal tubular reabsorption (>100 mg/day in urine during hypophosphatemia indicates excessive renal loss)
  - ▼ Primary (e.g., Fanconi syndrome, rickets [vitamin D deficient or dependent or familial], idiopathic hypercalciuria)
  - ▼ Secondary or acquired tubular disorders (e.g., hypercalcemia, excess PTH, primary hyperparathyroidism, hypokalemia, hypomagnesemia, diuresis, glycosuria, metabolic or respiratory acidosis, metabolic alkalosis, volume expansion, acute gout, dialysis)

- Intracellular shift of phosphate
  - ▼ Osteomalacia, steatorrhea
  - ▼ Growth hormone deficiency
  - ▼ Acute alcoholism
  - ▼ DM
  - ▼ Acidosis (especially DKA)
  - ▼ Hyperalimentation

▼ Nutritional recovery syndrome (rapid refeeding after prolonged starvation)
▼ IV administration of glucose (e.g., recovery after severe burns, hyperalimentation)
▼ Respiratory alkalosis (e.g., gram-negative bacteremia) or metabolic
▼ Salicylate poisoning
▼ Administration of anabolic steroids, androgens, epinephrine, glucagon, insulin
▼ Cushing syndrome (some patients)
▼ Prolonged hypothermia (e.g., open heart surgery)

■ TPN with inadequate phosphate supplementation
■ Refeeding after prolonged starvation (e.g., anorexia nervosa)
■ Thyrotoxic periodic paralysis
■ Sepsis
■ PTH-producing tumors
■ Familial hypocalciuric hypercalcemia
■ Severe malnutrition, malabsorption, severe diarrhea
■ Often more than one mechanism is operative, usually associated with prior phosphorus depletion.

❑ **Limitations**

■ Interference may occur with serum samples from patients diagnosed as having plasma cell dyscrasias and lymphoreticular malignancies associated with abnormal Ig synthesis, such as multiple myeloma, Waldenström macroglobulinemia, and heavy chain disease.
■ Should be measured in fasting morning specimens because of a diurnal variation. Phosphorus has a very strong biphasic circadian rhythm. Values are lowest in the morning, peak first in the late afternoon, and peak again in the late evening. The second peak is quite elevated, and results may be outside the reference range.
■ Levels are influenced by dietary intake, meals, and exercise.

PHOSPHATIDYLGLYCEROL (PG)

❑ **Definition**

■ This minor constituent of pulmonary surfactant begins to increase appreciably in AF several weeks after the rise in lecithin.
■ Because PG enhances the spread of phospholipids on the alveoli, its presence indicates an advanced state of fetal lung development and function.
■ PG determination is not generally affected by blood, meconium, or other contaminants.
■ PG can be performed by TLC, so it can be determined alone or in conjunction with lecithin-to-sphingomyelin testing.
■ It may be reported qualitatively as positive or negative, where positive represents an exceedingly low risk of respiratory distress syndrome (RDS), or in a quantitative fashion, in which a value 0.3 is associated with a minimal rate of respiratory distress.

16

- AmnioStat-FLM is an immunologic qualitative agglutination test for determining the presence of PG in AF. This test is specific, sensitive, and rapid. Results are not affected by moderate blood or meconium contamination. It requires <0.1 mL of specimen, which can be obtained by transabdominal amniocentesis or from a vaginal pool.
- **Normal range:**
  - ▼ Mature fetal lung: positive and weak positive
  - ▼ Immature fetal lung: negative

❏ **Use**

- Assessing fetal lung maturity
- Determining the ability of fetal lungs to produce sufficient quantities of pulmonary surfactant
- Predicting the likelihood of the development of respiratory distress syndrome if the fetus were delivered

❏ **Interpretation**

- Increased in mature fetal lungs
- Decreased in immature fetal lungs

❏ **Limitations**

- AmnioStat-FLM is not subject to artifacts associated with other lung surfactant tests.
- TLC test can produce false-positive test results with meconium contamination and vaginal fluid contamination.
- The absence of PG or low levels of PG cannot dependably predict the presence of RDS.
- Diabetes, regardless of glucose control, delays PG production.

PHOSPHOLIPIDS

❏ **Definition**

- Phospholipids are a class of lipids consisting of a hydrophilic polar head group and a hydrophobic tail. The polar head group contains one or more phosphate groups. The hydrophobic tail is made up of two fatty acyl chains. In an aqueous environment, the hydrophilic heads of the phospholipid molecules tend to face water and the hydrophobic tails bond together, forming a bilayer, which constitutes a major portion and function of cell membranes. Most of the phospholipids in human plasma are phosphatidyl choline (70–75%) or sphingomyelin (18–20%). The remaining phospholipids include phosphatidyl serine, phosphatidyl ethanolamine (3–6%), and lysophosphatidyl choline (4–9%).
- **Normal range:** 150–380 mg/dL.

❏ **Use**

- Aids in the diagnosis of obstructive jaundice, Tangier disease, beta- or hypobetalipoproteinemia, and lecithin cholesterol acyltransferase deficiency.
- Phospholipid analysis rarely provides added beneficial information in cases of dyslipoproteinemia.

❑ **Interpretation**

- Phospholipids are increased in hyperlipidemias and obstructive liver disease.
- They are decreased in Tangier disease.

Suggested Reading

McPherson RA, Pincus MR. Lipids and dyslipoproteinemia (estimation of plasma lipids). In: McPherson RA, Pincus MR (eds.). *Henry's Clinical Diagnosis and Management by Laboratory Methods*, 21st ed. Philadelphia, PA: Saunders Elsevier: 2007:200–218.

PHOSPHATE, URINE

❑ **Definition**

- Phosphate is a charged particle that contains mineral phosphorus. Extra phosphate is filtered through the kidneys and passes out of the body in the urine.
- **Normal range:**
  - ▼ Twenty-four–hour urine: 0.4–1.3 g/day
  - ▼ Random urine:
    - ● Male:
  - ▼ Less than 40 years: 36–1,770 mg/g creatinine
  - ▼ Greater than 40 years: 54–860 mg/g creatinine
    - ● Female:
  - ▼ Less than 40 years: 111–927 mg/g creatinine
  - ▼ Greater than 40 years: 105–1,081 mg/g creatinine

❑ **Use**

- Evaluation of calcium-to-phosphorus balance
- Evaluation of nephrolithiasis

❑ **Interpretation**

Increased In

- Primary hyperparathyroidism
- Humoral hypercalcemia of malignancy
- Vitamin D excess
- Paget disease
- Metastatic neoplasm of the bone
- Fanconi syndrome (renal tubular damage)
- Nonrenal acidosis (increased phosphate excretion as renal buffer)

Decreased In

- Hypoparathyroidism
- Pseudohypoparathyroidism
- Secondary hyperparathyroidism (renal rickets)
- Rickets and osteomalacia
- Parathyroidectomy

❑ **Limitations**

- Interpretation of urinary phosphorus excretion is dependent on the clinical situation and should be interpreted in conjunction with the serum phosphorus concentration.

16

- There is significant diurnal variation in excretion, with values highest in the afternoon.
- Urinary excretion depends on diet.
- Hypophosphatemia with normal serum calcium, high alkaline phosphatase, hypercalciuria, and low urinary phosphorus occurs with osteomalacia from excessive antacid ingestion. Children with thalassemia may have normal phosphorus absorption but high renal phosphaturia, leading to a deficiency of phosphorus.
- Increasing dietary intake of potassium has been reported to increase serum phosphate concentrations apparently by decreasing renal excretion of phosphate. During the last trimester of pregnancy, there is a sixfold increase in calcium and phosphorus accumulation as the fetus triples its weight.
- Plasma phosphorus concentrations and increased urinary phosphate may provide a useful means to assess response to phosphate supplements in the premature infants.

PLASMA RENIN ACTIVITY (PRA)

❏ Definition

- Renin activity is measured indirectly by the ability of the patient's plasma to generate angiotensin.
- **Normal range:**
  - ▼ **Cord blood:** 4.0–32.0 ng/mL/hour
  - ▼ **Newborn (1–7 days):** 2.0–35.0 ng/mL/hour
  - ▼ **Child, normal-sodium diet, supine:**
    - 1–12 months: 2.4–37.0 ng/mL/hour
    - 1–3 years: 1.7–11.2 ng/mL/hour
    - 3–5 years: 1.0–6.5 ng/mL/hour
    - 5–10 years: 0.5–5.9 ng/mL/hour
    - 10–15 years: 05–3.3 ng/mL/hour
  - ▼ **Adult, normal-sodium diet**
    - Supine: 0.2–1.6 ng/mL/hour
    - Standing: 0.7–3.3 ng/mL/hour
- Normal values depend on the laboratory and the patients prevailing Na and K, status of hydration, and posture. Only stimulated values are of practical value in evaluating hypertensive patients.

❏ Use

- Particularly useful to diagnose curable hypertension (e.g., primary aldosteronism, unilateral renal artery stenosis).
- May help differentiate patients with volume excess (e.g., primary aldosteronism) with low PRA from those with medium to high PRA; if latter group shows marked increase in PRA during captopril test, patients should be worked up for renovascular hypertension, but those with little or no increase are not likely to have curable renovascular hypertension.
- Captopril test criteria for renovascular hypertension: stimulated PRA ≥12 μg/L/hour, absolute increase PRA ≥10 μg/L/hour, increase PRA ≥150% (or ≥400% if baseline PRA <3 μg/L/hour).

- In children with salt-losing form of congenital adrenal hyperplasia due to 21-hydroxylase deficiency, severity of disease is related to degree of increase. PRA level may serve as guide to adequate mineralocorticoid replacement therapy.

❏ **Interpretation**

Increased In

- Secondary aldosteronism (usually very high levels), especially malignant or severe hypertension 50–80% of patients with renovascular hypertension (Table 16.66).
  - ▼ Normal or high PRA is of limited value to diagnose or rule out renal vascular hypertension.
  - ▼ Very high PRA is highly predictive but has poor sensitivity.
  - ▼ Low PRA using renin–sodium nomogram in untreated patients with normal serum creatinine is strongly against this diagnosis.
- Fifteen percent of patients with essential hypertension (high-renin hypertension)
- Renin-producing tumors of the kidney
- Reduced plasma volume due to low-sodium diet, diuretics, hemorrhage, Addison disease
- Some edematous normotensive states (e.g., cirrhosis, nephrosis, congestive heart failure)
- Sodium or potassium loss due to GI disease or in 10% of patients with chronic renal failure
- Normal pregnancy
- Pheochromocytoma
- Last half of menstrual cycle (twofold increase)
- Erect posture for 4 hours (twofold increase)
- Ambulatory patients compared to bed patients
- Bartter syndrome
- Various drugs (diuretics, ACE inhibitors, vasodilators; sometimes by calcium antagonists and alpha-blockers, e.g., diazoxide, estrogens, furosemide, guanethidine, hydralazine, minoxidil, spironolactone, thiazides)

Decreased In

- Ninety-eight percent of cases of primary aldosteronism. Usually absent or low and can be increased less or not at all by sodium depletion and ambulation in

TABLE 16–66. Differentiation of Primary and Secondary Aldosteronism Based on Blood Tests and Clinical Symptoms

	Primary Aldosteronism		Secondary Aldosteronism	
	Adenoma	**Hyperplasia**	**Hypertension**	**Edema**
Aldosterone	↑	↑	↑↑	↑
PRA	↓	N/↑	↑↑	↑
Serum sodium	N/↑	N	↑↑	↑
Serum potassium	↓	N/↓	↓	N/↓
Edema	0	0	0	Present
Hypertension	↑	↑	↑↑↑↑	N/↑

↑, increased; ↓, decreased; N, normal.

16

contrast to secondary aldosteronism. PRA may not always be suppressed in primary aldosteronism; repeated testing may be necessary to establish the diagnosis. Normal PRA does not preclude this diagnosis; it is not a reliable screening test.

▪ Hypertension due to unilateral renal artery stenosis or unilateral renal parenchymal disease.

▪ Increased plasma volume due to high-sodium diet, administration of salt-retaining steroids.

▪ Eighteen to twenty-five percent of essential hypertensives (low-renin essential hypertension) and 6% of normal controls.

▪ Advancing age in both normal and hypertensive patients (decrease of 35% from the third to the eighth decade).

▪ May also be decreased in CAH secondary to 11-hydroxylase or 17-hydroxylase deficiency with oversecretion of other mineralocorticoids.

▪ Rarely in Liddle syndrome and excess licorice ingestion.

▪ Use of various drugs (propranolol, clonidine, reserpine; slightly with methyldopa).

▪ Usually cannot be stimulated by salt restriction, diuretics, and upright posture that deplete plasma volume; therefore, measure before and after furosemide and 3–4 hours of ambulation.

❑ **Limitations**

▪ The plasma renin activity cannot be interpreted if the patient is being treated with spironolactone (Aldactone). Spironolactone should be discontinued for 4–6 weeks before testing.

▪ ACE inhibitors have the potential to "falsely elevate" PRA. Therefore, in a patient treated with an ACE inhibitor, the findings of a detectable PRA level or a low SA-to-PRA ratio do not exclude the diagnosis of primary aldosteronism. In addition, a strong predictor for primary aldosteronism is a PRA level undetectably low in a patient taking an ACE inhibitor.

▪ Not useful for determination of plasma renin concentration

▪ This test should not be requested in patients who have recently received radioisotopes, therapeutically or diagnostically, because of potential assay interference. A recommended time period before collection cannot be made, because it depends on the isotope administered, the dose given, and the clearance rate in the individual patient.

Suggested Reading

Mann SJ, Pickering TG. Detection of renovascular hypertension: State of the art. *Ann Intern Med.* 1992;117:845.

PLASMINOGEN*

❑ **Definition**

▪ Plasminogen is the inactive, circulating precursor of plasmin, the final product of the fibrinolytic system. Therapy with plasminogen activators results in the generation of plasmin and intended thrombolysis.

▪ **Normal range:** 70–113%.

---

*Submitted By Liberto Pechet, MD.

❑ **Interpretation**

Decreased In
- Congenital: rare reported cases; may result in a predisposition to thrombosis
- Acquired: severe DIC, pathologic fibrinolysis, or as the result of thrombolytic therapy, and in liver disease

PLASMINOGEN ACTIVATOR INHIBITOR 1 (PAI 1)*

❑ **Definition**
- PAI 1, an inhibitor of plasminogen activation is synthesized in endothelial cells, in platelets, and by the liver.
- **Normal range:** 0.0–22.0 IU/mL.

❑ **Use**
- This test may be used in rare cases with a tendency to thrombosis when no other cause is identified.

❑ **Interpretation**

Decreased Values
- Difficult to determine because the normal range can be as low as 0.0
- Cases with an increased fibrinolytic tendency (bleeding, rapid dissolution of hemostatic clots)

Increased Values
- May result in a tendency to arterial or venous thrombosis
- Acquired: during acute thrombotic episodes, pregnancy, sepsis
- Congenital: rare congenital elevations have been described

❑ **Limitations**
- This test is a biologic assay that is difficult to perform reproducibly.
- The inhibitor has diurnal variations, with highest levels during morning hours (blood should be drawn fasting between 8 AM and 12 PM).

PLATELET AGGREGATION†

❑ **Definition**
- Platelets participate in primary hemostasis by forming aggregates at the site of injury. In vivo the platelets are stimulated by chemical substances called agonists or by interaction with damaged endothelial surfaces in the presence of von Willebrand factor and collagen. These properties are used in vitro to study the change in optical density as the platelets aggregate under the effect of added agonists (ADP, collagen, epinephrine, arachidonic acid, thrombin).

16

---

*Submitted By Liberto Pechet, MD.
†Submitted By Liberto Pechet, MD.

Ristocetin is used to assess binding to von Willebrand factor, as reflected in platelets' agglutination. The aggregometers are photo optical instruments that require platelet-rich plasma. The more advanced equipment can use whole blood and can also assess ATP release by chemiluminescence methodology, thereby better determining platelet functionality.

- **Normal range:** decrease in optical density of ≥65% (represented by graphs waves generated by the aggregometer). The results are also interpreted in relation to the role of each agonist in platelet physiology. The normal response to various agonists of ATP release in chemiluminescence assays is measured in nanomoles and reported as normal or abnormal.

❏ Use

- Platelet aggregation studies are indicated in patients with a bleeding diathesis, especially mucocutaneous bleeding (but without acquired thrombocytopenia), when a platelet defect or von Willebrand disease is suspected. By varying the amount of the ristocetin reagent, subtype 2B or platelet type of von Willebrand disease can be diagnosed preliminarily.

❏ Interpretation

Causes of Decreased Values

- **Congenital conditions:**
  - ▼ The prototype for a severe platelet defect (thrombocytopathy) is Glanzmann thrombasthenia, where there is no aggregation with any agonists but positive agglutination with ristocetin.
  - ▼ Storage pool disease Bernard-Soulier syndrome.
  - ▼ Abnormal response to ristocetin may be due to von Willebrand disease.
- **Acquired conditions:**
  - ▼ Effect of drugs. Abnormalities in response to arachidonic acid reflect, in most cases, ingestion of aspirin or other NSAIDs
  - ▼ Myeloproliferative neoplasms and plasmacytic neoplasms with high globulins
  - ▼ Uremia

❏ Limitations

- Because of the short functional viability of platelets, the assay must be initiated within 2 hours from blood collection and completed within 4 hours.
- The blood must be kept at room temperature at all times.
- Platelet activation during blood drawing, such as traumatic draws with initiation of clotting, makes the assay invalid. Pneumatic tubes for delivering the blood should not be used.
- Lipemic or hemolyzed blood may affect the in vitro platelet response.
- Assays cannot be performed in severely thrombocytopenic patients.
- Platelet aggregation studies have not been standardized to test for aspirin or clopidogrel "resistance" or hyperaggregability.
- Platelet aggregation studies are labor intensive and require highly skilled, experienced technicians.

PLATELET ANTIBODY DETECTION*

❏ **Definition**

- Platelet antibodies can be divided into two categories: autoimmune and alloimmune. Autoimmune antibodies are part of an autoimmune condition, such as autoimmune thrombocytopenic purpura (ITP) or SLE, or they may develop following administration of certain drugs. Alloimmune antibodies develop as the result of immunization of transfused, incompatible, platelets.
- The development of platelet antibodies may result in shortened platelet survival and refractoriness to platelet transfusions (lack of adequate and sustained increment in platelet number). Therefore, from 20 to 70% of multitransfused thrombocytopenic patients become refractory to transfused platelets. Platelet antibodies in pregnant women may cause neonatal alloimmune thrombocytopenia. Platelet antibodies react with several antigenic groups on the platelet surface: ABO antibodies, HLA antibodies.
- The most common platelet antigen is known as HPA-1, also known as Pl^{A1}, present in 98% of the Caucasian population. Anti-HPA-1 are the most common clinically significant antibodies. The HPA-1b (PLA2) antigen occurs in 27% of the Caucasian population. Both reside on the platelet membrane protein GPIIIa.

❏ **Use**

- In refractory, multitransfused patients, the common approach is to determine the HLA type of the patient (ideally to be done before treatments that predictably result in the need for repeated platelet transfusions) and transfuse platelets from the best HLA-matched, ABO compatible, donor. Platelet cross-matching may also be used to select the best cross-matched compatible donors. Unfortunately, cross-matched platelets are effective in only 50% of transfused patients.
- Many hematologists used the platelet antibody assays to diagnose ITP. Because of the low specificity, this assay is presently not recommended.

❏ **Limitations**

- Attachment of antibodies to platelets is difficult to measure because platelets have normally cell-bound immunoglobulins attached to them. In addition, platelets do not lend themselves to agglutination methodology, as used for RBC antibody detection (see p. 884, DAT). The use of different proposed methodologies remains difficult to standardize, and practicality is limited. Solid-phase methodologies, such as those using ELISA immunoassays, are used by some laboratories to detect IgG antibodies against HLA, ABO, and HPA antigens.

PLATELET COUNT†

❏ **Definition**

- Platelets are small discoid blood corpuscles, the primary link in achieving hemostasis. They are counted by automated counters (rarely manually)

16

*Submitted By Liberto Pechet, MD.
†Submitted By Liberto Pechet, MD.

that also report mean platelet volume. Their morphology is studied on peripheral blood smear. Automated counters flag abnormal platelet count or appearance.

- **Normal range:** 140–440 ($\times$ 10^{-6} cells/L). Platelets can be estimated on peripheral blood smear (number of platelets/100$\times$ oil immersion field $\times$ 10,000); for accuracy, platelets in at least 10 different fields should be counted.

❑ **Interpretation**

Causes of Increases
- Clonal bone marrow disorders such as myeloproliferative neoplasms
- Reactive: after acute hemorrhage, in malignancies (about 50% of patients with "unexpected" thrombocytosis are found to have a malignancy), after splenectomy, severe trauma, infections, chronic inflammatory disorders, drug reactions, and many miscellaneous conditions

Causes of Decreases
- Immune destruction such as in ITP, reaction to certain drugs, neonatal alloimmune thrombocytopenia, aplastic anemia, leukemias, lymphoproliferative diseases, hypersplenism, DIC, or TTP/HUS and with extracorporeal circulation
- Following chemotherapy, posttransfusion thrombocytopenia
- Numerous congenital conditions, which may be associated with low platelet counts

❑ **Limitations**

- Interference and limitations of testing are more numerous with platelets than with RBC and WBC. Preanalytic errors occur if the blood was not admixed well with anticoagulant upon drawing; as soon as the clotting is activated, the platelets are consumed.
- Platelets cannot be accurately counted after being stored at 4°C for more than 24 hours. In some cases, and for no known reason, the EDTA used for anticoagulation of the CBC may clump platelets, reducing their number. In such situations, the blood must be drawn with a different anticoagulant, usually 3.2% sodium citrate. A similar situation resulting in low counts is platelet satellitism (platelet adherence to neutrophils).
- Other sources of error, especially in automated counters, are giant platelet (may be counted as RBC), white cell fragments, very small red cells, or red cell fragments, counted by automated counters as platelets.

PLATELET FUNCTION ASSAY, IN VITRO*

❑ **Definition**

- *Light transmittance aggregometry (LTA)* is based on platelet aggregation to ADP and other agonists and has traditionally been the most commonly used ex vivo assessment of platelet inhibition and activity. Due to the complexity of the assay and lack of standardization between institutions, LTA is a

---

*Submitted By Craig S. Smith, MD.

suboptimal test to monitor platelet activity in a clinical setting, and its use is increasingly limited to clinical trials.

- Point-of-care tests for platelet reactivity have become available for the *P2Y12* assay. The ADP-P2Y12 receptor plays a central role in the activation of platelets mediated through sustained activation of the GP IIb/IIIa platelet receptor. The assay measures ADP-induced platelet activation in citrated whole blood and reports results in P2Y12 reaction units (PRU). Initial versions of the assay also reported platelet reactivity to a thrombin receptor activation protein, which served as a measure of maximal platelet activation and reported a percentage of platelet inhibition. Increasingly, cardiovascular literature is defining platelet reactivity based on PRU alone and has defined a PRU of 235–240 as a threshold for increased ischemic events. Values at or above this level in patients on antiplatelet medications are referred to as "high on-treatment platelet reactivity" and may represent suboptimal dosing or intrinsic medication resistance.
- Other in vitro assays involve (1) measuring high shear-dependent platelet function across collagen/ADP-based cartridges. It requires only 0.8 mL of blood, and its results are obtained in a few minutes. It can be performed in the laboratory or as a POC test but lacks the reproducibility of other modalities. (2) Flow cytometric analysis of the vasodilator-stimulated phosphoprotein *(VASP)*, an intracellular marker of the residual P2Y12 reactor activity and has correlated with ischemic risk in clinical trials.

❑ Use

- In vitro platelet function assays are increasingly used in cardiovascular medicine to assess adequate inhibition to reduce ischemic events, or conversely, when platelet inhibition is low enough after cessation of antiplatelet medications to allow for invasive procedures that carry substantial bleeding risk (i.e., noncardiac procedures).
- Although no absolute consensus for a definition of a high-on treatment threshold for platelet activity exists, it is generally accepted as (1) >235–240 PRU by VerifyNow P2Y12 assay, (2) PRI >50% by VASP-P analysis, (3) >46% maximal 5 µmol/l ADP-induced aggregation, and (4) >468 arbitrary aggregation units/minute in multiplate analyzer.
- Functional platelet assays are also utilized for
  - ▾ von Willebrand disease types 1 (results may be inconclusive in mild type 1), 2A, 2B, 2M, and 3
  - ▾ Severe functional platelet defects
  - ▾ Rapid preoperative evaluation of patients with a bleeding history
  - ▾ Useful in detecting the effect of therapy with DDAVP (desmopressin acetate)
  - ▾ To detect improved hemostasis after platelet transfusions

❑ Limitations

- In vitro assays often do not detect mild platelet abnormalities.
- The in vitro results have a good negative (rule out) predictive value in cases with low or intermediate suspicion for a hemostatic defect. If, however, the results with the in vitro assay are negative, but the clinical suspicion

16

of a hemostatic defect is strong, more definitive studies are recommended (platelet aggregation assays or vWF panels [see p. 454]).

▪ If the results are positive, additional studies (platelet aggregation and/or vWF panels) are recommended for a definitive diagnosis.
▪ Several factors are known to effect in vitro platelet assays such as hematocrit and white cell count. Correction factors may need to be applied to ensure correct interpretation.

Suggested Readings

Bonello L, Tantry U, Marcucci R, et al. Consensus and future directions on the definition of high on-treatment platelet reactivity to adenosine diphosphate. *J Am Coll Cardiol.* 2010;56:919–933.

Kakouros N, Kickler TS, et al. Hematocrit alters VerifyNow P2Y12 assay results independently of intrinsic platelet reactivity and clopidogrel responsiveness. *J Thromb Haemost.* 2013;1:1–9.

PLEURA, NEEDLE BIOPSY (CLOSED CHEST)

❏ **Definition**

▪ Pleural diseases involve the parietal and visceral pleura and can be either inflammatory or malignant origin, resulting in pleural effusion. A needle biopsy of the pleura is performed to evaluate and exclusion of infectious etiologies such as tuberculosis malignant disease. Various biopsy techniques are available to diagnose pleural disease. The newer techniques include image-guided and thoracoscopic biopsy provide better diagnostic accuracy.

❏ **Use (see Chapter 13, "Respiratory, Metabolic and Acid–base Disorders," for more information about pleural effusions)**

▪ Evaluation of lymphocyte-predominant pleural effusion
▪ Diagnosis of an exudative pleural effusion that is undiagnosed after cytologic examination (diagnostic in 40–75% of cases)
▪ Recurrent pleural effusion of unknown etiology, pleural mass, or thickening

❏ **Interpretation**

▪ The test is positive for tumor in approximately 6% of malignant mesotheliomas and approximately 60% of other cases of malignancy.
▪ The test is positive for tubercles in two thirds of cases on first biopsy, with increased yield on second and third biopsies; therefore, repeat biopsy if suspicious clinically. Acid-fast stain or granulomas can be found in 50–80% of cases, and culture of biopsy material for TB is positive in ≤75% of cases. A fluid culture alone establishes a diagnosis of TB in 25% of cases.

POTASSIUM (K)

❏ **Definition**

▪ Potassium is a primary intracellular ion; <2% is extracellular. High intracellular concentrations are maintained by the Na–K ATPase pump, which continuously transports potassium into the cell against a concentration gradient. This pump is a critical factor in maintaining and adjusting the ionic gradients, on which nerve impulse transmission and contractility of cardiac and skeletal muscle depends. In acidemia, potassium moves out of cells; in alkalemia, potassium moves into cells. Hypokalemia inhibits aldosterone production; hyperkalemia stimulates aldosterone production. Plasma sodium and potassium control potassium reabsorption. Each 1 mmol/L decrease of serum potassium reflects a total deficit of <200–400 mmol; a serum potassium <2 mmol/L may reflect a total deficit >1,000 mmol.

- **Normal range:** see Table 16.67.

❑ Use

- Evaluation of electrolyte balance, cardiac arrhythmia, muscular weakness, hepatic encephalopathy, and renal failure
- Diagnosis and monitoring hyperkalemia and hypokalemia in various conditions (e.g., treatment of diabetic coma, renal failure, severe fluid and electrolyte loss, effect of certain drugs)
- Diagnosis of familial hyperkalemic periodic paralysis and hypokalemic paralysis

❑ Interpretation
Increased In
- Potassium retention
  - ▼ GFR <3–5 mL/minute
    - Oliguria caused by any condition (e.g., renal failure)
    - Chronic nonoliguric renal failure associated with dehydration, obstruction, trauma, or excess potassium
    - Drugs
    - Renal toxicity (e.g., amphotericin B, methicillin, tetracycline)
  - ▼ GFR >20 mL/minute
    - Decreased (aldosterone) mineralocorticoid activity
    - Addison disease
    - Hypofunction of the renin–angiotensin–aldosterone system
    - Hyporeninemic hypoaldosteronism with renal insufficiency (GFR, 25–75 mL/minute)
    - Various drugs (e.g., NSAIDs, ACE inhibitors, cyclosporine, pentamidine)
    - Decreased aldosterone production
    - Pseudohypoaldosteronism
    - Aldosterone antagonist drugs (e.g., spironolactone, captopril, heparin)
  - ▼ Inhibition of tubular secretion of potassium
    - Drugs (e.g., spironolactone, triamterene, amiloride)
    - Hyperkalemic type of distal RTA (e.g., sickle cell disease, obstructive uropathy)

TABLE 16–67. Normal Range for Potassium

From Age	Reference Range (mmol/L)	Critical Range (mmol/L)
0–4 mo	4.0–6.2	<2.6 >7.5
4 mo–1 y	3.7–5.6	<2.6 >7.5
>1 y	3.5–5.3	<3.0 >6.2

16

▼ Mineralocorticoid-resistant syndromes
  ● Primary tubular disorders
  ● Hereditary
  ● Acquired (e.g., SLE, amyloidosis, sickle cell nephropathy, obstructive uropathy, renal allograft transplant, chloride shift)
■ Potassium redistribution
  ▼ Familial hyperkalemic periodic paralysis (Gamstorp disease, adynamia episodica hereditaria)
  ▼ Acute acidosis (especially hyperchloremic metabolic acidosis; less with respiratory; little with metabolic acidosis due to organic acids) (e.g., diabetic ketoacidosis, lactic acidosis, acute renal failure, acute respiratory acidosis)
  ● Decreased insulin
  ● Beta-adrenergic blockade
  ● Drugs (e.g., succinylcholine, great excess of *Digitalis*, arginine infusion)
  ● Use of hypertonic solutions (e.g., saline, mannitol)
  ● Intravascular hemolysis (e.g., transfusion reaction, hemolytic anemia), rhabdomyolysis
  ● Rapid cellular release (e.g., crush injury, chemotherapy for leukemia or lymphoma, burns, major surgery)
■ Urinary diversion
  ▼ Ureteral implants into jejunum
  ▼ In neonates—dehydration, hemolysis (e.g., cephalohematoma, intracranial hemorrhage, bruising, exchange transfusion), acute renal failure, CAH, adrenocortical insufficiency

Decreased In
■ Excess renal excretion (in patients with hypokalemia, urine potassium, >25 mmol in 24 hours or >15 mmol/L implies at least a renal component)
  ▼ Osmotic diuresis of hyperglycemia (e.g., uncontrolled diabetes)
  ▼ Nephropathies
    ● Renal tubular acidosis (proximal and especially distal)
    ● Bartter syndrome
    ● Liddle syndrome
    ● Magnesium depletion due to any cause
    ● Renal vascular disease, malignant hypertension, vasculitis
    ● Renin-secreting tumors
  ▼ Endocrine
    ● Hyperaldosteronism (primary, secondary)
    ● Cushing syndrome especially caused by ectopic ACTH production
    ● CAH
    ● Hyperthyroidism (especially in Asian persons)
  ▼ Drugs
    ● Diuretics (e.g., thiazides, ethacrynic acid, furosemide); assay for diuretics should be done if urine chloride >40 mmol/L
    ● Mineralocorticoids (e.g., fluorocortisone)
    ● High-dose glucocorticoids
    ● High-dose antibiotics (e.g., penicillin, nafcillin, ampicillin, carbenicillin)

- Substances with mineralocorticoid effect (e.g., glycyrrhizic acid [licorice], carbenoxolone, gossypol)
- Drugs associated with magnesium depletion (e.g., aminoglycosides, cisplatin, amphotericin B, foscarnet)
▼ Acute myelogenous, monomyeloblastic, or lymphoblastic leukemia
- Nonrenal causes of excess potassium loss
  ▼ In patients with hypokalemia, urine potassium levels should be <25 mmol/24 hours. If levels drops to <15 mmol/L it implies extrarenal loss.
  ▼ GI
    - Vomiting
    - Diarrhea (e.g., infections, malabsorption, radiation)
    - Drugs (e.g., laxatives [phenolphthalein], enemas, cancer therapy)
    - Neoplasms (e.g., villous adenoma of the colon, pancreatic VIPoma that produces VIP >200 pg/mL, Zollinger-Ellison syndrome)
    - Excessive spitting (sustained expectoration of all saliva in neurotic persons and to induce weight loss in professional wrestlers)
  ▼ Skin
    - Excessive sweating
    - CF
    - Extensive burns
    - Draining wounds
  ▼ Cellular shifts
    - Respiratory alkalosis
    - Classic periodic paralysis
    - Insulin
    - Drugs (e.g., bronchodilators, decongestants)
    - Accidental ingestion of barium compounds
    - Treatment of severe megaloblastic anemia with vitamin B_{12} or folic acid
    - Physiologic (e.g., highly trained athletes)
  ▼ Diet
    - Severe eating disorders (e.g., anorexia nervosa, bulimia)
    - Dietary deficiency
  ▼ Delirium tremens
  ▼ In neonates—asphyxia, alkalosis, renal tubular acidosis, iatrogenic (glucose and insulin), diuretics
- Major causes of hypokalemia with hypertension:
  ▼ Diuretic drugs (e.g., thiazides)
  ▼ Primary aldosteronism
  ▼ Secondary aldosteronism (renovascular disease, renin-producing tumors)
  ▼ Cushing syndrome
  ▼ Malignant hypertension
  ▼ Renal tubular acidosis

❑ **Limitations**

- Laboratory artifacts
  ▼ Hemolysis during venipuncture, conditions associated with thrombocytosis or leukocytosis, incomplete separation of serum and clot, double spinning (respinning) of blood collection tubes

16

- ▼ Arm in upward position while collecting blood
- ▼ Betadine application
- ▼ Laboratory order of draw (lavender top tubes drawn before serum chemistry tubes)
- ▼ Drawing above IV site
- ▼ Vigorously mixed tubes
- ▼ Collection techniques
- ▼ Traumatic draw
- ▼ Pneumatic tube system issues: speed too high, unpadded canisters, excessive agitation
- ▼ Delay in processing
- ▼ Centrifuging at too high G force
- ▼ Increased heat exposure in centrifuge
- ▼ Chilling whole blood beyond 2 hours
- ▼ Prolonged tourniquet use and hand exercise when drawing blood
- ■ Potassium value can be elevated approximately 15% in slight hemolysis (Hb ≤50 mg/dL) and elevated approximately 30–50% in moderate hemolysis (Hb >100 mg/dL). Therefore, potassium status can be assessed in those with slight hemolysis but not in those with moderate hemolysis.
- ■ Excess dietary intake or rapid potassium infusion.
- ■ Drugs with high potassium content (e.g., 1 million units of penicillin G potassium contains 1.7 mmol of potassium).
- ■ Transfusion of old blood.

POTASSIUM, URINE

❏ Definition

- ■ Urinary potassium levels are helpful in the evaluation of patients with unexplained hypokalemia, electrolyte, and acid–base balance. In the presence of such hypokalemia, urine excretion is helpful to separate renal from nonrenal losses. Excretion <20 mmol/24 hours is evidence that hypokalemia is not from renal loss. Renal loss >50 mmol/L in a hypokalemic, and hypertensive patient not on a diuretic may indicate primary or secondary aldosteronism.
- ■ **Normal range:**
  - ▼ Twenty-four–hour urine:
    - ● Male:
      - • Less than 10 years: 17–54 mmol/day
      - • 10–14 years: 22–57 mmol/day
      - • Greater than 14 years: 25–125 mmol/day
    - ● Female:
      - • 6–10 years: 8–37 mmol/day
      - • 10–14 years: 18–58 mmol/day
      - • Greater than 14 years: 25–125 mmol/day
  - ■ Random urine:
    - ▼ Male: 13–116 mmol/g creatinine
    - ▼ Female: 8–129 mmol/g creatinine

❑ Use

- Evaluation of patients with unexplained hypokalemia, electrolyte, and acid–base balance.

❑ Interpretation

Increased In

- Dehydration
- Primary and secondary aldosteronism
- Diabetic acidosis
- Mercurial and thiazide diuretic administration
- Ammonium chloride administration
- Renal tubular acidosis
- Chronic renal failure
- Starvation
- Cushing syndrome

Decreased In

- Acute renal failure
- Malabsorption
- Chronic potassium deficiency states
- Addison disease
- Severe GN
- Pyelonephritis
- Nephrosclerosis

❑ Limitations

- Urinary potassium may be elevated with dietary (food and/or medicinal) increase, hyperaldosteronism, renal tubular acidosis, onset of alkalosis, and with other disorders.
- Urine chloride is often ordered with sodium and potassium as timed urine. The urinary anion gap $[Na^+ - (Cl^- + HCO_3^-)]$ or $[(Na^+ + K^+) - (Cl^-)]$ is useful in the initial evaluation of hyperchloremic metabolic acidosis.

PREALBUMIN

❑ Definition

- This 54-kDa protein tetramer is synthesized in the liver, choroid plexus, CNS, placenta, intestine, pancreas, and meninges. It contains two binding sites for thyroid hormones T_3 and T_4 and two binding sites for serum retinol-binding protein. These different binding sites do not overlap. As a thyroid hormone transport and binding protein, transthyretin binds 10–15% of serum T_3 and T_4 for transport in the blood. In the CSF, where there is typically no albumin or thyroglobulin present, transthyretin serves as the only CSF-binding protein for T_3 and T_4. The presence of high concentrations of transthyretin in the CSF makes it a key indicator of leakage of the CSF into the sinus cavities, eyes, and ears when cranial trauma has occurred. Prealbumin is a negative acute-phase reactant. Other names: prealbumin (PA), thyroxine-binding prealbumin (TBPA).
- **Normal range:** 18–40 mg/dL.

16

❏ **Use**

- Evaluation of nutritional status, total parenteral nutrition
- Clinical indicator of liver status

❏ **Interpretation**

Increased In

- Chronic renal failure
- Hodgkin disease

Decreased In

- Inflammation
- Hepatic dysfunction
- Protein deficiency states
- Cancer
- CF
- Chronic illness

❏ **Limitations**

- Anabolic steroids, corticosteroids, and androgens increase prealbumin levels.
- Estrogens and oral contraceptives decrease prealbumin levels.
- Zinc deficiency, acute alcohol intoxication, leakage of protein from damaged hepatic cells may cause a rise in the prealbumin levels.

 PRENATAL TESTING: SAMPLE COLLECTION PROCEDURES

AMNIOCENTESIS*

❏ **Definition**

- Invasive procedure to obtain amniotic fluid that contains cells sloughed from the fetus. Some biochemical tests can be performed directly on the fluid; most tests first require cell culture. It is generally not performed until 15 weeks of gestation; recent estimates of procedural risk of fetal loss are as low as 0.06%. Cell culture for chromosome analysis takes 5–7 days; slightly longer culture times are required to obtain material for biochemical or molecular genetic tests.

❏ **Use**

- Provides fetal material for chromosome (cytogenetic) testing, biochemical testing (metabolic disorders/inborn errors of metabolism), and molecular DNA–based testing for inherited disease (e.g., CF, fragile X).

---

*Submitted by Patricia Minehart Miron, PhD.

❏ **Limitations**

▪ Not performed until second trimester, which delays decisions regarding pregnancy termination.

CHORIONIC VILLUS SAMPLING*

❏ **Definition**

▪ Invasive procedure to obtain chorionic villus tissue generally performed between 10 and 12 weeks of gestation. Procedural risk of fetal loss (higher than for amniocentesis): approximately 1%.

❏ **Use**

▪ Provides placental material for chromosome (cytogenetic) testing, biochemical testing (metabolic disorders/inborn errors of metabolism), and molecular DNA-based testing for inherited disease (e.g., cystic fibrosis, fragile X).

▪ Primary advantage over amniocentesis is earlier time frame, allowing pregnancy termination in the first trimester or earlier relief of anxiety.

❏ **Limitations**

▪ Chromosome results may be ambiguous due to confined placental mosaicism (abnormal chromosome line limited to placental tissue) in approximately 2% of cases, requiring follow-up by amniocentesis

▪ Maternal cell contamination must be avoided for accurate diagnosis based on fetal chromosomes, enzyme assay, or DNA analysis

▪ Does not provide material to screen for neural tube defects

FETAL BIOPSY†

❏ **Definition**

▪ Invasive procedure to obtain fetal tissue such as skin, muscle, or liver.

❏ **Use**

▪ Diagnosis of specific inherited disorders when gene mutation is unknown

▪ Liver biopsy for specific inherited metabolic disorders (e.g., ornithine transcarbamylase deficiency, carbamoyl phosphate synthetase deficiency, G6PD [type 1a])

▪ Skin biopsy for specific genetic skin disorders (e.g., epidermolysis bullosa)

▪ Muscle biopsy for Duchenne muscular dystrophy

❏ **Limitations**

▪ High-risk procedures with value for a limited number of disorders

---

*Submitted by Patricia Minehart Miron, PhD.
†Submitted by Patricia Minehart Miron, PhD.

16

FETAL BLOOD SAMPLING (PERCUTANEOUS UMBILICAL BLOOD SAMPLING [PUBS], CORDOCENTESIS)*

❑ **Definition**

- Invasive procedure to obtain fetal blood generally performed after 18 weeks of gestation. Procedural risk of fetal loss is approximately 1–2%.

❑ **Use**

- Usually performed when diagnostic information cannot be obtained through amniocentesis, chorionic villus sampling (CVS), ultrasound examination, or following an inconclusive result from one of these tests
- Provides fetal material for chromosome (cytogenetic) testing, biochemical testing, and molecular DNA-based testing for inherited disease
- Chromosome analysis faster than with either amniocentesis or CVS because less culture time required; therefore, useful for late presentations
- Used to assess fetal isoimmunization (e.g., Rhesus factor, Kell), anemia, platelet count, hemolytic disease, and infection (e.g., toxoplasmosis, rubella, or CMV)
- May also be used to administer medication to the fetus

❑ **Limitations**

- Riskier procedure than amniocentesis of CVS performed late in pregnancy, limiting pregnancy termination options
- Does not assess neural tube defects

 # PRENATAL SCREENING

PRENATAL SCREENING, FIRST-TRIMESTER SCREENING†

❑ **Definition**

- Performed between 11 and 13 weeks of gestation, first-trimester screening combines maternal age plus two serum biochemical markers: pregnancy-associated plasma protein A (PAPP-A) and β-hCG. It also includes fetal nuchal translucency (NT) measurement.

❑ **Use**

- Risk assessment for trisomy 21

❑ **Interpretation**

- Increased NT associated with trisomy 13, trisomy 18, trisomy 21, 45,X, triploidy, and other chromosome aberrations.
- Trisomy 21 biochemical profile typically has increased β-hCG and decreased PAPP-A.
- Trisomy 18 has decreased β-hCG and decreased PAPP-A.

---

*Submitted by Patricia Minehart Miron, PhD.
†Submitted by Patricia Minehart Miron, PhD.

- Combining NT and maternal serum profile detects approximately 85% of affected trisomy 21 pregnancies with a 5% positive screening rate.

❏ **Limitations**

- Does not detect neural tube defects.
- Detects fewer affected pregnancies than combined first-semester plus second-trimester screening modalities.
- NT measurement requires experienced ultrasonographers.

NONINVASIVE PRENATAL TESTING (NIPT)*

❏ **Definition**

- The goal of noninvasive prenatal testing (NIPT) is to obtain information on genetic conditions (e.g., Down syndrome) of a pregnancy by analyzing cell-free fetal DNA circulating in maternal blood and maternal DNA using a blood sample drawn from the mother. The ACMG Policy Statement on "Noninvasive Prenatal Screening for Fetal Aneuploidy" emphasizes that "Positive results should be followed-up with an invasive diagnostic test before any decision is made regarding pregnancy termination." NIPT should not be used as a diagnostic testing but as a screening test.
- Counting method: sequenced DNA fragments are categorized by chromosome and recalculated for the proportion of each chromosome in the total genome; the proportion of DNA from a chromosome of interest is compared to the expected proportion (i.e., chromosome 21 should represent 1.5% of the total genome). Any deviation from the expected proportion is an indication of a possible aneuploidy. This method is looking for the excess of the chromosome in question (i.e., chromosome 21). Trisomy 21 would increase the amount of DNA from chromosome 21 from the expected 1.5–2.25%. One drawback of this method is that since maternal DNA is the majority of the sample, there is a very small change when the fetal and maternal DNAs are analyzed combined and not differentiated.
- Panorama method: differentiates fetal from maternal chromosomes. DNA is extracted from (1) maternal DNA from white blood cells and (2) cell-free DNA (**cf-DNA**) containing maternal and fetal cf-DNA from plasma. Panorama method tests for characteristic markers (**SNPs**) on both maternal chromosomes and on cell-free DNA (cf-DNA) containing both maternal and fetal DNA. Knowing which chromosomes originate from the mother, the Panorama method subtracts the maternal (and paternal if available) chromosome genotypes from the cell-free DNA (cf-DNA) genotypic information, thereby leaving only fetal chromosome genotypes. Additional analyses consider crossovers, frequency data, and possible fetal chromosome copy number to calculate the ploidy of the fetal sample.

16

*Submitted by Edward Ginns, MD and Marzena M. Galdzicka, PhD.

❏ **Use**

- Fetal screening testing—positive results should be followed up with an invasive diagnostic test before any decision is made regarding pregnancy termination
- Pretest information should be provided by a prenatal care provider, a trained designee or a genetic counselor to ensure that patients make informed decisions.

❏ **Limitations**

- Risk assessment is limited to specific fetal aneuploidies (trisomy 13, 18, and 21) at this time. Some platforms also screen for sex chromosome abnormalities. Other cytogenetic or genetic abnormalities (single gene mutations) or disorders will not be detected when trisomy 21, 18, and 13 are the only aneuploidies being screened.
- Chromosomal abnormalities such as unbalanced translocations, deletions, and duplications will not be detected by NIPS.
- NIPS is not able to distinguish specific forms of aneuploidy, an extrachromosome versus a Robertsonian translocation, or low-level mosaicism.
- Uninformative test results due to insufficient isolation of cell-free fetal DNA could lead to a delay in diagnosis or eliminate the availability of information for risk assessment.
- Providers should check turnaround time before offering patients NIPS if timing is important for reproductive decision making.
- NIPS does not replace the utility of a first-trimester ultrasound examination.
- Limited data are currently available on the use of NIPS in twins and higher-order pregnancies.
- NIPS has no role in predicting late-pregnancy complications.
- More information available: GREGG et al. ACMG statement on noninvasive prenatal screening for fetal aneuploidy.

PRENATAL SCREENING, SECOND-TRIMESTER SCREENING (MATERNAL SERUM SCREENING; QUAD SCREEN)*

❏ **Definition**

- Performed between 15 and 22 weeks of gestation, the quadruple screen combines maternal age plus four serum biochemical markers: hCG, inhibin A, AFP, and unconjugated estriol to assess the risk of trisomy 21 and trisomy 18.

❏ **Use**

- Risk assessment for trisomy 21 (Down syndrome), trisomy 18, and open neural tube defects

❏ **Interpretation**

- Trisomy 21 profile typically has high levels of hCG and inhibin A with low levels of AFP and unconjugated estriol.
- Trisomy 18 is associated with low levels of hCG, AFP, and estriol. (Inhibin A does not contribute to trisomy 18 risk profile.)

*Submitted by Patricia Minehart Miron, PhD.

- Different centers use different cutoffs, balancing detection rate against number of invasive procedures performed. A cutoff of 1:270 (approximately 5% positive screening rate) detects approximately 80% of trisomy 21 and trisomy 18 pregnancies.

❏ **Limitations**

- Detects fewer affected pregnancies than combined first-semester plus second-trimester screening modalities.
- Does not permit first-trimester decision making regarding termination of affected pregnancies.

COMBINED FIRST-TRIMESTER AND SECOND-TRIMESTER SCREENING (INTEGRATED/SEQUENTIAL SCREENING)*

❏ **Definition**

- Integrated screening combines first-semester and second-trimester screening to give one result after the second-trimester screen is completed.
- Sequential screening gives the risk after the first trimester if risk is higher than a specific cutoff and gives the combined risk after the second trimester if first-trimester risk was not higher than the cutoff. It can be further divided into stepwise and contingent.
  - ▼ Stepwise screening: Women with risk above a certain cutoff following the first-trimester screen are offered invasive diagnostic testing directly, whereas women below cutoff are offered second-trimester screening.
  - ▼ Contingent screening: Women with high risk are offered diagnostic testing, women with intermediate risk are offered second-trimester screening, and women with low risk have no further testing.
  - ▼ Some centers prefer to divide patients into two groups only: Those with high risk who will be offered invasive testing directing and those who will proceed to second-trimester testing.

❏ **Use**

- Risk assessment for trisomy 18, trisomy 21, and neural tube defects.
- Ultrasound in the first-trimester screen also contributes to detection of other chromosome abnormalities.

❏ **Interpretation**

- Approximately 95% detection of trisomy 21 with 5% screen-positive rate

❏ **Limitations**

- Noncompliant patients may not return for the second-semester screen.

Suggested Readings

American College of Obstetrics and Gynecology. Practice Bulletin, Clinical Management Guidelines for Obstetrician-Gynecologists #77, Screening for Fetal Chromosomal Abnormalities. 2007;109:217–227.
Driscoll DA, Gross S. Prenatal screening for aneuploidy. *N Engl J Med*. 2009;360:2556–2562.

16

---

*Submitted by Patricia Minehart Miron, PhD.

PRENATAL DIAGNOSTIC SCREENING

❏ Definition

- Noninvasive testing with goal of limiting invasive diagnostic procedures that carry risk to pregnancy.

❏ Use

- Screening modalities have been developed for Down syndrome/trisomy 21 detection because trisomy 21 is the most common viable autosomal chromosome abnormality. However, screening also provides specific risk assessment for trisomy 18 and neural tube defects.
- In addition, with inclusion of early ultrasound examination, increased fetal nuchal translucency may indicate other chromosome abnormalities including Turner syndrome (45,X), trisomy 13, and triploidy.
- Second-trimester measurement of AFP is used to assess risk of fetal neural tube defects.
- Screening is offered to all women, regardless of age, to provide more accurate risk information than provided by age alone.

❏ Limitations

- Risk for trisomy 13 is *not* calculated; however, trisomy 13 pregnancies are typically associated with ultrasound anomalies detectable with second-trimester ultrasound examination. By definition, screening is not diagnostic; most screen-positive pregnancies are chromosomally normal, and some affected pregnancies will be missed.

CYTOGENETICS: FLUORESCENCE IN SITU HYBRIDIZATION (FISH) AND CHROMOSOME ANALYSIS*

❏ Definition and Use

- **FISH**
  - ▼ Analysis of fetal tissue to detect targeted numeric or structural chromosome aberrations.
  - ▼ Interphase FISH performed on uncultured cells is used to provide a rapid (1 day) result for targeted chromosome enumeration. Typically, chromosomes 13, 18, 21, X, and Y are assessed. Metaphase FISH performed on cultured cells is used to assess chromosome aberrations too small to be detected by conventional chromosome analysis.
  - ▼ Generally used only in cases with specific risk (specific ultrasound anomalies, family history).
- **Chromosome analysis**
  - ▼ Analysis of fetal tissue to detect numeric and structural chromosome aberrations. Most chromosome aberrations are numeric (e.g., trisomies 13, 18,

*Submitted by Patricia Minehart Miron, PhD.

21 [Down syndrome], 45,X [Turner syndrome], 47,XXY [Klinefelter syndrome]).
▼ Principle indications:
  ● Increased risk determined from maternal screening
  ● Ultrasound anomaly
  ● Family history of chromosome anomaly (previous affect pregnancy, balanced rearrangement carrier parent)
  ● Fetal sexing for history of X-linked disorders

❏ **Limitations**
  ▪ **FISH**
    ▼ Targeted test that assesses only specific region on chromosome; does not ensure that entire chromosome is normal and does not assess every chromosome.
    ▼ Mosaicism may also confound results.
  ▪ **Chromosome analysis**
    ▼ Analysis cannot detect aberrations smaller than 5–10 megabases; requires cell culture to obtain actively dividing metaphase cells.
    ▼ Mosaicism, the presence of two cell lines, may be difficult to interpret, because chromosome anomalies can arise in vitro during specimen culture.

GENOMIC MICROARRAY ANALYSIS—ARRAY COMPARATIVE GENOMIC HYBRIDIZATION (aCGH)*

❏ **Definition**
  ▪ This technology uses probes covering the entire genome and can detect chromosome abnormalities up to 10 times smaller than those detectable by conventional chromosome analysis.

❏ **Use**
  ▪ Detection of chromosome abnormalities (copy number changes; e.g., deletion, duplication) up to 10 times smaller than can be detected by conventional chromosome analysis
  ▪ Detection of abnormalities that may be causal for developmental delay, autism, and congenital anomalies. Some laboratories are offering aCGH for prenatal diagnosis.
  ▪ Cancer-appropriate arrays are also in clinical use.

❏ **Interpretation**
  ▪ **Normal:** Two copies for all tested sequences in diploid cells
  ▪ **Abnormal:** Copy number < or >2

❏ **Limitations**
  ▪ aCGH *cannot* detect balanced rearrangements that may play a role in repeat pregnancy loss and cancer.

16

---

*Submitted by Patricia Minehart Miron, PhD.

- Interpretation of results is not always straightforward; some detected imbalances may be of no clinical significance. Variant databases are in development.

MOLECULAR GENETIC ANALYSIS (PRENATAL DNA ANALYSIS)*

❑ **Definition**

- Molecular testing on fetal DNA to test directly for specific mutations or to assess closely linked markers for an unknown mutation

❑ **Use**

- To assess mutational status for specific inherited diseases
- Typically performed only when parents are affected or known carriers for disease

❑ **Limitations**

- Direct testing assesses only particular targeted mutation(s) of interest
- Linkage analysis, testing of a nearby genetic marker used when the particular mutation is unknown, is limited by potential recombination between the tested marker and the causal mutation.
- Mitochondrial DNA testing may be problematic because the mutated mitochondrial mutation is likely to exist in combination with normal mitochondria (heteroplasmy).

PRETRANSFUSION COMPATIBILITY TESTING†

❑ **Definition and Use**

- Demonstration of RBC antigen–antibody reactions is the foundation for pretransfusion compatibility testing and the key to immunohematology. Agglutination is the end point for most of these tests (including performing the blood type, the antibody screen, and the crossmatch). Increased genetic knowledge has added a new approach to red cell antigen typing using DNA sequence determination, but these tests are currently not being used for routine blood bank testing, and the tests described in this chapter are based on the classical agglutination methodology.
- Three major requirements must be satisfied for safe RBC transfusions:
  - ▼ The RBCs to be transfused must be ABO compatible
  - ▼ RhD-positive RBCs should not be given to RhD-negative patients
  - ▼ Transfused RBCs should lack blood group antigens to which the patient has preexisting clinically significant antibodies
- To achieve these objectives, pretransfusion compatibility testing begins with the type and screen, where the recipient's ABO group and Rh (D) typing is determined. Antibodies to the ABO antigens are naturally occurring and are used to determine a person's ABO blood group. Next, the patient's serum is screened for the presence of clinically significant (non-ABO) antibodies

*Submitted by Edward Ginns, MD and Marzena M. Galdzicka, PhD.
†Submitted By Vishesh Chhibber, MD.

directed against other blood group antigens. If an antibody is detected by the antibody screen, an antibody identification panel must be performed to identify the antibody.

■ Safe transfusion can be ensured for most recipients by the correct ABO and Rh typing of patients and donors.

❑ ABO Group Determination

■ The forward and reverse ABO blood grouping of all patients must be determined prior to the transfusion of blood products using commercial reagents and the patient's red cells and serum (or plasma).

■ The forward ABO blood grouping is determined by checking the patient's (or donor's) red cells for the presence of A and B antigens using commercial anti-A and anti-B reagent antibodies.

■ The reverse ABO grouping is determined by checking the patient's (or donor's) serum for the presence of anti-A and anti-B antibodies using commercial reagent red cells.

■ The strength of the agglutination during testing is usually graded.

■ A group A individual has anti-B but not anti-A antibodies. A group B individual has anti-A but not anti-B antibodies. A group AB individual has neither anti-A nor anti-B antibodies. The serum of group O persons contains both anti-A and anti-B antibodies.

❑ Rh Typing

■ The Rh (D) type of all patients should be determined prior to transfusion or if the patient is pregnant in order to prevent immunization to the D antigen and production of the anti-D alloantibody. Anti-D is a clinically significant antibody that can cause hemolytic transfusion reactions and hemolytic disease of the fetus and newborn (HDFN).

■ The Rh typing is performed by testing the RBCs for the presence of D antigen using anti-D reagent antibodies and checking for agglutination.

■ Some patients may not show clear agglutination after centrifugation with anti-D but still have the D antigen. This is known as weak D and requires the addition of AHG for identification of the D antigen. These weak D patients are still considered Rh positive.

■ Weak D testing is not required for patients but is required for donors.

■ In practice, the terms Rh positive and Rh negative, respectively, refer to the presence or absence of the D antigen and routine pretransfusion tests only include testing for the D antigen. However, in addition to the D antigen, there are many other antigens in the Rh blood group system. When alloantibodies are present, it may be necessary to type patients and/or donors for these (other) Rh antigens, most commonly C, E, c, e.

■ Antibodies to Rh antigens are immune stimulated in most cases, mostly following pregnancy or transfusion.

❑ Antibody Screening

■ Antibody screening is used to detect the presence of unexpected alloantibodies in the recipient's serum, directed against non-ABO blood group antigens (e.g., Kell, Duffy, and Kidd). This is accomplished by using commercially

16

available screening RBCs. Generally, an IAT is performed using the patient's serum and two or three group O RBCs with known but varied blood group antigens.

■ If agglutination is detected in the antibody screen, the antibody must be identified and antigen-negative RBCs must be selected for transfusion.

❑ Crossmatching

■ The crossmatch assay involves testing the patient's serum with the donor RBC taken from a segment attached to the selected blood unit. Unless there is a very urgent need for blood, crossmatching is mandatory. The method used must be able to demonstrate incompatibility to ABO and other clinically significant RBC antibodies.

■ If the recipient/patient has a negative antibody screen, an abbreviated (immediate spin) crossmatch is adequate. However, if the patient has a positive antibody screen or there is a previous history of alloimmunization, antigen-negative donor units must be selected and a full Coombs crossmatch must be performed (by incubating the patient's plasma and the donor red cells at body temperature and then adding AHG).

■ An immediate spin crossmatch is one additional means of ensuring that the patient receives ABO compatible red cells as ABO antibodies will cause agglutination without incubation at body temperature and addition of AHG.

■ In order to detect many of the clinically significant non-ABO antibodies, a Coombs crossmatch is necessary as agglutination will not be seen without incubation at body temperature and addition of AHG.

❑ Limitations

■ Acquired antigens, such as "acquired B" antigens in group A individuals.

■ Forward and reverse typing discrepancies. When they occur, the cause must be immediately investigated. The most common cause is a patient who is a subgroup of A and who has formed anti-A_1 antibodies (80% of group A patients are subgroup A_1). Most of the remainder are A_2 and may develop anti-A_1 antibodies.

■ Warm and cold autoantibodies can interfere with pretransfusion testing.

■ Pretransfusion testing may be complicated in recently transfused and marrow transplant patients.

PROCALCITONIN (PCT)

❑ Definition

■ Procalcitonin (PCT) is a protein that can act as a hormone and a cytokine. It can be produced by several types of cells and many organs in response to proinflammatory stimuli, particularly bacterial infection. It is released under the stimulation of sepsis. PCT levels rise within 6 to 12 hours of bacterial infection with septic consequences.

■ **Procalcitonin (PCT) measurement is indicated:**

▼ On admission to the intensive care unit (ICU) in patients with a known or suspected respiratory infection, or sepsis with a probable bacterial source.

▼ In patients in the ICU with a suspicion of a new or relapsed respiratory infection or sepsis.
▼ On days 3 and 5 of a course of antimicrobial therapy being given to treat a respiratory infection, or potential sepsis for which a source has not been identified, to aid in assessing response to therapy and in clinical decisions of continuing versus discontinuing antimicrobial therapy.
- **Normal range:**
  ▼ Negative: <0.10 ng/mL

❑ **Use**

- Diagnosis of bacteremia and septicemia in adults and children (including neonates)
- Diagnosis, risk stratification, and monitoring of septic shock
- Differential diagnosis of bacterial versus viral meningitis
- Differential diagnosis of community-acquired bacterial versus viral pneumonia
- Monitoring of therapeutic response to antibacterial therapy

❑ **Interpretation**

- Procalcitonin levels above 2.00 ng/mL on the first day of ICU admission represent a high risk for progression to severe sepsis and/or septic shock.
- PCT for initiation of antimicrobial therapy
  ▼ PCT result <0.50 µg/L—initiation of antimicrobial therapy may not be indicated. Consider a noninfectious cause of the clinical syndrome. If antibiotics are withheld, may want to repeat PCT level in 6 hours to rule out an increase that would suggest antibiotic therapy is warranted
  ▼ PCT result 0.50–1 µg/L—initiation of antimicrobial therapy encouraged
  ▼ PCT result >1 µg/L—initiation of antimicrobial therapy strongly encouraged

❑ **Limitations**

- Procalcitonin levels in the serum are elevated in a variety of inflammatory conditions, including bacterial infection, malaria, burns, pancreatitis, and traumatic injury.
- Levels rise within 2–4 hours, peak generally in the 2nd day, and fall rapidly during recovery.
- Procalcitonin levels are generally not as high in fungal or viral infection.

PROGESTERONE

❑ **Definition**

- Natural steroid hormone that induces secretory changes in endometrium, promotes mammary gland development, relaxes uterine smooth muscles, blocks follicular maturation, and maintains pregnancy. Hormone synthesized by the ovary; low in follicular phase but increases to 10–40 mg/day during luteal phase and ≤300 mg/day if pregnancy occurs.
- **Normal range:** see Table 16.68.

16

TABLE 16–68. Normal Ranges of Progesterone			
Reference Group	n	Mean (ng/mL)	Range (ng/mL)
Male	50	0.36	0.14–2.06
Female			
Midfollicular phase	14	0.69	0.31–1.52
Midluteal phase	13	11.42	5.16–18.56
Postmenopausal	49	0.25	<0.08–0.78
Pregnancy			
First trimester	34	22.17	4.73–50.74
Second trimester	29	29.73	19.41–45.30

❑ **Use**

- Detection of ovulation in the evaluation of the function of the corpus luteum
- Monitoring patients having ovulation during induction with hCG, human menopausal gonadotropin, FSH/LH-releasing hormone, or clomiphene
- To evaluate patients at risk for early abortion

❑ **Interpretation**

Increased In

- Luteal phase of menstrual cycle
- Luteal cysts of the ovary; ovarian tumors (e.g., arrhenoblastoma)
- Adrenal tumors
- CAH caused by 21-hydroxylase, 17-hydroxylase, and 11-beta hydroxylase
- Molar pregnancy

Decreased In

- Amenorrhea
- Threatened abortion (some patients)
- Fetal death
- Toxemia of pregnancy
- Gonadal agenesis

PROINSULIN

❑ **Definition**

- Enzymatic process forms insulin in pancreatic secretory granules of beta cells. Proinsulin level is normally ≤20% of total insulin. Proinsulin has low biologic activity (10% insulin potency) and is the major storage form of insulin. Proinsulin is included in the immunoassay of total insulin, and separation requires special technique.
- **Normal range:** 2.0–2.6 pmol/L.

❑ **Use**

- Proinsulin: Insulin ratio is used as an indirect marker of beta cell function.

❑ **Interpretation**

- High proinsulin levels associated with benign or malignant beta cell tumors of the pancreas and endocrine pancreatic tumors associated with MEN-1.

- Elevated levels are positive risk factor for the development of NIDDM.
- Elevated levels in patients with chronic renal failure, cirrhosis, and hyperthyroidism.
- Proinsulin >30% of serum insulin after overnight fast suggests insulinoma.
- Proinsulin is increased in factitious hypoglycemia due to sulfonylurea.
- Proinsulin is increased in familial hyperproinsulinemia—heterozygous mutation affecting cleavage of proinsulin leading to secretion of excess amounts of proinsulin.
- Type 2 DM.

❏ **Limitations**

- Proinsulin may also be increased in renal disease.
- Elevation of proinsulin: insulin ratio correlates with a decreased acute illness response to glucose in patients with type 2 DM.

PROLACTIN

❏ **Definition**

- Prolactin is a single-chain polypeptide composed of 198 amino acids and is secreted by the anterior cells of the pituitary gland. Prolactin secretion is controlled by the hypothalamus primarily through the release of prolactin-inhibiting factor (dopamine) and prolactin-releasing factor (serotonin). TRH stimulates prolactin secretion and is useful as a provocative test to evaluate prolactin reserves and abnormal secretion of prolactin by the pituitary. The primary physiologic function of prolactin is to stimulate and maintain lactation in women.
- **Normal range:**
  - ▼ Males: 2.64–13.13 µg/L
  - ▼ Females <50 years (premenopausal): 3.34–26.72 µg/L
  - ▼ Females >50 years (postmenopausal): 2.74–19.64 µg/L

❏ **Use**

- Aiding in evaluation of pituitary tumors, amenorrhea, galactorrhea, infertility, and hypogonadism
- Monitoring therapy of prolactin-producing tumors

❏ **Interpretation**
Increased In

- Amenorrhea/galactorrhea
  - ▼ 10–25% of women with galactorrhea and normal menses
  - ▼ 10–15% of women with amenorrhea without galactorrhea
  - ▼ 75% of women with both galactorrhea and amenorrhea/oligomenorrhea
  - ▼ Cause of 15–30% of cases of amenorrhea in young women
- Pituitary lesions (e.g., prolactinoma, section of pituitary stalk, empty sella syndrome, 20–40% of patients with acromegaly, ≤80% of patients with chromophobe adenomas); concentrations are usually >200 ng/mL.
- Hypothalamic lesions (e.g., sarcoidosis, eosinophilic granuloma, histiocytosis X, TB, glioma, craniopharyngioma); concentrations are usually >200 ng/mL.

16

- Other endocrine diseases:
  - ▼ Approximately 20% of cases of hypothyroidism (second most common cause of hyperprolactinemia). Therefore, serum TSH and T_4 should always be measured.
  - ▼ Addison disease
  - ▼ Polycystic ovaries
  - ▼ Glucocorticoid excess—normal or moderately elevated prolactin
- Ectopic production of prolactin (e.g., bronchogenic carcinoma, renal cell carcinoma, ovarian teratomas, acute myeloid leukemia)
- Children with sexual precocity—may be increased into pubertal range
- Neurogenic causes (e.g., nursing and breast stimulation, spinal cord lesions, chest wall lesions such as herpes zoster)
- Stress (e.g., surgery, hypoglycemia, vigorous exercise, seizures)
- Pregnancy (increases to 8–20 times normal by delivery, returns to normal 2–4 weeks postpartum unless nursing occurs)
- Lactation
- Chronic renal failure (20–40% of cases; becomes normal after successful renal transplant but not after hemodialysis)
- Liver failure (due to decreased prolactin clearance)
- Idiopathic causes (some probably represent early cases of microadenoma too small to be detected by CT scan)
  - ▼ Drugs—most common cause; usually subsides a few weeks after cessation of using drug; these concentrations are usually 20–100 ng/mL
    - Neuroleptics (e.g., phenothiazines, thioxanthenes, butyrophenones)
    - Antipsychotic drugs (e.g., Compazine, Thorazine, Stelazine, Mellaril, Haldol)
    - Dopamine antagonists (e.g., metoclopramide, sulpiride)
    - Opiates (morphine, methadone)
    - Reserpine
    - Alpha-methyldopa (Aldomet)
    - Estrogens and oral contraceptives
    - Thyrotropin-releasing hormone
    - Amphetamines
    - Isoniazid

Decreased In

- Hypopituitarism: postpartum pituitary necrosis (Sheehan syndrome), idiopathic hypogonadotropic hypogonadism
- Drugs
  - ▼ Dopamine agonists
  - ▼ Ergot derivatives (bromocriptine mesylate, lisuride hydrogen maleate)
  - ▼ Levodopa, apomorphine, clonidine

❏ Limitations

- Normal prolactin secretion varies with time, which results in serum prolactin levels two to three times higher at night than during the day.
- The biologic half-life of prolactin is approximately 20–50 minutes. Serum prolactin levels during the menstrual cycle are variable and commonly exhibit slight elevations during the mid-cycle.

- Prolactin levels in normal individuals tend to rise in response to physiologic stimuli including sleep, exercise, nipple stimulation, sexual intercourse, hypoglycemia, pregnancy, and surgical stress.
- Prolactin values that exceed the reference values may be due to macroprolactin (prolactin bound to immunoglobulin). Macroprolactin should be evaluated if signs and symptoms of hyperprolactinemia are absent or pituitary imaging studies are not informative.

PROSTATE-SPECIFIC ANTIGEN (PSA), TOTAL AND FREE

❏ Definition

- PSA is a glycoprotein that is expressed by both normal and neoplastic prostate tissue and is prostate tissue specific and not prostate cancer specific. PSA is consistently expressed in nearly all prostate cancers, although its level of expression on a per cell basis is lower than in normal prostate epithelium. The absolute value of serum PSA is useful for determining the extent of prostate cancer and assessing the response to prostate cancer treatment; its use as a screening method to detect prostate cancer is also common, although controversial.
- PSA exists primarily as three forms in serum. One form of PSA is enveloped by the protease inhibitor, alpha-2 macroglobulin, and has been shown to lack immunoreactivity. A second form is complexed to another protease inhibitor, alpha-1 antichymotrypsin (ACT). The third form of PSA is not complexed to a protease inhibitor and is termed "free PSA." The latter two forms are immunologically detectable in commercially available PSA assays and are referred to collectively as "total PSA."
- Free PSA values alone have not been shown to be effective in patient management and should not be used. Both total PSA and free PSA concentrations should be determined on the same serum specimen and used to calculate the percentage of free PSA. Percent free PSA values are then used for patient management.

$$\frac{\text{free PSA}(\text{ng}/\text{mL})}{\text{total PSA}(\text{ng}/\text{mL})} \times 100\% = \text{percent free PSA}$$

- **Normal range:** see Table 16.69.

❏ Use

- Monitoring patients with a history of prostate cancer as an early indicator of recurrence and response to treatment
- Prostate cancer screening

❏ Interpretation
*Increased In**

- Prostate diseases
  - ▼ Cancer
  - ▼ Prostatitis, five to seven times

16

---

*Transient increases return to normal in 2–6 weeks.

TABLE 16–69. Normal Range

PSA Total: <4 ng/mL	
Probability of Cancer	**PSA Total Levels**
1%	0–2 ng/mL
15%	2–4 ng/mL
25%	4–10 ng/mL
>50%	>10 ng/mL
PSA Free: >25% of Total PSA	
Probability of Cancer	**Percent Free PSA**
56%	0–10%
28%	10–15%
20%	15–20%
16%	20–25%
8%	>25%

- ▼ Benign prostatic hyperplasia
- ▼ Prostatic ischemia
- ▼ Acute urinary retention five to seven times
- ■ Manipulations
  - ▼ Prostatic massage, ≤2 times
  - ▼ Cystoscopy: four times
  - ▼ Needle biopsy: >50 times for ≤1 month
  - ▼ Transurethral resection: >50 times
  - ▼ Digital rectal examination increases PSA significantly if initial value is >20 ng/mL and is not a confusing factor in falsely elevating PSA.
  - ▼ Radiation therapy
  - ▼ Indwelling catheter
  - ▼ Vigorous bicycle exercise: ≤2–3 times several days
- ■ Treadmill stress test: no change.
- ■ Drugs (e.g., testosterone).
- ■ Physiologic fluctuations: ≤30%.
- ■ PSA has no circadian rhythm, but 6–7% variation can occur between specimens collected on same day.
- ■ Ambulatory values are higher than sedentary values, which may decrease ≤50% (mean = 18%).
- ■ Ejaculation causes transient increase <1.0 ng/mL for 48 hours.
- ■ Analytic factors
  - ▼ Different assays yield different values
  - ▼ Antibody cross-reactivity
  - ▼ High titer heterophile antibodies
- ■ Other diseases/organs
  - ▼ Also found in small amounts in other cancers (sweat and salivary glands, breast, colon, lung, ovary) and in Skene glands of female urethra and in term placenta
  - ▼ Acute renal failure
  - ▼ Acute myocardial infarction

Decreased In

- Ejaculation within 24–48 hours
- Castration
- Antiandrogen drugs (e.g., finasteride)
- Radiation therapy
- Prostatectomy
- PSA falls 17% in 3 days after lying in hospital
- Artifactual (e.g., improper specimen collection; very high PSA levels)
- Finasteride (5-α-reductase inhibitor) reduces PSA by 50% after 6 months in men without cancer

❏ Limitations

- PSA has been recommended by the American Cancer Society for use in conjunction with a DRE for the early detection of prostate cancer starting at age 50 years for men with at least a 10-year life expectancy. Men at high risk, such as those of African descent or with a family history of the disease, may begin testing at an earlier age.
- PSA levels that are measured repeatedly over time may vary both because of imprecision in the analysis and biologic variability where the true PSA level in a given man is different on different measurements. This could potentially lead to an apparent rise in the PSA level, when no actual rise had occurred.
- It is highly recommended that the same assay method be used for longitudinal monitoring.
- A change in PSA of >30% in men with a PSA initially below 2.0 ng/mL was likely to indicate a true change beyond normal random variation.
- The acceptable PSA levels are less clear after radiation therapy, where values may not reach undetectable concentrations. With a nadir of <0.5 ng/mL, relapse is not likely with 5 years of treatment. Biochemical recurrence has been defined by the ASTRO as three consecutive increases in PSA above the nadir.
- The 5-α-reductase inhibitor drugs may affect PSA levels in some patients. Other drugs used to treat benign prostatic hyperplasia may also affect PSA levels. Drugs that decrease PSA levels include buserelin, finasteride, and flutamide. Care should be taken in interpreting results from patients taking these drugs.
- Although screening for prostate cancer with PSA can reduce mortality due to prostate cancer, the absolute risk reduction is small. ACS recommends providing sufficient information regarding risks and benefits of screening and treatment to men to make informed shared decision. For those who decide to screen PSA with or without DRE for average-risk men beginning 50 years of age. Screening should not be offered to men whose life expectancy is <10 years. Men who have >2.5 ng/mL level should undergo annual testing.
- AUA guidelines recommend screening against men younger than 40 years of age and does not recommend routine screening for average-risk men of 40–54 years of age, men older than 70 years, or men whose life expectancy of <10–15 years.

16

- USPSTF recommend that men not to be screened for prostate cancer. They did advise that men requesting screening be supported in making an informed decision.

PROTEIN (TOTAL), SERUM

❑ **Definition**

- Total serum protein is the sum of the concentration of the circulating proteins. A total serum protein test is a blood test that measures the amounts of total protein, albumin, and globulin in the blood. The amounts of albumin and globulin also are compared (albumin/globulin ratio). Normally, there is a little more albumin than globulin, and the ratio is >1. A ratio <1 or much >1 can give clues about problems in the body.
- **Normal range:**
  - ▼ 0–7 days: 4.6–7.0 g/dL
  - ▼ 7 days–1 year: 4.4–7.5 g/dL
  - ▼ 1–3 years: 5.5–7.5 g/dL
  - ▼ 3 years to adult: 6.0–8.0 g/dL

❑ **Use**

- Diagnosis and treatment of diseases involving the liver, kidney, or bone marrow, as well as other metabolic or nutritional disorders
- Screening for nutritional deficiencies and gammopathies

❑ **Interpretation**

Increased In

- Hypergammaglobulinemias (monoclonal or polyclonal; see following sections)
- Hypovolemic states

Decreased In

- Nutritional deficiency (e.g., malabsorption, Kwashiorkor, marasmus)
- Decreased or ineffective protein synthesis (e.g., severe liver disease, agammaglobulinemia)
- Increased loss
  - ▼ Renal (e.g., nephrotic syndrome)
  - ▼ GI disease (e.g., protein-losing enteropathies, surgical resection)
  - ▼ Severe skin disease (e.g., burns, pemphigus vulgaris, eczema)
  - ▼ Blood loss, plasmapheresis
- Increased catabolism (e.g., fever, inflammation, hyperthyroidism, malignancy, chronic diseases)
- Dilutional (e.g., IV fluids, SIADH, water intoxication)
- Third trimester of pregnancy

❑ **Limitations**

- Falsely elevated proteins (pseudohyperproteinemia) can be caused by hemoconcentration due to dehydration or sample desiccation.
- Upright posture for several hours after rising increases total proteins and several other analytes

PROTEIN (TOTAL), URINE

❑ **Definition**

- Normal urine contains up to 150 mg (1–14 mg/dL) of protein each day. This protein originates from ultrafiltration of plasma. Presence of increased amounts of proteins in urine is termed as proteinuria and is the first indication of renal disease. Proteinuria can be classified into three types:
    - ▼ Prerenal: overflow proteinuria, with an increase in plasma, low molecular weight proteins spill into urine (normal proteins, acute-phase reactants, light chain immunoglobulins)
    - ▼ Renal:
        - ● Glomerular proteinuria: defective glomerular filtration barrier. This could be selective or nonselective to different proteins.
        - ● Tubular proteinuria: defective tubular reabsorption; increase in low molecular weight proteins.
    - ▼ Postrenal: proteins produced by the urinary tract, during inflammation, malignancy, or injury
- **Normal range:**
    - ▼ Twenty-four–hour urine: <150 mg/day
    - ▼ Random urine: <200 mg/g creatinine

❑ **Use**

- Evaluation of proteinuria (see Table 16.70) (e.g., following urinalysis in which proteinuria is detected)
- Evaluation of renal diseases, including proteinuria complicating DM and the nephrotic syndromes.
- Workup of other renal diseases, including malignant hypertension, GN, TTP, collagen diseases, toxemia of pregnancy, drug nephrotoxicity, hypersensitivity reactions, and allergic reactions and renal tubular lesions
- Management of myeloma and evaluation of hypoproteinemia.

❑ **Interpretation**
Increased In

- Nephrotic syndrome
- Diabetic neuropathy
- Monoclonal gammopathies such as multiple myeloma and other myeloproliferative or lymphoproliferative disorders
- Abnormal renal tubular absorption
    - ▼ Fanconi syndrome
    - ▼ Heavy metal poisoning
    - ▼ Sickle cell disease
- Urinary tract malignancies
- Inflammatory, degenerative, and irritative conditions of the lower urinary tract
- After exercise

❑ **Limitations**

- Highly alkaline urine produces false-negative results.
- Not reliable to quantify urinary immunoglobulin light chains.

16

> **TABLE 16–70. National Kidney Foundation Guidelines for Assessment of Proteinuria**
>
> - Guidelines for adults and children
>   - Under most circumstances, untimed (spot) urine samples should be used to detect and monitor proteinuria in children and adults.
>   - It is usually not necessary to obtain a timed urine collection (overnight or 24 h) for these evaluations in either children or adults.
>   - First morning specimens are preferred, but random specimens are acceptable if first morning specimens are not available.
>   - In most cases, screening with urine dipsticks is acceptable for detecting proteinuria:
>   - Standard urine dipsticks are acceptable for detecting increased total urine protein.
>   - Albumin-specific dipsticks are acceptable for detecting albuminuria.
>   - Patients with a positive dipstick test (1+ or greater) should undergo confirmation of proteinuria by a quantitative measurement (protein-to-creatinine ratio or albumin-to-creatinine ratio) within 3 mo.
>   - Patients with two or more positive quantitative tests temporally spaced by 1–2 wk should be diagnosed as having persistent proteinuria and undergo further evaluation and management for chronic kidney disease.
>   - Monitoring proteinuria in patients with chronic kidney disease should be performed using quantitative measurements.
> - Specific guidelines for adults
>   - When screening adults at increased risk for chronic kidney disease, albumin should be measured in a spot urine sample using either:
>   - Albumin-specific dipstick
>   - Albumin-to-creatinine ratio
>   - When monitoring proteinuria in adults with chronic kidney disease, the protein-to-creatinine ratio in spot urine samples should be measured using:
>   - Albumin-to-creatinine ratio
>   - Total protein-to-creatinine ratio is acceptable if albumin-to-creatinine ratio is high (>500–1,000 mg/g)
> - Specific guidelines for children without diabetes
>   - When screening children for chronic kidney disease, total urine protein should be measured in a spot urine sample using either
>   - Standard urine dipstick
>   - Total protein-to-creatinine ratio
>   - Orthostatic proteinuria must be excluded by repeat measurement on a first morning specimen if the initial finding of proteinuria was obtained on a random specimen.
>   - When monitoring proteinuria in children with chronic kidney disease, the total protein-to-creatinine ratio should be measured in spot urine specimens.
> - Specific guidelines for children with diabetes
>   - Screening and monitoring of postpubertal children with diabetes of 5 or more years of duration should follow the guidelines for adults.
>   - Screening and monitoring other children with diabetes should follow the guidelines for children without diabetes.

Data from: http://www.kidney.org/professionals/kdoqi/guidelines_ckd/p5_lab_g5.htm

PROTEIN C*

❑ **Definition**

- Protein C is a vitamin K–dependent coagulation inhibitor which, in its activated form, activated protein C (APC), down-regulates the activity of factors

---

*Submitted By Liberto Pechet, MD.

V and VIII through proteolysis. It is produced mainly in the liver. Congenital deficiency leads to a high incidence of venous thrombosis. Because of its short half-life, measured in hours, initiation of vitamin K antagonist therapy results in very rapid decline in the protein C level in normal individuals. In heterozygous individuals, such therapy may lead to very low levels of protein C activity—approaching 0%, with a high risk for venous thrombosis and coumarin necrosis.

- **Normal range:** 70–140%.

❑ Use

- Protein C functional level is examined in cases of suspected congenital thrombophilia, such as suspected in patients with unprovoked venous thromboembolism, especially when in unusual sites.
- Determination of protein C antigen discriminates between type 1 protein C deficiency (concordant decrease of functional and immunologic assays) and type II deficiency, where the antigen level is normal. This difference has no known clinical implication.
- Protein C should not be assayed in patients taking vitamin K antagonists.

❑ Interpretation

Increased In

- Diabetes
- Nephrotic syndrome
- Ischemic heart disease
- Pregnancy
- Oral contraceptives
- Heparin therapy
- Increased age

Decreased In

- Congenital heterozygous deficiency of protein C, which is an autosomal trait with variable penetrance, with a prevalence of 1/500 individuals of European descent. Homozygous deficiency results in life-threatening massive thromboses in neonates (purpura fulminans).
- Acquired: liver disease, vitamin K deficiency or use of vitamin K antagonists, L-asparaginase therapy, DIC, acute-phase reaction (thrombotic, inflammatory, surgical).

❑ Limitations

- Highly elevated factor VIII levels falsely lower protein C measurements
- Lupus anticoagulant may falsely elevate reported protein C levels

PROTEIN S*

❑ Definition

- Protein S is a plasma protein synthesized in the liver and dependent on vitamin K for its functionality. It has an anticoagulant function, serving as a cofactor for activated protein C. Together they inhibit the activities of activated factors

16

*Submitted By Liberto Pechet, MD.

V and VIII. Protein S circulates in a free form, *free protein S* (about 40% of the protein), where the major cofactor function resides, and as bound to complement C4b, *bound protein S*. The bound form may also play a role in the natural anticoagulation mechanism, this possibility being under active investigation.

- **Normal range:** "free" or "total."
- Free protein S (measured functionally): 60–140% in males, slightly lower in females but increases with age.
- Total protein S (measured as antigen by enzyme immunoassay): 60–140%, lower in females but increases with age.
- During the first year of life, the total PS is low (free PS level is identical with that of adults). Adult levels of total PS are reached by 1 year of life.

❏ **Use**

- Protein S, both free and total, should be requested in patients with unprovoked venous thrombosis suspected of congenital thrombophilia.
- Protein S should not be performed in patients on vitamin K antagonist therapy. It is necessary to wait for 2 weeks after cessation of therapy.
- It is advisable to request protein S together with protein C, because both are affected by therapy with vitamin K antagonists, but they have different half-lives. Comparing the two facilitates the interpretation.
- If the functional assay for free protein S is decreased, an immunoassay for free protein S is recommended for confirmation.

❏ **Interpretation**

Decreased In

- Congenital condition. Prevalence of the congenital deficiency of protein S is 1 in 500 for the Caucasian population. It predisposes to venous thromboembolism. The rare homozygous type may cause severe neonatal purpura fulminans.
- Acquired: oral anticoagulants or vitamin K deficiency; pregnancy, hormone replacement therapy, oral contraceptives; young age; liver disease; acute-phase reaction situations (decreased free protein S but increased total protein S); proteinuria; DIC; and L-asparaginase therapy

❏ **Limitations**

- Very elevated (>250%) factor VIII decreases the activity of protein S.
- High titers of rheumatoid factor may lead to overestimation of protein S.
- Heparin (up to 1 IU/mL), high bilirubin, or hemolyzed blood do not interfere with measurements, but elevated values may be seen artificially during high-dose heparin therapy.

PROTEIN, CEREBROSPINAL FLUID

❏ **Definition**

- CSF protein concentration is one of the most sensitive indicators of pathology within the CNS.
- **Normal range:** 15–45 mg/dL.

❏ **Use**

- To detect increased permeability of the blood–brain barrier to plasma proteins
- To detect increased intrathecal production of immunoglobulins

❏ Interpretation

Increased In

- Bacterial meningitis
- Brain tumor
- Brain abscess
- Aseptic meningitis
- Multiple sclerosis
- Cerebral hemorrhage
- Epilepsy
- Acute alcoholism
- Neurosyphilis

Decreased In

- Repeated lumbar puncture or a chronic leak, in which CSF is lost at a higher than normal rate
- Some children between the ages of 6 months and 2 years
- Acute water intoxication
- Minority of patients with idiopathic intracranial hypertension

❏ Limitations

- CSF protein levels do not fall in hypoproteinemia.
- The normal reference ranges is somewhat technique dependent and vary from laboratory to laboratory.
- Excessive amounts of CSF proteins are seen in Froin syndrome, clotted specimens, xanthochromia, or the presence of free blood.
- In premature infants, values >130 mg/dL may occasionally be observed.

PROTHROMBIN G20210A MOLECULAR MUTATION ASSAY*

❏ Definition

- The prothrombin mutation *c.20210G>A* (*20210G>A*) in the *F2* gene is associated with increased plasma prothrombin levels and an increased risk of venous thrombosis (OMIM# 32790). Heterozygosity for the prothrombin *c.20210G>A* mutation is associated with an approximately threefold increased risk of venous thrombosis. Homozygosity for this mutation is rare, but the associated risk of venous thrombosis is likely to be higher than the heterozygous risk. Other factors can further increase the risk of thrombosis.
- **Normal values:** negative or no mutations are found.

❏ Use

- Prothrombin *c.20210G>A* testing should be performed in the following cases:
  - ▼ A first venous thrombotic embolism (VTE) before age 50 years
  - ▼ A first unprovoked VTE at any age
  - ▼ A history of recurrent VTE

16

*Submitted by Edward Ginns, MD and Marzena M. Galdzicka, PhD.

▼ Venous thrombosis at unusual sites such as the cerebral, mesenteric, portal, or hepatic veins

▼ VTE during pregnancy or the puerperium

▼ VTE associated with the use of oral contraceptives or hormone replacement therapy

▼ A first VTE at any age in an individual with a first-degree family member with a VTE before age 50 years

▼ Women with unexplained fetal loss after 10 weeks of gestation

■ Prothrombin c.20210G>A testing may be considered in the following cases:

▼ Women with unexplained early-onset severe preeclampsia, placental abruption, or significant intrauterine growth retardation

▼ A first VTE related to tamoxifen or other selective estrogen receptor modulators (SERM)

▼ Female smokers younger than 50 years with a myocardial infarction

▼ Individuals older than age 50 years with a first provoked VTE in the absence of malignancy or an intravascular device

▼ Asymptomatic adult family members of probands with one or two known c.20210G>A mutation in the F2 gene, especially those with a strong family history of VTE at a young age

▼ Asymptomatic female family members of probands with known prothrombin thrombophilia who are pregnant or who are considering oral contraception or pregnancy

▼ Women with recurrent unexplained first-trimester loss with or without second- or third-trimester loss

▼ Children with arterial thrombosis

❑ Limitations

■ The results of a genetic test may be affected by DNA rearrangements, blood transfusion, bone marrow transplantation, or rare sequence variations.

■ Genetic causes of thrombosis, other than the prothrombin c.20210G>A mutation, will not be detected.

PROTHROMBIN TIME (PT) AND THE INTERNATIONAL NORMALIZED RATIO (INR)*

❑ Definition

■ The PT assesses the coagulation activity of the extrinsic and common coagulation pathways.

■ Tissue thromboplastin (tissue factor) is used as a potent activator of the coagulation system in the presence of added calcium. Currently, recombinant tissue factor is used in most commercial reagents. The potency of tissue factor explains the shortness of clotting (in seconds) in the assay.

■ **Normal ranges:**

▼ PT: 9.6–12.4 seconds (may vary slightly from laboratory to laboratory)

▼ INR: 1.0 ratio (remains constant independent of equipment or reagent used)

*Submitted By Liberto Pechet, MD.

❏ Use

- Evaluation of clotting disorders that may involve the extrinsic coagulation mechanism (factor VII) and the common pathway (factors II, V, X and fibrinogen). In these situations, the PTT should be ordered in parallel with the PT. PT is not sensitive to clotting factors if they are modestly decreased (>30%). In addition, it is not sensitive to abnormalities in factors involved in the intrinsic coagulation pathway (factors XII, XI, IX, and VIII) or in protein C or S deficiencies.
- Evaluation of liver function reflecting abnormalities in factors VII, II, X, IX and V (but not VIII).
- To monitor long-term oral anticoagulant therapy with coumarin and indanedione derivatives. PT is prolonged >PTT, and more consistently so. Factor V is not affected by oral anticoagulants, whereas it may be decreased in liver disease.
  - ▼ INR is the preferred reporting to monitor patients on vitamin K antagonist therapy. In all other circumstances, the use of PT is encouraged rather than INR. The recommended range for INR during most indications for oral anticoagulants is 2–3, or 2.5–3.5 for patients with mechanical heart valves.

❏ Interpretation

- Marked prolongation of the PT in liver disease indicates advanced disease.
- Marked elevation of INR in patients receiving vitamin K antagonists is a marker of excessive anticoagulation and requires prompt action contrariwise, an INR below 2.0 reflects insufficient anticoagulation.
- Combined abnormal PT and PTT is found under two circumstances:
  - ▼ Medical: administration of oral anticoagulants, DIC, liver disease, vitamin K deficiency, massive transfusions
  - ▼ Coagulation factor abnormalities: dysfibrinogenemias; factors V, X, and II defects

❏ Limitations

- Preanalytic errors:
  - ▼ Partially clotted specimens due to poor mixture with the anticoagulant (3.2 sodium citrate, as offered by manufacturers' blue top vacuum tubes)
  - ▼ Over- or underfilled test tubes, altering the ratio of blood (9 parts) to anticoagulant (1 part)
- Analytic errors: Hemolyzed, lipemic, or icteric plasma may interfere with photoelectric measuring instruments (assay may have to be repeated on a mechanical clot measuring instrument)

PYRUVATE KINASE (PK), RED BLOOD CELL

❏ Definition

- PK is an enzyme involved in glycolysis. Genetic defects of this enzyme cause the disease known as PK deficiency. This deficiency is one of the most common enzymatic defects of the erythrocyte. The disorder manifests clinically as a hemolytic anemia, and the symptomatology is less severe than hematologic indices indicate. The clinical severity of this disorder varies widely, ranging from a mildly compensated anemia to severe anemia of childhood.

16

Most affected individuals do not require treatment. Individuals who are most severely affected may die in utero of anemia or may require blood transfusions or splenectomy, but most of the symptomatology is limited to early life and to times of physiologic stress or infection.

▪ **Normal range: 9.0–22.0 U/g Hb.**

❑ **Use**

▪ Evaluation of nonspherocytic hemolytic anemia
▪ Investigating families with PK deficiency to determine inheritance pattern and for genetic counseling

❑ **Interpretation**

▪ Increased in patients with younger erythrocyte population
▪ Decreased in congenital nonspherocytic hemolytic anemia

❑ **Limitations**

▪ Patients who have recently received transfusions have normal donor cells that may mask PK-deficient erythrocytes.
▪ Most PK-deficient patients have 5–25% of normal activity.
▪ Leukocytes also contain PK, that is not decreased by hereditary erythrocyte PK deficiency, freeing the blood of WBC is critical for accuracy.

QUANTITATIVE PILOCARPINE IONTOPHORESIS SWEAT TEST

❑ **Definition**

▪ The sweat test consists of the quantitative analyses of sweat chloride with or without sodium. This procedure, often referred to as the quantitative pilocarpine iontophoresis test, involves collection and quantification of sweat after pilocarpine iontophoresis with the use of gauze, filter paper, or Macroduct coils and quantitative analyses of sweat chloride. The sweat test entails three consecutive procedures: sweat stimulation, sweat collection, and sweat analysis.
▪ **Normal range** (sweat chloride):
  ▾ Less than 40 mmol/L (>3 months)
  ▾ Greater than 30 mmol/L (<3 months)
▪ **Borderline results:** sweat chloride 40–60 mmol/L
▪ A positive test is defined by sweat chloride >60 mmol/L in sweat from both arms, provided that a minimum of 15 µL of sweat is obtained from each site.

❑ **Use**

▪ Standard test for the diagnosis of CF

❑ **Interpretation**
Increased In

▪ CF (see Table 16.71)
▪ Endocrine disorders (e.g., untreated adrenal insufficiency, hypothyroidism, vasopressin-resistant diabetes insipidus, familial hypoparathyroidism, pseudohypoaldosteronism)

TABLE 16–71. Sweat Values in Cystic Fibrosis (mEq/L)

	Chloride		Sodium		Potassium	
	Mean	Range	Mean	Range	Mean	Range
Cystic fibrosis	115	79–148	111	75–145	23	14–30
Normal	28	8–43	28	16–46	10	6–17

- Metabolic disorders (e.g., malnutrition, glycogen storage disease type I, MPS I H [Hurler syndrome], MPS I S [Scheie syndrome], fucosidosis)
- GU disorders (e.g., Klinefelter syndrome, nephrosis)
- Allergic/immunologic disorders (e.g., hypogammaglobulinemia, prolonged infusion with prostaglandin E_1, atopic dermatitis)
- Neuropsychologic disorders (e.g., anorexia nervosa)
- Others (e.g., ectodermal dysplasia, G6PD deficiency)

Decreased In
- False-negative results if patient is edematous or if an inadequate quantity of sweat is collected and analyzed
- Methodologic and technical errors

❏ **Limitations**
- Values may be increased to CF range in healthy persons when sweat rate is rapid (e.g., exercise, high temperature), but pilocarpine test does not increase sweating rate.
- Mineralocorticoids decrease sodium concentration in sweat by approximately 50% in normal subjects and 10–20% in CF patients whose final sodium concentration remains abnormally high.
- Confirmation of a diagnosis of CF requires two positive sweat tests done on different days. Borderline results should be reported with the suggestion that the test be repeated if clinically indicated.
- The preferred patient age for testing is after 48 hours. During the first 24 hours after birth, sweat electrolytes are transiently elevated and rapidly decline on the 2nd day. Therefore, sweat testing should not be performed within 48 hours after birth.

Suggested Readings

Boat TF, Acton JD. Cystic fibrosis. In: Kliegman RM, Behrman RE, Jenson HB, et al. (eds.). *Nelson Textbook of Pediatrics*, 18th ed. Philadelphia, PA: Saunders Elsevier; 2007:1803–1817.
Farrell PM, Rosenstein BJ, White TB, et al. Guidelines for diagnosis of cystic fibrosis in newborns through older adults: cystic fibrosis consensus report. *J Pediatr.* 2008;153(2):S4–S14.

RED BLOOD CELLS (RBCs): COUNT AND MORPHOLOGY*

❏ **Definition and Use**
- The RBC count is part of the CBC as obtained by automated counters. It is less useful than the Hb or Hct.

16

*Submitted By Liberto Pechet, MD.

- **Normal range:** 4.2–5.4 cells/μL in women and 4.4–6.0 cells/μL in men (reported by automated counters in a random adult population)
  - ▼ Different values are reported for newborns, infants, and children until they reach adulthood.
  - ▼ Automated counters adjust normal values for age groups.

❏ **Interpretation**

- The RBC count is interpreted in conjunction with red cell indices, hemoglobin, and hematocrit.

Increased In

- Certain myeloproliferative neoplasms (e.g., polycythemia vera).
- Severe dehydration. RBC counts may be *appropriately* decreased or increased in certain physiologic states.

Decreased In

- Various types of anemia

Abnormal RBC Morphology

- It is flagged by automated counters, triggering microscopic examination of stained peripheral blood smears (see above).
- Abnormalities (see Tables 16.72 and 16.73) may be specific for certain conditions (e.g., spherocytes for hemolytic anemias, sickle cells for sickle cell anemias) or may be informative but not specific. *Anisocytosis* refers to variation in RBC size, *poikilocytosis* refers to variation in shape, and *polychromasia* refers to bluish discoloration of RBC reflecting high reticulocytes.

TABLE 16–72. Abnormal Shapes of Red Blood Cells

Shape	Description	Conditions
Acanthocytes (spur cells)	Pointed membrane spicules of uneven length	Hereditary: acanthocytosis in abetalipoproteinemia Acquired: postsplenectomy, fulminant liver disease, malabsorption
Bite cells (precipitated hemoglobin [Heinz bodies])	RBCs with a peripheral smooth semicircle fragment missing	Hemolysis due to certain drugs, with or without G6PD deficiency; unstable hemoglobin
Burr cells	Crenated RBCs with preserved central pallor	Uremia, liver disease, Rhesus factor null cells, phosphokinase deficiency, anorexia nervosa, hypophosphatemia, hypomagnesemia, hyposplenism
Echinocytes	Blunt uniform spicules	Similar to burr cells; may be artifacts
Elliptocytes/ovalocytes	Oval RBCs	Hereditary elliptocytosis, iron deficiency, sickle cell trait, thalassemias, HbC disease; megaloblastic anemias
HbC crystalloids	Rhomboid crystals inclusions in RBCs	HbC trait or disease

TABLE 16–72. Abnormal Shapes of Red Blood Cells (*Continued*)

Shape	Description	Conditions
Leptocytes	Flat, water-like, thin, hypochromic RBCs	Obstructive liver disease, thalassemia
Macrocytes	RBCs larger than normal, well filled with hemoglobin	Oval macrocytes in megaloblastic anemias; round macrocytes in liver disease Increased erythropoiesis
Microcytes	Decreased MCV (RBC smaller than normal)	Hypochromic anemias with defective iron stores
Microspherocytes		Artifacts; severe frostbite
RBC agglutination	Grouping together of RBCs due to IgM antibodies	Cold agglutinins, most commonly *Mycoplasma pneumoniae*; infectious mononucleosis
Rouleaux formation	Stack of coins appearance	Hyperproteinemias, especially multiple myeloma and plasmacytic lymphoma of IgM type; most frequently artifact
Schistocytes (mechanical destruction of RBC in the circulation)	Helmet-like or fragmented, distorted RBCs	Micro- or macroangiopathic (small or large arteries) hemolytic anemias, prosthetic heart valves, severe valvular disease or large atheromas, DIC, TTP, severe iron deficiency, megaloblastic anemias, severe burns, renal transplant rejection, postchemotherapy, snake bite, inherited abnormalities of RBC membrane spectrin
Sickle cells (drepanocytes)	Bipolar, spiculated RBCs, pointed at both ends (shaped like sickles)	Sickle cell anemia (absent in sickle cell trait, unless induced by oxygen reduction)
Spherocytes (loss of RBC membrane)	Increased MCHC, usually decreased MCV; spherical cells with dense appearance and without central pallor	Hereditary spherocytosis, autoimmune hemolytic anemias, recent RBC transfusion
Stomatocytes	Mouth-like deformity with slit-like central pallor	Hereditary stomatocytosis, Rhesus factor null disease, immune hemolytic anemia, acute alcoholism, certain drugs (phenothiazines); frequently artifacts
Target cells (increased ratio of RBC surface area to volume)	Target-like appearance, often hypochromic; decreased osmotic fragility	Thalassemias, HbC disease or trait, HbD and E, iron deficiency anemia, liver disease, postsplenectomy, artifacts
Teardrop cells (dacryocytes)	Distorted, teardrop-shaped RBCs	Primary myelofibrosis, myelophthisic anemia, other myeloproliferative neoplasms or myelodysplastic syndromes, β-thalassemia major, iron deficiency, conditions with Heinz bodies

16

TABLE 16–73. Red Blood Cell Inclusions

Red Cell Type	Description	Disease State Association
Basophilic stippling	Punctuate basophilic inclusions composed of precipitated ribosomes (RNA)	A variety of anemias, thalassemias; coarse in lead poisoning
Cabot rings	Circular, blue, thread-like inclusion with dots	Occasional in severe megaloblastic and hemolytic anemias, overwhelming infections, postsplenectomy
Heinz bodies	Precipitates of denatured hemoglobin attached to RBC membrane; require supravital stains (e.g., crystal violet) for visualization	G6PD deficiency, methemoglobin reductase, drug-induced hemolytic anemias, unstable hemoglobin (e.g., hemoglobin Zurich), postsplenectomy; can be artifactual
Howell-Jolly bodies	Nuclear remnants of DNA; one, rarely two, dark purple, nonrefractile spherical bodies located at periphery of RBCs	Postsplenectomy, megaloblastic anemias, thalassemia, myelodysplasia, lead poisoning
Organisms on smears, outside RBCs	Specific morphology	*Wuchereria bancrofti; Brugia malayi; Loa loa; Trypanosoma brucei gambiense, T. cruzi,* and *T. rhodesiense; Borrelia recurrentis*
Organisms within RBCs	Specific shapes	*Plasmodium* trophozoites, babesiosis, other organisms
Pappenheimer bodies	Siderotic, nonheme iron granules at periphery of RBC; seen best with Prussian blue stain	Sideroblastic anemias, iron load, thalassemia, lead poisoning, postsplenectomy

❏ **Limitations**

▪ Patient's circumstances (e.g., vomiting or diarrhea)
▪ Other preanalytic factors
  ▼ Marked leukocytosis marginally increases the RBC count.
  ▼ Inappropriate blood collection is a major source of preanalytic errors. For instance, inappropriate filling of test tube results in excess anticoagulant, thereby diluting the blood and decreasing the red cell parameters.
  ▼ Very low temperatures may lyse the red cells. Anticoagulated blood may be stored at 4°C for 24 hours, but beyond this interval, the results become increasingly altered.

RED CELL DISTRIBUTION WIDTH (RDW)*

❏ **Definition**

▪ RDW is a coefficient of variation of the distribution of individual RBC volume.
▪ **Normal range: 12.1–14 fL.**

❏ **Use**

▪ An elevation in RDW is useful in drawing attention to anisocytosis, a marker for various anemias.

---

*Submitted By Liberto Pechet, MD.

❏ Interpretation

- The RDW is particularly helpful in separating iron deficiency anemia (high RDW, normal to low MCV) from β-thalassemia trait (normal RDW, low MCV).
- Increased RDW is also useful in identifying red cell fragmentation, agglutination, or dimorphic cell populations.

❏ Limitations

- Very high WBC, numerous large platelets, and autoagglutination result in falsely elevated RDW.

REPTILASE TIME (RT)*

❏ Definition

- RT measures the conversion of fibrinogen to fibrin when added to plasma. The reagent is a thrombin-like enzyme derived from venom of *Bothrops atrox*. It is unaffected by heparin or hirudin.
- **Normal value:** <20 seconds.

❏ Use

- An abnormal RT indicates an abnormality of fibrinogen, whereas a normal RT suggests heparin or hirudin as the cause of an abnormal thrombin time.
- A RT evaluates prolonged PTT when heparin or hirudin contamination is suspected.
- It also excludes dysfibrinogenemia.

❏ Interpretation

Causes of Increased RT

- Hypofibrinogenemia or dysfibrinogenemia
- Slightly prolonged in the presence of fibrin degradation products as seen in severe DIC or pathologic fibrinolysis

❏ Limitations

- Preanalytic: partially clotted blood or hemolyzed blood, improperly filled or stored test tubes, specimens collected in wrong tubes
- Lipemic or icteric samples

RETICULOCYTES†

❏ Definition

- Reticulocytes are immature RBC without nuclei. The reticulocyte count provides an estimate of the rate of red cell production. To visualize the reticulum-like RNA and count reticulocytes as a separate group of RBC, a special stain is required. The reticulocytes can be counted manually (at the microscope) and reported as percent per 100 RBC, or by automated counters.

*Submitted By Liberto Pechet, MD.
†Submitted By Liberto Pechet, MD.

16

- **Normal range:** 0.3–2.3/100 RBCs with automated counters. However, this varies to some extent in the manual methodology. An absolute reticulocyte count or reticulocyte production index is more helpful than the percentage, and this can be calculated from the hematologic data.

❏ **Interpretation**

Causes of Increased Reticulocytes
- Reticulocytosis: Enhanced red cell production most marked in hemolytic anemias or during bone marrow regeneration

Causes of Decreased Reticulocytes
- Conditions with inadequate or ineffective hematopoiesis, despite the presence of anemia

❏ **Limitations**

- The manual counts result in great variability, being operator dependent. The automated counters provide better precision. Erythrocyte inclusions, other than the true reticulum, may falsely increase the reticulocyte count. Similar errors occur in sickle cell anemia and sickle/C hemoglobinopathies.

REVERSE T_3 (rT_3), TRIIODOTHYRONINE, REVERSE

❏ **Definition**

- Hormonally inactive isomer of T_3.
- **Normal range:**
  - ▼ Birth to 6 days: 600–2,500 pg/mL
  - ▼ ≥7 days: 90–350 pg/mL

❏ **Use**

- To distinguish low T_3 "sick thyroid" patients (usually increased) from true hypothyroidism

❏ **Interpretation**

Increased In
- Severe nonthyroidal illness except in some liver disorders, HIV, renal failure
- Usually in hyperthyroidism and increased serum TBG

Decreased In
- Often in hypothyroidism but overlaps with normal range

❏ **Limitations**

- Measurement is occasionally useful in hospitalized patients to distinguish between nonthyroidal illness and central hypothyroidism. Values are lower in central hypothyroidism, because of low production of T_4. In patients with mild hypothyroidism, rT_3 levels may be normal or even slightly higher limiting its usefulness.

RHEUMATOID FACTOR (RF)

❏ **Definition**

- RF is an immunoglobulin present in the serum of 50–95% of adults with RA. It appears in serum and synovial fluid several months after onset of RA and is present up to years after therapy. The autoantibodies are usually of IgM class, although approximately 15% of RA has IgG class. Most methods detect only the IgM class.

- **Normal range:** <20 IU/mL.

❑ **Use**

- Assisting in the diagnosis of RA, especially when clinical diagnosis is difficult

❑ **Interpretation**

Increased In

- Chronic hepatitis
- Chronic viral infections
- Cirrhosis
- Dermatomyositis
- Infectious mononucleosis
- Leishmaniasis
- Leprosy
- Malaria
- RA
- Sarcoidosis
- Scleroderma
- Sjögren syndrome
- SLE
- Syphilis
- TB
- Waldenström macroglobulinemia

❑ **Limitations**

- RF is not a finding isolated to RA and may be present in a number of connective tissue and inflammatory diseases, including infectious mononucleosis, SLE, scleroderma, and hepatitis.
- Older patients may have higher values.
- Recent blood transfusion, multiple vaccinations or transfusions, or an inadequately activated complement may affect results.
- Serum with cryoglobulin or high lipid levels may cause false-positive test results.

ROSETTE TEST*

❑ **Definition**

- The rosette test detects D-positive red cells in the blood of a D-negative mother, whose fetus or recently delivered baby is D positive.
- When anti-D reagent is added to the mother's blood, fetal D-positive red cells become coated with anti-D on incubation and exhibit mixed-field agglutination when antiglobulin (see p. 884) reagent is added. Because the mixed-field agglutination may be difficult to detect, D-positive RBCs are added to the

16

*Submitted By Vishesh Chhibber, MD.

mixture to demonstrate rosettes of several cells clustered against antibody-coated D-positive cells.

- **Normal value:** Absence of rosettes is considered negative for major fetomaternal hemorrhage in an Rh-negative mother with an Rh-positive fetus.

❑ **Use**

- The test is used to determine the presence of fetal–maternal hemorrhage by testing for the presence of D-positive fetal red cells in the circulation of a D-negative mother. If >30 mL of fetal (whole) blood or >15 mL of fetal red cells are present in the maternal circulation, the assay has a sensitivity of ≥99%.

❑ **Interpretation**

- The presence of a positive result indicates that the fetal blood is admixed with that of the mother. This happens when the fetus has hemorrhaged into the mother's circulation and may require intrauterine transfusion or obstetric intervention.

❑ **Limitations**

- The rosette test is a qualitative screening test. If it is positive, the amount of fetal blood in the maternal circulation must be quantified using flow cytometry or the Kleihauer-Betke (acid-elution) assay (see p. 1021).

Suggested Readings

Anstee DJ. Red cell genotyping and the future of pretransfusion testing. *Blood.* 2009;114:248–256.
Petrides M, Stack G. *Practical Guide to Transfusion Medicine*, 2nd ed. Bethesda, MD: AABB Press; 2007.
Roback J, Grossman B, Harris T, et al. (eds.). *Technical Manual*, 17th ed. Bethesda, MD: AABB Press; 2011.

SALICYLATES (ASPIRIN)*

❑ **Definition**

- An acidic drug that is rapidly metabolized to an active metabolite, salicylate; also known as acetylsalicylic acid (ASA). Included in aspirin, sodium salicylate, oil of wintergreen, methyl salicylate.
- **Normal therapeutic range (serum):**
  ▼ Analgesic/antipyretic use: <60 µg/mL
  ▼ Anti-inflammatory use: 150–300 µg/mL

❑ **Use**

- ASA and salicylate have analgesic, antipyretic, and anti-inflammatory properties; used in the treatment of RA.
- ASA also inhibits platelet aggregation and, therefore, prolongs bleeding time.

❑ **Interpretation**

- See discussion of salicylate poisoning in Chapter 14.

---

*Submitted By Amanda J. Jenkins, PhD.

❏ **Limitations**

■ Requires specific test request; not usually detected in routine screens:
  ▼ Color test:
    ● Limit of detection: 40–50 µg/mL
    ● Suitable for blood, serum, plasma, urine
    ● Not recommended for quantitative purposes due to interferences from metabolites, AND plasma constituents
■ Immunoassay
  ▼ Serum/plasma.
  ▼ With a Limit of quantitation: 50 µg/mL.
  ▼ Not whole blood.
  ▼ Anticoagulants (heparin, citrates, oxalates, EDTA) do not interfere.
  ▼ Do not use sodium azide in collection tubes.
  ▼ Hemolysis produces false-negative results.
  ▼ Hemoglobin concentrations >100 mg/dL may interfere.

■ Confirmation
  ▼ Sample pretreatment required
  ▼ Gas chromatography: derivatization may be necessary
  ▼ HPLC: preferred technique for distinguishing metabolites
  ▼ Limit of quantitation: 50 µg/mL

SCREENING FOR FETAL CHROMOSOME ABNORMALITIES AND NEURAL TUBE DEFECTS

❏ **Definition**

■ Noninvasive testing with goal of limiting invasive diagnostic procedures that carry risk to pregnancy

❏ **Use**

■ Screening modalities have been developed for Down syndrome/trisomy 21 detection because trisomy 21 is the most common viable autosomal chromosome abnormality. However, screening also provides specific risk assessment for trisomy 18 and neural tube defects.
■ In addition, with inclusion of early ultrasound examination, increased fetal nuchal translucency may indicate other chromosome abnormalities including Turner syndrome (45,X), trisomy 13, and triploidy.
■ Second-trimester measurement of AFP is used to assess risk of fetal neural tube defects.
■ Screening is offered to all women, regardless of age, to provide more accurate risk information than provided by age alone.

❏ **Limitations**

■ Risk for trisomy 13 is *not* calculated; however, trisomy 13 pregnancies are typically associated with ultrasound anomalies detectable with second-trimester ultrasound definition are chromosomally normal, and some affected pregnancies will be missed.

16

SECOND-TRIMESTER SCREENING (MATERNAL SERUM SCREENING; QUAD SCREEN)

❑ **Definition**

- Performed between 15 and 22 weeks of gestation, the quadruple screen combines maternal age plus four serum biochemical markers: hCG, inhibin A, AFP, and unconjugated estriol to assess the risk of trisomy 21 and trisomy 18.

❑ **Use**

- Risk assessment for trisomy 21 (Down syndrome), trisomy 18, and open neural tube defects.

❑ **Interpretation**

- Trisomy 21 profile typically has high levels of hCG and inhibin A with low levels of AFP and unconjugated estriol.
- Trisomy 18 is associated with low levels of hCG, AFP, and estriol. (Inhibin A does not contribute to trisomy 18 risk profile.)
- Different centers use different cutoffs, balancing detection rate against number of invasive procedures performed. A cutoff of 1:270 (approximately 5% positive screening rate) detects approximately 80% of trisomy 21 and trisomy 18 pregnancies.

❑ **Limitations**

- Detects fewer affected pregnancies than combined first-semester plus second-trimester screening modalities.
- Does not permit first-trimester decision making regarding termination of affected pregnancies.

SEDATIVE–HYPNOTICS*

See Alcohols (Volatiles, Solvents), Benzodiazepines.

❑ **Definition**

- This group of drugs includes those that reduce tension and anxiety, induce calm (sedative), or induce sleep (hypnotic). All have CNS depressant effects. Although other drugs may produce similar effects, the distinctive ability of these drugs is that they achieve their effects without altering mood or reducing sensitivity to pain.
- This class includes ethanol, chloral hydrate, glutethimide, ethchlorvynol (Placidyl), barbiturates, benzodiazepines, meprobamate (Miltown), methaqualone (Quaalude), buspirone (BuSpar), zolpidem (Ambien), and zopiclone (Imovane).
- **Therapeutic range (serum):**
  - ▼ Chloral hydrate (metabolite trichloroethanol [TCE]): 2–12 µg/mL serum
  - ▼ Ethchlorvynol: 2–8 µg/mL
  - ▼ Glutethimide: 1–5 µg/mL
  - ▼ Methaqualone: 1,000–4,000 ng/mL
  - ▼ Meprobamate: 5–25 µg/mL
  - ▼ Buspirone: 1–10 ng/mL

*Submitted By Amanda J. Jenkins, PhD.

▼ Zolpidem: 25–300 ng/mL

▼ Zopiclone: 50–150 ng/mL

- **Barbiturates:**
  ▼ Ultra–short acting (thiopental, methohexital) [approximate]: 40 µg/mL (thiopental); 3–10 µg/mL (methohexital for surgical anesthesia)
  ▼ Short acting (pentobarbital, secobarbital): 0.5–2.0 µg/mL
  ▼ Intermediate acting (amobarbital, butalbital, butabarbital): 1.0–5.0 µg/mL
  ▼ Long acting (phenobarbital): 5–15 µg/mL (sedative–hypnotic); 15–40 µg/mL (anticonvulsant)

❏ Use

- Treatment of sleeping disorders
- Reduction of anxiety

❏ Limitations

Specific Agents

- Chloral hydrate, ethchlorvynol, glutethimide, methaqualone (currently little used in the United States; requires specific request to test)
  ▼ **Chloral hydrate:** measure metabolite trichloroethanol (TCE) with gas chromatography, GC/MS, LC/MS
  ▼ **Ethchlorvynol:** color test, gas chromatography, GC/MS; measure parent
  ▼ **Glutethimide:** gas chromatography, GC/MS, liquid chromatography, LC/MS; measure parent and active metabolite hydroxyglutethimide
  ▼ **Methaqualone:** immunoassay screening test available for this agent
    • Target analyte—methaqualone
    • Cutoff concentration (urine)]—300 ng/mL
    • Confirmation by gas chromatography, GC/MS, liquid chromatography, LC/MS: limit of quantitation: 50–200 ng/mL
- **Meprobamate**
  ▼ Older CNS depressant
  ▼ Metabolite of muscle relaxant carisoprodol
  ▼ No immunoassay-based screening tests available
  ▼ Readily extracted in acidic neutral liquid–liquid or solid-phase extraction scheme: GC, GC/MS, liquid chromatography, LC/MS; limit of quantitation: 500–1,000 ng/mL
- **Buspirone**
  ▼ Newer antianxiety drug
  ▼ No immunoassay-based screening tests available
  ▼ Extracted in alkaline liquid–liquid or solid-phase extraction scheme
  ▼ GC/MS (SIM) due to low concentrations difficult to observe in full scan mode; LC/MS
  ▼ Active metabolite 1-(2-pyrimidinyl)piperazine (1-PP) may also be measured
  ▼ Limit of quantitation: 1 ng/mL
- **Zolpidem**
  ▼ Structurally similar to benzodiazepines
  ▼ No specific immunoassay-based screening tests available for clinical use (recently available for forensic applications)
    • Readily extracted in alkaline liquid–liquid or solid-phase extraction scheme
    • Gas chromatography, liquid chromatography, GC/MS, LC/MS
    • Limit of quantitation: 10–50 ng/mL

16

■ **Zopiclone**
  ▼ Newer hypnotic
  ▼ No immunoassay-based screening tests currently available for clinical use
  ▼ Readily extracted in neutral liquid–liquid or SPE extraction scheme
    ● Unstable in acidic and basic conditions
    ● Gas chromatography, GC/MS, liquid chromatography, LC/MS; may thermally degrade depending on gas chromatography, GC/MS operating parameters
    ● Limit of quantitation: 10–50 ng/mL

BARBITURATES

❏ Definition and Use

■ Older class of CNS depressants. Largely replaced by benzodiazepines and newer hypnotics such as zolpidem. Current main use as anticonvulsants, in treatment of migraines, and in reduction of cerebral edema and intracranial pressure resulting from head injury
  ▼ Screening
    ● Immunoassays for automated chemistry analyzers
    ● Urine
      • Target analyte—secobarbital
      • Cutoff concentration—200 or 300 ng/mL
      • Cross-reactivity—approximately 100% with amobarbital, 60–90% with butabarbital, butalbital, pentobarbital, and phenobarbital
    ● Serum/plasma/blood
      • EMIT, ELISA, FPIA
      • Target analyte—secobarbital
      • Cutoff concentration—10–50 ng/mL ELISA; 1,000 ng/mL EMIT
      • Cross-reactivity—manufacturer kit reagent dependent:
        ○ Low cross-reactivity with amobarbital, phenobarbital, butabarbital, and butalbital and high cross-reactivity with thiopental and pentobarbital
        ○ FPIA generally demonstrates more cross-reactivity than EMIT to other barbiturates
■ Confirmation: chromatography or UV–visible spectrophotometry
  ▼ Sample pretreatment required
  ▼ Gas chromatography
  ▼ HPLC
  ▼ GC/MS
    ● LC/MS
    ● Limit of quantitation: analyte dependent—0.5–5.0 µg/mL

SEMEN ANALYSIS*

❏ Definition

■ A complete semen analysis measures both macroscopic and microscopic characteristics of a semen specimen, all of which can provide clues in the workup of male infertility.

---

*Submitted by Charles R. Kiefer, PhD.

- Reference ranges (WHO):
  - ▼ pH: 7.2–7.8
  - ▼ Volume: 1.5 mL (95% CI 1.4–1.7)
  - ▼ Concentration: ≥15 million/mL (95% CI 12–16)
  - ▼ Total sperm number (count): 39 million per ejaculate (95% CI 33–46)
  - ▼ Progressive motility: 32% (95% CI 31–34)
  - ▼ Total motility (progressive + nonprogressive): 40% (95% CI 38–42)
  - ▼ Vitality: 58% live (95% CI 55–63)
  - ▼ Morphology: ≥ 30% normal forms (WHO criteria), or
  - ▼ ≥ 4% normal forms ("strict" Tygerberg criteria)

❏ Use

- Primary test for male factor infertility in the workup of infertility in a couple
- Confirmation of the effectiveness of vasectomy (sperm concentration alone)

❏ Interpretation

Increased In	Decreased In
■ No upper limit defined	■ Testicular disease (primary defects)
	■ Posttesticular defects (disorders of sperm transport)
	■ Hypothalamic–pituitary disease (secondary hypogonadism)

❏ Limitations

- Minimum specimen volume for microscopic analysis is 0.1 mL.
- Highly viscous specimens may affect accuracy of concentration results.
- A minimum of two analyses, preferably 1 month apart, are recommended to correct for cyclical variation in sperm concentration.
- Specimen collection should occur within a window of 48- to 72-hour abstinence to maximize average concentration of live cells.

Suggested Readings

Cooper TG, Noonan E, von Eckardstein S, et al. World Health Organization reference values for human semen characteristics. *Hum Reprod Update.* 2010;16:231–245.

World Health Organization Department of Reproductive Health and Research. *World Health Organization Laboratory Manual for the Examination and Processing of Human Semen*, 5th ed. Geneva, Switzerland: World Health Organization, 2010.

SEMEN FRUCTOSE*

❏ Definition

- The semen fructose test is a test for fructose in seminal plasma, which is a marker of seminal vesicle function.
- Reference range: ≥13 μmol per ejaculate.

❏ Use

- Workup of azoospermia, especially when ejaculate volume is <1 mL and fails to coagulate.

16

*Submitted by Charles R. Kiefer, PhD.

❏ Interpretation

Increased In	*Decreased In*
■ No upper limit defined	■ Seminal vesicle obstruction (in conjunction with low semen volume)
	■ Atresia distal to the seminal vesicles (in conjunction with low semen volume)

❏ Limitations
- Minimum specimen volume for analysis is 0.1 mL.

Suggested Reading
Dieudonné O, Godin PA, Van-Langendonckt A, et al. Biochemical analysis of the sperm and infertility. *Clin Chem Lab Med.* 2001;39:455–457.

SEROTONIN, BLOOD

❏ Definition
- Serotonin is an indole amine synthesized by the cells of the intestinal mucosa. It is stored in and transported by platelets but also found in many body tissues, including the CNS. Serotonin acts as a vasoconstrictor and neurotransmitter; stimulant of smooth muscle contraction, prolactin release, and GH release; and functions in hemocoagulation. Other names: 5-hydroxytryptamine.
- **Normal range:** 50–200 ng/mL.

❏ Use
- Confirming the diagnosis of carcinoid tumors.
- Adjunct test for 5-HIAA and chromogranin-A test to follow-up patients with carcinoid tumors.

❏ Interpretation
Increased In
- Metastasizing abdominal carcinoid tumors
- Dumpling syndrome
- Acute intestinal obstruction
- Cystic fibrosis
- AMI and nontropical sprue
- Oat cell carcinoma of the lung
- Pancreatic islet tumor
- Thyroid medullary carcinoma

Decreased In
- Down syndrome
- Severe depression
- Parkinson disease
- Phenylketonuria (treated and untreated)
- Renal insufficiency
- Teratomas

❑ Limitations

- Blood serotonin is very unstable.
- Medications that may affect serotonin concentrations include lithium, MAO inhibitors, methyldopa, morphine, and reserpine.
- In general, foods that contain serotonin do not interfere significantly.
- Slight increases may be seen in acute intestinal obstruction, acute MI, cystic fibrosis, dumping syndromes, and nontropical sprue.

SERUM PROTEIN ELECTROPHORESIS/IMMUNOFIXATION

❑ Definition

- Serum protein electrophoresis (SPE) is a method of physical separation of protein molecules based on their charge. Changes in both quality and nature of proteins determined by SPE allow clinicians to detect and monitor various pathophysiologic states. SPE, enhanced by follow-up procedures like protein quantification and immunofixation (IF), provides the best tools for general screening of human health state. The monoclonal gammopathies are a group of disorders characterized by the proliferation of a single clone of plasma cells that produces an immunologically homogeneous protein commonly referred to as a paraprotein or monoclonal protein (M-protein). SPE is usually done by the agarose gel electrophoresis or by the capillary zone electrophoretic method. It is the recommended method for the detection of an M-protein. The resulting M-protein, if found, can then be quantitated by means of a densitometer tracing of the gel. In the electrophoretic methodologies (agarose or capillary zone), proteins are classified by their final position after electrophoresis is complete into five general regions: albumin, alpha-1, alpha-2, beta, and gamma. The various immunoglobulin classes (IgG, IgA, IgM, IgD, and IgE) are usually of gamma mobility and make up most of the gamma region, but they may also be found in the beta-gamma and beta regions and may occasionally extend into the alpha-2 globulin area.
- Other names: serum protein electrophoresis (SPEP).
- **Normal range:**
  - ▼ SPE:
    - Albumin: 3.5–5.0 g/dL
    - Alpha-1 globulin: 0.1–0.3 g/dL
    - Alpha-2 globulin: 0.5–1.0 g/dL
    - Beta globulin: 0.5–0.9 g/dL
    - Gamma globulin: 0.6–1.4 g/dL
  - ▼ IF: no monoclonal protein detected

❑ Use

- Monitoring patients with monoclonal gammopathies
- Diagnosis of monoclonal gammopathies, when used in conjunction with immunofixation
- Assist in the diagnosis of hepatic disease, hypogammaglobulinemias and hypergammaglobulinemias, inflammatory states, neoplasms, renal disease, and GI disorders

16

- SPE should also be considered in any patient with an elevated total serum protein or otherwise unexplained signs and symptoms suggestive of the presence of a plasma cell disorder. These include any one or more of the following:
  - ▼ Elevated ESR or serum viscosity
  - ▼ Unexplained anemia, back pain, weakness, or fatigue
  - ▼ Osteopenia, osteolytic lesions, or spontaneous fractures
  - ▼ Renal insufficiency with a bland urine sediment
  - ▼ Heavy proteinuria in a patient older than 40 years of age
  - ▼ Hypercalcemia
  - ▼ Hypergammaglobulinemia
  - ▼ Immunoglobulin deficiency
  - ▼ BJ proteinuria
  - ▼ Unexplained peripheral neuropathy
  - ▼ Recurrent infections

❑ **Interpretation**
Increased In
- **Albumin**
  - ▼ Usually in hospitalized patients, hemoconcentration, albumin perfusion
  - ▼ Normal individuals: no clinical significance
  - ▼ Bisalbuminemia (double band), permanent
  - ▼ Bisalbuminemia, acquired, transient
    - High doses of beta-lactam antibiotics (complex formation)
    - Hyperbilirubinemia (jaundice, complexed with bilirubin)
    - Azotemia (urea and other N-compounds in blood)
    - Pancreatitis, pancreatic fistulas, or ascites (lysis of albumin by pancreatic enzymes)
- **Alpha-1 globulin**
  - ▼ Acute inflammatory disorders
  - ▼ Severe alcoholism
  - ▼ Some hepatic disorders
  - ▼ Double bands (AAT phenotypes)
- **Alpha-2 globulin**
  - ▼ Inflammatory syndromes
  - ▼ Nephrotic syndrome
  - ▼ Increased estrogen stimulation
  - ▼ Double bands in
    - Haptoglobin (Hp) phenotypes (no clinical significance)
    - Hemolysis (Hb-Hp complex)
    - Abnormal migrating beta-lipoproteins (aged samples)
- **Betaglobulin**
  - ▼ Primary and secondary hyperlipoproteinemias
  - ▼ Iron deficiency anemia
  - ▼ Estrogen, pregnancy, or anabolic steroids
  - ▼ Increase comigrates with transferrin, Hb (in excess to that bound in Hb-Hp complexes)
  - ▼ Acute inflammation (later phase)
  - ▼ Monoclonal immunoglobulins (IgA is frequent)

- ▼ Double bands
  - Transferrin phenotypes (different degrees of sialation)
  - Alcoholics
- ■ **Gammaglobulin**
  - ▼ Polyclonal gammopathy: chronic, subacute infections (AIDS, hepatic infections, chronic liver associated with beta–gamma bridging, autoimmune disorders)
  - ▼ Narrow band: monoclonal component, monoclonal gammopathy of undetermined significance, fibrinogen, CRP
  - ▼ Two narrow bands:
    - Biclonal or double gammopathies
    - Greater than two bands: oligoclonal hypergammaglobulinemia (present in low concentrations, transient, results in polyclonal processes); autoimmune, viral, bacterial, parasitic infections; restoration of immunoglobulin synthesis of immunosuppressants, 15% normal (no clinical significance)

Decreased In

- ■ **Albumin**
  - ▼ Congenital analbuminemia
  - ▼ Nutritional deficiency
  - ▼ Decreased synthesis
  - ▼ Hepatocellular insufficiency, damaged liver (cirrhosis, hepatitis)
  - ▼ Organ, tissue loss
  - ▼ Urinary (nephrotic syndrome), cutaneous (excessive burns) urinary excretion in pregnancy
  - ▼ Hypercatabolism
  - ▼ Endocrine disorders (thyrotoxicosis, Cushing syndrome)
- ■ **Alpha-1 globulin**
  - ▼ Hepatocellular insufficiency
  - ▼ Malnutrition, protein loss
  - ▼ Congenital deficiency of AAT
  - ▼ Tangier disease
- ■ **Alpha-2 globulin**
  - ▼ Hereditary deficiency of Hp phenotypes
  - ▼ Nutritional deficiency, hepatocellular insufficiency, protein loss, intravascular hemolysis (decreased Hp)
  - ▼ Pancreatitis
- ■ **Betaglobulin**
  - ▼ Chronic liver or renal disease
  - ▼ Hypobetalipoproteinemias
  - ▼ Thermal injuries
  - ▼ Acute inflammation
  - ▼ IgA deficiency
  - ▼ C3 degrades and eventually disappears in aged samples
- ■ **Gammaglobulin**
  - ▼ Physiologic (newborn)
  - ▼ Immunodeficiencies, induced (steroids, immunosuppressants, chemotherapy, radiotherapy)

16

▼ Suppressed synthesis caused by monoclonal gammopathies (multiple myeloma, light chain disease, amyloidosis)
▼ Lymphomas, leukemias

❑ **Limitations**

▪ The presence of a circulating monoclonal protein may interfere with one of more laboratory tests performed on liquid-based automated analyzers, either by precipitating during the analysis or by virtue of its specific binding properties.

▪ A small M-protein may be present even when quantitative immunoglobulin values, beta and gamma mobility components on SPEP, and total serum protein concentrations are all within normal limits.

▪ Fibrinogen (in plasma) is seen as a discrete band between the beta and gamma mobility regions. This is indistinguishable from an M-protein; the addition of thrombin to the specimen produces a clot if fibrinogen is present. The presence of fibrinogen is established if the discrete band is no longer detected when electrophoresis is repeated after the addition of thrombin.

▪ Hb-Hp complexes secondary to hemolysis may appear as a large band in the alpha-2 globulin region.

▪ High concentrations of transferrin in patients with iron deficiency anemia may produce a localized band in the beta region.

▪ Nephrotic syndrome is often associated with increased alpha-2 and beta bands, which can be mistaken for an M-protein. Serum albumin and gammaglobulin concentrations are usually reduced in this setting.

▪ Nonspecific increases in acute-phase reactants or certain hyperlipoproteinemias may result in increases in alpha-1 bands.

▪ Serum IF is more sensitive than SPE and also determines the heavy and light chain type of the monoclonal protein. However, unlike SPE, IF does not give an estimate of the size of the M-protein (i.e., its serum concentration) and thus should be done in conjunction with electrophoresis.

SEX HORMONE–BINDING GLOBULIN (SHBG)

❑ **Definition**

▪ A glycoprotein, synthesized in the liver, which binds testosterone and 5-dihydrotestosterone with high affinity, and estradiol with a somewhat lower affinity. SHBG typically circulates at higher concentrations in women than in men, due to the higher ratio of estrogens to androgens in women. Administration of androgens tends to be associated with decreased SHBG levels. Because variations in the carrier protein levels may affect the concentration of testosterone in circulation, SHBG levels are commonly measured as a supplement to total testosterone determinations. The "free androgen index" (FAI), calculated as the ratio of total testosterone to SHBG, has proved to be a useful indicator of abnormal androgen status in conditions such as hirsutism.

▪ **Normal range:** see Table 16.74.

TABLE 16–74. Normal Ranges of Sex Hormone–Binding Globulin		
Group	Central 95% (nmol/L)	Median (nmol/L)
Male	13–71	32
Female (nonpregnant)	18–114	51

❑ Use

- Diagnosis and follow-up of women with symptoms or signs of androgen excess (e.g., polycystic ovarian syndrome and idiopathic hirsutism)
- As an adjunct in monitoring sex steroid and antiandrogen therapy
- As an adjunct in the diagnosis of disorders of puberty
- As an adjunct in the diagnosis and follow-up of anorexia nervosa

❑ Interpretation

Increased In

- Hyperthyroidism
- Hepatic cirrhosis
- Pregnancy
- Drugs: estrogens (e.g., certain oral contraceptives, phenytoin [hepatic enzyme induction])
- Use of dexamethasone in the treatment of women with hyperandrogenic hirsutism

Decreased In

- Hirsutism
- Acne vulgaris
- Polycystic ovary syndrome
- Hypothyroidism
- Acromegaly
- Cushing disease
- Hyperprolactinemia

❑ Limitations

- SHBG can be increased with age, hyperestrogen states, marked weight loss and chronic exercise, HIV infection, cirrhosis.
- Decreased levels may also be due to obesity and protein losing nephropathies.

SICKLE SOLUBILITY TEST (SST)*

❑ Definition

- The SST (also called "sickle cell screen") was developed as a rapid screening for the presence of HbS. Red cells are lysed, and the released Hb is reduced by sodium hydrosulfite.

16

*Submitted By Liberto Pechet, MD.

❑ **Use**

- Patients with sickle cell trait are asymptomatic and do not present with sickle cells on the peripheral blood smear. The definitive diagnosis is made by hemoglobin variant studies. Reduced HbS is insoluble and forms a turbid suspension in the SST.
- HbA and most other hemoglobins are soluble under these conditions. Both sickle cell anemia (homozygous) and the sickle cell trait can be detected with this procedure.

❑ **Limitations**

- Recent transfusions may cause false-positive and false-negative results.
- False-negative results may occur with:
  - ▼ The patient's Hb <7 g/dL
  - ▼ Phenothiazine drugs
  - ▼ Unreliable for newborn screening because of high HbF and low percentage of HbS in the 1st year of life
- False-positive results may occur with
  - ▼ Increased turbidity (e.g., lipemic specimens)
  - ▼ Abnormal β-globulins
  - ▼ Polycythemia vera
  - ▼ Increased number of Heinz bodies (e.g., postsplenectomy)
  - ▼ Increased number of nucleated RBCs
  - ▼ Some rare Hb variants, such as HbC Harlem or C Georgetown

SODIUM (Na)

❑ **Definition**

- Sodium is the major extracellular cation and exerts a major influence on plasma osmolality. It plays a central role in maintaining the normal distribution of water and osmotic pressure. Changes in serum sodium most often reflect changes in water balance rather than sodium balance. It is adjusted by antidiuretic hormone (ADH) secretion and the thirst receptors to maintain plasma osmolality and volume. Aldosterone causes tubular reabsorption of sodium. Atrial natriuretic peptide hormone decreases sodium reabsorption.

❑ **Use**

- Diagnosis and treatment of dehydration and overhydration. If a patient has not received large load of sodium, hypernatremia suggests need for water, and values <130 mEq/L suggest overhydration.
- Electrolyte, acid–base balance; water balance; water intoxication.
- **Normal range:** 135–145 mmol/L.
- Critical values: <121 or >158 mmol/L.

Increased In

- Conditions associated with water loss in excess of salt loss through the skin, lungs, GI tract, and kidneys
- Dehydration—inadequate fluid intake to replace dermal, respiratory, or GI loss of fluid

- GI causes: vomiting or diarrhea
- Cutaneous causes: burns or excessive sweating
- Drugs: infusion of hypertonic sodium salts, hypertonic saline, Na-bicarbonate; hypertonic dialysis
- Hyperaldosteronism, Cushing syndrome—rare causes
- Diabetes insipidus (DI)
- Posttraumatic: caused by tumors, cysts, histiocytosis, TB, sarcoidosis
- Idiopathic: caused by aneurysms, meningitis, encephalitis, Guillain–Barre syndrome
- Renal failure and other renal causes: loop diuretics, osmotic diuresis (glucose, urea, mannitol), postobstructive diuresis, polyuric, phase of acute tubular necrosis, intrinsic renal disease

Decreased In

- Hyponatremia (defined as serum sodium <135 mmol/L after the exclusion pseudohyponatremia). This can be classified as three types depending upon extracellular fluid (ECF) status.
  - Hypovolemic hyponatremia (reduced ECF)
    - Renal loss of Na and water: caused by diuretic use, salt-wasting nephropathy, cerebral salt wasting, adrenal insufficiency, renal tubular acidosis
    - Extrarenal loss of Na and water with renal conservation: caused by burns, GI loss, pancreatitis, bowel obstruction, blood loss
  - Hypervolemic hyponatremia (expanded ECF and ICF but reduced effective arterial blood volume): caused by CHF, cirrhosis, nephrotic syndrome
  - Euvolemic hyponatremia (expanded ECF and ICF without edema: caused by thiazide diuretic use, hypothyroidism, adrenal insufficiency, SIADH secretion)

❑ Limitations and Interferences

- Plasma Na levels depend greatly upon the intake and excretion of water and to a somewhat lesser degree the renal regulation of Na.
- Determinations of blood sodium and potassium levels are not useful in diagnosis or in estimating net ion losses but are performed to monitor changes in sodium and potassium during therapy.
- Hyperglycemia—serum sodium decreases 1.7 mEq/L for every increase of serum glucose of 100 mg/dL.
- Hyperlipidemia and hyperproteinemia, which cause spurious results only with flame photometric but not with specific ion electrode techniques for measuring sodium.
- Pseudohyponatremia caused by "water exclusion effect" observed on indirect ISE (ion-selective electrode) measurements due to the dilution of samples and transfusion of blood products and due to infusion of IV immunoglobulins.

SODIUM, URINE

❑ Definition

- Urinary sodium determinations are usually performed to detect or confirm the presence of conditions that affect body fluids (e.g., dehydration, vomiting, and diarrhea) or disorders of the kidneys or adrenal glands.

16

■ **Normal range:**
  ▼ Twenty-four–hour urine:
    ● Male:
      • Less than 10 years: 41–115 mmol/day
      • 10–14 years: 63–177 mmol/day
      • Greater than 14 years: 40–120 mmol/day
    ● Female:
      • Less than 10 years: 20–69 mmol/day
      • 10–14 years: 48–168 mmol/day
      • Greater than 14 years: 27–287 mmol/day
  ▼ Random urine
    ● Male: 23–229 mmol/g creatinine
    ● Female: 26–297 mmol/g creatinine

❑ **Use**

■ Volume depletion: to determine the route of sodium loss. Low urinary sodium indicates extrarenal loss, and high value indicates renal salt wasting or adrenal insufficiency.
■ Differential diagnosis of acute renal failure: high values are consistent with acute tubular necrosis.
■ In hyponatremia, low urinary sodium indicates avid renal sodium retention, which may be attributable to either severe volume depletion or sodium-retaining states seen in cirrhosis, the nephrotic syndrome, and CHF. When hyponatremia is associated with urinary sodium excretion that equals or exceeds the dietary sodium intake, it is likely that SIADH is present.

❑ **Interpretation**
Increased In
■ Dehydration
■ Salicylate intoxication
■ Adrenocortical insufficiency
■ Diabetic acidosis
■ Mercurial and thiazide diuretic administration
■ Ammonium chloride administration
■ Renal tubular acidosis (<15 mmol/L are seen in prerenal acidosis)
■ Chronic renal failure
■ SIADH of different etiology
■ Any form of alkalosis and alkaline urine

Decreased In
■ Acute renal failure
■ Pulmonary emphysema
■ CHF
■ Excessive sweating
■ Diarrhea
■ Pyloric obstruction
■ Malabsorption

- Primary aldosteronism
- Premenstrual sodium and water retention
- Acute oliguria and prerenal azotemia

❏ **Limitations**

- Large diurnal variations exist in urine sodium levels. The rate of excretion during night is one fifth of the peak rate during the day.
- Levels are highly dependent on dietary intake and state of hydration.

TAY-SACHS DISEASE MOLECULAR DNA ASSAY*

❏ **Definition**

- Tay-Sachs disease (TSD; OMIM# 272800) molecular DNA testing identifies mutations in the hexosaminidase A gene but should be used concurrently with the hexosaminidase A (HEX A) enzyme activity assay to diagnose TSD. HEX A enzymatic activity is the primary method for diagnosing TSD or carrier identification. HEX A activity is determined by the ratio of HEX A to total hexosaminidase and can be measured in serum from women who are not pregnant and not using oral contraceptives, serum from male patients, or WBCs from individuals.
- **Normal values:** negative or no mutations are found.

❏ **Use**

- Confirmation of a clinical diagnosis.
- Carrier testing for Ashkenazi Jewish individuals.
- Carrier testing for at-risk family members of affected individuals.
- Confirmation that the reduced HEX A enzymatic activity is caused by a disease-causing allele rather than a pseudodeficiency allele, R247W or R249W. About 35% of non-Jewish individuals and 2–4% of Jewish individuals identified as heterozygotes by HEX A enzyme assay testing are carriers of a pseudodeficiency allele.
- Prenatal diagnosis: when both parental mutations are known.
- Identification for genetic counseling of specific disease-causing alleles in affected individuals and carriers.
- Available tests can be grouped as
  ▼ Targeted mutation analysis
    - A panel of six mutations comprising
      - *c.1274_1277dupTATC (+TATC1278), c.1421+1G>C (IVS12+1G>C), p.G269S (Gly269Ser), c.1073+1G>A (IVS9+1G>A)*
      - *p.R247W (Arg247Trp) and p.R249W (Arg249Trp):* the two pseudodeficiency alleles that do not cause TSD but reduce HEX A enzymatic activity as measured by the synthetic substrate
    - More extended panels include ethnic-specific mutations as *c.805+1G>A (IVS7+1G>A), del 7.6kb, p.R170Q (Arg170Gln), p.R170W (Arg170Trp), deltaF304/305 (c.915_917delCTT), c.571-2A>G (IVS5-2A>G)*

16

---

*Submitted by Edward Ginns, MD & Marzena M. Galdzicka, PhD.

▼ HEX A gene sequence analysis: analysis of the entire coding region and exon–intron boundaries useful for identifying rare mutant alleles associated with TSD

❑ **Limitations**

■ The results of a genetic test may be affected by DNA rearrangements, blood transfusion, bone marrow transplantation, or rare sequence variations.

TESTOSTERONE, TOTAL, FREE, BIOAVAILABLE

❑ **Definition**

■ Testosterone circulates in the blood of men and women in several forms. In healthy adults, approximately 44% of circulating testosterone is specifically bound to sex hormone–binding globulin (SHBG), 50% is nonspecifically bound to albumin, and 3–5% is bound to cortisol-binding globulin, indicating that only 2–3% is unbound and free. Current methods available to evaluate the androgen status include measurement of total testosterone, free testosterone by direct immunoassays, equilibrium dialysis, HPLC-MS, SHBG, calculated free (non–SHBG- and nonalbumin-bound) testosterone, and bioavailable (non–SHBG-bound) testosterone. In most, but not all clinical conditions, a measurement of total testosterone is adequate for the evaluation of a patient. It is widely believed that SHBG-bound testosterone is not readily available to most tissues, whereas albumin-bound and free testosterones are bioavailable. Because SHBG concentrations can be influenced by many factors (e.g., decreased by obesity, testosterone treatment, and hypoandrogenic female conditions such as polycystic ovary syndrome; increased by aging, pregnancy, and estrogen therapy), there are clinical situations in which measured concentrations of total testosterone may not reflect the bioavailable concentrations or the clinical status of the patient. In these circumstances, a supplemental test assessing bioavailable and free testosterone is helpful in clinical decision making.

■ **Normal range:** see Table 16.75.

❑ **Use**

■ Evaluation of gonadal hormonal function

❑ **Interpretation**

Increased In

■ Adrenal virilizing tumor causing premature puberty in boys or masculinization in women
■ CAH
■ Idiopathic hirsutism (inconclusive)
■ Stein-Leventhal syndrome: variable; increased when virilization is present
■ Ovarian stromal hyperthecosis
■ Use of certain drugs that alter thyroxine-binding globulins may also affect testosterone-binding globulins; however, the free testosterone level is not affected

TABLE 16–75. Normal Ranges of Testosterone

Age	Range
Testosterone, Total, Male	
Premature (26–28 wk)	59–125 ng/dL
Premature (3–35 wk)	37–198 ng/dL
Newborn	75–400 ng/dL
–7 mo	Levels decrease rapidly the 1st week to 20–50 ng/dL, and then increase to 60–400 ng/dL between 20 and 60 d. Levels then decline to prepubertal range levels of 3–10 ng/dL by 7 mo.
7–9 y	<9 ng/dL
10–11 y	2–57 ng/dL
12–13 y	7–747 ng/dL
14–15 y	33–585 ng/dL
16–17 y	185–886 ng/dL
18–39 y	400–1,080 ng/dL
40–59 y	350–890 ng/dL
≥60 y	350–720 ng/dL
Tanner stage I	<20 ng/dL
Tanner stage II	2–149 ng/dL
Tanner stage III	7–762 ng/dL
Tanner stage IV	164–854 ng/dL
Tanner stage V	194–783 ng/dL
Testosterone, Free Male	
1–6 y	<0.6 pg/mL
7–9 y	0.1–0.9 pg/mL
10–11 y	0.1–6.3 pg/mL
12–13 y	0.5–98.0 pg/mL
14–15 y	3–138.0 pg/mL
16–17 y	38.0–173.0 pg/mL
≥18 y	47–244 pg/mL
Tanner stage I	≤3.7 pg/mL
Tanner stage II	0.3–21 pg/mL
Tanner stage III	1.0–98.0 pg/mL
Tanner stage IV	35.0–169.0 pg/mL
Tanner stage V	41.0–239.0 pg/mL
Testosterone, Total, Female	
Premature (26–28 wk)	5–16 ng/dL
Premature (31–35 wk)	5–22 ng/dL
Newborn	20–64 ng/dL
–7 mo	Levels decrease during the first month to <10 ng/dL and remain at this level until puberty
7–9 y	<15 ng/dL
10–11 y	2–42 ng/dL
12–13 y	6–64 ng/dL
14–15 y	9–49 ng/dL
16–17 y	8–63 ng/dL
18–30 y	11–59 ng/dL
31–40 y	11–56 ng/dL
41–51 y	9–55 ng/dL
Postmenopausal	6–25 ng/dL
Tanner stage I	<17 ng/dL

16

(Continued)

TABLE 16–75. Normal Ranges of Testosterone (*Continued*)

Age	Range
Tanner stage II	4–39 ng/dL
Tanner stage III	10–60 ng/dL
Tanner stage IV	8–63 ng/dL
Tanner stage V	10–60 ng/dL
Testosterone, Free Females	
1–6 y	<0.6 pg/mL
7–9 y	0.6–1.8 pg/mL
10–11 y	0.1–3.5 pg/mL
12–13 y	0.9–6.8 pg/mL
14–15 y	1.2–7.5 pg/mL
16–17 y	1.2–9.9 pg/mL
18–30 y	0.8–7.4 pg/mL
31–40 y	1.3–9.2 pg/mL
41–51 y	1.1–5.8 pg/mL
Postmenopausal	0.6–3.8 pg/mL
Tanner stage I	<2.2 pg/mL
Tanner stage II	0.4–4.5 pg/mL
Tanner stage III	1.3–7.5 pg mL
Tanner stage IV	1.1–15.5 pg/mL
Tanner stage V	0.8–9.2 pg/mL
Testosterone, Male, Bioavailable	
1–6 y	<1.3 ng/dL
7–9 y	0.3–2.8 ng/dL
10–11 y	0.1–17.9 ng/dL
12–13 y	1.4–288.0 ng/dL
14–15 y	9.5–337.0 ng/dL
16–17 y	35.0–509.0 ng/dL
≥18 y	130–680 ng/dL
Tanner stage I	0.3–13.0 ng/dL
Tanner stage II	0.3–59.0 ng/dL
Tanner stage III	1.9–296.0 ng/dL
Tanner stage IV	40.0–485.0 ng/dL
Tanner stage V	124.0–596.0 ng/dL
Testosterone, Female, Bioavailable	
1–6 y	<1.3 ng/dL
7–9 y	0.3–5.0 ng/dL
10–11 y	0.4–9.6 ng/dL
12–13 y	1.7–18.8 ng/dL
14–15 y	3.0–22.6 ng/dL
16–17 y	3.3–28.6 ng/dL
18–30 y	2.2–20.6 ng/dL
31–40 y	4.1–25.5 ng/dL
41–51 y	2.8–16.5 ng/dL
Postmenopausal	1.5–9.4 ng/dL
Tanner stage I	0.3–5.5 ng/dL
Tanner stage II	1.2–15.0 ng/dL
Tanner stage III	3.8–28.0 ng/dL
Tanner stage IV	2.8–39.0 ng/dL
Tanner stage V	2.5–23.0 ng/dL

Decreased In

- Primary hypogonadism (e.g., orchiectomy)
- Secondary hypogonadism (e.g., hypopituitarism)
- Testicular feminization
- Klinefelter syndrome levels lower than in normal male individual but higher than in normal female and orchiectomized male
- Estrogen therapy
- Total (but not free) testosterone decreased due to decreased SHBG (e.g., cirrhosis, chronic renal disease)

❑ Limitations

- Due to the availability of many different forms of testosterone assays, as well as the confusion in the literature regarding their clinical relevance, there is a lack of consistency for its measurement in routine clinical situations. The earliest approaches to the measurement of free testosterone were equilibrium dialyses and ultrafiltration. These assays were very cumbersome for routine use.
- Indirect measurement of free testosterone using isotope-labeled testosterone was one of the earlier methods proposed and widely used. The endocrine society recently reported a review of the evidence that the analog-based free testosterone immunoassays should be avoided because of the problems with accuracy and sensitivity. Free testosterone measurements by calculation using algorithms based on the law of mass action, which requires total testosterone, SHBG, and albumin concentrations, have excellent correlations with physical separation measures.
- Testosterone exhibits significant circadian variations in young men, and early morning samples are recommended.

THEOPHYLLINE (1,3-DIMETHYLXANTHINE)*

❑ Definition

- A naturally occurring (tea) xanthine derivative with diuretic, cardiac stimulant, and smooth muscle relaxant properties. Other names: Theo-Dur, Uniphyl, Slo-bid, and Theolair.
- **Normal range:**
  - ▼ 0–5 months: 6–12 µg/mL
  - ▼ Greater than 6 months: 10–20 µg/mL

❑ Use

- As a bronchodilator to prevent and treat asthma

❑ Interpretation

- **Potentially toxic:** 20–25 µg/mL

❑ Limitations

- Serum: Quantitative immunoassay limitations
  - ▼ FPIA, chemiluminescence, EMIT, particle-enhanced turbidimetric inhibition immunoassay.

16

*Submitted By Amanda J. Jenkins, PhD.

▼ Do not use serum separator tubes or gels. Separate serum from cells as soon as possible.
▼ The incidence of patients having antibodies to *Escherichia coli* β-galactosidase is extremely low. However, some samples containing such antibodies may result in artificially high results that do not fit the clinical profile.
▼ Due to cross-reactivity with 1,3-dimethyluric acid (metabolite), the assay should not be used to quantitate samples from uremic patients.
▼ If mouse antibodies are utilized, the possibility exists for interference by human antimouse antibodies (HAMA) in the sample, which could cause falsely elevated results.

THROMBIN TIME (TT)*

❑ Definition

▪ TT measures the time of conversion of fibrinogen into fibrin once thrombin (used as a reagent) is added.
▪ **Normal range:** 14–21 seconds (may vary depending on reagent and equipment used).

❑ Use

▪ Detects decreased or abnormal fibrinogen.
▪ Detects unreported heparin use.
▪ Detects other thrombin inhibiting drugs, for example, hirudin, antithrombin agents such as argatroban, apixaban, and dabigatran. A new assay, the dilute thrombin time is now being offered commercially for the new antithrombin agents measurements.

❑ Interpretation

Causes of Increased (Prolonged) TT

▪ Very low fibrinogen (<80 mg/dL)
▪ Dysfibrinogenemia
▪ Interference with polymerization of fibrinogen
  ▼ Fibrin degradation products, such as DIC and pathologic or therapeutic fibrinolysis. TT is not recommended in the diagnosis of pathologic fibrinolysis or DIC because of very low specificity and low sensitivity
  ▼ High concentrations of monoclonal immunoglobulins
  ▼ Uremia
▪ Heparin therapy

❑ Limitations

▪ Preanalytic conditions may interfere with this test.
  ▼ Improper filling of blood collecting tube or use of wrong tubes (containing different anticoagulant than recommended or no anticoagulant)
  ▼ Clots in specimen
  ▼ Hemolysis

---

*Submitted By Liberto Pechet, MD.

▼ Heparin contamination of blood, such as drawings from IV lines with heparin flushes (when heparin contamination is suspected, a reptilase time can be performed instead [see above])

- Hyperlipidemia may artificially prolong the thrombin time obtained by optical equipment (most modern machines). In such cases, the assay can be done on equipment that uses mechanical clotting.
- Results are unreliable in patients with high fibrinogen (>500 mg/dL).
- Patients previously exposed to bovine thrombin to arrest bleeding may develop thrombin antibodies.
- Use of various radiocontrast agents may affect test results.

THROMBOELASTOGRAM (TEG)*

❑ **Definition**

- TEG uses equipment (TEG analyzer) that records the process of blood coagulation, including fibrinolysis and platelet defects. It measures in vitro the kinetics of clot formation and dissolution by a mechanical process, which monitors very low shear elasticity changes. The different parameters represent different aspects of the patient's hemostasis.

❑ **Use**

- The TEG is commonly used for cardiac bypass surgery, providing a rapid assessment of anticoagulation (heparin), restoration of coagulation with the use of protamine sulfate, excess fibrinolysis, and platelet function during the procedure.
- Its usefulness has been demonstrated since it reduces the number of red cell or platelet transfused during open heart surgery or shortly after its termination.

THYROGLOBULIN (Tg)

❑ **Definition**

- Heterogeneous iodoglycoprotein secreted only by thyroid follicular cells that is involved in iodination and synthesis of thyroid hormones. It is proportional to thyroid mass.
- **Normal value:** <55 ng/mL.

❑ **Use**

- To assess the presence and possibly the extent of residual or recurrent or metastatic follicular or papillary thyroid carcinoma after therapy. In patients with these carcinomas treated with total thyroidectomy or radioiodine and taking thyroid hormone therapy, Tg is undetectable if functional tumor is absent but is detected by sensitive immunoassay if functional tumor is present. Tg correlates with tumor mass with highest values in patients with metastases to bones and lungs.

16

*Submitted By Liberto Pechet, MD.

- To diagnose factitious hyperthyroidism: Tg is very low or not detectable in factitious hyperthyroidism and is high in all other types of hyperthyroidism (e.g., thyroiditis, Graves disease).
- To predict outcome of therapy for hyperthyroidism; higher remission rates in patients with lower Tg values. Failure to become normal after drug-induced remission suggests relapse after drugs are discontinued.
- To diagnose thyroid agenesis in newborn.

❏ **Interpretation**
- See Table 16.76.

Increased In
- Most patients with differentiated thyroid carcinoma but not with undifferentiated or medullary thyroid carcinomas
- Hyperthyroidism—rapid decline after surgical treatment; gradual decline after radioactive iodine treatment
- Silent (painless) thyroiditis
- Endemic goiter (some patients)
- Marked liver insufficiency

Decreased In
- Thyroid agenesis in newborns
- Total thyroidectomy or destruction by radiation

❏ **Limitations**
- A Tg test is not recommended for initial diagnosis of thyroid carcinomas. The presence of Tg in pleural effusions indicates metastatic differentiated thyroid cancer.
- A Tg test should not be used in patients with preexisting thyroid disorders.
- Tg autoantibodies: patients' serum must always first be screened for these antibodies (present in <10% of persons). In such cases, Tg mRNA can be measured using RT-PCR.
- Because Tg autoantibodies can interfere with both competitive immunoassays and immunometric assays for Tg, all patients should be screened for Tg autoantibodies by a sensitive immunoassay; recovery studies are not adequate for ruling out interference by these autoantibodies.
- Tg antibodies are present in the majority of patients with Hashimoto thyroiditis but also in approximately 3% of healthy individuals.
- At least 6 weeks should elapse after thyroidectomy or iodine-125 treatment before a Tg test. Some reports have indicated that Tg levels may remain elevated for several weeks following successful treatment. In this case, serial determinations assessed relative to a posttreatment baseline established for the patient may still be of value in monitoring.
- Many technical pitfalls in Tg measurement include between-method variability, in appropriate reference ranges, suboptimal functional sensitivity, hook effects, HAMA interferences. RIA method is relatively resistant to TGAB and HAMA influences.

- A newer HPLC-MS method is offered by many commercial labs and can be used in suspicious TGAB interference cases.

THYROID AUTOANTIBODY TESTS

❏ **Definition**

- Antithyroid peroxidase (TPO) antibodies are autoantibodies directed against the peroxidase enzyme. This enzyme catalyzes the iodination of tyrosine in thyroglobulin (Tg) during the biosynthesis of T_3 and T_4. Historically, these antibodies were referred to as antimicrosomal antibodies (AMAs) because the antibodies bind to the microsomal part of the thyroid cells. Recent research has identified thyroid peroxidase as the primary antigenic component of microsomes. Measurement of TPO antibodies has essentially replaced the measurement of antimicrosomal antibodies. In virtually all cases of Hashimoto disease and in the majority of cases of Graves disease, anti-TPO antibodies are elevated. High levels of anti-TPO antibodies, in the context of the clinical presentation of hypothyroidism, confirm the diagnosis of Hashimoto disease. Tg autoantibody measurements are most useful for evaluating samples submitted for Tg measurements because Tg autoantibodies can interfere with both competitive immunoassays and immunometric assays for Tg.
- **Normal range:**
  - ▼ Tg antibodies: <40 IU/mL
  - ▼ TPO antibodies: <35 IU/mL

❏ **Use**

- To assess the thyroid autoantibody status in patients with thyroid disease
- To distinguish subacute thyroiditis from Hashimoto thyroiditis, as antibodies are more common in the latter
- Occasionally useful to distinguish Graves disease from toxic multinodular goiter when physical findings are not diagnostic
- Thyroid receptor antibodies mainly used in Graves disease, especially as a predictor of relapse of hyperthyroidism

❏ **Interpretation**

- Positive in approximately 95% of cases of Hashimoto disease and approximately 85% of Graves disease. Very high titer is suggestive of Hashimoto thyroiditis but absence does not exclude Hashimoto thyroiditis. Less than 1:1,000 occurs virtually only in Graves disease or Hashimoto thyroiditis.

Increased In

- Significant titer of microsome antibodies indicates Hashimoto thyroiditis or postpartum thyroiditis.
- Significant titer of antibodies in euthyroid patient with unilateral exophthalmos suggests the diagnosis of euthyroid Graves disease. Elevated antibody titer in a patient with Graves disease should direct a surgeon to perform a more limited thyroidectomy to avoid late postthyroidectomy hypothyroidism.

16

TABLE 16–76. Thyroid Function Tests in Various Conditions

Condition	TSH	TT₄	FT₄	T₃	Tg	RAIU	Comment
Hypothyroidism							
Primary							
Clinical	I	D	D	D	N/I	D	Increased response to TRH administration
Subclinical	I	N	N	N	N	NA	No response to TRH administration
Secondary	N/D	D	D	D		NA	
Tertiary	N/D	D	D	D		NA	
Nonthyroidal illness*	V	N/D	N/D	D	D	NA	
Hyperthyroidism							
Primary							
Clinical	D	I	I	I	N	I	
Subclinical	D	N	N	N	N	NA	
T₃ thyrotoxicosis	D	N	N	I	N	NA	
TSH-secreting tumor	I	I	I	I	N	NA	
TRH-secreting tumor	I	I	I	I	N	NA	
Factitious							
T₄ ingestion	D	I	I	I	D/N	D	Augmented RAIU response to TSH administration
T₃ ingestion	D	D	D	I	D/N		
Pregnancy							
With hyperthyroidism	N	N	N	I	—	X	
With hypothyroidism	I	D	D	D	—	X	I T₄ and T₃ to normal range

Condition						Comments
Hereditary increased TBG	N	D	N	N		
Hereditary decreased TBG	V	V	V	V		
Hashimoto thyroiditis	N	N	N	N	V	Thyroid antibodies; biopsy
Goiter	N	N	N	N	A	Biopsy
Thyroid carcinoma	N	N	D	D	N	Serum calcitonin I in medullary CA; Tg I in differentiated
Nephrosis	N	D	N	D	VI	
Drug effects						
Thyroxine	D	—	I	D		
Inorganic iodine	I	—	—	—		
Radiopaque contrast media		—	—	—		
Estrogen; birth control pills	N	D	N	N		
Testosterone	N	D	D	D		D TBH
ACTH and corticosteroids	N	D	D	N		D TBH
Dilantin	V/I	—	D	D		Tissue resistance to T_4
Pituitary only	I	—	—	—		Tissue resistance to T_4
Generalized tissue	V/I	V/I	V/I	D	VI	T_4 administration does not suppress TSH

0, absent; A, abnormal; D, decreased; I, increased; N, normal; NA, not useful; TT_4, total thyroxine; V, variable; VD, variable decrease; VI, variable increase; X, contraindicated. Underlined test indicates most useful diagnostic change.

*Forms of nonthyroidal illness (euthyroid sick syndrome).

16

- Occasionally positive in papillary–follicular carcinoma of the thyroid, subacute thyroiditis (briefly), and lymphocytic (painless) thyroiditis (in approximately 60% of patients).
- Primary thyroid lymphoma often shows very high titers. This result should suggest need for biopsy in elderly patient with a firm enlarging thyroid.
- Low titers are present in >10% of normal population, increasing with age.
- Other autoimmune diseases (e.g., PA, RA, SLE, myasthenia gravis).

Decreased In
- In the absence of antibodies, Hashimoto thyroiditis is very unlikely cause of hypothyroidism.

❏ Limitations
- Tg antibodies may interfere with assay for serum Tg.

THYROID HORMONE–BINDING RATIO (THBR)

❏ Definition
- THBR values can be calculated according to the following equation proposed by the Committee on Nomenclature of the American Thyroid Association.

$$\text{THBR(FTI)} = \frac{T_4 \text{ value}(\mu g / dL) \times \text{thyroid uptake}(\%)}{\text{median of reference interval}(\%)^*}$$

- See Table 16.77.
- **Normal range:** 5.93–13.13 µg/dL.

❏ Use
- This calculated product permits correction of misleading results of T_3 and T_4 determinations caused by conditions that alter the thyroxine-binding protein concentration (e.g., pregnancy, estrogens, birth control pills).

TABLE 16–77. Free Thyroxine Index in Various Conditions

Condition	T_3	T_4	Free Thyroxine Index (T_7) $(T_3$ Uptake $\times$ $T_4)$
Normal			
Range	24–36	4–11	96–396
Mean	31	7	217
Hypothyroid	22	3	66
Hyperthyroid	38	12	456
Pregnancy, estrogen use (especially birth control pills)	20	12	240*

*Normal even though T_3 and T_4 alone are abnormal.

❑ **Interpretation**

Increased In

- Hyperthyroidism
- States with decreased TBG (e.g., androgen treatment, chronic liver disease), protein loss, or genetically low TBG

Decreased In

- Hypothyroidism
- States with increased TBG (e.g., estrogen treatment, pregnancy, acute hepatitis, genetically high TBG)

❑ **Limitations**

- Concordance values of T_4 and THBR tests suggest altered thyroid function.
- Discordant variance suggests primary change in TBG in a euthyroid state (e.g., pregnancy)

THYROID RADIOACTIVE IODINE UPTAKE (RAIU)

❑ **Definition**

- A tracer dose of radioactive iodine (^{131}I or ^{123}I) is administered orally, and the radioactivity over the thyroid is measured at specific time intervals.
- **Normal range:** 10–35% in 24 hours depending on local variations in iodine intake.

❑ **Use**

- Evaluation of hyperthyroidism associated with low RAIU (e.g., factitious hyperthyroidism, subacute thyroiditis, struma ovarii)
- Distinguish Graves disease from toxic nodular goiter
- Assess function of nodules ("hot" or "cold")
- Determine location and size of functioning thyroid tissue
- Detect metastases from differentiated thyroid cancers
- Evaluate use of radioiodine therapy
- Determine the presence of an organification defect in thyroid hormone production
- In combination with T_3 suppression test: Administration of triiodothyronine suppresses RAIU by >50% in the normal person but not in patients with Graves disease or toxic nodules; shows autonomy of TSH secretion. Infrequently used

❑ **Interpretation**

Increased In

- Graves disease (diffuse toxic goiter)
- Plummer disease (toxic multinodular goiter)
- Toxic adenoma (uninodular goiter)
- Thyroiditis (early Hashimoto; recovery stage of subacute thyroiditis)
- TSH excess
  - ▾ TSH administration
  - ▾ TSH production by pituitary tumor (TSH >4 µU/mL) or other neoplasm

16

▼ Defective thyroid hormone synthesis
▼ Human chorionic gonadotropin–mediated hyperthyroidism (e.g., chorio-carcinoma, hydatidiform mole, embryonal carcinoma of the testis, hyper-emesis gravidarum)

Decreased In

▪ Hypothyroidism (tertiary, secondary, late primary)
▪ Thyroiditis (late Hashimoto; active stage of subacute thyroiditis; RAIU does not usually respond to TSH administration)
▪ Thyroid hormone administration (T_3 or T_4)
  ▼ Therapeutic
  ▼ Factitious (RAIU is augmented after TSH administration)
▪ Antithyroid medication
▪ Iodine-induced hyperthyroidism (Jodbasedow)
▪ X-ray contrast media, iodine-containing drugs, iodized salt
▪ Graves disease with iodine excess
▪ Ectopic hypersecreting thyroid tissue
▪ Metastatic functioning thyroid carcinoma
▪ Struma ovarii
▪ Drugs (e.g., calcitonin, thyroglobulin, corticosteroids, dopamine)

❏ **Limitations**

▪ Contraindications: pregnancy, lactation, childhood.
▪ Not valid for 2–4 weeks after administration of antithyroid drugs, thyroid, or iodides; the effect of organic iodine (e.g., x-ray contrast media) may persist for a much longer period.
▪ Because of widespread dietary use of iodine in the United States, RAIU should not be used to evaluate euthyroid state.
▪ Increased by withdrawal rebound (thyroid hormones, propylthiouracil), increased iodine excretion (e.g., diuretics, nephrotic syndrome, chronic diarrhea), decreased iodine intake (salt restriction, iodine deficiency).

THYROID-STIMULATING HORMONE (TSH)

❏ **Definition**

▪ This glycoprotein hormone of 28–30 kDa is composed of alpha and beta sub-units. It is secreted by the anterior pituitary. TSH controls the biosynthesis and release of thyroid hormones T_4 and T_3.
▪ **Normal range:** 0.5–6.3 μIU/mL, depending on age and sex (Table 16.78).

❏ **Use**

▪ Sensitive measure of thyroid function. First line of test for suspected thyroid disorders
▪ Assessing true metabolic status
▪ Screening for euthyroidism
  ▼ Normal level in stable ambulatory patient not on interfering drugs excludes thyroid hormone excess or deficiency.
  ▼ TSH is recommended as the initial test rather than T_4.

TABLE 16–78. Normal Ranges of TSH According to Age and Sex

Age	TSH (μIU/mL)	
	Male	Female
0–1 mo	0.5–6.5	0.5–6.5 (same as in males)
1–11 mo	0.8–6.3	0.8–6.3 (same as in males)
1 y	0.7–6.0	0.7–5.9
6 y	0.7–5.4	0.6–5.1
11 y	0.6–4.9	0.5–4.4
16 y	0.5–4.4	0.5–3.9
18 y	0.28–3.89	0.28–3.89 (same as in males)

▼ Screening is not recommended for asymptomatic persons without suspicion of thyroid disease or for hospital patients with acute medical or psychiatric illness.

- Initial screening and diagnosis for hyperthyroidism (decreased to undetectable levels except in rare TSH-secreting pituitary adenoma) and hypothyroidism

- Especially useful in early or subclinical hypothyroidism before the patient develops clinical findings, goiter, or abnormalities of other thyroid tests

  ▼ Differentiation of primary (increased levels) from central (pituitary or hypothalamic) hypothyroidism (decreased levels)

  ▼ Monitoring of adequate thyroid hormone replacement therapy in primary hypothyroidism, although T_4 may be mildly increased (up to 6–8 weeks before TSH becomes normal). Serum TSH suppressed to the normal level is the best monitor of dosage of thyroid hormone for treatment of hypothyroidism

  ▼ Monitoring adequate thyroid hormone therapy in the suppression of thyroid carcinoma (should suppress to <0.1 μIU/mL) or goiter or nodules (should suppress to subnormal levels) with third- or fourth-generation assays

- Replacement of TRH stimulation test in hyperthyroidism, because most patients with euthyroid TSH level have a normal TSH response and patients with undetectable TSH level almost never respond to TRH stimulation

❏ Interpretation

Increased In

- Primary untreated hypothyroidism. The increase is proportionate to the degree of hypofunction, varying from 3 times normal in mild cases to 100 times normal in severe myxedema. A single determination is usually sufficient to establish the diagnosis.

- Patients with hypothyroidism receiving insufficient thyroid hormone replacement therapy.

- Patients with Hashimoto thyroiditis, including those with clinical hypothyroidism and about one third of those patients who are clinically euthyroid.

- Use of various drugs: amphetamines (abuse), iodine-containing agents (e.g., iopanoic acid, ipodate, amiodarone), and dopamine antagonists (e.g., metoclopramide, domperidone, chlorpromazine, haloperidol).

- Other conditions (test is not clinically useful).

16

▼ Iodide deficiency goiter or iodide-induced goiter or lithium treatment
▼ External neck irradiation
▼ Postsubtotal thyroidectomy
▼ Neonatal period; increased in first 2–3 days of life due to postnatal TSH surge
▼ Thyrotoxicosis due to pituitary thyrotroph adenoma or pituitary resistance to thyroid hormone
▼ Euthyroid sick syndrome, recovery phase
▼ TSH antibodies

Decreased In

■ Toxic multinodular goiter
■ Autonomously functioning thyroid adenoma
■ Ophthalmopathy of euthyroid Graves disease; treated Graves disease
■ Thyroiditis
■ Extrathyroidal thyroid hormone source
■ Factitious
■ Overreplacement of thyroid hormone in treatment of hypothyroidism
■ Secondary pituitary or hypothalamic hypothyroidism (e.g., tumor, infiltrates)
■ Euthyroid sick patients (some patients)
■ Acute psychiatric illness
■ Severe dehydration
■ Drug effect, especially large doses (use FT_4 for evaluation)
  ▼ Glucocorticoids, dopamine, dopamine agonists (bromocriptine), levodopa, T_4 replacement therapy, apomorphine, and pyridoxine; normal or low T_4
  ▼ Antithyroid drug for thyrotoxicosis, especially early in treatment; normal or low T_4
■ Assay interference (e.g., antibodies to mouse IgG, autoimmune disease)
■ First trimester of pregnancy
■ Isolated deficiency (very rare)

❑ Limitations

■ TSH may be normal in
  ▼ Central hypothyroidism: In the absence of hypothalamic or pituitary disease, normal TSH excludes primary hypothyroidism.
  ▼ Recent rapid correction of hyperthyroidism or hypothyroidism
  ▼ Pregnancy
  ▼ Phenytoin therapy
■ TSH may not be useful to evaluate thyroid status of hospitalized ill patients.
  ▼ Approximately 3 months of treatment of hypo- or hyperthyroidism; FT_4 is test of choice.
  ▼ Lag time of 6–8 weeks is required for normalization of TSH after initiation of thyroid hormone replacement therapy.
■ Dopamine or high doses of glucocorticoids may cause false normal values in primary hypothyroidism and may suppress TSH in nonthyroid illness.
■ Rheumatoid factor, human antimouse antibodies, heterophile antibodies, and thyroid hormone autoantibodies may produce spurious results, especially in patients with autoimmune disorders ($\leq 10\%$).

- Amiodarone may interfere with TSH.
- TSH is not affected by variation in thyroid-binding proteins.
- TSH has a diurnal rhythm, with peaks at 2:00–4:00 AM and troughs at 5:00–6:00 PM with ultradian variations. TSH levels vary diurnally by up to 50% and up to 40% variations on specimens performed serially during the same time of the day.
- Serum levels typically falls below 0.1 mIU/L during first trimester of pregnancy due to thyroid stimulatory effects of HCG and returns to normal in the second trimester.

THYROTROPIN-RELEASING HORMONE (TRH) STIMULATION TEST

❏ **Definition**

- TRH is a hormone produced in the hypothalamus; it can stimulate the release of TSH from the pituitary gland. TSH then further stimulates the production and the release of T_3 and T_4 from the thyroid gland. Therefore, the TRH stimulation test can evaluate the thyroid function status. However, TRH also stimulate the release of growth hormone (GH) as well as prolactin. Three blood specimens are collected for serum TSH testing: one immediately prior to TRH injection, and one 15 minutes and one 30 minutes after TRH injection. TRH is administrated IV (200–500 µg). Pharmacy consultation for TRH dosage is recommended (see Fig. 16.4).

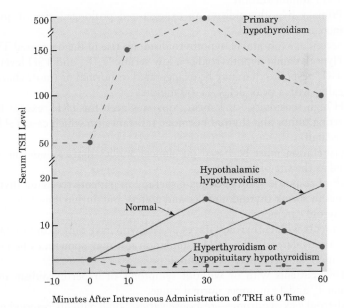

Figure 16–4 *Sample curves of serum thyroid-stimulating hormone (TSH) response to administration of thyrotropin-releasing hormone (TRH) in various conditions.*

16

❏ **Use**

■ Rarely used clinically for diagnosis of the thyroid diseases. Measurements of serum TSH and T_3 and T_4 levels are informative in evaluating thyroid function in most clinical situations. However, when the diagnosis is still unclear, the TRH stimulation test can be of help.

■ May be particularly useful in T_3 toxicosis in which the other test results are normal or in patients clinically suspicious for hyperthyroidism with borderline serum T_3 levels. TRH stimulation test is superior to the T_3 suppression test of RAIU. Abnormal TSH response to TRH administration does not definitely establish the diagnosis of hyperthyroidism (because autonomous production of normal or slightly increased amounts of thyroid hormones causes pituitary suppression). TRH test may remain abnormal even after successful therapy of Graves disease.

■ Helps differentiate two forms of thyrotropin-induced hyperthyroidism (whether or not due to tumor).

■ May help differentiate hypothalamic from pituitary hypothyroidism.

❏ **Interpretation**

■ Normally, a significant rise in serum TSH occurs from a basal level of 2–3 μU/mL, and this then returns to normal by 120 minutes. Response is usually greater in women than in men. A blunted response indicates hyperthyroidism but may occur in other conditions (e.g., uremia, Cushing syndrome, starvation, elevated levels of glucocorticoids, depression, some elderly patients). Largely replaced by sensitive TSH assays.

  ▼ Hyperthyroidism: ruled out by a normal increase of >2–3 μU/mL after TRH administration

  ▼ Primary hypothyroidism: an exaggerated prolonged rise of an already increased TSH level

  ▼ Secondary (pituitary) hypothyroidism: no rise in the decreased TSH level

  ▼ Hypothalamic hypothyroidism: low serum T_3, T_4, and TSH levels, with a TRH response that may be exaggerated or normal or (most characteristically) with a peak delay 45–60 minutes

■ TSH high sensitivity, <0.1 mU/L, obviates need for TRH, except for TSH-secreting tumor and thyroid hormone resistance (in which case TSH thyroxine is high).

■ Interpretation must be based on clinical studies that exclude the pituitary gland as the site of the disease.

■ Lack of response shows adequate therapy in patients receiving thyroid hormones to shrink thyroid nodules and goiters and during long-term treatment of thyroid carcinoma.

■ In patients with euthyroid Graves disease who have only exophthalmos (unilateral or bilateral), the TRH stimulation test may sometimes be normal. A T_3 suppression test may be required.

■ Elderly patients with or without symptoms of hyperthyroidism may have serum T_4 and T_3 in upper normal range.

■ Euthyroid sick syndrome—response varies. Some patients respond normally, whereas many have less than normal response.

❏ Limitations

- Contraindicated in pregnancy.
- No T_4 or T_3 should be given for 3 weeks prior to test.
- TRH can cause smooth muscle spasm; use with caution in asthma and ischemic heart disease.
- The TSH response to TRH is modified by antithyroid drugs, corticosteroids, estrogens, large amounts of salicylates, and levodopa.

THYROXINE, FREE (FT$_4$)

❏ Definition

- Both free and bound forms of T_4 and T_3 are present in the blood. More than 99% of the T_4 and T_3 circulates in the blood bound to carrier proteins, leaving <1% unbound. It is this level of unbound or free hormone that correlates with the functional thyroid state in most individuals. FT_4 is usually 0.02–0.04% of total T_4 (see Table 16.76).
- **Normal range** (adults): 0.58–1.64 ng/dL.
  - ▼ Pregnant women:
    - First trimester: 0.73–1.13 ng/dL
    - Second trimester: 0.54–1.18 ng/dL
    - Third trimester: 0.56–1.09 ng/dL

❏ Use

- FT_4 gives corrected values in patients in whom the total T_4 is altered on account of changes in serum proteins or in binding sites (e.g., pregnancy, drugs [such as androgens, estrogens, birth control pills, phenytoin], altered levels of serum proteins [e.g., nephrosis]).
- Monitoring restoration to normal range is the only laboratory criterion to estimate appropriate replacement dose of levothyroxine because 6–8 weeks are required before TSH reflects these changes.
- Not generally helpful unless pituitary/hypothalamic disease is suspected.

❏ Interpretation

Increased In

- Hyperthyroidism.
- Hypothyroidism treated with thyroxine.
- Euthyroid sick syndrome.
- Occasional patients with hydatidiform mole or choriocarcinoma with marked hCG elevations may show increased FT_4, suppressed TSH, and blunted TSH response to TRH stimulation; returns to normal with effective treatment of trophoblastic disease; severe dehydration (may be >6.0 ng/dL).

Decreased In

- Hypothyroidism
- Hypothyroidism treated with triiodothyronine
- Euthyroid sick syndrome

16

❏ Limitations

- FT_4 assays based on direct equilibrium dialysis are considered reference methods.
- FT_4 assays are prone to inaccurate readings in pregnant women. The studies have shown that FT_4 index measurement is more reliable than free T_4 immunoassays in pregnant women.
- Anticonvulsant drug therapy (particularly phenytoin) may result in decreased FT_4 levels due to an increased hepatic metabolism and secondarily to displacement of hormone from binding sites.

THYROXINE, TOTAL (T_4)

❏ Definition

- T_4 is major secretion of the thyroid. Bound to TBG, prealbumin, and albumin in blood. In tissues, it is deiodinated to T_3, which causes hormonal action and is responsible for hormonal action. See Tables 16.76 and 16.79 and Figure 16.5.

❏ Use

- Reflects secretory activity; useful in diagnosis of hyper- and hypothyroidism, especially when overt or due to pituitary or hypothalamic disease
- **Normal range:** 6.09–12.23 µg/dL

❏ Interpretation

- Not affected by
  - ▼ Mercurial diuretics
  - ▼ Nonthyroidal iodine

Increased In
- Hyperthyroidism.
- Pregnancy.
- Drugs (e.g., estrogens, birth control pills, D-thyroxine, thyroid extract, TSH, amiodarone, heroin, methadone, amphetamines, some radiopaque substances for x-ray studies [ipodate, iopanoic acid]).
- Euthyroid sick syndrome.
- Increase in TBG or abnormal thyroxine-binding prealbumin.
- Familial dysalbuminemic hyperthyroxinemia—albumin binds T_4 but not T_3 more avidly than normal, causing changes similar to thyrotoxicosis (total T_4 approximately 20 µg/dL, normal thyroid hormone–binding ratio, increased free T_4 index), but the patient is not clinically thyrotoxic.
- Serum T_4 >20 µg/dL usually indicates true hyperthyroidism rather than increased TBG.
- May be found in euthyroid patients with increased serum TBG.
- Much higher in first 2 months of life than in normal adults.

Decreased In
- Hypothyroidism
- Hypoproteinemia (e.g., nephrosis, cirrhosis)

TABLE 16–79. Free Thyroxine (FT$_4$) and Thyroid-Stimulating Hormone (TSH) Levels in Various Conditions

		Sensitive TSH	
	Normal	**Low**	**High**
T$_4$ **Normal**	Euthyroid	Subclinical/early hyperthyroidism[*] NTI Drug effects (e.g., L-dopa, glucocorticoids) Replacement therapy or excess T$_4$ therapy for hypothyroidism Rule out thyrotoxicosis	Subclinical/early hypothyroidism[†] NTI Drug effects (e.g., iodine, lithium, antithyroid drugs, amiodarone, interferon alfa) Insufficient T$_4$ therapy for hypothyroidism First 4–6 wk of therapy for hypothyroidism
Low	Secondary hypothyroidism Drug effects (e.g., T$_3$, phenytoin, androgens, salicylates, carbamazepine, rifampin)	Secondary hypothyroidism NTI Drug effects (e.g., dopamine, T$_3$, corticosteroids)	Primary hypothyroidism Drug effects (e.g., iodine, lithium, antithyroid drugs, amiodarone) Insufficient T$_4$ therapy for hypothyroidism
High	NTI (e.g., psychiatric and acute illness) Abnormal binding (excess TBG, familial dysalbuminemic hyperthyroxinemia, some monoclonal proteins) Thyroid hormone resistance Drug effects (e.g., estrogen, iodine drugs or contrast media, thyroxine [factitious])	T$_3$ hyperthyroidism (e.g., Graves disease, toxic goiter, thyroiditis, factitious/iatrogenic, hyperthyroidism, struma ovarii, thyroid carcinoma) NTI (e.g., psychiatric and acute illness) Primary hyperthyroidism[†]	TSH-secreting tumor Thyroid hormone resistance

T$_3$, triiodothyronine; T$_4$, thyroxine; NTI, nonthyroid illness.
[*]Low TSH with normal T$_4$.
[†]High TSH with normal T$_4$.
[‡]In 95% of cases of thyrotoxicosis. Serum T$_3$ is needed for diagnosis of T$_3$ thyrotoxicosis in the other 5% of cases of thyrotoxicosis.

16

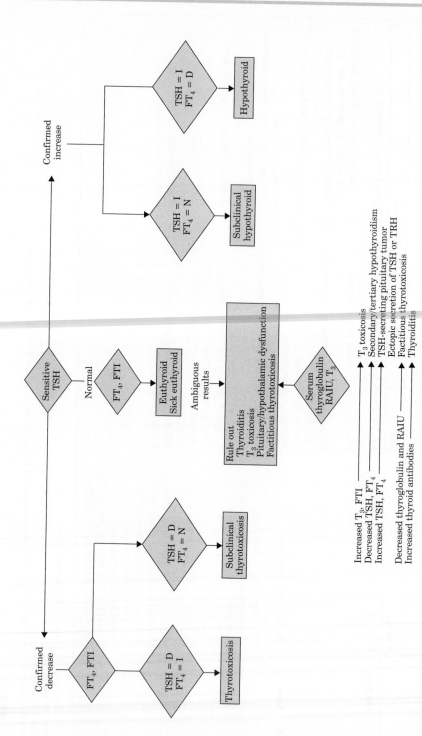

Figure 16–5 *Algorithm for thyroid function testing. (D, decreased; I, increased; N, normal.)*

- Certain drugs (phenytoin, triiodothyronine, testosterone, ACTH, corticosteroids)
- Euthyroid sick syndrome
- Decrease in TBG

Normal In

- Hyperthyroid patients with
  - ▼ T_3 thyrotoxicosis
  - ▼ Factitious hyperthyroidism owing to T_3 (Cytomel)
  - ▼ Decreased binding capacity due to hypoproteinemia or ingestion of certain drugs (e.g., phenytoin, salicylates)

❑ Limitations

- Various drugs can interfere with the test result.

THYROXINE-BINDING GLOBULIN (TBG)

❑ Definition

- This glycoprotein is the principal carrier for T_3 and T_4. It declines with age in parallel with total and free T_4 and T_3. The latter changes are accompanied by an increase in rT_3 and rT_3 index, suggesting a decrease in peripheral conversion of T_4 and T_3 rather than the change in secretory behavior of thyroid gland itself. With the availability of better free thyroid hormone tests, the TBG test is rarely used to assess the thyroid-binding hormone status.
- **Normal range:**
  - ▼ Male: 1.2–2.5 mg/dL
  - ▼ Female: 1.4–3.0 mg/dL

❑ Use

- Diagnosis of genetic or idiopathic excess TBG
- Sometimes used to detect recurrent or metastatic differentiated thyroid carcinoma, especially follicular type and where the patient has had an increased level due to carcinoma
- To distinguish increased/decreased total T_3 or total T_4 concentrations due to changes in TBG; same purpose as T_3 resin uptake and free thyroxine index

❑ Interpretation

Increased In

- Pregnancy.
- Certain drugs (e.g., estrogens, birth control pills, perphenazine, clofibrate, heroin, methadone).
- Estrogen-producing tumors.
- Systemic illness is increased early.
- Acute intermittent porphyria.
- Acute or chronic active hepatitis.
- Lymphocytic painless subacute thyroiditis.
- Neonates.
- Inherited.

16

▪ Idiopathic.
▪ An increased TBG is associated with increased serum T_4 and decreased T_3 resin uptake; a converse association exists for decreased TBG.

Decreased In

▪ Nephrosis and other causes of marked hypoproteinemia such as liver disease, severe illness (late), stress (thyroxine-binding prealbumin [TBPA] also decreased)
▪ Deficiency of TBG, genetic or idiopathic
▪ Acromegaly (TBPA also decreased)
▪ Severe acidosis
▪ Certain drugs (e.g., androgens, anabolic steroids; glucocorticoids [TBPA is increased])
▪ Testosterone-producing tumors
▪ Major illness, surgical stress, protein malnutrition, malabsorption resulting from various causes

❑ Limitations

▪ Decreased binding of T_3 and T_4 due to drugs (salicylates, phenytoin, Orinase, Diabinese, penicillin, heparin, barbital)

TISSUE TRANSGLUTAMINASE IgA ANTIBODY (tTG-IgA)

❑ Definition

▪ Celiac disease (CD) is an immune-mediated enteropathy caused by a permanent sensitivity to gluten in genetically susceptible individuals. Testing should begin with serologic evaluation, and the most sensitive and specific tests are tissue transglutaminase IgA antibody (tTG-IgA) and endomysial IgA antibody (EMA-IgA), which have equivalent diagnostic accuracy. Anti-tTG antibodies are highly sensitive and specific for the diagnosis of CD. The enzyme tTG is the major target antigen recognized by anti-endomysial antibodies. Based on the current evidence and practical considerations, including accuracy, reliability, and cost, measurement of tTG-IgA is recommended for initial testing for CD. Although as accurate as tTG, measurement of IEMA-IgA is observer dependent and, therefore, more subject to interpretation error and added cost. Because of the inferior accuracy of the antigliadin antibody (AGA) tests, the use of AGA IgA and AGA IgG tests is no longer recommended for detecting CD.
▪ **Normal range: <20 U (negative).**

❑ Use

▪ Diagnosis of certain gluten-sensitive enteropathies, such as CD and dermatitis herpetiformis
▪ Monitoring adherence to gluten-free diet in patients with dermatitis herpetiformis and CD
▪ Evaluating children with failure to thrive

❏ Interpretation

Increased In

- CD (20–30 U: weak positive; >30 U: moderate to strong positive)
- Autoimmune skin disease and dermatitis herpetiformis

❏ Limitations

- All testing should be performed while patients are on a gluten-containing diet.
- IgA deficiency is more common in CD (2–5%) than in the general population (<0.5%). The EMA-IgA and tTG-IgA serology tests will be falsely negative in untreated CD in patients with IgA deficiency. As a result, total serum IgA can be measured in addition to EMA-Ig A or tTG-IgA, especially when there is heightened clinical suspicion for CD and IgA markers are negative. If total IgA levels are abnormally low, an IgG-based assay should be used to test for CD.
- The IgG antigliadin assay has been traditionally used in this circumstance but is not ideal, since it yields frequent false-positive results. Therefore, serum IgG-tTG or IgG deamidated gliadin peptide (DPG) tests are preferable. Negative results on testing for HLA DQ2 or DQ8 can also help exclude the diagnosis in this setting.
- If serology is negative and/or there is substantial clinical doubt remaining, then further investigation should be performed with endoscopy and bowel biopsy. This is especially important in patients with frank malabsorptive symptoms, since many syndromes can mimic CD. For the patient with frank malabsorptive symptoms, bowel biopsy should be performed regardless of serologic test results.
- False-positive tests are rare but have been reported in patients with other autoimmune syndromes. Because the tTG antigen is derived from liver cells, false-positive results may be seen in patients with autoimmune liver disease.

Suggested Reading

Hill ID, Dirks MH, Liptak GS, et al. Guideline for the diagnosis and treatment of celiac disease in children: recommendations of the North American Society for Pediatric Gastroenterology, Hepatology and Nutrition. *J Pediatr Gastroenterol Nutr.* 2005;40(1):1–19.

TRANSFERRIN (TRF)

❏ Definition

- Transferrin transports circulating Fe^{3+} molecules. Normally only about one third of iron-binding sites are occupied (the remainder is called unsaturated iron-binding capacity). The half-life of transferrin is approximately 8–10 days. Plasma levels are regulated primarily by availability of iron, iron deficiency anemia. Plasma levels rise on successful treatment with iron and return to normal.
- **Normal range:** 202–336 mg/dL.

16

❑ Use

▪ Differential diagnosis of anemias

❑ Interpretation
Increased In

▪ Iron deficiency anemia; inversely proportional to iron stores
▪ Pregnancy, estrogen therapy, hyperestrogenism

Decreased In

▪ Hypochromic microcytic anemia of chronic disease
▪ Acute inflammation
▪ Protein deficiency or loss (e.g., burns, chronic infections, chronic diseases [e.g., various liver and kidney diseases, neoplasms], nephrosis, malnutrition)

❑ Limitations

▪ Transferrin in CSF appears in its desialated form, the Tau protein (beta-2-transferin). This form can be identified electrophoretically. The clinical application for identification of Tau protein is in the investigation of rhinorrhea or otorrhea, where its presence confirms the source of CSF leakage through a fracture or operative or traumatic site.
▪ Partly desialated transferrin is a marker for heavy alcohol ingestion.

TRIGLYCERIDES

❑ Definition

▪ Triglycerides are a form of fat and a major source of energy for the body. Most triglycerides are stored in adipose tissue as glycerol, monoglycerides, and fatty acids, and the liver converts these to triglycerides. Following eating, increased levels of triglycerides are found in the blood. Triglycerides move via the blood from the gut to adipose tissue for storage. Most triglycerides are carried in the blood by lipoproteins. Of the total triglycerides, about 80% are in VLDLs and 15% in LDLs, which play an important role in metabolism as energy sources and transporters of dietary fat.
▪ **Normal ranges:** see Table 16.80.

❑ Use

▪ Elevated levels of triglycerides in the blood are associated with an increased risk of developing cardiovascular disease and arteriosclerosis.

TABLE 16–80. National Cholesterol Education Program Guidelines for Triglycerides*

Triglyceride Level (mg/dL)	Category
<150	Normal
150–199	Borderline-high
200–499	High
≥500	Very high

*These values are based on fasting plasma triglyceride levels.

❏ **Interpretation**

- Concentrations associated with certain disorders:
  - ▼ Less than 150 mg/dL not associated with any disease state
  - ▼ 250–500 mg/dL associated with peripheral vascular disease; may be a marker for patients with genetic forms of hyperlipoproteinemias who need specific therapy
  - ▼ Greater than 500 mg/dL associated with high risk of pancreatitis
  - ▼ More than 1,000 mg/dL associated with hyperlipidemia, especially type I or type V; substantial risk of pancreatitis
  - ▼ Greater than 5,000 mg/dL associated with eruptive xanthoma, corneal arcus, lipemia retinalis, enlarged liver and spleen

Increased In
- Hyperlipoproteinemia types I, IIb, III, IV, and V
- Glycogen storage disease (von Gierke disease)
- Diabetes
- Hypothyroidism
- Nephrosis, chronic renal disease
- Pancreatitis
- Liver disease, alcoholism
- Werner syndrome
- Down syndrome
- Myocardial infarction
- Gout

Decreased In
- Abetalipoproteinemia
- Malnutrition
- Hyperthyroidism
- Hyperparathyroidism
- Malabsorption syndrome

❏ **Limitations**

- Factors that increase triglyceride levels include food and alcohol intake (should be 12-hour fast [24 hours for alcohol]); corticosteroids, protease inhibitors for HIV, beta blockers, and estrogens; pregnancy; acute illness; smoking; and obesity.
- Factors that decrease triglyceride levels include exercise and weight loss.
- Diurnal variation causes triglycerides to be lowest in the morning and highest around noon.

❏ **Other Considerations**

- Serum for triglyceride and for calculating LDL-C should follow a 12-hour fast.

Suggested Reading

National Institutes of Health, National Heart Lung and Blood Institute's National Cholesterol Education Program. http://www.nhlbi.nih.gov/about/ncep/. Accessed November 18, 2010.

16

TRIIODOTHYRONINE (T$_3$)

❑ **Definition**

- T$_4$ (thyroxine) is converted to T$_3$ in peripheral tissues; approximately 20% is synthesized by follicular cells. Most T$_3$ is transported bound to protein; only 0.3% is in free unbound state (see Table 16.76 and Fig. 16.5).
- **Normal range:**
  - ▼ Total T$_3$: 87–178 ng/dL
  - ▼ Free T$_3$: 2.5–3.9 pg/mL

❑ **Use**

- Diagnosis of T$_3$ thyrotoxicosis (when TSH is suppressed but T$_4$ is normal) or cases in which FT$_4$ is normal in the presence of symptoms of hyperthyroidism.
- Evaluating cases in which FT$_4$ is borderline elevated.
- Evaluating cases in which overlooking diagnosis of hyperthyroidism is undesirable (e.g., unexplained atrial fibrillation).
- Monitoring the course of hyperthyroidism.
- Monitoring T$_4$ replacement therapy—is better than T$_4$ or FT$_4$, but TSH is preferred to both.
- Predicting outcome of antithyroid drug therapy in patients with Graves disease.
- Evaluation of amiodarone-induced thyrotoxicosis.
- Good biochemical indicator of severity of thyrotoxicity in hyperthyroidism.
- Free T$_3$ gives corrected values in patients in whom the total T$_3$ is altered on account of changes in serum proteins or in binding sites (e.g., pregnancy), drugs (e.g., androgens, estrogens, birth control pills, phenytoin [Dilantin]), altered levels of serum proteins (e.g., nephrosis).

❑ **Interpretation**

Increased In

- Elevated concentrations of T$_3$ occur in Graves disease and most other classical causes of hyperthyroidism.

Decreased In

- Decreased concentrations occur in primary hypothyroid diseases such as Hashimoto thyroiditis and neonatal hypothyroidism or secondary hypothyroidism due to defects at the hypothalamohypophyseal level
- May decrease by ≤25% in healthy older persons while FT$_4$ remains normal

❑ **Limitations**

- Serum T$_3$ parallels FT$_4$; is early indicator of hyperthyroidism but TSH is better.
- Not recommended for diagnosis of hypothyroidism; decreased values have minimal clinical significance.
- More than 99% of the total concentration of T$_3$ and T$_4$ is bound by serum proteins, which is not available to elicit biologic activity. It is only the free fraction (<1%) that is readily available to bind its receptor and stimulate a response from the target organ or tissues.
- Values below the lower limit of the expected value range can be caused by a number of conditions, including nonthyroidal illness, acute and chronic stress, and hypothyroidism.

TRIIODOTHYRONINE (T₃) RESIN UPTAKE (RUR)

❑ **Definition**

- Measures unoccupied binding sites on TBG. Not a measure of T_3 concentration, which is assayed by other methods for diagnosis of T_3 thyrotoxicosis. Now replaced by free T_4 (see Table 16.77).
- **Normal range:** median value of 40.0% (0.40) with a 95% nonparametric range of 32.0–48.4%.

❑ **Use**

- Only with simultaneous measurement of serum T_4 to calculate T_7 in order to exclude the possibility that an increased total T_4 is due to an increase in TBG.
- RUR is inversely proportional to unsaturated hormone-binding sites.
- Total T_4 × RUR is proportional to free T_4 and inversely proportional to TSH.

❑ **Interpretation**

- Decreases when binding protein increases (pregnancy)
- Increases when binding protein decreases (hyperthyroidism)

❑ **Limitations**

- Normal in pregnancy with hyperthyroidism, nontoxic goiter, and in use of certain drugs (e.g., mercurials, iodine)
- In some cases of severe nonthyroid illness, RUR does not fully compensate and does not adjust the T_4 into the normal range.

TROPONINS, CARDIAC-SPECIFIC TROPONIN I AND TROPONIN T*

❑ **Definition**

- Cardiac troponin T and troponin I, also known as TnI, TnT, cTnI, cTnT, and cTn, are cardiac regulatory proteins specific to the myocardium that control the calcium-mediated interaction between actin and myosin. Troponin I remains increased longer than Ck-MB and is more specific, and cTnI is more sensitive but less specific.
- **Normal range:**
  ▼ Troponin T: 0.0–0.1 ng/mL
  ▼ Troponin I: 0.0–0.04 ng/mL

❑ **Use**

- Cardiac troponin is the preferred test for diagnosis of acute coronary syndrome (ACS). cTn establishes the diagnosis of irreversible myocardial necrosis (e.g., anoxia, contusion, inflammation), even when ECG changes or CK-MB are nondiagnostic (which occurs in ≤50% of patients with ACS). It is important to note that several distinct pathobiologic may cause elevated troponin, not all of which involve myocyte necrosis.

16

*Submitted By Craig S. Smith, MD.

- The diagnosis of myocardial infarction is predicated upon the rise and fall of cardiac troponin along with other clinical factors (see Chapter 3). However, serial normal cTn rules out myocardial necrosis.
  - ▼ In patients with a clinical syndrome consistent with ACS, a peak concentration exceeding the 99th percentile of values for a reference control group should be considered indicative of increased mortality, myocardial infarcts, and recurrent ischemic events.
  - ▼ Patients with ACS patients and cTnI and cTnT results above the decision limit should be labeled as having myocardial injury and a high-risk profile.
  - ▼ Troponin elevation above the 99th percentile due to pathobiologic mechanisms (below) other than myocardial necrosis also have an elevated risk profile for short- and long-term morbidity.
  - ▼ Troponin testing on hospital presentation followed by serial sampling with timing of sampling based on the clinical circumstances. cTnI may remain increased for ≤9 days, and cTnT may remain increased for ≤14 days.
  - ▼ The long duration of increased cTn provides a longer diagnostic window than CK-MB but may make it difficult to recognize reinfarction. Recurrent reinfarction is diagnosed if a 20% increase in troponin is observed with 3–6 hours after the initial assessment.
  - ▼ cTn is as sensitive as CK-MB during the first 48 hours after an AMI (>85% concordance with CK-MB); sensitivity is 33% from 0 to 2 hours, 50% from 2 to 4 hours, 75% from 4 to 8 hours, and approaching 100% from 8 hours after onset of chest pain. It may take ≤12 hours for all patients to show an increase. Sensitivity remains high for 6 days. Specificity is close to 100%.
- Serial cTn values may be indicator of cardiac allograft rejection. In selecting heart donors, cTnT >1.6 ng/mL predicts early graft failure with S/S = 73%/94%; cTnT >0.1 ng/mL predicts early graft failure with S/S = 64%/>98%.
- Troponin measurements are also useful in the differential diagnosis of skeletal muscle injury. Normal cTn values exclude myocardial necrosis in patients with increased CK of skeletal muscle origin (e.g., arduous physical exercise).
- Useful for diagnosis of perioperative AMI when CK-MB may be increased by skeletal muscle injury.
- Troponin may also be increased in <50% of patients with acute pericarditis. A value <0.5 ng/mL indicates no myocardial damage. A value >2.0 ng/mL indicates some myocardial necrosis.

❑ Interpretation
Increased In
- Myocardial infarction
- Cardiac trauma, including ablation, pacing, cardioversion, cardiac surgery
- CHF (acute and chronic)
- Aortic dissection, aortic valve disease, or hypertrophic cardiomyopathy
- Tachy- or bradyarrhythmias, or heart block
- Myocarditis

- Rhabdomyolysis with cardiac injury
- Hypotension
- Apical ballooning syndrome
- Renal failure
- Acute neurologic disease (stroke or subarachnoid hemorrhage)
- Infiltrative disease (amyloid, sarcoid)
- Drug toxicity (doxorubicin, 5-fluorouracil, trastuzumab, snake venom)
- Critically ill patients (especially ARDS and sepsis)
- Burns (particularly when >30% surface area)
- Technical lab error
- High concentrations of alkaline phosphate (interferes with some cTnI assays)

❑ Limitations

- cTnT may be increased in some patients with skeletal muscle injury and myotonic dystrophy but not in third-generation assays. cTnI is not increased by skeletal muscle injury, making it more highly specific for myocardial injury.
- Heterophile antibodies are one of the most common reasons for false-positive results due to interference with the immunoassay. Human antimouse antibodies, autoantibodies, rheumatoid factor also may cause false-positive results in addition to hemolysis of sample or fibrin clots in the specimen.
- Unfortunately, most point-of-care assays are not as sensitive as those performed in central laboratories. If a single value is out of proportion to others, it is recommended to respin the point-of-care sample and reanalyze.
- As troponin is able to detect very early stages of disease and confer a worse prognosis if elevated, if confounding factors for laboratory analysis of troponin are suspected, the use of other cardiac biomarkers in addition to direct cardiac imaging (or biopsy for transplant recipients) is strongly recommended.

Suggested Readings

Apple FS, Jesse RL, Newby LK, et al. National Academy of Clinical Biochemistry. National Academy of Clinical Biochemistry and IFCC Committee for Standardization of Markers of Cardiac Damage Laboratory Medicine Practice Guidelines: Analytical issues for biochemical markers of acute coronary syndromes. *Clin Chem.* 2007;53(4):547–551.

Jaffe AS. The clinical impact of the universal diagnosis of myocardial infarction. *Clin Chem Lab Med.* 2008;46(11):1485–1488.

Morrow DA, Cannon CP, Jesse RL, et al. National Academy of Clinical Biochemistry. National Academy of Clinical Biochemistry Laboratory Medicine Practice Guidelines: Clinical characteristics and utilization of biochemical markers in acute coronary syndromes. *Circulation.* 2007;115(13):e356–e375.

Roongsritong C, Warraich I, Bradley C. Common causes of troponin elevations in the absence of acute myocardial infarction incidence and clinical significance. *Chest.* 2004;125(5):1877–1884.

Starrow AB, Apple FS, Wu AH, et al. National Academy of Clinical Biochemistry Laboratory Medicine Practice Guidelines: point of care testing, oversight, and administration of cardiac biomarkers for acute coronary syndromes. *Point Care.* 2007;6(4):215–222.

Thygesen K, Alpert JS, White HD, Joint ESC/ACCF/AHA/WHF Task Redefinition myocardial infarction. *Eur Heart J.* 2007;28:2525–2538; *Circulation.* 2007;116:2634–2653; *J Am Coll Cardiol.* 2007;50:2173–2195.

16

Vafaie M, Biener M, Mueller M, et al. Analytically false or true positive elevations of high sensitivity cardiac troponin: a systematic approach. *Heart*. Online April 25. Doi: 10.1136/heart jnl-2012-303202

UREA NITROGEN, URINE

❑ **Definition**

▪ Urea is a low molecular weight substance that is freely filtered by glomeruli, and the majority is excreted into the urine, although variable amounts are reabsorbed along the nephron. Urine urea nitrogen is a measure of protein breakdown in the body. Urea is excreted by the kidneys, so excretion of urea can reflect kidney function. Approximately 50% of urinary solute excretion and 90–95% of total nitrogen excretion is composed of urea under normal conditions.

▪ **Normal range:**
  ▼ Twenty-four–hour urine: 2–20 g/day
  ▼ Random urine:
    ● Male: 2.8–9.8 g/g creatinine
    ● Female: 3.1–11.6 g/g creatinine

❑ **Use**

▪ Determination of a person's protein balance and the amount of dietary protein needed by severely ill patients

❑ **Interpretation**

Increased In

▪ Too much protein intake and/or increased protein breakdown in the body
▪ Hyperthyroidism

Decreased In

▪ Malnutrition
▪ Kidney damage and insufficiency from any cause
▪ Normal growing children and infants
▪ Pregnancy
▪ Low-protein and high-carbohydrate diet
▪ Liver disease

❑ **Limitations**

▪ Levels increase with age and protein content in the diet.
▪ Administration of GH, testosterone, and insulin decrease the urine levels.

URIC ACID (2,6,8-TRIOXYPURINE, URATE)

❑ **Definition**

▪ Uric acid is an end product of purine catabolism; it is released as DNA and RNA are degraded by dying cells. Most uric acid is synthesized in the liver and intestinal mucosa. Two thirds is excreted by the kidneys, and one third is excreted via the GI tract.

- **Normal range:**
  - ▼ Male: 2.5–8.0 mg/dL
  - ▼ Female: 1.9–7.5 mg/dL

❏ Use

- Monitor treatment of gout
- Monitor chemotherapeutic treatment of neoplasms to avoid renal urate deposition with possible renal failure (tumor lysis syndrome)

❏ Interpretation

Increased In

- Renal failure (does not correlate with severity of kidney damage; urea and creatinine should be used)
- Gout
- Twenty-five percent of the relatives of patients with gout
- Asymptomatic hyperuricemia (e.g., incidental finding with no evidence of gout; clinical significance is not known but people so afflicted should be rechecked periodically for gout); the higher the level of serum uric acid, the greater the likelihood of an attack of acute gouty arthritis
- Increased destruction of nucleoproteins
  - ▼ Leukemia, multiple myeloma
  - ▼ Polycythemia
  - ▼ Lymphoma, especially postirradiation; other disseminated neoplasms
  - ▼ Cancer chemotherapy (e.g., nitrogen mustards, vincristine, mercaptopurine, prednisone)
  - ▼ Hemolytic anemia
  - ▼ Sickle cell anemia
  - ▼ Resolving pneumonia
  - ▼ Toxemia of pregnancy (serial determinations to follow therapeutic response and estimate prognosis)
  - ▼ Psoriasis (one third of patients)
- Drugs (examples)
  - ▼ Intoxicants (e.g., barbiturates, methyl alcohol, ammonia, carbon monoxide); some patients with alcoholism
  - ▼ Decreased renal clearance or tubular secretion (e.g., various diuretics [thiazides, furosemide, ethacrynic acid] and all diuretics except spironolactone and ticrynafen)
  - ▼ Nephrotoxic effect (e.g., mitomycin C)
  - ▼ Low-dose salicylates (<4 g/day)
  - ▼ Other effects (e.g., levodopa, phenytoin sodium)
- Metabolic acidosis
- Diet
  - ▼ High-protein weight reduction diet
  - ▼ Excess nucleoprotein (e.g., sweetbreads, liver) may increase level ≤1 mg/dL
  - ▼ Alcohol consumption
- Miscellaneous
  - ▼ von Gierke disease
  - ▼ Chronic lead poisoning

16

- ▼ Lesch-Nyhan syndrome
- ▼ Maple syrup urine disease
- ▼ Down syndrome
- ▼ Polycystic kidneys
- ▼ Calcinosis universalis and circumscripta
- ▼ Hypoparathyroidism
- ▼ Primary hyperparathyroidism
- ▼ Hypothyroidism
- ▼ Sarcoidosis
- ▼ Chronic berylliosis
- ▼ Patients with arteriosclerosis and hypertension (serum uric acid is increased in 80% of patients with elevated serum triglycerides)
- ▼ Certain population groups (e.g., Blackfoot and Pima Indians, Filipinos, New Zealand Maoris)
- ▪ Most common causes in hospitalized men are azotemia, metabolic acidosis, diuretics, gout, myelolymphoproliferative disorders, other drugs, unknown causes.
- ▪ It is difficult to justify therapy in asymptomatic persons with hyperuricemia to prevent gouty arthritis, uric acid stones, urate nephropathy, or risk of cardiovascular disease.

Decreased In
- ▪ Drugs
  - ▼ ACTH
  - ▼ Uricosuric drugs (e.g., high doses of salicylates, probenecid, cortisone, allopurinol, coumarin)
  - ▼ Various other drugs (radiographic contrast agents, glyceryl guaiacolate, estrogens, phenothiazines, indomethacin)
- ▪ Wilson disease
- ▪ Fanconi syndrome
- ▪ Acromegaly (some patients)
- ▪ Celiac disease (slightly)
- ▪ PA in relapse (some patients)
- ▪ Xanthinuria
- ▪ Neoplasms (occasional cases) (e.g., carcinomas, Hodgkin disease)
- ▪ Healthy adults with isolated defect in tubular transport of uric acid (Dalmatian dog mutation)
- ▪ Decreased in approximately 5% of hospitalized patients; most common causes are postoperative state (GI surgery, coronary artery bypass), DM, various drugs, and SIADH in association with hyponatremia

Unchanged In
- ▪ Colchicine administration

❑ Limitations
- ▪ Methodologic interference (e.g., ascorbic acid, levodopa, methyldopa).
- ▪ A purine-rich diet (liver, kidney, sweetbread) as well as severe exercise, increases uric acid values.

- Rapid degradation of uric acid occurs at room temperature in the plasma of patients with tumor lysis syndrome who are treated with rasburicase. Blood should be collected in prechilled tubes containing heparin, immediately immersed in ice water bath, centrifuged in a precooled centrifuge, and the separated plasma maintained in an ice water bath, and it should be analyzed within 4 hours of collection.

URIC ACID, URINE

❑ **Definition**

- Uric acid is produced in the liver from the degradation of dietary and endogenously synthesized purine compounds. The normal male adult has a total body urate pool of approximately 1,200 mg, twice that of the female adult. This gender difference may be explained by an enhancement of renal urate excretion due to the effects of estrogenic compounds in premenopausal women. Under normal steady state conditions, daily turnover of 60% of the urate pool is achieved by balanced production and elimination of uric acid. Human tissues do not have the ability to metabolize urate. Therefore, to maintain homeostasis, urate must be eliminated by the gut and the kidney. The entry of urate into the intestine is most likely a passive process that varies with serum urate concentration. Intestinal tract bacteria are able to degrade uric acid. This breakdown process is responsible for approximately one third of total urate turnover and accounts for nearly all urate disposed of by extrarenal routes. Under normal conditions, uric acid is almost completely degraded by colonic bacteria, with little being found in the stool. Urinary uric acid excretion accounts for the remaining two thirds of the uric acid turned over daily.
- **Normal range:**
  - ▼ Twenty-four–hour urine: 250–750 mg/day
  - ▼ Random urine:
    - Male: 104–593 mg/g creatinine
    - Female: 95–741 mg/g creatinine

❑ **Use**

- Diagnosis of kidney stones
- Monitoring of people with gout, since many of these patients develop uric acid kidney stones

❑ **Interpretation**

Increased In

- Gout
- Renal failure
- Leukemia
- Multiple myeloma
- Lymphoma
- Toxemia of pregnancy

16

- Lesch-Nyhan syndrome
- Down syndrome
- Polycystic kidney disease
- Chronic lead nephropathy

Decreased In
- Wilson disease
- Fanconi syndrome
- Some malignancies
- Low-purine diet
- Folic acid deficiency

❑ Limitations

- Hyperuricosuria is present in patients with renal calculus formation. Even mild renal failure decreases uric acid excretion. Uric acid excretion is decreased with hypertension.
- Urine uric acid levels are elevated in states of uric acid overproduction such as in leukemia and polycythemia and after intake of food rich in nucleoproteins.
- High levels of bilirubin and ascorbic acid may interfere with measurement.
- Rasburicase (Elitek) causes enzymatic degradation of uric acid within blood samples left at room temperature resulting in spuriously low uric acid levels. To ensure accurate measurements in patients who have received rasburicase, blood must be collected into prechilled tubes containing heparin anticoagulant and immediately immersed and maintained in an ice bath; plasma samples must be assayed within 4 hours of sample collection.

URINALYSIS, COMPLETE

❑ Definition

- The dipstick reagent strip method is commonly used to assess the chemical evaluation of urine. The most frequently performed chemical tests using reagent test strips are specific gravity, pH, protein, glucose, ketones, blood, leukocyte esterase, nitrite, bilirubin, and urobilinogen.
- **Specific gravity:** Specific gravity is a measure of the dissolved substances present in the urine. It is a physical property of urine and an expression of concentration.
- **Color:** The color of the specimen is measured by comparison to four known wavelengths of light (red, violet, blue, and green), which are used to determine the color and hue of the sample.
- **Clarity:** The clarity or turbidity of the urine specimen is measured by passing a light beam through the sample and measuring the scattered light. The amount of scattered light increases as the specimen becomes more turbid. Clarity is reported as clear, turbid, or extremely turbid.
- **pH:** Along with the lungs, the kidneys are the major regulator of acid–base balance. pH testing provides valuable information for assessing and

managing disease and determines the suitability of a specimen for chemical testing. Freshly voided urine has a pH of 5.0–6.0. The pH of urine can be controlled by dietary regulation and medication.

- **Glucose:** Glucosuria is usually indicative of hyperglycemia due to diabetes but can also be seen in patients with other causes for hyperglycemia, in patients with renal tubular dysfunction, and in pregnancy due to increased glomerular filtration. In children especially younger than 2 years of age, it is important to perform a screening test for reducing sugar.
- **Protein:** The presence of protein in urine is mostly indicative of renal disease, but its appearance in the urine does not always signify renal disease. The strip is primarily sensitive to albumin.
- **Bilirubin:** The appearance of urinary bilirubin can be a sign of liver disease or extrahepatic or intrahepatic biliary obstruction.
- **Urobilinogen:** The normal urine has a small amount of urobilinogen. Increased amounts appear in hemolytic anemias and liver dysfunction.
- **Blood:** Equally specific for RBCs, Hb, or myoglobin present in the urine. Hematuria can be seen due to bleeding as a result of trauma or irritation. Hemoglobinuria occurs when there is lysis of RBCs in the urinary tract, intravascular hemolysis, or transfusion reactions. Very dilute or extremely alkaline urine can also lyse the cells. Myoglobinuria indicates muscular destruction that may appear in hypothermia, convulsions, and extensive exertions.
- **Ketones:** Ketonuria appears when there is an increased use of fat instead of carbohydrate for metabolism. Conditions of ketonuria include DM, vomiting, and inadequate intake of carbohydrates due to starvation or weight reduction, or pregnancy.
- **Nitrite:** Bacteria, specifically gram-negative bacteria, are detected. This analysis provides a rapid and economical means of detecting significant bacteriuria caused by nitrate reducing bacteria. It is limited by various factors, including

TABLE 16–81. Reference Values for Urinalysis

Test	Reference Range
Color	Yellow
Appearance	Clear
Specific gravity	1.005–1.030
pH	4.6–8.0
Protein	Negative
Glucose	Negative
Ketone	Negative
Bilirubin	Negative
Occult blood	Negative
Nitrite	Negative
Urobilinogen	Normal
Leukocyte esterase	Negative
White blood cells	0–2/HPF
Red blood cells	0–2/HPF
Hyaline casts	0–2/LPF
Bacteria	None

16

TABLE 16–82. Interferences Which May Cause False-Positive or False-Negative Test Results

Analyte	Causes of False-Positive Results	Causes of False-Negative Results
Specific gravity	High protein concentrations between 100 and 500 mg/dL and presence of keto acids	>1 g/dL glucose and urea concentrations
pH	No interferences known	
Blood	Menstrual contamination, microbial peroxidases, strong oxidizing agents (soap and detergents)	Ascorbic acid, high specific gravity, captopril
	Dehydration, exercise	
Leukocyte esterase	Highly colored substances mask results, beets, drugs (phenazopyridine), vaginal contamination of urine	High specific gravity, increased glucose, protein, strong oxidizing agents, drugs such as gentamicin, cephalosporins, presence of lymphocytes
Nitrite	Highly colored substances mask results, beet ingestion, drugs (phenazopyridine), improper storage with bacterial proliferation, exposure of dipstick to air	Ascorbic acid, various factors that inhibit nitrite formation despite bacteriuria
Protein	Alkaline urine, alkaline drugs, improperly preserved specimen, contamination with quaternary ammonium compounds; highly colored substances mask results, beet ingestion, drugs (phenazopyridine)	Presence of protein other than albumin
Glucose	Strong oxidizing agents such as bleach, peroxidase contaminants	Ascorbic acid, improperly stored specimens (glycolysis)
Ketones	Compounds containing free sulfhydryl groups such as captopril, N-acetylcysteine, highly pigmented urine, atypical colors with phenylketones and phthaleins, large amounts of levodopa metabolites, acidic urine, elevated specific gravity	Improper storage, resulting in volatilization, bacterial breakdown
Bilirubin	Drug-induced color changes such as phenazopyridine, indicant-indoxyl sulfate, large amounts of chlorpromazine metabolites	Ascorbic acid, high nitrite concentrations, improper storage resulting in oxidation or hydrolysis to nonreactive biliverdin and free bilirubin, light exposure, chlorpromazine (Thorazine), selenium
Urobilinogen	Atypical colors caused by sulfonamides, p-aminobenzoic acid, p-aminosalicylic acid, substances that induce color mask results, beet ingestion, elevated nitrite levels	Formalin, improper storage resulting in oxidation to urobilin

characteristics of microorganisms, dietary factors, urinary retention time, and specimen storage.
- **Leukocytes:** The presence of WBCs is an indicator of inflammation; lysed and intact WBCs are detected.
- **Normal range:** see Table 16.81.

❏ **Use**
- Frequently performed screening test for metabolic and kidney disorders and for UTIs.

❏ **Interpretation**
- For specific causes of increased and decreased values of constituents, see individual tests.

❏ **Limitations**
See Table 16.82.

Suggested Reading
Brunzel NA. *Fundamentals of Urine and Body Fluid Analyses*, 2nd ed. Philadelphia, PA: Saunders; 2004.

URINE PROTEIN ELECTROPHORESIS/IMMUNOFIXATION

❏ **Definition**
- Urine protein electrophoresis (UPEP) is analogous to the serum protein electrophoresis test and is used to detect monoclonal proteins (M-proteins) in the urine by an electrophoretic method. A 24-hour urine collection is necessary for determination of the total amount of protein excreted in the urine per day. The quantity of M-protein excreted is determined by measuring the size (percent) of the M-spike in the densitometer tracing and multiplying it by the total 24-hour urinary protein excretion. The amount of protein can be expressed as mg/dL or mg/L, but it is much more useful to report the M-protein in g/24 hours because of wide variability in the daily urinary volume. On UPEP, a urinary M-protein is seen as a dense localized band on agarose or a tall narrow peak on the densitometer tracing. Generally, the amount of urinary monoclonal protein correlates directly with the size of the plasma cell burden, as long as renal function is relatively normal. Other names: Bence-Jones protein test.
- **Normal range:** negative or no monoclonal free light chains detected.

❏ **Use**
- All patients with a diagnosis of a plasma cell dyscrasia should have a baseline UPEP (and immunofixation) of an aliquot from a 24-hour urine collection. This test is essential for detection of the presence of potentially nephrotoxic concentrations of urinary light chains.
- UPEP testing is subsequently required to detect progression and to monitor response to therapy in patients who have urinary monoclonal proteins at baseline.
- UPEP (and immunofixation) has been used also as a standard screening test for patients in whom there is clinical suspicion for a monoclonal plasma cell

16

proliferative disorder such as myeloma or primary amyloidosis. The serum free light chain assay can be used as an alternative method.

■ Quantitative determination of M-protein is useful in the response to chemotherapy or progression of disease.

❑ Interpretation

Increased In

■ Various proteinuria states
■ Monoclonal plasma cell proliferative disorders such as myeloma or primary amyloidosis

❑ Limitations

■ The 24-hour urine specimen requires no preservative and may be kept at room temperature during collection.
■ Immunofixation should be performed in these patients even if the routine urine analysis is negative for protein, 24-hour urine protein concentration is within normal limits, and electrophoresis of a concentrated urine specimen shows no globulin peak.
■ If the patient has nephrotic syndrome, the presence of a monoclonal light chain strongly suggests either primary amyloidosis (AL) or light chain deposition disease in almost all instances.

UROVYSION™ FISH FOR BLADDER CANCER*

❑ Definition

■ The UroVysion™ FISH test for bladder cancer is designed to detect, in cells shed into urine, the presence of aneuploidy for chromosomes 3, 7, 17, and loss of the 9p21 locus, using fluorescence in situ hybridization. These chromosomal abnormalities are commonly associated with urothelial carcinoma.
■ Reference ranges:
  ▼ (Negative) absence of cells identified with numeric chromosomal aberrations associated with urothelial carcinoma
  ▼ (Positive) presence of cells identified with numeric chromosomal aberrations associated with urothelial carcinoma

❑ Use

■ The UroVysion™ FISH test is intended to be used in conjunction with standard diagnostic procedures for the primary diagnosis of bladder cancer in patients with hematuria and in subsequent monitoring for tumor recurrence.

❑ Interpretation

Negative	Positive
Lack of evidence for the presence of numeric chromosomal abnormalities commonly associated with urothelial carcinoma, within the cells collected in the urine specimen.	Presence of one or more numeric chromosomal abnormalities commonly associated with urothelial carcinoma, within the cells collected in the urine specimen.

*Submitted by Charles R. Kiefer, PhD.

❏ **Limitations**

- Mutations or genetic defects other than amplification of chromosomes 3, 7, or 17; or other than deletion of the 9p21 locus, will not be detected.
- Minimum specimen volume ≥35 mL.
- Specimens are stable to 72 hours only if fixed with Saccomanno or PreservCyt® fixative.

VANILLYLMANDELIC ACID (VMA), URINE

❏ **Definition**

- Major metabolite of catecholamine, historically has been used to screen pheochromocytoma. The current recommended test now is fractionated plasma free metanephrines.
- Other names: 3-methoxy-4-hydroxymandelic acid and 4-hydroxy-3-methoxymandelic acid.
- **Normal range:** 0–7 mg/day.

❏ **Use**

- Screening for catecholamine-secreting tumors in children when accompanied by HVA
- Supporting a diagnosis of neuroblastoma
- Monitoring neuroblastoma treatment

❏ **Interpretation**

Increased In

- Pheochromocytoma
- Paraganglioma
- Neuroblastoma

❏ **Limitations**

- Patients should avoid salicylates, caffeine, phenothiazine, and antihypertension agents, as well as coffee, tea, chocolate, and fruit (especially bananas and any vanilla-containing substances for 72 hours prior to collection).
- Some neuroblastoma patients are positive for urinary homovanillic acid abnormality but do not excrete increased VMA. Twenty to thirty-two percent of patients with neuroblastoma do not have elevation of VMA. Many have other laboratory abnormalities such as increased metanephrines, HVA, or dopamine.

VASOACTIVE INTESTINAL POLYPEPTIDE (VIP)

❏ **Definition**

- A member of the secretin–glucagon family; highest levels in the gut and nervous system. A neuropeptide that functions as a neuromodulator and neurotransmitter. A potent vasodilator that regulates smooth muscle activity, epithelial cell secretion, and blood flow in the gastrointestinal tract. Functions as a neurohormone and paracrine mediator, being released from nerve terminals and acting locally on receptor-bearing cells
- **Normal range:** 0–60 pg/mL

16

❑ **Use**

- Detection of VIP-secreting tumors
- To detect occult metastases
- To evaluate the success of surgical or drug therapies

❑ **Interpretation**

Increased In

- VIPomas
- Neural crest tumors in children (ganglioneuroblastoma, ganglioneuroma, and neuroblastoma)
- Pancreatic islet cell hyperplasia
- Liver disease
- MEN type I, pheochromocytoma
- MTC
- Branchiogenic carcinoma
- Retroperitoneal histiocytoma
- CHF

❑ **Limitations**

- This test should not be requested in patients who have recently received radioisotopes, therapeutically or diagnostically, because of potential assay interference.

VISCOSITY, SERUM

❑ **Definition**

- Blood viscosity is a measure of the resistance of blood to flow due to any stress. Changes in the concentration of one or more blood protein fractions will result in a change in viscosity. Blood or serum viscosity can, therefore, be used both as a diagnostic tool for the presence of diseases known to alter the proteins and as a measure of the extent of the condition.
- **Normal range:** 1.10–1.80 cP (relative to water).

❑ **Use**

- Evaluate hyperviscosity syndrome associated with monoclonal gammopathy states (myeloma, Waldenström macroglobulinemia, and other dysproteinemias), including RA, SLE, and hyperfibrinogenemia.

❑ **Interpretation**

Increased In

- Increased leukocyte count
- Thrombocytosis
- Hyperlipoproteinemia
- Macroglobulinemia
- Sjögren syndrome
- SLE
- Lymphoproliferative disorders

- Hyperglobulinemia associated with cirrhosis
- Chronic active hepatitis
- Acute thermal burns

Decreased In
- No clinical significance

❏ **Limitations**
- Whole blood measurement is of limited use because of differences in shear rates between instrumentation and in vivo conditions.
- Clinical symptoms do not correlate well with test results.

VITAMIN A (RETINOL, CAROTENE)

❏ **Definition**
- Vitamin A is a subclass of a family of lipid-soluble compounds referred to as retinoic acids. There are essentially three forms of vitamin A: retinols, beta-carotenes, and carotenoids. Retinol, also known as preformed vitamin A, is the most active form and is mostly found in animal sources of food. Beta-carotene, also known as provitamin A, is the plant source of retinol from which mammals make two thirds of their vitamin A. Carotenoids, the largest group of the three, contain multiple conjugated double bonds and exist in a free alcohol or in a fatty acyl ester form. Vitamin A promotes normal vision and prevents night blindness; contributes to growth of bone, teeth, and soft tissues; supports thyroxine formation; maintains epithelial cell membranes, skin, and mucous membranes; and acts as an anti-infection agent.
- **Normal range:** see Table 16.83.

❏ **Use**
- Assist in the diagnosis of night blindness
- Evaluate skin disorders
- Investigate suspected vitamin A deficiency

❏ **Interpretation**
Increased In
- Chronic kidney disease
- Idiopathic hypercalcemia in infants
- Vitamin A toxicity

TABLE 16–83. Normal Ranges for Vitamin A by Age

Age	Reference Interval (mg/L)
0–1 mo	0.18–0.50
2 mo–12 y	0.20–0.50
13–17 y	0.26–0.70
≥18 y	0.30–1.20

16

Decreased In
- Abetalipoproteinemia
- Carcinoid syndrome
- Chronic infections
- CF
- Disseminated TB
- Hypothyroidism
- Infantile blindness
- Liver, GI, or pancreatic disease
- Night blindness
- Protein malnutrition
- Sterility and teratogenesis
- Zinc deficiency

❑ **Limitations**
- Alcohol (moderate intake), oral contraceptives, and probucol increase vitamin A levels.
- Alcohol (chronic intake, alcoholism), allopurinol, cholestyramine, colestipol, mineral oil, and neomycin decrease vitamin A levels.
- Serum retinol is typically maintained until hepatic stores are almost depleted. Values >0.30 mg/L represent adequate liver stores, whereas values <0.10 mg/L indicate deficiency.
- Samples that come in contact with plastic tubing or have been exposed to excessive light may show low results.

VITAMIN A RELATIVE DOSE–RESPONSE (RDR) TEST

❑ **Definition**
- Retinol (vitamin A) measurements in blood have several disadvantages. It is decreased only in severe vitamin A deficiency, when liver stores are nearly exhausted. In addition, infection can decrease serum vitamin A levels in blood, leading to misclassification of individuals. Because the majority of vitamin A is stored in liver, RDR test/calculation was developed to reliably measure vitamin A storage. Retinyl palmitate is given either as a water miscible solution of 1,000 µg administered IV over 30 minutes or as 450 µg diluted in corn oil and administered orally. Fasting and 5 hours after-dose plasma specimens should be drawn. RDR is calculated as 5-hourvitamin A fasting (0 hour)/vitamin A 5 hour × 100.
- **Normal range:** <10%.

❑ **Use**
- Identify subjects with marginal liver vitamin A stores
- As a tool for estimation of total body stores of vitamin A

❑ **Interpretation**
Increased In
- RDR values of >20% indicate depleted liver vitamin A stores.

❑ **Limitations**

- The vitamin A RDR oral dose test has the similar limitations of other absorption tests. It decreases in malabsorption, cirrhosis, cholestasis, hepatocellular disease, protein–calorie malnutrition, and zinc deficiency.

VITAMIN B₁ (THIAMINE)

❑ **Definition**

- Thiamine, first named "the antiberiberi factor" in 1926, has a historical value due to the very early description of beriberi in the Chinese medical texts, as far back as 2697 BC. Thiamine is found in larger quantities in food products such as yeast, legumes, pork, rice, and cereals. Milk products, fruits, and vegetables are poor sources of thiamine. The thiamine molecule is denatured at high pH and high temperatures. Hence, cooking, baking, and canning of some foods as well as pasteurization can destroy thiamine. Thiamine is an essential vitamin required for carbohydrate metabolism, brain function, and peripheral nerve myelination. Thiamine deficiency has been associated with three disorders: Beriberi (infantile and adult), Wernicke-Korsakoff syndrome, and Leigh syndrome.
- **Normal range: 70–180 nmol/L.**

❑ **Use**

- Assessment of thiamine deficiency: Thiamine measurement is appropriate in patients with behavioral changes, eye signs, gait disturbances, delirium, and encephalopathy; or in patients with questionable nutritional status, especially those who appear at risk and who also are being given insulin for hyperglycemia.
- Investigation of suspected beriberi.
- Monitoring the effects of chronic alcoholism.

❑ **Interpretation**
Increased In
- Leukemia
- Polycythemia vera
- Hodgkin disease

Decreased In
- Alcoholism with and without liver disease
- Deficient diet
- Chronic febrile infections
- Prolonged diarrhea
- Diabetes
- Carcinoid syndrome
- Hartnup disease
- Pellagra

❑ **Limitations**

- Whole blood is the preferred specimen for thiamine assessment. Approximately 80% of thiamine present in whole blood is found in RBCs.

16

- Drugs that may decrease vitamin B₁ levels include glibenclamide, isoniazid, and valproic acid.
- Diets high in freshwater fish and tea, which are thiamine antagonists, may cause decreased vitamin B₁ levels.
- Thiamine deficiency can be assessed by measuring the blood thiamine concentration, erythrocyte thiamine transketolase (ETKA), or transketolase urinary thiamine excretion (with or without a 5-mg thiamine load). Most laboratories now measure blood thiamine concentration directly, in preference to the ETKA method. The ETKA method is a functional test, and results are influenced by the hemoglobin concentration.

VITAMIN B₁₂ (CYANOCOBALAMIN, COBALAMIN)

❑ Definition

- Vitamin B₁₂ is essential in DNA synthesis, hematopoiesis, and CNS integrity. Its absorption depends on the presence of intrinsic factor (IF) and may be due to lack of IF secretion by gastric mucosa (e.g., gastrectomy, gastric atrophy) or intestinal malabsorption (e.g., ileal resection, small intestinal diseases). Vitamin B₁₂ deficiency frequently causes macrocytic anemia, glossitis, peripheral neuropathy, weakness, hyperreflexia, ataxia, loss of proprioception, poor coordination, and affective behavioral changes. These manifestations may occur in any combination; many patients have the neurologic defects without macrocytic anemia. PA is a macrocytic anemia caused by B₁₂ deficiency that is due to a lack of IF secretion by gastric mucosa. Serum methylmalonic acid (MMA) and homocysteine levels are also elevated in vitamin B₁₂ deficiency states. A significant increase in RBC MCV may be an important indicator of vitamin B₁₂ deficiency.
- **Normal range:** 180–914 pg/mL.
  - ▼ Indeterminate range: 145–180 pg/mL
  - ▼ Deficient range: <145 pg/mL

❑ Use

- Investigation of macrocytic anemia
- Workup of deficiencies seen in megaloblastic anemias
- Assistance in the diagnosis of CNS disorders
- Evaluation of alcoholism
- Evaluation of malabsorption syndromes

❑ Interpretation
Increased In
- Chronic granulocytic leukemia
- COPD
- Chronic renal failure
- Diabetes
- Leukocytosis
- Liver cell damage (hepatitis, cirrhosis)
- Obesity
- Polycythemia vera

- Protein malnutrition
- Severe CHF
- Some carcinomas

Decreased In
- Abnormalities of cobalamin transport or metabolism
- Bacterial overgrowth
- Crohn disease
- Dietary deficiency (e.g., in vegetarians)
- Diphyllobothrium (fish tapeworm) infestation
- Gastric or small intestine surgery
- Hypochlorhydria
- Inflammatory bowel disease
- Intestinal malabsorption
- Intrinsic factor deficiency
- Late pregnancy
- PA

❏ Limitations
- Serum samples should be protected from light at room temperature (15–30°C) for no longer than 1 hour. If the assay will not be completed within 2 hours, samples should be frozen and be protected from light exposure.
- Drugs such as chloral hydrate increase vitamin B_{12} levels. On the other hand, alcohol, aminosalicylic acid, anticonvulsants, ascorbic acid, cholestyramine, cimetidine, colchicine, metformin, neomycin, oral contraceptives, ranitidine, and triamterene decrease vitamin B_{12} levels.
- Many other conditions are known to cause an increase (vitamin C, vitamin A, estrogens, hepatocellular injury, myeloproliferative disorders, uremia) or decrease (pregnancy, smoking, hemodialysis, multiple myeloma) serum B_{12} levels.
- The evaluation of macrocytic anemia requires measurement of both vitamin B_{12} and folate levels; ideally, they should be measured simultaneously.
- Specimen collection soon after blood transfusion can falsely increase vitamin B_{12} levels.
- Patients taking vitamin B_{12} supplementation may have misleading results.
- A normal serum concentration of B_{12} does not rule out tissue deficiency of vitamin B_{12}. The most sensitive test for B_{12} deficiency at the cellular level is the assay for MMA. If clinical symptoms suggest deficiency, measurement of MMA and homocysteine should be considered, even if serum B_{12} concentrations are normal.

VITAMIN B₂ (RIBOFLAVIN)

❏ Definition
- Vitamin B_2, or riboflavin, is one of the water-soluble vitamins. It is synthesized in plants and microorganisms and occurs naturally in three forms: the physiologically inactive riboflavin and the physiologically active coenzymes flavin mononucleotide (FMN) and flavin adenine dinucleotide (FAD). The latter accounts for about 90% of the total riboflavin in whole blood. Because

16

of their capacity to transfer electrons, FAD and FMN are essential for proton transfer in the respiratory chain, for the dehydration of fatty acids, the oxidative deamination of amino acids, and for other redox processes.

- **Normal range:** 3–15 µg/L.
  - ▼ Marginally low: 2 µg/L
  - ▼ Diminished: <2 µg/L

❑ Use

- Evaluation of persons who present the signs of ariboflavinosis
- Detect riboflavin deficiency

❑ Interpretation

Decreased In

- Patients with anorexia nervosa
- Individuals who avoid dairy products (such as people with lactose intolerance) because dairy products are a good source of riboflavin
- Patients with malabsorptive syndromes such as celiac sprue, malignancies, and short bowel syndrome
- Rare inborn errors of metabolism in which there is a defect in riboflavin synthesis
- Long-term use of phenobarbital and other barbiturates, which may lead to oxidation of riboflavin and impair its function

❑ Limitations

- Testing of nonfasting specimens or the use of dietary vitamin B_2 supplementation can result in elevated plasma vitamin B_2 concentrations.
- Sample should be frozen immediately to reduce the stability of B_2 in serum.

Suggested Reading

Russell RM, Suter PM. Vitamin and trace mineral deficiency and excess. In: Fauci AS, Kasper DL, Braunwald E, et al. (eds.). *Harrison's Principles of Internal Medicine*, 17th ed. New York, NY: McGraw-Hill; 2008:441–449.

VITAMIN B_6 (PYRIDOXINE)

❑ Definition

- Vitamin B_6 is a complex of six vitamers: pyridoxal, pyridoxol, pyridoxamine (pyridoxine), and their 5′-phosphate esters. Because of its role as a cofactor in a number of enzymatic reactions, pyridoxal phosphate (PLP) has been determined to be the biologically active form of vitamin B_6. Vitamin B_6 is important in heme synthesis and functions as a coenzyme in amino acid metabolism and glycogenolysis. Vitamin B_6 deficiency is associated with symptoms of irritability, weakness, depression, dizziness, peripheral neuropathy, and seizures. In the pediatric population, deficiencies have been characterized by diarrhea, anemia, and seizures.
- **Normal range:** 5–50 µg/L.

❑ Use

- Determining vitamin B_6 status
- Investigating suspected malabsorption or malnutrition

- Determining the overall success of a vitamin B$_6$ supplementation program
- Diagnosis and evaluation of hypophosphatasia

❏ **Interpretation**

Increased In

- Hypophosphatasia

Decreased In

- Alcoholism
- Asthma
- Carpal tunnel syndrome
- Gestational diabetes
- Lactation
- Malabsorption
- Malnutrition
- Neonatal seizures
- Normal pregnancies
- Occupational exposure to hydrazine compounds
- Pellagra
- Preeclamptic edema
- Renal dialysis
- Uremia

❏ **Limitations**

- In addition to PLP, the following methods can be used to assess for vitamin B$_6$ deficiency:
  - Erythrocyte transaminase activity with and without PLP added has been used as a functional test of pyridoxine status.
  - Urinary 4-pyridoxic acid excretion >3.0 mmol/day can be used as an indicator of adequate short-term vitamin B$_6$ status.
  - Urinary excretion of xanthurenic acid is normally <65 mmol/day following a 2-g tryptophan load.
- Drugs that may decrease vitamin B$_6$ levels include amiodarone, anticonvulsants, cycloserine, disulfiram, ethanol, hydralazine, isoniazid, levodopa, oral contraceptives, penicillamine, pyrazinoic acid, and theophylline.
- B$_6$ may be decreased with pregnancy, lactation, alcoholism, DM, and in an uncommon B$_6$ dependency state, vitamin B$_6$–responsive neonatal convulsions. There is evidence of significant neurotoxicity associated with pyridoxine megavitaminosis; tingling, numbness, clumsiness, gait disturbances, and pseudoathetosis, with doses >2 g/day.

VITAMIN C (ASCORBIC ACID)

❏ **Definition**

- Ascorbic acid is essential for the enzymatic amidation of neuropeptides, production of adrenal cortical steroid hormones, promotion of the conversion of tropocollagen to collagen, and metabolism of tyrosine and folate. It also plays a role in lipid and vitamin metabolism and is a powerful reducing agent or antioxidant. Specific actions include activation of detoxifying enzymes in the liver, antioxidation, interception and destruction of free radicals, preservation

16

and restoration of the antioxidant potential of vitamin E, and blockage of the formation of carcinogenic nitrosamines. Vitamin C promotes collagen synthesis, maintains capillary strength, facilitates release of iron from ferritin to form hemoglobin, and functions in the stress response. In addition, vitamin C appears to function in a variety of other metabolic processes in which its role has not been well characterized.

▪ **Normal range:** 0.4–2.0 mg/dL.

❑ **Use**

▪ Investigate suspected metabolic or malabsorptive disorders
▪ Investigate suspected scurvy

❑ **Interpretation**

Decreased In

▪ Alcoholism
▪ Anemia
▪ Cancer
▪ Hemodialysis
▪ Hyperthyroidism
▪ Malabsorption
▪ Pregnancy
▪ Rheumatoid disease
▪ Scurvy

❑ **Limitations**

▪ Drugs and substances that may decrease vitamin C levels include acetylsalicylic acid, aminopyrine, barbiturates, estrogens, heavy metals, oral contraceptives, nitrosamines, and paraldehyde.
▪ Chronic tobacco smoking decreases vitamin C levels.
▪ Testing of nonfasting specimens or the use of vitamin supplementation can result in elevated plasma vitamin concentrations. Reference values were established in patients who were fasting.
▪ After consuming vitamin C, plasma values rapidly rise within 1–2 hours and reach peak concentration within 3–6 hours after ingestion.

VITAMIN D, 1,25-DIHYDROXY

❑ **Definition**

▪ It is the active form of vitamin D and is produced primarily in the kidney by the hydroxylation of 25-hydroxyvitamin D. Other names: calcitriol and 1,25-dihydroxycholecalciferol (1,25-OHD).
▪ **Normal range:** 15–75 pg/mL.

❑ **Use**

▪ As a second-order test in the assessment of vitamin D status, especially in patients with renal disease
▪ Investigation of some patients with clinical evidence of vitamin D deficiency (e.g., vitamin D–dependent rickets due to hereditary deficiency of renal 1-alpha hydroxylase or end-organ resistance to 1,25-dihydroxyvitamin D)
▪ Differential diagnosis of hypercalcemia

❏ Interpretation
Increased In
- Sarcoidosis (synthesized by macrophages within granulomas).
- Non-Hodgkin lymphoma (approximately 15% of cases). Returns to normal after therapy.

Decreased In
- Renal failure
- Hyperphosphatemia
- Vitamin D–dependent rickets, types 1 and 2

Normal In
- HPT
- Humoral hypercalcemia of malignancy

❏ Limitations
- The level of 1,25-OHD is maintained despite significant vitamin D depletion, because secondary hyperparathyroidism stimulates increased conversion of 25-OHD to 1,25-OHD in this situation.
- Although 1,25-OHD is the biologically active form of vitamin D, its level in the body provides *no* useful information about a patient's vitamin D status. The kidney tightly controls serum 1,25-OHD levels, which are often normal or even elevated in vitamin D deficiency. Therefore, a patient with normal or high levels of 1,25-OHD is vitamin D deficient despite high serum levels of the active hormone. At this time, there is consensus that serum 1,25-OHD is a measure of only the endocrine function of vitamin D and not an indicator of the body stores or the ability of vitamin D to perform its pleiotropic autocrine functions.

VITAMIN D, 25-HYDROXY

- Other names: 25-hydroxy D2; 25-hydroxy D3; 5-hydroxy vitamin D; 25-hydroxycholecalciferol; 25-hydroxyergocalciferol; 25-OH vitamin D; calcidiol.

❏ Definition
- A steroid hormone that has long been known for its important role in regulating body levels of calcium and phosphorus and in the mineralization of bone. The term "vitamin D" specifically refers to two biologically inert precursors, vitamin D_3 (cholecalciferol) or D_2 (ergocalciferol). Neither vitamin D_3 nor vitamin D_2 has significant biologic activity; rather they must be metabolized within the body to the hormonally active form. Vitamin D_3 is generated in the skin when light energy is absorbed (UV radiation in the UVB spectrum 290–320 nm) by a precursor molecule 7-dehydrocholesterol (7-DHC; provitamin D_3). However, cutaneous vitamin D_3 production after single prolonged UVB exposure is capped at approximately 10–20% of the original epidermal 7-DHC concentration, a limit achieved with suberythemogenic UV exposures. Vitamin D_2 is plant derived, produced exogenously by irradiation of ergosterol, and enters the circulation through diet. Vitamin D_3 from the skin and vitamin D_3 and D_2 from the diet enter the blood and are

16

TABLE 16–84. Normal Ranges of 25-OH Vitamin D

Vitamin D Status	25-OH Vitamin D (ng/mL)
Deficiency	<10
Insufficiency	10–30
Sufficiency	30–100
Toxicity	>100

metabolized to their 25-hydroxy counterparts. Once formed, 25-hydroxyvitamin D (25-OHD) is metabolized in the kidney to 1,25-dihydroxyvitamin D (1,25-OHD).

- **Normal range:** see Table 16.84.

❑ **Use**

- Diagnosis of vitamin D deficiency
- Differential diagnosis of causes of rickets and osteomalacia
- Monitoring vitamin D replacement therapy
- Diagnosis of hypervitaminosis D

❑ **Interpretation**

Increased In

- Vitamin D intoxication
- Excessive exposure to sunlight

Decreased In

- Malabsorption
- Steatorrhea
- Dietary osteomalacia, anticonvulsant osteomalacia
- Biliary and portal cirrhosis
- Thyrotoxicosis
- Pancreatic insufficiency
- Celiac disease
- Inflammatory bowel disease
- Rickets
- Alzheimer disease

❑ **Limitations**

- More recently, it has become clear that receptors for vitamin D are present in a wide variety of cells and that this hormone has biologic effects extending beyond the control of mineral metabolism.
- Vitamin D deficiency is not clear. Levels needed to prevent rickets and osteomalacia (15 ng/mL) are lower than those that dramatically suppress parathyroid hormone levels (20–30 ng/mL). In turn, those levels are lower than levels needed to optimize intestinal calcium absorption (34 ng/mL). Neuromuscular peak performance is associated with levels approximately 38 ng/mL. A recent study states that increasing mean baseline levels from 29 to 38 ng/mL was associated with a 50% lower risk for colon cancer and levels of 52 ng/mL with a 50% reduction in the incidence of breast cancer.

- Various methods for measuring circulating concentrations 25-OHD are available. Current methods include RIA, CIA, HPLC, and LCMS/MS tandem mass spectrometry. Immunoassays measure total 25-OHD, which includes levels of both 25-OHD$_2$ and 25-OHD$_3$. The antibodies cross-react 100% with both D$_2$ and D$_3$ to give the total 25-OHD. Some commercial laboratories use LCMS/MS technology and report 25-OHD$_2$ and 25-OHD$_3$ separately and add both values to get the total 25-OHD. The studies report reasonable correlations between methods, but with significant differences, the reasons for which are not well understood. There could be many reasons for these variations, including drifts in the reagents being manufactured, and there is an urgent need for harmonization and standardization.
- The reference ranges discussed in the preceding are related to total 25-OHD; as long as the combined total is 30 ng/mL or more, the patient has sufficient vitamin D. The Institute of Medicine 3, 4 and the Endocrine Society 5 announced that levels <20 ng/mL (50 nmol/L) are considered deficient, which is lower than in previous guidelines. Given the absence of assay standardization and lack of consensus regarding clinical cutoff values, vitamin D levels must be interpreted within the clinical context of each patient and one should not rely solely on cutoff values based on so-called normal values.

VITAMIN E (ALPHA-TOCOPHEROL)

❑ **Definition**

- Tocopherol is a fat-soluble vitamin with antioxidant properties; it protects cell membranes from oxidation and destruction. Vitamin E is found in a variety of foods, including oils, meat, eggs, and leafy vegetables. Serum vitamin E levels are strongly influenced by concentration of serum lipids and do not accurately reflect tissue vitamin levels. Effective vitamin E levels are calculated as the ratio of serum alpha-tocopherol per gram total lipids. Vitamin E reserves in lung tissue provide a barrier against air pollution and protect red blood cell membrane integrity from oxidation. Oxidation of fatty acids in red blood cell membranes can result in irreversible membrane damage and hemolysis. Studies are in progress to confirm the suspicion that oxidation also contributes to the formation of cataracts and macular degeneration of the retina. Because vitamin E is found in a wide variety of foods, a deficiency secondary to inadequate dietary intake is rare.
- **Normal range:** see Table 16.85.

TABLE 16–85. Normal Ranges for Vitamin E

	Range (mg/L)
Age: 0–17 y	3.8–18.4
Age: ≥18 y	5.5–17.0
Significant deficiency	<3.0
Significant excess	>40

16

❏ Use

- Evaluate neuromuscular disorders in premature infants and adults
- Evaluate patients with malabsorption disorders
- Evaluate suspected hemolytic anemia in premature infants and adults
- Monitor patients on long-term parenteral nutrition
- Evaluation of individuals with motor and sensory neuropathies
- Monitoring vitamin E status of premature infants requiring oxygenation

❏ Interpretation

Increased In

- Obstructive liver disease
- Hyperlipidemia
- Vitamin E intoxication

Decreased In

- Abetalipoproteinemia
- Hemolytic anemia
- Malabsorption disorders, such as biliary atresia, cirrhosis, CF, chronic pancreatitis, pancreatic carcinoma, and chronic cholestasis

❏ Limitations

- As previously stated, serum vitamin E levels are strongly influenced by concentration of serum lipids and do not accurately reflect tissue vitamin levels. Therefore, effective vitamin E levels are calculated as the following ratio:
  - ▼ Effective serum vitamin E level = alpha-tocopherol/(cholesterol + triglycerides)
  - ▼ A normal ratio is >0.8 mg alpha-tocopherol/gram total lipids.
  - ▼ For patients with normal levels of serum lipids, serum alpha-tocopherol levels provide an adequate estimate of vitamin E sufficiency. Alpha-tocopherol levels of <0.5 mg/dL (5 μg/mL) are considered deficient.
- Drugs that may increase vitamin E levels include anticonvulsants (in women).
- Drugs that may decrease vitamin E levels include anticonvulsants (in men).
- Exposure of the specimen to light decreases vitamin E levels, resulting in a falsely low result.
- Platelet tocopherol is suggested to be a better measure of vitamin E nutritional status than plasma tocopherol because it is more sensitive to vitamin E intake and is not dependent on circulating lipid levels.

von WILLEBRAND DISEASE (VWD) ASSAYS*

❏ Definition

- VWD is a bleeding disorder manifested by mucocutaneous bleeding.

❏ Use

- No single laboratory test can detect all forms of VWD, hence the following four-assay panel is recommended: von Willebrand factor (vWF) activity by a ristocetin (RCoF) or an immunoassay, von Willebrand factor (VWF)

*Submitted by Liberto Pechet, MD.

antigen, factor VIII activity which is decreased in parallel to VWF levels, and ristocetin-induced platelet aggregation (RIPA); once a diagnosis of vWD is established with this panel, VWF multimer analysis is recommended to distinguish various subtypes.

- Determination of the blood group is also helpful in interpreting low values since patients with group 0 run 20–30% lower values that those established for a random normal population.
- *RCoF.* A quantitative test for VWF is used whenever a history of mucocutaneous bleeding suggests VWD. In the presence of ristocetin, the VWF causes agglutination of platelets, measured in an aggregometer by the change in optical density. It is unaffected by anticoagulants.
- *Normal range for* RCoF: 48–172%.

Decreased In
- Various types of VWD
- Platelet-type VWD
- Hypothyroidism
- Acquired inhibitors to VWF

Increased In
- Acute inflammatory conditions (VWF is an acute-phase reactant).
- High levels are seen in some patients with thromboembolic events. There is some evidence that patients with very elevated VWF levels may be predisposed to thromboembolism.

❏ Limitations of Assay
- Great variability in results (see above the broad range for normal values).
- Therapy with factor VIII concentrates that contain VWF, or with DDAVP, raise the RCoF levels.
- Interfering substances: Lipemia, clotted or hemolyzed blood, blood collected in wrong anticoagulant, or improperly filled test tube.
- **VWF antigen:** normal values: 60–150. The antigen values may be higher than the vWF activity in certain subtypes with qualitative defects, resulting in a ratio <0.7 of activity/antigen.
- **Factor VIII coagulant:** normal range: 70–150%
- **RIPA** is a semiquantitative assay for VWF, used when there is a strong suspicion for VWD. It uses ristocetin as the platelet agglutinating agent in the presence of VWF. The changes in optical density (OD) are recorded in an aggregometer. Abnormal response to ristocetin is the result of von Willebrand disease or of the platelet receptors responsible for binding von Willebrand factor

❏ Use of RIPA
- To estimate VWF activity and rule in or out type 2B VWD (see below.)

RESULTS

- Two concentrations of ristocetin are used in the RIPA assay: a high concentration results in *65% or more change in OD* if normal VWF is present. A lower concentration of ristocetin is also used: it will not agglutinate platelets

16

in cases with normal (or low) VWF but will result in agglutination in cases of type 2B VWD, which represent a gain of function in the factor. A similar pattern is found when platelets form patients with platelet-type VWD (pseudo-VWD) are used.

❏ **Limitations**

- The assay is labor intensive and requires highly trained technologists.
- The quantitation of VWF by this assay is imprecise.
- Clotted blood or blood obtained in an appropriate anticoagulant invalidates results.

WATER DEPRIVATION TEST

❏ **Definition**

- Normal physiologic response to the water deprivation will increase plasma osmolality, which will then lead to a progressive elevation in ADH release and an increase in urine osmolality. Once the plasma osmolality reaches 295–300 mOsm/kg (normal: 275–290 mOsm/kg), the effect of endogenous ADH on the kidney is maximal. At this point, administering ADH does not further elevate the urine osmolality unless endogenous ADH release is impaired (e.g., the patient has central diabetes insipidus [DI]). This test is also known as the water restriction test.
- **Normal response:** Water deprivation causes kidney to increase urine osmolality to 1,000–1,200 mmol/kg. ADH does not cause further increase in urine osmolality because endogenous ADH is already at maximum.

❏ **Use**

- To distinguish the major forms of DI—neurogenic, nephrogenic, and polydipsic.
- Steps:
  - ▼ Have the patient should stop drinking 2–3 hours before coming to the office or clinic; overnight fluid restriction should be avoided, because potentially severe volume depletion and hypernatremia can be induced in patients with marked polyuria.
  - ▼ Collect 7–10 mL of heparinized blood for immediate measurements of serum sodium concentration and osmolality. Also ask the patient to void his/her bladder, record the urine volume, and send urine specimen for immediate measurement of osmolality.
  - ▼ Repeat step 2 every hour until (a) plasma sodium concentration or osmolality rises above the upper limit of normal range or (b) urine osmolality rises above 300 mOsm/kg H_2O.
    - If (a) occurs before (b), primary polydipsia, partial neurogenic, and partial nephrogenic DI are excluded, and a dDAVP (synthetic analog of ADH) challenge test should be done as follows:
      - Inject 2 μg of dDAVP subcutaneously.
      - Ask the patient to empty bladder at 1 and 2 hours after the injection; measure the urine osmolality. Also measure the patient's plasma ADH level.

- ○ If either urine samples has an osmolality >50% higher than the value immediately before injection, the patient probably has complete neurogenic DI.
- ○ If both urine samples have osmolality increase of <50% than the value immediately before injection, the patient is very likely to have complete nephrogenic DI.
- ▼ If (b) occurs before (a), complete neurogenic and nephrogenic DI are excluded. Further differentiate among partial nephrogenic DI, partial neurogenic DI, and primary polydipsia will require trained personnel and specialized measurements.

❑ **Interpretation**

- **Complete DI:** Water deprivation increases plasma osmolality but urine osmolality stays <290 mmol/kg and does not increase following dDAVP challenge.
- **Partial DI:** Water deprivation causes some increase in urine osmolality to 400–500 mmol/kg (less than normal).
- **Complete or partial nephrogenic DI or psychogenic polydipsia:** Increased ADH levels. Giving ADH does not increase urine osmolality in complete nephrogenic DI.
- **Complete or partial neurogenic DI:** Low ADH relative to plasma osmolality. Giving ADH increases urine osmolality approximately 200 mmol/kg but not in partial nephrogenic DI.

❑ **Limitations**

- Some nonosmotic stimuli, such as smoking, hypotension, and nausea, can increase ADH release. If a transient episode of hypotension and nausea occurs, the entire test is invalid and it needs to be repeated in another day.
- Complete emptying of the bladder during each collection is important because incomplete emptying may dilute the urine of the next collection.
- The plasma sample for osmolality measurement should be from heparinized blood, and EDTA should be avoided because it artificially increases the osmolality by 3–10%.
- The plasma for ADH measurement should be collected without disturbing the buffy coat in order to minimize the contamination from platelets.
- The test should be performed only when the patient's basal plasma sodium concentration is within the normal range, otherwise it may cause potential harm to the patient.
- The test should not be performed in patients with renal insufficiency, uncontrolled DM, or hypovolemia of any cause or uncorrected adrenal or thyroid hormone deficiency.
- Patients should be observed for the entire duration of the test.
- For pregnant patients, the blood sample for ADH measurement should be drawn into a tube that contains 6 mg of 1,10-phenanthroline to prevent the degradation of ADH by placental vasopressinase. The results should be evaluated in the context of altered relationship between the plasma osmolality/sodium concentration and the plasma ADH concentration.

16

WHITE BLOOD CELL: INCLUSIONS AND MORPHOLOGIC ABNORMALITIES*

❑ **Definition**

■ The WBC morphology may present with unusual inclusions (Table 16.86) or with other abnormalities in granules or morphology (Table 16.87). Some are associated with congenital syndromes; some are acquired. These morphologic abnormalities may or may not be associated with functional abnormalities.

TABLE 16–86. White Blood Cell Inclusions in Peripheral Blood

Inclusions	Morphology and Conditions
Howell-Jolly bodies	Cytoplasmic chromatin remnants; seen in granulocytic series in splenectomized patients
Auer rods	Linear azurophilic granules; seen in immature myeloid or monocytic cells of acute leukemias
Döhle bodies	Small, oval inclusions in the peripheral cytoplasm of neutrophils, remnants of ribosomes or endoplasmic reticulum; seen in infections, burns, aplastic anemia, following administration of toxic agents
Toxic granulation	Primary granules in bands and neutrophils; seen in infections, especially with leukemoid reactions, toxic conditions, and after therapy with granulocyte colony–forming unit drugs
Chédiak-Higashi syndrome granules	Coarse, deeply staining, peroxidase-positive fused large granulations in cytoplasm of granulocytes; characteristic of Chédiak-Higashi syndrome
May-Hegglin anomaly	Basophilic and pyroninophilic inclusions in neutrophils, eosinophils, basophils, and monocytes; accompanied by variable thrombocytopenia with giant platelets containing few granules; rare, dominantly inherited anomaly, without clinical consequences in most affected subjects
Alder-Reilly anomaly bodies	Dense azurophilic granules in all WBC lines on peripheral blood smear (inconstant) and marrow (always present in white cells and macrophages); seen in genetic mucopolysaccharidoses
Jordan anomaly (familial vacuolization of leukocytes)	Presence of vacuoles in the cytoplasm of granulocytes, monocytes, and occasionally lymphocytes and plasma cells; vacuoles with lipids; familial disorder
Batten (Batten-Spielmeyer-Vogt) granules	Azurophilic hypergranulation of WBCs in patients with Batten disease (autosomal recessive type of juvenile amaurotic idiocy) and members of their families
Organisms (especially pneumococcal sepsis), *Neisseria meningitides*, *Staphylococcus aureus*, *Ehrlichia chaffeensis*, *Histoplasma capsulatum*, candidiasis, CMV	It usually means overwhelming sepsis; frequently found in splenectomized or immunodeficient patients

*Submitted By Liberto Pechet, MD.

TABLE 16–87. White Cell Morphologic Abnormalities

Abnormalities	Morphology and Condition
Pelger-Huet anomaly	Nuclei of >80% of granulocytes show hyposegmentation (2 pince-nez eyeglass lobes); hereditary in heterozygotes for an autosomal dominant mutation at chromosome 1q42.1 and of no clinical consequence (neutrophils are functionally normal); acquired (pseudo–Pelger-Huet anomaly) in myelodysplastic syndromes, acute and chronic myeloproliferative neoplasms, myxedema, transient in some infections or with certain drugs
Hereditary hypersegmentation of neutrophils and hereditary hypersegmentation of eosinophils	Most neutrophils (or eosinophils) have 4 or more lobes; rare, harmless autosomal dominant condition; ≥5 lobes in >10% of heterozygotes and >30% in homozygotes
Acquired hypersegmentation of neutrophils	Normally only 10–20% of neutrophils have 4 lobes, and no more than 5% have 5 lobes; increases found in patients with megaloblastic anemias and chronic renal disease with BUN 30 mg/dL for >3 mo
Giant bands and metamyelocytes	Patients with megaloblastic anemias
Hereditary giant neutrophilia	1–2% of neutrophils are ≤2 times normal size and contain 6–10 nuclear lobes; innocuous dominant anomaly

WHITE BLOOD CELL COUNTS AND DIFFERENTIALS*

❏ **Definition**

- WBC counts refer to numerical reporting of the total number of WBCs as well as to describing and classifying the white cell components: neutrophils (which include bands), lymphocytes, monocytes, eosinophils, and basophils (Table 16.88).
- **Normal range** (adults): $4.3–10.3 \times 10^3$ cells/μL. Different values are reported for infants and children, separated by age groups. Automated counters report results in percentages or as absolute counts of each WBC population. The absolute differential counts are considered more relevant in evaluating WBC abnormalities.

TABLE 16–88. Normal Values for White Blood Cell Counts*

White Cells	% of 100 White Cells	Absolute Count $\times 10^3$ cells/μL
Neutrophils	43–72	1.6–7.5
Lymphocytes	18–43	0.9–3.4
Reactive lymphocytes	0–6 (manual differentials only)	
Monocytes	4–12	0.0–1.2
Eosinophils	0–8	0.0–0.6
Basophils	0–2	0.0–0.3

*Note that the normal values described in the table do not reflect differences related to age or race.

16

*Submitted By Liberto Pechet, MD.

❏ **Use**

- Most automated WBC counters separate the white cells into five categories. Immature white cells are flagged as abnormal, requiring direct examination of the peripheral blood smears. Recent machines do a six-part differential, the sixth parameter being "immature fraction."
- Abnormalities are discussed separately for each population (see Leukocytosis and Leukopenia and Leukemoid).

❏ **Limitations**

- Poorly prepared stains (mostly the manual ones) may corrupt the ability of the technician to report accurate differentials.
- Because in most laboratories the technician examines only 100 randomly selected cells, there is an inherent bias in the report, and rare, but important, abnormal WBCs may be missed, especially in leukopenic conditions. With the recent introduction of automated equipment for reporting differential counts this bias is minimized.

XYLOSE ABSORPTION TEST

❏ **Definition**

- D-xylose is a monosaccharide that does not require digestion by pancreatic enzymes or bile acids prior to absorption. In this test, 25 g of D-xylose is given orally and blood xylose levels are measured at 1 and 3 hours later and urinary excretion of xylose is measured for 5 hours. Abnormal D-xylose test suggests a mucosal problem as the cause of malabsorption.
- Normal range:
  ▼ Serum: ≥25 mg/dL (adult, 1 hour, 25-g dose, normal renal function)
  ▼ Urine: ≥4 g/5 hours (5-hour urine collection in adults >12 years [25-g dose])

❏ **Use**

- Diagnose conditions that presents with malabsorption due to defects in the integrity of gastrointestinal mucosa.

❏ **Interpretation**

Increased In
- NA.

Decreased In
- Malabsorption syndromes, such as Celiac or Crohn disease
- Small intestine bacterial overgrowth
- Whipple disease

❏ **Limitations**

- D-xylose results can be normal in malabsorption syndromes caused by pancreatic insufficiency.
- False-positives can occur with decreased renal function, dehydration/ hypovolemia, surgical blind loops, decreased gastric emptying, vomiting.

- Patients should not eat foods containing high levels of pentose, including fruits, jams, jellies, and pastries for 24 hours prior to test.
- Low values can also be caused by inflammation of the lining of the intestine, short bowel syndrome, and infection with parasites, like giardiasis or hookworm.
- Blood D-xylose levels are generally considered more reliable than urine levels in children younger than 12 years old.

ZINC (Zn)

❑ Definition

- Zinc, an essential trace element, is the intrinsic metal component or activating cofactor for more than 70 important enzyme systems, including carbonic anhydrase, the ALPs, dehydrogenases, and carboxypeptidases. It is involved in the regulation of nucleoproteins and the activity of various inflammatory cells and plays a role in growth, tissue repair and wound healing, carbohydrate tolerance, and synthesis of testicular hormones. Zinc intake is closely related to protein intake; as a result, it is an important component of nutritionally related morbidity worldwide. Symptoms attributable to severe zinc depletion include growth failure, primary hypogonadism, skin disease, impaired taste and smell, and impaired immunity and resistance to infection. Subclinical zinc deficiency may significantly increase the incidence of and morbidity and mortality from diarrhea and upper respiratory tract infections. Along with iron, iodine, and vitamin A, zinc deficiency is one of the most important micronutrient deficiencies globally. Several studies have now demonstrated that supplementation of high-risk populations can have substantial health benefits.
- **Normal range:** (see Table 16.89).

❑ Use

- Detecting zinc deficiency
- Assist in confirming acrodermatitis enteropathica
- Evaluate nutritional deficiency
- Evaluate possible toxicity
- Monitor replacement therapy in individuals with identified deficiencies
- Monitor therapy of individuals with Wilson disease

TABLE 16–89. Normal Range for Zinc by Age	
Age	**Conventional Units (µg/dL)**
Newborn to 6 mo	26–141
6–11 mo	29–131
1–4 y	31–115
4–5y	48–119
6–9y	48–129
10–13y	25–148
14–17y	46–130
Adult	70–120

16

❑ **Interpretation**

Increased In
- Anemia
- Arteriosclerosis
- Coronary heart disease
- Primary osteosarcoma of the bone

Decreased In
- Acrodermatitis enteropathica
- AIDS
- Acute infections
- Acute stress
- Burns
- Cirrhosis
- Conditions that decrease albumin
- Diabetes
- Long-term TPN
- Malabsorption
- Myocardial infarction
- Nephrotic syndrome
- Nutritional deficiency
- Pregnancy
- Pulmonary TB
- Ulcerative colitis, Crohn disease
- Regional enteritis, sprue, intestinal bypass, neoplastic disease
- Increased catabolism induced by anabolic steroids

❑ **Limitations**

- Plasma levels of zinc do not necessarily correlate with tissue levels and do not reliably identify individuals with zinc deficiency. Although plasma levels are generally a good index of zinc status in healthy individuals, these levels are depressed during inflammatory disease states.
- Erythrocyte concentrations of zinc may provide a more useful measure of zinc status during acute or chronic inflammation. Several functional indices also can be used to indirectly assess zinc status. Serum superoxide dismutase and erythrocyte alkaline phosphatase activities have been proposed as indirect markers of zinc status, but these tests are not widely available.
- The conditions of anorexia and starvation also result in low zinc levels.
- Hemolyzed specimens cause false elevation of serum zinc levels.
- Specimens should be collected in metal-free specimen containers.
- Auranofin, chlorthalidone, corticotropin, oral contraceptives, and penicillamine increase zinc levels.
- Anticonvulsants, cisplatin, citrates, corticosteroids, estrogens, interferon, and oral contraceptives decrease zinc levels.

CHAPTER 17

Infectious Disease Assays

Michael J. Mitchell and Lokinendi V. Rao

This chapter presents the most commonly ordered infectious diseases–related tests arranged in alphabetical order. For pathogen-specific tests, the entry is grouped under the pathogen name. The test methods in this chapter include general cultures by source, targeted cultures to rule out specific pathogens, direct antigen assays, antibody assays, macroscopic and microscopic detection, as well as molecular methods.

It is important to consider the limitations for each of these methods. In general, cultures are considered the gold standard for pathogen detection; however, testing typically takes 24–48 hours for completion and longer for fastidious pathogens (like anaerobes) or slow growing organisms (like mycobacteria). Targeted cultures are available and requested when pathogens cannot be efficiently detected by routine culture methods. Nevertheless, it is important to consider that (1) selective culture conditions may also inhibit some individual strains of the target pathogen; (2) nonselective media should also be inoculated along with selective media; and (3) cultures for specific pathogens may not detect other significant pathogens when used for evaluation of infected patient samples. Submission of routine bacterial cultures appropriate for the specimen type is usually recommended in addition to targeted cultures.

Direct antigen detection assays are widely available and provide quick turnaround time; however, they often have low sensitivity. Molecular methods are becoming common in detecting pathogens due to the high sensitivity and shorter turnaround time than conventional cultures, yet these assays are currently costly. See Chapter 11 for additional information regarding the basis of microbiology identification methods and pathogen-specific diseases.

ACID-FAST BACILLUS (AFB) SMEAR

❑ **Definition and Use**

- Smears of patient specimens are stained and examined for the presence of mycobacteria. They may provide early evidence of TB or other mycobacterial diseases. Certain dyes bind to the thick, mycolic acid–rich cell walls of mycobacteria. The lipids of the cell wall make the cells resistant to decolorization with acid–alcohol solutions. AFB staining should be undertaken for most specimens that are submitted for mycobacterial culture.
- **Methods:**
  - ▼ There are two types of AFB stains: chromogenic (carbol-fuchsin stains [hot: Ziehl-Neelsen; cold: Kinyoun]) and fluorogenic (auramine O + rhodamine). After staining, the smear is destained with an acid–alcohol solution, typically HCl in ethanol. Mycobacteria retain the stain.
    - In chromogenic methods, slides are examined using a 100× oil immersion objective with light microscopy. Nonmycobacterial cells are

17

counterstained with methylene blue. Mycobacteria appear red, whereas other bacteria and background are stained blue.

▼ In fluorogenic methods, auramine-stained slides are examined by fluorescence microscopy using a 25× or 40× objective. Mycobacteria are yellow-orange against a dark background. The improved signal-to-noise of auramine fluorochrome staining, allowing scanning with lower power objective, results in examination of a greater area of the slide at a given time, and therefore greater sensitivity. Any detected organisms should be confirmed by examination for typical morphology using the 100× objective. Some laboratories confirm positive fluorochrome smears with a carbol-fuchsin–based stain.

■ Specimens should be collected and transported to the laboratory according to recommendations for mycobacterial cultures.

■ **Turnaround time:** <24 hours

❏ **Interpretation**

■ **Expected results:** Negative. Detection of mycobacteria requires 10,000 or more organisms per milliliter or gram of sample for consistent detection. Sensitivity may be improved by concentration of specimen, such as by centrifugation, and by examination of multiple specimens. Rapidly growing mycobacteria, such as *Mycobacterium fortuitum*, have relatively thin layers of cell wall mycolic acid and may decolorize with acid–alcohol decolorizing solutions. These organisms may be stained using a weaker acid in aqueous solution.

■ **Positive results:** Positive specimens are very likely (>90%) to yield growth of mycobacteria in culture. In a minority of patients, usually with cavitary or extensive tuberculosis, sputum AFB stains may remain persistently positive for weeks after patients have converted to negative cultures. Nonviable organisms may be detected by AFB stains. *Nocardia* and related species are weakly acid fast and may give false-positive results if staining protocols are not followed closely.

❏ **Limitations**

■ Standardized protocols, such as those published by the American Thoracic Society, should be followed carefully to ensure sensitive detection and accurate interpretation of smears.

■ **Common pitfalls:** Care must be taken to avoid contaminating slides with acid-fast organisms. Common causes of slide contamination are use of tap water for solution preparation, carryover between slides with immersion oil, and use of common staining chambers.

ACID-FAST STAIN, MODIFIED

❏ **Definition and Use**

■ This stain may be used for detection of *Nocardia* in patient specimens or culture isolates when nocardiosis is suspected on the basis of clinical presentation or because of typical morphology in culture isolates. The Gram stain is very sensitive for detection of *Nocardia* in patient specimens.

- The modified acid-fast stain is typically used to confirm nocardioform organisms detected by Gram stain. The modified acid-fast stain is useful for differentiating *Nocardia* (positive) from *Streptomyces* (negative), especially in culture isolates. The modified acid-fast stain is similar to the carbol-fuchsin–based acid-fast stains (Ziehl-Neelsen or Kinyoun stains) except that a less active decolorizer is used (1% H_2SO_4 or 3% HCl in aqueous solution). Specimens should be collected and transported as appropriate for routine bacterial cultures for the specimen type.
- **Turnaround time:** 24–72 hours

❏ **Interpretation**

- **Expected results:** Negative. Negative stains do not rule out nocardiosis. Rapidly growing mycobacteria, such as *M. fortuitum*, may be negative by routine acid-fast staining but positive by modified acid-fast staining.
- **Positive results with *Nocardia*:** Delicate, branching filaments that retain the carbol-fuchsin stain.

❏ **Limitations**

- *Nocardia* may stain poorly in direct staining of patient specimens. Other species of aerobic actinomycetes, such as *Rhodococcus equi* and occasionally coryneform bacteria, may be modified acid-fast stain positive.

Suggested Readings

Al-Moamary M, Black W, Bessuille E, et al. The significance of the persistent presence of acid-fast bacilli in sputum smears in pulmonary tuberculosis. *Chest* 1999;116:726–731.
Winn WC Jr, Allen SD, Janda WM, et al. *Koneman's Color Atlas and Textbook of Diagnostic Microbiology*, 6th ed. Baltimore, MD: Lippincott Williams & Wilkins; 2006.

AEROBIC CULTURE

❏ **Definition and Use**

- Aerobic cultures are indicated for the detection of common aerobic bacterial pathogens in patient specimens taken from sites with signs and symptoms of bacterial infection (e.g., swelling, redness, heat, pus, or exudate). Site-specific bacterial cultures (e.g., sputum culture, genital culture) are recommended, if available. Specimens may be inoculated on several types of aerobic culture plates and broth media and may include selective and enriched media. Typical media for aerobic cultures include
  - ▼ Supportive media to isolate nonfastidious organisms, like sheep blood agar (SBA).
  - ▼ Enriched media to isolate organisms with special nutritional requirements, like chocolate agar.
  - ▼ Selective media to suppress the growth of specific types of bacteria. Selective media are often formulated so that colonies of different types of organisms that are able to grow on the media have different appearances. MacConkey is an example: Selective: nonfastidious gram-negative bacilli are able to grow. Differential: lactose fermenters are distinguished from lactose nonfermenters.
  - ▼ Solid versus Broth Media

- Culture media may be prepared in a solid or broth phase.
- Solid media (culture plates) are inoculated with a small amount of specimen. Mixed cultures are recognized by differences in colony morphology. The amount of each type of organism (and relative proportions in mixed cultures) can be estimated (e.g., rare, light, moderate, or heavy).
- Pyogenic infections are usually associated with growth of a single (or predominant) pathogen in moderate or heavy amounts.
- Broth media can be inoculated with a larger volume of specimen than agar plates, which may improve detection of infections with low concentrations of pathogens, but the amount of bacteria in the specimen cannot be estimated from broth cultures.
- Broth media may allow detection of some relatively aerotolerant anaerobic pathogens. Broth cultures have been associated with an increased rate of contamination.

■ **Expected results:** No pathogen isolated
■ **Turnaround time:** 48–72 hours
  ▼ In positive cultures, additional time is required for isolation, identification, susceptibility testing, and further characterization, as appropriate.

❑ Special Collection and Transport Instructions

■ Standard precautions apply. Ensure that material from the site of infection is collected.
■ Decontaminate skin or mucous membranes that must be crossed to obtain the specimen.
■ Use appropriate sterile supplies to collect the specimen. Place the specimen in a sterile, leak-proof container for transport. Ensure that the lid is firmly tightened, but avoid overtightening. Use specific transport medium and/or procedures as required for suspected pathogens (described below) or if transport to the lab will be prolonged (>2 hours). Apply a label to the specimen with information to identify the patient and type of specimen, as described below. Transport the specimen to the lab as quickly as possible, avoiding extremes of temperature. Note that collection protocols for some types of specimens require specific training and/or certification of the health care professional performing the collection. Examples include collection of bone marrow and CSF specimens.

❑ Limitations

■ Anaerobic culture is recommended for infections at sites likely to be infected by anaerobic pathogens. Examples include pelvic infections, intra-abdominal infections, abscesses, and traumatic and surgical wounds. Certain aerobic pathogens, such as *Legionella* species, require special processing or culture techniques for detection.
■ **Common pitfalls:**
  ▼ Specimens may be collected from sites that are not the primary site of active infection (even though there may be signs of inflammation at the site).
  ▼ Inadequate site preparation may result in false-positive cultures due to specimen contamination with endogenous flora. Contaminated specimens may also mask the recognition of slow-growing or fastidious pathogens in the culture.

ANAEROBIC CULTURE

❏ **Definition and Use**
- Anaerobic cultures are indicated for evaluation of patient specimens taken from sites with signs and symptoms of bacterial infection (e.g., swelling, redness, heat, pus, or exudate). Infections associated with anaerobic pathogens include surgical and traumatic wounds, sinusitis and pararespiratory infections, pelvic and intra-abdominal infections, osteomyelitis, myositis, gangrene, and necrotic wounds, abscesses, and actinomycosis and infections associated with fistula formation.
- Anaerobic cultures are used for the detection of common anaerobic bacterial pathogens from patient specimens. Site-specific aerobic bacterial cultures (e.g., tissue culture, abscess culture, wound culture) are recommended, if available. Specimens are inoculated on several types of anaerobic culture media. (see "Aerobic Culture" for a general discussion about media). Media should be fresh and prereduced. Typical media for aerobic cultures include
  - ▼ Supportive agar media, like Schaedler agar or CDC anaerobic blood agar
  - ▼ Selective/differential agar media:
    - Phenylethyl alcohol or CNA agar for anaerobic gram-positive pathogens
    - Kanamycin–vancomycin–laked blood agar, for anaerobic gram-negative bacilli
    - Bacteroide bile–esculin agar, for *Bacteroides fragilis* group
    - Egg yolk agar, for characterization of *Clostridium* species
    - Cycloserine–cefoxitin–egg yolk–fructose agar (CCFA), for *Clostridium difficile*
  - ▼ Broth, like enriched thioglycolate medium or chopped meat broth
- **Turnaround time:** Incubation for 5–7 days
  - ▼ Additional time is required for positive cultures for additional testing required for isolation, confirmation as anaerobic (aerotolerance testing), identification, susceptibility testing, and further characterization, as needed. Anaerobic infections are frequently polymicrobial; final results may require several weeks for full laboratory evaluation, if needed.

❏ **Special Collection and Transport Instructions**
- See "Aerobic Culture" for a general discussion of collection and transport instructions
- Because of the anaerobic endogenous flora, specimens from the following sites should not be submitted for anaerobic culture: sputum or bronchoscopically collected lower respiratory specimens, swabs from skin or mucosal surfaces, specimens from the GI tract (including fistulae, stoma surfaces, and so on), superficial ulcers or eschars, including decubitus ulcers, vaginal or cervical swabs or urine (except suprapubic aspirate urine).
  - ▼ When submitting samples, ensure that sufficient specimen is collected for all of the diagnostic testing required (e.g., aerobic, fungal, and/or mycobacterial cultures and stains). Minimize exposure to atmospheric oxygen and transport in an anaerobic transport system. Do not refrigerate or freeze specimens for anaerobic culture. Note the following: Specimens

collected and transported for anaerobic culture are also acceptable for aerobic bacterial, fungal, or mycobacterial culture, provided a sufficient volume of specimen is provided.

❑ **Interpretation**

▪ **Expected results:** No anaerobic pathogen isolated.

❑ **Limitations**

▪ Anaerobic infections are frequently polymicrobial. Initial isolation and aerotolerance testing may require repeated subculture of the primary culture media. Many anaerobic pathogens are slow growing and biochemically indolent, making identification, susceptibility testing, and further characterization of isolates in the laboratory much slower than most aerobic bacterial pathogens. Therefore, patient care decisions must often be made before results of testing are available, limiting the clinical utility of extensive workup of mixed anaerobic cultures.

▪ **Common pitfalls**

▼ Anaerobic culture may be significantly compromised by collection and transport conditions that are not strictly anaerobic or because of refrigeration during transport. Inadequate site preparation may result in false-positive cultures due to specimen contamination with endogenous flora. Contaminated cultures may also mask the recognition of slow-growing or fastidious anaerobic pathogens in the culture.

BACTERIAL ANTIGEN DETECTION

❑ **Definition and Use**

▪ This test in intended for the rapid initial detection of *Streptococcus pneumoniae*, *Haemophilus influenzae* type b, group B beta-hemolytic *Streptococcus* (GBS), or *Neisseria meningitidis* in CSF. The indication for this test is limited. Published reports have demonstrated limited sensitivity for the detection of patients with meningitis caused by common pathogens, and test results rarely result in changes to the management or therapy of patients. There may be some utility in patients who have been treated with antibiotics prior to CSF collection. There is some evidence that the performance for initial detection of GBS meningitis in neonates is acceptable.

▪ Latex particles are coated with antibodies directed against specific antigens of the pathogens noted above. Agglutination should occur if the antigen is present in CSF, as either a free antigen or intact bacterial cells. Specimens are collected and transported according to directions for CSF culture.

▪ **Turnaround time:** <4 hours

❑ **Interpretation**

▪ **Expected results:** Negative; no agglutination means that a CSF infection caused by specific pathogen is less likely. Positive agglutination for specific latex reagent: CSF infection caused by the specific pathogen is more likely.

❏ Limitations

- The sensitivity and specificity are too low to be recommended for routine use. Results are unlikely to change patient therapy or management.

Suggested Readings

Perkins MD, Mirrett S, Reller LB. Rapid bacterial antigen detection is not clinically useful. *J Clin Microbiol*. 1995;30(06):1486–1491.
Ringelmann R, Heym B, Kniehl E. Role of immunologic tests in diagnosis of bacterial meningitis. *Antibiot Chemother*. 1992;45:68–78.

BLOOD CULTURE, FUNGAL

❏ Definition and Use

- Fungal blood cultures are used for detection of bloodstream infection caused by fungi, especially when dimorphic species and uncommon pathogens are suspected. Identification, susceptibility, and further testing can be performed on culture isolates. The culture is indicated primarily for patients with cancer, extensive therapy with broad-spectrum antibiotics, trauma, and HIV and other immunocompromising conditions and symptoms that suggest sepsis, like fever, chills, malaise, hypotension, poor perfusion, toxicity, tachycardia, and hyperventilation. Biphasic and lysis–centrifugation methods have demonstrated improved isolation of dimorphic and filamentous fungi.
- **Turnaround time:** 4 weeks

❏ Special Collection and Transport Instructions

- Inoculate blood culture system according to the manufacturer's recommendations. Alert the laboratory if infection due to *Malassezia furfur* is suspected. Special culture processing is needed for isolation of this lipophilic yeast. Transport to the laboratory at room temperature.

❏ Interpretation

- **Expected results:** No growth
- Most commonly isolated pathogens in positive cultures:
  - ▼ Yeasts: *Candida albicans*, nonalbicans *Candida* species, and *Cryptococcus neoformans*. (*Candida* and other commonly isolated yeasts may be efficiently detected using routine blood cultures.)
  - ▼ Dimorphic fungus: *Histoplasma capsulatum*.
  - ▼ Mold: *Fusarium* and *Scedosporium* species.

❏ Limitation

- *Aspergillus* species are rarely isolated by blood culture even in the presence of acute systemic infection.

Suggested Reading

CLSI. *Principles and Procedures for Blood Cultures; Approved Guideline*. CLSI document M47-A. Wayne, PA: Clinical and Laboratory Standards Institute; 2007.

17

BLOOD CULTURE, MYCOBACTERIAL

❑ **Definition and Use**

■ The mycobacterial blood culture is used for the detection of bloodstream infection due to *Mycobacterium* species. Mycobacteremia is most commonly seen in patients with AIDS, although it may occur in other congenital and acquired immunocompromising conditions, including patients taking chronic corticosteroid therapy, and malignancies. Growth of mycobacteria in culture requires the use of specialized, supplemented media with prolonged incubation time. Lysis of blood cells improves detection, by releasing phagocytized organisms, and is used in most methods (e.g., lysis–centrifugation methods).

■ **Turnaround time:** 4–8 weeks

❑ **Special Collection and Transport Instructions**

■ Collect 5–10 mL of blood in sodium polyanethol sulfonate (SPS) or heparin, or directly inoculate specific mycobacterial blood culture media. Inoculate the blood culture media or collection system according to the manufacturer's instructions. Transport to the laboratory at room temperature.

❑ **Interpretation**

■ **Expected results:** No growth

■ **Positive results:** *Mycobacterium avium* complex (MAC) is the most commonly isolated mycobacterial pathogen. *M. tuberculosis* may be isolated at the time of hematogenous spread associated with severe primary or reactivation disease. Rapidly growing mycobacteria, such as *M. fortuitum*, have been associated with chronic indwelling vascular catheters and other prosthetic material.

❑ **Limitations**

■ Some mycobacterial infections are rarely associated with mycobacteremia. EDTA or acid citrate dextrose (ACD)-anticoagulated blood should not be used for mycobacterial blood culture inoculum.

Suggested Reading

CLSI. *Principles and Procedures for Blood Cultures; Approved Guideline.* CLSI document M47-A. Wayne, PA: Clinical and Laboratory Standards Institute; 2007.

BLOOD CULTURE, ROUTINE

❑ **Definition and Use**

■ The routine blood culture is used for detection of bloodstream infections (BSIs) due to common aerobic and anaerobic bacterial and yeast pathogens. Potentially pathogenic isolates are identified, and susceptibility testing is performed, as appropriate. Special testing is required for the detection of mycobacteria, parasites, viruses, and certain fungal pathogens.

■ Indications:

▼ Sepsis syndrome, fever, chills, malaise, hypotension, poor perfusion, toxicity, tachycardia, hyperventilation.

▼ Evaluation of serious localized infections, such as pneumonia, UTIs, and meningitis. Classic signs and symptoms may be absent in infants, the elderly and patients with certain medical or surgical conditions.

■ **Methods:**
  ▼ Most commercially available blood culture systems recommend inoculation of blood into two broth media: one aerobic and one anaerobic. Lysis–centrifugation methods may be used for routine detection of BSIs due to bacteria or yeast but are more typically used for detection of mycobacteremia or fungemia.

■ **Turnaround time:** Generally, incubation for 5–7 days. Most true-positive blood cultures become positive within 24–48 hours after inoculation.

❏ **Special Collection and Transport Instructions**

■ Decontamination of the collection site is the most important factor in preventing false-positive (contaminated) blood cultures. Inoculate media according to the manufacturer's instructions. Usually, 8–10 mL of blood is inoculated into each blood culture bottle. A smaller inoculum volume, based on weight or age, is recommended for small children. Submission of two or three independently drawn (different venipuncture sites) blood cultures is recommended for the initial evaluation of patients with suspected BSI. Transport blood cultures to the laboratory at room temperature.

❏ **Interpretation**

■ **Expected results:** No growth
■ **Positive results:** Bacteremia or fungemia present. Positive blood cultures must be carefully evaluated to assess the possibility of false-positive culture, usually due to specimen contamination at the time of collection. Organisms, like viridans *Streptococci*, that are most commonly isolated as contaminants may also cause true BSI, usually in patients with some compromise in immune function. Interpret all positive blood cultures in the context of number of positive blood cultures as well as clinical and laboratory signs and symptoms. In patients with clinically relevant BSIs (true positive), the pathogen is typically isolated from a majority of cultures/bottles. In patients with contaminated blood cultures (false positive), a common contaminant is typically isolated in a single culture or bottle, whereas other cultures are drawn during evaluation remain negative.
■ **Negative results:** Bacteremia and fungemia at the time of specimen collection are unlikely. False-negative results may be seen in patients with prior antimicrobial therapy. False-negative results may be caused by inoculation of blood culture bottles with less than the recommended volume of blood. Because clinically significant bacteremia may be intermittent, collection of two or three blood cultures is recommended to rule out bacteremia.

❏ **Limitations**

■ The significance of positive blood cultures must be evaluated in terms of several factors, including patient signs and symptoms, the intrinsic pathogenicity of the blood culture isolate, number of positive cultures, number of isolates in culture (mixed cultures typically represent contamination), and cultures positive at other infected sites for the blood culture isolate.

17

- Routine blood cultures are optimized for detection of the pathogens most frequently associated with BSIs. Clinically relevant BSIs may be associated with pathogens for which special blood cultures are required (e.g., mycobacteria, dimorphic fungi, fastidious bacteria).
- **Common pitfalls:**
  - ▼ Decreased sensitivity because of such factors as a low volume of blood inoculated into blood culture media. Decreased specificity because of contamination due to poor preparation of collection site.

Suggested Readings

CLSI. *Principles and Procedures for Blood Cultures; Approved Guideline.* CLSI document M47-A. Wayne, PA: Clinical and Laboratory Standards Institute; 2007.

Katidis AG, et al. *Pediatric Infect Dis J.* 1996;15:615–620.

Yakoe DS, Anderson J, Chambers R, et al. Simplified surveillance for nosocomial bloodstream infections. *Inf Control Hosp Epidemiol.* 1998;19:657–660.

BLOOD PARASITE EXAMINATION

❏ Definition and Use

- This test is used to detect parasites circulating in peripheral blood. It should be ordered in patients when infection caused by *Plasmodium* species (malaria), *Babesia* species (babesiosis), *Trypanosoma* species (sleeping sickness, Chagas disease), or certain microfilaria species or systemic infection with *Leishmania* species is suspected. Thin and thick blood smears are prepared from free-flowing capillary blood or EDTA-anticoagulated blood. Smears are inspected after staining with Giemsa, Wright, or Wright-Giemsa stain. For positive smears, the level of parasitemia should be determined for each specimen.
- **Turnaround time:**
  - ▼ Preliminary examination should be performed "STAT" if malaria is suspected (turnaround time <4 hours). Final report for positive smears: <24 hours.

❏ Special Collection and Transport Instructions

- Preparation of smears at the bedside, from free-flowing capillary blood if possible, yields the best morphology. Alternatively, EDTA-anticoagulated blood may be collected. For microfilariae, the diurnal circulation of some species must be taken into account in timing specimen collection (*Loa loa*: 10 AM–2 PM; *Wuchereria* or *Brugia* species: 8 PM–4 AM). Transport specimens to the laboratory and prepare smears as soon as possible. In general, collect specimens on each of 3 successive days. Collect specimens every 6–8 hours (until positive) for optimal detection in suspected cases. Blood should be examined in treated patients after 24, 48, and 72 hours to determine effectiveness of therapy.

❏ Interpretation

- **Expected results:** Negative. Sensitive detection of parasitemia may require the examination of several specimens, as recommended above.
- **Positive result:** Disease caused by specific parasite identified.

❏ Limitations

- Low level of parasitemia may require the examination of multiple specimens for detection. Examination of smears prepared from buffy coat preparations may improve the sensitivity of detection for some parasites, like microfilaria and trypanosomes. The efficient detection of microfilaria requires specimen collection during the specific hours when circulation of the parasite is expected.
- **Common pitfalls:** Include the collection of too few specimens for examination.

❏ Other Considerations

- In effectively treated patients, the level of parasitemia should drop very quickly. In patients with drug-resistant parasites, the level may remain stable, or even increase.

Suggested Readings

Garcia LS. *Diagnostic Parasitology*, 5th ed. Washington, DC: ASM Press; 2007.
NCCLS document M15-A. *Laboratory Diagnosis of Blood-borne Parasitic Diseases*; Approved Guideline. 2000. Clinical and Laboratory Standards Institute.

BODY FLUID CULTURE

❏ Definition

- Sterile fluid-filled spaces are present at a number of anatomic sites and are subject to infection. Examples of sterile fluids include peritoneal, pleural, pericardial, and synovial/joint fluid. Infections associated with CSF are life threatening and associated with a different etiology of bacterial pathogens, so these cultures are typically processed differently than other sterile fluids. Urine is also processed with different culture techniques because of its connection with the external environment, via the urethra, and pathogenesis of infection. A broad etiology of bacterial pathogens may cause infections of sterile sites, and culture methods are optimized for recovery of organisms present in low concentrations.

❏ Use

- Collect sterile fluid cultures from sites associated with signs and symptoms of inflammation, including redness, swelling, pain, heat, fluid accumulation, and pus formation.
- **Method:** Supportive and enriched solid agar (SBA and chocolate agar) and broth media (blood culture media) are typically inoculated; selective/differential agar media, such as MacConkey agar (gram-negative bacilli), CNA, or phenylethyl alcohol agar (gram-positive organisms), should be inoculated for specimens likely to show polymicrobial infection (e.g., peritonitis) or contamination by endogenous flora (e.g., cul-de-sac aspirates). Anaerobic media should be inoculated if there is a significant possibility of anaerobic pathogens. If infection with an uncommon, fastidious pathogen is suspected, the laboratory should be informed so that special cultures may be inoculated.
- **Turnaround time:** Cultures are incubated for up to 7 days. Additional time is required for isolation, identification, susceptibility testing, and further characterization, as needed.

❑ **Special Collection and Transport Instructions**

■ Fluid aspiration is performed after preparation of the puncture site in a manner consistent with a preparation of a surgical site. Submission of specimens from drainage devices is discouraged because of the high incidence of contamination with endogenous flora; direct collection of the sterile fluid is recommended.

■ Collection of the maximum amount of fluid from the infected site is recommended. Blood culture bottles may be inoculated and is recommended for patients with spontaneous bacterial peritonitis, but a small amount of fluid should be retained for Gram stain and for special culture inoculation, if needed.

■ Swabs should not be used for fluid collection.

■ Place fluid into sterile transport tubes; small-volume specimens, or several milliliters from large-volume specimens, should be placed into an anaerobic transport tube. Note: Specimens transported under anaerobic conditions are acceptable for inoculation of cultures for aerobic bacterial, mycobacterial, and fungal cultures.

■ Submission of several specimens prior to antibiotic therapy may significantly improve sensitivity of culture detection.

■ The use of anticoagulants is discouraged because of possible inhibition of some pathogens. If anticoagulation is required, heparin or SPS is recommended.

■ Transport specimens at room temperature; do not refrigerate or freeze specimens.

❑ **Interpretation**

■ **Expected results:** No growth. Infection is not excluded by a negative culture, especially after initiation antibiotic therapy. Uncommon, fastidious pathogens may not be isolated in culture without inoculation of special media.

■ **Positive cultures** indicate infection of the sterile site, but cultures that may be contaminated with endogenous flora must be interpreted with caution in the context of quantity or bacterial growth, purity of culture, Gram stain findings, and clinical signs and symptoms. Infected peritoneal fluid may yield numerous aerobic and anaerobic pathogens. Extensive identification and susceptibility testing are usually not clinically useful: final results are often not available until well into therapy, and empirical treatment is usually effective.

Suggested Readings

Atkins BL, Athanasou N, Deeks JJ, et al.; the Osiris Collaborative Study Group. Prospective evaluation of criteria for microbiologic diagnosis of prosthetic-joint infection at revision arthroplasty. *J Clin Microbiol.* 1998;36:2932–2939.

Baselski V, Beavis KG, Bell M, et al. *Clinical Microbiology Procedures Handbook*, 3rd ed. Editor in Chief: Lynne S. Garcia, Washington, DC: ASM Press; 2010.

Bernard L, Pron B, Vaugnat A, et al.; the Groupe d'Etude sur l'Osteite. The value of suction drainage fluid culture during aseptic and septic orthopedic surgery: a prospective study of 901 patients. *Clin Infect Dis.* 2002;34:46–49.

BORDETELLA PERTUSSIS CULTURE (RULE OUT)

❑ **Definition and Use**

■ This test is used to detect acute infection caused by the slow-growing, fastidious pathogen *B. pertussis*, the cause of pertussis or whooping cough.

Nasopharyngeal specimens should be submitted for *B. pertussis* culture; aspirates are preferred. Anterior nares or throat specimens are unacceptable. Transport medium (e.g., Regan-Lowe) is recommended. Specimens are typically inoculated onto an enriched, selective agar, like Regan-Lowe.

- **Turnaround time:** Most cultures are positive in 7–10 days, although some cultures are incubated for up to 14 days. Additional time is required for final identification and further characterization.

❏ **Interpretation**

- **Expected results:** Negative. A negative culture does not exclude the diagnosis of pertussis, especially when a specimen is collected after the early, acute phase of infection.
- **Positive results:** Confirm the diagnosis of pertussis.

❏ **Limitations**

- The sensitivity of culture for *B. pertussis* falls significantly after the first 7–14 days after onset of symptoms. Poor specimen collection, submission of specimens other than nasopharyngeal specimens, and submission of specimens during the chronic phase of disease are associated with poor sensitivity of culture.

❏ **Other Considerations**

- PCR methods have been described for diagnosis of pertussis. Cross-reactions have been described (e.g., *Bordetella holmesii*) and may limit the utility of molecular diagnostic testing. The sensitivity of PCR is greatest in the early acute phase of infection, but *B. pertussis* DNA may be detectable for weeks after resolution of acute disease. A number of serologic assays are commercially available, including assays for IgM and IgA. Variable sensitivity and specificity have limited the clinical utility of these assays.

BORDETELLA PERTUSSIS SEROLOGY IgG

❏ **Definition**

- *Pertussis* is a respiratory tract infection caused by the gram-negative coccobacillus *Bordetella pertussis*. It is characterized clinically by a severe and prolonged cough. Coughing fits may be paroxysmal and, usually in infants, followed by an inspirational "whoop." A clinical diagnosis will form the basis of most pertussis diagnosis and treatment decisions. The CDC provides the following clinical case definition for pertussis: A cough illness lasting at least 2 weeks with one of the following: paroxysms of coughing, inspiratory "whoop," or post-tussive vomiting, without other apparent cause. This test is used to detect acute infection caused by the slow-growing, fastidious pathogen *B. pertussis*, the cause of pertussis or whooping cough. Because of the contagiousness of the infection, specific laboratory testing may be needed to confirm the diagnosis when pertussis is suspected clinically. Laboratory diagnosis of pertussis is complicated by the limitation of available tests. Options for diagnostic and confirmatory testing, when required, depend on the age of the patient and the phase of illness.
- **Expected result:** Negative.

❏ Use

- Aids in the detection of *B. pertussis* infection. Serologic testing for *B. pertussis* infection involves the detection of antibodies to pertussis antigens using standardized assays. Pertussis toxin (PT) and filamentous hemagglutinin (FHA) are the most widely used antigens and to a lesser extent pertactin (PRN) and fimbriae (FIM). Only PT is specific for *B. pertussis*; FHA and pertactin antigens cross-react with antibodies arising from infection by other *Bordetella* species and possibly by other bacteria. Serum antibodies have been measured by ELISA, complement fixation, agglutination, and toxin neutralization; ELISA is the detection method of choice due to its wide availability and ease of performance.
- Although *B. pertussis* serology is most useful in epidemiologic investigations or vaccine trials, it does have some utility in the diagnosis of pertussis in some patients, particularly in adolescents, adults, and previously vaccinated individuals. Serologic testing may also be useful for patients with cough >2–3 weeks in duration. Antibodies can be detected against *B. pertussis* antigens 1–2 weeks after the onset of the symptoms of pertussis in nonvaccinated individuals. Both IgG and IgA isotypes are produced in response to infection, whereas IgG is the predominant isotype detected after vaccination. However, no single antigen or isotype can be used to distinguish between infection and a response to vaccination with certainty. IgM responses are usually not measured for pertussis and have questionable diagnostic significance.
- The most reliable serologic approach to diagnosis of pertussis is with simultaneous testing of paired acute and convalescent sera. A significant increase (fourfold or greater) in IgG or IgA antibody titers to PT or FHA, comparing convalescent to acute sample, suggests recent *B. pertussis* infection in patients with a clinical illness compatible with pertussis. Paired sera, however, are not practical in most clinical settings. Single-sample serology tests for antipertussis toxin IgG must be collected at least 2 weeks after symptom onset. A high antibody titer >2 years following vaccination supports the diagnosis of pertussis.

❏ Interpretation

- **Positive:** IgG antibody to *B. pertussis* detected, which may indicate a current or past exposure/immunization to *B. pertussis*.

❏ Limitations

- The CDC does not currently accept serology as laboratory verification of pertussis; cases that meet the clinical case definition with a positive serology but a negative culture or PCR are considered probable cases. Single serology tests are used for the diagnosis of pertussis by the state laboratory in Massachusetts and in selected countries in the European Union.
- The IgG serology test results are not interpretable in children younger than 11 years of age because of interference due to persistent antibody formed by childhood vaccination. The test also cannot be interpreted in older patients who have received the Tdap vaccination in the previous 3 years.

BORRELIA BURGDORFERI (LYME DISEASE)—ANTIBODY SCREEN

❏ **Definition**

- A sensitive serum serology screening test for the detection of IgG and/or IgM antibodies to *Borrelia burgdorferi*.

❏ **Use**

- This test is used if Lyme disease is suspected in at-risk patients. Testing is not necessary if a patient presents with a tick bite and erythema migrans.

❏ **Interpretation**

$$<1.00 = \text{negative}$$
$$1.00-1.19 = \text{equivocal}$$
$$>1.19 = \text{positive}$$

Note: Current CDC recommendations state that equivocal and positive results should be confirmed with Western blot prior to reporting screen results. If testing is negative, consider other tick-borne diseases (i.e., *Babesia*, *Ehrlichia*).

❏ **Limitations**

- Should not be used to screen general population. False-negative results can occur if the patient is tested too early; repeat testing in 2–4 weeks. The IgG antibody response is usually not detectable until 4–6 weeks after infection; the IgM antibody response usually not detected during the first 2 weeks of infection, peaking 3–6 weeks following infection. False-positive results may occur from other spirochetal diseases, autoimmune diseases, or other infections (EBV, HIV, syphilis, infectious mononucleosis, etc.). IgG antibodies can be detected as early as 2 weeks, and both IgM and IgG antibodies can remain detectable for years. Diagnosis depends on clinical features, combined with available laboratory tests.

Suggested Reading

FDA Public Health Advisory: Assays for Antibodies to Borrelia burgdorferi; Limitations, Use, and Interpretation for Supporting a Clinical Diagnosis of Lyme Disease. July 7, 1997. http://www.fda.gov/MedicalDevices/Safety/AlertsandNotices/PublicHealthNotifications/UCM062429

BORRELIA BURGDORFERI (LYME DISEASE)—WESTERN BLOT*

❏ **Definition**

- The western blot assay for antibodies to *Borrelia burgdorferi*, the etiologic agent of Lyme disease, is a qualitative method of categorizing specific immunoreactivities in serum or plasma to *B. burgdorferi* proteins that have been formatted according to molecular weight into discrete bands on nitrocellulose strips.
- **Normal range:** Negative.

❏ **Use**

- The western blot assay for *B. burgdorferi* is used as a second-tier test to characterize the specificity of an individual's immune response to the component

---

*Submitted by Charles R. Kiefer, PhD.

proteins of B. *burgdorferi* by identifying the presence, relative level, and pattern of reactivities to the complete set of the bacterial proteins. The assay is used routinely to provide supportive serologic evidence of infection following a more sensitive but less specific screening test (such as EIA) for general reactivity to B. *burgdorferi*. Both IgM and IgG reactivities to the bacterial proteins are assayed to provide information on the evolution of the immune response relative to the stage of infection (i.e., early localized, early disseminated, or late disseminated). A caveat to this use is that IgM testing is not recommended in patients with symptoms lasting greater than 1–2 months. For such patients, IgG testing alone should be performed.

❑ **Interpretation**

▪ Reactivity scores: Specimen reactions with protein bands are first scored in terms of relative reaction intensity versus a cutoff control or minimally positive ("+") band reaction intensity by a positive control specimen.

▪ **Test interpretation (IgM class reactivities)**
   ▼ **Positive:** Reactivity scores of "+" or greater for at least two of three clinically significant proteins at the early stage of the disease (2–3 weeks after infection): 41, 39, 23 kDa
   ▼ **Negative:** Absence of any band reactivity on the test strip or reactivity for only one of the three clinically significant proteins

▪ **Test interpretation (IgG class reactivities)**
   ▼ **Positive:** Reactivity scores of "+" or greater for at least 5 of 10 clinically significant proteins at the later stages of the disease (weeks to months after infection): 93, 66, 58, 45, 41, 39, 30, 28, 23, 18 kDa
   ▼ **Negative:** Absence of any band reactivity on the test strip or reactivity for <5 of the 10 clinically significant proteins

❑ **Limitations**

▪ Minimum specimen volume is 40 μL (20 μL each for the IgM and IgG tests).

▪ Like any second-tier test, the positive predictive value for a western blot assay is a function of the a priori likelihood of the disease by clinical and epidemiologic criteria, whereas the negative predictive value is not as well defined because of the variability of the immune response among infected individuals. Cross-reactive diseases are most frequently evidenced by reactivity to the 41-kDa flagellar protein and at much lower frequency to the 66-kDa heat shock protein. Specimens from patients diagnosed with *Ehrlichia* or *Babesia* infections can show other *Borrelia*-specific bands.

Suggested Reading

Branda JA, Aguero-Rosenfeld ME, Ferraro MJ, et al. 2-tiered antibody testing for early and late Lyme disease using only an immunoglobulin G blot with the addition of a VisE band as the second-tier test. Clin Infect Dis. 2010;50:20–26.

BRONCHIAL CULTURE (BAL OR BRUSH), QUANTITATIVE

❏ **Definition**

- Quantitative bacterial cultures of specimens collected bronchoscopically (BAL or protected brush) are usually submitted for the evaluation for ventilator-associated pneumonia (VAP). The diagnosis of VAP is challenging, requiring a combination of clinical, imaging, and laboratory studies. Cultures are assessed in comparison to thresholds established by the laboratory in collaboration with clinicians.

❏ **Special Collection and Transport Instructions**

- Protected brush and BAL specimens are collected by a trained physician using standard procedures.
- Brush:
  - ▼ The brush is inserted through a plugged catheter via the biopsy channel of the bronchoscope. After expulsion of the plug, the brush is used to collect cells and secretions from the distal airways.
  - ▼ The brush end should be removed, using sterile technique, and placed in a small volume (1 mL) of nonbacteriostatic saline for transport.
- BAL:
  - ▼ BAL specimens are collected by a trained physician using standard procedures. The procedure and placement of the tip may be done under direct visualization or "blindly" through an endotracheal tube (mini-BAL).
  - ▼ The bronchoscope should be wedged in the terminal airways to ensure sampling of alveolar contents; return from the procedure should be 10–100 mL, sampling approximately 1 mL of alveolar secretions.
  - ▼ Samples should be transported to the laboratory as quickly as possible, using standard protocols for bacterial cultures.

❏ **Use**

- Method:
  - ▼ Known volumes of the specimen (or specimen dilutions) are inoculated onto solid agar media, including SBA, chocolate, and MacConkey agar (and other media as required for uncommon pathogens, such as *Legionella*); quantitative results are reported on the basis of the number of colonies isolated.
  - ▼ Protected brush: The brush is vigorously agitated in the saline transport fluid to release trapped microorganisms. The saline is then used to prepare dilutions for media inoculation.
  - ▼ BAL: A measured aliquot of BAL fluid is used to prepare dilutions for media inoculation.
  - ▼ After incubation, the concentration of each type of organism is calculated using the colony count on the solid media, volume inoculated onto the solid media, and the dilution of the original specimen. Cultures are interpreted on the basis of the isolate identification, quantity of isolate in culture, and the presence of other flora, especially endogenous flora of low pathogenicity.
- **Turnaround time:** Incubation for 48 hours. Additional time is required for pathogen isolation, identification, susceptibility testing, and further characterization, if needed.

17

❏ **Interpretation**

■ **Expected results:** A low quantity of endogenous upper respiratory flora is often seen.

■ **Positive results:** In patients with pneumonia, growth of a respiratory pathogen is expected at a concentration of $>10^3$ CFU/mL for bronchial brush. Growth of a respiratory pathogen is expected at a concentration of $>10^4$ CFU/mL for visually guided BAL or $>10^5$–10^6 for blind mini-BAL.

■ **Negative results:** False-negative cultures may be caused by prior antimicrobial therapy. Detection of pneumonia caused by certain fastidious pathogens may require inoculation of special media. Heavy contamination of the specimen with endogenous flora may mask the growth of the causative pathogen.

❏ **Limitations**

■ Quantitative culture of protected brush specimens has only moderate to good performance, with the PPV and NPV of 74% and 85%, respectively. Quantitative culture of BAL has only moderate to good performance, with a PPV of 83–91% and NPV of 87–89%. The presence of intracellular organisms in $>5\%$ of cells is associated with higher specificities. Tissue histopathology and quantitative culture of biopsy are considered the "gold standard" for diagnosis.

■ **Common pitfalls:**

▼ The predictive value of cultures is markedly decreased for patients with any antibiotic therapy prior to the procedure.

▼ *Candida* species are common contaminants and should not routinely be identified to species level.

Suggested Readings

Carroll KC. Laboratory diagnosis of lower respiratory tract infections: controversy and conundrums. *J Clin Microbiol.* 2002;40:3115–3120.

Koenig SM, Truwit JD. Ventilator-associated pneumonia: diagnosis, treatment, and prevention. *Clin Microbiol Rev.* 2006;19:637–657.

BRUCELLA CULTURE (RULE OUT)

❏ **Definition**

■ Human infection may be caused by several species of the genus *Brucella*. These organisms are fastidious, slow-growing gram-negative bacilli capable of producing severe localized and systemic infection. Infections have typically been acquired by zoonotic transmission, primarily related to livestock and dairy industries. There is great concern regarding the use of this organism for a bioterror-related attack. The organism is easily transmissible, so it is critical that the laboratory be informed whenever brucellosis is suspected.

❏ **Use**

■ This culture is used to isolate *Brucella* species from clinical specimens. Because of the risk of laboratory-acquired infection and because isolation of *Brucella* species may represent a sentinel event in a bioterror attack, most clinical microbiology laboratories limit the workup of suspected isolates to simple tests to rule out suspicious colonies, referring isolates that fail to "rule out" to their local public health laboratory for identification and further characterization. Final results for testing, therefore, may be delayed compared to common bacterial isolates.

- **Method:** Specimens are inoculated onto a blood agar (such as *Brucella* blood agar), chocolate agar, and Thayer-Martin agar (if contamination with endogenous flora is suspected). Specimens for *Brucella* are also inoculated onto MacConkey agar.
- **Turnaround time:** Isolation and preliminary identification for routine cultures are usually available in 3–7 days. Additional time is required for transfer to the local public health laboratory, confirmation of identification, and further testing.

❏ **Special Collection and Transport Instructions**

- The organisms primarily infect the reticuloendothelial system, so bone marrow and blood are the specimens of choice for patient evaluation. Specimens from other infected tissue or sites should also be submitted for culture. Serologic testing is recommended for diagnosis in patients with suspected brucellosis.

❏ **Interpretation**

- **Expected results:** Negative.
- **Positive:** Isolation of *Brucella* in culture is diagnostic for brucellosis.

❏ **Limitations**

- *Brucella* may be difficult to detect by Gram stain in primary specimens.
- **Common pitfalls:** Because brucellosis may present after a prolonged incubation period, or present with nonspecific symptoms and an indolent onset, the diagnosis may not be considered until progression into the chronic phase of illness. Clinicians may fail to request specific cultures for brucellosis, or alert the laboratory of their clinical suspicion.

❏ **Other Considerations**

- Brucellosis is a reportable disease. Patients with a diagnosis of brucellosis must be reported to the local department of health.

CEREBROSPINAL FLUID (CSF) CULTURE

❏ **Definition and Use**

- CSF culture is used for specific diagnosis of bacterial meningitis. Patients commonly present with severe headache, fever, neck stiffness, and meningeal signs, mental status changes, and signs of systemic toxicity.
- Method
  - ▼ CSF is inoculated onto sheep blood and chocolate agar, incubated aerobically. Broth media may be inoculated. Special media or culture conditions may be used for non–community-acquired meningitis, such as infections associated with trauma and prosthetic implants.
- **Turnaround time:** Cultures are incubated for 96 hours. Additional time is required for isolate identification, susceptibility testing, and further characterization, as needed.

17

❑ **Special Collection and Transport Instructions**

■ CSF is collected by needle aspiration after preparation of the puncture site in a manner consistent with a surgical site preparation.
■ Fluid is transported in a sterile container or tube with a tight-fitting lid.
■ CSF should be transported at room temperature; do not refrigerate or freeze for transport.
■ Specimens submitted for bacterial culture are also acceptable for fungal or mycobacterial stains and culture, antigen testing, and VDRL, if sufficient volume of fluid is submitted.

❑ **Interpretation**

■ **Expected results:** No growth. False-negative cultures may be caused by low pathogen concentration in CSF, especially when low-volume samples are submitted, or prior antibiotic therapy.
■ **Positive results:** Positive CSF culture supports a specific diagnosis of meningitis. False-positive cultures may be caused by contamination with endogenous skin flora. For most bacterial pathogens, CSF samples in patients with acute bacterial meningitis usually show increased WBCs (PMNs predominate), increased protein, and decreased glucose.

❑ **Limitations**

■ A broad etiology, which may require a number of different tests for diagnosis, may be considered for patients presenting with signs and symptoms of meningitis. The volume of CSF submitted is often insufficient for optimal sensitivity for the range of tests requested.

CHLAMYDIA TRACHOMATIS, AMPLIFIED NUCLEIC ACID DETECTION

See: Sexually Transmitted Infections, Molecular Diagnosis (*Chlamydia trachomatis, Neisseria gonorrhoeae, Trichomonas vaginalis*)

CHLAMYDIA TRACHOMATIS CULTURE

❑ **Use**

■ *C. trachomatis* is an obligate intracellular pathogen, and this culture may be used to diagnose *C. trachomatis* infections. Although tests based on nucleic acid amplification have emerged as the most sensitive methods for diagnosis of *Chlamydia* genital infections, *Chlamydia* culture is still required for specimen types for which molecular diagnostic tests have not been validated. *Chlamydia* cultures should also be performed in cases that may have legal implications, such as rape and child abuse.
■ Method:
   ▼ Infected cells from patient specimens are inoculated onto cultured eukaryotic cells, most commonly McCoy cells.
   ▼ Cultures are incubated for 48–72 hours.
   ▼ Positive cultures are now most commonly detected by staining fixed monolayers with specific anti–*C. trachomatis* antibodies; positive cultures

show staining of intracellular inclusions. The sensitivity of cultures for *C. trachomatis* detection is improved by blind subculture of a primary culture after the initial incubation.

- **Turnaround time:** Cultures are incubated for 72 hours. An additional 48–72 hours are required if primary cultures are subcultured prior to final examination.

❑ **Special Collection and Transport Instructions**

- It is critical to collect infected epithelial cells from infected sites using toxicity-tested swabs or other device. Swabs may be premoistened with sterile nonbacteriostatic saline before specimen collection. Scrapings or biopsy specimens may be submitted for some specimen types. (See specimens below.)
- Place specimens into a *Chlamydia* transport medium, such as 2-SP, and transport to the laboratory at 4°C. Deliver to the laboratory as quickly as possible.
- Specimens commonly submitted for *Chlamydia* culture come from the following sites:
  - ▼ **Cervix:** Remove excess mucus from the exocervix. Insert a new swab approximately 1 cm into the cervical canal and gently rotate for 10–15 seconds.
  - ▼ **Urethra:** Clean the distal urethra and meatus with a swab. Insert a new thin-shafted swab 2–4 cm into the urethra and gently rotate for 10–15 seconds.
  - ▼ **Conjunctiva:** Remove excess purulent discharge with a swab. With a new swab, gently rotate over the affected conjunctival surface.
  - ▼ **Anus:** Insert a premoistened swab into the anorectal juncture and rotate gently. The swab should not be heavily stained with feces.
  - ▼ **Fallopian tube or epididymis:** Place aspirate into an equal volume of *Chlamydia* transport media.
  - ▼ **Respiratory tract (neonate):** Place aspirate or wash into an equal volume of *Chlamydia* transport media.
- Biopsies (lymph node, endometrium, fallopian tube, lung) may be taken. Place the biopsy specimen in a sterile container with the *Chlamydia* transport medium.

❑ **Interpretation**

- **Expected results:** No growth
- **Positive results:** *Chlamydia* culture is very specific for infection caused by *C. trachomatis*.
- **Negative results:** *Chlamydia* infection is not ruled out by a negative culture. Repeat testing, using a nucleic acid amplification test if appropriate for the site, is recommended for patients with a high suspicion for chlamydial infection.

❑ **Limitations**

- *Chlamydia* culture is intrinsically less sensitive than molecular diagnostic techniques. *Chlamydophila* species, *C. psittaci*, and *C. pneumoniae*, are not isolated by *C. trachomatis* culture. The following specimens are not recommended for *Chlamydia* culture:
  - ▼ Peritoneal fluid
  - ▼ Urethral discharge
  - ▼ Urine
  - ▼ Cul-de-sac fluid

17

▼ Vagina or vaginal fluid
▼ Throat
- **Common pitfalls:**
  ▼ Poor specimen collection (sample selection or collection technique) or loss of viability during transport. Swabs may be toxic for *C. trachomatis*. Specific types and lots of swabs should be tested for toxicity before releasing before clinical use. Urethral specimens should not be collected within 1 hour after the patient has urinated.

CLOSTRIDIUM DIFFICILE DETECTION

❑ **Definition and Use**

- *Clostridium difficile* is a major cause of antibiotic-associated diarrhea and pseudomembranous colitis, and it represents a significant and serious agent of nosocomial infection. *C. difficile* infection (CDI) may be mild and self-limited after discontinuation of antibiotics, but a significant number of patients have persistent and/or severe diarrheal illness that may progress to pseudomembranous colitis or toxic megacolon. *C. difficile* is an anaerobic, spore-forming, gram-positive bacillus. It forms several toxins (toxins A and B) that have been used as the basis for detection. *C. difficile* detection is recommended for patients in whom diarrheal illness develops after antibiotic therapy or during hospitalization, especially when colitis (increased fecal leukocytes) is a prominent feature.
- **Methods**
  ▼ **Cytotoxicity:** In this method, a suspension of stool, passed through a membrane filter to remove bacteria, is inoculated on cultured eukaryotic cells (e.g., WI-38). The cell monolayer is examined for 48 hours for evidence of typical "actinomorphic" cytotoxicity (disruption of the normal cellular morphology in the monolayer). In order to exclude nonspecific cytotoxicity that may be seen with stool filtrates, neutralization of the cytotoxic effect, using anti–*C. difficile* antiserum, must be demonstrated.
  ▼ **Toxigenic culture:** *C. difficile* may be isolated from stool using a spore selection technique (by heat shock or alcohol pretreatment of a stool suspension prior to medium inoculation) and selective media. Because not all *C. difficile* isolates produce the toxins associated with disease, culture supernatants must be tested for toxin production to make a diagnosis of *C. difficile*–associated disease.
  ▼ **Toxin detection using immunodiagnostic procedures:** A number of commercially available latex agglutination or EIA kits have been developed for the detection of *C. difficile* toxin A and/or toxin B in stool samples. These assays provide a more rapid turnaround time, but lower sensitivity and specificity, compared to culture or cytotoxicity assays.
  ▼ *C. difficile* **glutamate dehydrogenase antigen detection:** Detection of *C. difficile* glutamate dehydrogenase antigen may be used to screen stool for the presence of *C. difficile*. Because glutamate dehydrogenase is not specific for toxigenic *C. difficile*, positive specimens must be tested for toxin to confirm the diagnosis of *C. difficile*–associated disease.

▼ **Molecular diagnostic methods:** Molecular diagnostic methods for detection of the *C. difficile* are commercially and provide the most sensitive assay for CDI. The test is very specific when used on patients with typical clinical signs and symptoms of *C. difficile* disease.

■ **Turnaround time:**
  ▼ Molecular diagnostic, immunodiagnostic assays, and the glutamate dehydrogenase assays: 24 hours
  ▼ Cytotoxicity assays: 24–72 hours
  ▼ Culture: 96 hours
■ Liquid stool specimens collected in clean containers with tight-fitting lids should be transported to the laboratory at room temperature within 2 hours. If transport will be prolonged, the specimen should be held at refrigerator temperature. Do not freeze.

❏ **Interpretation**
  ■ **Expected results:** Negative

❏ **Limitations**
  ■ The available assays vary somewhat in sensitivity and specificity for diagnosis of *C. difficile* disease. The choice of diagnostic methods must take cost, assay performance, turnaround time, and other factors into consideration. Positive *C. difficile* test results must be interpreted with caution in infants; toxin may be detected in the stool of healthy infants without signs of diarrheal illness or colitis.

CORYNEBACTERIUM DIPHTHERIAE CULTURE (RULE OUT)

❏ **Definition and Use**
  ■ This culture is used to detect *Corynebacterium diphtheriae* in clinical specimens. It should be considered in patients who present with signs and symptoms consistent with diphtheria, which is caused by local infection, most commonly respiratory or cutaneous infection, or by systemic disease caused by the action of diphtheria toxin, primarily on the heart, central or peripheral nervous system, liver, and kidney. Diphtheria is now uncommon in countries that have implemented widespread vaccination programs against this pathogen.
  ■ **Method:**
    ▼ Specimens must be inoculated onto special media, including selective, enriched and differential media, for isolation of *C. diphtheriae*.
    ▼ Respiratory or cutaneous specimens are inoculated onto SBA or CNA agar (to detect other pathogens), and agar-enriched media containing cystine and tellurite, such as cystine–tellurite blood agar or modified Tinsdale agar for *C. diphtheriae* detection.
    ▼ On cystine–tellurite agar, *C. diphtheriae*, *Corynebacterium ulcerans*, and *Corynebacterium pseudodiphtheriae* produce black colonies surrounded by a dark halo.
    ▼ The identification of suspect colonies must be confirmed. Toxin-producing and non–toxin-producing strains of *C. diphtheriae* may be isolated from clinical specimens. *C. diphtheriae* isolates should be referred for toxin production testing.

17

■ **Turnaround time:** 48–72 hours for initial isolation. Additional time is required for confirmation of the identity, toxin testing, and further characterization of suspicious isolates.

❏ **Special Collection and Transport Instructions**

■ The laboratory should be alerted before specimen submission to ensure that appropriate medium is available for culture inoculation.
■ Swab specimens are collected from multiple inflamed sites of the pharynx or other respiratory mucosal surfaces. Collection of specimens from near or under any diphtheritic membrane is recommended.
■ Aspirate, swab, or tissue samples for detection of cutaneous diphtheria are collected following general collection recommendations for skin lesions.
■ Routine transport media can be used for transport.

❏ **Interpretation**

■ **Expected results:** No growth.
■ **Positive results:** Isolation of toxigenic strains of C. *diphtheriae* from upper respiratory or cutaneous lesions is diagnostic of diphtheria.
■ **Negative results:** Submission of multiple specimens may be required for C. *diphtheriae* isolation.

CRYPTOCOCCUS ANTIGEN TEST

❏ **Use**

■ This test may be ordered for the early diagnosis of infections caused by *Cryptococcus neoformans*. It is usually appropriate for immunocompromised patients presenting with clinical signs of meningitis. Testing is most sensitive when testing CSF for cryptococcal meningitis. Testing serum has a lower sensitivity for confirmation of infection at other sites. Determination of antigen titer (testing twofold serial dilutions of the specimen) is recommended for positive CSF specimens to monitor response to treatment.
■ Method:
  ▼ There are several formats for commercially available cryptococcal antigen tests, most commonly latex agglutination assays. In these assays, latex particles are coated with polyclonal or monoclonal antibodies against C. *neoformans* antigens.
  ▼ Agglutination at dilutions of 1:8 or greater indicates active disease. Approximately 95% of patients with cryptococcal meningitis are detectable by cryptococcal antigen testing of the CSF.
  ▼ The sensitivity for CSF is 93–100%, and for serum, it is 83–97%. Specificity for both specimen types is typically >95%.
■ **Turnaround time:** <24 hours

❏ **Interpretation**

■ **Expected results:** Negative.
■ **Positive results:** Cryptococcal infection very likely. Positive results should be confirmed by culture.
■ **Negative results:** Cryptococcal infection unlikely. Use fungal culture to definitively rule out cryptococcal infection.

❑ **Limitations**

- False-negative reactions may occur, especially due to a prozone effect in serum samples. (Pronase treatment of serum samples decreases the incidence of the prozone phenomenon.) Some isolates from profoundly immunocompromised patients may produce very little polysaccharide capsular material, resulting in false-negative tests.
- There are several sources of false-positive reactions. Positive reactions caused by rheumatoid factor (RF) may be reduced by pretreatment of the specimen with pronase, EDTA, or reducing agents. The syneresis fluid from agar media can cause false-positive results; an aliquot of the specimen for cryptococcal antigen testing should be removed before medium inoculation. Finally, several uncommon pathogens, including *Trichosporon beigelii* and *Capnocytophaga canimorsus*, can cause false-positive cryptococcal agglutination reactions.
- **Common pitfalls:**
  - ▼ Positive cryptococcal antigen titers should be confirmed by culture to document active infection and rule out false-positive reactions. Some infected patients may have very low antigen titers. All specimens submitted for cryptococcal antigen testing should be accompanied by cultures of spinal fluid, blood, or other potentially infected material for fungal isolation.

❑ **Other Considerations**

- Antigen titers are usually higher in patients with AIDS compared to those seen in HIV-negative patients with cryptococcal infection. In patients with AIDS, baseline CSF antigen titers <1:2,048 are associated with improved prognosis. Antigen titers should fall with effective antifungal therapy. Steady or increasing cryptococcal antigen titers, even with sterilization of cultures, are an indication of likely treatment failure and recurrence of infection.

CRYPTOSPORIDIUM ANTIGEN DETECTION

❑ **Use**

- This test is used to evaluate diarrheal disease in patients at risk for cryptosporidiosis, specifically for the identification of *Cryptosporidium parvum* in stool specimens.
- **Method:**
  - ▼ Enzyme immunoassays are used. EIAs have very high sensitivity (near 100%) and specificity (near 100%) compared with a series of stool O & P examinations. For information about microscopic *Cryptosporidium* detection, see the test *Ova and Parasite Examination, Stool*.
  - ▼ Different EIA assays for fecal parasite detection have different specimen requirements (fresh vs. preserved) and transport conditions. Laboratories should provide assay-specific information for their providers.
- **Turnaround time:** 24–48 hours

❑ **Interpretation**

- **Expected results:** Negative.

17

❑ Limitations

- Examination of several specimens improves detection in patients with light infection. A series of O & P examinations is recommended in patients with repeatedly negative immunoassays in whom parasitic infection is still suspected.

Suggested Readings

CLSI. *Procedures for the Recovery and Identification of Parasites from the Intestinal Tract; Approved Guideline*, 2nd ed. CLSI document M47-A. Wayne, PA: Clinical and Laboratory Standards Institute; 2005.

Garcia LS. *Diagnostic Parasitology*, 5th ed. Washington, DC: ASM Press; 2007.

CYTOMEGALOVIRUS (CMV) CULTURE (RULE OUT)

❑ Definition and Use

- CMV is a ubiquitous viral pathogen. Most infections in immunocompetent patients are asymptomatic or mildly symptomatic, including a self-limited mononucleosis syndrome. In immunocompromised patient populations, including neonates, patients with AIDS, and transplant patients, serious localized (e.g., retinitis, colitis, polyradiculopathy, encephalopathy) or systemic infection may occur.
- Method:
  - ▼ Specimens for CMV culture are usually inoculated onto monolayers of human fibroblasts (e.g., foreskin, fetal lung). Tube cultures should always be inoculated for CMV cultures. The shell vial cultures may also be inoculated. Shell vial cultures provide a more rapid turnaround time than tube cultures but are somewhat less sensitive for detection.
  - ▼ Presumptive CMV infection may be inferred by typical cytopathic effect, but positive cultures should be confirmed by immunologic techniques, such as DFA staining with CMV-specific reagents.
- **Turnaround time:** Specimens with high viral loads, such as urine, may give positive results within several days, but negative cultures may require incubation for up to 4 weeks before signing out as negative. Shell vial cultures are processed for growth at 48–72 hours after inoculation.

❑ Special Collection and Transport Instructions

- Specimens should be collected according to general recommendations for virus culture of the specimen type.
- Specimens should be collected early in acute infection.
- Urine is most often recommended for evaluation of neonates with suspected CMV infection. For evaluation of patients with suspected viremia, heparinized whole blood or isolated buffy coat cells are used to inoculate cultures.
- CMV is a fastidious virus and should be delivered to the laboratory as quickly as possible. Most specimens should be placed in a viral transport medium and transported at 4°C; do not freeze.

❑ Interpretation

- **Expected results:** Negative.
- **Negative results:** Negative cultures do not rule out CMV infection; they may be due to loss of viability after collection or low viral load in the specimen submitted.

- **Positive results:** Positive cultures usually indicate active CMV infection. Occasionally, positive cultures represent asymptomatic shedding of virus not associated with disease.

❏ **Limitations**

- Positive cultures may be due to asymptomatic shedding during latent infection; correlation with histopathology, and other clinical signs and symptoms may be needed to ensure specific diagnosis.

❏ **Other Considerations**

Viral culture may be used to provide a patient isolate for antiviral susceptibility testing or further characterization. CMV antigenemia studies or CMV viral load determination is more effective than viral culture for identification of early, preclinical CMV infection in transplant and other immunocompromised patients.

CYTOMEGALOVIRUS (CMV) QUANTITATIVE MOLECULAR ASSAY*

❏ **Definition**

- The CMV quantitative assay uses real-time PCR to quantitate CMV DNA extracted from plasma of CMV-infected individuals. The test quantifies CMV DNA over different ranges depending on the laboratory and assay methodology—for example 50–4,200,000 copies/mL. The first WHO International Standard for human cytomegalovirus (HCMV), NIBSC code 09/162, will help with standardization of nucleic acid amplification technique (NAT)-based assays for human CMV. The FDA-approved COBAS® AmpliPrep/ COBAS® TaqMan® CMV Test has a range 1.37E+02–9.10E+06 IU/mL.
- **Normal values:** Not detected when the result is below the level of detection of the assay.

❏ **Use**

- Management of CMV-infected individuals undergoing antiviral therapy
- Individuals at risk of severe CMV infection
- Confirmation of the presence CMV infection

❏ **Limitations**

- Caution should be taken when interpreting results obtained by different laboratories or assay methodologies. Use of IU/mL units is intended to make comparison possible. PCR inhibitors in the patient specimen may lead to underestimation of viral quantitation or in rare cases, false-negative results.

CYTOMEGALOVIRUS (CMV) SEROLOGY IGG AND IGM

❏ **Definition**

- Human CMV is a herpes virus. It is ubiquitous, species specific, and spread by close human contact. Primary infection may be acquired through different transmission routes and in different periods of life (e.g., congenital, perinatal

*Contributed by Marzena M. Galdzicka, PhD.

and postnatal infections). Serologic diagnosis of CMV infection relies on the detection of IgG and IgM antibodies. CMV IgM appears within 2–4 weeks and persists for several weeks. In addition, CMV IGM may reappear during secondary CMV infection. CMV IgG can be detected typically after 4 weeks and persists for years to life. Unequivocal diagnosis of CMV primary infection is achieved by documenting a CMV IgG seroconversion on acute convalescent pair of serum samples.

❑ **Use**

- ▪ Aids in the diagnosis of mononucleosis-like illness in immunocompetent patients
- ▪ Discriminates between current (IgM) and prior infections (IgG). Suspected CMV infection based on presentation in immunocompromised patients. Congenital syndrome that presents with symptoms of CMV

❑ **Interpretation**

- ▪ **Normal range:** Negative.
- ▪ Serology reporting is done as qualitative (negative, equivocal or positive) based on the cutoff values established by manufacturer-specific clinical trials. A negative result, however, does not always rule out acute hCMV infection. The IgM response may not be detectable in the very early stage of the infection or if the patient is immunocompromised. If clinical exposure to hCMV is suspected despite a negative finding, a second sample should be collected and tested no <1 or 2 weeks.

❑ **Limitations**

- ▪ Screening of the general population should not be performed. The positive predictive value depends on the likelihood of the virus being present. Testing should only be performed on patients with clinical symptoms or when exposure is suspected. Diseases such as Epstein-Barr viral syndrome, toxoplasmosis, and hepatitis may cause symptoms similar to CMV infection and must be excluded before confirmation of diagnosis.

EPSTEIN-BARR VIRUS (EBV) MOLECULAR TESTING*

❑ **Definition**

- ▪ Epstein-Barr virus (EBV) quantitative PCR detects the presence of EBV DNA in clinical specimens, most commonly plasma or serum. Normal adults usually do not have detectable EBV DNA in their plasma/serum, although normal adults previously infected with EBV will have low levels of EBV DNA in their lymphocytes.

❑ **Use**

- ▪ Monitoring the level of viral reactivation and/or disease activity, particularly in the posttransplant and chemotherapy patients.
- ▪ In diagnosis, prognosis, prediction, and prevention of diseases as mononucleosis, lymphoma, sarcoma, and carcinoma.

---

*Contributed by Marzena M. Galdzicka, PhD.

- EBV viral load in whole blood reflects clinical status in patients with infectious mononucleosis, allogeneic transplant, and nasopharyngeal carcinoma.
- The EBV DNA level in healthy carriers is low and restricted to the intracellular compartment of the blood. The high level is characteristic of EBV-related disease.
- Patients with active infection or EBV-related cancer tend to have high levels of EBV DNA in the plasma or serum.

❏ Limitations

- Currently, there is no international standard available for calibration of this assay. Therefore, caution should be taken when interpreting results obtained by different laboratories or assay methodologies. PCR inhibitors in the patient specimen may lead to underestimation of viral quantitation or in rare cases, false-negative results. Proper storage and timely separation serum or plasma are necessary for obtaining reliable results. EBV DNA released from the intracellular compartment may cause false-positive EBV results in plasma or serum. False-negative results can be obtained due to nuclease activities.
- http://www.fda.gov/MedicalDevices/ProductsandMedicalProcedures/ InVitroDiagnostics/ucm330711.htm

EPSTEIN-BARR VIRUS (EBV) SEROLOGY SCREEN ANTIBODY PROFILE

❏ Definition

- EBV is the etiologic agent of infectious mononucleosis (IM) and is a widely disseminated herpesvirus that is spread by intimate contact between susceptible persons and EBV shedders. EBV spreads primarily via passage of saliva but is not a particularly contagious disease. The virus can persist in the oropharynx of patients with IM for up to 18 months following clinical recovery. EBV has also been isolated in both cervical epithelial cells and in male seminal fluid, suggesting that transmission may also occur sexually. This test comprises four serologic markers: EBV-NA (nuclear antigen IgG); EBV-VCA (viral capsid antigen) IgG and IgM; infectious mononucleosis antibody; and EBV-EA IgG (early antigen IgG).
- **Normal range:** Negative.
- **Tests for EBV:**
  - ▼ **IgG-VCA:** Indicates past infection and immunity. May be present early in illness, usually before clinical symptoms are present. Detected at onset in 100% of cases; only 20% show a fourfold increase in titer after visiting a physician. Decreases during convalescence but detectable for many years after illness; therefore, not helpful in establishing diagnosis of IM.
  - ▼ **IgM-VCA:** Detected at onset in 100% of cases; high titers present in serum 1–6 weeks after onset of illness, starts to fall by 3rd week and usually disappear in 1–6 months. Sera are often taken too late to be detected. It is almost always present in active EBV infection and, thus, most sensitive and specific to confirm acute IM. May be positive in other herpes virus infections (especially CMV); therefore, confirmation with IgG and EBV-NA assays is recommended.

17

▼ **Early antigen:** IgG antibodies to early antigen are present at the onset of clinical illness. There are two subsets of EA IgG: anti-D and anti-R. The presence of anti-D antibodies is consistent with recent infection, since titers disappear after recovery; however, their absence does not exclude acute illness because the antibodies are not expressed in a significant number of patients. Anti-R antibodies are only occasionally present in IM.

▼ Early antigen anti-D titers rise later (3–4 weeks after onset; is transient) in course of IM than AB-VCA and disappear with recovery; combined with IgG-VCA suggests recent EBV infection; only found in 70% of patients with IM due to EBV. High titers are found in nasopharyngeal carcinoma due to EBV. Early antigen anti-R antibodies occur rarely in primary EBV infection, 2 weeks to months after onset, and may persist for a year; more often in atypical or protracted cases. No clinical significance; high titers are found in chronic active EBV infection or Burkitt lymphoma.

▼ **Epstein-Barr nuclear antigen:** Last antibodies to appear and are rare in acute phase; develops 4–6 weeks after onset of clinical illness and rises during convalescence (3–12 months) and persists for many years after illness. Absence when IgM-VCA and anti-D are present implies recent infection. Appearance early in illness excludes primary EBV infection. Appearance after previous negative test evidences recent EBV infection.

❏ **Use**

■ Diagnosing IM. In patients with suspected IM and a negative heterophile test.

❏ **Interpretation**

Table 17-1

❏ **Limitations**

■ EBV serology testing should not be performed as a screening procedure for the general population. The predictive value of a positive or negative result depends on the prevalence of analyte in a given patient population. Testing should only be done when clinical evidence suggests the diagnosis of EBV-associated infectious mononucleosis.

TABLE 17–1. Interpretation of Epstein-Barr Virus (EBV) Serologic Status

Serologic Status	EBV VCA IgM	EBV VCA IgG	EBV-NA IgG	EBV-EA IgG
Primary acute	Positive	Positive	Negative	Positive
	Positive	Negative	Negative	Positive
	Positive	Negative	Negative	Negative
Acute primary/late	Positive	Positive	Negative	Negative
Late acute	Positive	Positive	Positive	Positive
	Positive	Positive	Positive	Negative
	Negative	Positive	Positive	Positive
Primary acute/recover	Negative	Positive	Negative	Positive
Previous infection	Negative	Positive	Negative	Negative
	Negative	Positive	Positive	Negative
Susceptible	Negative	Negative	Negative	Negative

- Antibodies to EBV have been demonstrated in all population groups with a worldwide distribution; approximately 90–95% of adults are eventually EBV seropositive. EBV acquired during childhood years is often subclinical; <10% of children develop clinical infection despite the high rates of exposure.
- The false-negative rates are highest during the beginning of clinical symptoms (25% in the first week; 5–10% in the 2nd week, 5% in the 3rd week).
- Approximately 10% of mononucleosis-like cases are not caused by EBV. Other agents that produce a similar clinical syndrome include CMV, HIV, toxoplasmosis, HHV-6, hepatitis B, and possibly HHV-7.
- IgM and IgG antibodies directed against viral capsid antigen have high sensitivity and specificity for the diagnosis of IM (97% and 94%, respectively).

ESCHERICHIA COLI (ENTEROHEMORRHAGIC, SHIGA TOXIN–PRODUCING *E. COLI*, STEC, *E. COLI* O157:H7) CULTURE (RULE OUT)

❏ Definition

- This test is a specialized stool culture for the detection of GI infection caused by *Escherichia coli* strains associated with enterohemorrhagic infection. These strains produce a Shiga toxin and are most commonly, but not exclusively, associated with *E. coli* O157:H7 strains. Enterohemorrhagic *E. coli* O157:H7 gastroenteritis commonly presents with abdominal pain with vomiting and diarrhea. Stool may become bloody with signs of colitis. Low-grade fever may be present. In most patients, the symptoms resolve within a week. Rare patients, usually the elderly or very young patients, develop HUS with onset commonly occurring 7 days or more after onset of diarrheal symptoms.

❏ Use

- This culture is used to diagnose GI infection caused by Shiga toxin–producing *E. coli*. (Stool may be tested directly for the presence of Shiga toxin as an alternative to culture isolation). Special medium (sorbitol–MacConkey agar) is used to screen stool. Suspicious isolates are confirmed by serotyping and/or Shiga toxin production. *E. coli* O157:H7 strains are almost all sorbitol negative.
- **Turnaround time:** 24–48 hours. Additional time is needed for positive cultures to confirm final identification.

❏ Special Collection and Transport Instructions

- Specimens are collected and transported according to recommendation for routine stool culture.

❏ Interpretation

- **Expected results:** Negative.
- **Negative results:** Infection is unlikely, but a single-negative culture does not rule out infection by enterohemorrhagic *E. coli*.
- **Positive results:** A positive test indicates infection by *E. coli* O157:H7 in patients with a compatible clinical presentation.

❏ Limitations

- Cultures are usually positive only in acute, early infection. The use of stool culture for evaluation of patients with HUS is limited. The use of

17

sorbitol–MacConkey agar is not sensitive for the detection of non–O157 Shiga toxin–producing strains of *E. coli*; alternative testing methods should be used in areas where toxigenic non-O157 strains are prevalent or during outbreaks caused by non-O157 strains. Antibiotic therapy of *E. coli* O157:H7 infection is not routinely recommended; treatment may induce Shiga toxin production and increase disease severity.

ENTEROVIRUS CULTURE (RULE OUT)

❑ **Definition**

- Poliovirus, coxsackie viruses (A and B), and echoviruses are enteroviruses (EVs). As the name implies, EVs most commonly replicate in the GI tract, and fecal–oral transmission is typical. Most clinical manifestations of EV infection are outside the GI tract. EV infection is most commonly considered in children who present with signs and symptoms of aseptic meningitis in summer months. EVs also cause a severe sepsis syndrome in neonates (<2 weeks of age), pleurodynia, myocarditis and cardiomyopathy, and respiratory and oral mucosal diseases. Except for neonatal sepsis syndrome and endemic or vaccine-related poliomyelitis, EV infection is usually followed by complete recovery.

❑ **Use**

- This test is used to detect viral infections caused by EVs. A number of different cell lines are susceptible to EV infection. Different EVs show differing infectivity for specific cell lines, so a number of different lines are typically inoculated for EV isolation. Monkey kidney cells may be used for poliovirus, coxsackie B virus, and echoviruses. WI-38 and human embryonic lung fibroblast cells may be used for coxsackie A virus.
- **Turnaround time:**
  - ▼ Tube cultures may be incubated for up to 4 weeks before signing out as negative.
  - ▼ CSF cultures are usually positive within 7 days (when positive).
  - ▼ Stool cultures, or other specimen types with higher concentrations of virus, are often positive within several days.

❑ **Special Collection and Transport Instructions**

- Specimens should be collected within the first week after onset of symptoms.
- Specimens should be collected according to general recommendations for virus culture of the specimen type. For patients with aseptic meningitis, CSF should be transported to the laboratory on wet ice (4°C). Submission of stool for viral culture may improve the detection of EV CNS infection.

❑ **Interpretation**

- **Expected results:** Negative.

❑ **Limitations**

- Submission of specimens >7 days after onset of acute infection is associated with decreased sensitivity. Cell culture is negative in 25% or more of patients presenting with typical EV infection. EVs may grow slowly in culture.

Coxsackie A isolates grow poorly in culture; sensitivity for detection is fairly low. Commercially available RT-PCR methods have emerged as the most sensitive and specific tests for the detection of EV aseptic meningitis.

FECAL LEUKOCYTES EXAMINATION

❑ **Definition**

- The presence of fecal leukocytes is an indication of an inflammatory process of the colon, including colitis caused by invasive enteric pathogens. A number of GI infections are typically associated with the presence of fecal leukocytes: Infections caused by *Shigella* spp., *Salmonella* spp., *Campylobacter* spp., *Yersinia* spp., enteroinvasive *E. coli*, and *C. difficile*, and amebic dysentery.

❑ **Use**

- This test is used to detect leukocytes in stool. A fecal leukocyte examination may be indicated for patients with a clinical diarrheal syndrome and signs of colitis. A fixed smear or wet mount of diarrheal stool is stained with methylene blue and examined for the presence of PMNs using a high-power objective.
- **Turnaround time:** <24 hours.
- Stool is collected according to recommendations for stool culture and transported to the laboratory within 2 hours.

❑ **Interpretation**

- **Expected results:** Negative.
- Negative fecal leukocyte examination does not rule out significant bacterial enteric infection.
- Positive results support a diagnosis of invasive gastrointestinal infection. Enteroinvasive GI infections are usually associated with 3+ to 4+ fecal leukocytes (1–4 PMN/HPF or >5 PMN/HPF) with sensitivity >50% for specimens with results of 3+ or greater. The positive predictive value increases with increasing numbers of PMN/HPF.

❑ **Limitations**

- Significant infections caused by a number of enteric pathogens, including *Vibrio* spp., enterohemorrhagic *E. coli*, and viral agents, do not show an increase in fecal leukocytes. An increase in fecal leukocytes is not specific for infection and may be caused by other conditions, such as inflammatory bowel disease.

FRANCISELLA TULARENSIS CULTURE (RULE OUT)

❑ **Definition**

- *Francisella tularensis* is a slow-growing, fastidious, gram-negative bacillus capable of producing severe infection, including localized and systemic disease. Infections have typically been acquired by zoonotic tick-borne transmission or direct contact. The common reservoir for organisms includes rabbits, rodents, deer, squirrels, and other wild mammals. Domestic animals may harbor the organism. This organism is easily transmissible, so it is critical that the

17

laboratory be informed whenever tularemia is suspected. Typical disease syndromes include glandular, oculoglandular, and ulceroglandular tularemia; oropharyngeal tularemia; typhoidal tularemia; and pneumonic tularemia. There is great concern regarding the use of this organism for a bioterror-related attack.

❏ **Use**

- This culture is used to isolate *F. tularensis* from clinical specimens.
- **Method:**
  - ▼ Specimens for *F. tularensis* isolation should be inoculated onto cysteine-enriched agar media. Blood–cysteine–glucose agar is recommended; most clinical isolates will grow on chocolate, Thayer-Martin, and nonselective buffered charcoal–yeast extract (BCYE) agar. Enriched broth media, such as thioglycollate broth, should also be inoculated. Blood agar and MacConkey agar are typically inoculated for clinical specimens for isolation of other possible pathogens.
  - ▼ Because of the risk of laboratory-acquired infection and because isolation of *F. tularensis* may represent a sentinel event in a bioterror attack, most clinical microbiology laboratories limit the workup of suspected isolates to simple tests to rule out suspicious colonies, referring isolates that fail to "rule out" to their local public health laboratory for identification and further characterization. Final results for testing, therefore, may be delayed compared to common bacterial isolates.
- **Turnaround time:** Isolation and a preliminary identification are usually available within 3–6 days. Additional time is required for transfer to the local public health laboratory, confirmation of identification, and further testing.

❏ **Special Collection and Transport Instructions**

- Lymph node aspirate, ulcerative lesions, sputum, BAL, or other localized specimens, depending on the clinical presentation, are usually submitted for diagnosis.
- Culture of multiple specimens from different infected tissues may improve detection.
- Blood cultures are recommended for evaluation of patients with suspected tularemia.
- Serologic testing is recommended for diagnosis in patients with suspected tularemia.

❏ **Interpretation**

- **Expected results:** Negative. After the acute phase of infection, cultures may become negative. Tularemia cannot be confidently ruled out by negative cultures.
- **Positive:** Isolation of *F. tularensis* is diagnostic of tularemia. Tularemia is a reportable disease; positive cultures must be reported to the local department of health.

❏ **Limitations**

- Because *F. tularensis* organisms are tiny and faintly staining, direct detection by Gram stain of clinical specimens is uncommon. Cultures late in infection may be negative. Serologic diagnosis may be helpful in patients with disease consistent with tularemia, but negative cultures.

- **Common pitfalls:**
  - ▼ The diagnosis of tularemia may not be entertained until after the most acute phase of illness, a time when cultures are less likely to be positive.
  - ▼ Clinicians may fail to request specific cultures for tularemia or alert the laboratory of their clinical suspicion.

FUNGAL ANTIGEN, BETA-D-GLUCAN

❑ **Definition**

- (1-3)-β-D-glucan (BG) is a cell wall component of most fungi, except *Zygomycetes* and *Cryptococcus* species. BG has been used as a biomarker for invasive fungal infections (IFI), including candidemia and *Pneumocystis* pneumonia; an FDA-approved test for quantitative BG detection is available. In patients with ILI or *Pneumocystis* pneumonia, significant levels of BG may be detected in the serum significantly earlier than clinical signs and symptoms or detection of infection by laboratory or imaging studies. Decreasing BG levels have been associated with treatment success.

❑ **Special Collection and Transport Instructions**

- Blood samples are collected and transported according to standard protocol. Samples are allowed to clot and serum separated for testing (minimum 0.5 mL).

❑ **Use**

- BG testing may be submitted for early evaluation of patients at risk for IFI or *Pneumocystis* pneumonia, or to monitor the effectiveness of therapy.

❑ **Interpretation**

- **Expected result:** Not detected.
- **Positive result:**
  - ▼ For IFI in neutropenic patients, BG levels ≥80 pg/mL are consistent with emerging or active infection (sensitivity approximately 65%; specificity approximately 95%).
  - ▼ For *Pneumocystis* pneumonia, a higher cutoff value (≥100 pg/mL) has been recommended, yielding sensitivity approximately 95% with approximately 99% specificity.
- **Indeterminate result:** Detectable BD levels below cutoff values do not establish or reject a diagnosis. Repeat testing is recommended.
- **Negative result:** Fungal infection or *Pneumocystis* pneumonia is unlikely, but infection with *Cryptococcus* species or Zygomycetes is not ruled out.

❑ **Limitations**

- The BG assay is not specific for any specific fungal pathogen. Additional testing is required for identification of the infecting species. Evaluation of patients at risk for IFI or *Pneumocystis* pneumonia should not be evaluated by BD as the sole diagnostic testing. Fungal culture, wet mount, imaging studies, histopathology and other relevant diagnostic evaluations should be performed as relevant.

17

FUNGAL ANTIGEN, GALACTOMANNAN

❏ Definition

■ Galactomannan is an *Aspergillus* antigen that may be detected in the serum of patients with invasive aspergillosis (AI). The most sensitive galactomannan detection uses monoclonal specific antibodies in an EIA format. Detection of *Aspergillus* galactomannan has been shown to provide good sensitivity and specificity for AI. Galactomannan testing may improve patient management of patients at risk for AI because culture and histopathologic methods have limited sensitivity for specific detection, and *Aspergillus* culture isolates may represent contamination or patient colonization.

❏ Special Collection and Transport Instructions

■ Serum is most commonly collected for testing; standard laboratory procedures for collection and transport are used. Other specimens may be acceptable and are collected and transported according to instructions of the assay manufacturer.

❏ Use

■ Specimens may be collected from patients at risk for invasive aspergillosis. Sequential testing may improve detection in patients with emerging AI. Testing is not recommended for patients receiving antifungal prophylaxis because this treatment markedly decreases sensitivity of the assay.

❏ Interpretation

■ **Expected result:** Not detected.
■ **Positive results:** Positive results support a diagnosis of invasive aspergillosis, but two consecutive positive results are required for a positive patient evaluation. A second specimen should be collected, before initiation of antifungal treatment, from patients to confirm initially positive galactomannan results. False-positive results may be caused by cross-reactive antigens from non-aspergillus species. Positive reactions, even persistently positive reactions, should be interpreted in the context of clinical presentation and other signs and symptoms.
■ **Negative results:** The probability of invasive *Aspergillus* is reduced, but AI is not excluded. Repeat testing in high-risk patients may improve detection of early AI. False-negative reactions may be caused by collection of specimens after initiation of antifungal treatment, low fungal load in serum (e.g., localized infection), high galactomannan antibody titers, or other factors.

❏ Limitations

■ Sensitivity of assays may be limited early in active infection. False positive results may be seen in up 18% of patients without AI. Attempts to confirm positive results by culture or histopathology should be attempted to minimize the possibility of false-positive diagnosis. Evaluation of patients at risk for invasive aspergillosis should not be evaluated with galactomannan as the sole diagnostic testing. Fungal culture, wet mount, imaging studies, histopathology and other relevant diagnostic evaluations should be performed as relevant.

FUNGAL CULTURE (MOLD, YEAST, DIMORPHIC, AND DERMATOPHYTE PATHOGENS)

❑ **Definition and Use**

- Fungal cultures are indicated when clinically significant fungal infection is suspected. Symptomatic fungal infections commonly can be characterized as follows:
  - ▼ Superficial (skin/nail/hair)
  - ▼ Subcutaneous (chromoblastomycosis, mycetoma, phaeohyphomycotic cyst, sporotrichosis)
  - ▼ Systemic mycosis (e.g., coccidiomycosis)
  - ▼ Opportunistic mycosis (e.g., aspergillosis)
- Fungal cultures are used as the most sensitive routine laboratory method for detection of fungal infections.

Method

- The media inoculated vary, depending on the specimen submitted and type of pathogen suspected.
- Direct examination, such as wet mount or calcofluor white staining, should be performed for most specimen types; see *Fungal Wet Mount*. Specimens for routine fungal culture are inoculated onto nonselective media, such as BHI or Sabouraud dextrose–BHI agar. For specimens likely to be contaminated, selective media, such as inhibitory mold agar, are inoculated. An enriched medium, such as BHI blood agar, is inoculated to improve recovery of dimorphic fungal pathogens.
- Special media may be inoculated for some types of specimens or suspected pathogen, like Bird (niger) seed agar for *Cryptococcus neoformans*, chromogenic agar for differentiation of *Candida* isolates, or dermatophyte test medium for dermatophytes. If *Malassezia furfur* is suspected, medium supplemented with a source of long-chain fatty acids (like olive oil) is inoculated.
- Inoculated media are typically incubated at 25–30°C in room air for up to 4 weeks. Cultures for isolation of systemic, dimorphic pathogens may be incubated at 35–37°C, but the incremental yield, versus 30°C incubation, is minimal. Cultures for fastidious pathogens are incubated for up to 8 weeks.
- Media inoculated for aerobic bacterial culture will support the growth of the common yeast pathogens, *Candida* species, so specific culture for yeast is not usually required.
- See *Blood Culture, Fungal* for information regarding the detection of fungemia.

Turnaround Time

- Cultures for yeast are incubated for 7 days. Routine fungal cultures are incubated for up to 4 weeks. Cultures for systemic dimorphic pathogens are incubated for up to 8 weeks. Additional time is needed for isolation and identification of isolates.

❑ **Special Collection and Transport Instructions**

- Specimens are collected using sterile technique and transported in a sterile container within 2 hours. Store specimens at 4°C if transport will be delayed.

17

- Most specimens for fungal culture are collected following standard specimen collection instructions.
  - ▼ Collection of specimens using swabs is not recommended, except for samples from mucous membranes for the diagnosis of candidiasis.
  - ▼ SPS anticoagulation is recommended for blood and bone marrow specimens.
  - ▼ Pluck multiple hairs (10 or more) and scrape scalp from involved areas.
  - ▼ Wipe affected nail with 70% alcohol. Submit nail clippings and scrapings from beneath nails in a clean container.
  - ▼ Wipe affected skin lesions with 70% alcohol. Scrape the advancing margin to remove superficial cells and keratinized material; submit in a clean container.

❏ **Interpretation**

- **Expected results:** No growth.
- **Positive:** Positive cultures must be carefully interpreted to ensure that endogenous fungal flora and culture contaminants are recognized.

❏ **Limitations**

- The results of fungal cultures may not be available when decisions regarding therapy of acute infection are required. Empiric therapy may be required.
- **Common pitfalls:** Isolation of endogenous *Candida* species or environmental mold contaminants may result in unneeded treatment.

❏ **Other Considerations**

- Clinical information, such as travel history, immune status, and animal exposure, should be included on the requisitions for fungal cultures.
- Histopathologic testing and immunologic testing are important methods for diagnosis of invasive fungal infections. Specific molecular diagnostic testing shows promise for sensitive and specific diagnosis with short turnaround time.
- A diagnosis of vaginal and oral candidiasis (thrush) can be made reliably by direct microscopic examination (Gram stain or wet mount) of scrapings of mucosal surfaces without need for fungal culture.
- Detection of antigen or fungal products, such as cryptococcal antigen, histoplasma antigen, β-D-glucan, or galactomannan, may be useful for diagnosis.
- The India ink wet mount is less sensitive than cryptococcal antigen testing for meningitis caused by *C. neoformans*.

FUNGAL WET MOUNT (KOH, CALCOFLUOR)

❏ **Definition**

- A direct examination for fungal elements may provide a rapid detection of fungal infection and is recommended for most types of specimens submitted for fungal culture.

❏ **Use**

- This test is used for the direct detection of fungal forms in patient specimens. The specimen is processed to form a liquid suspension of the patient sample.

▼ Solid specimens, such as tissues, should be minced to facilitate suspension.
▼ The specimen may be suspended in saline or a 10% KOH solution. KOH may improve liquefaction of the specimen and also lyses host cells and keratin; fungal cells are resistant to KOH digestion.
▼ A cover slip is added for examination with regular or phase-contrast light microscopy.
▼ Calcofluor white, a fluorogenic dye that binds to specific polysaccharide bonds found in fungal cell walls, may be added to the KOH solution to improve microscopic visualization of fungi.
- **Turnaround time:** 24 hours.
- Specimens should be collected and transported according to guidelines for fungal culture of the specimen type.

❑ **Interpretation**
- **Expected result:** Negative.
- **Positive:** Provides evidence of fungal infection. Fungal elements may be characterized on the basis of morphology (e.g., budding yeast, aseptate hyphae, conidia-forming structures consistent with *Aspergillus* species).
- **Negative:** Fungal infection is not ruled out by a negative wet mount examination.

❑ **Limitations**
- The morphology of objects must be examined carefully to exclude artifacts or nonspecific absorption of calcofluor dye to nonfungal objects, such as capillaries.

GENITAL CULTURE

❑ **Definition**
- Genital cultures should be collected from patients with signs and symptoms of localized genital tract infection or sexually transmitted disease, including discharge, dysuria, or lower abdominal pain.

❑ **Use**
- This culture is used to detect common bacterial pathogens from genital specimens. Target pathogens typically include *N. gonorrhoeae*, yeast, group A and B β-hemolytic streptococci, *Staphylococcus aureus*, and *Listeria monocytogenes*. *Gardnerella vaginalis* should be reported if predominant and isolated in moderate to heavy growth. Invasively collected specimens should be cultured for isolation of these, as well as a broad range of other bacterial pathogens.
- **Method:**
  ▼ A Gram stain should be prepared from specimens submitted for genital culture. In male patients, the presence of many intracellular gram-negative diplococci is consistent with a diagnosis of gonorrhea. In female patients, a vaginal Gram stain may be used to identify "clue cells"; the absence of lactobacilli may be a marker of disruption of the normal vaginal flora, as with bacterial vaginosis.

17

▼ Specimens are plated onto selective and nonselective media that support growth of fastidious pathogens. Examples include
  ● Blood and chocolate agar
  ● CNA and MacConkey agar, or comparable selective agar for gram-positive and gram-negative isolation
  ● Selective agar for *N. gonorrhoeae*, such as Thayer-Martin, Martin-Lewis, NYC, or comparable media

▪ **Turnaround time:** Routine genital cultures are incubated for up to 72 hours. Additional time is required in positive cultures for isolation, final identification, and further testing.

❑ **Special Collection and Transport Instructions**

▪ **Male:** An urethral swab should be collected. It may be possible to collect discharge expressed from the penile urethra. Collection of urethral discharge after prostatic massage may improve detection in patients with symptoms of prostatitis.

▪ **Female:**
  ▼ Urethral swabs or swabs from the cervical os are recommended. The cervix is visualized using a speculum lubricated only with water. Prior to collection of cervical specimens, mucus from the exocervix should be removed by use of a cleaning swab.
  ▼ Vaginal specimens are not recommended for routine genital cultures. Vaginal specimens may be useful for diagnosis of vaginal candidiasis, *Trichomonas vaginalis* infection, or *S. aureus* superinfection.
  ▼ Other specimens usually require more invasive sampling techniques, such as endometrial curettage, Bartholin gland aspiration, and culdocentesis.

❑ **Interpretation**

▪ **Expected results:** Cultures should yield only endogenous flora for the specimen submitted.

▪ **Positive:** The interpretation of positive cultures may depend on the organism isolated and the quantity. *N. gonorrhoeae* is never normal flora and indicates gonorrhea.

▪ **Negative:** A single negative culture does not rule out infection with *N. gonorrhoeae* or other genital pathogen. Sampling several sites, like the cervix and urethra, and serial sampling may improve detection.

❑ **Limitations**

▪ The symptoms related to genital infections may overlap with those of UTI, so urine cultures are recommended for most patients for whom genital cultures are submitted. Routine genital cultures are most often submitted for diagnosis of an STD caused by *N. gonorrhoeae*. A number of STDs will not be detected by routine bacterial genital culture, including *C. trachomatis*, *Treponema pallidum*, *Haemophilus ducreyi*, *Ureaplasma urealyticum*, *T. vaginalis*, HSV, and HPV. Special cultures or procedures are needed for detection of infections with these pathogens. See *Group B Streptococcus Rectovaginal Culture Screen* for detection of group B beta-hemolytic *Streptococcus* carriage during pregnancy.

- Additional information:
  - ▼ Special cultures are required to detect *N. gonorrhoeae* infections of non-genital sites, such as the rectum or throat.
  - ▼ Molecular diagnostic techniques provide improved sensitivity for diagnosis of genital infections caused by *N. gonorrhoeae* and *C. trachomatis*.
  - ▼ Isolation of a sexually transmitted pathogen from a child must be investigated as a sign of possible abuse.

GIARDIA ANTIGEN DETECTION

❏ **Definition and Use**

- The *Giardia* antigen detection test is used for the identification of *Giardia lamblia* in stool specimens. It is used to evaluate diarrheal disease in patients at risk for giardiasis. Giardia EIA has a very high sensitivity (near 100%) and specificity (near 100%) compared with a series of stool O & P examinations.
- **Turnaround time:** 24–48 hours.

❏ **Interpretation**

- **Expected results:** Negative.

❏ **Limitations**

- Several specimens may be required in patients with light infection. Repeat testing improves sensitivity of detection. A series of O & P examinations is recommended in patients with repeatedly negative immunoassays in whom parasitic infection is still suspected.
- **A common pitfall** is submission of the incorrect type of specimen for the assay. To perform immunoassays accurately, the correct specimen type (preserved or fresh) and procedures, as specified in kit instructions, must be followed exactly.

Suggested Readings

CLSI. *Procedures for the Recovery and Identification of Parasites from the Intestinal Tract; Approved Guideline*, 2nd ed. CLSI document M28-A2. Wayne, PA: Clinical and Laboratory Standards Institute; 2005.
Garcia LS. *Diagnostic Parasitology*, 5th ed. Washington, DC: ASM Press; 2007.

GRAM STAIN

❏ **Definition and Use**

- Indications:
  - ▼ This test should be routinely performed for certain specimen types submitted to the laboratory for bacterial culture (e.g., lower respiratory, wound, tissue, abscess and drainage, sterile fluids, CSF, genital samples).
  - ▼ Because Gram stain is less sensitive than culture for detection of bacteria, culture should always be performed with Gram stains with a few possible exceptions. Gram stain without culture may provide accurate detection of vaginal and oropharyngeal candidiasis.

17

- The Gram stain is used for the direct detection and initial presumptive identification of bacteria and yeast in patient specimens. Specimens should be collected and transported according to instructions for specific specimen types. Patient specimens are used to make smears on glass microscope slides. After fixation, slides are sequentially stained with crystal violet followed by iodine solution. The intracellular crystal violet–iodine complexes formed are too large to escape through the thick peptidoglycan cell wall of gram-positive organisms by alcohol decolorization, rendering them dark blue. But the crystal violet–iodine complexes can be rinsed through the thinner, fenestrated cell wall of gram-negative organisms, leaving them colorless. After the rinsing step, gram-negative organisms are counterstained with safranin, resulting in mild to intense pink staining.
- The Gram stain is a differential staining technique. Staining characteristics (e.g., pink or blue) and morphology (e.g., cocci or bacilli) and other characteristics of the primary pathogens are reported. This information may contribute to informed decisions regarding initial empirical therapy.
- The Gram stain may demonstrate host PMNs and other evidence of inflammation. Epithelial cells, derived from mucosal or cutaneous surfaces, predict contamination of the specimen with the patient's endogenous flora.
- **Turnaround time:** <4 hours.

❑ **Interpretation**

- **Expected results:**
  - ▼ Specimens from sterile sites should be negative for microorganisms. Smears from nonsterile sites, such as mucosal surfaces, usually demonstrate organisms of various morphologies typical for the endogenous flora of the site (e.g., respiratory, vaginal, GI).
  - ▼ PMNs and other signs of an inflammatory reaction are not typical for normal tissue specimens and suggest infection (or other inflammatory condition) at the site of collection.
- **Positive results:**
  - ▼ Microorganisms (usually a single morphotype), in moderate or heavy amounts, with PMNs, and other inflammatory markers are typical of pyogenic infections.
  - ▼ Pathogens present in the specimen in concentrations greater than approximately 10^3–10^4 organisms per milliliter should be detected by Gram stain and will typically yield moderate or heavy growth in culture. Concentration of CSF and sterile fluid specimens, using techniques such as centrifugation, improves detection of microorganisms by Gram stain.
  - ▼ Any type of organisms seen by Gram stain should be isolated by culture after appropriate processing. Monitoring the correlation of Gram stain and bacterial culture results, therefore, may be used as an important quality assurance (QA) tool. Detection of an organism by Gram stain for which culture yields no comparable isolate suggests that additional cultures, like anaerobic or mycobacterial, may be required.
- **Negative results:**
  - ▼ Infections may be associated with low concentrations of pathogens (<10^3 organisms/mL). For example, in adults with overwhelming bacteremia and sepsis, the concentration of organisms in the bloodstream is typically

approximately 1–10 organism/mL, well below the detection level by Gram stain microscopy.

▼ PMNs and other signs of inflammation may increase suspicion of infection in smears negative for microorganisms.

❏ **Limitations**

■ Some pathogenic microorganisms fail to stain avidly by the Gram stain technique. Special modifications or stains may improve detection, like the use of fuchsin as a counterstain for the Gram stain, or acridine orange as a fluorogenic alternative to the Gram stain. Poor specimen collection, such as not sampling the site of infection, may give false-negative or misleading results.

Suggested Reading

Winn WC Jr, Allen SD, Janda WM, et al. *Koneman's Color Atlas and Textbook of Diagnostic Microbiology*, 6th ed. Baltimore, MD: Lippincott Williams & Wilkins; 2006.

GROUP B STREPTOCOCCUS VAGINAL–RECTAL CULTURE SCREEN

❏ **Definition**

■ Group B *Streptococcus* (GBS) infection is the leading cause of early-onset neonatal sepsis. Bacteremia, multiorgan disease, and meningitis are all possible manifestations of neonatal GBS infection. Maternal GBS carriage in the GU or GI tract is the primary risk factor for neonatal infection. The CDC and relevant professional organizations have recommended screening pregnant women for GU and GI carriage of GBS and using culture results as primary guidance for the use of intrapartum antimicrobial prophylaxis for prevention of neonatal infection.

❏ **Special Collection and Transport Instructions**

■ Swab specimens should be collected at 35–37 weeks' gestation.

■ Swab the lower vagina/vaginal introitus, followed by the rectum (i.e., through the anal sphincter). Two swabs or a single swab may be used. If two swabs are used, they should be submitted to the laboratory together as a single specimen.

■ Transport to the laboratory within 24 hours in a nonnutritive transport medium; transport and store the specimen at 4°C prior to laboratory processing. Note if the patient is at risk for anaphylaxis to penicillin, an indication for susceptibility testing for GBS-positive specimens.

❏ **Use**

■ Enrichment culture: Swabs are inoculated into selective broth medium, like Todd-Hewitt broth with gentamicin (8 µg/mL) and nalidixic acid (15 µg/mL) [TransVag broth], or colistin (10 µg/mL) and nalidixic acid (15 µg/mL) [Lim broth]. Commercially available enriched chromogenic broths may be used for the enrichment culture. Incubate broth cultures for 18–24 hours at 35–37°C in room air or 5% CO_2.

■ For TransVag and Lim broth, subculture to an appropriate agar medium (e.g., SBA, CNA, GBS chromogenic agar). Examine subculture plates for colonies suggestive of GBS and perform confirmatory testing.

■ Process chromogenic broth according to the manufacturer's instructions.

17

- Broth enrichment is the most common method. Alternative testing of the broth enrichment culture includes specific latex agglutination or nucleic acid probe or PCR.
- Susceptibility testing should be performed on GBS isolates for patients with significant penicillin allergy; D-testing for inducible clindamycin resistance should be performed on isolates that are clindamycin sensitive but erythromycin resistant by routine testing.
- Direct plating of swabs may be performed in urgent circumstances, like when an unscreened woman presents in active labor, but enrichment culture should also be performed to ensure optimal sensitivity.
- History of early-onset neonatal GBS infection in a prior pregnancy and GBS bacteriuria or UTI at any time during a current pregnancy are indications for intrapartum prophylaxis, regardless of screening test results; screening is not recommended for these patients.

❏ **Interpretation**

- **Expected results:** 10–30% of pregnant women are vaginal or rectal carriers of GBS. Carriage may be transient, intermittent, or persistant.
- **Positive results:** In the absence of intrapartum prophylaxis, 1–2% of infants born to GBS-colonized mothers develop early-onset neonatal infection.
- **Negative results:** The risk of early-onset GBS neonatal infection is markedly reduced but not eliminated in patients with negative vaginal–rectal carriage screens.

❏ **Limitations**

- GBS carriage may be intermittent and may fall below the level of detection at the time of screening culture. Optimal detection depends on the quality of specimen collection. Both rectal and lower vaginal specimens should be submitted. Specimens unacceptable for culture: cervical, perianal, perirectal, and perineal specimens; a speculum should not be used for collection. Nonhemolytic GBS may be missed if colonies with consistent morphology are not ruled out by additional specific testing.

Suggested Reading

Prevention of Perinatal Group B Streptococcal Disease. Revised Guidelines from CDC, 2010. *MMWR* November 19, 2010;59(RR-10).

HELICOBACTER PYLORI SEROLOGY SCREEN (H. PYLORI ANTIBODY [IgG, IgA, AND IgM] SCREEN)

❏ **Definition**

- *H. pylori* is a bacterium that is found in the stomach of about two thirds of the people in the world, although most infected people will never develop disease. *H. pylori* infection is a major risk factor for peptic ulcer disease. These bacteria are responsible for the large majority of gastric ulcers and upper duodenal ulcers. Research studies indicate that infection with *H. pylori* increases the risk of gastric cancer, gastric mucosa-associated lymphoid tissue (MALT) lymphoma, and possibly pancreatic cancer.
- **Normal range:** Negative.

❑ Use

- Screening for *H. pylori* infection.
- Laboratory-based serologic testing to detect *H. pylori* IgG antibodies is inexpensive and noninvasive. This is the predominant serologic test available for clinical use, and it is well suited to primary care practice. However, concerns over its accuracy have limited its use. Large studies have found that it has high sensitivity (90–100%) but variable specificity (76–96%); the accuracy has ranged from 83 to 98%.
- Some studies found that IgA antibodies may detect cases that were negative by IgG testing. However, a number of studies have demonstrated that IgA testing is overall less sensitive and less specific than IgG testing. Some laboratories also offer IgM tests, which if elevated would indicate an acute infection. IgM assays have little or no role in clinical practice for the diagnosis or management of what is almost always a long-standing condition by the time *H. pylori* infection is considered.

❑ Interpretation

- **Positive result:** Indicates that *H. pylori* IgG antibodies were detected in the sample. The presence of IgG antibodies to *H. pylori* is an indication of previous exposure to the organism.
- **Negative result:** Indicates that *H. pylori* IgG antibodies were not detected in the sample. Negative results by this test do not preclude recent primary infection.

❑ Limitations

- The ACG guidelines recommend that testing for *H. pylori* should be performed only if the clinician plans to offer treatment for positive results.
- Testing is indicated in patients with active peptic ulcer disease, a past history of documented peptic ulcer, or gastric MALT lymphoma.
- The test-and-treat strategy for *H. pylori* (i.e., test and treat if positive) is a proven management strategy for patients with uninvestigated dyspepsia who are younger than 55 years of age and have no "alarm features" (bleeding, anemia, early satiety, unexplained weight loss, progressive dysphagia, odynophagia, recurrent vomiting, family history of GI cancer, previous esophagogastric malignancy).
- Deciding which test to use in which situation relies heavily on whether a patient requires evaluation with upper endoscopy and an understanding of the strengths, weaknesses, and costs of the individual test.
- General population screening of asymptomatic patients not recommended.
- Patients with family history of GI cancer should have screening if symptomatic (endoscopy with biopsy).
- Patients without "alarm" symptoms, a dyspepsia that does not respond to antireflux treatment, may be candidates for *H. pylori* testing.

HELICOBACTER PYLORI STOOL ANTIGEN DETECTION

❑ Definition

- *H. pylori* is a bacterium that is found in the stomach of about two thirds of the people in the world, although most infected people will never develop disease. *H. pylori* infection is a major risk factor for peptic ulcer disease.

17

These bacteria are responsible for the large majority of gastric ulcers and upper duodenal ulcers. Research studies indicate that infection with *H. pylori* increases the risk of gastric cancer, gastric mucosa-associated lymphoid tissue (MALT) lymphoma, and possibly pancreatic cancer. *H. pylori* infection may be diagnosed by invasive (e.g., histopathology) or noninvasive (e.g., serology, breath urea test, stool antigen) tests. Most tests use an EIA format. Tests using monoclonal antibodies against *H. pylori* have reported the best accuracy.

❑ **Use**

▪ Testing is requested for evaluation of patients with dyspepsia or other upper GI symptoms suggesting *H. pylori* infection. Stool specimens, collected and transported using standard laboratory methods. Testing may be submitted to monitor effect of treatment for *H. pylori* infection. Stool antigen become undetectable with effective therapy.

❑ **Interpretation**

▪ **Expected result:** Negative.
▪ **Positive result:** Active *H. pylori* infection. False-positive results may be seen in approximately 5% of tests.
▪ **Negative result:** The patient is unlikely to have active infection with *H. pylori*. False-negative results may be seen in 5–7% of patients; repeat testing or testing with other types of assays for infection should be considered in patients with high suspicion for *H. pylori* infection.

Suggested Reading

Choi J, Kim CH, Kim D, et al. Prospective evaluation of a new stool antigen test for the detection of *Helicobacter pylori*, in comparison with histology, rapid urease test, ^{13}C-urea breath test, and serology. *J Gastroenterol Hepatol.* 2011;26:1053–1059.

HEPATITIS A VIRUS (HAV) ANTIBODIES (IgM AND TOTAL)

❑ **Definition**

▪ The detection of HAV-specific antibodies, both IgG and IgM, occurs early in the acute infection, with IgG persisting for years. Diagnosis of HAV infection requires positivity for IgM. HAV never causes chronic infection, but acute relapses occasionally occur.
▪ **Normal range:** Negative.

❑ **Use**

▪ Indicated, in conjunction with other serologic and clinical information, as an aid in the clinical laboratory diagnosis of individuals with acute or past hepatitis A virus infection aids in the identification of HAV-susceptible individuals prior to HAV vaccination.

❑ **Limitations**

▪ The total assay detects the presence of anti-HAV total (both IgG and IgM combined). A positive result indicates that the patient had hepatitis A either recently or in the past. IgM antibodies against HAV are detected soon after the onset of symptoms. Persistence of the IgM response is extremely variable, with specific IgM detected for <1 month in some cases to >1 year in others. In most cases, IgM antibodies against HAV persist for a period of 3–6 months, after which they decline to levels that are below detection.

HEPATITIS B CORE ANTIBODY (HBcAb; TOTAL AND IgM)

❏ **Definition**

- Hepatitis B core antibodies appear shortly after the onset of symptoms of hepatitis B infection and soon after the appearance of HBsAg and persists for life. Initially, anti-HBcAb consists almost entirely of the IgM class, followed by appearance of anti-HBc IgG, for which there is no commercial diagnostic assay. The anti-HBc total antibodies test, which detects both IgM and IgG antibodies and is the test for anti-HBc IgM antibodies, may be the only markers of a recent hepatitis B infection detectable in the "window period." The window period begins with the clearance of HBsAg and ends with the appearance of antibodies to HBsAg.
- **Normal range:** Negative.

❏ **Use**

- Differential diagnosis of hepatitis; diagnosis of recent or past resolved hepatitis B infection.

Determination of occult hepatitis B infection in otherwise healthy HBV carriers with negative test results for HBsAg, anti-HBs Ab, anti-HBc IgM Ab, HBeAg, and antibodies to HBeAg.

❏ **Interpretation**

Increased In

- HBcAb total assay: Acute, chronic, or past resolved hepatitis B infection
- HBcAb IgM assay: Recent infection with hepatitis B virus (≤ 6 months)

Decreased In

- Normal finding.

❏ **Limitations**

- Not produced after hepatitis B immunization.
- Positive anti-HBc total antibody test results should be correlated with the presence of other HBV serologic markers, elevated liver enzymes, clinical signs and symptoms, and a history of risk factors.
- Low levels of IgM core antibodies can sometimes be present in chronic hepatitis B, particularly during flares of activity and at times of conversion from positive antigen to positive antibody.
- Neonates (<1-month-old) with positive anti-HBc total antibody results from this assay method should be tested for anti-HBc IgM antibody to rule out possible maternal anti-HBc total antibody causing false-positive results. Repeat testing for anti-HBc total antibody within 1 month is also recommended in these neonates.

17

HEPATITIS B SURFACE ANTIBODY (HBsAB)

❏ **Definition**

■ The presence of HBsAb in the serum generally indicates recovery and immunity from hepatitis B infection. With naturally occurring hepatitis infections, anti-HBs usually appear in serum several weeks after disappearance of HBsAg; also known as HBsAb, anti-HBs, Australia Bs antibody, and HBV antibody.

■ **Normal range:**
  ▼ <5.00 mIU/mL: Negative
  ▼ ≥5.00 mIU/mL and <12.0 mIU/mL: Indeterminate
  ▼ ≥12.0 mIU/mL: Positive

❏ **Use**

■ Identifying current and previous exposure to HBV. Determining adequate immunity from hepatitis B vaccination

❏ **Interpretation**

Increased In

■ Recovery from acute or chronic HBV infection, or acquired immunity from HBV vaccination.

■ Positive results (quantitative anti-HBs levels of ≥12 mIU/mL) indicate an adequate immunity to hepatitis B from previous HBV infection or HBV vaccination.

■ Screen for individuals at high risk for exposure, such as hemodialysis patients, persons with multiple sex partners, persons with a history of other STDs, IV drug abusers, infants born to infected mothers, individuals residing in long-term residential facilities or correctional facilities, recipients of blood- or plasma-derived products, allied health care workers, and public service employees who come in contact with blood and blood products.

Decreased In

■ Inadequate immune response to HBV vaccination.

❏ **Limitations**

■ Passively acquired anti-HBs (i.e., transfusion of whole blood or plasma, recent immune globulin treatment) can yield positive results without indicating permanent immunity to HBV infection.

■ Anti-HBs levels from previous hepatitis B or HBV vaccination may fall below detectable levels over time.

■ Not useful for diagnosis of acute HBV infection. Does not differentiate between vaccine-induced immunity and immunity after recovery from hepatitis B infection without further tests like hepatitis B core total antibodies.

■ Coexistence of HBsAg/HBsAb reported in 24% patients. In most cases, the antibodies are unable to neutralize circulating virions. These are regarded as carriers.

HEPATITIS B SURFACE ANTIGEN (HBsAg)

❑ **Definition**

- Serologic hallmark of HBV infection. First serologic marker to appear (1–10 weeks of acute exposure). Patients who subsequently recover; undetectable after 4–6 months. Persistent for >6 months in chronic infection.
- **Normal range:** Negative.

❑ **Use**

- Diagnosis of acute, recent, or chronic hepatitis B infection. Determination of chronic hepatitis B carriage.

❑ **Limitations**

- Vaccination for HBV can produce transiently detectable levels of HBsAg in patients (≤14 days). Most commonly occurs in hemodialysis patients, neonates, and children.
- Some rare mutations result in false-negative test results. In these suspected cases, the presence of virus can be deduced by testing for HBcAb, surface antigen antibodies, and HBV DNA.
- Specimens with initially reactive test result but negative (not confirmed) by HBsAg confirmation test are likely to contain cross-reactive antibodies from other infectious or immunologic disorders. Repeat testing is recommended at a later date when clinically indicated.

HEPATITIS BE ANTIGEN AND ANTIBODY (HBeAg AND HBeAb)

❑ **Definition**

- Presence of HBeAg in the serum indicates active replication of virus and is usually associated with HBV DNA. HBeAg to HBeAb seroconversion occurs early in patients with acute infection, prior to HBsAg-to-HBsAb seroconversion. However, HBeAg seroconversion may be delayed for years to decades in chronic infection. HBeAg-to-HBeAb seroconversion usually associated with disappearance of HBV DNA in serum. Presence of HBeAb in the serum usually indicates that the virus is no longer replicating. Limited use clinically.
- **Normal range:** Negative.

❑ **Use**

- Diagnosis and monitoring of HBV infectivity. Recognition of resolution of hepatitis B infection with seroconversion of HBeAg to HBeAb.

❑ **Interpretation**

- Presence indicates highly infective stage of hepatitis B.

❑ **Limitations**

- Persistence of HBeAg is associated with chronic liver disease.
- Presence of HBeAg implies infective HBV present in the serum, but its absence on conversion to HBeAb does not rule out infectivity, especially in persons infected with genotypes other than A.

17

- During the HBeAg-positive state, usually 3–6 weeks, hepatitis B patients are at increased risk of transmitting the virus to their contacts, including babies born during this period. Exposure to serum or body fluid positive for HBeAg and HBsAg is associated with three to five times greater risk of infectivity than when HBsAg positivity occurs alone.
- HBeAg may be negative in the "precore mutant" form of hepatitis B and can be highly infectious. HBeAg-negative strains respond similarly to antiviral treatment.
- Measurement of HBV DNA is now recommended, especially in persons with increased ALT but negative HBeAg.

HEPATITIS C VIRUS (HCV) ANTIBODY

❏ **Definition**

- HCV is now known to be the causative agent for most, if not all, blood-borne non-A, non-B hepatitis. The presence of anti-HCV indicates that an individual may have been infected with HCV and may be capable of transmitting HCV infection. Also known as HCV antibody, non-A, non-B hepatitis.
- **Normal range:** Negative.

❏ **Use**

- Screening for past (resolved) or chronic hepatitis C.

❏ **Interpretation**

Increased In

- Hepatitis C infection: Current and past exposure.

❏ **Limitations**

- Presence of HCV antibodies in serum does not imply protective immunity. False-positive anti-HCV results are rare in certain clinical settings, because the majority of persons being tested have evidence of liver disease, and the sensitivity and specificity of the screening assays are high. However, among populations with a low prevalence of HCV infection, false-positive results do occur. This is of concern when testing is performed on asymptomatic persons for whom no clinical information is available, when persons are being tested for HCV infection for the first time, and when testing is being used to determine the need for postexposure follow-up.
- All HCV antibody–positive samples should be followed by nucleic acid testing for HCVRNA according to the testing algorithm recommended by the CDC (MMWR, May 7, 2013).
- If HCVRNA is detected, that indicates current infection. If HCVRNA is not detected, that indicates either past, resolved HCV infection or false-positive HCV antibody test.
- HCV serologic testing is not useful for detection of early/acute HCV infection, and it is not useful for differentiating between past (resolved) and chronic hepatitis C. In most infected people, antibodies will show up in blood within 6 weeks to 3 months.

- Infants born to HCV-infected mothers may have false-reactive HCV antibody test results due to transplacental passage of maternal HCV IgG antibodies. HCV antibody testing is not recommended until at least 18 months of age in these infants.
- May remain negative in immunosuppression and renal failure, although it appears to be a rare finding.

HEPATITIS C VIRUS (HCV) ANTIGEN

❑ **Definition**

- This test, based on detection of a 21-kDa protein made by a stable region of the HCV genome, may be used in research settings to aid in the diagnosis of HCV infection. It is a major component of the viral capsid. It is not clear whether it circulates freely or is only in viral particles. A commercial immunoassay to detect HCV antigen is available for research use only. Level strongly correlates with HCV RNA.
- **Normal range:** Negative.

❑ **Use**

- To predict a sustained virologic response early during therapy (4 weeks), reaching an optimal performance at month 3. The determination of total HCV core antigen levels in serum constitutes an accurate and reliable alternative to HCV RNA for monitoring and predicting treatment outcome in patients receiving PEG–interferon/ribavirin combination therapy.

❑ **Interpretation**

- Increased in hepatitis C exposure.

❑ **Limitations**

- Lacks sensitivity in early detection. HCV antigen has similar sensitivity in infection with all genotypes of HCV.

HEPATITIS C VIRUS (HCV) GENOTYPING ASSAY

❑ **Definition**

- The HCV genotyping assay identifies HCV genotypes 1–6 in human serum or EDTA plasma samples. Availability of subtype information depends on the method used for testing. The methods may differ in their ability to genotype samples with low viral load or mixed infection.
- **Normal range:** Negative.

❑ **Use**

- Methods:
  - ▼ Invader (Third Wave)
  - ▼ True Gene (Bayer)
  - ▼ LiPA (Innogenetics)
  - ▼ TaqMan (Abbot Diagnostics)
  - ▼ "Home brew" sequencing

17

- ■ The HCV genotyping assay should be used in the management of HCV-infected individuals undergoing antiviral therapy

❑ **Limitations**

- ■ Samples with low viral load may be untypable. Sequencing methods are less effective than hybridization methods in genotyping samples with mixed genotypes.

HEPATITIS C VIRUS (HCV) RNA, QUANTITATIVE VIRAL LOAD: MOLECULAR ASSAY

❑ **Definition**

- ■ The HCV viral load assay quantifies HCV RNA in the plasma of HCV-infected individuals. The HCV test is standardized against the first WHO International Standard for HCV RNA for nucleic acid amplification technology assays (NIBSC code 96/790).
- ■ **Normal range:** Not detected when the result is below the level of detection of the assay.

❑ **Use**

- ■ Methods
  - ▼ Branched DNA assay (bDNA; Siemens): A signal amplification technology that detects the presence of specific nucleic acids by measuring the signal generated by branched, labeled DNA probes; a reliable method that provides consistent results in the higher range of the assay.
  - ▼ Real-time PCR: Reverse transcription followed by amplification and quantification of the targeted DNA molecule; generally offers both a wider range of quantification and a lower limit of detection than the bDNA method.
- ■ Used in the management of HCV-infected individuals undergoing antiviral therapy.

❑ **Limitations**

- ■ PCR inhibitors in the specimen may lead to underestimation of viral quantitation or false-negative results in rare cases. However, current technologies include internal controls which if not amplified during the PCR, will not give a result rather than a false-negative result.

HEPATITIS D VIRUS (HDV; DELTA HEPATITIS) ANTIBODY

❑ **Definition**

- ■ HDV is a subviral agent that is dependent on the HBV virus for its life cycle; therefore, HDV infection cannot occur in the absence of HBV infection.
- ■ **Normal range:** Negative.

❑ **Use**

- ■ Diagnosis of concurrent HDV infection in patients with fulminant acute HBV infection (acute coinfection), chronic HBV infection (chronic coinfection), or acute exacerbation of known chronic HBV infection (HDV superinfection).

❑ **Interpretation**

 ▪ Increased in previous or current hepatitis D infection.

❑ **Limitations**

 ▪ The role of HDV antibody testing is controversial because the incidence of infection with HDV has declined markedly in the United States with use of HBV vaccine.
 ▪ Interferon treatment may decrease the antibody levels.
 ▪ This testing should be ordered only when the patient has an acute or chronic hepatitis B infection.

HEPATITIS E VIRUS (HEV) ANTIBODY (IgM AND IgG)

❑ **Definition**

 ▪ HEV is a small nonenveloped virus that causes an acute, usually self-limited, infection that is spread by the fecal–oral route. HEV is endemic in Southeast and Central Asia, with several outbreaks observed in the Middle East, northern and western parts of Africa, and Mexico. In developed countries, HEV infection occurs mainly in persons who have traveled to disease endemic areas.
 ▪ Transmission of HEV may also occur parenterally. Direct person-to-person transmission is rare. Unusually high mortality (approximately 20%) occurs in patients infected in the third trimester of pregnancy. There is no carrier state associated with HEV.
 ▪ Viremia and virus shedding occur in the preicteric phase and last up to 10 days into the clinical phase. After an incubation period ranging from 15 to 60 days, HEV-infected patients develop symptoms of hepatitis with appearance of anti-HEV IgM antibody in serum, followed by detectable anti-HEV IgG antibody within a few days. Anti-HEV IgM remains positive for up to 6 months after onset of symptoms, whereas anti-HEV IgG levels usually persist for years after infection. Anti-HEV IgG is the serologic marker of choice for diagnosis of past HEV infection.
 ▪ **Normal range:** Negative.

❑ **Use**

 ▪ HEV antibody IgM: diagnosing acute or recent (<6 months) hepatitis E infection
 ▪ HEV antibody IgG: diagnosis of past hepatitis E

❑ **Interpretation**

 ▪ Increased in previous or current hepatitis E infection

HERPES SIMPLEX VIRUS (HSV) CULTURE (RULE OUT)

❑ **Definition and Use**

 ▪ HSV infection usually involves vesicular rashes of the oropharyngeal or genital sites, although HSV is capable of causing serious disseminated disease,

17

including infection of multiple organ systems. Vertical transmission may result in neonatal infections, involving localized disease (skin, eyes, and mouth), systemic infection, or encephalitis. Other sites of infection in normal or immunocompromised patients include skin, conjunctiva, and the CNS. HSV can cause severe disseminated disease in immunocompromised patients, resulting in multiorgan dysfunction and failure.

■ This test may be used to isolate HSV when specific diagnosis is required for patient management.

■ Patient specimens are inoculated onto cultured eukaryotic cells, like human foreskin fibroblast or Vero cells. Tube or shell vial cultures may be used for HSV isolation. Cytopathic effect is usually manifested within 24–48 hours in specimens with heavy virus loads, such as vesicular lesions.

■ Specific HSV-1 and HSV-2 antibody reagents may be used to further characterize HSV culture isolates, as needed.

■ **Turnaround time:** Most positive cultures are detected within 2 days. Negative tube cultures are typically incubated for up to 7 days. Shell vial cultures are usually finalized within 48–72 hours.

❑ **Special Collection and Transport Instructions**

■ General recommendations for viral culture apply.

■ Specimens should be collected early in acute infection.

■ Specimens should be collected according to general recommendations for virus culture of the specimen type. Specimens from cutaneous or mucous membranes are most commonly submitted for viral culture to rule out HSV. Samples should be taken from fresh, wet lesions, ideally from intact vesicles after unroofing.

■ Most specimens should be placed in a viral transport medium and transported at 4°C.

❑ **Interpretation**

■ Expected results:
   ▼ **Positive:** Cell cultures positive for HSV indicate probable active infection. Occasionally, positive cultures represent asymptomatic shedding of virus that may be clinically insignificant.
   ▼ **Negative:** Negative cell cultures do not rule out HSV infection, especially for CSF and other nonvesicular lesions.

❑ **Limitations**

■ There may be poor sensitivity for certain specimen types, such as CSF. Molecular diagnostic testing may improve detection from these specimens.

■ **Common pitfalls:** Collection of specimens from dried, crusted lesions.

■ HSV-specific DFA, performed on cells from the base of vesicles or wet ulcers, provides rapid and specific identification of HSV infection.

■ PCR is the most sensitive method for HSV detection and is most useful for diagnosis of CNS infections.

■ Culture isolates may be typed, but clinical management decisions can generally be made without typing results. Typing is used mainly for epidemiologic purposes.

HERPES VIRUS (HSV OR VZV) DIRECT DETECTION DIRECT FLUORESCENT ANTIBODY (DFA)

❑ **Definition and Use**

- These tests may be ordered in patients presenting with a vesicular rash in whom specific and rapid diagnosis of HSV or VZV infection is important for therapy or management. Infection is diagnosed by detection of antigens in specimens by staining with fluorescently labeled virus-specific antibodies.
- Cells are collected from the base of wet ulcers or vesicles (after unroofing) using a swab or edge of a scalpel. Slides are prepared by gently rolling the swab or spreading cells collected by scalpel onto the slide surface.
- After fixation, the smear is stained with an HSV- or VZV-specific antibody reagent tagged with a fluorescent label. After washing away excess reagent, the slide is examined by fluorescence microscopy for the presence of cells showing specific staining.
- **Turnaround time:** <24 hours.

❑ **Interpretation**

- **Expected results:** Negative, with no cells showing fluorescent staining
- **Positive result:** The presence of any cells showing +2 or greater specific fluorescent staining

❑ **Limitations**

- The slide must be assessed to ensure cells are present in the smear. If no cells are present, the slide is uninterpretable.
- The number of staining cells drops with evolution of the skin lesion from vesicle to crusted/healing ulcer.
- Faint staining may be an indication of problems with the staining technique or reagents.

HERPES SIMPLEX VIRUS (HSV) SEROLOGY TESTS, TYPE 1 AND TYPE 2–SPECIFIC ANTIBODIES, IgG AND IgM

❑ **Definition**

- HSV is a common STD worldwide. Although HSV type 2 (HSV-2) remains the main causative agent for the preponderance of virologically confirmed infections, HSV type 1 (HSV-1) is associated with an increasing proportion of cases of genital herpes.
- HSV-1 generally infects the mucous membrane of the eye, mouth, and mucocutaneous junctions of the face, and it is also one of the most common causes of severe sporadic encephalitis in adults.
- HSV-2 is usually associated with mucocutaneous genital lesions. Recently, an increasing number of genital herpes infections have been shown to be due to HSV-1. HSV-1 causes primary episodes indistinguishable from HSV-2, but with less frequent recurrence.
- Pregnant women who develop genital herpes near the time of delivery are at high risk for transmission to the neonate. Transmission of HSV

17

infection to neonates is associated with high morbidity and mortality rates if untreated.

- Because HSV-1 and HSV-2 share common antigenic determinants, antibody detected against one viral type may cross-react with the other viral type. Truly type-specific antibody tests are based on glycoprotein G1 (from HSV-1) and glycoprotein G2 (from HSV-2), as these proteins exhibit very limited homology. The CDC recommends the use of type-specific glycoprotein G based assays when serology is performed.
- Other names: Herpes simplex serology, HSV antibody titer.
- **Normal range:** Negative.

❏ Use

- To diagnose a patient with a history of genital lesions who did not have a diagnostic workup, diagnose a past or present HSV infection in a patient with an atypical presentation, determine susceptibility of a sexual partner of a patient with documented genital HSV infection, and identify asymptomatic HSV infection in pregnant women who are at risk for shedding at the time of delivery with potential transmission to the infant or help predict the risk of recurrence.

❏ Interpretation

- HSV IgM–combined positive result (i.e., the presence of IgM class HSV 1 and/or 2 antibodies) indicates recent infection. The presence of HSV 1 and/or 2 antibodies may indicate a primary or reactivated infection but cannot distinguish between them.
- The IgG antibody assay differentiates between type 1 and 2 HSV antibodies. The presence of IgG antibodies specific for HSV type 1 or 2 indicates previous exposure to the corresponding serotype of the virus.

❏ Limitations

- A clinical diagnosis of genital herpes should be confirmed with laboratory testing. The diagnosis can be made by viral culture, PCR, DFA, Tzanck preparation, and type-specific serologic tests. The choice of test varies with the clinical presentation.
- Both the CDC and the International Union against Sexually Transmitted Infections (IUSTI) recommend using molecular methods for typing all patients with first-episode genital herpes.
- The prevalence of HSV antibodies can vary depending on a number of factors such as age, gender, geographic location, socioeconomic status, race, sexual behavior, testing method used, specimen collection and handling procedures, and the clinical and epidemiologic history of individual patients.
- A negative result does not necessarily rule out a primary or reactivated infection, since specimens may have been collected too early in the course of disease, when antibodies have not yet reached detectable levels, or too late, after IgM levels have declined below detectable levels.
- False-positive test results may occur in patients infected with EBV, in primary or reactivated varicella virus infection, and in the presence of rheumatoid factor antibodies.

HUMAN IMMUNODEFICIENCY VIRUS 1/2 ANTIBODY SCREEN

❏ **Definition**

- HIV is a highly variable virus that mutates readily, and numerous virus strains may be classified into types, groups, and subtypes. There are two types of HIV: HIV-1 and HIV-2. Both types are transmitted by sexual contact, through blood, and from mother to child, and they appear to cause clinically indistinguishable AIDS. However, it seems that HIV-2 is less easily transmitted, and the period between initial infection and illness is longer in the case of HIV-2.

- The diagnosis of HIV infection is established by one of the following methods: detecting antibodies to the virus; detecting the viral p24 antigen; detecting viral nucleic acid (NAT); or culturing HIV. The most widely used test is the detection of IgG antibody against HIV-1 and HIV-2 antigens in serum. HIV-1 antigens include p24 (a nucleocapsid protein) and gp 120 and gp 41 (envelope proteins). Antibodies to gp41 and p24 antigens are the first detectable serologic markers following HIV infection. IgG antibodies appear 6–12 weeks following HIV infection in the majority of patients and by 6 months in 95% of patients. IgG antibodies to HIV generally persist for life. Positive tests should be confirmed with repeat antibody testing, testing to differentiate HIV-1 and HIV-2, and confirmatory testing (e.g., type-specific HIV RNA, western blot assays). Assays for IgM antibodies are not used because they are relatively insensitive.

- Fourth-generation HIV tests can detect both antibody and p24 antigen. The main advantage of these assays is the ability to detect HIV infection during the "window period," where antibody may not be detected.

- HIV has evolved into several groups: M, N, O, and P. Group M ("main") is considered the pandemic strain and comprise most strains of HIV. Group O ("outlier") represents far fewer strains from Cameroon, Gabon, and Equatorial Guinea. Group N ("non-M/non-O") and group P are represented by very few isolates and have only been documented in Cameroon. Viruses from group M are subsequently divided into 10 distinct subtypes (A–J). HIV testing was originally developed to detect HIV subtype B, the most common subtype in the United States and Europe. The estimated frequency of non-B subtypes in the United States is approximately 2%. The CDC does not recommend routine testing for HIV-2 in settings other than blood centers.

- **Normal range:** Negative.

❏ **Use**

- Screening of HIV-1 and/or HIV-2 infection, organ transplant donors, testing individuals who have documented and significant exposure to other infected individuals, and testing exposed high-risk individuals for detection of antibody (e.g., persons with multiple sex partners, persons with a history of other STDs, IV drug users, infants born to infected mothers, allied health care workers, and public service employees who have contact with blood and blood products) (Figure 17-1)

17

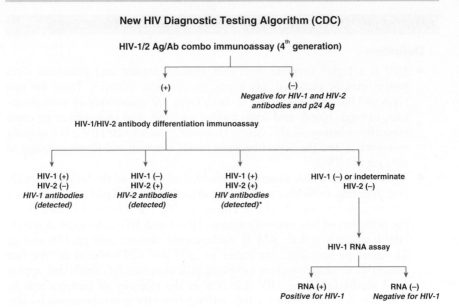

Figure 17−1 *HIV diagnostic testing algorithm. (From Morbidity & Mortality Weekly Report. June 21, 2013, 62:490–494.)*

❏ Interpretation

- Positive in HIV infection; a positive screen test is considered "preliminary" and requires confirmation by definitive, specific testing, like HIV-1 RNA or Western blot assay. The patient with a positive test should be told of the result and advised on avoiding risk of transmitting HIV.
- A negative screen test is regarded as a true negative, and requires no confirmation; the patient may be informed that the test is negative.

❏ Limitations

- Common causes of false-negative results can occur due to acute infection and failure to detect certain HIV subtypes.
- Rare causes of false-negative results include immune dysfunction due to defective humoral response or agammaglobulinemia, immunosuppression due to malignancy or medications, delay in seroconversion following early initiation of antiretroviral therapy, and fulminant HIV infection.
- False-positive test results for HIV infection have been documented after participation in an HIV vaccine trial.
- Indeterminate results may occur due to partial seroconversion during acute HIV infection, advanced HIV infection with decreased titers of p24 antibodies, or infection with HIV-2.
- Other causes for an indeterminate test result in persons who are not infected with HIV include

▼ Cross-reacting alloantibodies from pregnancy
▼ Autoantibodies (collagen–vascular diseases, autoimmune diseases, and malignancy)
▼ Receipt of an experimental HIV-1 vaccine
▼ Influenza vaccination

Suggested Reading

CLSI. *Criteria for Laboratory Testing and Diagnosis of Human Immunodeficiency Virus Infection; Approved Guideline.* CLSI document M53-A. Wayne, PA: Clinical and Laboratory Standards Institute; 2011.

HUMAN IMMUNODEFICIENCY VIRUS (HIV-1) CONFIRMATORY WESTERN BLOT ASSAY

❏ Definition

- The Western blot (WB) assay is a method in which individual proteins of an HIV-1 lysate or recombinant HIV proteins allow the determination of antigenic specificity of the antibodies in the patients' serum. This is considered a confirmation test for HIV serology.
- Western blot assays are specific for different HIV species and subtypes.
- HIV-1 antibodies present in the specimen bind to HIV-1 antigens (p15, p17, p24, p31, gp41, p51, p66, p55, gp120, gp160).
- Alternative confirmation testing algorithms have been described, including use of a second, different EIA, IFA, line immunoassay, or nucleic acid amplification test.

❏ Use

- The Western blot is used for confirmation of repeatedly reactive HIV antibody screen or rapid HIV antibody results.
- Western blots specific for HIV-2 or HIV-1 subtypes other than M should be considered for patients at epidemiologic risk for such infections, or when HIV-1 WB gives indeterminate or negative results. HIV-2 is most commonly acquired in West Africa.

❏ Interpretation

- **Positive result:** As established by CDC, the interpretive criterion for HIV-1 is defined by the presence of any two of the following bands: p24, gp41, and gp120/160.
- **Indeterminate results:** HIV infection is neither confirmed nor ruled out; additional testing is required.
- Indeterminate results may be caused by factors related to HIV infection, including a weak titer of anti–HIV-1 antibodies (e.g., early seroconversion), advanced AIDS, or infection with HIV-2 or HIV-1 subtype O. Nonspecific causes include autoantibodies, hemodialysis, hypergammaglobulinemia, or recent vaccination.
- Additional testing for indeterminate results may include HIV-1 RNA testing, WB for HIV-2 or HIV-1 subtype O, or repeat HIV serology and WB in 4–6 weeks.
- **Negative result:** Negative results do not exclude the diagnosis of HIV infection; further testing is required.

17

- Additional testing for negative results may include HIV-1 RNA testing, WB for HIV-2 or HIV-1 subtype O, or repeat HIV serology and WB in 4–6 weeks.
- Persistent reactivity of the antibody screening assay on repeat testing with negative confirmation by WB pattern suggests nonspecific reactivity and the absence of HIV infection.

❏ **Limitations**

- HIV WB testing should be ordered only on sera that are repeatedly reactive by HIV screening EIA or rapid HIV antibody tests.
- Patients with HIV-2 infection may give indeterminate results for HIV-1 Western blots. For HIV-2 WB test, no single standard can currently be applied to all tests. The CDC recommends that each test be interpreted by the criteria suggested by the kit manufacturer.
- HIV-2 cross-reacts with HIV-1 in serologic tests. A positive screen test for HIV 1 and 2 antibodies with a repeated negative or indeterminate HIV-1 WB suggests positive HIV-2 infection and need to be confirmed HIV-2–specific test.

HUMAN IMMUNODEFICIENCY VIRUS TYPE 1 (HIV-1) GENOTYPE (MOLECULAR ASSAY)*

❏ **Definition**

- HIV-1 genotyping detects HIV genomic mutations that confer resistance to specific types of antiretroviral drugs. Current sequence-based assays detect resistance mutations in the protease (PR) and part of the reverse transcriptase (RT) genes. Two Food and Drug Administration (FDA)-approved genotyping methods are commercially available: the ViroSeq HIV-1 genotyping system, version 2.0 (Celera Diagnostics) and the Trugene HIV-1 genotyping system for drug resistance (Siemens Healthcare Diagnostics).

❏ **Use**

- As an aid in monitoring and treating HIV-1–infected individuals:
  - ▼ At initial presentation, before initial drug therapy
  - ▼ At drug therapy failure

❏ **Limitations**

- Viral load not <1,000 copies/mL for TrueGene and 2,000 copies/mL for ViroSeq.
- The FDA-approved tests are specific for analysis of subtype B HIV-1 only. For analysis of non–B HIV-1 strains that represent up to 90% of HIV-1 variants circulating worldwide, lab-developed tests should be used.

HUMAN IMMUNODEFICIENCY VIRUS TYPE 1 (HIV-1) RNA, QUANTITATIVE VIRAL LOAD (MOLECULAR ASSAY)*

❏ **Definition**

- The HIV-1 viral load assay quantifies HIV-1 RNA in the plasma of HIV-1 infected individuals. Result of HIV-1 RNA testing are reported in copies/mL

*Contributed by Marzena M. Galdzicka, PhD.

and/or International Units/mL (IU/mL). Results reported in IU/mL can be compared between laboratories independently which platform was used to obtained results.

- **Normal range:** Not detected when the result is below the level of detection of the assay.

❑ **Use**

- Methods
  - ▼ Branched DNA assay (bDNA; Siemens): A signal amplification technology that detects the presence of specific nucleic acids by measuring the signal generated by branched, labeled DNA probes; a reliable method that provides consistent results in the higher range of the assay.
  - ▼ Real-time PCR (Cobas AmpliPrep/Cobas TaqMan, Roche): Reverse transcription is followed by PCR amplification and quantification of the targeted DNA molecule; generally offers both a wider range of quantification and a lower limit of detection than the bDNA method.
- Used in the management of HIV-1–infected individuals undergoing antiviral therapy.

❑ **Limitations**

- PCR inhibitors in the specimen may lead to underestimation of viral quantitation or false-negative results in rare cases.
- For consistency in interpretation of patient results, the same methodology should be used in patient management.

HUMAN PAPILLOMAVIRUS (HPV) MOLECULAR TESTING*

❑ **Definition**

- HPV test provides information to clinicians on a patient's risk for developing cervical cancer. There are currently five FDA-approved HPV assays that are detecting high-risk (HR) genital HPV types that are commonly associated with cervical cancer. Hybrid Capture 2 High Risk HPV DNA Test (Digene, Qiagen) detects 13 HR-HPV types; Cervista™ HPV HR (Third Wave Technologies, Hologic) detects 14 HR genital HPV types; Cervista HPV 16/18 identifies DNA types 16 and 18; Cobas HPV Test (Roche) specifically identifies types HPV 16 and HPV 18 while concurrently detecting the rest of the high risk types. These four tests detect HPV viral DNA in cervical cells collected during the liquid-based Pap test ("pap smear"). APTIMA HPV assay with the TIGRIS DTS System (Gen-Probe) is the first FDA-approved assay that detects the messenger RNA of two HPV viral oncogenes, E6 and E7. Although HPV infection is very common, and usually self-resolving, if HPV RNA is present, the patient is in a higher risk category for developing cervical cancer than if HPV is not detected.

---

*Contributed by Marzena M. Galdzicka, PhD.

❑ **Use**

▪ Guidelines for cervical cancer screening that include HPV DNA testing issued by the American Society for Colposcopy and Cervical Pathology (ASCCP), the Centers for Disease Control and Prevention, and the American College of Obstetricians and Gynecologists recommend that

▼ HPV molecular testing is not used for evaluation of women younger than 21 years—most HPV infections in this age group are transient and will be cleared by the immune system.

▼ HPV molecular testing is performed as a reflex test for women older than 21 with atypical cells of undetermined significance (ASC-US) Pap test result,

▼ HPV molecular testing is performed concurrently with a Pap test for women 30 years and older.

❑ **Limitations**

▪ Test results may be affected by improper specimen collection, storage, or specimen processing.

▪ Cervista™ HPV HR HPV tests, Cobas HPV Test, and TIGRIS DTS detect high-risk HPV types 16, 18, 31, 33, 35, 39, 45, 51, 52, 56, 58, 59, 66 (with exception of Hybrid Capture 2 HR HPV), and 68 but not HPV low-risk types.

▪ Testing of alternate specimen types (rectal and oropharyngeal) is not currently FDA approved; however, some laboratories have conducted validation studies to offer testing.

LEGIONELLA ANTIGEN SCREEN

❑ **Definition**

▪ Legionellosis refers to two clinical syndromes caused by bacteria of the genus *Legionella*—Legionnaires disease and Pontiac fever. Legionnaires disease is considered an atypical pneumonia. *Legionella pneumophila* is responsible for approximately 90% of infections. Most cases are caused by *L. pneumophila*, serogroup 1. Although a number of prominent clinical manifestations are distinctive for *Legionella* infection, none of them are pathognomonic or highly specific. Therefore, laboratory testing using specialized tests for *Legionella* should be considered for all patients hospitalized with community-acquired pneumonia.

▪ Culturing for *Legionella* species is the single most important laboratory test. Urinary antigen testing is rapid, sensitive, and specific, but it is only useful for the diagnosis of *L. pneumophila* type 1 infection. The combination of culture of an appropriate respiratory specimen and urinary antigen testing is optimal as a diagnostic approach. Serologic tests are generally far less useful for the diagnosis of an individual patient. Although PCR-based tests exist, to date they do not exceed the sensitivity of culturing the organism.

▪ **Normal range:** Negative.

❑ **Use**

▪ In conjunction to culture for the presumptive diagnosis of past or current Legionnaire disease (*L. pneumophila* serogroup 1), patients suspected of health care–associated pneumonia, patients who have failed outpatient antibiotic therapy, and patients with a travel history within 2 weeks before the onset of illness.

❑ **Interpretation**

- **Positive:** Presumptive positive for *L. pneumophila* serogroup 1 antigen in urine, suggesting current or past infection.
- **Negative:** Presumptive negative for *L. pneumophila* serogroup 1 antigen in urine, suggesting no recent or current infection. Infection due to *Legionella* cannot be ruled out, since other serogroups and species may cause disease, antigen may not be present in urine in early infection, and the level of antigen present in the urine may be below the detection limit of the test.

❑ **Limitations**

- There is no single confirmatory laboratory test for Legionnaire disease. Culture results, serology, and antigen detection methods may all be useful, in conjunction with clinical findings, for diagnosis.
- The *Legionella* antigen test will not detect infections caused by other *L. pneumophila* serogroups and by other *Legionella* species. Culture is recommended for suspected pneumonia to detect causative agents other than *L. pneumophila* serogroup 1 and to recover *L. pneumophila* serogroup 1 when antigen is not detected.
- Excretion of *Legionella* antigen in urine may vary depending on the individual patient. Antigen excretion may begin as early as 3 days after onset of symptoms and persist for up to a year afterward.
- A positive *Legionella* urinary antigen test result can occur due to current or past infection and, therefore, is not definitive for infection without supporting evidence.

LEGIONELLA CULTURE (RULE OUT)

❑ **Definition**

- This test is requested for diagnosis of legionellosis by culture of patient specimens, usually of the lower respiratory tract. Testing is recommended on patients with pneumonia who fail treatment, have severe pneumonia, are immunocompromised, or have epidemiologic risk for legionellosis. Special testing, usually performed outside of clinical microbiology laboratories, is needed for evaluation of environmental cultures for isolation of *Legionella* species.

❑ **Special Collection and Transport Instructions**

- Specimens should be submitted early in the acute phase of infection.
- Sputum (expectorated or induced), BAL, bronchial brush, lung biopsy, or tracheal aspirate specimens are usually submitted for culture to rule out *Legionella*.
- Submission of multiple specimens is recommended to improve sensitivity of detection because shedding may be intermittent for this intracellular pathogen.
- Blood, cardiac valve, or other specimen types are occasionally submitted when extrapulmonary legionellosis is suspected. (If *Legionella* endocarditis is suspected, alert the laboratory because special processing and culture techniques are required.)

17

❑ **Use**

- Culture Method:
  - ▼ All specimens should be inoculated onto supplemented BCYE agar, both nonselective and selective.
  - ▼ Specimens may be diluted 1:10 in tryptic soy broth to prepare culture inoculum. For specimens that are likely to be heavily contaminated by endogenous flora, a 1:10 dilution of specimen in 0.2M KCl acid wash (pH = 2.2) is recommended to improve isolation of *Legionella*. The specimen is incubated at room temperature for 4 minutes, and then aliquots are inoculated onto selective and nonselective BCYE media as for unwashed specimens.
  - ▼ Cultures are incubated at 35–37°C in a humidified incubator. CO_2 supplementation (2–5%) may be used.
- **Turnaround time:** Cultures are inspected for up to 5 days after inoculation. Additional time is required after isolation for confirmation and further characterization.

❑ **Interpretation**

- **Expected results:** Negative.
- **Positive results:** Positive cultures confirm a diagnosis of legionellosis. Isolates from *Legionella* cultures must be confirmed as *Legionella* species by further testing and characterization.
- **Negative results:** Because *Legionella* may be shed intermittently, a negative culture does not rule out legionellosis.

❑ **Limitations**

- *Legionella* are typically present in low concentrations in patient specimens. Isolation of *Legionella* from infected extrapulmonary specimens is inconsistent.
- Diagnosis of legionellosis may require multiple testing modalities, including culture, serology, PCR, and antigen detection methods, in conjunction with clinical findings.
- **Common pitfalls:**
  - ▼ The rejection criteria applied to sputum specimens for routine bacterial cultures should not be applied to specimens submitted for *Legionella* culture.
  - ▼ *Legionella* may be present in very low concentrations in respiratory secretions. Therefore, BAL and bronchial brush specimens should be directly inoculated onto BCYE media before dilutions are prepared for quantitative bacterial cultures.

MACROSCOPIC EXAMINATION, ARTHROPOD

❑ **Use**

- This test is used to identify arthropods by visual examination. This test is indicated for identification of ticks, mites, fleas, spiders, lice, maggots, and other insects that may be associated with human infection, infestation, disease, or disease transmission.

- **Method**
  - ▼ These agents are submitted in clean containers with tight-fitting lids. Specimens for scabies detection may be collected by skin scraping.
  - ▼ Plucked hair may be submitted for identification of nits and the eggs of lice. Maggots may be expelled spontaneously, surgically, by vacuum extraction, or by other methods.
  - ▼ The submitted arthropods and insects are inspected by the naked eye or with low-power microscopy. Identification is based on morphologic features.
- **Turnaround time:** 24–48 hours.

❏ **Interpretation**
- **Expected results:** Negative.

MACROSCOPIC EXAMINATION, PARASITES

❏ **Definition and Use**
- Large parasitic pathogens, or fragments, may be isolated from patients. Examples include single proglottids or chains of tapeworm segments, pinworms, or ascarid worms.
- This test is used for identification of parasites by visual inspection.
- The submitted parasite is inspected by the naked eye or with low-power microscopy. Identification is based on specific morphologic features. Speciation of *Taenia* proglottids may be attempted by techniques for evaluation of lateral uterine branches, like injection of India ink through the genital pore.
- The eggs of *T. solium* can infect humans. Therefore, great care must be taken in the laboratory when examining *Taenia* proglottids.
- **Turnaround time:** 24–48 hours.

❏ **Interpretation**
- **Positive result:** A human parasitic pathogen is identified.
- **Negative result:** A nonhuman pathogen or artifact is identified.

❏ **Limitations**
- Limited material available for examination. The specimen may have been fragmented or damaged during collection or transport so that specific identification is impossible.
- **Common pitfall:** Nonhuman pathogens, like earthworms, may be submitted for examination.

MEASLES SEROLOGY SCREEN (MEASLES [RUBEOLA] IgG AND IgM)*

❏ **Definition**
- Measles is a highly contagious, acute, exanthematous disease caused by the measles (rubeola) virus. It is generally self-limiting and without serious consequences, although complications such as bronchopneumonia and otitis

---

*Contributed by Marzena M. Galdzicka, PhD.

17

media do occur. The most serious consequence is encephalomyelitis (about 1 in 10,000 cases). Natural infection with measles virus confers permanent immunity. Measles infection poses a serious threat to immunosuppressed or immunocompromised patients. For these reasons, the laboratory diagnosis of measles has become increasingly important, notwithstanding the reduction in the incidence due to the introduction of vaccines.

■ The usual means of laboratory diagnosis of acute measles is serologic, by the demonstration of either a fourfold or greater rise in virus-specific IgG antibody in acute and convalescent serum pairs, or by the detection of virus-specific IgM antibody in a single, early serum specimen.

■ **Normal range:** Negative.

❏ Use

■ To assist in the diagnosis of acute-phase infection with rubeola (measles) virus and assist in identifying nonimmune individuals.

❏ Interpretation

■ Positive IgM results, with or without positive IgG results, indicate a recent infection with measles virus.

■ Positive IgG results coupled with a negative IgM result indicate previous exposure to measles virus and immunity to this viral infection.

■ Negative IgG and IgM results indicate the absence of prior exposure to rubeola and nonimmunity.

■ Equivocal results should be followed up with a new serum specimen within 10–14 days.

■ False-positive measles IgM results can occur due to cross reactivity with rheumatoid factor, parvovirus, rubella and roseola antibodies.

❏ Limitations

■ If the assay is used with cord blood as the specimen source, positive results should be interpreted with caution. The presence of IgG antibodies to measles in cord blood may be the result of passive transfer of maternal antibody to the fetus. A negative result, however, may be helpful in ruling out infection.

METHICILLIN-RESISTANT *STAPHYLOCOCCUS AUREUS* CULTURE (RULE OUT)*

❏ Definition and Use

■ This test is usually ordered to detect methicillin-resistant *S. aureus* (MRSA) carriage in asymptomatic patients for infection control purposes. It is indicated to screen patients at risk for MRSA self-infection or transmitting MRSA to close contacts, such as other hospitalized patients. The test may also be requested to document clearance of MRSA carriage.

■ Patient specimens are plated onto selective agar, typically containing 4–6 μg/ mL of oxacillin. A base agar selective for gram-positive organisms (like PEA) or staphylococci (mannitol–salt agar) is often used to improve sensitivity of

*Contributed by Marzena M. Galdzicka, PhD.

detection of MRSA. Selective chromogenic agar is commercially available to screen for MRSA carriage. These agars provide increased sensitivity and decreased turnaround time for detection of MRSA carriage.

- **Special collection and transport instructions:** Swab specimens of the anterior nares, throat, axilla, perineum, and/or umbilicus (neonates) are usually submitted for MRSA screening cultures.
- **Turnaround time:** 48–72 hours.

❑ **Interpretation**

- **Expected results:** Negative.
- Any growth of *S. aureus* likely represents MRSA; confirmation of isolate identification and oxacillin resistance by standardized susceptibility testing is recommended.

❑ **Limitations**

- **Common pitfall:** The MRSA screening culture is not recommended for evaluation of potentially infected material. Because only selective media are used, other potential pathogens would be missed if MRSA screening culture only is performed. MRSA isolates grow well in routine bacterial cultures submitted for evaluation of patient specimens.
- Commercially available molecular diagnostic methods have been developed for detection of MRSA carriage. These assays have been shown to be more sensitive for detection of MRSA carriage, but the clinical implication for detection of very low level MRSA carriage has not been clearly defined.

MICROSPORIDIA EXAMINATION

❑ **Definition and Use**

- This test is submitted for the evaluation of stool specimens in patients with diarrhea and risk for enteric parasite infection. It is used for the direct detection of the intracellular microsporidial parasitic pathogens.
- Permanent smears of diarrheal stool are stained with modified trichrome stains (chromotrope 2R) or similar stains.
- Fresh and preserved specimens are collected and transported to the laboratory according to recommendations for stool submitted for routine O & P examination.
- **Turnaround time:** 24–72 hours.

❑ **Interpretation**

- **Expected results:** Negative.
- **Positive results:** Confirms a diagnosis of microsporidiosis in patients with compatible signs and symptoms.
- **Negative results:** A negative result does not rule out microsporidiosis. Multiple specimens may be required for diagnosis in infected patients.

Suggested Readings

CLSI. *Procedures for the Recovery and Identification of Parasites From the Intestinal Tract; Approved Guideline*, 2nd ed. Wayne, PA: Clinical and Laboratory Standards Institute; 2005.
Garcia LS. *Diagnostic Parasitology*, 5th ed. Washington, DC: ASM Press; 2007.

MUMPS SEROLOGY SCREEN (MUMPS IgG AND IgM)

❑ Definition

- Mumps is a generalized illness characterized by fever and by inflammation and swelling of the salivary glands, particularly the parotid glands. Mumps is usually not severe in children, but in the adults, the inflammation may involve the ovaries or testes (orchitis).
- Inflammation and swelling of the parotid glands (parotitis) in mumps infection are usually sufficiently diagnostic to preclude serologic confirmation. However, inasmuch as one third of mumps infections are subclinical, viral isolation, and/or some other serologic procedure may be required.
- **Normal range:** Negative.

❑ Use

- Virus isolation is cumbersome and time consuming and is usually an impractical procedure for the typical clinical laboratory. Serodiagnosis of mumps infection has been accomplished by neutralization, hemagglutination inhibition (HI), indirect immunofluorescence, and complement fixation (CF). These methods lack specificity, which limits their usefulness in determining immune status. The HI test also requires pretreatment of test sera to remove nonspecific inhibitors of hemagglutination.
- Enzyme immunoassays (EIA, ELISA) are sensitive and specific, and their sensitivity equals that of the neutralization test and is greater than CF or HI. They are, therefore, reliable tests for the determination of immune status. Serum IgM antibody testing should be obtained no earlier than 3 days following initial onset of symptoms. The test typically remains positive for up to 4 weeks but may be negative in up to 50–60% of specimens from individuals with acute disease who were previously immunized. A negative IgM titer in vaccinated individuals, therefore, does not rule out mumps. Immunity to mumps is established by demonstrating IgG antibodies on ELISA.
- The test is used to assist in the diagnosis of acute-phase infection with mumps virus and to assist in identifying nonimmune individuals.

❑ Interpretation

- Positive IgM results, with or without positive IgG results, indicate a recent infection with mumps virus.
- Positive IgG results coupled with a negative IgM result indicate previous exposure to mumps virus and immunity to this viral infection.
- Negative IgG and IgM results indicate the absence of prior exposure to mumps and nonimmunity.
- Equivocal results should be followed up with a new serum specimen within 10–14 days.

❑ Limitations

If the assay is used with cord blood as the specimen source, positive results should be interpreted with caution. The presence of IgG antibodies to mumps in cord blood may be the result of passive transfer of maternal antibody to the fetus.

A negative result, however, may be helpful in ruling out infection. Salivary mumps IgM testing is standard in the United Kingdom. The pattern of response and accuracy is very similar to that for serum IgM.

MYCOBACTERIA (AFB, TB) CULTURE

❑ **Definition**
- Mycobacteria may cause acute and chronic infections. Infections may be localized or systemic, and there is significant overlap with signs and symptoms of fungal and other bacterial infections. Isolation of mycobacteria requires special culture techniques.
- Mycobacteria are usually acquired via the respiratory route, and the lower respiratory tract is the site of most serious mycobacterial infections. *M. tuberculosis* is the most common pathogen associated with these infections. Other mycobacterial species, including other species in the *M. tuberculosis* complex and *M. avium* complex (MAC), may cause chronic pulmonary infections.
- Organisms may disseminate from the site of primary infection to cause localized or systemic infection. Virtually all organ systems may be involved. The CNS, bone, and urinary tract are common sites of extrapulmonary infection. Mycobacteria may be isolated from stool, most commonly in HIV-infected patients, but the role of mycobacteria as a cause of GI infection has been questioned.
- Superficial mycobacterial infections, such as "swimming pool granuloma" caused by *M. marinum* and wound infections caused by rapidly growing mycobacteria, may be caused by direct inoculation of environmental non–*M. tuberculosis* species.

❑ **Use**
- Mycobacterial culture is used to detect mycobacterial pathogens and to provide isolates for susceptibility testing and further characterization.

❑ **Special Collection and Transport Instructions**
- Collect specimens using procedures that minimize the contamination with the patient's endogenous flora.
- Because routine bacterial, fungal, and other types of infections may be in the differential diagnosis when mycobacterial infection is suspected, ensure that a sufficient volume of infected material is collected to ensure that all testing can be performed.
- For the diagnosis of TB, a minimum of three sputum specimens should be submitted for culture. Patients must be carefully instructed in the proper technique for sputum collection.
- Early-morning specimens are preferred because of pooling of secretions at night. A minimum of 5–10 mL of sputum should be submitted for each specimen.
- Collection of sputum induced by inhalation of nebulized hypertonic saline or BAL specimens improve detection of pulmonary TB.
- Twenty-four–hour sputum collections should not be submitted.

17

- First-morning gastric aspirates may be collected for patients unable to produce sputum, like small children and the frail elderly.
- Up to five, first-morning urine specimens should be submitted for patients with suspected renal TB.
- Lysis–centrifugation, biphasic, and automated mycobacterial culture techniques are optimal for blood and bone marrow specimens submitted for detection of systemic mycobacterial disease.
- Specimens should be transported to the laboratory as soon as possible in sterile containers with tight-fitting lids.
- If same-day AFB stain results are needed, the specimen should arrive in the laboratory early enough in the day to allow enough time for specimen processing (decontamination and concentration) and smear interpretation.
- Specimens for mycobacterial culture should not be collected using swabs.

❑ **Use**

- Patients with tuberculosis, and specimens collected from them, are a significant risk for health care–acquired infection. Appropriate safety precautions must be followed through all aspects of TB diagnosis.
- AFB smears should be performed on all specimens submitted for mycobacterial culture. See *ACID-FAST BACILLUS (AFB) SMEAR.*
- Large-volume liquid specimens should be concentrated, usually by centrifugation, and specimens likely to be contaminated by endogenous flora should be decontaminated and concentrated prior to medium inoculation.
- Specimens are inoculated into liquid (e.g., Middlebrook 7H9) media and at least one type of solid media. Special media may be required for fastidious mycobacterial pathogens, like *M. haemophilum*, or special incubation temperature for agents causing superficial infection, like *M. marinum.*
- Most cultures are incubated at 37°C; cultures from skin or superficial lesions should also be incubated at 30–32°C to improve isolation of mycobacteria that are common pathogens at these sites, such as *M. marinum* and *M. haemophilum.* Cultures are incubated in 3–10% CO_2. Broth media may be monitored on automated platforms, allowing earlier detection time and providing organisms for identification using molecular genetic tests. Clear, agar-based solid media, like Middlebrook media, provide sensitive isolation of *M. tuberculosis*, early detection of "microcolonies," and preliminary, presumptive identification by microcolony morphology. Selective media, which contain a variety of antibiotic agents, may be inoculated for specimens when heavy contamination is likely. Because pathogenic mycobacteria may be inhibited by selective media, nonselective media must always be included. If *M. haemophilum* infection is suspected, media supplemented with blood, hemin (X factor strip), or ferric ammonium citrate should be inoculated. Inoculation of parallel cultures, with one culture exposed to light during the early growth phase, and one incubated in the dark only, can be used to determine characteristics of pigment formation.
- Gram and AFB staining is performed on growth from positive AFB cultures; further testing for identification and susceptibility, as appropriate, is performed.
  - ▼ Growth rate and pigment formation, including photoreactivity, are used to initially characterize non–*M. tuberculosis* mycobacterial species (NMTB)

and help to determine the panel of tests required for full identification. Rapidly growing mycobacterial species yield mature colonies within 10 days after subculture.

▼ Newer technologies for definitive identification of isolates have replaced biochemical and phenotypic testing in many laboratories. The NAP (*p*-nitro-acetylamino-hydroxypropiophenone) test may be used to rapidly identify *M. tuberculosis*. Nucleic acid probes are available for identification of *M. tuberculosis* complex, *M. avium* complex (MAC), *Mycobacterium kansasii*, and *M. gordonae*. Nucleic acid sequencing technology is emerging as an important tool for identification of mycobacteria in reference laboratories.

Turnaround Time
- Cultures are incubated for 6–8 weeks. Specimens with a positive AFB smear or direct molecular test result should be incubated for an additional 4 weeks before signing out as negative.
- In positive cultures, several additional weeks may be required for isolation, identification, susceptibility testing, and further characterization, as needed.
- Antimicrobial susceptibility testing should be performed on initial isolates, if *M. tuberculosis*, as well as isolates from cultures, positive longer than 3 months after initiation of therapy. Susceptibility testing should also be performed on most NMTB isolates.
- The primary panel for TB isolates include isoniazid, rifampin, ethambutol, and pyrazinamide. For isolates resistant to rifampin or any other two drugs from the primary panel, a secondary panel is performed, including amikacin; capreomycin; cycloserine; ethionamide; kanamycin; PAS; and streptomycin at a low level and a high level.
- Various species-specific drug panels are used for significant NMTB isolates.
- Using optimal growth, identification, and susceptibility testing systems, complete identification and susceptibility testing should be completed for the majority of *M. tuberculosis* isolates within 4 weeks of submission of specimen to the lab.

❑ Interpretation
- **Expected results:** No growth.
- **Positive:** Growth of *M. tuberculosis* in culture is usually very specific for mycobacterial infection. Because of their wide distribution in the environment, cultures positive for NMTB species must be interpreted carefully, taking into consideration factors such as the species, number of positive cultures, and the patient's clinical presentation. *M. gordonae* (tap water bacillus) is often isolated from patient specimens, but is rarely associated with disease; its growth is most likely caused by contamination of the specimen, or transient contamination of the patient, with organisms from external water sources.
- **Negative:** The post-test probability of mycobacterial infection is significantly diminished if cultures are negative, but additional cultures and specimens collected from different patient sites may be needed in patients with continued suspicion for mycobacterial disease in spite of initial negative cultures.

❑ **Limitations**

- Three or more specimens, and specimens from different sites, may be required for sensitive detection; invasive collection techniques may be needed. The final results of testing may not be available for up to 2 months after collection; decisions regarding empirical therapy and management may be required before culture results are available.

❑ **Other Considerations**

- The following mycobacterial species are most commonly associated with human disease:
    - ▼ *M. tuberculosis* complex: *M. tuberculosis*, *M. africanum* (rare), *M. bovis*, including BCG, and *M. microti* (rare)—pulmonary and other localized infections and systemic disease
    - ▼ *M. avium* complex (MAC)—systemic infection in immunocompromised patients, like patients with AIDS or chronic pulmonary disease
    - ▼ *M. kansasii*—pulmonary disease
    - ▼ Rapid growers: *M. fortuitum*, *M. chelonae*, *M. abscessus*—wound infections, localized and systemic infection
    - ▼ *M. scrofulaceum*—cervical lymphadenitis
    - ▼ *M. marinum*, *M. ulcerans*, *M. haemophilum*—skin and superficial infections
    - ▼ *M. xenopi*—pulmonary
    - ▼ *M. genavense*—disseminated and GI disease in immunocompromised patients
    - ▼ *M. malmoense*—pulmonary

MYCOBACTERIUM TUBERCULOSIS SCREENING INTERFERON-GAMMA RELEASE ASSAY

❑ **Definition and Use**

- *M. tuberculosis* infection may present with a range of disease syndromes, including acute infection, active infection, latent infection, and reactivation disease. Patients are evaluated on the basis of clinical presentation, epidemiologic risk assessment, radiographic studies, and evidence of host response by screening tests; diagnosis is established by detection of *M. tuberculosis* by culture or molecular diagnostic methods.
- In the past, the tuberculin skin test (TST) was used to detect host response, but the recent development of FDA-approved interferon-gamma release assays (IGRAs) has provided an alternative method for detecting immunologic response to *M. tuberculosis* antigens. IGRAs may be used in the evaluation of patients for latent or active (acute or reactivation) TB.

Method

- Three FDA-approved IGRAs are currently available.
- IGRAs measure immune reactivity of a patient's WBCs when challenged with synthetic antigens that are present in all strains of *M. tuberculosis* but absent in BCG strains. Immune reactivity is measured by the interferon-gamma

concentration, or number of interferon-gamma–producing cells, after exposure of viable WBCs to these antigens.

- Advantages of IGRAs include
  - ▼ IGRAs require only a single patient visit to conduct the test.
  - ▼ Results are available within 24 hours, which may facilitate patient evaluation and contact investigation.
  - ▼ IGRA testing does not boost the immunologic response in subsequent tests.
  - ▼ Prior BCG vaccination does not cause false-positive reaction in IGRAs.
- The assessment of IGRA test accuracy depends on the populations studied, the comparator method, and other factors. In general, the sensitivity of the IGRAs is high and comparable to TSTs. Studies suggest that the specificity of IGRAs is slightly higher than the specificity of TSTs. IGRAs may be used and considered acceptable medical and public health practice in all situations in which the CDC recommends TST to aid in the diagnosis of TB.
- IGRA assays (and TSTs) are recommended only for patients with a significant prior probability of tuberculosis; routine patient testing is not recommended. If indicated, either TST or IGRA may be used.
- IGRA testing may be recommended after initial TST in special circumstances:
  - ▼ If the initial, primary test is negative, and
    - The risk for poor patient outcome (severe or progressive disease) is high, as for young children or HIV-infected patients.
    - The clinical suspicion for TB, based on other criteria, is high.
    - A positive result from a second test would be interpreted as increased sensitivity for detection of infection.
  - ▼ If the initial, primary test is positive, and
    - Additional evidence of infection may encourage a patient's acceptance of the diagnosis and compliance with therapy.
    - A negative result would establish a false-positive TST result in patients with a low probability of tuberculosis based on other factors.
    - Initial TST indeterminate or equivocal test result is seen in patients in whom TB cannot be ruled out by other factors.

❑ **Special Collection and Transport Instructions**

- Specimens must be collected into tubes specified by the manufacturer.
- Specimens must be collected strictly following the manufacturer's instructions.
- Specimens must be inverted or shaken vigorously according to the manufacturer's instructions.
- Transport at room temperature. Specimens should not be refrigerated or frozen during transport.

❑ **Interpretation**

- **Expected results:** Negative.
- **Positive results:** Positive results suggest that infection with *M. tuberculosis* is likely, but cannot determine the stage of infection. Reactive specimens support a diagnosis of acute, active or, latent infection, or reactivation TB.
- **Negative results:** Infection with *M. tuberculosis* is unlikely.
- **Indeterminate or borderline:** *M. tuberculosis* infection is not established. Alternative or sequential testing may resolve the diagnosis.

❑ **Limitations**

■ The performance of IGRAs has not been adequately evaluated in certain patient populations, like pregnant women, children, patients with malignancies and other chronic infections, patients treated with medications that affect immune response, and patients with extended therapy with antituberculous agents.

■ Negative test results cannot exclude a diagnosis of TB.

■ Results, especially negative responses, must be interpreted in the context of the patient's state of immunocompetence.

■ TSTs are preferred for the evaluation of children, especially those younger than 5 years of age.

■ For patients with latent TB, IGRAs cannot be used to predict which patients will progress to reactivation disease.

■ The use of IGRAs versus TSTs, as a first-line screening tool, must be determined on the basis of several factors, including cost, patient population served, likely compliance of patients with return visits, prior vaccination with BCG, and access to laboratory processing in a timely manner.

■ The effect of recent live-virus vaccination on the performance of IGRAs has not been well studied. IGRAs may be performed prior to or on the same day as live-virus vaccination. Otherwise, the IGRA should be delayed for 4–6 weeks after vaccination.

■ The effect of lymphopenia on IGRAs is unknown.

  ▼ The antigens used in IGRAs (ESAT-6 and CFP-10) are present in *Mycobacterium kansasii, M. szulgai, M. marinum,* and several other non–*M. tuberculosis* species. Infection with other mycobacterial species should be considered, and ruled out as appropriate, in patients with positive IGRA test results.

■ Common pitfalls:

  ▼ IGRAs (and TSTs) may be submitted for patients at very low risk for infection with *M. tuberculosis.*

  ▼ Delayed transport or improper specimen handling during transport may decrease the viability of lymphocytes and result in false-negative results.

Suggested Reading

Centers for Disease Control and Prevention. Updated guidelines for using interferon gamma release assays to detect mycobacterium tuberculosis infection—United States, 2010. *MMWR Morbid Mortal Wkly Rep.* 2010;59(RR-5).

NEISSERIA GONORRHOEAE, AMPLIFIED NUCLEIC ACID DETECTION

See: Sexually Transmitted Infections, Molecular Diagnosis (*Chlamydia trachomatis, Neisseria gonorrhoeae, Trichomonas vaginalis*)

OVA AND PARASITE EXAMINATION, STOOL

❑ **Definition**

■ This test is ordered for diagnosis of common enteric parasitic pathogens in fecal specimens.

- Parasitic infections present with a remarkable diversity of signs and symptoms. Indications for testing for endemic parasitic infections may be fairly straightforward. Clinicians must have a high index of suspicion for parasitic infection when patients present with symptoms after travel to regions where other parasites are endemic.

❏ Use

- Specimens should be examined visually to identify any macroscopic parasitic forms, like pinworms or tapeworm proglottids. The routine O & P examination of stool includes three components: a direct wet mount (unpreserved liquid stool only), wet mount of stool concentrate (formalin-fixed specimen), and preparation of a permanent stained smear (polyvinyl alcohol [PVA]-fixed specimen).
  - ▼ The direct wet mount may provide a rapid diagnosis and demonstrate motility of trophozoites in heavily infected patients.
  - ▼ The concentrated stool wet mount, prepared from the formalin-fixed stool specimen by sedimentation or flotation, provides for detection of protozoal cyst forms, oocyst of coccidian parasites, microsporidia, and helminth eggs and larvae.
  - ▼ The permanent smear, made from the PVA-preserved stool specimen, provides the best morphology for identification of parasites and recognition of artifacts as well as providing a permanent slide that can be referred for identification, if necessary. Permanent stains should be used to confirm the identification of any parasite detected by wet mount.
- **Turnaround time: 48–72 hours.**

❏ Special Collection and Transport Instructions

- Stool should be submitted in clean containers with tight-fitting lids. It is not necessary to use sterile containers. Stool specimens collected by swab, from the toilet, or on toilet paper are not appropriate. The detection of parasites may be inhibited by intestinal contrast (barium sulfate), mineral oil, bismuth medications, antidiarrheals, and medications with antiparasitic action. Delay specimen collection for 1–2 weeks after the use of these agents.
- Submit stool during the diarrheal phase of disease. Trophozoite forms may be detected only in diarrheal stool; cyst forms are more common in formed stool.
- At least three stool specimens, collected on separate days, should be submitted within 10 days. A purgative agent, such as magnesium sulfate, improves the detection of intestinal parasites. Six specimens, collected on different days over a 2-week period, should detect more than 90% of amebic infections.
- Stool specimens should be transported to the laboratory as quickly as possible. Stool must be examined within 1 hour of passage (30 minutes for liquid or semiliquid stool) if direct wet mount is needed for detection of motile forms. If the transport to the laboratory will be delayed, the stool should be placed into preservative. Stool collection kits generally contain a vial of 10% formalin and a vial of PVA solution. The PVA vial is inoculated to give a 3:1 ratio of fixative to stool. The ratio for formalin should be 3:1 or greater. The stool must mixed be thoroughly with the preservative to ensure that parasitic elements do not degrade with storage. The formalin suspension is used to prepare a direct wet mount from concentrated material. The PVA-fixed material is used to prepare smears for permanent stains.

- Three O & P examinations should be performed after therapy: 3 or 4 weeks after treatment for protozoal infection and 5 or 6 weeks after treatment for *Taenia* infection.
- Special techniques are required for collection of duodenal specimens or specimens collected by endoscopy or other invasive techniques.

❑ **Interpretation**

- **Expected results:** Negative.
- **Positive results:** Positive O & P examinations are associated with a high probability of parasitic infection or colonization. Identification of nonpathogenic parasites suggests exposure to unsanitary conditions; repeat testing should be considered in symptomatic patients.
- **Negative:** A single negative test does not effectively rule out enteric parasitic infection. Sensitive detection of the infecting parasite may require additional testing of alternative techniques, like duodenal aspiration.

❑ **Limitations**

- For some enteric parasitic infections, specimens other than stool, like duodenal contents, may be required for diagnosis. Special techniques, like egg-hatching techniques, may be needed for sensitive detection of certain parasites.
- **Common pitfalls:**
   ▼ The submission of too few specimens limits the performance of stool O & P examination.
   ▼ Special staining techniques are required for effective detection of certain enteric parasitic pathogens, like use of a modified acid-fast stain for detection of *Cryptosporidium parvum* or microsporidia.

PINWORM EXAMINATION

❑ **Definition**

- This test should be considered in patients, most often children, who present with pruritus ani. Sleep disturbances are common.

❑ **Use**

- This test is used to diagnose enteric infection with the parasitic pathogen *Enterobius vermicularis* (pinworm). Eggs or adult female worms are identified in specimens collected from skin of the perianal area. Specimens are collected with clear cellophane tape or a commercial pinworm collection device. The sticky side of the tape or collection device is pressed onto the perianal skin. Because the female worm emerges from the anus to lay eggs during the night, specimens should be collected in the early morning, before the patient passes a bowel movement, and ideally before arising.
- **Turnaround time:** 24–48 hours.

❑ **Interpretation**

- **Expected results:** Negative.
- **Positive results:** Typical ova of *E. vermicularis* are usually seen. An adult female *E. vermicularis*, identified by characteristic structures, is occasionally seen.

❏ **Limitations**

- The sensitivity of a single examination is fairly low. The examination of multiple specimens is typically required for diagnosis; empirical treatment for enterobiasis may be a cost-effective alternative to therapy based on specific diagnosis.
- **Common pitfall:** The examination of only one or two specimens will often result in a false-negative diagnosis.

PNEUMOCYSTIS JIROVECII (FORMERLY PNEUMOCYSTIS CARINII), MICROSCOPIC DETECTION

❏ **Definition**

- *Pneumocystis jirovecii*, a fungal pathogen, is ubiquitous in nature, with low pathogenic potential. In severely immunocompromised patients, especially patients with AIDS, however, it is responsible for potentially fatal respiratory disease.

❏ **Use**

- This test is used to detect infection with the fungal pathogen *P. jirovecii* in lower respiratory specimens. This test may be used to evaluate immunocompromised patients who present with severe atypical pneumonia.
- Method:
  ▼ Direct examination of respiratory specimens for *P. jirovecii* can be performed using several staining methods. Detection is based on the identification of organisms with typical morphology; different reagents may stain the "cyst" form, "trophozoite" form, or both.
  ▼ Giemsa-based stains are convenient but may be difficult to read because of staining of background material. Sensitivity is approximately 50%. Stains using tagged monoclonal antibody reagents provide the highest sensitivity, approximately 91%. Calcofluor white staining has sensitivity approximately 74%. GMS staining provides sensitivity approximately 79%. Staining techniques have excellent specificity when interpreted by experienced microbiologists.

❏ **Special Collection and Transport Instructions**

- Acceptable specimens include material obtained by BAL or sputum induced using nebulized hypertonic saline.
  ▼ Transbronchial or surgical biopsy specimens are acceptable specimens for *Pneumocystis* detection.
  ▼ Expectorated sputum and respiratory secretions obtained by suction through an endotracheal tube or after percussive respiratory therapy are not acceptable for *Pneumocystis* testing.

❏ **Limitations**

- The performance of tests for direct detection of *P. jirovecii* depends on numerous factors, including the prior probability of infection, type of specimen submitted, specimen processing, and staining method used.

17

- Submission of expectorated sputum, tracheal aspirates, or specimens other than induced sputum, BAL, or biopsy specimens results in poor detection of *P. jiroveci*.

Suggested Readings

Cruciani M, Marcati P, Malena M, et al. Meta-analysis of diagnostic procedures for *Pneumocystis carinii* pneumonia in HIV-1-infected patients. *Eur Respir J.* 2002;20:982–989.

Procop GW, Haddad S, Quinn J, et al. Detection of *Pneumocystis jiroveci* in respiratory specimens by four staining methods. *J Clin Microbiol.* 2004;42(7):3333–3335.

Thomas CF Jr, Limper AH. *Pneumocystis* pneumonia. *N Engl J Med.* 2004;350:2487–2498.

RESPIRATORY ADENOVIRUS CULTURE (RULE OUT)

❑ Definition

- Adenovirus respiratory infections most commonly occur in young children and typically present with nonspecific findings of febrile viral respiratory tract infection. Immunocompromised, especially bone marrow transplant, patients may present with severe disease. Respiratory adenovirus infections do not show as strong a seasonal variability (winter months) as the other common respiratory viral pathogens.

❑ Use

- This test is used to detect respiratory viral infections caused by adenoviruses. Respiratory specimens for adenovirus are inoculated onto human cell lines; A549, HeLa, HEp-2, and MRC-5 cell lines are commonly used. Tube cultures or shell vial culture technique may be used. A presumptive diagnosis may be made on the basis of typical cytopathic effect and then confirmed by immunologic techniques. Adenovirus detection may be included in virus culture or molecular test panels for respiratory virus detection. Children with respiratory adenovirus infection frequently demonstrate leukocytosis (>15,000/mm^3) and increased ESR and CRP, in contrast to the lack of these signs in other common viral respiratory tract infections.
- **Turnaround time:** Most cultures are positive within 2 weeks. Tube cultures may be incubated for up to 4 weeks before signing out as negative. Shell vial cultures are stained within 3 days of incubation.

❑ Special Collection and Transport Instructions

- Specimens should be collected in the first week after onset of symptoms.
- Nasopharyngeal swabs or aspirates are recommended; other respiratory tract specimens may be acceptable for culture.
- It is recommended that specimens be inoculated into a viral transport medium and transported to the laboratory at 4°C.

❑ Interpretation

- **Expected results:** Negative.

❑ Limitations

- Submission of specimens >7 days after onset of acute infection is associated with decreased sensitivity.

Suggested Reading

Carr MJ, Kajon AE, Lu X, et al. Deaths associated with human adenovirus-14p1 infections, Europe, 2009–2010. *Emerg Infect Dis.* [serial on the Internet]. 2011 Aug [date cited]. http://dx.doi.org/10.3201/1708.101760

RESPIRATORY CULTURE, RULE OUT BACTERIAL PATHOGENS

❏ **Definition**

- Structures adjacent to the respiratory tract, like the sinuses, are usually sterile or only transiently contaminated. They may become infected, often as a superinfection complicating upper respiratory viral infection. Cultures may be considered in patients who present with unusually severe signs and symptoms consistent with sinusitis, otitis media, or other pararespiratory infection, or when symptoms persist for more than 7 days.
- The common bacterial pathogens are most commonly derived from the endogenous flora, including *Moraxella catarrhalis, Streptococcus pneumoniae, Haemophilus influenzae,* and *Staphylococcus aureus.* Anaerobic bacteria have been implicated, but usually with chronic infection or acute infection associated with trauma. Opportunistic molds, such as *Mucor* species, may cause severe, invasive upper respiratory tract infections in immunocompromised patients, especially in patients with DM.

❏ **Special Collection and Transport Instructions**

- Swab specimens should be considered unacceptable for culture, except for those collected by direct visualization by an otolaryngologist. Swab specimens are not optimal for isolation of anaerobic pathogens in chronic infections or acute abscesses.
- Pus collected by surgical aspiration or drainage or by sinus aspiration should be transported to the laboratory under anaerobic transport conditions as quickly as possible.

❏ **Use**

- Specimens are typically inoculated onto SBA and chocolate and MacConkey agar. Anaerobic media are inoculated if requested.
- **Turnaround time:** Cultures are examined for at least 48 hours. Several days are required for isolation and identification, susceptibility testing, and further characterization of isolates.

❏ **Interpretation**

- **Expected results:** No growth, but light growth of endogenous respiratory flora is common.
- **Positive:** Because common causes of pararespiratory infections are usually derived from upper respiratory tract endogenous flora, positive culture must be interpreted in the context of quantity or bacterial growth, purity of culture, Gram stain findings, and clinical signs and symptoms.

17

❑ **Limitations**

■ **Common pitfall:** Noninvasively collected specimens, which are more likely to represent endogenous rather than pathogenic flora, are often submitted for patient evaluation.

RESPIRATORY CULTURE, RULE OUT VIRAL PATHOGENS

❑ **Definition**

■ Most respiratory viral syndromes are relatively mild and self-limited. Occasionally, severe disease develops for which specific diagnosis is needed to optimize therapeutic and management decisions. Viral culture may be used to provide isolates for antiviral susceptibility testing or further characterization for epidemiologic reasons. This test may be ordered to make a specific diagnosis for severe seasonal respiratory viral illness. Agents cultured typically include influenza virus A and B, RSV, and parainfluenza virus types 1, 2, and 3; adenovirus may be included.

❑ **Special Collection and Transport Instructions**

■ Specimens should be collected according to general recommendations for virus culture of the specimen type.
■ Specimens should be collected early in acute infection.
■ Nasopharyngeal specimens are often optimal for diagnosis.
■ RSV is a fastidious virus and should be delivered to the laboratory as quickly as possible. This virus may not survive freezing if prolonged transport is needed. Most specimens should be placed in a viral transport medium and transported on wet ice (4°C).
■ Specimens for molecular diagnostic, DFA, EIA, or other diagnostic testing for respiratory viruses should be submitted according to laboratory recommendations.

❑ **Use**

■ Method:
  ▼ Nasopharyngeal wash specimens, or swabs, are usually associated with the best sensitivity of culture.
  ▼ Specimens are typically inoculated onto several different types of cell lines to help ensure growth of all of the target pathogens. Shell vial cultures may be inoculated in addition to tube cultures. Positive cultures are determined by cytopathic effect or by staining with virus-specific tagged monoclonal antibodies.
■ **Turnaround time**
  ▼ Shell vial cultures may be positive within 48–72 hours.
  ▼ Most respiratory viral pathogens can be detected in tube cultures by blind staining with immunologic reagents after 7 days of inoculation.

❑ **Interpretation**

■ **Expected results:** Negative.
■ **Positive results:** Positive cultures for specific viruses indicate active infection with that agent.

- **Negative results:** Negative viral culture significantly decreases the possibility but does not rule out respiratory virus infection. Molecular diagnostic techniques should be considered in patients with severe disease.

❑ **Limitations**

- Negative cultures may be caused by numerous factors, including poor specimen collection technique, collection of specimens after acute disease when virus concentrations are below the level of detection, or infection caused by a viral pathogen not included in the respiratory virus culture panel used.
- Coinfection with two or more respiratory viral pathogens is relatively common. The impact of coinfection with specific viral pathogens, such as human metapneumovirus, awaits further study.

RESPIRATORY VIRUS DIRECT DETECTION BY ENZYME IMMUNOASSAY (EIA) AND DIRECT FLUORESCENT ANTIBODY (DFA) TESTS

❑ **Definition**

- Tests for the direct detection of respiratory viral pathogens, like influenza, RSV and human metapneumovirus; they may provide results significantly sooner than results from respiratory virus culture or molecular diagnostic testing and serve a critical role in early patient management and infection control activities. EIA tests have only moderate sensitivity, but high specificity, for detection of influenza virus infection; they are commonly used for screening. DFA tests have high sensitivity and specificity compared to respiratory viral culture, and they may be a cost-effective definitive diagnostic technique.

❑ **Use**

- EIA and DFA tests are commonly used to provide early screening for influenza virus infection. Assays vary in terms of sensitivity; specimens with negative results by EIA should be submitted for sensitive testing, like molecular assays, for patients at risk for complicated respiratory viral infection.
- Method:
  - ▼ **EIA:** There are a number of kit formats for EIA tests. Antibodies directed at specific virus antigens are immobilized on the surface of a membrane of a test device. The specimen is added to the reaction surface, allowing virus antigen in the specimen to react with the bound antibodies. After washing, a second tagged virus-specific antibody reagent is added. After washing away excess detection antibody, a label-specific detection reagent is added and the test read as positive or negative.
  - ▼ **DFA:** Cells collected by nasopharyngeal swab or wash are fixed onto a microscopic slide. The slide is dried, fixed, and stained with a reagent containing labeled antibodies directed against specific virus antigens. The label is typically fluorogenic. Stained slides are examined by fluorescence microscopy using excitation and barrier filter appropriate for the specific fluorogenic label.
- **Special collection and transport instructions:** Specimens are collected as recommended for samples for viral culture. Nasopharyngeal specimens,

17

especially nasopharyngeal wash specimens, typically provide specimens with the greatest sensitivity for detection of infected patients.

▪ **Turnaround time:** 24–48 hours. Some EIA kits allow testing with a turnaround time <4 hours.

❏ **Interpretation**

▪ **Expected results:** Negative.
▪ **Positive results:**
   ▼ EIA: The specificity of EIA assays is high; a diagnosis is established in patients with compatible signs and symptoms of influenza; additional diagnostic testing is generally not required.
   ▼ DFA: Specimens showing a significant number of cells with 2+ or greater fluorescence are considered positive, establishing a diagnosis of influenza in patients with compatible signs and symptoms. Slides must be examined to ensure that the specimen contains enough respiratory epithelial cells to provide informative testing. Laboratories should establish a lower limit of cells present below which the test is considered uninterpretable. Specimens that demonstrate only few, faintly staining cells should be considered equivocal; repeat testing may provide clear positive or negative results.
▪ **Negative results:**
   ▼ EIA: A negative result does not exclude respiratory virus infection.
   ▼ DFA: A cellular specimen without staining by the labeled reagent is reported as negative. Infection with the specific viral pathogen is unlikely.

❏ **Limitations**

▪ The sensitivity for different commercially available EIA tests is variable. Sensitivities commonly range from 50% to 80%. Clinically, test performance depends on the type of specimen and quality of specimen collection. Only specimen types acceptable for the kit, collected according to kit instructions, should be accepted.
▪ The PPV of antigen detection tests depends on the prevalence of viral pathogen in the region. Testing results should be interpreted with caution, if performed at all, during periods when there is a low prevalence of the pathogen circulating in the region.
▪ **Common pitfall:** Poor test performance may be seen when specimens are submitted that have not been validated for the platform/kit used for testing. Anterior nasal swabs, for example, may be submitted instead of nasopharyngeal swabs, resulting in an increased number of false-negative results.

RESPIRATORY VIRUS PANEL (RVP) MOLECULAR ASSAY*

❏ **Definition**

▪ The RVP assay is a comprehensive panel of tests for the detection of multiple viral strains and subtypes. Various molecular assays differ in the specific list of respiratory viruses tested, but most include influenza A (and subtypes), influenza B, parainfluenza, adenovirus, metapneumovirus (HMPV), RSV, and rhinovirus.

---

*Contributed by Marzena M. Galdzicka, PhD.

■ **Normal range:** Not detected.

❏ **Use**

■ The RVP molecular assay tests for the major respiratory viruses commonly tested for surveillance and patient management. In addition, the RVP molecular assay is frequently used for the confirmation of negative results obtained by other methods, such as the rapid antigen assay, direct immunofluorescence, or EIA.

❏ **Limitations**

■ The low limit of detection varies depending on the methods and viruses tested.

ROTAVIRUS FECAL ANTIGEN DETECTION

❏ **Definition and Use**

■ This test is used for the diagnosis of enteric infections caused by Rotavirus.
■ This test may be ordered for patients, usually young children, who present with a sudden onset of watery diarrhea, which is often preceded by vomiting.
■ Unpreserved stool is submitted for testing.
■ Rotavirus antigen in stool is detected by immunologic techniques using rotavirus-specific antibodies. LA and EIA formats are typically used. Sensitivity and specificity of commercial EIA assays are reported in the high 90% range.
■ **Turnaround time:** <24 hours.

❏ **Interpretation**

■ **Expected results:** Negative.

❏ **Limitations**

■ LA tests have reported sensitivities less than the sensitivities of EIA assays. Assays may be less reliable in neonates.

RUBELLA SEROLOGY SCREEN (RUBELLA IgG AND IgM)

❏ **Definition**

■ Rubella virus causes German measles, a mild subclinical infection with a characteristic exanthem that affects both children and adults. Rubella is transmitted directly by contact or by droplets from the nasopharynx of infected individuals and can cause significant birth defects if disease occurs early in fetal life. It has an incubation period of 14–21 days. Individuals may shed virus for up to 2 weeks prior to the outbreak of rash; therefore, patients are typically infectious for some time before the infection becomes clinically obvious. Virus shedding decreases significantly after the appearance of the rash, a period coinciding with the development of neutralizing antibodies. Rubella is no longer endemic in the United States as a result of an intensive vaccination campaign. Minor epidemics occurred in the United States every 5–7 years and major epidemics every 10–30 years.
■ **Normal range:** Negative.

❏ **Use**

- Determination of rubella immune status assists in the diagnosis of rubella infection or determines susceptibility to rubella, particularly in pregnant women.

❏ **Interpretation**

- **Positive** ($\geq$10 IU/mL): Indicative of past infection or vaccination
- **Equivocal** ($\geq$5 to $\leq$10 IU/mL): Considered to be "indeterminate"
- **Negative** (<5 IU/mL): Does not preclude recent primary infection

❏ **Limitations**

- In general, 90% of the US population has been either vaccinated or exposed to rubella, with rubella IgG values of $\geq$10 IU/mL.
- The presence of IgG antibodies in a single specimen is not sufficient to distinguish between active infection and past infection. The results of the test must be taken within the context of the patient's clinical history, symptomatology, and other laboratory findings.
- Patients suspected of having primary, active infection should be tested for the presence of IgM antibodies to rubella virus.

SEXUALLY TRANSMITTED INFECTIONS, MOLECULAR DIAGNOSIS (CHLAMYDIA TRACHOMATIS, NEISSERIA GONORRHOEAE, TRICHOMONAS VAGINALIS)

❏ **Definition**

- Amplified nucleic acid techniques (NAATs) are the most sensitive tests for detection of common sexually transmitted infections (STI), *C. trachomatis*, *N. gonorrhoeae*, and *T. vaginalis*, in urine and urogenital specimens. Culture techniques for detection of these pathogens require specialized culture, long turnaround time, and transport conditions that are often not realized in clinical practice.

❏ **Special Collection and Transport Instructions**

- Commercially available NAATs may be validated for use with urine and urogenital specimens (including Pap thin-prep solutions). They are not validated for use with other types of specimens.
- NAATs should not be used for the sole testing technique in the evaluation of rape or child abuse.
- Specimens must be collected according to the manufacturer's instructions, including specimen type and materials. Use collection kits provided by the manufacturer for swab and urine specimen; transfer vials may be provided for thin-prep specimens. Ensure that vials for liquid specimens are filled with the appropriate volume.
- Care must be taken to prevent cross-contamination of specimens, for example, at the area used for transfer of urine into a transfer vial.
- Transport to the laboratory at refrigerator or room temperature.

❏ **Use**

- Specimens may be submitted for evaluation of sexually active adult patients with symptoms consistent with STDs. Commercially available NAATs for detection of *C. trachomatis*, *N. gonorrhoeae*, and *T. vaginalis* have very high sensitivity and specificity (>95%).

■ **Turnaround time:** 24–72 hours.

❏ **Interpretation**

■ **Expected results:** Negative.
■ **Positive results:** A positive result establishes a diagnosis in patients with compatible symptoms and risk for STD. Positive results must be interpreted with caution in patients with low risk for STD. Repeat testing, ideally performed on a repeat specimen using a different test platform or target sequence, is recommended if a false-positive result is suspected.
■ **Negative results:** Infection is unlikely. Poor collection technique, low target levels, or other factors may cause false-negative results.

❏ **Limitations**

■ **Common pitfalls:** Test results must be interpreted in the context of the clinical impression and prior probability of infection. Repeat testing should be performed if false-positive or false-negative test results are suspected.
■ There is significant overlap in the signs and symptoms of these and other urogenital infections, like bacterial vaginitis, or noninfectious conditions. Laboratory testing for these STIs does not replace physical examination and other testing appropriate for the patient's presentation.
■ Accuracy depends on proper specimen collection: the use of incorrect swabs for specimen collection, improper filling of urine transport tubes, and submission of inappropriate specimen types may result in false-negative results.
■ Amplified nucleic acid tests should not be used for test of cure evaluations (within 4 weeks of treatment), because DNA may be detectable even after viable organisms have been eliminated.

❏ **Other Considerations**

■ As part of routine quality assurance practices, laboratories that perform amplified nucleic acid tests should routinely perform "wipe tests" of surfaces in the laboratory where NAATs are performed, and perform further evaluation and maintenance according to the test manufacturer's instructions. Laboratories should also monitor their reported rates of *C. trachomatis*, *N. gonorrhoeae*, and *T. vaginalis* infections; increasing positivity rates not explained by changes in patient populations tested may be an indication of laboratory contamination; careful evaluation of laboratory procedures should be performed.

SPUTUM CULTURE (ROUTINE)

❏ **Definition**

■ Lower respiratory tract (LRT) infections may involve any of the anatomic areas inferior to the larynx. Infections include tracheobronchitis (large airway disease), bronchiolitis (small airway disease), and pneumonia (alveolar disease). The common etiologies depend on the site of infection, age and underlying health of the patient, season, and other factors.

17

■ Patients with LRT infections typically present with a constellation of symptoms of varying severity, including fever, cough, sputum production, difficulty breathing, and shortness of breath. Common bacterial pathogens are less commonly associated with coryza and rhinorrhea than are respiratory viruses and mycoplasmas. Symptoms and clinical examination may help distinguish tracheobronchitis, bronchiolitis, and pneumonia from one another.

❑ **Special Collection and Transport Instructions**

■ For expectorated sputum samples, patient instruction is critical for collection of a good-quality, informative sample.
■ Specimens must be collected in sterile transport containers with tight-fitting lids.
■ First-morning specimens are usually most sensitive because of pooling of secretions during sleep.
■ Contamination is reduced for patients who brush their teeth and gargle with water or saline just before specimen collection.
■ The patient must understand that sputum from a deep cough is needed, and saliva should not be spit into the collection cup.
■ Sputum production may be improved by chest wall percussive techniques.
■ Specimens obtained by more invasive procedures, such as sputum induction, BAL, tracheal aspirate, and lung puncture, are collected by physicians or respiratory therapists trained with specific collection protocols.
■ Specimens must be transported to the laboratory as quickly as possible at room temperature.

❑ **Use**

■ These cultures are used to identify bacterial pathogens responsible for LRT infections by culture of sputum. A variety of human pathogens may cause lower respiratory infections; there is a large overlap in the clinical signs and symptoms.
■ Method:
  ▼ Gram stain examination of sputum should be performed to ensure that poor-quality specimens are not processed for routine sputum culture. A number of screening strategies have been proposed. Sputum specimens are scored on the basis of the presence and quantity of PMNs and SECs.
  ▼ Acceptable specimens are usually inoculated onto SBA, chocolate and MacConkey agar.
  ▼ If anaerobic infection is suspected, specialized techniques, like needle aspiration, are required to exclude contamination by the patient's endogenous flora.
■ **Turnaround time**
  ▼ Cultures are incubated for 48–72 hours.
  ▼ Additional time is required for isolation, identification, susceptibility, and other testing, as required.

❑ **Interpretation**

■ **Expected results:** Light or rare growth of normal endogenous respiratory tract flora (or no growth).

- **Positive results:** Positive cultures must be interpreted carefully in the context of Gram stain results and other laboratory findings, imaging studies, and clinical presentations.
- **Negative results:** A negative culture does not exclude LRT infection. Poor specimen quality and transport conditions, or heavy contamination, may prevent the isolation of fastidious pathogens. Uncommon fastidious LRT pathogens, such as *Bordetella pertussis*, are not detected reliably by routine sputum culture.

❑ **Limitations**

- Noninvasive and minimally invasive techniques for specimen collection may result in contamination of the specimen with the patient's endogenous upper respiratory flora. Because LRT infections are commonly caused by a patient's flora, such contamination may compromise the interpretation of sputum cultures.
- The sensitivity and specificity of routine sputum cultures are relatively low for diagnosis of LRT infections. Diagnoses may be improved by submission of blood cultures, urinary antigen tests (e.g., *S. pneumoniae*), serology, and molecular diagnostic techniques and tests for other types of LRT pathogens, such as *Mycoplasma* species.
- **Common pitfalls**
  - ▼ Poor specimen collection and transport are the major causes for compromised information from sputum cultures. Rejection criteria may be not be applied appropriately.

STAPHYLOCOCCUS AUREUS (SA) AND METHICILLIN-RESISTANT STAPHYLOCOCCUS AUREUS (MRSA)*

❑ **Definition**

- The MRSA/SA molecular assay is a qualitative diagnostic test for the rapid detection of *Staphylococcus aureus* (SA) and methicillin-resistant *Staphylococcus aureus* (MRSA). Staphylococcal resistance to oxacillin/methicillin occurs when an isolate carries an altered penicillin-binding protein, PBP2a, which is encoded by the mecA gene. Most MRSA infections occur in people who have been in hospitals or other health care settings. These infections are known as health care–associated MRSA (HA-MRSA). HA- MRSA isolates often have multiply resistant to commonly used antimicrobial agents, including all β-lactam agents, erythromycin, clindamycin, and tetracycline. Community-associated MRSA (CA-MRSA) infection increases. CA-MRSA isolates are often resistant only to β-lactam agents and erythromycin. If clinically indicated susceptibility testing should be ordered.

❑ **Use**

- Diagnostic test—skin and soft tissue, surgical wound infections, many people who have a staph skin infection often mistake it for a spider bite; less commonly MRSA can cause the urinary tract infection, pneumonia, or infection of the bloodstream.

---

*Contributed by Michael Mitchell, MD & Marzena M. Galdzicka, PhD.

17

- Preoperative testing—screening of patients for MRSA is associated with a significant reduction in subsequent MRSA surgical site infections.
- Target screening—elective admissions, ICU admissions, neonatal units, trauma and burn units, patients with previous positive MRSA cultures, transfers from residential care facilities, and patients from specific high-risk wards (e.g. cardiothoracic, neurosurgery, orthopedic, renal).
- Universal screening—at hospital admission; identified MRSA-colonized individuals are managed to prevent transmission and reduce MRSA prevalence in the patient population.
- Nucleic acid amplification tests, such as the polymerase chain reaction (PCR), can be used to detect the mecA gene, which mediates oxacillin resistance in staphylococci.

❏ **Limitations**

- A negative MRSA or *Staphylococcus aureus* result should not be used as the sole basis for diagnosis, treatment or management decisions. Negative test results may occur from improper specimen collection, handling or storage, or presence of inhibitors, or because the number of bacteria in the specimen is below the analytical sensitivity of the test.

❏ **Considerations**

- Specimens should be kept between 2°C and 25°C during transport and protected against freezing or exposure to excessive heat.
- Specimens can be stored up to 48 hours at 15–25°C or 5 days at 2–8°C before testing.
- PCR test can be affected by genetic rearrangements or the presence of rare bacterial DNA variants.
- Mutations or polymorphisms in primer- or probe-binding regions may affect detection of new or unknown MRSA/SA variants resulting in a false-negative result with the PCR assay.

STOOL CULTURE (ROUTINE)

❏ **Definition**

Routine stool culture should be considered for patients with acute diarrheal illness who are producing frequent, loose stools. Nausea, abdominal pain, and vomiting may be present. Fever may be present, but is not a prominent feature in uncomplicated enteric infection. Fluid loss, especially in infants and small children, may be severe and associated with complications including electrolyte imbalance and cardiovascular instability.

❏ **Special Collection and Transport Instructions**

- Acceptable specimens: liquid stool (feces), rectal swab.
- Sterile collection containers are not required. Specimens may be collected in clean containers. The container should be free of detergent or preservative.
- Specimens should be transported promptly to the laboratory. If transport will be delayed >2 hours, use of a transport medium, like Cary-Blair, is recommended.

- Three specimens, collected on consecutive days, are recommended for sensitive detection of enteric pathogens, especially for patients at risk for complication or at increased risk for transmission of enteric pathogens, like food handlers.
- Specimens collected on toilet paper or diapers are not acceptable. Specimens contaminated by urine are not acceptable.

❏ **Use**

- The routine stool culture is used to detect GI infections caused by enteric bacterial pathogens. The target pathogens identified by routine stool culture may vary somewhat among laboratories, but all should be capable of detecting *Salmonella*, *Shigella*, and *Campylobacter* species. Other pathogens may be included, like Shiga toxin–producing *E. coli*, depending on local prevalence. Detection of other enteric pathogens may require special testing.
- Method: Stool specimens are typically inoculated onto several agar media, including a nonselective medium (e.g., SBA), a mildly selective differential medium (e.g., MacConkey agar), and a moderately selective differential medium (e.g., Hektoen enteric agar). Some laboratories have used selective broth enrichment (e.g., Selenite broth) prior to plate inoculation, but the cost-effectiveness of these strategies has been questioned. Selective agar media and incubation at increased temperature (42°C) and microaerophilic conditions are used for isolation of enteric *Campylobacter* species.
- **Turnaround time:** Cultures are examined for growth at 24 and 48 hours. Suspicious colonies are isolated and confirmatory testing performed.

❏ **Interpretation**

- **Expected results:** Negative.
- **Positive results:** Any growth of *Salmonella*, *Shigella*, *Campylobacter* or other enteric pathogen.
- **Negative results:** The probability infection is decreased but is not excluded. Additional stool cultures or testing for other enteric pathogens should be considered.

❏ **Limitations**

- Effective detection of enteric infection due to enterohemorrhagic *E. coli* (e.g., *E. coli* O157:H7), *Yersinia enterocolitica*, *Vibrio* species, *Aeromonas* species, *C. difficile*, or other bacterial pathogens requires special cultures for sensitive detection.
- Diarrheal illness caused by parasitic or viral pathogens requires special test methods.
- *C. difficile* testing should be considered as an alternative to routine enteric pathogen testing for inpatients.
- Stool culture may be negative in invasive enteric infections, like typhoid fever. Blood cultures are recommended for primary gastrointestinal infections that progress to significant fever associated with signs of systemic infection.
- *Shigella* species may not survive broth enrichment techniques.
- **Common pitfalls:**
  ▼ Rectal swabs can collect only a small amount of feces; their use should be restricted to infants.

17

▼ *Shigella* species are fastidious and may not survive changes in stool pH that occur after passage. Rapid transport and/or the use of transport media is important for reliable isolation by culture.

❏ **Other Considerations**

■ Direct detection of *Campylobacter* antigen in stool is an alternative to culture for diagnosis of enteric campylobacteriosis. Sensitivity of antigen testing is 80–96% with specificity approximately 98%.

■ Absence of normal fecal flora or the presence of predominant growth of yeast, *S. aureus*, or *Pseudomonas aeruginosa* can be recognized by inspection of the SBA plate, providing clinically relevant information about alternative diagnoses.

■ Oxidase testing may be performed on SBA isolated with heavy growth to screen for unexpected enteric infection caused by *Vibrio*, *Aeromonas*, or *Plesiomonas* species.

STREPTOCOCCUS, GROUP A, DIRECT DETECTION (ANTIGEN, NUCLEIC ACID)

❏ **Definition**

■ The results of direct tests for group A streptococci may guide early therapy. In antigen tests, the group A cell wall polysaccharide is extracted from a throat swab.

❏ **Use**

■ Direct detection tests for group A beta-hemolytic streptococci (*Streptococcus pyogenes*) are used for direct diagnosis of streptococcal pharyngitis. Patients present with symptoms including sore throat, fever, headache, and abdominal pain.

■ Method:

▼ Extracted antigen is detected by specific antibodies using standard immunologic techniques, such as LA or EIA. The sensitivity of antigen tests varies by technique and specific kit used, ranging from 60% to 95%; the specificity of most tests exceeds 95%. Therefore, throat culture has been recommended to confirm negative antigen tests, but is not needed to confirm positive tests.

▼ The Group A Streptococcus Direct Test (Gen-Probe, San Diego, CA) is an FDA-approved molecular diagnostic assay for the detection of *S. pyogenes* in pharyngeal specimens. Group A streptococci are detected using a specific DNA probe directed against specific *S. pyogenes* rRNA sequences. Sensitivity of the assay is 88–95% with specificity of 98–99.7%. The high sensitivity and specificity for this test allow test results to stand without the need for confirmation of positive or negative tests.

■ **Special collection and transport instructions:** Throat swab specimens are collected as recommended for throat cultures.

■ **Turnaround time:** <4 hours for antigen tests; <24 hours for molecular tests.

❏ **Interpretation**

■ **Expected results:** Negative.

■ **Positive results:** Positive results are diagnostic of group A streptococcal pharyngitis in patients with consistent clinical findings.

- **Negative results:** Negative antigen tests decrease the likelihood of group A streptococcal pharyngitis but must be confirmed by a more sensitive technique, such as throat culture or molecular detection.

❏ **Limitations**

- Only swabs specified by the manufacturer may be used for the Gen-Probe assay.

STREPTOCOCCUS PNEUMONIAE URINE ANTIGEN TEST

❏ **Definition**

- Streptococcus *pneumoniae* is a leading bacterial cause of pneumonia globally and is the most common agent leading to hospitalization in all age groups. *S. pneumoniae* are gram-positive, typically lancet-shaped diplococci. It is the most frequently encountered bacterial agent of community-acquired pneumonia (CAP). Because of the significant morbidity and mortality associated with pneumococcal pneumonia, septicemia, and meningitis, it is important to have diagnostic test methods available that can provide a rapid diagnosis.

❏ **Use**

- Rapid diagnosis of pneumococcal pneumonia. This is a rapid immunochromatographic membrane assay that detects soluble C-polysaccharide cell wall pneumococcal antigen common to all *S. pneumoniae* strains. It is intended, in conjunction with culture results and clinical findings, to aid in the presumptive diagnosis of pneumococcal pneumonia.

❏ **Interpretation**

- **Negative result:** Does not exclude *S. pneumoniae* infection.
- **Positive result:** Indicative of pneumococcal pneumonia. A diagnosis of *S. pneumoniae* infection must take into consideration all test results, culture results, and the clinical presentation of the patient.

❏ **Limitations**

- *S. pneumoniae* vaccine may cause false-positive results, especially in patients who have received the vaccine within 5 days of having the test performed. This test has sensitivity of 74% and specificity of 94%. Unfortunately, the test has poor specificity in children due to detection of pneumococcal nasopharyngeal colonization. Pneumococcal pneumonia is best diagnosed by sputum culture.

STREPTOZYME, ANTISTREPTOCOCCAL ANTIBODIES, ANTISTREPTOLYSIN O [ASO], ANTI–DNASE-B [ADB]

❏ **Definition**

- There are several disease-causing strains of streptococci (groups A, B, C, D, and G), which are identified by their behavior, chemistry, and appearance. Each group causes specific types of infections and symptoms. Group A streptococci are the most virulent species for humans and are the cause of "strep"

17

throat, tonsillitis, wound and skin infections, blood infections, scarlet fever, pneumonia, RF, Sydenham chorea (formerly called St. Vitus dance), and GN. Although symptoms may suggest a streptococcal infection, the diagnosis must be confirmed by tests. The best procedure, and one that is used for an acute infection, is to take a sample from the infected area for culture. However, cultures are useless about 2–3 weeks after initial infection, so the ASO, streptozyme, and ADB screen tests are used to determine if a streptococcal infection is present.

■ High titers of these antibodies have been associated with PANDAS (Pediatric Autoimmune Neuropsychiatric Disorder Associated with Streptococcal Infections) and with autism, Tourette syndrome, tic disorder, Parkinson disease, and OCD.

■ Streptococcal infections are probably a significant environmental trigger for narcolepsy.

■ *Streptozyme:*
  ▼ The streptozyme test is often used as a screening test for antibodies to the streptococcal antigens NADase, DNase, streptokinase, streptolysin O, and hyaluronidase. This test is most useful in evaluating suspected poststreptococcal disease following *S. pyogenes* infection, such as rheumatic fever. Streptozyme has certain advantages over ASO and ADB. It can detect several antibodies in a single assay, it is technically quick and easy, and it is unaffected by factors that can produce false positives in the ASO test.
  ▼ The disadvantages are that, although it detects different antibodies, it does not determine which one has been detected, and it is not as sensitive in children as in adults. In fact, borderline antibody elevations, which could be significant in children, may not be detected at all.

■ *ASO titer*
  ▼ The ASO titer is used to demonstrate the body's reaction to an infection caused by group A beta-hemolytic streptococci. Group A streptococci produce the enzyme streptolysin O, which can destroy (lyse) red blood cells.
  ▼ ASO appears in the blood serum 1 week to 1 month after the onset of a strep infection. A high titer is not specific for any type of poststreptococcal disease, but it does indicate if a streptococcal infection is or has been present. Serial ASO testing is often performed to determine the difference between an acute or convalescent blood samples. The diagnosis of a previous strep infection is confirmed when serial titers of ASO rise over a period of weeks and then fall slowly. ASO titers peak during the 3rd week after the onset of acute symptoms of a streptococcal disease; at 6 months after onset, approximately 30% of patients exhibit abnormal titers.
  ▼ Elevated titers are seen in 80–85% patients with acute RF and 95% in acute GN.

■ *Anti–DNase B or ADB*
  ▼ This test also detects antigens produced by group A streptococcus and is elevated in most patients with RF and poststreptococcal GN.
  ▼ This test is often done concurrently with the ASO titer. When ASO and ADB are performed concurrently, 95% of previous strep infections are detected.

- **Normal values** may vary with season of the year, age, and geographic location of the patient. **Expected values** for normal adults as reported in the literature are typically <100 IU/mL. The ULN ASO titer for pediatrics is <100 IU/mL; in school-age children or young adults, it is between 166 and 250 IU/mL. A twofold increase in the ASO value, using serial analysis, within 1–2 weeks of the initial result is supportive of a prior streptococcal infection. In the absence of complications or reinfection, the ASO level usually falls to preinfection activity within 6–12 months.
- **Normal range:** ULN, 116 IU/mL.

❑ Use

- Direct diagnostic value in scarlet fever, erysipelas, and streptococcal pharyngitis and tonsillitis. Indirect diagnostic value in RF, GN, detection of subclinical streptococcal infection, and differential diagnosis of joint pains of RF and RA.

❑ Interpretation

- Increased in pyoderma, postimpetigo nephritis caused by GAS, RF, and pharyngitis.

❑ Limitations

- When evaluating patients with acute RF, the American Heart Association recommends the ASO titer rather than ADB. Even though the ADB is more sensitive than ASO, its results are too variable. It also should be noted that, although ASO is the recommended test, when ASO and ADB are done together, the combination is better than either ASO or ADB alone.
- With the ASO test, false-positive results are observed with increased levels of serum beta lipoproteins produced in liver disease and contamination of serum with *Bacillus cereus* or *Pseudomonas* species. In addition, these titers are not formed as a result of streptococcal pyoderma. Technically, false-positive results occur due to the oxidation of reagents.
- A single ASO analysis may not be meaningful due to the variability of ASO values within the normal population. Both clinical and laboratory findings should be considered in reaching a diagnosis.
- Streptococcal infections already treated with antibiotics may not produce increased results.

SYPHILIS SEROLOGY TESTS

❑ Definition

- Syphilis is an STD caused by the bacterium *Treponema pallidum.* Symptoms of infection are often subtle and easily confused with other STDs such as genital herpes infection. Syphilis is passed from person to person through direct contact with infectious exudates from obvious or concealed, moist, early lesions of skin and mucous membranes of infected people during sexual contacts. Exposure almost always occurs during oral, anal, or vaginal intercourse. A pregnant woman with the disease can pass it to her newborn child.

17

- The diagnosis of syphilis is most commonly made by serologic testing and is typically performed in two settings: screening of patients at increased risk and evaluation of patients with suspected disease.
- There are two types of serologic tests for syphilis: nontreponemal tests such as the rapid plasma reagin (RPR) test and Venereal Disease Research Laboratory (VDRL) test, and specific treponemal tests such as the *Treponema pallidum* particle agglutination assay (TP-PA), fluorescent treponemal antibody absorption (FTA-ABS) test, and the microhemagglutination test for antibodies to *Treponema pallidum* (MHA-TP).
- **Normal range:** Negative.

❑ **Use**

- An aid in the diagnosis of active or past *T. pallidum* infection. Nontreponemal tests are based upon the reactivity of serum from patients with syphilis to a cardiolipin–cholesterol–lecithin antigen. These tests measure IgG and IgM antibodies and are used as the screening test for syphilis in most settings. Positive tests are usually reported as a titer of antibody, and they can be used to follow the response to treatment in many patients. Treponemal tests are more complex and are usually used as confirmatory tests when the nontreponemal tests are reactive. These tests all use *T. pallidum* antigens and are based upon the detection of antibodies directed against treponemal cellular components. These tests are qualitative and are reported as reactive or nonreactive.

❑ **Interpretation**
❑ **Limitations**

- A nonreactive result does not totally exclude a recent (within the last 2–3 weeks) *T. pallidum* infection. Therefore, results need to be interpreted with caution.
- Detection of treponemal antibodies may indicate recent, past, or successfully treated syphilis infections and, therefore, cannot be used to differentiate between active and cured cases.
- False-positive tests for syphilis can occur with both nontreponemal and treponemal tests. A false-positive test result may be identified by a reactive nontreponemal test followed by a nonreactive treponemal test. It is estimated that 1–2% of the US population has false-positive nontreponemal test results. False-positive tests are particularly common during pregnancy.
- The syphilis serology tests may be reactive with sera from patients with yaws (*T. pallidum* subspecies pertenue) or pinta (*Treponema carateum*).
- With nontreponemal tests, biologic false-positive reactions have been reported in diseases such as infectious mononucleosis, leprosy, malaria, SLE, vaccinia, narcotic addiction, autoimmune diseases, and viral pneumonia.
- Despite active syphilis serologic tests may be negative in severely immune-compromised patients.
- CDC recommends standard (traditional) testing algorithm where initial screening with a nontreponemal test such as the RPR; a reactive specimen is then confirmed as a true positive with a treponemal test such as the TP-PA test. When results are reactive to both treponemal and RPR tests, persons should be considered to have untreated syphilis unless this is ruled out

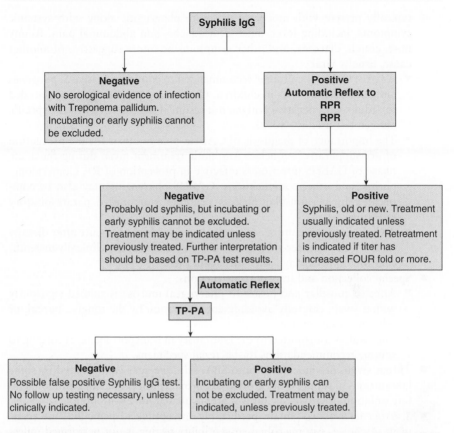

Figure 17–2 *Nontraditional algorithm for syphilis testing. RPR, rapid plasma reagin (test); TP-PA, Treponema pallidum particle agglutination (test).*

by treatment history. Persons who were treated in the past are considered to have a new syphilis infection if quantitative testing on an RPR test (or another nontreponemal test) reveals a fourfold or greater increase in titer.

- Nontraditional testing algorithm: When reverse sequence screening (Figure 17-2) is used, all appropriate reflexing criteria should be used. FTA-ABS test should not be used to confirm discordant treponemal screening results.

Suggested Reading

Discordant results of reverse sequence syphilis screening-Five laboratories; United States 2006–2010. *MMWR Morb Mortal Wkly Rep.* 2011;60:133.

THROAT CULTURE (ROUTINE)

❑ Definition and Use

- This culture is primarily used to detect group A beta-hemolytic *Streptococcus* (GABHS, *S. pyogenes*) from throat swabs. This test is used, usually in children, who present with symptoms of streptococcal pharyngitis. Patients typically present with moderate to severe pharyngitis along with systemic symptoms, including fever, malaise, headache, and abdominal pain. Runny nose, cough, diarrhea, and other symptoms are more suggestive of another cause, usually viral.

▼ A GABHS throat culture is recommended to confirm negative *S. pyogenes* antigen screening tests in children. Confirmatory cultures are not needed for adults with negative antigen test results if the sensitivity of the specific antigen test used is >80%.

▼ The importance of diagnosis of GABHS pharyngitis is for the prevention of nonsuppurative sequelae. Antibiotic treatment given during the acute phase of GABHS infection is effective in prevention of RF, glomerulonephritis, and other complications. GABHS pharyngitis may also be complicated by peritonsillar abscess or other suppurative pararespiratory infections.

▼ A GABHS throat culture is not recommended for test of cure after therapy for documented strep throat; cultures may demonstrate clinically insignificant low-level carriage after successful therapy.

▪ **Special collection and transport instructions:**
   ▼ Affected tonsillar and posterior pharyngeal mucosa is rubbed vigorously with a swab, carefully avoiding contamination by the tongue, buccal, or other mucosal surface.
   ▼ The swab is transported to the laboratory in transport media according to routine recommendations for bacterial specimens.

▪ Throat swabs are inoculated onto SBA; selective agar is inoculated by some laboratories to suppress the growth of normal endogenous flora and to facilitate isolation of GABHS. Cultures are incubated for 24–48 hours.

▪ *S. pyogenes* isolates remain predictably susceptible to penicillin, the treatment of choice. Antimicrobial susceptibility testing is not performed unless requested because of penicillin allergy.

▪ **Turnaround time:** Cultures are examined for 24–48 hours. An additional day may be required for isolation and identification of suspected isolates from heavily contaminated specimens.

❑ **Interpretation**

   ▪ **Expected results:** No growth of group A beta-hemolytic *Streptococcus*.
   ▪ **Positive result:** Positive cultures, in the setting of a clinical diagnosis, are diagnostic of GABHS pharyngitis. In the absence of symptoms, positive cultures may indicate carriage and not infection.
   ▪ **Negative results:** Throat cultures are sensitive to rule out streptococcal pharyngitis, but may be negative if there is poor specimen collection.

❑ **Limitations**

   ▪ Cultures are typically negative in patients presenting with symptoms consistent with nonsuppurative complications of GABHS infection. Serologic tests, like ASO, may provide support for the diagnosis.
   ▪ **Common pitfall:** A throat culture is not optimized for the detection of organisms other than *S. pyogenes*. (Group C and G beta-streptococci and/or *A. hemolyticum* are identified in throat cultures in some laboratories.)

- Submission of a throat culture is not recommended for detection of carriage or infection by other organisms. To determine the cause of sinusitis or other pararespiratory infections, special procedures for collection and culture (e.g., respiratory tract bacterial culture) are required.

❑ **Other Considerations**

- Other causes of pharyngitis include viruses (most common), mycoplasmas, group C and G beta-hemolytic streptococci, and *Arcanobacterium hemolyticum*. *N. gonorrhoeae* may be considered in patients at risk. *C. diphtheriae* is uncommon in the United States, but should be considered in patients at risk. Special testing is usually required to detect pathogens other than *S. pyogenes* from throat cultures.
- GABHS may cause infection at other sites, especially cellulitis. Routine bacterial cultures appropriate for these sites should be requested.

THROAT AND PHARYNGEAL CULTURE, PATIENTS WITH CYSTIC FIBROSIS

❑ **Use**

- This culture is used to screen for the bacterial pathogens that commonly cause lower respiratory tract infections in patients with CF. Pharyngeal specimens are most useful to document carriage/chronic infection, whereas lower respiratory specimens are recommended for the evaluation of clinically evident, acute infection.
- Pneumonia is a cause of significant morbidity and mortality in patients with CF. The etiology of these infections is different than that seen in other patient groups. *P. aeruginosa* (including mucoid variants), *Burkholderia cepacia* complex organisms, *Stenotrophomonas maltophilia*, *H. influenzae*, and other glucose-fermenting and nonfermenting gram-negative bacilli, as well as mycobacteria, *S. aureus*, and *S. pneumoniae*, are commonly isolated from lower and upper respiratory tract specimens submitted from patients with CF.
- Sputum from patients with CF should not be screened by Gram stain, as recommended for routine sputum cultures submitted from patients without CF.
- Special collection and transport instructions:
  - ▼ Posterior pharyngeal swabs may be submitted.
  - ▼ Expectorated sputum or invasively obtained lower respiratory specimens are recommended for evaluation of chronic carriage/infection and acute exacerbation of pulmonary infection.
  - ▼ Specimens are transported as for routine sputum specimens.
- Method:
  - ▼ A variety of supportive, selective, and differential agar media are inoculated. Commonly inoculated media include
    - ● SBA as a supportive medium capable of supporting the growth of many pathogens, including *S. pneumoniae*.
    - ● CNA agar for gram-positive pathogens; mannitol–salt agar for isolation of *S. aureus*.
    - ● MacConkey agar for nonfastidious gram-negative bacilli, including *P. aeruginosa* and *S. maltophilia*.

- ● *B. cepacia*–selective agar.
- ● Chocolate agar for isolation of *H. influenzae*.
- ▼ Cultures for mycobacterial, fungal, viral, or other respiratory pathogens are also recommended in addition to bacterial cultures.
- ■ **Turnaround time:** Cultures are examined daily for 96 hours. Several days are required for isolation, susceptibility testing, and identification of suspected isolates.

❑ **Interpretation**

- ■ Patients with CF often show respiratory tract colonization that changes little over time, even in response to antimicrobial therapy. The interpretation of cultures demonstrating such "abnormal flora" may be challenging; clinical and therapeutic decisions must be based on a variety of clinical and other factors, in addition to culture results.
- ■ The workup and interpretation of CF respiratory cultures are typically based on several factors, including type of specimen submitted, organism(s) isolated, and the predominance of a specific pathogen compared to other flora.

❑ **Limitations**

- ■ Although rapidly growing mycobacteria and mold may be isolated with CF respiratory cultures, special cultures are needed for sensitive detection of nontuberculous mycobacteria, *Aspergillus* species and other molds, and viruses that may cause acute respiratory infections in these patients. It is difficult to differentiate isolates that represent chronic colonization versus acute exacerbation on the basis of laboratory criteria.
- ■ **Common pitfalls:**
  - ▼ Clinicians must order special throat or lower respiratory cultures specifically designed for evaluation of patients with CF; routine cultures are not optimized for evaluation of the flora typically isolated from such specimens. Laboratories should not apply sputum rejection criteria based on Gram stain screening recommended for routine sputum cultures submitted from other patients.

TOXOPLASMA SEROLOGY SCREEN (*TOXOPLASMA GONDII*, IgG AND IgM)

❑ **Definition**

- ■ *Toxoplasma gondii* is an obligate intracellular parasite capable of infecting most mammals, including humans. Toxoplasmosis usually is asymptomatic, but primary infection during pregnancy can result in congenital disease. The domestic cat is the only definitive host for *T. gondii* and is the reservoir of the infective oocysts that are passed in the feces. Human infection may be acquired by consuming cysts in uncooked or undercooked meat of infected animals or by contact with oocysts from the feces of an infected cat.
- ■ Acute *Toxoplasma* infection can pose a serious threat to immunocompromised individuals and newborns who acquire the infection in utero. Immunosuppressed patients may develop encephalitis, myocarditis, or pneumonitis. Congenital infections usually result as a consequence of asymptomatic acute maternal

infection. This infection can cause premature delivery, spontaneous abortion, or stillbirth.

- Management of toxoplasmosis requires serologic monitoring of infected individuals, as the organism is not readily available for culture.
- **Normal range:** Negative.

❏ Use

- Aids in the diagnosis of toxoplasmosis.
- First-line test in endemic areas for identifying *T. gondii* infection in pregnant women.
- Testing for the presence of *Toxoplasma* IgG can be useful to determine prior infection and indicate reactivation of the infection.
- Testing for the presence of *Toxoplasma* IgM is useful to determine acute infection.

❏ Interpretation

- Positive in *Toxoplasma* infection.
- Individuals infected with the *Toxoplasma* organism typically exhibit detectable levels of IgM antibody immediately before or soon after the onset of symptoms. IgM titers normally decline within 4–6 months but may persist at low levels up to a year. Patients with active *Toxoplasma* chorioretinitis usually have undetectable levels of IgM.

❏ Limitations

- IgG is not useful for diagnosing infection in infants <6 months of age, because they are usually the result of passive transfer from the mother.
- Low levels of IgM antibodies may occasionally persist for >12 months postinfection. For the determination of seroconversion from nonreactive to reactive, two serum samples should be drawn 3–4 weeks apart, during the acute and convalescent stages of the infection. The acute-phase sample should be stored and tested in parallel with the convalescent sample.
- CDC suggests equivocal or positive results should be retested using a different assay from another reference laboratory specializing in toxoplasmosis testing (IgG dye test, IgM ELISA, reflex to avidity, and/or other tests).
- In a pregnant patient, if both IgG/IgM positive, an IgG avidity test should be performed. A high avidity result in 12–16 weeks of pregnancy essentially rules out an infection acquired during gestation.
- A low IgG avidity result should not be interpreted as recent infection, because some individuals have persistent low IgG avidity for many months after infection.
- Newborn infants suspected of congenital toxoplasmosis should be tested by both an IgM- and an IgA-capture EIA (CDC recommendation). Detection of *Toxoplasma*-specific IgA antibodies is more sensitive than IgM detection in congenitally infected babies.

TRICHOMONAS VAGINALIS MOLECULAR DETECTION

See: Sexually Transmitted Infections, Molecular Diagnosis (*Chlamydia trachomatis, Neisseria gonorrhoeae, Trichomonas vaginalis*)

URINE CULTURE (ROUTINE)

❏ Definition

- Urine culture is used for the detection of UTI caused by common uropathogenic bacteria and yeast. The range of UTI syndromes is broad, including asymptomatic bacteriuria through pyelonephritis with systemic symptoms. Patients with uncomplicated UTIs often present with dysuria and frequency, whereas pyelonephritis may be associated with signs of sepsis, including fever, flank pain, and nausea. The risk of UTI, including complicated UTI, is increased in patients with urinary tract prosthetic materials, like stents, GU tract malformations, history of GU surgery, and medical conditions, such as pregnancy, neurologic disorders, and DM.

❏ Special Collection and Transport Instructions

- **Acceptable specimens:** Clean-catch midstream urine, straight catheterization ("in and out"), newly placed indwelling catheters, and suprapubic aspirates are commonly submitted and should be associated with low contamination rates.
  - ▼ Urine collected from an indwelling catheter or from pediatric collection bags is frequently contaminated. Negative cultures may be helpful in ruling out UTI; positive cultures should be interpreted with caution. Urine for culture should never be taken from a collection bag attached to an indwelling catheter.
  - ▼ Collection of urine from ileal conduits or by invasive procedures (like percutaneous nephrostomy or by cystoscopy) is obtained by personnel specifically trained in these techniques.
- The specimen should be transported to the laboratory within 2 hours after collection. If transport is delayed, the specimen should be refrigerated.
  - ▼ Alternatively, urine may be inoculated into a preservative collection system, allowing transport up to 48 hours. Preservative systems must be inoculated according to the manufacturer's instructions. Preserved specimens are transported at room temperature.
  - ▼ There are several commercially available systems that allow culture media to be directly inoculated at the site of collection. These systems may be incubated prior to transport to the laboratory.

❏ Use

- Urine is cultured quantitatively. For most patients, 1 µL of urine is inoculated onto SBA and onto a selective, differential agar for isolation of gram-negative bacilli. Urine specimens with fewer than 10^3 organisms per milliliter of urine yield no growth on the media.
  - ▼ For patients at risk for clinically significant UTI at lower concentrations of uropathogens, 10 µL of urine may be inoculated, resulting in a lower detection level of 10^2 organisms per milliliter. Uropathogens present in concentrations between 10^2 and 10^3 organisms per milliliter may be clinically significant in symptomatic patients. Repeat culture has shown that these patients may rapidly progress to higher concentrations of bacteria.

▼ The extent of workup and susceptibility testing is determined by the type of specimen submitted, concentration and species isolated, and patient risk factors. Workup of mixed cultures, which usually represent specimen contamination with endogenous flora, should be limited.

■ Potentially pathogenic isolates are identified and susceptibility testing performed, as appropriate.

■ **Turnaround time:** Urine cultures from patients at low risk for complicated UTI should be incubated for a minimum of 16 hours. Cultures from patients at risk for complicated UTI should be incubated for a minimum of 48 hours before signing out as negative. Several additional days may be required for final identification and susceptibility testing in positive cultures.

❏ **Interpretation**

■ **Expected results:** $<10^3$ colonies/mL for routine urine cultures; $<10^2$ colonies/mL for special cultures taken from patients at high risk for complicated UTI. A low concentration of genital flora is commonly seen.

■ **Positive results:** Isolation of a common uropathogen at concentrations $>10^4$ colonies/mL ($>10^3$ colonies/mL for high-risk patients), when present as the sole or predominant isolate, is considered positive.

■ **Negative results:** Urine culture is sensitive for ruling out UTI, but prior antimicrobial therapy can inhibit the growth of uropathogens, resulting in false-negative cultures.

❏ **Limitations**

■ **Common pitfalls:**

▼ Contamination, due to poorly collected or transported urine samples, limits the value of a significant proportion of specimens submitted to the laboratory.

▼ Clinically significant polymicrobial UTI is uncommon ($<5\%$). Interpret mixed cultures with caution—they most likely indicate contaminated specimens.

▼ Urine is frequently transported in collection cups on which the caps are not firmly tightened, resulting in leakage and possible contamination.

▼ Urethritis and vaginitis may be associated with pyuria and clinically mimic cystitis.

Suggested Reading

McCarter YS, Burd EM, Hall GS, et al. *Cumitech 2C, Laboratory Diagnosis of Urinary Tract Infections.* Washington, DC: ASM Press, 2009.

VAGINITIS PANEL, MOLECULAR PROBE

❏ **Definition and Use**

■ Symptoms of vaginitis and vaginosis are seen frequently in clinical practice. The most common causes are bacterial vaginosis (BV), trichomoniasis, and vulvovaginal candidiasis. Because of significant clinical overlap in the symptoms, specific diagnostic testing may be required to guide appropriate antimicrobial therapy and patient management.

- This test is based on pathogen detection by nucleic acid probe hybridization. The testing includes probes for the detection *Gardnerella vaginalis* (a marker for the disruption of the normal vaginal flora seen in BV), *Candida* species (for candidiasis), and *Trichomonas vaginalis* (for trichomoniasis).
- The assessment of test accuracy depends on the populations studied, the comparator method, and other factors.
  - ▼ Sensitivity and specificity for detection of candidiasis in symptomatic women: 82% and 95%, respectively.
  - ▼ Sensitivity and specificity for detection of BV in symptomatic women: 98% and 100%, respectively.
  - ▼ Sensitivity and specificity for detection of trichomoniasis, compared to wet mount detection: 93% and 99%, respectively.
- **Turnaround time:** 24 hours.

❏ **Specimen Collection and Transport Instructions**

- Vaginal fluid specimens should be collected only from patients with symptoms consistent with vaginosis or vaginitis.
- Use only supplies provided in the Affirm VPIII transport system, sample collection set, or test kit for specimen collection.
- Samples are collected from the posterior vaginal fornix, using an unlubricated (no water or jelly) speculum, ensuring that the entire circumference of the swab has been inoculated with vaginal secretions.
- Place the swab into sample collection tube and snap on cap following the kit instructions.
- Transport specimens according to kit instructions. Specimens may be transported at room temperature or refrigerated.

❏ **Interpretation**

- **Expected results:** Negative for all three pathogens. Negative results for a specific pathogen suggest that infection with that pathogen is unlikely.
- **Positive results:** If one or more of the pathogens tested indicate infection when consistent signs and symptoms are present. Infection with more than one of the pathogens is not uncommon.

❏ **Limitations**

- Specimens must be collected, transported, tested, and interpreted using protocols described in the package insert of the kit used.
- Performance of the test depends on optimal specimen collection.
- Negative results do not exclude the possibility of infection with any of the specific pathogens.
- Alternative testing, like pH, "amine test," and microscopic examination of vaginal fluid may be considered for the evaluation of patients.
- The Affirm VPIII test does not detect infection by *Neisseria gonorrhoeae* or *Chlamydia trachomatis*; these pathogens and other possible causes of the patient's symptoms should be considered, and ruled out as appropriate, in women presenting with vaginal discharge or other compatible symptoms.
- The test cannot be used as a test of cure because DNA from nonviable pathogens may be detectable after resolution of infection.

VANCOMYCIN-RESISTANT ENTEROCOCCUS (VRE) SCREEN CULTURE

❑ **Definition and Use**

- This test is usually ordered to detect VRE carriage in asymptomatic patients for infection control purposes. It is indicated to screen patients at risk for self-infection or for transmitting VRE to close contacts. The test may also be requested to document clearance of VRE carriage. A patient specimen is plated onto selective agar, typically containing 6 μg/mL vancomycin. Any growth of *Enterococcus* likely represents VRE, but vancomycin resistance and identification should be confirmed by subsequent testing of the isolate. Swab specimens of the rectum or perianal skin are recommended for VRE screening cultures.
- **Turnaround time:** 48 hours.

❑ **Interpretation**

- **Expected results:** Negative.

❑ **Limitations**

- Detection of VRE carriage may require submission of several samples, and collection from several potentially colonized sites.
- **Common pitfall:** The VRE screening culture is usually not indicated for evaluation of potentially infected material. Because only selective media is used for screening, other potential pathogens would be missed if VRE screening culture only is requested. VRE grow well in wound and other cultures submitted for evaluation of infected specimens.

VARICELLA-ZOSTER VIRUS (VZV) CULTURE (RULE OUT)

❑ **Definition**

- VZV causes chickenpox and shingles. Clinical diagnosis is usually straightforward for these infections. Occasionally, specific diagnosis may be needed for unusual, serious infections, including disseminated disease, or infections in pregnant, immunocompromised, and other high-risk patients.

❑ **Special Collection and Transport Instructions**

- General recommendations for viral culture apply. Specimens should be collected early in acute infection. Specimens from cutaneous or mucous membranes are most commonly submitted. Samples should be taken from fresh, wet lesions, ideally from intact vesicles after unroofing. Most specimens should be placed in a viral transport medium and transported on wet ice (4°C).

❑ **Use**

- This test may be used to isolate VZV when specific diagnosis is required. Patient specimens are usually inoculated onto human lung fibroblast cell cultures, like WI-38. Cell morphology is monitored; cultures showing cytopathic

17

effect typical for VZV should be confirmed using specific immunologic techniques, like staining with tagged monoclonal anti-VZV antibodies.

- **Turnaround time:** Up to 4 weeks. Most positive cultures are detected within 7 days.

❑ **Interpretation**

- **Expected results:** Negative.
  - ▼ **Positive result:** Cell cultures positive for VZV indicate active infection.
  - ▼ **Negative result:** Negative cell cultures decrease the likelihood of VZV infection, but cannot absolutely rule out VZV infection, especially for CSF and mucosal surface samples.

❑ **Limitations**

- There may be poor sensitivity for certain specimen types.
- **Turnaround time** for VZV culture may be prolonged, limiting their utility for acute management of critically ill patients.
- **Common pitfall:** Collection of specimens from dried, overcrusted lesions.

VARICELLA-ZOSTER VIRUS (VZV) DIRECT DETECTION (DFA)

See Herpes Virus (HSV or VZV) Direct Detection (DFA)

VARICELLA-ZOSTER VIRUS (VZV) SEROLOGY SCREEN (IgG AND IgM)

❑ **Definition**

- VZV infection causes two clinically distinct forms of disease. Primary infection with VZV results in varicella (chickenpox), characterized by vesicular lesions in different stages of development on the face, trunk, and extremities. Herpes zoster, also known as "shingles," results from reactivation of endogenous latent VZV infection within the sensory ganglia. This clinical form of the disease is characterized by a painful, unilateral vesicular eruption, which usually occurs in a restricted dermatomal distribution. The diagnosis of these two diseases is usually made clinically. However, the use of diagnostic assays may be important in specific situations.
- Other names include chickenpox serology testing.

❑ **Use**

- To assist in the diagnosis of acute-phase infection with varicella virus
- To assist in identifying nonimmune individuals

❑ **Interpretation**

- **Normal range:** Negative.
- A positive IgG result coupled with a positive IgM result indicates recent infection with VZV.
- A positive IgG result coupled with a negative IgM result indicates previous exposure to VZV and immunity.

- A negative IgG result coupled with a negative IgM result indicates the absence of prior exposure to VZV and no immunity. However, a negative result does not rule out a VZV infection. Negative results in suspected early VZV infections should be followed by testing a new serum specimen in 2–3 weeks.
- Equivocal results should be followed up with testing a new serum specimen within 10–14 days.

❏ Limitations

- Test for VZV IgG antibodies is of use when clinical symptoms are present or infection suspected. Screening of the general population leads to no appreciable diagnostic advantage. Results from immunosuppressed patients should be interpreted with caution.
- Many different antibody tests are available with a wide range of performance standards. The fluorescent antibody to membrane antibody (FAMA) is the most extensively validated assay and correlates best with susceptibility to and protection against varicella. However, this test is not widely used because it is labor intensive and requires expert interpretation.
- Many commercially available ELISAs are available that are considered generally less sensitive than FAMA, although specificities are comparable.
- Commercial ELISA assays are suitable for screening for VZV susceptibility among health care workers. The rationale for this is that the risk of vaccinating an adult with a false-negative test result is much lower than the risk of natural infection in an individual falsely identified as seropositive.
- Routine screening for varicella in individuals born in the United States before 1980, who are not health care workers, is not recommended because of extremely high rates of seropositivity in this population.

VIBRIO CULTURE OF STOOL (RULE OUT)

❏ Definition

- *Vibrio* species are an uncommon cause of bacterial enteric infections in this country, but endemic infections occur in many countries. Epidemic outbreaks are well described, generally associated with inadequately treated sewage or contaminated water. *Vibrio* species are halophilic, and brackish water and shellfish serve as an important reservoir for organisms. Although infection may be relatively mild and self-limited, some patients develop cholera: severe disease with vomiting and profuse watery diarrhea (rice water stools). The severe diarrhea may rapidly lead to life-threatening dehydration and electrolyte imbalance. Stool culture to rule out *Vibrio* species should be considered for patients who develop diarrhea, especially severe watery diarrhea, after travel to an endemic area, ingestion of contaminated sea food, or exposure to brackish water.

❏ Use

- This culture is used to detect enteric infection caused by *Vibrio cholerae* or related *Vibrio* species. Specimens are inoculated on the thiosulfate citrate bile sucrose (TCBS) medium, a differential and selective medium for *Vibrio* isolation. Broth enrichment using alkaline peptone water may be used to improve isolation. Colonies from routine stool culture may be screened for cytochrome oxidase–positive isolates, which should be further tested to rule out *Vibrio* species.

■ **Turnaround time:** Cultures are incubated for 48 hours. Additional time is required for isolation and identification.

❏ **Interpretation**

■ **Expected results:** No growth.

❏ **Limitations**

■ *Vibrio* enteric infection may be missed if specific cultures are not requested.

WEST NILE VIRUS (WNV) SEROLOGY

❏ **Definition**

■ WNV is a mosquito-transmitted Flavivirus of the family Flaviviridae. It is maintained in a cycle between birds and mosquitoes mostly belonging to the *Culex* genus. Besides horses and humans, several other mammals are dead-end hosts of WNV. About 80% of humans infected with WNV develop no or only very mild symptoms. In about 20% of the cases, patients develop more severe symptoms such as fever, myalgia, and lymphadenopathy. Furthermore, in a small proportion of cases, the infection progresses to life-threatening neuroinvasive forms characterized by meningitis, encephalitis, and/or flaccid paralysis. The risk of developing lethal forms is increased in the elderly or in immunocompromised patients. WNV is most widely spread in temperate areas: isolated in parts of Europe, Middle East, Africa, Asia, America, and Australia. The IgM enzyme immunoassay (EIA) on CSF and/or serum is currently the most sensitive screening test for West Nile virus in humans.

❏ **Use**

■ As an aid to the diagnosis of West Nile virus encephalitis.

❏ **Interpretation**

■ Following infection with WNV, IgM antibodies are produced and can be detected within 4–7 days after exposure and may persist for about 1 year, while IgG antibodies can be reliably detected from day 8 after infection.

❏ **Limitations**

■ There are several types of serologic tests routinely used for WNV diagnostics: enzyme-linked immunosorbent assay (ELISA), immunofluorescence assay (IFA), neutralization test (NT), and the hemagglutination inhibition assay.

■ Because West Nile IgM may not be positive until up to 8 days following onset of illness, specimens collected <8 days after onset may be negative for IgM, and testing should be repeated.

■ A positive West Nile IgG in the absence of a positive West Nile IgM is consistent with past infection with a Flavivirus and does not by itself suggest acute West Nile virus infection.

- If acute West Nile virus infection is suspected, it is best to collect both acute and convalescent sera. Convalescent specimens should be collected 2–3 weeks after acute specimens.
- A major issue in WNV diagnostics is cross-reactivity with antibodies against heterologous flaviviruses, for example, dengue virus (DENV), Japanese encephalitis virus (JEV), tick-borne encephalitis virus (TBEV), or yellow fever virus, which is especially true for IgG antibodies.

WOUND CULTURE

❑ Definition

- Wound cultures are used to identify pathogenic bacteria causing wound infections. Traumatic injury of tissue may be complicated by infection. Infections may be caused by organisms introduced from the external environment, like bite and surgical and traumatic wounds, or by organisms derived from the patient's endogenous flora, like peritonitis associated with a ruptured appendix. Wound culture should be considered when a wound shows signs and symptoms typical of infection: swelling, redness, exudate or pus formation, sinus tract formation, pain, swelling, or other.

❑ Special Collection and Transport Instructions

- Specimens should be collected from the site of active infection. Adjacent areas may show "sympathetic" signs of inflammation, but may not yield relevant pathogens.
- Wash and decontaminate the collection site, typically using a soap and 70% alcohol.
- Collection of infected tissue or aspirate, at least 1 g, is recommended. Collection using swabs is not recommended.
- Collection and transport under anaerobic conditions are recommended, especially for closed wounds. Specimens should be transported to the laboratory within 2 hours. Specimens may be held at 4°C for a short time if transport is delayed.

❑ Use

- Most specimens for bacterial wound cultures should be examined by Gram staining. Specimens from superficial wounds showing a significant numbers of epithelial cells are likely to be contaminated by endogenous flora unrelated to the infection.
- Specimens are inoculated onto supportive, enriched, and selective/differential media.
- Specimens are inoculated onto supportive and enriched nonselective media, like SBA and chocolate agar media, and selective media, like MacConkey, PEA, and CNA agar. Some laboratories include a broth medium, like thioglycollate broth, to routine cultures. Anaerobic medium is inoculated for appropriate specimens collected and submitted under anaerobic conditions.
- **Turnaround time:** Cultures are incubated for 48–72 hours. Additional time is required for isolation, identification, susceptibility testing, and further characterization, as needed.

17

❑ **Interpretation**

- **Expected results:** No growth.
- **Positive results:** Cultures of infected wounds often show growth of several types of organisms. Cultures must be interpreted carefully: Mixed cultures may be caused by colonization by endogenous flora or contamination due to poor specimen collection technique. However, mixed cultures may represent synergistic polymicrobial infections, especially when anaerobes are isolated.
- **Negative results:** Negative culture decreases the likelihood of active bacterial infection.

❑ **Limitations**

- Negative cultures may be caused by prior antimicrobial treatment, infection caused by a fastidious pathogen, or collection of the sample from a site other than that of active infection.
- Significant pathogens may not be recognized in mixed cultures.
- Submission of multiple cultures or cultures of several affected sites may be required for detection, especially in chronic infections. The structure and milieu of abscesses may prevent effective antibiotic treatment. They are avascular spaces, and their outer capsule may prevent entry of antimicrobial agents. In addition, antibiotics may be inactivated by the acidic environment and degradative enzymes present. Adjunctive surgical therapy may be required, especially for large collections of pus.
- **Common pitfall:** Collection of specimens from sites other than the active site of infection, such as sinus tracts, often yields growth of endogenous flora unrelated to the infection.

❑ **Other Considerations**

- Pyogenic infections are usually associated with heavy growth (10^5 CFU/mL) of the responsible pathogen.
- Polymicrobial infections are often treated successfully with surgical and/or empirical antimicrobial therapy. Extensive culture analysis with identification and susceptibility of multiple isolates is usually not clinically indicated.
- Certain pathogens are associated with specific types of wound infections, such as *P. aeruginosa* with penetrating foot wounds through sneakers and *P. multocida* with cat bites. These infections may require special laboratory techniques for optimal detection; alert the laboratory when suspected.

YERSINIA ENTEROCOLITICA CULTURE (RULE OUT)

❑ **Definition**

- *Yersinia enterocolitica* is an infrequent cause of bacterial diarrheal infection, usually in children. Infection has been associated with ingestion of undercooked pork, dairy products, and tainted water. Infection can also be transmitted by the fecal–oral route. Symptoms are fairly nonspecific: fever, abdominal pain, and diarrhea, which may be bloody. Abdominal pain in adults may mimic appendicitis. This test is a specialized stool culture for the detection of GI infection caused by *Y. enterocolitica*.

❑ **Use**

- Cold enrichment, holding stool suspended in buffered saline at 4°C prior to subculture onto enteric media, may improve recovery in heavily contaminated specimens. *Y. enterocolitica* may be isolated using a selective medium, like MacConkey agar. Many laboratories use a more selective medium, like CIN agar (cefsulodin–ingrasan–novobiosin), to improve recovery. *Y. enterocolitica* isolation may be improved by culture incubation at 25°C.

- **Turnaround time:** Cultures are examined for 48 hours. Several days are required for isolation and identification of suspected isolates.

❑ **Interpretation**

- **Expected results:** No growth.

❑ **Limitations**

- The symptoms of yersiniosis are not specific, and this enteric pathogen may not be suspected unless specific risk factors or epidemiologic evidence suggests this infection. Isolates are sucrose positive, so isolates may be missed by laboratories using EMB agar for enteric cultures. (The EMB medium contains sucrose so isolates will look similar to normal enteric flora.)

17

APPENDIX

Abbreviations and Acronyms

A/G	albumin-to-globulin ratio	BJ protein	Bence-Jones protein
AA	amyloid A, atomic absorption	BPH	benign prostatic hyperplasia
		BT	bleeding time
ABG	arterial blood gas	BUN	blood urea nitrogen
ACE	angiotensin-converting enzyme	CA-125	cancer antigen 125
		CAD	coronary artery disease
Ach	acetylcholine	CAH	congenital adrenal hyperplasia
AChR	acetylcholine receptor		
ACTH	adrenocorticotropic hormone	cAMP	cyclic adenosine monophosphate
ADH	antidiuretic hormone	CBC	complete blood count
AF	amniotic fluid	CDC	Centers for Disease Control and Prevention
AFB	acid-fast bacillus		
AFP	α-fetoprotein	CEA	carcinoembryonic antigen
AG	anion gap	CF	complement fixation, cystic fibrosis
AHF	antihemophilic factor		
AIDS	acquired immunodeficiency syndrome	CFU	colony forming unit
		CHD	congenital heart disease, coronary heart disease
ALA	aminolevulinic acid		
ALL	acute lymphoblastic leukemia	ChE	cholinesterase
		CHF	congestive heart failure
ALP	alkaline phosphatase	CIE	counter (-current) immunoelectrophoresis
ALT	alanine aminotransferase (see SGPT)		
		CK	creatine kinase
AMI	acute myocardial infarction	CK-MB	creatine kinase MB band
AML	acute myeloblastic leukemia acute myelocytic leukemia acute myelogenous leukemia	CK-MM	creatine kinase MM band
		CLL	chronic lymphocytic leukemia
ANA	antinuclear antibody	CMV	cytomegalovirus
ANCA	anti–neutrophil cytoplasmic antibody	CNS	central nervous system
		COPD	chronic obstructive pulmonary disease
ARC	AIDS-related complex (see AIDS)		
		CRH	corticotropin-releasing hormone
ARDS	acute respiratory distress syndrome		
		CRP	C-reactive protein
ASOT	antistreptolysin-O titer	CSF	cerebrospinal fluid
AST	aspartate aminotransferase (see SGOT)	CT	computed tomography
		CVA	cerebrovascular accident
ATP	adenosine triphosphate	d	day
BAL	bronchoalveolar lavage	Da	dalton
BCG	bacillus Calmette-Guérin	DFA	direct fluorescent antibody

DHEA	dehydroepiandrosterone
DHEA-S	dehydroepiandrosterone sulfate
DI	diabetes insipidus
DIC	disseminated intravascular coagulation
DKA	diabetic ketoacidosis
dL	deciliter
DM	diabetes mellitus
DNA	deoxyribonucleic acid (also see the Glossary)
DOC	deoxycorticosterone
EBV	Epstein-Barr virus
ECG	electrocardiogram
EDTA	edetic acid (ethylenediaminetetraacetic acid)
EIA	enzyme immunoassay
ELISA	enzyme-linked immunosorbent assay
EM	electron microscopy
EMIT	enzyme-multiplied immunoassay technique
ENA	extractable nuclear antigen
EPA	Environmental Protection Agency
ERCP	endoscopic retrograde cholangiopancreatography
ESR	erythrocyte sedimentation rate
Fab	antigen-binding fragment of immunoglobulin
FAB	French-American-British classification for acute leukemias
FBS	fasting blood sugar
Fc	crystallizable fragment of immunoglobulin
FDA	Food and Drug Administration
FISH	fluorescence in situ hybridization (also see the Glossary)
fL	femtoliter
FNA	fine needle aspiration
FPIA	fluorescence polarization immunoassay
FSH	follicle-stimulating hormone
FT_4	free thyroxine
FTA	fluorescent treponemal antibody
FTA-ABS	fluorescent treponemal antibody absorption test
FTI	free thyroxine index
g	gram

GC/MS	gas chromatography/mass spectrometry
GFR	glomerular filtration rate
GGT	γ-glutamyl transferase
GI	gastrointestinal
GN	glomerulonephritis
G6PD	glucose-6-phosphate dehydrogenase
GTT	glucose tolerance test
GU	genitourinary
HA	hemagglutination
HAA	hepatitis-associated antigen
HAI	hemagglutination inhibition
HAV	hepatitis A virus
Hb	hemoglobin (may be followed by types: HbC, HbD, HbE, HbF, HbH, HbS)
HbA_{1c}	glycosylated hemoglobin, hemoglobin A1c
HBcAb	hepatitis B core antibody
HBcAg	hepatitis B core antigen
HBeAb	hepatitis B e antibody
HBeAg	hepatitis B e antigen
HBIG	hepatitis B immune globulin
HBsAb	hepatitis B surface antibody
HBsAg	hepatitis B surface antigen
HBV	hepatitis B virus
hCG	human chorionic gonadotropin
Hct	hematocrit
HCV	hepatitis C virus
H&E	hematoxylin and eosin (stain)
HDL	high-density lipoprotein
HDN	hemolytic disease of the newborn
HDV	hepatitis delta virus
HELPP	hemolysis, elevated liver enzymes, low platelets [syndrome]
HEV	hepatitis E virus
hGH	human growth hormone
HI	hemagglutination inhibition
HIAA	hydroxyindole acetic acid
HIV	human immunodeficiency virus
HLA	human leukocyte antigen
HPF	high-power field
HPLC	high performance liquid chromatography
HPV	human papillomavirus
HSV	herpes simplex virus
HTLV	human T-cell leukemia virus human T-cell lymphotropic virus

HUS	hemolytic uremic syndrome	MRI	magnetic resonance imaging
HVA	homovanillic acid	mRNA	messenger RNA (also see the Glossary)
ICDH	isocitric dehydrogenase		
ICU	intensive care unit	N	normal
IEP	immunoelectrophoresis	NANB	non-A, non-B hepatitis (hepatitis C)
IF	immunofluorescence		
IFA	indirect immunofluorescent assay	NBT	nitroblue tetrazolium
		NIDDK	National Institute of Diabetes and Digestive and Kidney Diseases
Ig	immunoglobulin (can be found as IgA, IgD, IgE, IgG, IgM)		
		NPV	negative predictive value
IHA	indirect hemagglutination	NSAID	nonsteroidal anti-inflammatory drug
IM	infectious mononucleosis, intramuscular		
		5'-NT	5'-nucleotidase
INH	isoniazid	OGTT	oral glucose tolerance test
INR	international normalized ratio	17-OHKS	17-hydroxyketosteroids
IRMA	immunoradiometric assay	O & P	ova and parasites
ITP	idiopathic thrombocytopenic purpura	PA	pernicious anemia
		Pap	Papanicolaou smear
IU	international unit	PAP	prostatic acid phosphatase
IV	intravenous	PBS	peripheral blood smear
17-KGS	17-ketogenic steroids	pCO_2	partial pressure of carbon dioxide
KOH	potassium hydroxide		
17-KS	17-ketosteroids	PCR	polymerase chain reaction (also see Glossary)
L	liter		
LA	latex agglutination, lupus anticoagulant	PCV	packed cell volume
		PDW	platelet distribution width
LAP	leucine aminopeptidase/ Leukocyte Alkaline Phosphatase	pg	picogram
		Ph	Philadelphia chromosome
		PK	pyruvate kinase
LC/MS	liquid chromatography/mass spectrometry	PKU	phenylketonuria
		PMN	polymorphonuclear neutrophil
LD, LDH	lactate dehydrogenase		
LDL	low-density lipoprotein	PNH	paroxysmal nocturnal hemoglobinuria
LE	lupus erythematosus		
LH	luteinizing hormone	PO	by mouth (Latin, *per os*)
LUTS	lower urinary tract symptoms	pO_2	partial pressure of oxygen
		POC	point of care
MAO	monoamine oxidase	POCT	point-of-care testing
MCH	mean corpuscular hemoglobin	ppm	parts per million
		PPV	positive predictive value
MCHC	mean corpuscular hemoglobin concentration	PRA	plasma renin activity
		PSA	prostate-specific antigen
MCV	mean corpuscular volume	PSP	phenolsulfonphthalein
MEN	multiple endocrine neoplasia (syndrome)	PT	prothrombin time
		PTH	parathyroid hormone
mEq	milliequivalent	PTT	partial thromboplastin time
mg	milligram	RA	refractory anemia, rheumatoid arthritis
MHA-TP	microhemagglutination test (for *Treponema pallidum*)		
		RAIU	thyroid uptake of radioactive iodine
mm Hg	millimeters of mercury		
mmol	millimole	RAST	radioallergosorbent test
mol	mole	RBC	red blood cell
MoM	multiples of the median (also see the Glossary)	RDW	red cell distribution width
		RE	reticuloendothelial

RF	rheumatic fever, rheumatoid factor	TLC	thin-layer chromatography
Rh	Rhesus factor	TMP/SMX	trimethoprim and sulfamethoxazole
RIA	radioimmunoassay	TORCH	toxoplasma, others, rubella, cytomegalovirus, herpes simplex
RNA	ribonucleic acid		
ROC	receiver-operating characteristic (curve, or ROC curve)	TP	total protein
		TPN	total parenteral nutrition
RSV	respiratory syncytial virus	TRH	thyrotropin-releasing hormone
rT3	reverse triiodothyronine (T3)	TSH	thyroid-stimulating hormone
SBE	subacute bacterial endocarditis	TSI	thyroid-stimulating immunoglobulin
SD	standard deviation	TT	thrombin time
SGOT	serum glutamic oxaloacetic transaminase (see aspartate aminotransferase, AST)	TTP	thrombotic thrombocytopenic purpura
		TTP/HUS	thrombotic thrombocytopenic purpura hemolytic uremic syndrome
SGPT	serum glutamic pyruvic transaminase (see alanine aminotransferase, ALT)		
		U	unit
SI	Systeme Internationale d'Unites	UIBC	unsaturated iron-binding capacity
SIA	strip immunoblot assay	ULN	upper limit of normal
SIADH	syndrome of inappropriate antidiuretic hormone secretion	URI	upper respiratory infection
		UTI	urinary tract infection
SLE	systemic lupus erythematosus	UV	ultraviolet
		V	variable
S/S	sensitivity/specificity	VCA	viral capsid antigen
STD	sexually transmitted disease	VDRL	Venereal Disease Research Laboratory (test for syphilis)
T_3	triiodothyronine		
T_4	thyroxine	VIP	vasoactive intestinal polypeptide
TB	tuberculosis		
TBG	thyroxine-binding globulin	VLDL	very-low-density lipoprotein
TDM	therapeutic drug monitoring	VMA	vanillylmandelic acid
TGT	thromboplastic generation time	vWF	von Willebrand factor
		VZV	varicella-zoster virus
THC	marijuana (delta-9-tetrahydrocannabinol)	WBC	white blood cell
		WHO	World Health Organization
TIBC	total iron-binding capacity	Z-E	Zollinger-Ellison (syndrome)

Glossary

Chromosome: an individual portion of DNA containing some or all genes of a cell or virus. Humans have 23 pairs of chromosomes.

DNA: deoxyribonucleic acid: double-helix strands composed of nucleotides (A, C, G, and T) with A on one strand paired with T and C paired with G on the other strand. The order of nucleotides determines genetic information.

FISH: fluorescent in situ hybridization: technique for fluorescent staining of molecules (e.g., used for gene mapping and to identify chromosome abnormalities).

gene: functional unit in genome of cells and viruses that encode RNA and proteins.

genotype: an individual's genetic makeup indicated by his or her DNA sequence.

haplotype: group of adjacent alleles inherited together.

heterozygous: two different alleles at a specific autosomal gene locus (or X chromosome in a female).

homozygous: two identical alleles at a specific autosomal gene locus (or X chromosome in a female).

MoM: multiples of the median: unit used to express marker concentrations in maternal serum that allows for variations in concentration during gestation and between laboratories (see α-fetoprotein).

mRNA: messenger RNA: template for protein synthesis. Sequence of a strand of mRNA is based on sequence of a complementary strand of DNA.

mutation: permanent change in structure of DNA.

nucleic acids: chains of nucleotides that form DNA and RNA.

oncogene: gene with ability to convert a noncancer cell to a cancer cell. Protooncogenes are genes able to contribute to formation of cancer due to mutations in nucleotide sequence or organization; for example, retroviral oncogenes are derived from protooncogenes.

PCR: polymerase chain reaction: quick way to make unlimited number of copies of any piece of DNA.

phenotype: clinical expression of specific genes and/or environmental factors, for example, hair color, presence of a disease.

retrovirus: class of viruses—including HIV and RNA tumor viruses—that replicate by copying RNA genome into DNA form by reverse transcriptase.

reverse transcriptase: enzyme that copies RNA into DNA carried by retroviruses. transcriptase

RNA: ribonucleic acid: delivers DNA messages to cytoplasm of cell where proteins are made. Similar to a single strand of DNA but uracil (U) is substituted for (T) in genetic code. Order of nucleotides is usually determined by a corresponding sequence in DNA.

Southern blot: named for Dr. Southern. Procedure used to identify and locate DNA sequences that are complementary to another piece of DNA (called a *probe*).

tyrosine kinase: enzymes that add phosphate to tyrosine in proteins (many encoded by protooncogenes). Some (e.g., *ABL* and *EGF* receptor tyrosine kinases) are inhibited by anticancer drugs (e.g., Gleevec).

WB (Western blot): procedure used to identify and locate proteins using specific antibodies that bind to these proteins.

Symbols

>	greater than
≥	equal to or greater than
<	less than
≤	equal to or less than; up to
×	times (e.g., 4× increase = fourfold increase)
±	plus or minus
~	approximately
↑ to ↑↑↑↑	increased to markedly increased
↓ to ↓↓↓↓	decreased to markedly decreased

Index

Note: Page numbers followed "f" indicates figures, "t" indicates tables.